T0192588

Second Edition

Nutrition for the Critically Ill Patient

A Guide to Practice

Second Edition

Nutrition for the Critically Ill Patient

A Guide to Practice

Edited by Gail A. Cresci

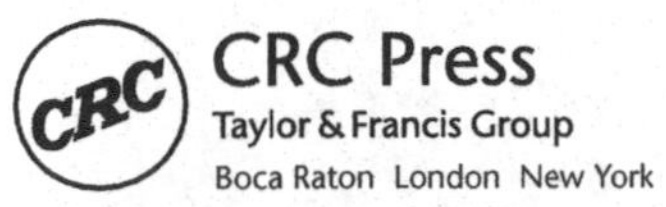

CRC Press is an imprint of the
Taylor & Francis Group, an **informa** business

CRC Press
Taylor & Francis Group
6000 Broken Sound Parkway NW, Suite 300
Boca Raton, FL 33487-2742

First issued in paperback 2021

Version Date: 20150325

ISBN 13: 978-1-03-209870-8 (pbk)
ISBN 13: 978-1-4398-7999-3 (hbk)

Visit the Taylor & Francis Web site at
http://www.taylorandfrancis.com

and the CRC Press Web site at
http://www.crcpress.com

Contents

SECTION V Nutrition Therapy for Special Interests Groups

SECTION VI Specific Organ System Failure

SECTION VII General Systemic Failures

SECTION VIII Professional Issues

Foreword

During the latter half of the twentieth century and to the present day, critical care of seriously ill or injured patients has evolved to become the highest priority for most, especially skilled, health-care teams in most hospitals in the United States and throughout the world. Indeed, we are rapidly approaching the point at which hospitalized patients will consist of those requiring highly specialized intensive care services in various critical care units by highly talented and motivated comprehensive teams of health-care professionals, using state-of-the-art knowledge and technology, and those with complex acute or chronic disorders or conditions that cannot be treated adequately or practically on an ambulatory basis, or in an alternate health maintenance and care facility, or at home. The vast majority of patients requiring medical and/or surgical services will be treated in same-day or short-stay facilities and discharged promptly to their homes or to appropriate assisted living facilities for recovery, convalescence, and rehabilitation. Many of the hospitalized patients will belong to opposite ends of the life cycle, that is, the pediatric and geriatric age groups, especially the latter group, which is the most rapidly increasing segment of the population in this country. Not only do these cadres of hospitalized patients experience the highest incidences of critical illnesses, complications, and collateral conditions, but a majority of them will also exhibit some form of undernutrition or malnutrition prior to, or at, admission or will develop nutritional deficiencies or aberrations during the course of their diagnostic and therapeutic interventions throughout their hospitalization. The adage that "No disease process, injury, or major disorder can be expected to respond as favorably to therapeutic medical and/or surgical treatments when the patient is malnourished or undernourished as when the patient is optimally nourished" remains as true today as when it was first uttered, perhaps by Hippocrates, centuries ago. This fact alone justifies the production of this second edition of *Nutrition Therapy for the Critically Ill Patient: A Guide to Practice* by Gail A. Cresci, PhD, RD, and the distinguished cast of colleagues and authors that she has assembled to share their vast expertise, in depth and in a broad field of nutrition-related topics. Moreover, in more than three dozen chapters, the editor and her contributors have conscientiously and effectively addressed and dealt with the most important of the myriad complex aspects of nutrition therapy in critically ill patients, which is highly essential to their survival and subsequently to the quality of their lives.

The advancements in the field of both critical care and nutrition therapy during the past 50 years have been truly phenomenal, have occurred in symbiosis with each other, have revolutionized the care and management of critically ill patients, have saved countless lives, have changed the practice of medicine forever, and will undoubtedly improve the morbidity, mortality, and other outcomes in this vital arena of health-care endeavor as progress continues in the future. During the past 55 years of my education, training, and practice of medicine, surgery, and nutrition support, I have been privileged to witness and/or participate in a virtual revolution in the care of critically ill patients, which, in retrospect, borders on the unbelievable. When I was a medical student from 1957 to 1961 at the University of Pennsylvania School of Medicine, the only formal nutrition taught in the curriculum was a one-hour lecture on vitamin deficiencies; clinical *intravenous therapy* consisted of peripherally administered 5% dextrose in water, saline, or lactated Ringers solution with added vitamin C and the B complex vitamins, and some potassium; tube feedings were used rarely and usually consisted of blenderized house diets infused into the stomach by a large nasogastric tube or occasionally through a large gastrostomy tube; jejunostomy tube feedings, usually consisting of blenderized foods, were highly problematic, and no special partially digested food substrates acceptable for infusion into the duodenum or jejunum had yet been developed; and no intensive care, critical care, or special care units were available in the Hospital of the University of

Pennsylvania, which comprised largely multiple 40-bed *Florence Nightingale Wards*, and some semiprivate two-bed rooms and private single-bed rooms. Caring for critically ill patients at that time was difficult and frustrating, without adequate designated special space, special skilled nurses, special dieticians/nutritionists, and special equipment, supplies, resources, and access. Moreover, it was well known among the medical students and house officers that a critically ill patient was more likely to receive more, better, and more effective care in an open ward than in a relatively isolated and confined private or semiprivate room.

Several events during my senior year in medical school and my internship transformed both me and the hospital as health-care providers. The Department of Surgery acquired limited amounts of experimental intravenous protein hydrolysate solutions and intravenous cottonseed oil emulsion for limited patient use, and I was privileged to participate in some clinical trials of these new, revolutionary, intravenous nutritional substances. Early in my internship year (1961–1962), I became acutely aware of, and deeply disturbed by, the lethal effect of severe malnutrition and undernutrition upon the outcomes of major surgical patients, especially those with complex problems requiring multiple operative procedures. Even more disconcerting to me was our inability to provide adequate nutrition to patients with major disabilities of, or other impediments to, the use of the gastrointestinal tract. This stimulated me to undertake basic and clinical investigations, which eventually led to the development of the first successful technique of long-term total parenteral nutrition (TPN).

During the same time period, the hospital remodeled a small area to create its first four-bed surgical intensive care unit (SICU) and another similar area to create an acute coronary care unit (CCU). I was actually the first house officer assigned to the rudimentary SICU that had four beds, each having access to an oxygen supply for delivery by mask or nasal cannula, suction apparatus, a 4 in. diameter continuous EKG monitor, and a skilled nurse (the most important feature). I was the indwelling house officer, and I had a reclining chair in which I could rest or even nap occasionally during the month of my rotation while attending to the continual needs of the most critically ill surgical patients in the hospital. Such was critical care in the early 1960s—but it was a giant step forward in the right direction. By the time I was the chief resident in surgery in 1966–1967, the hospital had added three 12-bed special care units, each individually designed and equipped to provide critical care specifically for patients with surgical, cardiac, or pulmonary problems. Modern monitoring equipment, ventilators, respirators, defibrillators, external cardiac pacing units, supplies and equipment for emergency tracheostomy, venous cutdowns, arterial lines, insertion of chest tubes, ostomy care, and portable fluoroscopic and x-ray equipment were added to the armamentarium of the critical care team.

Although these units were the premier care stations for critically ill patients, they also served as a source of invaluable new information and knowledge as we studied the effects of our efforts upon the patients' clinical courses and outcomes. However, perhaps the most profound advance in this critical area was the acquisition of the first extramural NIH Clinical Research Center in the United States by the Department of Medicine faculty of the Hospital of the University of Pennsylvania. It was there that I was able to carry out the most finite and elegant nutritional and metabolic studies in critically ill patients, with the help and support of an elite, skilled, motivated, conscientious staff of nurses, dietitians, technicians, and physicians who were dedicated to practicing their professions with utmost precision and proficiency in a most collegial and collaborative manner. Intravenous infusion pumps, central venous catheters and infusion lines, laminar airflow areas, and regimens for long-term continuous central venous infusion of TPN were introduced and perfected there to the point that our results could be evaluated, validated, and shared with the critical care community, not only of the United States but also of the world. Principles, practices, and procedures were developed, tested, and standardized as much as possible to ensure their optimal safety and effectiveness with minimal complications, morbidity, and mortality. Special nutrient solutions were developed for patients with renal, liver, and pulmonary failures and metabolic lipodystrophies. Our most notable achievement, however, occurred in the neonatology intensive care unit of our Children's Hospital of Philadelphia, where a severely malnourished infant with multiple congenital anomalies, including extremely short bowel syndrome (and near death), was nourished entirely by central venous TPN for 45 days. She was the first infant to exhibit normal growth and development long term while being fed exclusively intravenously. This demonstration revolutionized the care of premature infants and all critically ill infants with severely compromised gastrointestinal tracts and secondary malnutrition—and changed the practice of neonatology forever.

The relevance of nutrition therapy for the critically ill patient was obvious, largely as a result of these basic studies, and has spawned myriad investigations in virtually all aspects of nutritional and metabolic support, orally, enterally, parenterally, and in various combinations. Nonetheless, many questions remain to be answered and many problems beg resolution in this vital area of health care as we strive to achieve perfection in nutrition and metabolic support. This textbook, by virtue of the many important areas addressed by the many expert clinician-scientists, will serve to provide the most up-to-date, state-of-the-art data, information, experience, technology, and techniques to help keep both novices and experts informed and aware of the continuous accrual of knowledge applicable to the optimal care of the critically ill patient. However, the reader will also be aware that controversies still exist regarding nutrition therapy, especially in critically ill patients. Among them are optimal dietary composition, early feeding to target goals, hyperglycemia and insulin use, maintenance of euglycemia, early enteral versus parenteral feeding, overfeeding and refeeding syndrome, and the composition and prudent use of lipid emulsions. Additionally, the compositions of amino acid, vitamin, trace element, and immune-enhancing formulations, and their appropriate use, are still controversial. Problems persist relevant to obesity prevention, arrest, and reversal, on one hand, and to the management of various cachexia problems on the other. Persistent areas of special feeding problems include cancer patients, geriatric patients, premature neonates and surgical infants, and patients with severe short bowel syndrome, especially those with associated liver failure. Obviously, much remains to challenge our interests, talents, and ingenuity (and especially, our motivation, persistence, and resilience) as we strive to provide optimal nutrition to all patients under all conditions at all times. As we do so, we will find this guide to practice to be an invaluable asset in our quest to craft and provide optimal nutrition therapy for the critically ill patient. For that, we are deeply indebted to nutritionist and editor Gail A. Cresci and her collaborating authors for so generously sharing with us their expertise, experience, knowledge, counsel, skills, and wisdom.

Stanley J. Dudrick, MD, FACS, FACN, CNS
Department of Surgery
School of Medicine
Yale University
New Haven, Connecticut

Editor

Gail A. Cresci, PhD, RD, LD, is an associate staff in the Department of Gastroenterology, Hepatology and Pathobiology at the Cleveland Clinic and assistant professor of medicine at the Cleveland Clinic Lerner College of Medicine, Cleveland, Ohio. She has more than 25 years of clinical experience practicing in critical care with a focus on surgery and gastrointestinal disorders. Dr. Cresci is the author of numerous peer-reviewed journal articles, book chapters, abstracts, and videos and currently serves on the editorial boards of several journals. She lectures extensively, both nationally and internationally and has held numerous positions within the American Society for Parenteral and Enteral Nutrition (ASPEN), the Academy of Nutrition and Dietetics, and the Society of Critical Care Medicine.

Dr. Cresci is the past chair of Dietitians in Nutrition Support, a practice group within the Academy of Nutrition and Dietetics. She has served on multiple national and state society conference planning committees, serving as chair for the ASPEN planning committee. She is the recipient of numerous honors and awards, including the American Dietetic Association Excellence in Practice of Clinical Nutrition, the ASPEN Distinguished Nutrition Support Dietitian Advanced Clinical Practice Award, the ASPEN Promising New Investigator Award, and the Academy of Nutrition and Dietetics Excellence in Practice Dietetics Research Award.

Contributors

Mazen Albeldawi
Department of Gastroenterology and Hepatology
NCH Healthcare System
Naples, Florida

Jill Barsa
Fairview Hospital
Cleveland Clinic Health System
Cleveland, Ohio

Amy Berry
University of Virginia Health System
Charlottesville, Virginia

Jatinder Bhatia
Division of Neonatology
Department of Pediatrics
Georgia Regents University
Augusta, Georgia

Britta Brown
Medical Nutrition Therapy
Hennepin County Medical Center
Minneapolis, Minnesota

Rex O. Brown
Department of Pharmacy
University of Tennessee Health Science Center
and
Regional Medical Center at Memphis
Memphis, Tennessee

Deborah A. Carpenter
Akron Children's Hospital
Akron, Ohio

Ronni Chernoff
Arkansas Geriatric Education Center
and
Reynolds Department of Geriatrics
University of Arkansas for Medical Sciences
Little Rock, Arkansas

Dian J. Chiang
Cleveland Clinic
Cleveland, Ohio

Srinath Chinnakotla
Transplantation
Baylor University Medical Center
Dallas, Texas

Michael Christensen
University of Tennessee Health Science Center
Memphis, Tennessee

Maria Isabel Toulson Davisson Correia
Medical School
Federal University of Minas Gerais
Belo Horizonte, Brazil

Mandy L. Corrigan
Center for Human Nutrition
Cleveland Clinic
Cleveland, Ohio

Gail A. Cresci
Gastroenterology and Center for Human Nutrition
Cleveland Clinic
Cleveland, Ohio

Letícia De Nardi
Department of Gastroenterology
Medical School
University of Sao Paulo
Sao Paulo, Brazil

Roland N. Dickerson
Department of Clinical Pharmacy
University of Tennessee Health Science Center
and
Regional Medical Center at Memphis
Memphis, Tennessee

Lindsay M. Dowhan
Center for Gut Rehabilitation and Transplant
Digestive Disease Institute
Cleveland Clinic
Cleveland, Ohio

Stanley J. Dudrick
Department of Surgery
School of Medicine
Yale University
New Haven, Connecticut

Arlene Escuro
Cleveland Clinic
Cleveland, Ohio

David Frankenfield
Milton S. Hershey Medical Center
Hershey, Pennsylvania

Vanessa Fuchs-Tarlovsky
Oncology Department
Hospital General de Mexico
Mexico City, Mexico

Kendra Glassman Perkey
Rocky Mountain Hospital for Children at PSL
Denver, Colorado

Michele M. Gottschlich
Shriners Hospitals for Children
Cincinnati, Ohio

and

Department of Surgery
College of Medicine
University of Cincinnati
Cincinnati, Ohio

Jesse Gutnick
Administrative Chief Resident
Department of General Surgery
Cleveland Clinic
Cleveland, Ohio

Katherine Hall
Medical Nutrition Therapy
Hennepin County Medical Center
Minneapolis, Minnesota

Jeanette Hasse
Transplantation
Baylor University Medical Center
Dallas, Texas

Peggy Hipskind
Center for Human Nutrition
Cleveland Clinic
Cleveland, Ohio

A. Christine Hummell
Cleveland Clinic
Cleveland, Ohio

Elizabeth Isenring
Faculty of Health Sciences and Medicine
Bond University
Brisbane, Australia

Gerri Keller
Akron Children's Hospital
Akron, Ohio

Joe Krenitsky
Digestive Health Center of Excellence
University of Virginia Health System
Charlottesville, Virginia

Kavitha Krishnan
Clinical Dietitian
Fairview Hospital
Cleveland Clinic Health System
Cleveland, Ohio

Kenneth A. Kudsk
Department of Surgery
University of Wisconsin Medical Center
Madison, Wisconsin

Joy Lehman
The Ohio State University Wexner Medical Center
Columbus, Ohio

Mary E. Leicht
Department of Nutrition
John Peter Smith Hospital
Fort Worth, Texas

Maria R. Lucarelli
Division of Pulmonary, Allergy, Critical Care, and Sleep Medicine
Department of Internal Medicine
The Ohio State University Wexner Medical Center
Columbus, Ohio

Ainsley M. Malone
Mount Carmel West Hospital
Columbus, Ohio

William Manzanares
Faculty of Medicine
Department of Critical Care
University of the Republic
Montevideo, Uruguay

Mary Marian
Colleges of Agriculture and Life Sciences/Medicine
The University of Arizona
Tucson, Arizona

Robert Martindale
General Surgery Division
Oregon Health Sciences University
Portland, Oregon

Alfredo A. Matos
Faculty of Medicine
Dr. AAM Social Security Hospital
University of Panama
Panama City, Panama

Theresa Mayes
Division of Nutrition Therapy
Cincinnati Children's Hospital Medical Center
Cincinnati, Ohio

John E. Mazuski
School of Medicine
Barnes-Jewish Hospital
Washington University
St. Louis, Missouri

Mary S. McCarthy
Center for Nursing Science and Clinical Inquiry
Madigan Army Medical Center
Fort Lewis, Washington

Tom Stone McNees
Holston Valley Medical Center
Wellmont Health System
Kingsport, Tennessee

Jeffrey I. Mechanick
Division of Endocrinology, Diabetes, and Bone Diseases
Icahn School of Medicine at Mount Sinai
New York, New York

R.F. Meier
Department of Gastroenterology, Hepatology and Nutrition
Kantonsspital Baselland
Medical University Clinic
Liestal, Switzerland

Jay M. Mirtallo
College of Pharmacy
The Ohio State University
Columbus, Ohio

Cynthia Mundy
Division of Neonatology
Department of Pediatrics
Georgia Regents University
Augusta, Georgia

Víctor Sánchez Nava
Monterrey Institute of Technology and Higher Education
Monterrey, Mexico

Mark H. Oltermann
John Peter Smith Hospital
Fort Worth, Texas

Neha Parekh
Center for Gut Rehabilitation and Transplantation
Cleveland Clinic
Cleveland, Ohio

Carol Rees Parrish
Digestive Health Center of Excellence
University of Virginia Health System
Charlottesville, Virginia

Lindsay Pell Ryder
Department of Pharmacy
The Ohio State University Wexner Medical Center
Columbus, Ohio

Cassandra Pogatschnik
Center for Human Nutrition
and
Center for Gut Rehabilitation and Transplantation
Cleveland Clinic
Cleveland, Ohio

Mary Rath
Cleveland Clinic
Cleveland, Ohio

Susan Roberts
Nutrition Department
Baylor University Medical Center
Dallas, Texas

Mary Krystofiak Russell
Baxter Healthcare Corporation
Deerfield, Illinois

Rifka C. Schulman
Division of Endocrinology, Metabolism and Diabetes
Long Island Jewish Medical Center
New Hyde Park, New York

Denise Baird Schwartz
Food and Nutrition Services
Providence Saint Joseph Medical Center
Burbank, California

Mary Beth Shirk
Department of Pharmacy
The Ohio State University Wexner Medical Center
Columbus, Ohio

Krishnan Sriram
Cook County Health and Hospital Systems
John H. Stroger, Jr. Hospital
Chicago, Illinois

Ezra Steiger
Department of General Surgery
Digestive Disease Institute
Cleveland Clinic
Cleveland, Ohio

Beth Taylor
Barnes-Jewish Hospital
St. Louis, Missouri

and

American College of Critical Care Medicine
Mt. Prospect, Illinois

Michael D. Taylor
Department of Surgery
Fairview Hospital
Cleveland Clinic Health System
Cleveland, Ohio

Raquel S. Torrinhas
Department of Gastroenterology
Medical School
University of São Paulo
São Paulo, Brazil

Christina J. Valentine
Cincinnati Children's Hospital
Cincinnati, Ohio

Carol L. Wagner
The Medical College of South Carolina
Charleston, South Carolina

Dan L. Waitzberg
Department of Gastroenterology
University of São Paulo
São Paulo, Brazil

Malissa Warren
Portland VA Medical Center
Portland, Oregon

Jodi Wolff
Rainbow Babies and Children's Hospital
Cleveland, Ohio

Section I

Metabolic Alterations in the Critically Ill: Comparison of Nonstressed and Stressed States

1 Organic Response to Stress

Maria Isabel Toulson Davisson Correia

CONTENTS

INTRODUCTION

The organic response to stress—first described as the metabolic response to trauma, in 1942, by Sir David Cuthbertson—is a physiologic phenomenon secondary to any insult to the body. Cuthbertson [1] introduced the terms *ebb* and *flow* to describe the phases of hypo- and hypermetabolism that follow traumatic injury. Such phenomenon is triggered by multiple stimuli, including arterial and venous pressure derangements, changes in volume, osmolality, pH, and arterial oxygen content. Also, pain, anxiety, and toxic mediators from tissue injury and infection trigger the organic response (Table 1.1). These stimuli reach the hypothalamus stimulating the sympathetic nervous system and the adrenal medulla. This physiological response to an insult might become pathological depending on the intensity and duration of injury. The organic response can be seen as the *fight or flight* response to adverse phenomena that can become highly associated with increased morbidity and mortality if perpetuated for long periods. The ultimate goal of the organic response is to restore homeostasis. Intermediate goals are to limit further blood loss; to increase blood flow, allowing greater delivery of nutrients and elimination of waste products; and to debride necrotic tissue and to initiate wound healing.

Currently, with the development of medical sciences, the once *simple* metabolic response to stress (represented by the ebb and flow phases) has evolved into a complicated and intricate web of responses. Therefore, a better appropriate denomination such as the organic response to stress that encompasses several body compartments should be used. Although, one cannot fully go against

TABLE 1.1
Organic Response to Stress: Triggering Factors

- Body temperature (hypo- and hyperthermia)
- Excessive bleeding (shock)
- Fluid and electrolyte derangements
- Infection
- Inflammation
- Pain
- Poor nutritional status
- Prolonged fasting
- Psychological problems

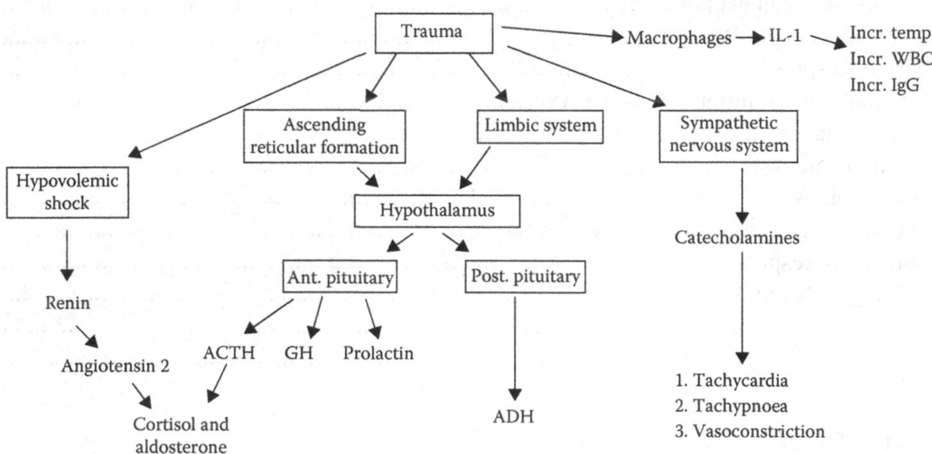

FIGURE 1.1 Organic response to stress.

its development, recognizing its magnitude and knowing its different particularities might help minimize the risks of perpetuating its duration, leading to the reduction of morbidity and mortality related to it. In surgical stress, especially under major elective conditions, it's important for surgeons to be aware that a perfect anatomic operation maybe followed by a disastrous outcome if patients are not metabolically conditioned. Undernutrition, pain control, and fluid and electrolyte balance, among others, are of paramount importance and should be dealt in a multimodal approach to decrease the organic response to trauma [2–6]. Therefore, it is extremely important to be acquainted with the complex mechanisms of the organic response (Figure 1.1) in order to act early and, maybe, prevent some of its deleterious effects.

The magnitude of the response and the adequate initial approach are determinant factors that might influence the patient's outcome [2,5,7–9]. The severity of the hypermetabolic phenomena thereafter might lead to the systemic inflammatory response syndrome (SIRS), the amplified generalized body response, which may culminate with multiorgan dysfunction and death.

STRESS

Stress is a term applied to the fields of physiology and neuroendocrinology and refers to those forces or factors that cause disequilibrium to an organism and therefore threaten homeostasis [10]. The stressors might be a consequence of physical injury, mechanical disruptions, chemical changes, or emotional factors. The body's response to these factors will depend on their magnitude, duration, as well as the nutritional status of the patient. Complex sensory systems trigger reflex nervous system responses to the stressors that alert the central nervous system (CNS) of the disturbance. In the CNS, neurons of the paraventricular nucleolus of the hypothalamus elaborate corticotropin-releasing hormone (CRH) and activate the hypothalamic–pituitary–adrenal axis (HPA). In addition, other areas of the brain also signal the peripheral autonomic nervous system. These two latter systems elicit an integrated-response, referred to collectively as the *stress response*, which primarily controls bodily functions such as arousal, cardiovascular tone, respiration, and intermediate metabolism [1]. Other functions such as feeding and sexual behavior are suppressed, while cognition and emotion are activated. In addition, gastrointestinal activity and immune/inflammatory responses are altered.

HISTORICAL PERSPECTIVE

Sir David Cuthbertson, a chemical pathologist in Glasgow, was the first physician studying the metabolic response to injury in the early part of the twentieth century, by following patients with long bone fractures [1]. However, long before Cuthbertson's studies, John Hunter, in his *Treatise on the Blood, Inflammation and Gunshot Wounds* [11], was the first to question the paradox of the response to injury by saying, "Impressions are capable of producing or increasing natural actions and are then called *stimuli*, but they are likewise capable of producing too much action, as well as depraved, unnatural, or what we commonly call diseased action." He must have intuitively perceived that nature might have created these responses in order to have some advantages in terms of recovery, but he also noticed that if the responses were overexaggerated, life could be jeopardized.

The concept that illness was associated with an increased excretion of nitrogen leading to negative nitrogen balance was defined in the late nineteenth century. During the First World War, studies carried out by DuBois [12] showed that an increase in 1°C in temperature was associated with a 13% increase in the metabolic rate.

Cuthbertson's findings were derived from questions aroused by orthopedic surgeons who were eager to find out why patients with fractures of the distal third of the tibia were slow to heal. His studies were negative in the sense that he could not offer the exact explanation to the question, but at the same time, he came up with something much more interesting and fundamental. He measured the excretion of calcium, phosphorus, sulfate, and nitrogen in the urine and found that the amount of excreted phosphorous and sulfate in relation to calcium was higher than expected if all these elements had come from the bone. He went on to show that this was a catabolic phenomenon related to breakdown of protein, reflecting an increase in metabolic rate. The association between the systemic metabolic response and hormonal elaboration was soon sought, but this approach was initially hampered by methodological problems. The investigations carried out by Cannon [13] on the autonomic nervous system suggested the increased catecholamine response to illness as one of the explanations of the physiologic responses seen by Cuthbertson. Later, Selye proposed corticosteroids as the main mediators of the protein catabolic response [14]. However, the following question still remained unanswered: what was the signal that initiated and propagated the immediate elaboration of the adrenal cortical hormones? Hume [15] and Egdahl [16] showed that in injured dogs (operative injury or superficial burn to the limbs) with intact sciatic nerves or spinal cords, there was an increase of adrenal hormones, contrary to what happened in those animals with transected nerves or spinal cords, in whom the response was abated. From the investigated setting, it was possible to identify afferent nervous signals as essential components to trigger the HPA stress response.

Allison et al. [17] showed that such organic response was also associated with suppression of insulin release, followed by a period of insulin resistance and with high glucagon and growth hormone (GH) levels. Recently, the organic response has been associated not only with neuroendocrine alterations but it is also accompanied by inflammatory responses and mediators as well as immunologic dysfunctions.

ORGANIC RESPONSE TO STRESS (TABLE 1.2)

EBB AND FLOW PHASES

Cuthbertson [1] originally divided the organic response into an ebb and a flow phase. The ebb phase begins immediately after injury and typically lasts 12–24 h, if the initial injury is under control. However, this phase may last longer depending on the severity of trauma and the adequacy of resuscitation. The ebb phase may equate with prolonged and untreated shock, a circumstance that is more often seen in experimental animals than in clinical practice. It is characterized by tissue hypoperfusion and a decrease in overall metabolic activity. In order to compensate this, catecholamines are discharged with norepinephrine being the primary mediator of the ebb phase. Norepinephrine is released from peripheral nerves and binds to beta$_1$ receptors in the heart and alpha and beta$_2$ receptors in peripheral and, to a lesser degree, splanchnic vascular beds. The most important effects are the cardiovascular, because norepinephrine is a potent cardiac stimulant, causing increased contractility and heart rate and vasoconstriction. These phenomena are attempts to restore blood pressure and increase cardiac performance and maximal venous return.

Hyperglycemia may be seen during the ebb phase. The degree of hyperglycemia parallels the severity of injury. Hyperglycemia is promoted by hepatic glycogenolysis secondary to catecholamine release and by direct sympathetic stimulation of glycogen breakdown.

Some authors have investigated the ebb phase in experimental animals and human beings [18] and have noticed important aspects, such as that after sustained long fractures, with concomitant great loss of blood, there is an impairment of vasoconstriction, which is not seen in bleeding events alone, such as that seen in duodenal ulcer bleeding. In another study, Childs et al. [19] showed an effect of injury on impairing thermoregulation in injured subjects who presented with reduced vasoconstriction in response to cold stimulus.

The onset of the flow phase that encompasses the catabolic and anabolic phases is signaled by high cardiac output with the restoration of oxygen delivery and metabolic substrate. The duration of this phase depends on the severity of injury or the presence of infection and development of complications (Table 1.3). It typically peaks around the third to the fifth day, subsides by 7–10 days, and merges into an anabolic phase over the next few weeks. During this hypermetabolic phase, insulin release is high but elevated levels of catecholamines, glucagon, and cortisol counteract most of its metabolic effects.

TABLE 1.2
Organic Response to Stress

The organic response is related to

- Magnitude (severity)
- Duration (the longer the more severe)
- Nutritional status of the patient (malnourished patients do worse)
- Associated diseases (increase morbidity and mortality)
  - Diabetes
  - Heart disease
  - Pulmonary
  - Immunologic
  - Others

TABLE 1.3
Metabolic Response to Stress

- The ebb and flow phases
  - Glucose and protein metabolism
- Fluid and electrolyte response
- Endocrine response
  - HPA
  - Thyrotropic axis
  - Somatotropic axis
  - Lactotropic axis
  - Luteininizing hormone-testosterone axis
- Inflammatory response
- Immunologic response

Increased mobilization of amino acids and free fatty acids from peripheral muscles and adipose tissue stores result from this hormonal imbalance. Some of these released substrates are used for energy production—either directly as glucose or through the liver as triglyceride. Other substrates contribute to the synthesis of proteins in the liver, where humoral mediators increase production of acute phase reactants. Similar protein synthesis occurs in the immune system for the healing of damaged tissues. While this hypermetabolic phase involves both catabolic and anabolic processes, the net result is a significant loss of protein, characterized by negative nitrogen balance and also decreased fat stores. This leads to an overall modification of body composition, characterized by losses of protein, carbohydrate, and fat stores, accompanied by enlarged extracellular (and, to a lesser extent, intracellular) water compartments.

Glucose and Protein Metabolism

Glucose is always fundamental independently of which organic response phase the patient is in. Dr. Jonathan Rhoads pointed out that providing 100 g of glucose guarantees energy to cells that solely rely on this substrate such as neurons and red cells and allows the body to use fat stores and some muscle protein for the remaining energy needs [20]. During simple starvation without any stress condition, glucose infusion inhibits hepatic gluconeogenesis, but after injury, despite the high concentration of circulating glucose, gluconeogenesis prevails.

The amino acids released from protein catabolism in muscle are largely taken up by the liver for new glucose production, rather than being used as fuel to meet energy demands. The latter are provided by the fat reserve (about 80%–90%) [21]. The reason why injured patients need such a high rate of endogenous glucose production may be explained by the high demand of injured tissues for glucose. Wilmore et al. showed that patients with severe burns in one leg and with minor injury to the other had a fourfold increase of glucose uptake by the burnt limb [22]. At the same time, the burnt leg produced higher amounts of lactate, suggesting anaerobic respiration. The lactate is then returned to the liver for gluconeogenesis, in the so-called Cori cycle, which is metabolically expensive. One mole of glucose yields two ATP through glycolysis, but via gluconeogenesis costs three ATP. This may contribute to the underlying increase in the metabolic rate (Figure 1.2).

Insulin has an anabolic or storage effect by synthesizing large molecules from small molecules and inhibiting catabolism. It also promotes glucose oxidation and glycogen synthesis, whereas it inhibits glycogenolysis and gluconeogenesis. On the other hand, the catabolic hormones, such as catecholamines, cortisol, and glucagons, enhance glycogenolysis and gluconeogenesis.

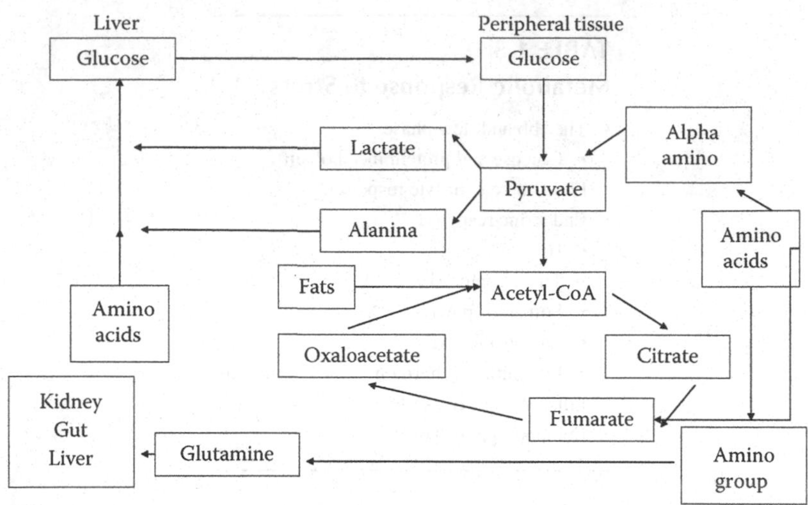

FIGURE 1.2 Aerobic glycolysis and Cori cycles.

Fluid and Electrolyte Response

Hypovolemia prevails in the ebb phase and is entirely reversible with appropriate fluid administration. However, in the absence of volume resuscitation, within 24 h, mortality is nearly uniform [23]. The patient's initial response to hypovolemia is targeted to keep adequate perfusion to the brain and the heart in detriment of the skin, fat tissue, muscles, and intra-abdominal structures. The oliguria, which follows injury, is a consequence of the release of antidiuretic hormone (ADH) and aldosterone. Secretion of ADH from the supraoptic nuclei in the anterior hypothalamus is stimulated by volume reduction and increased osmolality. The latter is mainly due to increased sodium content of the extracellular fluid. Francis Moore coined the terms *the sodium retention phase* and *sodium diuresis phase* of injury to describe the antidiuresis of both salt and water in the flow phase [24]. Volume receptors are located in the atria and pulmonary arteries, and osmoreceptors are located near ADH neurons in the hypothalamus. ADH acts mainly on the connecting tubules of the kidney but also on the distal tubules to promote reabsorption of water. Aldosterone acts mainly on the distal renal tubules to promote reabsorption of sodium and bicarbonate and increase excretion of potassium and hydrogen ions. Aldosterone also modifies the effects of catecholamines on cells, thus affecting the exchange of sodium and potassium across all cell membranes. The release of large quantities of intracellular potassium into the extracellular fluid is a consequence of protein catabolism and may cause a rise in serum potassium, especially if renal function is impaired. Retention of sodium and bicarbonate may produce metabolic alkalosis with impairment of the delivery of oxygen to the tissues. After injury, urinary sodium excretion may fall to 10–25 mmol/24 h and potassium excretion may rise to 100–200 mmol/24 h. Intracellular fluid and exogenously administered fluid accumulate preferentially in the extracellular third space because of increased vascular permeability and relative increase in interstitial oncotic pressure. This is the reason most patients become so edematous after the first days following injury and resuscitation.

Endocrine Response

Hypothalamic–Pituitary–Adrenal Axis

The hypothalamus secretes CRH in response to the stress stimuli. CHR stimulates the production, by the pituitary, of adrenocorticotropic hormone (ACTH), also known as corticotropin, which as its name implies, stimulates the adrenal cortex. More specifically, it triggers

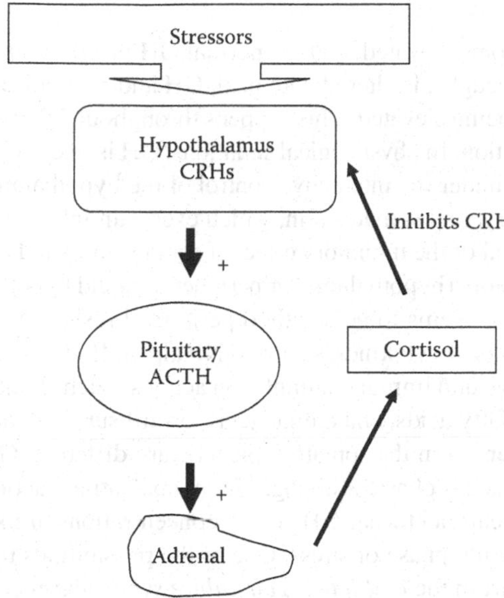

FIGURE 1.3 The hypothalamic–pituitary–adrenal axis.

the secretion of glucocorticoids, such as cortisol, and has little control over the secretion of aldosterone, the other major steroid hormone from the adrenal cortex. CRH itself is inhibited by glucocorticoids, making it part of a classical negative feedback loop (Figures 1.1 and 1.3). It seems that the secretion of aldosterone is most likely under the control of an activated renin–angiotensin system.

Hypercortisolism acutely shifts carbohydrate, fat, and protein metabolism, so that energy is instantly and selectively available to vital organs such as the brain, and anabolism is thus delayed. Intravascular fluid retention and the enhanced inotropic and vasopressor response to catecholamines and angiotensin II offer hemodynamic advantages in the *fight and flight* response. This hypercortisolism can be interpreted as an attempt of the organism to mute its own inflammatory cascade, thus protecting itself against over-responses [25].

Serum ACTH was found to be low in chronic critical illness, while cortisol concentrations remained elevated, suggesting that cortisol release may be driven through alternative pathways, possibly involving endothelin [26].

Thyrotropic Axis

Serum levels of T3 decrease, within 2 h after surgery or trauma, whereas T4 and Thyroid stimulating hormone (TSH) briefly increase. Apparently, low levels of T3 are due to a decreased peripheral conversion of T4. Subsequently, circulating levels of TSH and T4 often return to *normal* levels, whereas T3 levels remain low. It is important to mention that the magnitude of T3 decrease has been found to reflect the severity of illness. Several cytokine mediators, mainly tumor necrosis factor (TNF), interleukin-1 (IL-1), and interleukin-6 (IL-6), have been investigated as putative mediators of the acute low T3 levels [27]. Teleologically, the acute changes in the thyroid axis may reflect an attempt to reduce energy expenditure, as in starvation.

A somewhat different behavior is seen in patients remaining in intensive care units for longer periods. It has been seen that there is a low-normal TSH values and low T4 and T3 serum concentrations. This seems to be reduced due to reduced hypothalamic stimulation of the thyrotropes, in turn leading to reduced stimulation of the thyroid gland. Endogenous dopamine and prolonged hypercortisolism may play a role in this phenomenon. When exogenous dopamine and glucocorticoids are given, hypothyroidism is provoked or aggravated, in critical illness [28].

Somatotropic Axis

Circulating levels of GH become elevated, and the normal GH profile, consisting of peaks alternating with virtually undetectable troughs, is altered with peak GH and interpulse concentrations being high and the GH pulse frequency being elevated. This happens throughout the first hours or days of an insult, be it surgery, trauma, or infection. In physiological situations, GH is released from the pituitary somatotropes in a pulsatile fashion, under the interactive control of the hypothalamic GH-releasing hormone (GHRH), which is stimulatory, and somatostatin, which exerts an inhibitory effect. Apparently, after stress, it seems that withdrawal of the inhibitory effect of somatostatin and the increased availability of stimulatory GH-releasing factors (hypothalamic or peripheral) could hypothetically be involved. It has also been suggested that there seems to be acquired peripheral resistance to GH, and these changes are brought about by the effects of cytokines, such as TNF alpha, IL-1, and IL-6 [29]. GH exerts direct lipolytic, insulin-antagonizing, and immune-stimulating actions. Such changes prioritize essential substrates such as glucose, free fatty acids, and amino acids toward survival rather than anabolism.

In chronic illness, the changes in the somatotropic axis are different. GH secretion is chaotic and reduced compared with the acute phase. Although the nonpulsatile fraction is still elevated and the number of pulses is high, mean nocturnal GH serum concentrations are scarcely elevated and substantially lower than in the acute phase of stress. One of the possibilities that explain this situation is that the pituitary is taking part in the *multiple organ failure syndrome* becoming unable to synthesize and secrete GH [29]. Another explanation could be that the lack of pulsatile GH secretion is due to increased somatostatin tone or to reduced stimulation by endogenous releasing factors, such as GHRH.

Lactotropic Axis

Prolactin was among the first hormones known to have increased serum concentrations after acute physical or psychological stress [29]. This increase might be mediated by oxytocin, dopaminergic pathways, or vasoactive intestinal peptide (VIP). Inflammatory cytokines may be the triggering factor. Changes in prolactin secretion in response to stress might contribute to altered immune function during the course of critical illness. In mice, inhibition of prolactin release results in impaired lymphocyte function, depressed lymphokine-dependent macrophage activation, and death from normally nonlethal exposure to bacteria [30]. It remains unclear if hyperprolactinemia contributes to the vital activation of the immune cascade, after the onset of critical illness. In the chronic setting of critical illness, serum prolactin levels are no longer as high as in the acute phase.

Luteinizing Hormone–Testosterone Axis

Testosterone is the most important endogenous anabolic steroid hormone. Therefore, changes within the luteinizing hormone–testosterone axis in the male may be relevant for the catabolic state in critical illness, in which there are low testosterone levels. The exact cause is unclear, but cytokines may once again be enrolled in this phenomenon [31]. Hypothesizing over the low testosterone levels, it may be important to switch off anabolic androgen secretion, in acute stress, in order to conserve energy and metabolic substrates for vital functions [32].

In chronic states, circulating testosterone levels become extremely low, in fact almost undetectable. Endogenous dopamine, estrogens, and opiates might be the cause for the low levels.

Inflammatory Response

The local inflammatory response is part of the body's attempt to restore homeostasis, particularly healing, which in most situations after injury is successful (Figure 1.4). However, at times, this is not the case and deviations occur, leading to a perpetuated response that may jeopardize survival such as in the SIRS. In the latter, inflammation is triggered at sites remote from the site of initial injury. In some cases, SIRS progresses to multiple organ dysfunction syndrome (MODS), which is associated with high mortality rates.

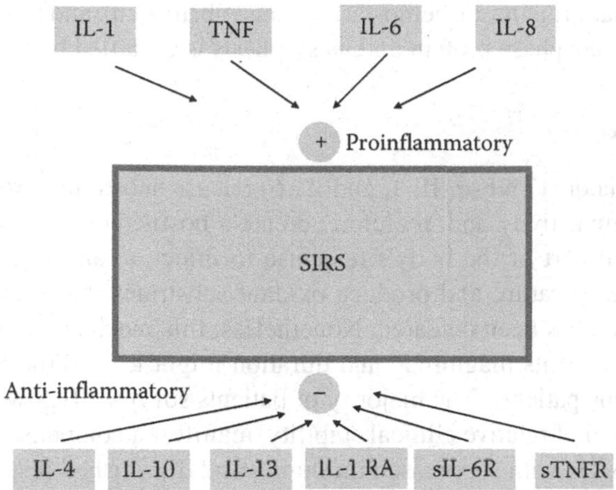

FIGURE 1.4 Most common cytokes produced in SIRS.

The physiologic inflammatory response to trauma is a complex cellular and molecular event, in which inflammatory cells such as polymorphonuclear cells (PMNs), macrophages, and lymphocytes are recruited to the site of injury and secrete inflammatory mediators. The endothelium at the site of injury also participates. PMNs are the first cells arriving at the site of injury and release potent oxidizing molecules, including hydrogen peroxide, hypochlorous acid, oxygen-free radicals, proteolytic enzymes, and vasoactive substances, such as leukotrienes, eicosanoids, and platelet-activating factor (PAF). There is evidence that PAF is partially responsible for the increased permeability in sepsis and shock [33]. Oxygen-free radicals are proinflammatory molecules causing lipid peroxidation, inactivation of enzymes, and consumption of antioxidants. PMNs release proteolytic enzymes, which activate the kinin/kallikrein system. In turn, this system stimulates the release of angiotensin II, bradykinin, and activated plasminogen. Bradykinin causes vasodilatation and mediates increased vascular permeability.

Macrophages are activated by cytokines and engulf invading organisms. They also debride necrotic host tissue and elaborate additional cytokines. TNF alpha (synthesized by macrophages) and IL-1 beta (synthesized by macrophages and endothelial cells) are the proximal proinflammatory mediators. These cytokines initiate the elaboration and release of other cytokines, such as IL-6. Monocytes, macrophages, neutrophils, T and B cells, endothelial cells, smooth muscle cells, fibroblasts, and mast cells secrete this cytokine. It is probably the most potent inductor of acute phase response, although its exact role in the inflammatory response remains unclear. On the other hand, it is considered to be the most reliable prognostic indication of outcome, particularly in sepsis because it reflects the severity of injury [34].

Il-8 belongs to a group of mediators known as chemokines because of their ability to recruit inflammatory cells to the sites of injury. It is synthesized by monocytes, macrophages, neutrophils, and endothelial cells. It is also used as an index of magnitude of systemic inflammation and it seems to be able to identify those patients who will develop MODS [35]. High levels of IL-6 and IL-8 in alveolar washouts, 2 h after injury, have been reported, suggesting that the alveoli might be the first structures suffering with the metabolic response to stress [36]. These high levels might be used, in the future, as prognostic factors to the development of multiorgan dysfunction syndrome.

IL-4 and IL-10 are anti-inflammatory cytokines, synthesized by lymphocytes and monocytes and exert similar effects. They inhibit the synthesis of TNF alpha, IL-1, IL-6, and IL-8.

Nitric oxide (NO) is elaborated by various cell types, including endothelial cells, neurons, macrophages, smooth muscle cells, and fibroblasts. NO mediates vasodilatation and regulates vascular tone. NO is probably a key mediator in the pathophysiology of stress and shock.

Acute-phase reactants are produced in the liver in response to injury in order to maintain homeostasis. Its production is induced by cytokines. These proteins function as opsonins (C-reactive protein), protease inhibitors (alpha$_1$-proteinase), hemostatic agents (fibrinogen), and transporters (transferring). Albumin is a negative acute phase protein and its synthesis is curtailed by inflammation.

Immunologic Response

The inflammatory mediators (TNF-α, IL-1, and IL-6) release substrates, from host tissues, to support T and B lymphocyte activity and, therefore, create a hostile environment for invading pathogens. This is an integral part of the body's response to infection and injury. Such inflammatory mediators raise body temperature and produce oxidant substrates that initiate downregulation of the process once invasion has been defeated. Nonetheless, this mechanism poses considerable cost to the host and according to its magnitude and duration might lead to the SIRS. The latter might cause the MODS, in some patients. The majority of patients survive SIRS without developing early MODS and, after a period of relative clinical stability, manifest a compensatory anti-inflammatory response syndrome (CARS) with suppressed immunity and diminished resistance to infection.

The interaction between the innate and adaptive immune systems seems to be important inductor of both SIRS and CARS. T cells from the adaptive immune system play a role in the early SIRS response to injury and in CARS. Other possible mediators of CARS include prostaglandins of the E series. Also, products of complement activation seem to induct TNF alpha production. In summary, the SIRS, which regularly occurs after serious injury and in some cases proves fatal to the individual, has been partially characterized by both clinical and animal researches. However, the triggering mechanisms and signaling systems involved in inducing and maintaining it are incompletely understood and defined.

CONCLUSIONS

The organic response consists of the complex hydroelectrolytic, hematological, hormonal, metabolic, inflammatory, and immunologic changes that follow injury or trauma. It is the body's life-saving process that will definitely impact on patients' outcomes according to the way it is approached. Therefore, it is currently accepted that the best way to face such situation is by providing a series of multimodal attitudes, which encompass good nutrition status, short preoperative fasting time, intraoperative body temperature control, adequate fluid administration, pain control and early oral or enteral nutrition, as well as early mobilization among others. Most of these recommendations are easily accomplished at very low cost.

In summary, the organic response is a physiological phenomenon that tries to protect the body against any aggression. However, when it is too intense and lasts for longer periods, it is associated with higher morbidity and mortality. In order to avoid such situation, it is of utmost importance to be aware of the different facets and comply with the several attitudes that might be able to decrease the magnitude of the response. Nonetheless, these interventions, especially those that have tried to abrogate it, should be seen with caution and under protocol control because attenuating or abolishing the organic response may not be without risk, with the latter placing responsibility on the care provider to be fully aware of the possible side effects. Future research, especially in the area of genetics and molecular biology, will no doubt help understand several aspects not currently known.

REFERENCES

1. Cuthbertson D. Effect of injury on metabolism. *Biochemical Journal*. 1930;2:1244.
2. Ahmed J, Khan S, Lim M, Chandrasekaran TV, Macfie J. Enhanced recovery after surgery protocols—Compliance and variations in practice during routine colorectal surgery. *Colorectal Disease: The Official Journal of the Association of Coloproctology of Great Britain and Ireland*. September 2012;14(9):1045–1051. PubMed PMID: 21985180.
3. da Fonseca LM, Profeta da Luz MM, Lacerda-Filho A, Correia MI, Gomes da Silva R. A simplified rehabilitation program for patients undergoing elective colonic surgery—Randomized controlled clinical trial. *International Journal of Colorectal Disease*. May 2011;26(5):609–616. PubMed PMID: 21069355.

4. Fearon KC, Ljungqvist O, Von Meyenfeldt M, Revhaug A, Dejong CH, Lassen K et al. Enhanced recovery after surgery: A consensus review of clinical care for patients undergoing colonic resection. *Clinical Nutrition*. June 2005;24(3):466–477. PubMed PMID: 15896435.
5. Gustafsson UO, Hausel J, Thorell A, Ljungqvist O, Soop M, Nygren J et al. Adherence to the enhanced recovery after surgery protocol and outcomes after colorectal cancer surgery. *Archives of Surgery*. May 2011;146(5):571–577. PubMed PMID: 21242424.
6. Yamada T, Hayashi T, Cho H, Yoshikawa T, Taniguchi H, Fukushima R et al. Usefulness of enhanced recovery after surgery protocol as compared with conventional perioperative care in gastric surgery. *Gastric Cancer: Official Journal of the International Gastric Cancer Association and the Japanese Gastric Cancer Association*. January 2012;15(1):34–41. PubMed PMID: 21573918.
7. Abraham N, Albayati S. Enhanced recovery after surgery programs hasten recovery after colorectal resections. *World Journal of Gastrointestinal Surgery*. January 27, 2011;3(1):1–6. PubMed PMID: 21286218. PubMed Central PMCID: 3030737.
8. Huibers CJ, de Roos MA, Ong KH. The effect of the introduction of the ERAS protocol in laparoscopic total mesorectal excision for rectal cancer. *International Journal of Colorectal Disease*. June 2012;27(6):751–757. PubMed PMID: 22173714. PubMed Central PMCID: 3359461.
9. Lassen K, Coolsen MM, Slim K, Carli F, de Aguilar-Nascimento JE, Schafer M et al. Guidelines for perioperative care for pancreaticoduodenectomy: Enhanced Recovery After Surgery (ERAS®) Society recommendations. *Clin Nutr*. December 2012;31(6):817–830.
10. Wilmore DW. From Cuthbertson to fast-track surgery: 70 Years of progress in reducing stress in surgical patients. *Annals of Surgery*. November 2002;236(5):643–648. PubMed PMID: 12409671. PubMed Central PMCID: 1422623.
11. Moore W, Hunter J. Learning from natural experiments, 'placebos', and the state of mind of a patient in the 18th century. *J R Soc Med*. September 1, 2009;102(9):394–396.
12. DuBois EF. *Basal Metabolism in Health and Disease*. Philadelphia, PA: Lea & Febiger, 1924.
13. Cannon WB. *The Wisdom of the Body*, 2nd edn. New York: Norton Co., 1932.
14. Selye HT. The general adaptation syndrome and the diseases of adaptation. *Journal of Clinical Encocrinology*. 1946;6:117.
15. Hume DM. The neuro-endocrine response to injury: Present status of the problem. *Annals of Surgery*. 1953;46:548.
16. Egdahl RH. Pituitary-adrenal response following trauma to the isolated leg. *Surgery*. 1959;46:9.
17. Allison SP, Hinton P, Chamberlain MJ. Intravenous glucose tolerance, insulin, and free fatty acid levels in burned patients. *Lancet*. 1968;2:1113.
18. Little RA, Stoner HB. Effect of injury on the reflex control of pulse rate in man. *Circulatory Shock*. 1983;10(2):161–171. PubMed PMID: 6839425.
19. Childs C, Stoner HB, Little RA, Davenport PJ. A comparison of some thermoregulatory responses in healthy children and in children with burn injury. *Clinical Science*. October 1989;77(4):425–430. PubMed PMID: 2805601.
20. Blackburn GL. Metabolic considerations in management of surgical patients. *The Surgical Clinics of North America*. June 2011;91(3):467–480. PubMed PMID: 21621691.
21. Kinney JM, Duke Jr. JH, Long CL, Gump FE. Tissue fuel and weight loss after injury. *Journal of Clinical Pathology Supplement*. 1970;4:65–72. PubMed PMID: 4950033. PubMed Central PMCID: 1519990.
22. Wilmore DW, Aulick LH, Mason AD, Pruitt Jr. BA. Influence of the burn wound on local and systemic responses to injury. *Annals of Surgery*. October 1977;186(4):444–458. PubMed PMID: 907389. PubMed Central PMCID: 1396291.
23. Boyd JH, Forbes J, Nakada TA, Walley KR, Russell JA. Fluid resuscitation in septic shock: A positive fluid balance and elevated central venous pressure are associated with increased mortality. *Critical Care Medicine*. February 2011;39(2):259–265. PubMed PMID: 20975548.
24. Moore FD. *The Metabolic Care of the Surgical Patient*. Philadelphia, PA: Saunders, 1959.
25. Gold PW, Kling MA, Khan I, Calabrese JR, Kalogeras K, Post RM et al. Corticotropin releasing hormone: Relevance to normal physiology and to the pathophysiology and differential diagnosis of hypercortisolism and adrenal insufficiency. *Advances in Biochemical Psychopharmacology*. 1987;43:183–200. PubMed PMID: 3035886.
26. Vermes I, Haanen C, Steffens-Nakken H, Reutelingsperger C. A novel assay for apoptosis. Flow cytometric detection of phosphatidylserine expression on early apoptotic cells using fluorescein labelled Annexin V. *Journal of Immunological Methods*. July 17, 1995;184(1):39–51. PubMed PMID: 7622868.

27. Celic-Spuzic E. Effect of anesthesia on the changes in the hormones levels during and after transvesical prostatectomy. *Medicinski Arhiv*. 2011;65(6):348–353. PubMed PMID: 22299297.
28. Van den Berghe G. Endocrine changes in critically ill patients. *Growth Hormone & IGF Research: Official Journal of the Growth Hormone Research Society and the International IGF Research Society*. April 1999;9(Suppl. A):77–81. PubMed PMID: 10429886.
29. Weinmann M. Stress-induced hormonal alterations. *Critical Care Clinics*. January 2001;17(1):1–10. PubMed PMID: 11219222.
30. Shelly S, Boaz M, Orbach H. Prolactin and autoimmunity. *Autoimmunity Reviews*. May 2012;11(6–7): A465–A470. PubMed PMID: 22155203.
31. Oertelt-Prigione S. The influence of sex and gender on the immune response. *Autoimmunity Reviews*. May 2012;11(6–7):A479–A485. PubMed PMID: 22155201.
32. Van den Berghe G. Dynamic neuroendocrine responses to critical illness. *Frontiers in Neuroendocrinology*. October 2002;23(4):370–391. PubMed PMID: 12381331.
33. Suematsu M, Tsuchiya M. Platelet-activating factor and granulocyte-mediated oxidative stress. Strategy for in vivo oxyradical visualization. *Lipids*. December 1991;26(12):1362–1368. PubMed PMID: 1668122.
34. Dalla Libera AL, Regner A, de Paoli J, Centenaro L, Martins TT, Simon D. IL-6 polymorphism associated with fatal outcome in patients with severe traumatic brain injury. *Brain Injury*. 2011;25(4):365–369. PubMed PMID: 21314275.
35. Rhodes J, Sharkey J, Andrews P. Serum IL-8 and MCP-1 concentration do not identify patients with enlarging contusions after traumatic brain injury. *The Journal of Trauma*. June 2009;66(6):1591–1597; discussion 8. PubMed PMID: 19509619.
36. Ware LB, Koyama T, Billheimer DD, Wu W, Bernard GR, Thompson BT et al. Prognostic and pathogenetic value of combining clinical and biochemical indices in patients with acute lung injury. *Chest*. February 2010;137(2):288–296. PubMed PMID: 19858233. PubMed Central PMCID: 2816641.

2 Carbohydrate Metabolism
A Comparison of Stress and Nonstress States

Mary Marian and Susan Roberts

CONTENTS

INTRODUCTION

Carbohydrates (CHOs) are the primary source of energy for human cells and usually comprise 45%–65% of energy consumed yielding 4 kcal/g substrate. Glucose is an essential fuel for the brain and central nervous tissue. Additionally, CHOs are vital to the composition of RNA and DNA, coenzymes, glycoproteins, and glycolipids. There are several forms of CHO including monosaccharides, disaccharides and oligosaccharides, and polysaccharides such as starch and fibers.[1,2]

CHOs are defined chemically as an aldehyde or ketone derivative of polyhydric alcohol or compounds that yield such molecules on hydrolysis.

Tightly regulated, glucose concentration in the blood is maintained within a narrow range (70–105 g/dL) that ensures a steady source of glucose to the brain.[1] Blood glucose levels are regulated by both metabolic and hormonal mechanisms. The major hormones controlling blood glucose levels are insulin, glucagon, and epinephrine, but glucocorticoids, thyroid hormone, and growth hormone can also play a role.[1]

FED STATE

CHO metabolism during the fed state is characterized by an increase in blood glucose levels, fats, amino acids, and their metabolites. Following ingestion, CHO is digested by a variety of enzymes including salivary and pancreatic amylase, maltase, sucrose, and lactase. The latter three enzymes break down disaccharides and oligosaccharides further into monosaccharides (glucose, galactose, and fructose), which are then absorbed in the proximal intestine. The absorption of glucose occurs through sodium-dependent glucose transporters.[3] Glucose uptake into tissues requires a number of facilitated glucose transporter molecules and/or insulin, and glucose transporters are expressed on glucose-requiring tissues (e.g., the liver, brain, skeletal muscle, kidneys, adipocytes, skin, and blood cells). Glucose is then phosphorylated and either oxidized by the tissues for energy or stored as glycogen or triacylglycerols, depending on the metabolic state of the host. Both storage forms of glucose can both serve as an available energy source for use when needed.[4]

Glucose not needed for immediate energy is stored in the liver and muscle as glycogen, through a process called glycogenesis.[2] Glycogen plays a principle role in metabolism serving as a ready source of glucose to maintain blood glucose levels. A larger amount (approximately three to four times) of glycogen is stored in the muscle compared to that stored in the liver. Muscle glycogen is used only by the myocytes for energy, whereas hepatic glycogen can be released into the systemic circulation for glucose homeostasis and use by other body tissues.[2]

Glucose is metabolized in the cells through glycolysis, an anaerobic process that occurs in the cell cytoplasm.[2] During glycolysis, glucose is converted to pyruvate resulting in the production of adenosine triphosphate (ATP) (see Figure 2.1).[5] Pyruvate can be metabolized under anaerobic conditions to form lactate. During anaerobic metabolism, six molecules of ATP are formed. Additionally, pyruvate can be transaminated to the amino acid alanine, carboxylated to oxaloacetate, or decarboxylated to acetyl CoA (see Figure 2.2).[6] The Krebs cycle, as illustrated in Figure 2.3, serves as the final common pathway for the oxidation of many fuel molecules. CHOs, amino acids, and lipids can enter the Krebs cycle after being converted to acetyl CoA.[6]

Following an increase in the blood glucose level as well as certain amino acids and fatty acids, the β-cells in the islets of Langerhans in the pancreas secrete the anabolic hormone insulin, which promotes the storage of nutrients. Incretins (gastrointestinal hormones), glucose-dependent insulinotropic polypeptide (GIP), and glucagon-like peptide-1 (GLP-1) also play a role in glucose homeostasis. Like insulin, they are released in response to a meal and act on the pancreatic β-cells, thereby stimulating insulin secretion.[1] Insulin secretion results in the

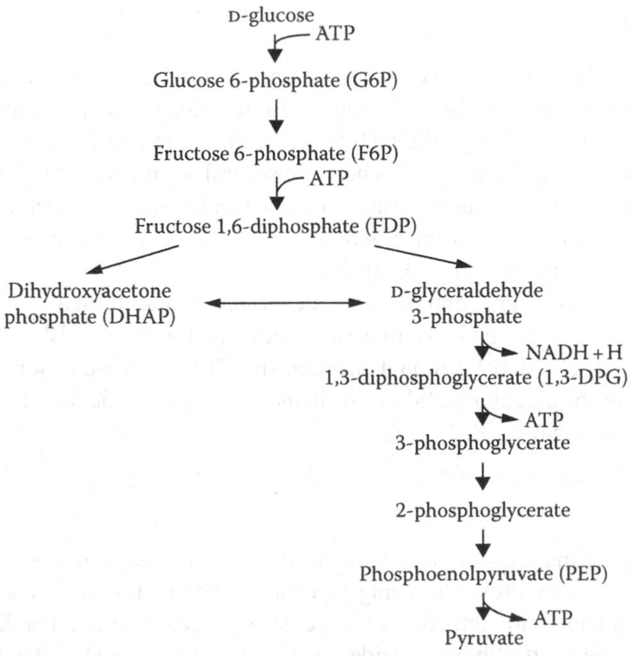

FIGURE 2.1 Two stages of glycogen. (Reprinted with permission from Welborn, M.B. and Moldawer, L.L., Glucose metabolism, in: Rombeau, J.L. and Rolandelli, R.H. (eds.), *Clinical Nutrition Enteral and Tube Feeding*, 3rd edn., WB Saunders Co., Philadelphia, PA, 1997, pp. 61–80.)

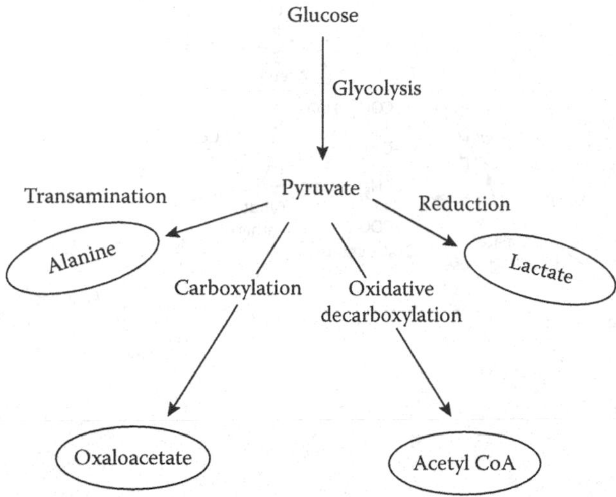

FIGURE 2.2 Possible fates of pyruvate. (Reprinted with permission from DeLegge, M.H. and Ridley, C., Nutrient digestion, absorption, and excreation, in: Gottschlich, M.M., Fuhrman, M.P., Hammond, K.A., Holcombe, B.J., and Seidner, D.L. (eds.), *The Science and Practice of Nutrition Support: A Case-Based Core Curriculum*, Kendall/Hunt Publishing Co., Dubuque, IA, 2001, pp. 1–16.)

disposal of glucose within the tissues as glycogen in the liver and muscle, triglyceride synthesis, and amino acid transport and synthesis into proteins in the insulin-sensitive peripheral tissues, primarily the skeletal muscle. Following cellular uptake, the majority of glucose is metabolized to pyruvate via glycolysis to provide energy for cellular processes, while some is stored as glycogen (see Figure 2.1).[2,5]

A decrease in the blood glucose level, or hypoglycemia, is the main stimulus for the secretion of glucagon from the α-cells of the islets of Langerhans in the pancreas. Glucagon, the major counter-regulatory hormone of insulin, is primarily responsible for signaling the production of glucose from endogenous sources through the activation of hepatic glycogenolysis (the breakdown of glycogen stores) and gluconeogenesis and mobilization of fatty acids from the adipose tissue.[1] The glucocorticoids such as cortisol, secreted by the adrenal cortex, also stimulate the secretion of glucagon as well as secretion of gluconeogenic precursors from the peripheral tissues. Glucocorticoids also inhibit glucose utilization by extrahepatic tissues.[1]

Gluconeogenesis, which entails the use of non-CHO substrates (amino acids and fat) for conversion to glucose, serves as a mechanism to ensure a steady source of glucose is always available. The liver is the major site of gluconeogenesis, but the kidney is also able to produce glucose and release it into the circulation via gluconeogenesis.[7] Gluconeogenesis occurs during stress when inadequate glucose substrate is available. The hormones, glucagon, cortisol, and epinephrine stimulate the process, while insulin suppresses it. Gluconeogenesis can also be inhibited by hyperglycemia independent of hormonal levels. During times of stress, enhanced gluconeogenesis persists despite elevated serum glucose and insulin levels.[2]

During the postabsorptive state, the body relies on endogenous fuel production to meet metabolic requirements. This state is characterized by the release, interorgan transfer, and oxidation of endogenous fatty acids and the continued release of glucose from liver glycogen stores and skeletal release of amino acids. Glycogen stores within the muscle serve as a ready source of glucose within the muscle, and circulating insulin levels remain low.[1,2]

Healthy adults require approximately 200 g of CHO per day to meet metabolic demands and provide the brain with adequate glucose (the adult brain requires approximately 140 g/day).[1,2] When blood glucose levels fall below a critical level, headache, slurred speech, confusion, seizures, unconsciousness, coma, and death can result if energy substrate for brain activity is reduced.[7] To avoid

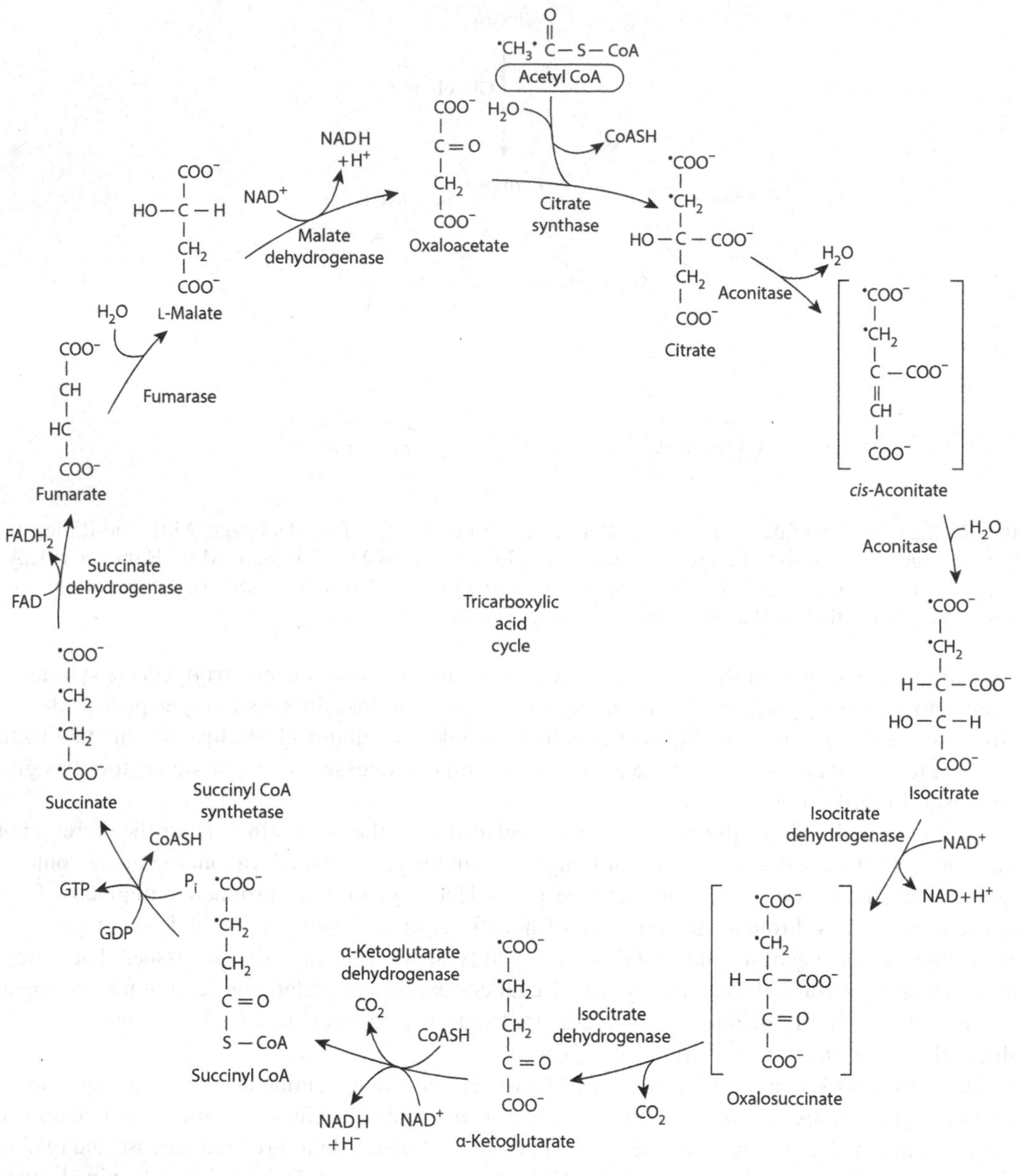

FIGURE 2.3 Krebs cycle. (Reprinted with permission from DeLegge, M.H. and Ridley, C., Nutrient digestion, absorption, and excreation, in: Gottschlich, M.M., Fuhrman, M.P., Hammond, K.A., Holcombe, B.J., and Seidner, D.L. (eds.), *The Science and Practice of Nutrition Support*: *A Case-Based Core Curriculum*, Kendall/Hunt Publishing Co., Dubuque, IA, 2001, pp. 1–16.)

these circumstances, glucose levels are generally tightly controlled by a variety of physiological controls, including glycogenolysis and gluconeogenesis, with each providing approximately 50% of endogenously produced glucose in the postabsorptive state.[2]

Blood glucose and insulin levels start declining with blood glucagon levels increasing approximately an hour after meal consumption. During the fasted state, both blood glucose and serum insulin levels continually decline. Glucose transport into the muscle and fat stores also decrease as a result. Due to changes in the plasma glucose-to-glucagon ratio, glycogenolysis ensues resulting in inhibition of hepatic glycogen synthesis. Figure 2.4 summarizes the substrate fluxes associated with both the fasted and fed states.[8]

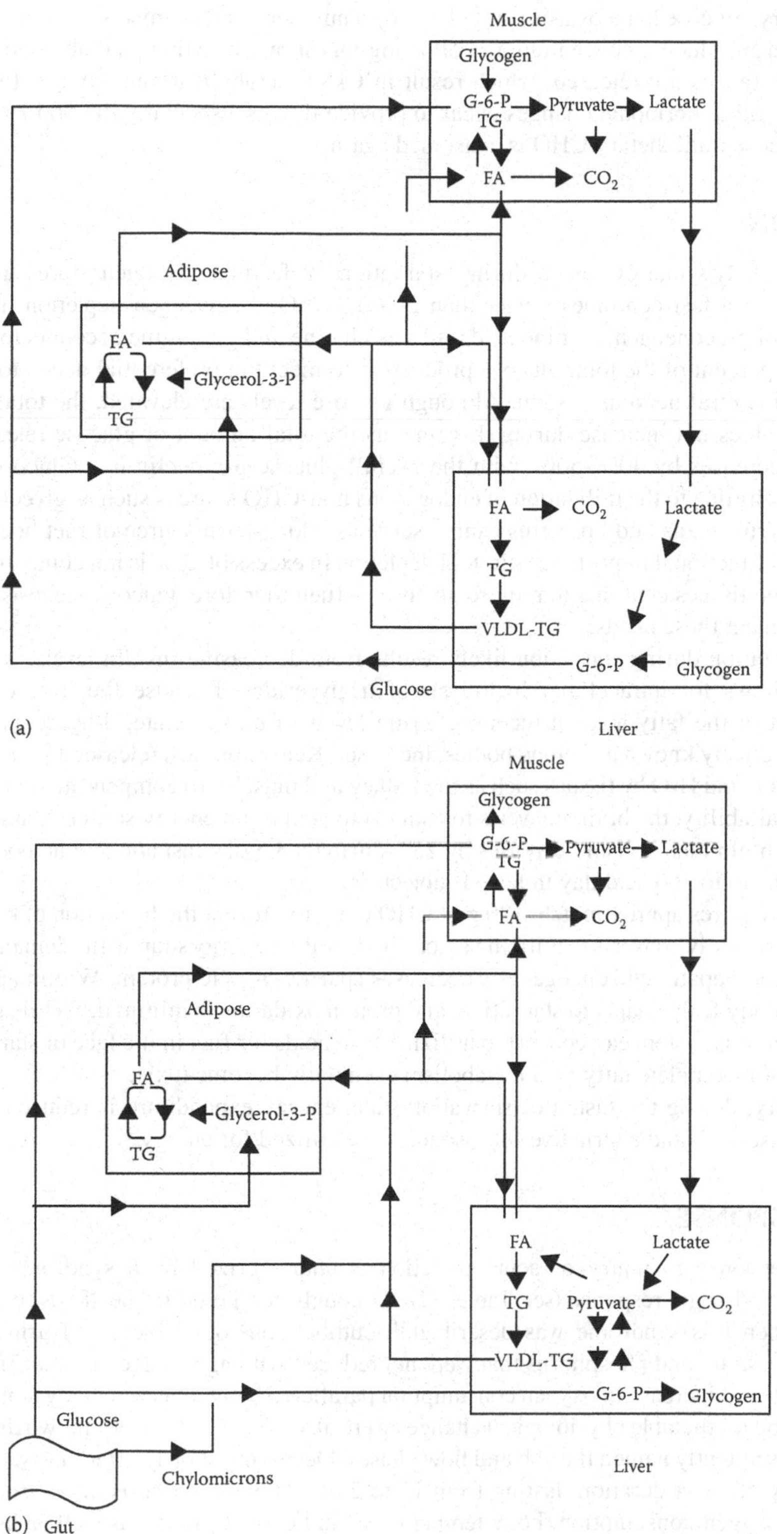

FIGURE 2.4 Substrate fluxes in fasted (a) and fed (b) critically ill patients. (Reprinted with permission from Wolfe, R.R. and Martini, W.Z., *World J. Surg.*, 24, 639, 2000.)

In summary, glucose homeostasis is regulated by a number of mechanisms, designed to maintain an optimal serum glucose concentration. Following ingestion, digestion, and absorption of CHOs, hormonal substances are released, which result in CHO metabolism and storage. In the postabsorptive state, other hormonal changes occur to provide tissues, especially the brain, with a steady supply of glucose until dietary CHO is consumed again.

STARVATION

To meet the body's energy needs during starvation or fasting, glycogen stores are gradually exhausted when a fast continues longer than 2–3 days.[9] Once glycogen depletion has occurred, deamination of gluconeogenic amino acids such as alanine and glutamine accounts for an increasingly greater percent of the total glucose production to meet the preferential needs for glucose by the brain and central nervous system. Although glucose levels are elevated, the total rate of gluconeogenesis does not increase during this time as the total amount of glucose released into the circulation decreases by 40%–50%, with the overall glucose use declining.[9] Glucose production thereafter results due to the utilization of endogenous non-CHO sources such as glycerol, as well as lactate and pyruvate, as body proteins cannot serve as a long-term source of fuel because of their structural and functional importance. Protein depletion in excess of 20% is not compatible with life. However, some tissues continue to require glucose as fuel; therefore, gluconeogenesis continues at low levels to meet these needs.

Fat mobilization during starvation likely results from decreasing insulin levels, which inhibits lipase and allows for intracellular hydrolysis of triglycerides. Because the liver only partially oxidizes most of the fatty acids it receives, serum levels of acetoacetate, β-hydroxybutyrate, and acetone, collectively known as ketone bodies, increase.[9] Ketone bodies, released by the liver, can be oxidized to CO_2 and H_2O by tissues such as the kidney and muscle. To compensate for this reduction in glucose availability, the brain converts to using keto acid as an energy source. Hasselbalch et al. reported that brain metabolism decreases by 25% during a 3.5 day fast and ketone body utilization increases from 16 to 160 kcal/day in fasted subjects.[10]

The body requires approximately 100 g of CHO daily to prevent the formation of ketone bodies. As the body gradually converts to utilizing ketone bodies as an energy source, the demand for glucose diminishes, and hepatic gluconeogenesis decreases sparing muscle protein. Within approximately 2 weeks, the body fully adapts to starvation, and protein oxidation is minimal.[9] While the brain and the central nervous system can convert to utilizing keto acids for fuel in the face of starvation, these by-products of incomplete fatty acid metabolism eventually become toxic.

In summary, during the fasted or starvation state, energy expenditure is reduced, and protein stores are conserved, and alternative fuels sources are utilized for energy.

STRESS RESPONSE

The stress response to injury or acute infection is characterized by a syndrome exhibiting a predictable physiologic response (see Table 2.1). Although first noted in the 1860s, it was not until the 1930s when this syndrome was described.[11] Cuthbertson found increased urinary losses of nitrogen, potassium, and phosphorus that were not reduced with aggressive oral nutrition following injury.[11] A gradual increase in oxygen consumption paralleled by increases in body temperature was also noted. The predictable physiological changes were also observed to occur in two distinct phases that were subsequently named the ebb and flow phases. Occurring shortly after injury, the ebb phase was generally of short duration, lasting from 12 to 24 h. The ebb phase is also associated with a reduction in oxygen consumption, body temperature, and cardiac output as well as hypoperfusion and lactic acidosis.[11]

Following resuscitation, the ebb phase gradually gives way to the flow phase that is characterized by hypermetabolism, alterations in glucose, protein and fat metabolism, and a hyperdynamic

TABLE 2.1
Clinical Manifestations of the Stress Response

Ebb Phase	Flow Phase
Reduced oxygen consumption	Increased oxygen consumption
Reduced body temperature	Body temperature increased
Reduced cardiac output	Increased cardiac output
Elevated blood glucose levels	Normal or slightly increased glucose
Glucose production normal	Glucose production increased
Increased free fatty acids	Release of free fatty acids increased
Low insulin levels	Insulin levels increased
Increased catecholamine levels	Elevated catecholamine levels
Increased glucagon levels	Elevated glucagon levels
Increased blood lactate levels	Normal blood lactate levels

cardiovascular response (see Table 2.1). Elevated ADH and aldosterone levels also result in sodium and fluid retention leading to increases in body weight. Generally, the stress response peaks several days following insult and slowly diminishes as recovery ensues. During the recovery phase, excess fluid and sodium accumulations are also excreted resulting in body weight.

The duration of the flow phase depends on the severity of injury, presence of infection, and development of complications but typically peaks around 3–5 days, subsides by 7–10 days, and abates with transition into the anabolic phase.[11] Although this stress response is a fundamental physiologic response to preserve organ function and repair damaged tissue and occurs following uncomplicated procedures such as elective surgery, with trauma and severe infections, the response can be prolonged having a deleterious impact on health as protein and fat mass is depleted resulting in malnutrition. If allowed to continue unabated, multiorgan failure and death follow. The intensity of the stress response generally parallels the severity of illness and injury.

Alterations in Glucose Metabolism

As discussed, alterations in CHO metabolism are commonly associated with trauma, sepsis, burns, and surgery. Although the precise mechanisms leading to the hypermetabolic response are not completely understood, a predictable milieu mediated by a variety of hormones and cytokines generally results in hypercatabolism (see Figure 2.5).[12]

This stress response results in major metabolic alterations as the body shifts from an anabolic state of storing glucose as glycogen to a catabolic state and significant increases in energy expenditure. To meet the increased demands in energy, body nutrient stores are mobilized to provide substrates to meet the increased energy demands. The body's glycogen stores are quickly depleted in the first 24 h.[15] Fat and protein mass serve as energy sources thereafter. Although adipose stores are mobilized and oxidized for energy, they do not inhibit the catabolism of protein. Similarly to simple starvation, the hypercatabolism leads to the loss of lean body mass but quicker and to a greater extent.

The alterations in CHO metabolism commonly associated with the hypermetabolic response include stress-induced hyperglycemia, enhanced peripheral glucose uptake and utilization, hyperlactatemia, increased glucose production via glyconeolysis and gluconeogenesis, suppressed glycogenesis, glucose intolerance, and insulin resistance (IR) as reflected by persistent hyperglycemia in spite of elevated insulin levels.[14] Moreover, the production of reactive oxygen species (ROS) may also indirectly alter glucose metabolism through modifications in DNA that activate signaling cascades (e.g., nuclear enzyme poly-ADP-ribose polymerase 1) that diminish glycolysis and ATP synthesis.[14]

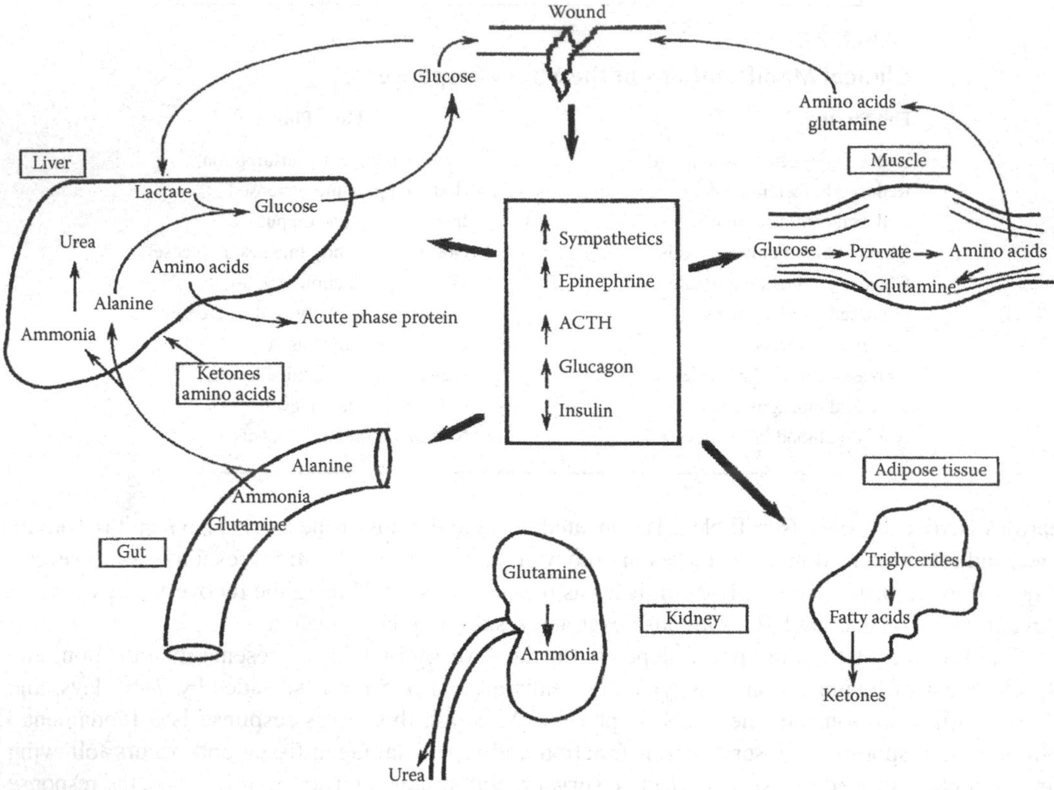

FIGURE 2.5 Neuroendocrine and metabolic consequences of injury. (Reprinted with permission from Smith, M.K. and Lowry, S.F., The hypercatabolic state, in: Shils, M.E., Olson, J.A., Shike, M., and Ross, A.C. (eds.), *Modern Nutrition in Health and Disease*, 9th edn., Williams & Wilkins, Baltimore, MD, 1999, pp. 1555–1568.)

Initially during the ebb phase, glucose production is slightly increased with low insulin levels.[15] While insulin levels increase during the flow phase, glucose levels continue to be elevated as characterized by hyperglycemia suggesting an alteration in the relationship between insulin sensitivity and glucose disposal. Studies involving trauma patients reflect that hepatic glucose production results from utilization of three-carbon precursors including glycerol, pyruvate, lactate, and amino acids, primarily glutamine and alanine.[16] Lactate, produced as a result of anaerobic metabolism, released from the skeletal muscle and other tissues, is recycled to glucose via the Cori cycle, whereas glucose is reconstituted from alanine in the glucose–alanine cycle.[18] The utilization of lactate for gluconeogenesis via the Cori cycle is metabolically expensive as 1 mol of glucose yields two ATP through glycolysis but costs three ATP via gluconeogenesis.[12] This may also contribute to the increased energy requirements associated with the flow phase. Elevated serum lactate levels are frequently associated with hypotension, hypoperfusion, and hypoxia.[19]

In spite of this built-in protective mechanism, it appears that during times of sepsis, hypoglycemia can result. Wilmore observed that in burn patients who developed septic complications, glucose production decreased, whereas production was maintained in patients with thermal injuries without sepsis.[18] It thus appears that a factor inhibiting glucose production is present during sepsis that is not apparent during nonseptic stress.

Elevated glucose levels typically parallel the severity of the illness or injury. Stress-induced hyperglycemia is commonly associated with surgery, trauma, sepsis, and myocardial infarction.[14] While glucose utilization by the central nervous system appears normal in the injured patient, the kidneys and the wound appear to be the primary consumers of glucose.[15] Souba and Wilmore reported that patients with severe burns to one leg compared with minor injuries sustained by the other leg experienced a fourfold uptake of glucose by the burned limb.[16] Furthermore, the wound released large amounts of lactate due to the significant amounts of glucose consumed. Although, as previously described, lactate is converted back to glucose, this again results in greater utilization of energy.

A marked rise in the counterregulatory hormones glucagon, glucocorticoids, and catecholamines accompanies all phases of injury. With the onset of the flow phase and hypermetabolism, these hormones exert a constellation of metabolic effects as exhibited in Figure 2.5.

Glucagon, epinephrine, and norepinephrine are the catabolic hormones primarily responsible for stimulating endogenous glucose production and pro-inflammatory cytokine release (e.g., tumor necrosis factor [TNF]-alpha and interleukins [IL] IL-1, IL-6, and IL-12).[20] In clinical studies, administration of these hormones, singly or in combinations, mimics the metabolic alterations associated with critical illness.[21] Glucagon is known as the primary hormone responsible for producing hepatic gluconeogenesis and glycogenolysis, while epinephrine is the primary culprit in stimulating glycogenolysis.[18,21] Cortisol mobilizes amino acid efflux from the skeletal muscle thereby providing substrate for hepatic gluconeogenesis. The catecholamines stimulate hepatic gluconeogenesis and glycolysis, increase lactate production from the peripheral tissues, and increase metabolic rate and lipolysis.[15]

Many of the hormonal changes manifested with injury or infection appear to be mediated by a variety of cytokines. TNF, IL-1, IL-2, and IL-6 and interferon-γ are the cytokines most studied, with TNF thought to be the primary initiator of many of the subsequent responses that occur following injury and infection.[15] IR results with increased hepatic glucose production, decreased glycogen deposition, and alterations in insulin cell signaling due to the influence of elevated cytokine levels.[14] IR is further promoted through the inhibition of insulin receptor phosphorylation by TNF-α and reductions in the expression of GLUT4.[22] Overall, glucose uptake is increased in the gut, liver, spleen, and lung, while alternatively glucose uptake is diminished in the skeletal muscle due to IR.[22] Cortisol, in addition to pro-inflammatory cytokines (primarily IL-6 and TNF-α), also supports IR by reducing pancreatic β-cell insulin production.[14]

IMPLICATIONS FOR NUTRITION SUPPORT

When starvation is superimposed on injury or critical illness, the metabolic alterations commonly associated with starvation (discussed in the section "Starvation") that result in a reduction in energy expenditure and protein sparing do not occur. Conversely, due to the physiological changes that occur during the stress response (also discussed in the section "Starvation"), lean body mass is catabolized as an energy source to meet the increased energy needs. Hyperglycemia is a common complication in the critically ill patient, even in those without a prior history of diabetes mellitus.[23,24] Therefore, clinicians must take the alterations in glucose metabolism into consideration when making recommendations for or prescribing administration of exogenous glucose provided via parenteral or enteral nutrition, as well as other glucose-containing solutions. In healthy individuals, the exogenous provision of glucose or insulin results in suppression of glucose production. In contrast, studies in the critically ill have found IR (central or hepatic and peripheral) is prevalent and contributes to endogenous glucose production (gluconeogenesis) and poor glycemic control.[25–28]

Insulin Resistance and Glycemic Control

IR and subsequent hyperglycemia are associated with adverse effects such as suppression of immune function, increased release of inflammatory cytokines, elevated oxidative stress (which can lead to more endothelial and platelet dysfunction and vascular constriction), hypercatabolism, hypertriglyceridemia, and prolonged gastric emptying.[23,27] Zauner et al. compared IR in medical ICU patients on their second ICU day with healthy controls. The researchers found the ICU patients to have severe IR compared to the healthy controls ($p < 0.001$). IR was associated with APACHE III score, body mass index (BMI), and resting energy expenditure. Factors that did not impact IR in this study were age, basal glucose level, diagnosis, and respiratory quotient.[25] Saberi et al. studied IR in both surgical and medical ICU patients. This study found upon admit to the ICU, 67% of patients had overt IR and ~10% had nonovert IR, while 24% were sensitive to insulin. Additional patients developed IR during the ICU course, and only 10% of patients remained insulin sensitive.[27] Duška and Anděl studied IR in multiple trauma patients on nutrition support (enteral feedings + supplemental parenteral feedings to reach the goals of 1.5 g protein/kg and caloric provision at 80% of measured energy expenditure).[28] The glucose dose was 192 ± 57 g/day and was constant throughout the 13-day study, and all the patients required exogenous insulin for glycemic control. These investigators demonstrated that IR and exogenous insulin requirements are more pronounced during the first week following injury and that by 14 days post-trauma, insulin sensitivity improves and stabilizes.[28] IR is present in all types of ICU patients and appears to correlate with severity of illness. The underlying causes of IR are complex and could be related to a decrease and inhibition of insulin receptors.[29]

Despite a large body of evidence that suggests hyperglycemia leads to worse outcomes, ongoing controversy exists about how to intervene in the critically ill patient with IR and subsequent hyperglycemia. The van den Berghe prospective randomized trials demonstrated tight glycemic control (target blood glucose: 80–110 mg/dL) versus conventional therapy (target blood glucose: 180–200 mg/dL) led to better outcomes, including less organ failure and lower mortality.[30,31] More recent research, including the normoglycaemia in intensive care evaluation and survival using glucose algorithm regulation (NICE-SUGAR) trial and a meta-analysis, did not confirm these findings and found intensive insulin therapy associated with more hypoglycemic events and higher mortality.[32,33] The NICE-SUGAR study compared tight glycemic control (target blood glucose: 81–108 mg/dL) to conventional therapy (target blood glucose: 140–180 mg/dL). Methodological differences do exist between these studies that may explain their conflicting results, including predominant routes of nutrition support. The subjects in the van den Berghe trials received a higher proportion of calories from parenteral nutrition than those in the NICE-SUGAR trial. Additionally, the target blood glucose levels and methods of insulin administration delivery were not the same.[34] After reviewing and grading the evidence available, The American Society of Parenteral and Enteral Nutrition (ASPEN) released guidelines for patients on nutrition support with hyperglycemia. ASPEN's recommendation, which takes into account not only the evidence but also patient safety, for the optimal target blood glucose is 140–180 mg/dL.[35]

Another intriguing and important consideration in the debate surrounding the optimal blood glucose target involves critically ill patients with and without preexisting diabetes. A multicenter retrospective study by Lanspa et al. evaluated 30-day mortality in patients with and without diabetes receiving moderate (90–140 mg/dL) versus tight glycemic control (80–100 mg/dL). Not surprisingly, the patients with diabetes, compared to those without, had a higher average glucose level (132 vs. 124 mg/dL) and more glycemic variability (41 vs. 29 mg/dL). Both types of patients who were treated for tight glycemic control had a higher incidence of hypoglycemia compared to those with the moderate target. The 30-day mortality risk in the moderate control patients, evaluated by a multivariate analysis, was decreased in those with diabetes but increased in those without diabetes.[36] A retrospective study by Schlussel et al. compared outcomes (primary, mortality; secondary, hospital and ICU length of stay [LOS], days on mechanical ventilation, and readmission to the ICU) in 395 medical and surgical ICU patients (235 patients with preexisting diabetes) with controlled (80–140 mg/dL) versus uncontrolled blood glucose levels (>140 mg/dL). They conducted three different analyses of the patients: nondiabetic versus diabetic, diabetic patients with controlled versus uncontrolled blood glucose levels, and diabetic survivors versus nonsurvivors. A majority of the patients (59%) had a history of diabetes. There were no differences in outcomes between the nondiabetic and diabetic patients except for ICU LOS (patients with diabetes were in the ICU ~ 3 days less than nondiabetic patients, $p = 0.01$). The outcome data for controlled versus uncontrolled diabetic patients were not different. Several parameters (presence of one hypoglycemic event, minimum blood glucose, ventilator days, and ICU LOS) were worse in nondiabetic survivors than diabetic survivors.[37] This study, like the one by Lanspa, suggests that patients with a history of diabetes are particularly vulnerable to worse outcomes with tight glycemic control and increased risk of hypoglycemia.

Recommendations for Glucose Provision

Changes in glucose metabolism in the critical care setting impact the nutrition support prescription leading to patient variability in CHO dosing. Clinicians should evaluate patients' glycemic control and factors that predispose the patient to hyperglycemia prior to initiation of nutrition support and determine the appropriate amount of CHO to provide in the initial nutrition support prescription. And, as a patient's clinical status and medications change (e.g., corticosteroids, intravenous fluids, other medications that can influence serum glucose levels), the CHO dose may need to be adjusted. Excess administration of CHO has been associated with hyperglycemia, which is more common with parenteral versus enteral nutrition, hepatic dysfunction, and increased carbon dioxide production. In general, the ideal amount of CHO is that which spares the use of protein for energy while also avoiding hyperglycemia. The recommended dose of CHO is no more than 4–5 mg/kg/min and should not exceed 7 mg/kg/min in adults. To minimize the potential for hyperglycemia associated with parenteral nutrition (PN), others recommend initiating support with approximately half of the CHO needs, approximately 150–200 g for the first 24 h. In patients who are hyperglycemic prior to initiation of PN, an even lower dose of 100 g of CHO is appropriate.[38]

A study by Rosmarin and colleagues demonstrates why a CHO dose of 4–5 mg/kg/min is recommended. In a relatively small retrospective study (not exclusively in ICU patients), 102 patients receiving PN were evaluated to determine if those who received a dextrose infusion rate >4–5 mg/kg/min had more hyperglycemia (defined as >200 mg/dL). Patients were excluded if they were obese, were significantly underweight, or had a condition that made them more likely to develop hyperglycemia. Patients who received PN for <3 days and those who received >500 cal via enteral nutrition by the third day of PN were also excluded. Of the patients (N = 19) who received dextrose provision ≤4 mg/kg/min, none experienced hyperglycemia; 5 patients experienced hyperglycemia with glucose provision of 4.1–5.0 mg/kg/min, and hyperglycemia was experienced by 18/19 (~95%) of patients receiving dextrose ≥5 mg/kg/min. A multivariate analysis found the relationship between PN dextrose infusion rate and glucose concentration was statistically significant ($p < 0.001$).[39] This study attempted to control for confounding factors by eliminating patients that are more likely to experience hyperglycemia. Despite the exclusion criteria, the impact of the dextrose dose on serum glucose levels was significant. Another retrospective study by Lee and associates investigated the relationship between the dextrose provided in the PN during the first week in the ICU and development of hyperglycemia (defined as ≥140 mg/dL) and impact on clinical outcomes (infections, acute renal failure, cardiac complications, and mortality) in 88 ICU patients. Fifty-nine (67%) of the patients were designated to the hyperglycemia group. The average intravenous dextrose dose from both PN and IV fluids for all patients was 2.3 ± 1.4 g/kg/day. Patients with hyperglycemia received significantly more dextrose (from IV sources) than those with normal glucose levels (2.6 ± 1.4 vs. 1.8 ± 1.3 g/kg/day, $p = 0.013$). The majority (75/88 or 85%) of the patients were also provided enteral nutrition (EN) within the first week of their ICU stay. The total dose of CHO (between 3 and 4 g/kg/day that translates into ~2–2.8 mg/kg/min) from all sources was not different between the hyperglycemia and normoglycemia groups. However, the route of delivery, parenteral versus enteral, was important as those patients receiving more CHO via EN had lower rates of hyperglycemia compared to patients receiving more CHO from PN. This study found mortality to be significantly higher in the hyperglycemia group (42.4% vs. 13.8%, $p = 0.008$). Other complications were not different. The retrospective design and relatively small sample size may have affected this outcome. Nonetheless, this study demonstrates the high incidence of hyperglycemia in ICU patients, particularly those who receive more dextrose via a parenteral route.[40] In contrast, a retrospective study by Dan et al. did not find a difference in hyperglycemia between 96 ICU patients fed enterally compared to 2 different parenteral formulas (dextrose based or dextrose + lipid based). Despite higher caloric intake in the patients on PN, there was not a difference in mean blood glucose or daily insulin dose between the groups. They attribute the lack of difference to their intensive insulin therapy protocol.[41] Based on the evidence to date, avoiding excessive dextrose as well as overfeeding in general, along with effective insulin therapy, can assist in better glycemic control and promote better outcomes. To promote optimal glycemic control, the dextrose provision for critically ill patients should not exceed 4–5 mg/kg/min that can be calculated as follows:

$$\text{mg/kg/min dextrose load} = \frac{\text{Dextrose (mg)}}{\text{Body weight (kg)} \times (1440\ \text{min}^{*})}$$

$$^{*}24\ \text{h} = 1440\ \text{min}$$

Preoperative Carbohydrate Loading

Because the fasted state changes the hormonal milieu, researchers have been investigating whether avoidance of the traditional fasting period prior to elective surgery impacts outcomes. Earlier research in animal models demonstrates that short-term fasting affects survival following hemorrhage. The mechanism behind the fed state improving survival is related to the availability of hepatic glycogen as a source of glucose and the subsequent hyperglycemic state. Hyperglycemia leads to hyperosmolality in the extracellular space, followed by a shift of water from the intracellular space to the extracellular space, which includes plasma. The ability to replenish the plasma volume was essential for survival in these animal studies. Further studies found that the fasted state at the time of insult was the factor that led to a heightened stress response compared to animals in the fed state, and the availability of glycogen was the crucial element. Based on these animal data, researchers began investigating CHO loading in humans undergoing elective surgery and its effect on IR and outcomes.[42]

An initial small study in patients undergoing elective cholecystectomy evaluated the use of preoperative intravenous 20% glucose solution infused overnight (~300 g CHO in 1500 mL infused at 5 mg/kg/min) compared to fasting on postoperative IR, which was decreased by 50% in those who received the treatment compared to the controls. However, this concentration of dextrose was not well tolerated via a peripheral vein.[43] Therefore, the focus shifted to the development of an oral CHO drink that would empty out of the stomach quickly enough to avoid safety concerns prior to surgery, which contains adequate CHO content to stimulate insulin release (which then leads to glycogen storage). A drink comprised of ~12% complex CHO/50 g CHO (with a low osmolality) was created and has been utilized safely in many clinical trials and clinical practice to date.[42] A meta-analysis by Awad and colleagues evaluated whether preoperative carbohydrate loading (PCL) affected clinical outcomes (LOS, postoperative IR, complications, nausea, and vomiting). The meta-analysis included randomized prospective studies evaluating nondiabetic adults who received PCL (≥50 g oral CHOs 2–4 h preanesthesia) versus being fasted or receiving a placebo. Over 1600 patients from 21 studies were included in the meta-analysis that found no difference in LOS for all patients as well as subgroups with an expected hospital stay ≤2 days or those undergoing orthopedic surgical procedures. The patients that seemed to benefit from the PCL were those undergoing major abdominal surgery as these patients did have a shorter LOS. The PCL compared to controls did have less postoperative IR, but there was not any effect on complications. The researchers noted significant heterogeneity among the studies and stated the evidence is of low to moderate quality in this meta-analysis.[44]

While PCL is not possible for all ICU patients due to the situations, often emergent, which lead to their need for a surgical procedure and ICU admission, preliminary research suggests it may play a role in reducing IR in elective surgical cases. While PCL seems to improve postoperative IR, more research is needed to establish that clinical outcomes are improved as well.

REFEEDING SYNDROME

Refeeding syndrome (RFS) occurs after reintroduction of nutrition, particularly CHO (from oral, EN, PN, or dextrose-containing IVFs) in starved and/or malnourished individuals. RFS is characterized by a shift in fluid and electrolytes and can lead to cardiac, pulmonary, neurologic, muscular, and hematologic complications.[45,46] While nutrition support (EN or PN) is commonly associated with RFS, clinicians should remember that oral nutrition as well as intravenous dextrose can also precipitate this potentially fatal condition. RFS was first recognized after World War II (WWII) when malnourished prisoners of war were released and provided food in an effort to help them recover and died suddenly. These were extreme cases of malnutrition and starvation. RFS can occur in less severe cases of starvation in hospitalized patients than what was seen following WWII. In the ICU patient population, where EN and PN are common place, it is important during assessment and when designing a nutrition support regimen to determine if the patient possesses risk factors for RFS. The common conditions that place patients at risk for RFS are listed in Table 2.2.[45,47]

During starvation, fat and protein mass is tapped for energy once glycogen stores are depleted (see the section "Starvation"). Once nutrition is reinstated, a change in metabolism occurs, namely, a shift from using fat stores for energy to using CHO. The presence of glucose stimulates insulin release and leads to cellular uptake of glucose and electrolytes to support anabolic activities in the cells. Circulating levels of potassium, phosphorus, and magnesium can drop precipitously. Other possible RFS manifestations include hyperglycemia, fluid and sodium retention, and thiamine deficiency. Thiamine deficiency can occur because patients at risk for RFS may already be deficient in thiamine, and it is a necessary cofactor for CHO metabolism and can be rapidly depleted with CHO refeeding. The combination of these can lead to muscle weakness, cardiac arrhythmias, poor cellular oxygenation, cardiac failure, respiratory failure, Wernicke's encephalopathy, anemia, and infections.[48]

A prospective cohort study by Rio et al. aimed to identify which risk factors best predict the development of RFS.[49] They studied 243 patients who were started on EN or PN in the hospital (both ICU and non-ICU units). The risk factors were based on criteria set by the England's National

TABLE 2.2
Conditions/Patient Populations Associated with RFS

- Prolonged fasting
- Post-bariatric surgery
- Hunger strikers
- Oncology patients
- Postoperative patients
- Uncontrolled diabetes
- Severely malnourished
- Anorexia nervosa
- Chronic alcoholism
- Elderly with decreased reserves and other comorbidities
- Hospitalized patients who go without nutrition for >7 days
- Malabsorptive conditions (short bowel syndrome, inflammatory bowel diseases, chronic pancreatitis)
- Long-term users of antacids (due to binding of phosphate)
- Long-term users of diuretics (due to electrolyte losses)

Sources: Mehanna, H.M. et al., *Brit. Med. J.*, 336, 1495, 2008; Kraft, M.D. et al., *Nutr. Clin. Pract.*, 20, 625, 2005.

TABLE 2.3
NICE Criteria for Identifying Risk for RFS

Patients are considered at risk if one of the following is present:	Patients are considered at risk if two of the following are present:
• BMI <16 kg/m^2	• BMI <18.5 kg/m^2
• Unintentional weight loss >15% in the preceding 3–6 months	• Unintentional weight loss >10% in the preceding 3–6 months
• Very little or no nutritional intake for more than 10 days	• Very little or no nutritional intake for more than 5 days
• Low levels of serum potassium, phosphate, or magnesium prior to feed	• History of alcohol or drug abuse

Source: NICE guideline—Nutrition support in adults, The National Institute for Health and Clinical Excellence, http://www.nice.org.uk, Accessed February 5, 2013.

Institute for Health and Clinical Excellence (NICE) and are found in Table 2.3.[50] They found 133 (55%) patients with RFS risk factors and 44 (18%) of these were ICU patients. The majority (87.2%) of the patients were provided EN, while 9.5% were on PN and 3.3% were given EN + PN. Patients at risk for RFS were initially fed 50% of estimated energy requirements. The researchers used preset criteria for confirmation of RFS: severely low electrolyte levels, peripheral edema or acute circulatory fluid overload, and organ dysfunction (respiratory failure, cardiac failure, or pulmonary edema). Only three patients, all fed with EN, were diagnosed with RFS based on this criteria, and RFS was not deemed the cause of death in any patients. They found that of the potential predictors of RFS, both starvation (poor intake for >10 days) and a low magnesium level at baseline are independent predictors for RFS. They also noted that IV dextrose infusion given prior to the initiation of nutrition support could have triggered the RFS.

A retrospective study by Zeki et al. examined the incidence of RFS in 321 patients fed with EN or PN. They also utilized the NICE risk criteria (Table 2.3) and evaluated whether these predicted the development of RFS as well as the sensitivity and specificity of the NICE guidelines.[51] RFS was defined by the presence of hypophosphatemia (a drop from a normal level to a level <0.6 mmol/L within 1 week of nutrition support initiation) in this study. Ninety-two (29%) patients were classified as being at risk for RFS, and 49 patients (15%) developed RFS. Thirty-three percent (54/168) of patients fed with EN were deemed at risk, and 18/54 (33%) did develop RFS. In EN patients, there was a significant relationship between being at risk and development of RFS ($p < 0.02$). Among patients fed with PN ($n = 153$), 25% (38/153) were at risk and only 5 (13%) developed RFS. In contrast to the EN patients, there was not a significant association between being at risk and developing RFS ($p = 0.31$). Eighteen EN and eight PN patients, who were not identified at risk by the NICE guidelines, did develop RFS. In this study, EN patients were more likely to develop RFS than PN patients ($p < 0.03$). The authors hypothesized that this could be due to the incretin effect associated with enteral glucose intake and poorer enteral absorption of phosphorus. While more patients on EN versus PN (13% vs. 0%) died during the first 7 days of feeding, death was not associated with RFS ($p = 0.73$). They found the NICE guidelines to have a moderate specificity but poor sensitivity for the development of RFS when identified as being at risk.[51]

Skipper analyzed 27 published cases of RFS reported between 2000 and 2011.[52] The majority of the patients were given EN but six received some PN. All cases had a low BMI or poor nutritional intake for more than 48 h prior to the introduction of nutrition. The incidence of electrolyte abnormalities was common, especially hypophosphatemia (96%), hypomagnesemia (51%), and hypokalemia (46%). Hypocalcemia (27%) and hyponatremia (8%) were less common, and thiamine deficiency was confirmed in only one patient. There were not any cases reported with all the characteristics used to define RFS (hypophosphatemia, hypomagnesemia, hypokalemia, hyperglycemia, fluid overload, and thiamine deficiency) during the time period of 2000–2011. Skipper et al. propose that the overall incidence of RFS is either very low or is not being detected and reported. Also suggested is that RFS and refeeding hypophosphatemia (which is what many clinicians use to diagnose RFS) may need to be defined as two distinct problems. Skipper concludes, based on this review of case reports, additional research including adequate follow-up, careful monitoring, and accurate information on nutritional intake is needed to help define and identify the incidence of RFS.[52]

Because RFS can be harmful, prevention of its development is the best practice to undertake, and overzealous feeding with nutrition support in patients at risk for RFS, both EN and PN, should be avoided. Prior to initiating nutrition support in patients at risk for RFS, electrolyte levels (including potassium, phosphate, magnesium, and calcium) should be checked and abnormalities corrected.[45] Thiamine supplementation is also recommended (200–300 mg enterally daily). Nutrition support should be initiated at a maximum of 10 kcal/kg/day and advanced slowly to full dose over 4–7 days. In severe cases of malnutrition (extremely low BMI or almost no intake for >15 days), nutrition should be provided at 5 kcal/kg/day initially. These patients' fluid balance and overall clinical status (including cardiac rhythm) should be monitored very closely. Usually, RFS will develop within the first 4–5 days of refeeding, and close monitoring of electrolytes, serum glucose, and fluid and clinical status should occur during the first 2 weeks of nutrition therapy.[45,50] Identification of patients at high risk and proactive interventions are key to prevention and appropriate management of RFS.

CONCLUSION

CHOs typically constitute the primary energy substrate in human diets. A thorough understanding of the differences between CHO metabolism in starvation and fed states versus a stress state is critical when designing nutrition support regimens for critically ill patients. This will minimize the potential complications associated with glucose administration and promote positive clinical outcomes.

REFERENCES

1. Keim NL, Levin RJ, Havel PJ. Carbohydrates. In Shils ME, Shike M, Ross CA et al. (eds.), *Modern Nutrition in Health and Disease*. Philadelphia, PA: Lippincott, Williams, & Wilkins, pp. 62–82, 2006.
2. Ling P, McCowan KC. Carbohydrates. In Gottschlich MM (ed.), *The A.S.P.E.N. Nutrition Support Core Curriculum: A Case-Based Approach—The Adult Patient*. Silver Spring, MD: American Society for Parenteral and Enteral Nutrition, pp. 33–47, 2007.
3. Colaizzo-Anas T. Nutrient intake, digestion, absorption, and excretion. In Gottschlich MM (ed.), *The A.S.P.E.N. Nutrition Support Core Curriculum: A Case-Based Approach—The Adult Patient*. Silver Spring, MD: American Society for Parenteral and Enteral Nutrition, pp. 3–18, 2007.
4. Triplitt CL. Examining the mechanisms of glucose regulation. *Am J Manag Care*., 18:S4–S10, 2012.
5. Welborn MB, Moldawer LL. Glucose metabolism. In Rombeau JL, Rolandelli RH (eds.), *Clinical Nutrition Enteral and Tube Feeding*, 3rd edn. Philadelphia, PA: WB Saunders Co., pp. 61–80, 1997.
6. DeLegge MH, Ridley C. Nutrient digestion, absorption, and excretion. In Gottschlich MM, Fuhrman MP, Hammond KA, Holcombe BJ, Seidner DL (eds.), *The Science and Practice of Nutrition Support: A Case-Based Core Curriculum*. Dubuque, IA: Kendall/Hunt Publishing Co., pp. 1–16, 2001.
7. Triplitt CL. Understanding the kidneys' role in blood glucose regulation. *Am J Manag Care*., 18:S11–S16, 2012.
8. Wolfe RR, Martini WZ. Changes in intermediary metabolism in severe surgical illness. *World J Surg*., 24:639–647, 2000.
9. Wolfe R, Allsop J, Burke J. Glucose metabolism in man: Responses to intravenous glucose infusion. *Metabolism*, 28:210–220, 1979.
10. Hasselbalch SG, Knudsen GM, Jakobsen J et al. Brain metabolism during short-term starvation in humans. *J Cereb Blood Flow Metab*., 14:125–131, 1994.
11. Cuthbertson DP. Observations on disturbance of metabolism produced by injury to the limbs. *Q J Med*., 25:233–246, 1932.
12. Smith MK, Lowry SF. The hypercatabolic state. In Shils ME, Olson JA, Shike M, Ross AC (eds.), *Modern Nutrition in Health and Disease*, 9th edn. Baltimore, MD: Williams & Wilkins, pp. 1555–1568, 1999.

13. Zhang XF, Kunkel KR, Jahoor F, Wolfe RR. Role of basal insulin the regulation of protein kinetics and energy metabolism in septic patients. *J Parenter Enteral Nutr*., 15:394–399, 1991.
14. Losser MR, Damoisel C, Payen D. Bench-to-bedside review: Glucose and stress conditions in the intensive care unit. *Crit Care*, 14:231, 2010.
15. Wilmore DW, Goodwin CW, Aulick LH et al. Effect of injury and infection on visceral metabolism and circulation. *Ann Surg*., 192:491–504, 1980.
16. Souba W, Wilmore D. Diet and nutrition in the care of the patient with surgery, trauma, and sepsis. In Shils ME, Olson JA, Shike M, Ross AC (eds.), *Modern Nutrition in Health and Disease*, 9th edn. Baltimore, MD: Williams & Wilkins, pp. 1589–1641, 1999.
17. Fischer JE. Nutrition support: We have failed in our ability to support patients with sepsis and cancer. *Surg Clin N Am*., 91:641–651, 2011.
18. Wilmore D. Nutrition and metabolism following thermal injury. *Clin Plast Surg*., 1:603–619, 1974.
19. Chu CA, Sindelar DK, Neal DW et al. Comparison of the direct and indirect effects of epinephrine on hepatic glucose production. *J Clin Invest*., 99:1044–1056, 1997.
20. Calcagni E, Elenkov I. Stress system activity, innate and T-helper cytokines and susceptibility to immune-related diseases. *Ann N Y Acad Sci*., 1069:62–79, 2006.
21. Desbough JP. The stress response to trauma and surgery. *Br J Anaesth*., 85(1):109–117, 2000.
22. Thompson LH, Kim HT, Ma Y, Kokorina NA, Messina JL. Acute, muscle-type specific insulin resistance following injury. *Mol Med*., 14:715–723, 2008.
23. Krenitsky J. Glucose control in the intensive care unit: A nutrition support perspective. *Nutr Clin Pract*., 26:31–43, 2011.
24. Farrokhi F, Smiley D, Upmierrez GE. Glycemic control in non-diabetic critically ill patients. *Best Pract Res Clin Endocrinol Metab*., 25:813–824, 2011.
25. Zauner A, Nimmerrichter P, Anderwald C et al. Severity of insulin resistance in critically ill medical patients. *Metabolism*, 56:1–5, 2007.
26. Van Cromphaut SJ. Hyperglycemia as part of the stress response: The underlying mechanisms. *Best Pract Res Clin Anaesthesiol*., 23:375–386, 2009.
27. Saberi F, Heyland D, Lam M, Rapson D, Jeejeebhoy K. Prevalence, incidence, and clinical resolution of insulin resistance in critically ill patients: An observational study. *J Parenter Enteral Nutr*., 32:227–235, 2008.
28. Duška F, Anděl M. Intensive blood glucose control in acute and prolonged critical illness: Endogenous secretion contributes more to plasma insulin than exogenous insulin infusion. *Metabolism*, 57:669–671, 2008.
29. Brealey D, Singer M. Hyperglycemia in critical illness: A review. *J Diabetes Sci Technol*., 3:1250–1260, 2009.
30. van den Berghe G, Wouters P, Weekers F et al. Intensive insulin therapy in critically ill patients. *N Engl J Med*., 345:1359–1367, 2001.
31. van den Berghe G, Wilmer A, Hermans G et al. Intensive insulin therapy in the medical ICU. *N Engl J Med*., 354:449–461, 2006.
32. Finfer S, Chittock DR, Su SY et al. Intensive versus conventional glucose control in critically ill patients. *N Engl J Med*., 360:1283–1297, 2009.
33. Ling Y, Li X, Gao X. Intensive versus conventional glucose control in critically ill patients: A meta-analysis of randomized controlled trials. *Eur J Intern Med*., 23:564–574, 2012.
34. van den Berghe G, Schertz M, Vlasselaers D et al. Intensive insulin therapy in critically ill patients: NICE-SUGAR or Leuven blood glucose target? *J Clin Endocrinol Metab*., 94:3163–3170, 2009.
35. Lanspa MJ, Hirshberg EL, Phillips GD, Holmen J, Stoddard G, Orme J. Moderate glucose control is associated with increased mortality compared to tight glucose control in critically ill non-diabetics. *Chest*, 143:1226–1234, 2013.
36. Schlussel AT, Holt DB, Crawley EA, Lustik MB, Wade CE, Uyehara CFT. Effect of diabetes mellitus on outcomes of hyperglycemia in a mixed medical surgical intensive care unit. *J Diabetes Sci Technol*., 5:731–740, 2011.
37. McMahon MM, Nystrom E, Braunschweig C et al. A.S.P.E.N. clinical guidelines: Nutrition support of adult patients with hyperglycemia. *J Parenter Enteral Nutr*., 37:23–36, 2013.
38. Kumpf VJ, Gervasio J. Complications of parenteral nutrition. In Gottschlich MM (ed.), *The A.S.P.E.N. Nutrition Support Core Curriculum: A Case-Based Approach—The Adult Patient*. Silver Spring, MD: American Society for Parenteral and Enteral Nutrition, pp. 323–339, 2007.
39. Rosmarin DK, Mirtallo JM, Wardlaw GM. The relationship between TPN dextrose infusion rate and incidence of hyperglycemia. *Nutr Clin Pract*., 11:72, 1996.

40. Lee H, Koh SO, Park MS. Higher dextrose delivery via TPN related to the development of hyperglycemia in non-diabetic critically ill patients. *Nutr Res Pract.*, 5:450–454, 2011.
41. Dan A, Jacques TC, O'Leary MJ. Enteral nutrition versus glucose-based or lipid-based parenteral nutrition and tight glycemic control in critically ill patients. *Crit Care Resusc.*, 8:283–288, 2006.
42. Ljungqvist O. Modulating postoperative insulin resistance by preoperative carbohydrate loading. *Best Pract Res Clin Anaesthesiol.*, 23:401–409, 2009.
43. Ljungqvist O, Thorell A, Guniak M, Häggmark T, Efendic S. Glucose infusion instead of preoperative fasting reduces postoperative insulin resistance. *J Am Coll Surg.*, 178:329–336, 1994.
44. Awad S, Varadhan KK, Ljungqvist O. A meta-analysis of randomized controlled trials on preoperative oral carbohydrate treatment in elective surgery. *Clin Nutr.*, 32:34–44, 2013.
45. Mehanna HM, Moledina J, Travis J. Refeeding syndrome: What it is, and how to prevent and treat it. *Brit Med J.*, 336:1495–1498, 2008.
46. Kraft MD, Btaiche IF, Sacks GS. Review of the refeeding syndrome. *Nutr Clin Pract.*, 20:625–633, 2005.
47. Khan LUR, Ahmed J, Khan S, MacFie J. Refeeding syndrome: A literature review. *Gastroenterol Res Pract.*, 2011:410971, 2011. doi: 10.1155/2011/410971. Accessed February 5, 2013.
48. Byrnes MC, Stangenes J. Refeeding in the ICU: An adult and pediatric problem. *Curr Opin Clin Nutr Metab Care*, 14:186–192, 2011.
49. Rio A, Whelan K, Goff L, Reidlinger DP, Smeeton N. Occurrence of refeeding syndrome in adults started on artificial nutrition support: Prospective cohort study. *BMJ Open*, 3:e002173, 2013. doi:10.1136/bmjopen-2012–002173. Accessed February 5, 2013.
50. NICE guideline—Nutrition support in adults. The National Institute for Health and Clinical Excellence. http://www.nice.org.uk, Accessed February 5, 2013.
51. Zeki S, Culkin A, Gabe SM, Nightingale JM. Refeeding hypophosphatemia is more common in enteral than parenteral feeding in adult patients. *Clin Nutr.*, 30:365–368, 2011.
52. Skipper A. Refeeding syndrome or refeeding hypophosphatemia: A systematic review of cases. *Nutr Clin Pract.*, 27:34–40, 2012.

3 Protein and Amino Acid Metabolism

Stress versus Nonstress States

Gail A. Cresci

CONTENTS

> ... there is a circumstance attending accidental injury which does not belong to a disease, namely that the injury done has in all cases a tendency to produce both, the disposition and means of cure
>
> **John Hunter**
> *Blood, Inflammation and Gunshot Wounds, 1794.*

INTRODUCTION

Critical illness due to trauma, injury, or infections is a major health problem in industrialized society: some 8% of the population die each year as the result of injuries [1,2]. Since trauma affects young people disproportionately, it claims as many years of productive life as cardiovascular diseases and cancer combined [3].

The care of injured patients has improved over the past decade. Some of the responsible factors include effective management of shock, fluid and electrolyte balance, and new nutritional means.

As both common and specific mechanisms for alterations in substrate metabolism are being covered, there arise unique opportunities to intervene in the disease process [4]. Undoubtedly, the efficacy of providing substrate to the injured, immunocompromised, and/or malnourished host has caused a renaissance in the clinical application of dietary intervention in the treatment and prevention of disease [5,6]. Presently, it has become feasible to employ specialized nutritional support and to modify the metabolic response to stress by using pharmacological doses of specific nutrients, especially those related to protein metabolism. Pharmacological nutrition is a novel concept that has introduced a new dimension into the fascinating field of modern clinical nutrition. The explosion of new information related to this exciting approach is certainly only a prelude to its use in routine clinical settings [7].

Indeed, aggressive nutritional support plays a major role in the comprehensive care of injured or critically ill patients [8,9]. The purpose of this chapter is to present a general approach to protein (amino acid) metabolism of severely injured and critically ill patients. The approach is based on our current understanding of biochemical and physiological alterations that occur in such patients and that are known as the metabolic response to trauma, injury, and infection.

NEUROENDOCRINE AND METABOLIC RESPONSE TO STRESS AND THEIR EFFECT ON PROTEIN METABOLISM

Trauma, injury, and infection are insults to a living body caused by certain external forces and may range from minor elective surgery to massive damage, such as severe burns or multiple-system injury. The pathophysiological and biochemical responses from moderate to severe trauma exhibit a very complex picture, influenced by the local effect and the systemic response.

In the majority of cases, the local effects are more easily resolved with adequate treatment. In contrast, the systemic effects are highly dependent on the nature and magnitude of the local injury and thus represent a stereotyped response, which is difficult to treat and stands for the factor that frequently may jeopardize survival [10]. After a variety of insults (e.g., shock, trauma, burns, sepsis, or pancreatitis), patients develop a systematic inflammatory response that is presumably beneficial and resolves as the patient recovers. However, if it is exaggerated or perpetuated, severe disturbances in protein metabolism may arise. The resulting hypermetabolism and catabolism can cause acute protein malnutrition, with impairment in immune function, and subclinical multiple-organ dysfunction, including acute renal failure [11].

The florid protein-wasting response seen early after injury or burns [12], which appears to require adrenaline as well as cortisol and growth hormone, is obviously a catabolic response. Nevertheless, catecholamines also possess general anabolic effects, which appear to be mediated through β-receptors of an unusual kind [13–15]. The anabolic effects of catecholamines are not well understood, and there is a substantial amount of confusion in the literature concerning the exact mechanisms of these effects. Consequently, at present, it is difficult to come to a satisfactory integrated view of the role of catecholamines in the regulation of protein metabolism and lean body mass (LBM).

The hypermetabolism of the stressed patient, whether from injury or infection, is associated with increases in muscle proteolysis, hepatic ureagenesis associated with enhanced glucose production, together with increased mobilization of fat. Both injured and septic patients reveal an increased rate of whole-body protein catabolism, with a more modest increase in protein synthesis leaving a negative nitrogen (N) balance. Infusion with adequate amount of amino acids partially improved the synthesis rate, but the extent of protein catabolism was insensitive to intravenous nutrition [16,17]. Metabolic rate and nitrogen excretion are related to the extent of injury. The two responses generally parallel each other as shown in Figure 3.1.

It has been demonstrated that the infusion of a combination of cortisol, epinephrine, and glucagon could produce the hyperglycemia seen in stress, as well as the increased thermogenesis and N loss, a catabolic picture not shown with the administration of any single hormone [18]. However,

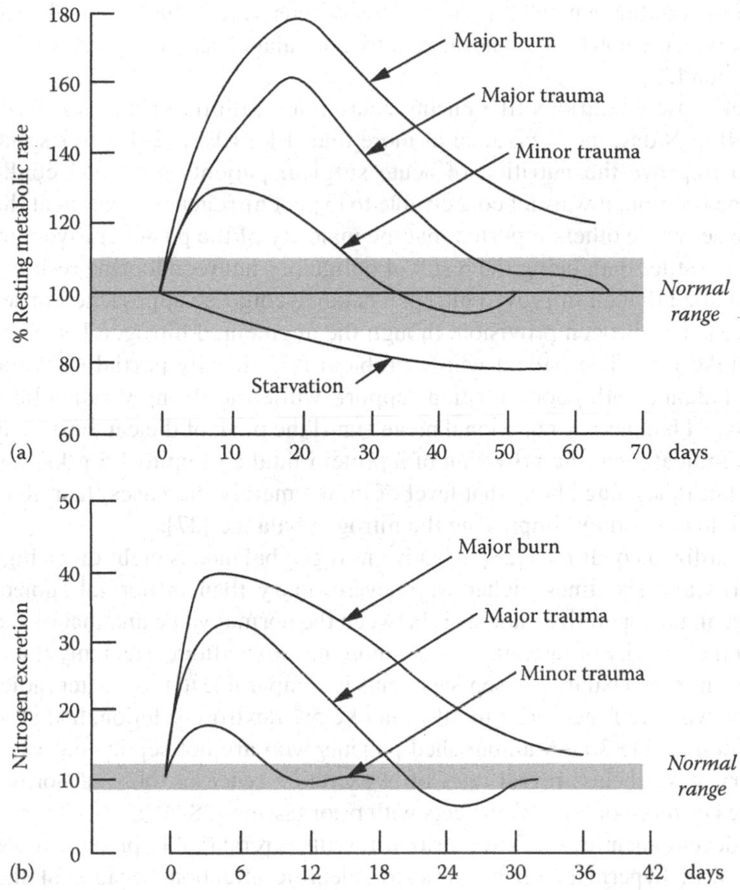

FIGURE 3.1 Metabolic rate (a) and nitrogen excretion (b) are related to the extent of injury. The two responses generally parallel each other (patients received 12 g nitrogen daily). (From Wilmore, D.W., *The Metabolic Management of the Critically Ill*, Plenum Medical Book, New York, 1977. With permission.)

some important inflammatory features of the metabolic response could not be reproduced by the hormone infusion [19]. Frayn questioned the importance of the counterregulatory hormones in stress, emphasizing that the high levels of these hormones occurred early after injury and returned to essentially normal values before the peak of the catabolic response [20].

The cascade of alterations in neuroendocrine control mechanisms resulting from critical illness influences profoundly protein and amino acid metabolism and thus body protein components.

EFFECT OF CRITICAL ILLNESS ON BODY PROTEIN MASS: THE NEGATIVE NITROGEN BALANCE

Following an acute injury without a low-flow state, LBM is first mobilized and then lost. The major reservoir is skeletal muscle. Superimposed on these are effects of other organ disease such as the kidney, liver, or intestinal tract, which are considered more specifically in Chapters 26, 28, and 29. Loss of LBM or more specifically body cell mass (BCM) can result in impaired host defense and increased morbidity and mortality with critical illness [17,21]. The clinical impressions of muscle loss after injury were placed on a quantitative basis by the early work of Cuthbertson, who reported the increase in resting metabolism and the excretion of nitrogen, sulfur, phosphorous, and creatine following leg-bone fracture in man [22]. These observations were extended by subsequent metabolic balance studies, which emphasized a negative nitrogen balance as the hallmark of the response to injury and infection [23].

In severe traumatic conditions like during acute renal failure, urinary excretion of nitrogen may reach 35–40 g N/day, the equivalent of more than 1 kg LBM [24]. Efforts made by various investigators to improve the nutrition of acute surgical patients produced conflicting results. According to one opinion, it was not conceivable to expect nitrogen utilization at the height of the catabolic response, while others reported that the majority of the postoperative nitrogen loss was due to starvation, rather than being the result of obligatory neuroendocrine responses [25]. Later on, it was established that an improved nitrogen balance could be approached in severe catabolic states with increasing nitrogen provision, though the augmented nitrogen loss is not reduced by the nitrogen intake [26]. The patient whose problem is primarily partial starvation can be put into positive N balance with good nutrition support, while the strongly catabolic patient cannot achieve a positive N balance by nutritional means until the peak of the catabolic drive has passed. Kinetic studies indicate that the provision of a protein intake of up to 1.5 g/kg/day can improve the N balance, but that going above that level of intake merely increases the rate of protein synthesis and breakdown, without improving the nitrogen balance [27].

During standardized conditions [28], negative nitrogen balance is eight times higher in patients with severe burns and six times higher with severe injury than in normal subjects (Table 3.1). Nitrogen balance in postoperative patients is between the normal value and that of accidental injury and depends on the severity of operation, being more negative after cystectomy than after total hip replacement. The nitrogen balance of septic patients is comparable to those after radical cystectomy. Normal subjects, who are fasted prior to infusion of a 5% dextrose solution, had about 50% reduction in N excretion (Table 3.1). Malnourished patients who are not septic, and were remote from injury or surgery, nevertheless reveal rates of N excretion twice of those of normal subjects and about three times of those of normal subjects with prior fasting [28–31].

Indeed, the development of clinical nutrition reveals a remarkable picture. Increased nitrogen loss associated with hypermetabolism attracted scientific attention because of the new interest devoted to adrenocortical hormones and the possibility that injury induced cortisol secretion, which then caused muscle breakdown and negative nitrogen balance [32]. This argument was repeatedly

TABLE 3.1
Nitrogen Balance (Mean ± SD) during 5% Dextrose Infusion

	Nitrogen Balance	
Pathophysiological State	**mg/kg/day**	**g/70 kg/day**
Severe burns	−380 ± 70	−27.0 ± 5.0
Severe injury	−260 ± 90	−18.0 ± 6.0
Post radical bladder cystectomy	−172 ± 47	−12.0 ± 1.3
Sepsis	−162 ± 84	−11.4 ± 5.9
Post total hip replacement	−96 ± 25	−6.7 ± 1.8
Malnourished	−90 ± 20	−3.2 ± 0.2
Normal subjects	−45 ± 3	−3.2 ± 0.2
Normal subjects after a 10–14-day fast	−30 ± 1	−2.1 ± 0.1

Sources: Takala, J. and Klossner, J., *Clin. Nutr.*, 5, 167, 1986; Kinney, J.M. et al., The intensive care patient, in: *Nutrition and Metabolism in Patient Care*, Kinney, J.M. et al., eds., W.B. Saunders, Philadelphia, PA, 1988, pp. 656–671; Rodriguez, D.J. et al., *JPEN*, 15, 319, 1991; Takala, J. et al., Nutrition support in trauma and sepsis, in: *Artificial Nutrition Support in Clinical Practice*, Payne-James, J., Grimble, G., and Silk, D., eds., Greenwich Medical Media Limited, London, U.K., 2001, pp. 511–522.

used to emphasize the futility of providing extra nutrition when the metabolic response had been shown to be obligatory. When protein hydrolysates were given to surgical patients, however, the N loss seemed to remain high, although the N balance was somewhat improved depending upon the severity of the stress. Later, Wretlind produced an improved protein hydrolysate for intravenous use but felt that the utilization of such a material would always be limited, until more calories could be administered than could be given by glucose solutions in a peripheral vein. The majority of presently available preparations are lacking glutamine, tyrosine, and cysteine. This might seriously limit optimum protein synthesis. Short-chain synthetic dipeptides containing these amino acids are available, enabling optimum composition and proportion of amino acids for support of the critically ill, catabolic patients (c.f. vide infra).

CHANGES IN PROTEIN TURNOVER

The manner in which net protein catabolism takes place is a subject of great debate. While the classic text by Waterlow et al. contains a detailed account of the underlying theory [33], more recent reviews discuss the difficulties identified as a result of modern work [16,34,35]. Unidirectional rates of protein synthesis and degradation might be measured by using the following methods:

1. Whole-body turnover studies in which isotopic amino acids are given by bolus or constant infusion and the specific activity of precursor and degradation products (CO_2, urea, ammonia) are determined as a function of time in blood, urine, and breath
2. Measurement of synthesis rates in muscle and blood by sampling protein from these tissues in studies similar to whole-body studies
3. Measurement of 3-methylhistidine excretion in urine, or arteriovenous difference of 3-methylhistidine, as a measure of the unidirectional rate of muscle protein breakdown

Older data indicate that changes in both protein synthesis and catabolism depend on the severity of injury. Severe burn [36], skeletal trauma, and sepsis [37] appear to cause increases in both synthesis and catabolism. Mild burns [36] and elective operation [38–40] result in only minimal changes. These early studies unfortunately have not been corrected for nutrient intake, which is a major factor influencing protein synthesis [7].

More recent patterns are summarized in Figure 3.2. Critical illness or endocrine diseases, which result in lean tissue wasting over a long period of time, also depress muscle protein turnover through reduced protein synthesis and protein breakdown. Whole-body protein turnover is, therefore, also depressed, although in some circumstances, visceral protein turnover may be elevated (e.g., liver and kidney disease). Under these circumstances, it makes sense that any attempts to replenish depleted cell mass should *aim to increase muscle protein synthesis* rather than to decrease muscle protein breakdown [16]. In circumstances where there is an excessive muscle wasting associated with increased whole-body energy expenditure, such as in severe injury, after burns of more than about 10% of body surface area [41–44], in polymyositis [45], during infection [46], and with some kinds of cancer [45,47], whole-body nitrogen balance is markedly negative probably because of changes that include an increase of protein breakdown in different tissues. Whether muscle protein synthesis also falls, as might be expected, or rises (possibly as an adaptive response to the rise in protein breakdown) is not known. The major change is a marked acceleration of lean tissue proteolysis [48], probably including muscle proteolysis.

3-Methylhistidine excretion has been measured during burn injury and sepsis, and both indicate marked increase in muscle catabolism [49–51]. Patients after minor operative procedures and with hyperketonuria after trauma had slightly increased or normal rates of 3-methylhistidine excretion [51,52]. In traumatized patients, the response of nitrogen balance and 3-methylhistidine excretion to exogenously administered amino acids is of interest. Parenteral nutrition with adequate levels of amino acids and energy markedly improves nitrogen balance, compared to administration of

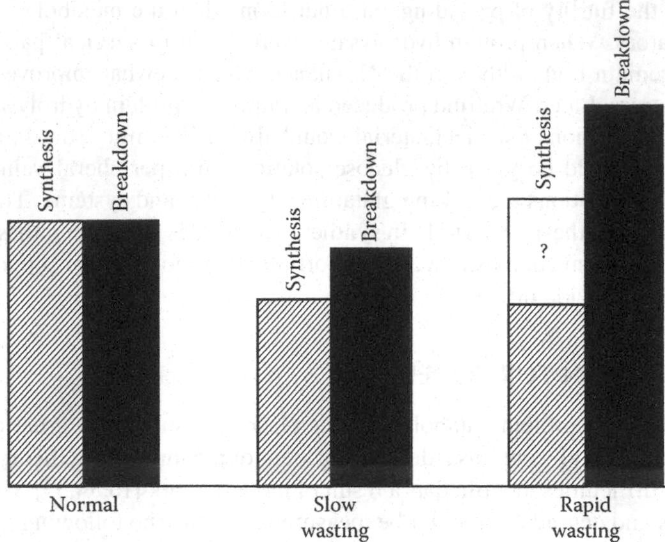

FIGURE 3.2 Extent of protein synthesis and protein breakdown. The slow wasting condition is found in mild injury, malnutrition, cancer, immobilization, etc. Rapid wasting occurs after severe injury, burns, and infection. The responses are for the most part well grounded in observations in patients. It is not certain to what extent protein synthesis can rise in injury associated with inflammatory disease. (Reproduced from Rennie, M.J. and Cuthbertson, D.J.R., Protein and amino acid metabolism in the whole body and in the tissue, in: *Artificial Nutrition Support in Clinical Practice*, Payne-James, J.J., Grimble, G., and Silk, D.B.A., eds., Greenwich Medical Media Limited, London, U.K., 2002, pp. 25–50. With permission.)

energy substrate alone. Measurement of 3-methylhistidine excretion under each of these conditions, however, indicates no difference in skeletal muscle catabolic rates [52]. These data suggest that exogenous nutritional support is effective in increasing protein synthesis in the presence of increased protein catabolism, and that increased protein synthesis results in improved nitrogen balance [52]. Urinary 3-methylhistidine excretion must be interpreted with caution, since under some conditions, the gut may be a major contributor. It is now also realized that myofibrillar and sarcoplasmic protein are regulated separately [16,53,54]. Nevertheless, these considerations do not restrict the usefulness of the method for specific measurement of myofibrillar protein breakdown. It is to remember that all the implicated methods rely on many assumptions that have not yet been verified, and the problem of precursors and their measurements is still a vexed question. Currently, the implication of mass isotopomer analysis has been advocated [55,56]. The use of this novel theoretical approach to the analysis of tracer appearance in polymeric molecules (such as proteins) may, in future, render the need to measure precursor labeling redundant [16].

PLASMA AND MUSCLE AMINO ACID CHANGES IN RESPONSE TO INJURY AND INFECTION

Plasma Amino Acids

Although the circulating plasma amino acids constitute a small fraction of the free amino acid pool in the body, they are important because of their role in the transport of nitrogen to body organs and because their concentration pattern reflects the net amino acid metabolism. In the 1940s, Man et al. monitored plasma α-amino acid nitrogen in patients undergoing operative procedures. They observed decline following the operation, and the values returned slowly to normal during convalescence [57]. Interestingly, malnourished patients exhibited lower preoperative α-amino nitrogen concentrations;

the values remaining depressed for a longer period of time following the operation. At this early time, very little attention was paid to nutritional factors. However, in recent carefully conducted studies, the aforementioned postoperative decline of most plasma free amino acids has been confirmed, although with time certain essential amino acids showed an increase [58,59]. In patients following severe injury, amino acid concentrations have been reported to rise, fall, and/or remain within normal limits [60]. Only in reports in which the measurements were obtained during the flow phase and under defined conditions, a more consistent response emerged [61]. In burn patients receiving rigorous nutritional support during their hospitalization, the majority of plasma free amino acid levels were found to be decreased, although phenylalanine was elevated [62].

It is notable that the branched-chain amino acid concentrations were not distinguishable from control values. Other investigators noted similar results, but except for the elevation of phenylalanine, enhanced concentrations of glutamic acid, methionine, aspartic acid, and hydroxyproline were occasionally noted. Profound hyperaminoacidemia is noted during the radiation period in patients who have undergone bone marrow transplantation [63]. Thermal injury induces time-dependent variations in plasma amino acids, that is, an initial hyperaminoacidemia reflecting proteolysis in the wounded areas, a decrease in gluconeogenic amino acids as a consequence of excessive usage in the liver, and a progressive return to normal [64,65]. There is also a durable hyperphenylalaninemia, reflecting increased protein turnover and specific alterations of sulfur amino acids. The finding of high levels of aromatic (phenylalanine and tyrosine) and sulfur-containing (methionine and cysteine) amino acids in sepsis and severe trauma certainly suggests impaired liver function (vide infra) [66,67].

Intracellular Muscle Free Amino Acids

It is obvious that the maintenance of the plasma amino acid steady state is dependent upon the net balance of the released amino acids from endogenous protein stores, as well as being contingent upon their subsequent utilization in the peripheral tissues. It is further to be expected that the extent of proteolysis in various tissues will be influenced by the catabolic stimuli and thereby contributes to the characteristic changes of circulating amino acids and their turnover during the catabolic state.

In carefully conducted flux studies, it could be demonstrated that amino acid release by the skeletal muscle in severely ill patients highly exceeded that observed in a healthy control group [68]. This augmented influx of amino acids into the extracellular compartment is accompanied by a corresponding influx of amino acids from plasma to the visceral tissues. This means that amino acids released from peripheral tissue (skeletal muscle) compare favorably with the uptake in splanchnicus and confirm the marked translocation of amino acid nitrogen from carcass to viscera. In other words, changes in the extracellular compartment are dependent upon amino acids derived from the free intracellular pool, the concentration of this pool being determined by muscle protein breakdown, by intracellular intermediary metabolic pathways, and by the efflux to the plasma compartments. Consequently, changes in plasma compartment must be evaluated on the basis of the magnitude of intracellular oxidation, the rate of gluconeogenesis, and the extent of intracellular reutilization. It is conceivable to assume that the study of the intracellular compartment will promote the understanding of amino acid metabolism in catabolic states. Skeletal muscle contains the largest pool of intracellular free amino acids. In normal man, the majority of the amino acids have a much higher concentration in intracellular water than in plasma [69].

The pattern of changes in amino acid concentration in muscle shows many similarities during catabolism [70]. In all cases, there is an increase in branched-chain amino acid (BCAA), aromatic amino acids, and methionine and a decrease in glutamine and basic amino acids (lysine and arginine). Regarding the changes observed in neutral amino acids, there is a graduation of response, with minimal changes seen in muscle with bed rest and maximal changes in sepsis [71].

A uniform reduction of approximately 50% of free muscular glutamine associated with negative nitrogen balance seems to be one of the most typical features of the response to trauma and

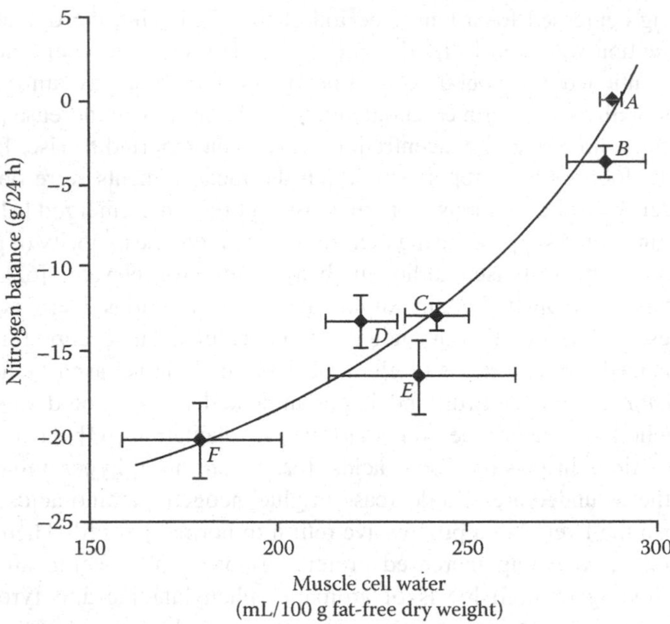

FIGURE 3.3 Trauma-induced intracellular glutamine depletion in human muscle tissue (mean ± SEM). (Combined data from Fürst, P., *Proc. Nutr. Soc.*, 42, 451, 1983; Fürst, P. and Stehle, P., Glutamine and glutamine-containing dipeptides, in: *Metabolic and Therapeutic Aspects of Amino Acids in Clinical Nutrition*, Cynober, L., ed., CRC Press, Boca Raton, FL, 2004, pp. 613–631. With permission.)

infection (Figure 3.3). The marked intracellular glutamine depression has been demonstrated after elective operation [72], major injury [61,73], burns [60,61], infections [73–75], and pancreatitis [76], irrespective of nutritional attempts of repletion. Reduction of the muscle free glutamine pool thus appears to be a hallmark of the response to injury, and its extent and duration is proportional to the severity of the illness. Recent studies underlined that the tissue glutamine depletion is mainly caused by stress-induced alterations in the interorgan glutamine flow [77]. Muscles, and probably lung glutamine effluxes, are accelerated to provide substrate for the gut, immune cells, and the kidneys [78,79], explaining at least in part the profound decline in muscle free glutamine concentration.

Most of the liver free amino acid concentrations are lower in critically ill patients than in the control group, the BCAA levels being decreased by 35% [80]. In nonsurviving patients, the hepatic concentrations of total amino acids, BCAA, gluconeogenic amino acids, and basic amino acids are lower than in surviving patients. The liver amino acid pattern reflects rather the plasma than the muscle amino acid patterns [80]. The elevated hepatic phenylalanine levels are in agreement with muscle and plasma data and may indicate that, during critical illness, the liver cannot metabolize the amount of phenylalanine released by muscle tissue. In experimental studies, a remarkably uniform response of decreased levels in all intestinal amino acids was elicited by trauma. Glutamine, which is one of the major amino acid components of the muscle (27%) and liver (22%), reveals relatively low contents in the intestine (3.3%). This low level in the intestine may be due to high GDH activity of the mucosa. The BCAA contents in rat liver and intestine are 2.6 and 6.4 times, respectively, of those present in the muscle. Trauma elicits a minor reduction (6%) in muscle BCAA but a marked increase (22%) in liver BCAA and a decrease (27%) in intestinal BCAA [80,81].

Human adipose tissue in vivo is a consistent net exporter of both alanine and glutamine and a consumer of glutamate [82]. After an overnight fast, adipose tissue seems to contribute about one-third as much as muscle to whole-body alanine and glutamine production and more than one-half as much as muscle to glutamate uptake. No data are available for the influence of injury on the adipose tissue amino acid content and release, which may play a substantial role in whole-body production during episodes of stress.

Similarly, little is known about the altered amino acid concentrations due to injury of the actively metabolizing leukocyte cells [83] and cerebrospinal fluid (CSF) [84]. Trauma, remote from the brain, enhances the total amino acid levels in CSF in contrast to the well-known decline in plasma. Glutamine and glutamate account for 73% of this increase in CSF. The systemic trauma enhances the levels of excitatory neurotransmitters—glutamate and aspartate in CSF [84].

CELLULAR HYDRATION

In a fascinating recent hypothesis, the essential importance of cellular hydration state as determinant of protein catabolism in health and disease is emphasized [85]. It is postulated that an increase in cellular hydration (swelling) acts as an anabolic proliferate signal, whereas cell shrinkage is catabolic and antiproliferative. The authors put forward the hypothesis that changes in cellular hydration state might be the variable linking muscle glutamine content with protein turnover and, because of the large muscle mass, the whole-body nitrogen balance. Data from previous studies of the relation between intracellular glutamine content and catabolism in patients with various underlying disorders enabled the evaluation of the relation between muscle-cell water content and whole-body nitrogen balance, showing an inverse relation (Figure 3.4). The concentrative uptake of glutamine into muscle and liver cells would be expected to increase cellular hydration, thereby triggering a protein anabolic signal. Indeed, glutamine (dipeptides) supplementation may facilitate aggressive therapeutic interventions, in order to improve cellular hydration state and subsequently modify, or reverse, catabolic changes [86].

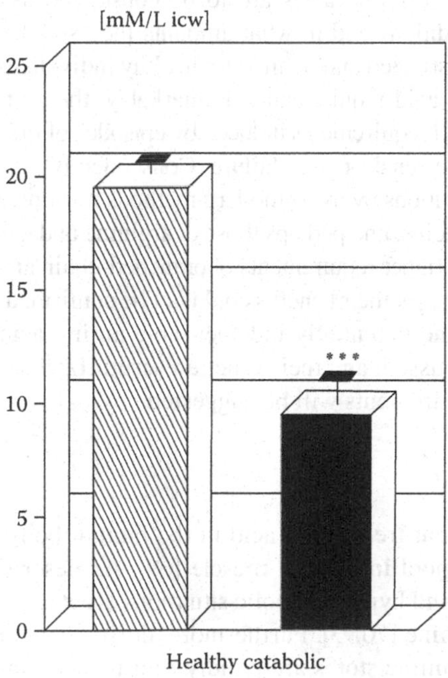

FIGURE 3.4 Whole-body nitrogen balance and cellular hydration of skeletal muscle. (a) Healthy subjects (n = 17); other subjects are patients with (b) liver tumors (n = 5); (c, d) polytrauma, day 2 (c) and day 9 (d) after trauma (n = 11); (e) acute necrotizing pancreatitis (n = 6); (f) burns (n = 4). Skeletal muscle-cell water was measured in a needle biopsy sample from quadriceps femoris by the chloride distribution method. Extra-/intracellular distribution was calculated by the chloride method, assuming normal membrane potential of 87.2 mV. (Reproduced from Häussinger, D. et al., *Lancet*, 341, 1330, 1993. With permission.)

CONCEPT OF CONDITIONALLY ESSENTIAL AMINO ACID IN CRITICAL ILLNESS: REQUIREMENTS

During episodes of various acute and chronic wasting diseases, the classical definition of the essentiality of amino acids is seriously challenged. In 1962, Mitchell pointed out in the first volume of his treatise *Comparative Nutrition of Man and Domestic Animals* that an "amino acid may be a dietary essential even if an animal is capable of synthesizing it, provided that the demand for it exceeds the capacity for synthesis" [87]. Thus, the strict nutritional classification of the common amino acids formulated by Rose and later by Jackson, Chipponi, and others is not acceptable as we attempt to understand how dietary protein serves to meet our nutritional needs in disease [86,88].

Grimble proposes that, regardless of the definition used, a final judgment about the usefulness of an essential amino acid will be on the ground of clinical and nutritional efficacy [89]. A more general proposition is that "a possible and useful direction might put more emphasis on metabolic control and its regulation of tissue and organ function and nutritional status." This definition offers suggestions as to how certain shared metabolic characteristics might be used to differentiate the various nutritionally important amino acids. It also implies that the dietary *essentiality* of a given amino acid is dependent on the ratio of supply to demand; the distinction between *essential* and *nonessential* largely disappears because it is dependent on conditions [86,88]. In this context, chronic and acute wasting diseases are associated with particular amino acid deficiencies and imbalances causing specific changes in amino acid requirements. Thus, the new approach categorizes amino acids as indispensable, conditionally indispensable, or dispensable according to their functional and physiological properties as well as considering the ratio of supply to demand under various pathological conditions [86]. Indeed, administration of the required conditionally indispensable amino acid might greatly facilitate an anabolic response to life-threatening disease [90].

The major question is which amino acids are to be considered as conditionally essential (indispensable) during diseased conditions and in what amounts they should be administered. Amino acid requirements are carefully investigated and defined for healthy individuals [91]. Critical illness, however, considerably influences amino acid requirements. Remarkably, there are no conclusive data available relative to changes of amino acid requirements induced by episodes of infection, injury, trauma, multiple-organ failure (MOF), and acute renal or liver failure. Consequently, future research evaluating amino acid requirements in these conditions by using modern methods must receive a high priority. Indeed, the requirements of glutamine, cysteine, and perhaps those of arginine and taurine are apparently very different in critically ill patients [7]. Higher requirements of branched-chain amino acids have been repeatedly claimed in controversial debates, yet their benefits could not be confirmed in well-controlled studies [92].

In the following section, the potentially indispensable amino acids (glutamine, cysteine, arginine, and taurine) will be discussed, and their function scrutinized as well as their possible clinical application, and tentative requirements will be suggested.

GLUTAMINE

Glutamine is the most prevalent free amino acid in the human body, constituting more than 60% of the total free amino acid pool in skeletal muscle [69]. As described previously, there is much evidence that hypercatabolic and hypermetabolic situations are accompanied by marked depression of muscle intracellular glutamine [70,93]. Furthermore, during catabolic stress or when tumors are proliferating, peripheral glutamine stores are rapidly diminished, and the amino acid is preferentially shunted as a fuel source toward visceral organs or tumor tissue. This creates a glutamine-depleted environment, the consequences of which include enterocyte and immunocyte starvation [94]. Consequently, glutamine is considered conditionally indispensable and should be endogenously administered during episodes of catabolic stress and undernutrition.

Two unfavorable chemical properties of free glutamine hamper its use as a nutritional substrate in routine clinical settings: (1) instability, especially during heat sterilization and prolonged storage, and (2) limited solubility (~3 g/100 mL at 20°C). The rate of breakdown of free glutamine depends on temperature, pH, and anion concentration. The decomposition of free glutamine yields the cyclic product pyroglutamic acid and ammonia. All these drawbacks can be overcome by the use of synthetic glutamine-containing dipeptides [93,95].

Leaving aside such considerations, several studies show that free glutamine may be provided by adding the crystalline amino acid to a commercially available amino acid solution before administration. However, appropriate preparation of such a solution requires a daily procedure at +4°C, under strictly aseptic conditions in a local pharmacy, followed by laborious sterilization through membrane filtration [96]. In addition, to diminish the risk of precipitation, glutamine concentrations in such solutions should not exceed 1%–2%.

Many clinical investigations showed improved nitrogen economy and maintained intracellular glutamine concentration with glutamine or glutamine-containing dipeptide supplementation. More importantly, numerous well-controlled clinical studies directed to investigate primary endpoints such as morbidity, mortality, and length of hospital stay demonstrated obvious improvements in clinical outcome in both surgical and critically ill patients (c.f. Refs. [7,93]).

In a comprehensive meta-analysis, Novak et al. examined the relationship between glutamine supplementation and length of hospital stay and morbidity and mortality in patients undergoing surgery and experiencing critical illness [97]. They reviewed 550 titles, abstracts, and papers. There were 14 randomized trials showing lower risk ratio with glutamine supplementation, the rate of infectious complications being also lower and shorter hospital stay with glutamine nutrition. With respect to mortality, the treatment benefit was observed in studies of parenteral glutamine and high-dose glutamine compared to studies of enteral glutamine and low-dose glutamine, respectively. With respect to length of hospital stay, all of the treatment benefit was observed in surgical patients compared to critically ill patients (–3.5 vs. 0.9 day). That a longer period on the control and treatment and parenteral feeds is required to effect survival has been emphasized by a study involving 144 ICU patients [98]. Consistent with previous results, there was no difference in clinical outcomes in those patients fed for a shorter period, but for those fed for more than 9 days, the survival measured at 6 months was significantly better, 22 out of 33 versus 13 out of 35 (Figure 3.5).

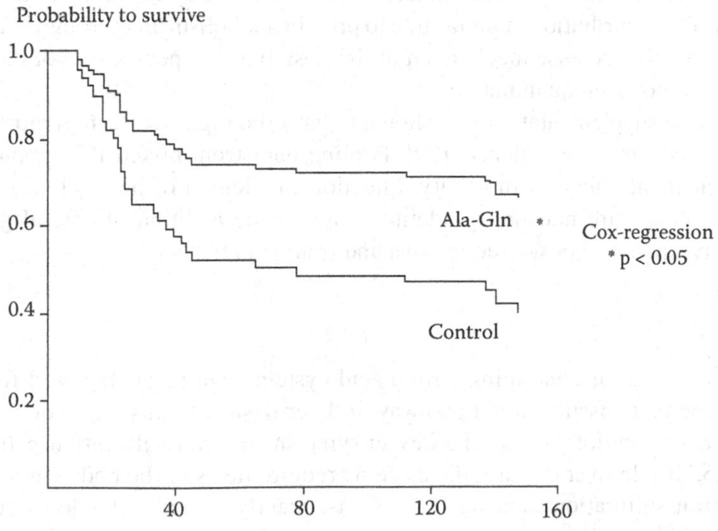

FIGURE 3.5 Survival plot of a subgroup of parenterally fed patients treated for 9 days and longer under standardized conditions. Ala-Gln: 1.2 g of standard amino acid solution per kilogram of body weight plus 0.3 g of alanyl-glutamine per kilogram of body weight per day. Control: 1.5 g of standard amino acid solution per kilogram of body weight. (Reproduced from Goeters, C. et al., *Crit. Care Med.*, 30, 2032, 2002. With permission.)

However, several recent trials and meta-analysis have raised the issue of safety and efficacy of providing parenteral glutamine to critically ill patients. In a large prospective randomized controlled trial involving 1223 critically ill adults in 40 ICU's worldwide, patients were randomized to one of four groups: placebo, glutamine (enteral and parenteral), antioxidant cocktail (intravenous selenium with oral selenium, zinc, beta-carotene, vitamin E, and vitamin C), and combined glutamine with antioxidant cocktail [99]. Patients receiving glutamine experienced higher mortality, in-hospital and 6-month postdischarge (37.2% vs. 31%, p = 0.02 and 43.7% vs. 37.2% and p = 0.02, respectively). Another study also failed to demonstrate mortality or infectious complication benefits with parenteral glutamine provision [100]. Similarly, a recent meta-analysis of prospective randomized controlled trials evaluated the effect of glutamine supplementation in critically ill patients; 17 trials (n = 3383) had mortality events reported [101]. There was no difference in mortality between groups that received glutamine compared to those that did not. Higher doses of glutamine (>0.5 g/kg/day) were associated with a higher mortality (relative risk [RR] 1.18; 95% confidence interval [CI], 1.02–1.38; p = 0.03). In 15 trials, glutamine supplementation was associated with a lower incidence of nosocomial infections (RR 0.85; 95% CI, 0.74–0.97; p = 0.02). Compared to control patients, nosocomial infection risk was lower in surgical ICU patients receiving glutamine (RR 0.70; 95% CI, 0.52–0.94; p = 0.04), as well as those receiving parenteral glutamine (RR 0.83; 95% CI, 0.70–0.98; p = 0.03). In the 14 trials (n = 2777) in which length of stay was reported, glutamine had no effect.

The SCCM/ASPEN critical care nutrition guidelines do not recommend parenteral glutamine supplementation be used in the critical care setting [102].

There is limited data on beneficial effects of enteral glutamine supplementation. Since glutamine is absorbed in the upper part of the small intestine and subsequently metabolized in the liver, glutamine might thus not be available for the target mucosal tissue at the lower sites of the intestine [103]. Other reasons in critically ill might be the presence of bacterial overgrowth; the bacteria are preferentially consuming glutamine [103]. The underlying mechanisms of supplemental glutamine (dipeptide) might be due to support of the mucosa, the immune system, and the hepatic biosynthesis of glutathione [104–106]. According to another proposal, glutamine plays a more global regulatory role by modifying the endogenous inflammatory responses. These mechanisms might be due to attenuation of the elaboration of pro-inflammatory mediators and upregulation of anti-inflammatory factors [107,108]. The contribution of glutamine to protein anabolism and through acid–base homeostasis may elicit a further defense mechanism of the host, but the specific role of these functions to the host defense has not been quantitated.

Enteral glutamine supplementation was shown to have the highest effect on mortality in a small but high-quality study in burn patients [109]. Pooling data from mixed ICU populations showed no significant beneficial effect on mortality, infections, or length of hospital stay [109–114]. The SCCM/ASPEN critical care nutrition guidelines suggest the addition of enteral glutamine to an enteral nutrition regimen be considered in burn and trauma patients [102].

Cysteine

In healthy adults, the sulfur-containing amino acid cysteine can be synthesized from methionine using the liver-specific transsulfuration pathway. In liver tissue of fetuses and of preterm and term infants, the activity of cystathionase, the key enzyme in the transsulfuration pathway, is low or undetectable [115,116]. In liver disease, the cysteine requirements of the body cannot be met due to the diminished transsulfuration capacity [117]. Consequently, cysteine should be considered as an essential amino acid in immature infants and a conditionally essential amino acid in liver disease. In both cases, it should be provided exogenously. The tentative requirements are estimated to be 20 mg/kg [91].

Cyst(e)ine is a potent antioxidant per se and a precursor for glutathione [118,119]. Glutathione and cysteine inhibit the expression of the nuclear transcription factor in stimulated T-cell lines [118,119].

This might provide an interesting approach in the treatment of AIDS, as the transcription factor enhances HIV mRNA expression. In fact, in vitro studies show that the stimulatory effects of TNF, induced by free radicals, on HIV replication in monocytes can be inhibited by sulfur-containing antioxidants [120]. These basic studies indicate that treatment of inflammatory diseases and AIDS with sulfhydryl antioxidants may be beneficial, and powerful arguments have been advanced in favor of such treatment [121,122]. Clinical studies using this strategy are not yet available.

Route of administration seems to influence the rate of hepatic cysteine synthesis by altering the delivery of cysteine precursors to the liver. Stegink and Den Besten [123] demonstrated in healthy men that intravenous infusion of solutions containing methionine but not cyst(e)ine resulted in depressed concentrations of all three forms of circulating cysteine (free cysteine, free cystine, and protein-bound cysteine). This result suggests that parenteral solutions should not only contain methionine but additional amounts of cyst(e)ine. Supplementation with cyst(e)ine may also improve taurine concentrations during long-term TPN. However, addition of cyst(e)ine to TPN solutions is problematic. At neutral or slightly alkaline pH, cysteine is rapidly oxidized during heat sterilization, and storage of cysteine yields the dimer cystine, which itself is very poorly soluble and which precipitates in the solution. Acidic conditions may lead to a reduction of the sulfhydryl group and the formation of hydrogen sulfide.

N-acetyl-cysteine is proposed to be used at the ICU as a cysteine replacement, especially in the treatment of sepsis. Nevertheless, the results are strikingly poor [124]. The reason is that humans lack tissue acylases, except in the kidney [7,93]. Consequently, following long-term infusion, the compound will accumulate in body fluids and/or excreted in the urine [7,93]. A recent study confirmed that *N*-acetyl-cysteine metabolism is disturbed in sepsis resulting in impaired cardiac performance [125].

Future use of synthetic cysteine-containing dipeptides will be the solution. Studies with highly soluble cysteine peptides (L-cysteine–L-alanine and L-cysteine–glycine) provided evidence that they are well utilized in experimental animals [126,127]. Their synthesis in industrial scale and subsequent human studies are still warranted [108].

Arginine

Arginine is a precursor of polyamine and nucleic acid synthesis, a promoter of thymic growth, and an endocrinologic secretagogue stimulating release of growth hormone, prolactin, insulin, and glucagons [128]. It is metabolized within the enterocyte by the arginase pathway to ornithine and urea and by the arginine deaminase pathway to citrulline [129]. Arginine metabolism in enterocytes may participate in the support of gut morphology and function by acting as a substrate for nitric oxide synthesis [130]. Inhibition of nitric oxide synthesis increases intestinal mucosal permeability in experimental models of ischemia/reperfusion intestinal injury [131] and acute necrotizing enterocolitis [132]. In addition, administration of arginine reverses the effect of nitric oxide synthase inhibition [131]. These results suggest that basal nitric oxide production is important in minimizing the mucosal barrier dysfunction in these models.

During major catabolic insults such as trauma or surgery, an increase in urinary nitrogen, excreted largely as urea, represents the end products of increased lean body tissue catabolism and reprioritized protein synthesis. Arginine during these stress situations is claimed to become conditionally essential in that demand is greater than endogenous supply [133]. Arginine may be of significance in the critically ill because of its potential role in immunomodulation [134,135], and it is hypothesized that (high-dose) arginine enhances the depressed immune response of individuals suffering from injury, surgical trauma, malnutrition, or sepsis. On the basis of animal and in vitro experiments, however, the results derived from critically ill patients are controversial. This is due to the theory that septic hemodynamically unstable critically ill patients may be at risk for further compromise if provided arginine due to its ability to upregulate inducible nitric oxide synthase (iNOS) leading to an increase in nitric oxide and vasodilation [136]. However, clinical trials in which arginine was provided to septic patients failed to corroborate this theory but show that arginine may promote tissue perfusion increasing cardiac output [137].

Recent human trials suggest an imbalance between arginine and asymmetric dimethylarginine (ADMA), a catabolic end product of protein, is associated with altered endothelial and cardiac dysfunction. Visser et al. reported elevated arginine and lower ADMA levels resulted in improved mortality in septic patients, which is attributed to better organ perfusion and cardiac output [138]. Similarly, comparing patients with severe sepsis to those without sepsis, a low arginine to high ADMA ratio was independently associated with increased mortality [139].

Clinical studies on enteral arginine administration have shown moderate net nitrogen retention and protein synthesis compared with isonitrogenous diets in critically ill and injured patients. After surgery for certain malignancies in elderly postoperative patients, supplemental arginine (25 g/day) enhanced T-lymphocyte responses to phytohemagglutinin and concanavalin A and increased the CD4 phenotype number [135]. Interestingly, insulin-like growth factor 1 levels were increased by about 50%, reflecting the growth hormone secretion induced by arginine supplementation. A large oral arginine intake (30 g/day) improved wound healing [140] and enhanced the blastogenic response to several mitogens [141]. Overall, there was, however, no improvement in patient outcome or length of hospital stay [142].

Taurine

Taurine (2-aminoethanesulfonic acid) is the most abundant free amine in the intracellular compartment [69]. Taurine has functional roles in stabilizing the membrane potential, in bile salt formation, growth modulation, osmoregulation, antioxidation, promotion of calcium transport, and calcium binding to membranes. It exerts positive ionotropic effects of the heart, as well as having antiarrhythmic and antihypertensive effects. It is involved in many metabolic responses in the central nervous system, has an anticonvulsant action, may have an insulinogenic action, and is required for eye function [143]. Taurine is capable of influencing programmed cell death in various cell types depending upon the initiating apoptotic stimulus [144] and of affecting Fas (CD95/APO-1)-mediated neutrophil apoptosis through the maintenance of calcium homeostasis [145].

There is some evidence that taurine might be indispensable during episodes of catabolic stress. We and others found low extracellular and intracellular taurine concentrations after trauma and infection [70]. Low taurine concentrations in plasma, platelets, and urine have been described in infants and children and also in adult trauma patients undergoing taurine-free long-term parenteral nutrition [146–148]. Plasma taurine deficiency after intensive chemotherapy or radiotherapy is more severe in patients receiving taurine-free parenteral nutrition than in orally fed patients [149]. Low intracellular taurine concentrations in muscle are typical feature in patients with chronic and acute renal failure, probably because of impaired metabolic conversion of cysteine sulfinic acid to taurine [150,151]. Intracellular taurine depletion may be associated with the well-known muscle fatigue and arrhythmic episodes that occur in uremia.

Taurine Supplementation

Taurine has been characterized as a conditionally essential amide in preterm infants and neonates and is currently incorporated in most neonatal dietary regimens [152]. Our understanding of the role of taurine in various pathological functions is largely based upon animal studies. More recently, however, there have been a few human studies that provide some insight into possible therapeutic applications. Taurine is obviously important in several medical conditions such as sepsis, ischemia–reperfusion states, postoperative states, pulmonary fibrosis, cardiac failure, and other conditions [152].

The question arises as whether taurine supplementation could be beneficial in acute and chronic renal failure, during episodes of catabolic stress, and in other conditions in which it might have a beneficial effect on morbidity or outcome. Free crystalline taurine is available for inclusion in intravenous or enteral preparations. However, we hypothesize that the extremely high intracellular to extracellular transmembrane gradient (250:1) might limit the cellular uptake of taurine. We proposed a novel binding of taurine to a suitable amino acid carrier in the form of a synthetic taurine conjugate [153]. Experimental data strongly suggest improvement in transmembrane transport and intracellular utilization with this conjugate [154].

Taurine might possess biological properties that enable it to act as a potent molecule in the regulation of inflammatory and immunological processes as well as serving as a powerful antioxidant. It is worthwhile considering taurine as a future important member in the growing family of pharmacological nutrients.

CONCLUSION

More than 300 years ago, John Hunter summarized the paradox of the response to injury: "Impressions are capable of producing or increasing natural actions and are than called *stimuli*, but they are likewise capable of producing too much action, as well as depraved, unnatural, or what we commonly call diseased action" [155]. Presumably, he perceived that nature must have designed these responses to promote healing and recovery but realized that in case responses exceeding normal limits, they threatened and jeopardized the life of the host. Therefore, one of the major goals of modern clinical nutrition is indeed to modify stress response below extreme and thereby positively influence recovery.

Optimum nutrition support with proteins (amino acids) should be adjusted to the undergoing metabolic state of the patient. The metabolic state is the result of some bland of the response to starvation and the response to injury (insult), infection, or a specific disease. In all cases, adequate energy and protein (nitrogen substrates) is provided to meet the increased requirements of hypercatabolic, hypermetabolic, malnourished (depleted) patients. With current techniques, appropriate nutritional support may be provided with a low incidence of complication. Improved understanding of regulatory mechanisms may lead to novel means of therapies that could modify the intensity or nature of the injury response and thus alter the consequent metabolic demands. Specific modifications of the composition of amino acid intake might have clinical benefit in certain disease states; such modification is known as disease-specific therapy.

The main focus of this chapter concerns the evaluation of the clinical use of protein and amino acids as well as new nitrogen-containing substrates (dipeptides, conjugates) exerting specific actions on immune system, maintaining of gut integrity, and modifying the metabolic response to trauma, thereby reducing morbidity and mortality. This compilation may well illustrate how far we have advanced in our knowledge of the importance of changed composition and new nitrogen-containing substrates in modern artificial nutrition. An attempt was also made to highlight directions that hold promise for advancing conditionally essential amino acids in future patient care. There is little question that efforts made to modify the response to disease by nutritional means will be rewarded with improved patient outcome. Surprising and exciting medical progress of yesterday today belongs to the daily medical exercise.

ACKNOWLEDGMENT

Professor Dr. Peter Fürst, an outstanding scientist who made invaluable contributions to the field of clinical nutrition with a specialty area in protein and amino acid metabolism, who wrote this chapter for the first edition of this book.

REFERENCES

1. Trunkey, D.D., On the nature of things that go bang in the night, *Surgery*, 92, 123–132, 1982.
2. Trunkey, D.D., In search of solutions, *J. Trauma*, 53, 1189–1191, 2002.
3. Deaths, H.M., Leading Causes for 2010. National Vital Statistics Reports 62, 1–95, 2013.

4. Suchner, U., Kuhn, K.S., and Fürst, P., The scientific basis of immunonutrition, *Proc. Nutr. Soc.*, 59, 553–563, 2000.
5. Abbott, W.C. et al., Nutritional care of the trauma patient, *Surg. Gynecol. Obstet.*, I 57, 1–13, 1983.
6. Biffl, W.L., Moore, E.E., and Haenel, J.B., Nutrition support of the trauma patient, *Nutrition,* 18, 960–965, 2002.
7. Fürst, P. and Stehle, P., Parenteral nutrition substrates, in *Artificial Nutrition Support in Clinical Practice*, Payne-James, J., Grimble, G., and Silk, D., eds., Greenwich Medical Media Limited, London, U.K., 2001, pp. 401–434.
8. Bessey, P.Q., What's new in critical care and metabolism, *J. Am. Coll. Surg.*, 184, 115–125, 1997.
9. Bessey, P.Q., Parenteral nutrition and trauma, in *Parenteral Nutrition*, Rombeau, J.L. and Caldwell, M.D., eds., W.B. Sanders, Philadelphia, PA, 1986, pp. 471–488.
10. Hasselgren, P.O., Catabolic response to stress and injury: Implications for regulation, *World J. Surg.*, 24, 1452–1459, 2000.
11. Trujillo, E.B., Robinson, M.K., and Jacobs, D.O., Feeding critically ill patients: Current concepts, *Crit. Care Nurs.*, 21, 60–69, 2001.
12. Wernerman, J. and Vinnars, E., The effect of trauma and surgery on interorgan fluxes of amino acids in man, *Clin. Sci.*, 73, 129–133, 1987.
13. Martinez, J.A., Portillo, N.I.P., and Larralde, J., Anabolic actions of a mixed beta-adrenergic agonist on nitrogen retention and protein turnover, *Horm. Metab. Res.*, 23, 590–593, 1991.
14. Mantle, D., Delday, M.I., and Maltin, C.A., Effect of clenbuterol on protease activities and protein levels in rat muscle, *Muscle Nerve*, 15, 471–478, 1992.
15. Mantle, D. and Reedy, V.R., Adverse and beneficial functions at proteologic enzymes in skeletal muscle: An overview, *Adverse Drug React. Toxicol. Rev.*, 21, 31–49, 2002.
16. Rennie, M.J. and Cuthbertson, D.J.R., Protein and amino acid metabolism in the whole body and in the tissue, in *Artificial Nutrition Support in Clinical Practice*, Payne-James, J.J., Grimble, G., and Silk, D.B.A., eds., Greenwich Medical Media Limited, London, U.K., 2002, pp. 25–50.
17. Douglas, R.G. and Shaw, J.H., Metabolic response to sepsis and trauma, *Br. J. Surg.*, 7, 281–289, 1989.
18. Bessey, P.Q. et al., Combined hormonal infusion simulates the metabolic response to injury, *Ann. Surg.*, 200, 264–281, 1984.
19. Watters, J.M. et al., Introduction of interleukin-l in humans and its metabolic effects, *Surgery*, 98, 298–306, 1985.
20. Frayn, K.N., Hormonal control of metabolism in trauma and sepsis, *Clin. Endocrinol.*, 24, 577–599, 1986.
21. Cunha, H.F., Rocha, E.E., and Hissa, M. Protein requirements, morbidity and mortality in critically ill patients: Fundamentals and applications. *Rev. Bras. Ter. Intensiva.*, 25, 49–55, 2013.
22. Cuthbertson, D.P., The distribution of nitrogen and sulfur in the urine during conditions of increased catabolism, *Biochem. J.*, 25, 236–244, 1931.
23. Cuthbertson, D.P., Observation on the disturbances of metabolism produced by injury to the limbs, *Q. J. Med.*, 1, 223–230, 1932.
24. Duke, J.H. et al., Contribution of protein to caloric expenditure following injury, *Surgery*, 68, 168–174, 1970.
25. Moore, F.D. and Brennan, M.R., Intravenous amino acids, *N. Engl. J. Med.*, 293, 194–195, 1975.
26. Shenkin, A. et al., Biochemical changes associated with severe trauma, *Am. J. Clin. Nutr.*, 33, 2119–2127, 1980.
27. Shaw, J.H.F., Wildbore, M., and Wolfe, R.R., Whole body protein kinetics in severely septic patients, *Ann. Surg.*, 205, 288–294, 1987.
28. Takala, J. and Klossner, J., Branched chain enriched parenteral nutrition in surgical patients, *Clin. Nutr.*, 5, 167–170, 1986.
29. Kinney, J.M. et al., The intensive care patient, in *Nutrition and Metabolism in Patient Care*, Kinney, J.M. et al., eds., W.B. Saunders, Philadelphia, PA, 1988, pp. 656–671.
30. Rodriguez, D.J. et al., Obligatory negative nitrogen balance following spinal cord injury, *JPEN,* 15, 319–322, 1991.
31. Takala, J., Suojaranta-Ilinen, R., and Pitkänen, O., Nutrition support in trauma and sepsis, in *Artificial Nutrition Support in Clinical Practice*, Payne-James, J., Grimble, G., and Silk, D., eds., Greenwich Medical Media Limited, London, U.K., 2001, pp. 511–522.
32. Kinney, J.M. and Elwyn, D.H., Protein metabolism and injury, *Annu. Rev. Nutr.*, 3, 433–466, 1983.
33. Waterlow, J.C., Garlick, P.J., and Millward, D.J., *Protein Turnover in Mammalian Tissues and in the Whole Body*, Elsevier-North Holland, Amsterdam, the Netherlands, 1978.

34. Bier, D.M., Intrinsically difficult problems, the kinetics of body proteins and amino acid in man, *Diabetes Metab.*, 5, 111–132, 1989.
35. Pacy, P.J. et al., Stable isotopes as tracers in clinical research, *Ann. Nutr. Metab.*, 33, 65–78, 1989.
36. Kien, C.L. et al., Increased rates of whole body protein synthesis and breakdown in children recovering from burns, *Ann. Surg.*, 187, 383–391, 1978.
37. Long, C.L. et al., Whole body protein synthesis and catabolism in septic man, *Am. J. Clin. Nutr.*, 30, 1340–1344, 1977.
38. Crane, C.W. et al., Protein turnover in patients before and after elective orthopaedic operations, *Br. J. Surg.*, 64, 129–133, 1977.
39. Tashiro, T. et al., Whole body turnover, synthesis and breakdown in patients receiving parenteral nutrition before and after recovery from surgical stress, *JPEN*, 9, 452–455, 1985.
40. O'Keefe, S.J.D., Sender, P.M., and James, W.P.T., Catabolic loss of body nitrogen in response to surgery, *Lancet*, 2, 1035–1037, 1974.
41. Golden, M., Waterlow, J.C., and Picou, D., The relationship between dietary intake, weight change, nitrogen balance and protein turnover in man, *Am. J. Clin. Nutr.*, 30, 1345–1350, 1977.
42. Biolo, G. et al., Mechanisms of altered protein turnover in chronic diseases. A review of human kinetic studies, *Curr. Opin. Clin. Nutr. Metab. Care*, 6, 55–63, 2003.
43. Donati, L. et al., Nutritional and clinical efficacy of ornithine-α-ketoglutarate in severe burn patients, *Clin. Nutr.*, 18, 307–311, 1999.
44. Wolfe, R.R., Relation of metabolic studies to clinical nutrition—The example of burn injury, *ASCN*, 64, 800–808, 1996.
45. Rennie, M.J., Muscle protein turnover and the wasting due to injury and disease, *Br. Med. Bull.*, 41, 257–264, 1985.
46. Tomkins, A.M. et al., The combined effects of infection and malnutrition on protein metabolism in children, *Clin. Sci.*, 65, 313–324, 1983.
47. Mitchell, L.A. and Norton, L.W., Effect of cancer plasma on skeletal muscle metabolism, *J. Surg. Res.*, 47, 423–426, 1989.
48. Arnold, J. et al., Increased whole-body protein breakdown predominates over increased whole-body protein synthesis in multiple organ failure, *Clin. Sci.*, 84, 655–661, 1993.
49. Blazes, C. et al., Quantitative contribution by skeletal muscle on elevated rates of whole-body protein breakdown in burned children as measured by 3-methylhistidine output, *Metabolism*, 27, 671–676, 1978.
50. Long, C.L. et al., Urinary excretion of 3-methylhistidine: An assessment of muscle protein catabolism in adult normal subjects and during malnutrition, sepsis and skeletal trauma, *Metabolism*, 30, 765–776, 1981.
51. Williamson, D.H. et al., Muscle-protein catabolism after injury in man, as measured by urinary excretion of 3-methylhistidine, *Clin. Sci. Mol. Med.*, 52, 527–533, 1977.
52. Neuhäuser, M. et al., Urinary excretion of 3-methylhistidine as an index of muscle protein catabolism in postoperative trauma: The effect of parenteral nutrition, *Metabolism*, 29, 1206–1213, 1980.
53. Kettelhut, I.C., Wing, S.S., and Goldberg, A.L., Endocrine regulation of protein breakdown in skeletal muscle, *Diabetes Metab. Rev.*, 4, 751–772, 1988.
54. Hasselgren, P.O., Muscle protein metabolism during sepsis, *Biochem. Soc. Trans.*, 23, 1019–1025, 1995.
55. Hellerstein, M.K. and Neese, R.A., Mass isotopomer distribution analysis: A technique for measuring biosynthesis and turnover of polymers, *Am. J. Physiol.*, 263, E988–E1001, 1992.
56. Hellerstein, M.K. and Neese, R.A., Mass isotopomer distribution analysis at eight years: Theoretical analytic and experimental considerations, *Am. J. Physiol.*, 276, E1146–E1170, 1999.
57. Man, E.B. et al., Plasma α-amino acid nitrogen and serum lipids of surgical patients, *J. Clin. Invest.*, 25, 701–708, 1946.
58. Askanazi, J. et al., Muscle and plasma amino acids after injury: Hypocaloric glucose vs. amino acid infusion, *Ann. Surg.*, 191, 465–472, 1980.
59. Dale, G. et al., The effect of surgical operation on venous plasma free amino acids, *Surgery*, 81, 295–301, 1977.
60. Stinnett, J.D. et al., Plasma and skeletal muscle amino acids following severe burn injury in patients and experimental animals, *Ann. Surg.*, 195, 75–89, 1982.
61. Fürst, P. et al., Influence of amino acid supply on nitrogen and amino acid metabolism in severe trauma, *Acta Chir. Scand.*, 494, 136–138, 1979.
62. Aulick, L.H. and Wilmore, D.W., Increased peripheral amino acid release following burn injury, *Surgery*, 85, 560–565, 1979.
63. Hutchinson, M.L., Clemans, G.W., and Detter, F., Abnormal plasma amino acid profiles in patients undergoing bone marrow transplant, *Clin. Nutr.*, 3, 133, 1984.

64. Cynober, L., Amino acid metabolism in thermal burns, *JPEN*, 13, 196–205, 1989.
65. Cynober, L. et al., Plasma and urinary amino acid pattern in severe burn patients—Evolution throughout the healing period, *Am. J. Clin. Nutr.*, 36, 416–425, 1982.
66. Woolf, L.I. et al., Arterial plasma amino acids in patients with serious postoperative infection and in patients with major fractures, *Surgery*, 79, 283–292, 1976.
67. Jeevanandam, M., Trauma and sepsis, in *Amino Acid Metabolism and Therapy in Health and Nutritional Disease*, Cynober, L., ed., CRC Press, Boca Raton, FL, 1995, pp. 245–255.
68. Wilmore, D.W. et al., Effect of injury and infection on visceral metabolism and circulation, *Ann. Surg.*, 192, 491–504, 1980.
69. Bergström, J. et al., Intracellular free amino acid concentration in human muscle tissue, *J. Appl. Physiol.*, 36, 693–697, 1974.
70. Fürst, P., Intracellular muscle free amino acids—Their measurement and function, *Proc. Nutr. Soc.*, 42, 451–462, 1983.
71. Fürst, P., Alvestrand, A., and Bergström, J., Branched-chain amino acids and branched-chain keto acids in uremia, in *Branched Chain Amino Acids: Biochemistry, Physiopathology and Clinical Science,* Schauder, P. et al., eds., Raven Press Ltd., New York, 1992, pp. 173–186.
72. Askanazi, J. et al., Muscle and plasma amino acids after injury. The role of inactivity, *Ann. Surg.*, 188, 797–803, 1978.
73. Askanazi, J. et al., Muscle and plasma amino acids following injury. Influence of intercurrent infection, *Ann. Surg.*, 192, 78–85, 1980.
74. Milewski, P.J. et al., Intracellular free amino acids in undernourished patients with and without sepsis, *Clin. Sci.*, 62, 83–91, 1982.
75. Roth, E. et al., Metabolic disorders in severe abdominal sepsis: Glutamine deficiency in skeletal muscle, *Clin. Nutr.*, 1, 5–41, 1982.
76. Roth, E. et al., Amino acid concentrations in plasma and skeletal muscle of patients with acute hemorrhagic necrotizing pancreatitis, *Clin. Chem.*, 31, 1305–1309, 1985.
77. Souba, W.W., Glutamine: A key substrate for the splanchnic bed, *Annu. Rev. Nutr.*, 11, 285–308, 1991.
78. Rennie, M.J. et al., Skeletal muscle glutamine transport, intramuscular glutamine concentration, and muscle protein turnover, *Metabolism*, 38, 47–51, 1989.
79. Plumley, D.A., Souba, W.W., and Hautamaki, R.D., Accelerated lung amino acid release in hyperdynamic septic surgical patients, *Arch. Surg.*, 125, 1761, 1990.
80. Roth, E. et al., Liver amino acids in sepsis, *Surgery*, 97, 436–442, 1985.
81. Jeevanandam, M. and Ali, M.R., Altered tissue amino acid levels in traumatized, growing rats due to ornithine-alpha-ketoglutarate supplemented oral diet, *J. Clin. Nutr. Gastroenterol.*, 6, 23–28, 1991.
82. Caballero, B., Gleason, R.E., and Wurtman, R.T., Plasma amino acid concentrations in healthy elderly men and women, *Am. J. Clin. Nutr.*, 53, 1249–1252, 1991.
83. Wells, F.E. and Smits, B., Leucocyte amino acid concentrations and their relationships to changes in plasma amino acids, *JPEN*, 4, 264–268, 1980.
84. Ali, R. et al., Altered amino acid (AA) levels due to remote trauma in cerebrospinal fluid (CSF), *FASEB J.*, 7, A646, 1993.
85. Häussinger, D. et al., Cellular hydration state: An important determinant of protein catabolism in health and disease, *Lancet*, 341, 1330–1332, 1993.
86. Fürst, P., Old and new substrates in clinical nutrition, *J. Nutr.*, 128, 789–796, 1998.
87. Mitchell, H.H., *Comparative Nutrition of Man and Domestic Animals*, Vol. 1, Academic Press, New York, 1962.
88. Young, V.E. and Tharakan, J.F., Nutritional essentiality of amino acids and amino acid requirements in healthy adults, in *Metabolic and Therapeutic Aspects of Amino Acids in Clinical Nutrition*, Cynober, L., ed., CRC Press, Boca Raton, FL, 2004, pp. 439–464.
89. Grimble, G.K., The significance of peptides in clinical nutrition, *Annu. Rev. Nutr.*, 14, 419–447, 1994.
90. Wilmore, D.W., The practice of clinical nutrition: How to prepare for the future, *JPEN*, 13, 337–343, 1989.
91. Fürst, P., What are the essential elements needed for the determination of amino acid requirements in humans, *J. Nutr.*, 134(6 Suppl.):1558S–1565S, 2004.
92. Brennan, M.F. et al., Report of a research workshop: Branched chain amino acids in stress and injury, *JPEN*, 10, 446–452, 1986.
93. Fürst, P. and Stehle, P., Glutamine and glutamine-containing dipeptides, in *Metabolic and Therapeutic Aspects of Amino Acids in Clinical Nutrition*, Cynober, L., Ed., CRC Press, Boca Raton, FL, 2004, pp. 613–631.
94. Bode, B.P. and Souba, W.W., Modulation of cellular proliferation alters glutamine transport and metabolism in human hepatoma cells, *Ann. Surg.*, 220, 411–424, 1994.

95. Fürst, P., New developments in glutamine delivery, *J. Nutr.*, 131, 2562S–2568S, 2001.
96. Khan, K. et al., The stability of L-glutamine in total parenteral nutrition, *Clin. Nutr.*, 10, 193, 1991.
97. Novak, F. et al., Glutamine supplementation in serious illness: A systematic review of the evidence, *Crit. Care Med.*, 30, 2022–2029, 2002.
98. Goeters, C. et al., Parenteral L-alanyl-L-glutamine improves 6-month outcome in critically ill patients, *Crit. Care Med.*, 30, 2032, 2002.
99. Heyland, D. et al., A randomized trial of glutamine and antioxidants in critically ill patients, *N. Eng. J. Med.*, 368, 1489, 2013.
100. Wernerman, J. et al., Scandinavian glutamine trial: A pragmatic multicentre randomised clinical trial of intensive care unit patients, *Acta Anaesthesiol. Scand.*, 55, 812, 2011.
101. Chen, Q.H. et al., The effect of glutamine therapy on outcomes in critically ill patients: A meta-analysis of randomized controlled trials, *Crit. Care*, 18, R8, 2014.
102. McClave, S. et al., Guidelines for the provision and assessment of nutrition support therapy in the adult critically ill patient: Society of Critical Care Medicine and the American Society for Parenteral and Enteral Nutrition, *J. Parenter. Enteral Nutr.*, 33, 277, 2009.
103. Fürst, P., Conditionally indispensable amino acids in enteral feeding and the dipeptide concept, in *Proteins Peptides and Amino Acids in Enteral Nutrition*, Fürst, P. and Young, V., eds., Karger, Basel, Switzerland, 2000, pp. 199–219.
104. Harward, T.R. et al., Glutamine preserves gut glutathione levels during intestinal ischemia/reperfusion, *J. Surg. Res.*, 56, 351, 1994.
105. Yun, J.C. et al., Alanyl-glutamine preserves hepatic glutathione stores after 5-FU treatment, *Clin. Nutr.*, 15, 261, 1996.
106. Fläring, U.B. et al., Glutamine attenuates post-traumatic glutathione depletion in human muscle, *Clin Sci.* (Lond), 104, 275–282, 2003.
107. Wilmore, D.W., Glutamine saves lives! What does it mean? *Nutrition*, 13, 375, 1997.
108. Fürst, P., A thirty-year odyssey in nitrogen metabolism: From ammonium to dipeptides, *JPEN*, 24, 197–209, 2000.
109. Garrel, D. et al., Decreased mortality and infectious morbidity in adult burn patients given enteral glutamine supplements: A prospective, controlled, randomized clinical trial, *Crit. Care Med.*, 31, 2444, 2003.
110. Hondijk, A.P. et al., Randomized trial of glutamine-enriched enteral nutrition on infections morbidity in patients with multiple trauma, *Lancet*, 352, 772–776, 1998.
111. Peng, X. et al., Analysis of the therapeutic effect and the safety of glutamine granules per os in patients with severe burns and trauma, *Zhonghua Shao Shang Za Zhi*, 20, 206, 2004.
112. Zhou, Y.P. et al., The effect of supplemental enteral glutamine on plasma levels, gut function, and outcome in severe burns: A randomized, double-blind, controlled clinical trial, *JPEN J. Parenter. Enteral Nutr.*, 27, 241, 2003.
113. Hall, J.C. et al., A prospective randomized trial of enteral glutamine in critical illness, *Intensive Care Med.*, 29, 1710, 2003.
114. Jones, C., Palmer, T.E., and Griffiths, R.D., Randomized clinical outcome study of critically ill patients given glutamine-supplemented enteral nutrition, *Nutrition*, 15, 108, 1999.
115. Gaull, G., Sturman, J.A., and Räihä, N.C.R., Development of mammalian sulphur metabolism: Absence of cystathionase in human fetal tissues, *Pediatr. Res.*, 6, 538–547, 1972.
116. Di Buono, M. et al., Dietary cysteine reduces methionine requirement in men, *Am. J. Clin. Nutr.*, 74, 761–766, 2001.
117. Chawla, R.K. et al., Plasma cysteine, cystine and glutathione in cirrhosis, *Gastroenterology*, 87, 770–776, 1984.
118. Mihm, S. and Dröge, W., Intracellular glutathione level controls DNA binding activity of NFκB-like proteins, *Immunobiology*, 181, 245–247, 1990.
119. Mihm, S., Ennen, J., and Pessagra, U., Inhibition of HIV-1 replication and NFκB activity by cysteine and cysteine derivatives, *AIDS*, 5, 497–503, 1991.
120. Grimble, R.F. and Grimble, G.K., Immunonutrition: Role of sulphur amino acids, related amino acids, and polyamines, *Nutrition*, 14, 605–610, 1998.
121. Roederer, M. et al., N-acetylcysteine: Potential for AIDS therapy, *Pharmacology,* 46, 121–129, 1992.
122. Dröge, W., Cysteine and glutathione deficiency in AIDS patients: A rationale for the treatment with N-acetyl-cysteine, *Pharmacology*, 46, 612–615, 1993.
123. Stegink, L.D. and Den Besten, L., Synthesis of cysteine from methionine in normal adult subjects: Effect of route of alimentation, *Science*, 178, 514–516, 1972.
124. Griffiths, R.D., Nutrition support in critically ill septic patients, *Curr. Opin. Clin. Nutr. Metab. Care*, 6, 203–210, 2003.

125. Spapen, H.D. et al., N-acetylcysteine and cardiac dysfunction in human septic shock, *Clin. Intensive Care*, 13, 27–32, 2002.
126. Fürst, P. et al., Design of parenteral synthetic dipeptides for clinical nutrition: In vitro and in vivo utilization, *Ann. Nutr. Metab.*, 41, 10–21, 1997.
127. Stehle, P. et al., Intravenous dipeptide metabolism and the design of synthetic dipeptides for clinical nutrition, in *Peptides in Mammalian Protein Metabolism*, Grimble, G.K. and Backwell, F.R.C., eds., Portland Press Ltd., London, U.K., 1998, pp. 103–118.
128. Barbul, A., Arginine: Biochemistry, physiology and therapeutic implications, *J. Parenter. Enteral Nutr.*, 10, 227–238, 1986.
129. Blachier, F. et al., Arginine metabolism in rat enterocytes, *Biochem. Biophys. Acta*, 1092, 304–310, 1991.
130. Cynober, L., Can arginine and ornithine support gut functions? *Gut*, 35, S42–S45, 1994.
131. Kubes, P., Ischemia-reperfusion in feline small intestine: A role for nitric oxide, *Am. J. Physiol.*, 264, G143–G149, 1993.
132. Miller, M.J. et al., Nitric oxide release in response to gut injury, *Scand. J. Gastroenterol.*, 28, 149–154, 1993.
133. Schmidt, M. and Martindale, R., Nutraceuticals in critical care nutrition, in *Nutrition and Critical Care*, Cynober, L. and Moore, F.A., eds., Karger, Basel, Switzerland, 2003, pp. 245–265.
134. Kirk, S.S. and Barbul, A., Role of arginine in trauma, sepsis and immunity, *JPEN*, 14, 226–229, 1990.
135. Evoy, D. et al., Immunonutrition: The role of arginine, *Nutrition,* 14, 611–617, 1998.
136. Visser, M. et al., Imbalance of arginine and asymmetric dimethylarginine is associated with markers of circulatory failure, organ failure and mortality in shock patients, *Br. J. Nutr.*, 107, 1458, 2012.
137. Luiking, Y.C., Engelen, M.P., and Deutz, N.E., Regulation of nitric oxide production in health and disease, *Curr. Opin. Clin. Nutr. Metab. Care*, 13, 97–104, 2010.
138. Visser, M. et al., Nutrition before, during, and after surgery increases the arginine: Asymmetric dimethylarginine ratio and relates to improved myocardial glucose metabolism: A randomized controlled trial, *Am. J. Clin. Nutr.*, 99, 1440, 2014.
139. Gough, M.S. et al., The ratio of arginine to dimethylarginines is reduced and predicts outcomes in patients with severe sepsis, *Crit. Care Med.*, 39, 1351, 2011.
140. Daly, J.M., Reynolds, J., and Thom, A., Immune and metabolic effects of arginine in the surgical patient, *Ann. Surg.*, 298, 512–523, 1988.
141. Barbul, A. et al., Arginine enhances wound healing and lymphocyte response in humans, *Surgery*, 108, 331–337, 1990.
142. Lin, E., Goncalves, J.A., and Lowry, S.F., Efficacy of nutritional pharmacology in surgical patients, *Curr. Opin. Clin. Nutr. Metab. Care*, 1, 41–50, 1998.
143. Huxtable, R.I., Physiological actions of taurine, *Physiol. Rev.*, 72, 101–163, 1992.
144. Wang, J.H. et al., The beneficial effect of taurine on the prevention of human endothelial cell death, *Shock*, 6, 331–338, 1996.
145. Condron, C., Taurine attenuates calcium-dependent, Fas-mediated neutrophil apoptosis, *Shock*, 19, 564–569, 2003.
146. Geggel, H.S. et al., Nutritional requirement for taurine in patients receiving long-term parenteral nutrition, *N. Engl. J. Med.*, 312, 142–146, 1985.
147. Heird, W.C. et al., Pediatric parenteral amino acid mixture in low birth weight infants, *Pediatrics*, 81, 41–50, 1988.
148. Kopple, J.D. et al., Effect of intravenous taurine supplementation on plasma, blood cell and urine taurine concentrations in adults undergoing long-term parenteral nutrition, *Am. J. Clin. Nutr.*, 52, 846–853, 1990.
149. Desai, T.I.C. et al., Taurine deficiency after intensive chemotherapy and/or radiation, *Am. J. Clin. Nutr.*, 55, 708–711, 1992.
150. Bergström, J. et al., Sulphur amino acids in plasma and muscle in patients with chronic renal failure: Evidence for taurine depletion, *J. Intern. Med.*, 226, 189–194, 1989.
151. Suliman, M.E., Anderstam, B., and Bergström, J., Evidence of taurine depletion and accumulation of cysteinesulfinic acid in chronic dialysis patients, *Kidney Int.*, 50, 1713–1717, 1996.
152. Redmond, H.P. et al., Immunonutrition: The role of taurine, *Nutrition*, 14, 599–604, 1998.
153. Fürst, P. et al., Reappraisal of indispensable amino acids. Design of parenteral synthetic dipeptides: Synthetic and characterization, *Ann. Nutr. Metab.*, 41, 1–9, 1997.
154. Hummel, M. et al., Intestinal taurine availability from synthetic amino acid-taurine conjugates: An in vitro perfusion study in rats, *Clin. Nutr.*, 16, 137–139, 1997.
155. Turk , J.L., Inflammation: John Hunter's "A treatise on the blood, inflammation and gun-shot wounds," *Int J Exp Pathol.*, 175(6), 385–395, 1994.

4 Lipid Metabolism

Stress versus Nonstress States

Dan L. Waitzberg, Raquel S. Torrinhas, and Letícia De Nardi

CONTENTS

BASIC CONCEPTS

DEFINITION

The word *lipid* is derived from the Greek *lipos* meaning fat. The lipids are products of biological origin, consisting of groups of fatty acids (FAs)—carboxylic acids with long unbranched chains, formed by an even number of carbon atoms connected by simple or double bonds. They can be found in various forms, as described in Table 4.1.

TABLE 4.1
Various Forms of Fats

Form	Examples
Oils	Esters formed from fatty acids (FAs) and which present in liquid form
Fats	Esters formed from FA and which present in solid form
Waxes	The principle components are esters formed from FA and long-chain alcohols
Steroids	Cholesterol and sex hormones
Others	Soaps, detergents, and biliary salts

Source: Holum, R.J., Lipids, in: *Fundamentals of General, Organic and Biological Chemistry*, Holum, J.R., (ed.) John Wiley & Sons Inc., 1994, pp. 566–582.

Nomenclature/Classification

FAs are characterized by the following:

1. The number of atoms in the carbon chain: (long chain, 14–20 carbon atoms; medium length chain, 6–12 carbon atoms; and short chain, up to 6 carbon atoms).
2. The number of double bonds: (saturated fats, no double bonds; monounsaturated fats, one double bond; and polyunsaturated, more than one double bond).
3. In the case of unsaturated FAs by the position of the first double bond counting from the methyl radical (represented by the Greek letter omega—ω) or starting from its functional group (represented by the letter delta—Δ).[2] See example in Figure 4.1.

The various types of FAs and their principal sources are described briefly in Table 4.2.[3]

The lipids can be further classified into simple, composite, or variable, according to their composition.[4]

Simple: FA, neutral fats (steroids of FA with glycerol, e.g., triglycerides [TGs]), and waxes (steroids of FA with alcohols, e.g., cholesterol esters).

Composite: Phospholipids (composed of phosphoric acid, FA, and a nitrogenated base), glycolipids (composed of FA, monosaccharide, and a nitrogenated base), and lipoprotein (lipid particles and protein).

Variable: Steroids (such as cholesterol, vitamin D, biliary salts) and vitamins A, E, and K.

Function

In basic terms, the lipids are a source of energy with a high caloric density (9.3 kcal/g). They also have a role in the synthesis of hormones and cellular structures, in the transportation of liposoluble vitamins, in intracellular and extracellular signaling, and in the supply of essential FAs.[3] The main functions of the lipids are outlined in Table 4.3.

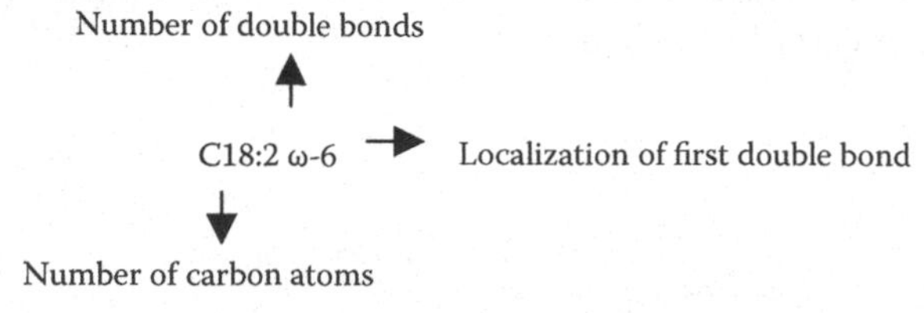

FIGURE 4.1 C, carbon and ω, omega.

TABLE 4.2
Types of Fatty Acids and Their Principal Sources

Saturated			Monounsaturated	Polyunsaturated	
Short Chain	**Medium Chain**	**Long Chain**	**ω-9**	**ω-6**	**ω-3**
Acetic	Capric	Myristic	Oleic	Linoleic 18:2	α-linolenic 18:3
Propionic	Caprylic	Palmitic	Palmitoleic		
Butyric	Capric	Stearic		γ-linolenic 18:3	EPA 20:5
	Lauric	Arachidic		DHA 22:6	
				Arachidonic 20:4	
Sources					
Butter	Coconut	Animal fat	Olive oil	Safflower oil	Fish oil
Fibers	Palms	Cocoa	Rapeseed oil	Soybean oil	Nut oil
				Corn oil	Rapeseed oil
				Cotton oil	Soybean oil

Source: Borges, V. and Waitzberg, D.L., Gorduras, in: *Nutrição enteral e parenteral na prática clínica*, Waitzberg, D.L., ed., Atheneu, São Paulo, Brazil, 1995, pp. 21–32.

TABLE 4.3
Main Functions of Lipids

Principal functions

Energy supply through foods (9.3 kcal/g), essential fatty acids, and liposoluble vitamins (A, D, E, K)

Stored combustible energy (where 95% is in the form of triglycerides), principally for periods of fasting

Mechanical protection (bones and organs) and maintenance of body temperature

Synthesis of cellular structures, such as phospholipid membrane synthesis of hormones

Transport or liposoluble vitamins

Intra- and extracellular mediators of immune response

Participation in inflammatory process and in oxidative stress

Source: Calder, P.C., *Braz. J. Med. Biol. Res.*, 36, 433, 2003.

BASIC HUMAN PHYSIOLOGY AND LIPID BIOCHEMISTRY

INGESTION

The daily energy requirement of humans is generally provided by FA ingested in the diet. However, when necessary, FAs (saturated or monounsaturated) can be synthesized from glucose and amino acids through enzymatic elongation reactions (by adding units of two carbons) and desaturation (creation of new double bonds).[3] The desaturation mechanism is stimulated by insulin and inhibited by glucose, adrenaline, and glucagon.[3]

However, we do not produce specific desaturating enzymes (Δ-12 and Δ-15 desaturase) responsible for adding a double bond before the ninth carbon at the end of the methyl (distal) extremity. Consequently, the long-chain polyunsaturated FAs (PUFA), namely, ω-6 (linoleic acid) and ω-3 (α-linolenic acid), cannot be produced endogenously. These are obtained exclusively from diet and are therefore denominated essential.[3]

The daily requirements of ω-6 and ω-3 essential FAs are 3% and 5%, respectively, of the total caloric ingestion. However, the diet typical of Western nations and other industrialized countries is rich in ω-6 PUFAs (7%–10%) and contains little ω-3 PUFAs, which explains the great predominance of the former in the cellular membrane structures.

By sequential enzymatic processes of elongation and desaturation, linoleic acid forms γ-linolenic acid that is in turn converted into arachidonic acid. By the same metabolic pathway and in a competitive manner, α-linolenic acid is converted into eicosapentaenoic acid (EPA) and docosahexaenoic acid (DHA), as shown in Figure 4.2. These FAs participate in the composition of cellular membranes and are precursors of eicosanoids that regulate the immune and inflammatory functions.[5]

Certain derivatives of essential FAs, such as arachidonic acid (ω-6) and EPA (ω-3), are especially important since they are precursors of lipid mediators involved in many physiological functions.[5]

Insufficient ingestion of essential FAs can cause immunological dysfunction, dermatitis, alopecia, thrombocytopenia, and poor cicatrization. The main symptoms and clinical signs of ω-6 and ω-3 deficiency are given in Table 4.4.

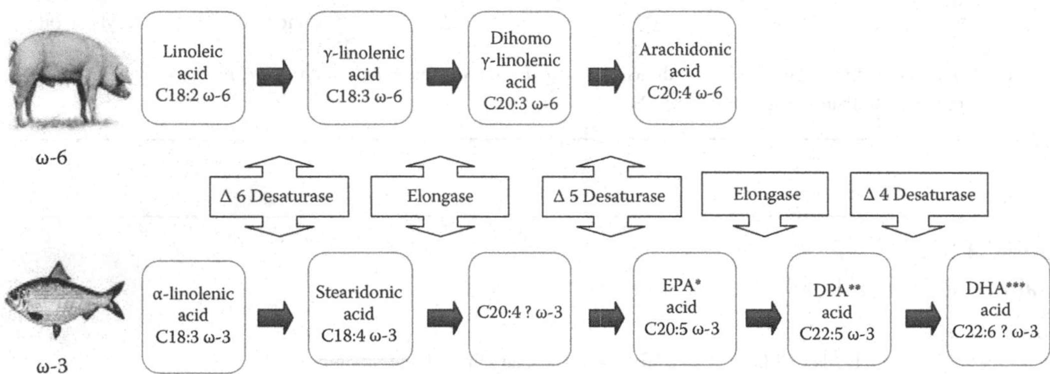

FIGURE 4.2 Formation of new long-chain ω-6 and ω-3 PUFAs from α-linoleic and α-linolenic essential FAs. *Notes:* *, Eicosapentaenoic acid; **, Docosapentaenoic acid; and ***, Docosahexaenoic acid.

TABLE 4.4
Clinical Symptoms of the Deficiency of Essential Fatty Acids

Deficiency	Clinical Symptoms
ω-6 fatty acids	Skin lesions
	Anemia
	Augmented platelet aggregation
	Thrombocytopenia
	Hepatic steatosis
	Delayed cicatrization
	Increased susceptibility to infections
	In children: growth retardation and diarrhea
ω-3 fatty acids	Neurological symptoms
	Reduction in visual acuity
	Skin lesions
	Growth retardation
	Impaired learning capacity
	Abnormal electroretinogram

Digestion

Fats are frequently consumed in the form of TGs (three molecules of FAs and one of glycerol). Due to their molecular complexity and hydrophobic nature, TGs require the action of various enzymes and mechanical movement in order to be broken down and absorbed by the digestive system.

The process of digesting lipids begins in the stomach with emulsification by physical movements (propulsion, retropropulsion, and mixing) and by enzymatic action (through the lingual and gastric lipases). The lingual and gastric lipases are efficient in the emulsification and breaking down of medium-chain FAs (MCFAs).[6]

The digestion of food and nutrients principally takes place in the small bowel, where the secretion of cholecystokinin (CCK) occurs in response to the presence of fats and proteins. CCK stimulates the secretion and release of bile by the liver and gall bladder. The bile (rich in biliary salts and phospholipids) intensifies the emulsification process, thereby increasing the surface area and favoring the enzymatic action on the fats.[7]

The principal enzymes involved in the duodenal digestion of lipids are as follows: pancreatic lipase, phospholipase-A_2, and cholesterol esterase.[7]

Absorption

The absorptive process of FAs varies in relation to the length of their carbon chains. The long-chain FAs (LCFAs) are absorbed in the brush border of the enterocytes and migrate to the smooth endoplasmic reticulum, where the resynthesis of the TGs occurs. The TGs are incorporated into the apolipoproteins, resynthesized phospholipids, and cholesterol, forming the lipoproteins that reach the circulation through the lymphatic system.

The MCFAs, after passing through the enterocytes, bind to albumin. Most of the MCFA are conducted to the liver by means of the blood stream, and not by lymphatic transport, which is used mainly by the LCFAs.[3] The short-chain FAs (SCFAs) can be produced via the bacterial fermentation of fibers, especially the soluble ones; they are absorbed directly in the large intestine and used as a source of energy. The SCFA produced in the intestine are acetic, butyric, and propionic acid.[8] SCFAs absorbed in the intestinal lumen do not necessarily reach the circulation, since in general they are used in the metabolism of the colonocytes. The absorption of the liposoluble vitamins A, D, E, K, all the fats, and cholesterol occurs in the ileum.

Transport

After their intestinal absorption, the FAs are transported in the bloodstream to be used by the liver and peripheral tissues or for storage in the adipose tissue.

The FAs are conducted in various forms: as free FAs (bonded to albumin), chylomicrons, and lipoproteins (composed of cholesterol esters, phospholipids, and TGs). The transportation pathway can be either exogenous (transport of the dietary lipids from the intestine to the liver) or endogenous (transport of the lipoproteins synthesized in the hepatocytes to the peripheral tissues).[9,10]

The LCFAs have a strong affinity for binding with albumin, unlike MCFAs and SCFAs that do not need to bind with this protein in order to be transported.

The FAs can be transported through the bloodstream by lipoproteins of various densities, depending on the local of production: when originating from intestinal absorption, they are transported in the form of chylomicrons (lipoprotein rich in dietary TGs—density: 0.92–0.96 g/L) or when produced by the liver through very-low-density lipoproteins (VLDLs—density, 0.95–1.0 g/L), low-density lipoproteins (LDLs—density, 1.0–1.06 g/L), and high-density lipoproteins (HDLs—density, 1.06–1.21 g/L).[11]

The VLDLs are formed in the liver and transported to the adipocytes, where hydrolysis, reesterification, and storage of TGs occur. Hepatic lipase action transforms VLDLs into LDLs by removal of TGs.

The LDLs are a part of the metabolic pathway of cholesterol-rich lipoproteins. They remain longer in the vascular compartment and are responsible for the distribution of cholesterol to the extrahepatic tissues.

Cholesterol released by LDLs is incorporated into the cellular membranes and stored in the form of cholesterol ester or used for synthesis of steroid hormones. In hypercholesterolemia, elevated levels of LDL favor the generation of an oxidized form (LDL-ox) that is extremely atherogenic.

HDLs play a fundamental role in the reverse transport of cholesterol, by removing excess from the peripheral tissues and transporting it to the liver, where it is then metabolized and eliminated in the form of acid and biliary salts.[12]

The principal function of the chylomicrons is to supply energy to the peripheral tissues, through the release of free FA. Contact with the capillary endothelium stimulates the lipoprotein lipase (LPL) enzyme that releases TGs and generates free FAs that are used as energy substrate or stored.[13]

Recently, a family of proteins known as fatty-acid-binding proteins (FABPs) has been identified that seems to have an important role in the transfer of these acids through the membrane, besides making them available for metabolizing. When managing the distribution of FAs through the organelles, FABPs modulate their utilization as metabolites of energy and storage.[14] Furthermore, they have an effect on cellular differentiation and functionality, besides the proliferation and regulation of genetic transcription.[15,16]

Cellular Utilization of the Lipids

The lipids can be used as an energy source through a β-oxidation reaction within the mitochondria. Upon reaching the cells to be oxidized, the FAs pass through the cellular membrane to the cytosol. However, before oxidation can effectively take place in the matrix, they must also cross the barrier represented by the mitochondrial membrane. For this, LCFAs need the aid of carnitine that is activated by specific enzymes (Figure 4.3). The MCFAs are more soluble in water than LCFAs and

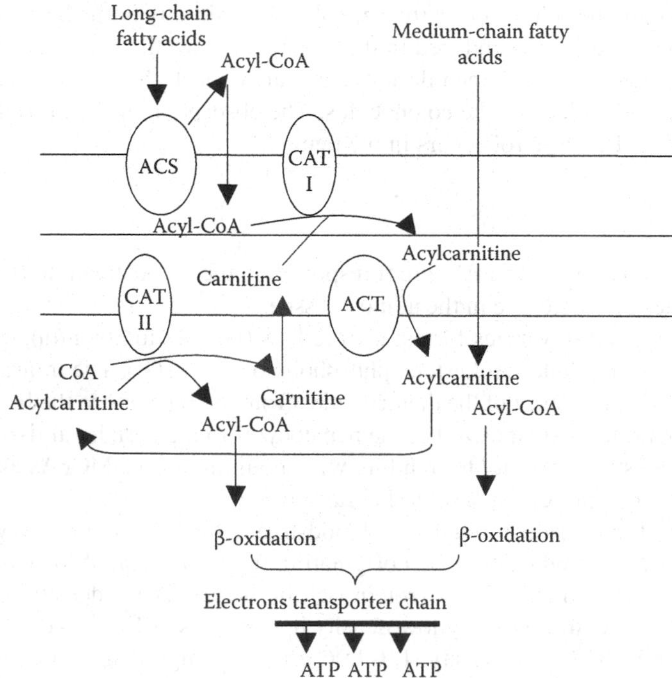

FIGURE 4.3 ACS, acyl-CoA synthase; CAT, carnitine translocase; TCA, tricarboxylic acid; and ATP, adenosine triphosphate.

can get into the mitochondria with partial independence from the aid of carnitine (only 10%–20%); nevertheless, in muscle tissue, they are totally dependent on the activity of carnitine as a carrier. Once inside the mitochondria, the FAs serve as substrata for β-oxidation and energy synthesis.[3]

The FA can also be useful, in a selective manner, in the synthesis of the phospholipids of cellular and organelle membranes. In humans, the predominant FA incorporated in the membranes are EPA and DHA (ω-3), arachidonic acid (ω-6), and oleic acid (ω-9).[17] The lipids cellular distribution is generally specific, but it can be altered by the availability of fats in the diet and especially PUFA.[18]

The essential FAs can cause structural and functional alterations in the phospholipidic membrane (including immune system cells), modifying their stability, their permeability, the activity of receptors and enzymes, their transport, regulatory functions, and cellular metabolism.[19,20] In addition, they can activate intracellular routing of signals by the formation of biologically active molecules that act as secondary messengers and inflammatory mediators called eicosanoids.[17,21]

There are two pathways for the synthesis of eicosanoids: cyclooxygenase and lipoxygenase, which respectively produce prostanoids (thromboxane, prostaglandin) and leukotriene and lipoxin (Figure 4.4).

The eicosanoids participate in various cellular and physiological events, modulating processes such as platelet aggregation, smooth muscle contraction, leukocyte chemotaxis, inflammatory cytokine production, and immune functions.[22] In an inflammatory picture, there is an increase in the even-number series eicosanoids, produced by the metabolism of ω-6 FA. High levels of some of these eicosanoids are also found in patients with inflammatory conditions or sepsis and in critically ill patients.

The eicosanoids modulate the inflammatory response in a varying manner. Eicosanoids originating from the metabolism of PUFAs type ω-6 are potent inflammatory mediators, but those of the odd number series, originating from the metabolism of ω-3 PUFAs, result in an attenuated inflammatory response.[23] This indicates that ω-3 FAs have the capacity to inhibit an acute inflammatory response induced or aggravated by eicosanoids derived from the metabolism of ω-6 FAs. The role of eicosanoids, resulting from the metabolism of arachidonic acid and EPA, on phagocytic cells is depicted in Figure 4.5.

The eicosanoids regulate the production of several cytokines involved in inflammation. Prostaglandin 2, originating from ω-6 FAs, produces several proinflammatory effects that include fever, increased vascular permeability, and vasodilatation but inhibits the production of IL-1, IL-2,

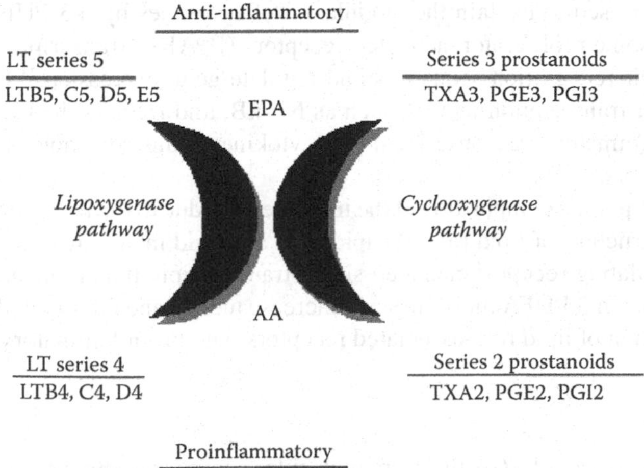

FIGURE 4.4 LT, leukotriene; TX, thromboxane; PG, prostaglandin; EPA, eicosapentaenoic acid; and AA, arachidonic acid.

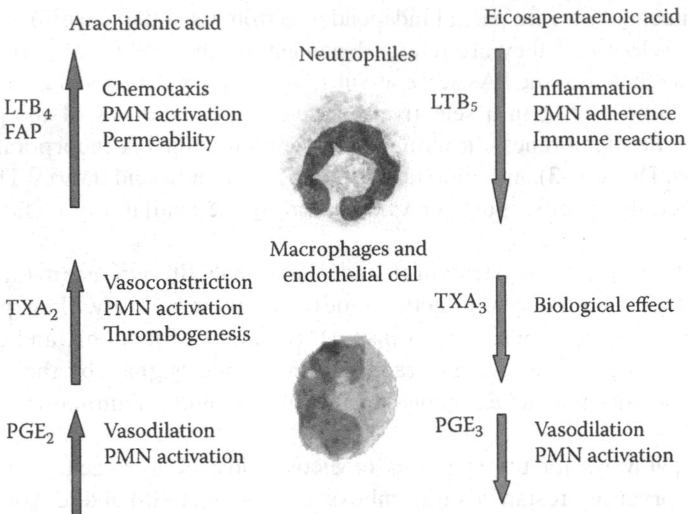

FIGURE 4.5 LT, leukotriene; TX, thromboxane; PG, prostaglandin; and PAF (FAP), platelet activating factor.

IL-6, and TNF-alpha (TNF-α).[24] On the other hand, leukotrienes of series −4 increase the production of IL-1, IL-2, and IL-6 and augment lymphocyte proliferation.[24] With the increased offer of ω-3 PUFAs in relation to ω-6 PUFAs, the synthesis of prostaglandins and leukotrienes of the even-number series is reduced, thereby modulating the inflammatory cytokines, particularly in humans.[25–27]

The capacity of ω-3 FAs in antagonizing the production of eicosanoids derived from the metabolism of ω-6 FAs constitutes a key point in the anti-inflammatory effect attributed to ω-3 FAs, but they also exert other effects that seem to be independent of the modulation of eicosanoids production.

Currently, another class of immune mediators derived from n-3 PUFAs was identified, the so-called resolvins.[28] These lipid mediators are released during cell-to-cell communication via transcellular biosynthesis and participate in the local endogenous control of the inflammation, inhibiting the activation and migration of polymorphonuclear (PMN) leukocytes during the resolution phase and then enabling inflamed tissues to return to homeostasis.[28]

Experimental and human studies have shown that n-3 PUFAs can also affect cytokines release, by inhibiting the synthesis of proinflammatory cytokines, such as TNF-α and interleukins (ILs) IL-1β and IL-6, and positively modulating the production of the anti-inflammatory cytokine IL-10.[28] The mechanisms proposed to explain the modulation of cytokines by n-3 PUFA include the activation of the peroxisome proliferator–activated receptors (PPARs), transcription factors that once activated bind to their recognition sequences and regulate gene expression.[28] PPAR-γ was shown to bind directly other transcription factors, such as NF-κB, and inhibits the transcription of genes involved in the inflammatory response including cytokines, adhesion molecules, and other proinflammatory mediators.[29–33]

Changes in the membrane composition of the immune cells due to the incorporation of n-3 PUFAs can also affect the structure of lipid rafts.[28] Lipid rafts are rigid membrane microdomains that are responsible for modulating receptor-mediated signal transduction, thus influencing cell activation. The highly unsaturated n-3 PUFA molecules can increase membrane fluidity and disrupt lipid rafts, impairing the activation of lipid raft–associated receptors (i.e., proinflammatory receptors).[28]

Storage

Lipids are stored in the form of TGs; these are molecules comprising three esters of FAs (saturated, monounsaturated, or polyunsaturated) and an alcohol (glycerol). The deposit of TGs occurs mainly in the adipose tissue, a specialized type of connective tissue that acts primarily as a major fat deposit. In humans, adipose tissue accounts for approximately 15% of the body weight of a normal adult male and is equivalent to about 2 months of energy reserve.

There are two types of adipose tissue: white and brown. Brown, tan, or multilocular adipose tissue has a special function in the regulation of the body temperature in newborns, while in adults, deposits of this tissue are practically nonexistent.[34] White, yellow, or unilocular adipose tissue is widely distributed in the subcutaneous tissues. The blood flow for this tissue varies depending on the body weight and nutritional state, since it increases during fasting. It also possesses nerve fibers comprising part of the sympathetic nervous system (SNS).[35] The ingested TGs in the food are the main components of the fat deposits; however, excess carbohydrate and dietary proteins can also be converted into FAs in the liver through lipogenesis.

Under certain metabolic circumstances, a breaking down of TGs (lipolysis) can occur, with the release of FAs from the adipose tissue for cellular use in the synthesis of energy. This process prevails over lipogenesis when there is a greater demand for energy. Lipolysis in the adipose tissue can occur through the action of the LPL enzyme or of a lipase sensitive to a hormone, through the stimulation of lipolytic hormones: adrenocorticotropic hormone (ACTH), catecholamines (adrenaline and noradrenaline), growth hormone (GH), glucagon, cortisol, and leptin.

Lipolytic hormones bind to receptors present in the cellular membrane of the adipocytes, triggering a cascade of activation, through adenosine cyclic monophosphate (cAMP), which transports them to the activation of the enzyme hormone-sensitive lipase and consequent hydrolysis of the FAs (see schematic representation in Figure 4.6). Their concentrations are directly related to the degree of activation of the SNS. The antilipolytic hormone is insulin.

In this way, hormones released by nerve stimulation can stimulate lipolysis, through the activation of the hormone-sensitive lipase in the adipocytes and thereby influence the regulation of the lipid metabolism.

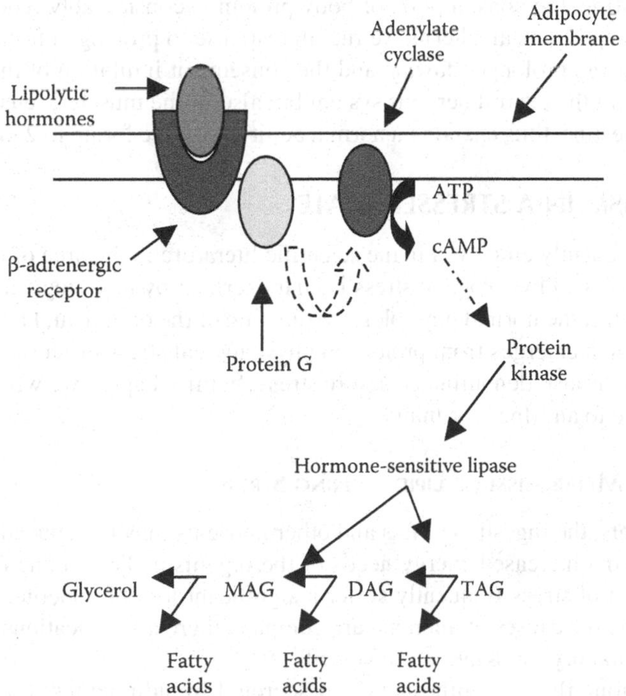

FIGURE 4.6 ATP, adenosine triphosphate; cAMP, cyclic adenosine monophosphate; MAG, monoacylglycerol; DAG, diacylglycerol; and TAG, triacylglycerol.

ALTERATIONS IN METABOLISM DURING FASTING WITHOUT COMPLICATIONS

The response to chronically inadequate alimentary ingestion (fasting) aims to preserve fat-free body mass. It is characterized by a decrease in the expenditure of energy, the use of alternative sources of fuel, and a reduced expenditure of protein. Low seric glucose levels (between 60 and 80 mg/dL) triggers a signal to the brain notifying a hypoglycemia state. In response, counterregulating hormones are released, that is, cortisol, glucagon, GH, and adrenaline.[13]

A reduction of the plasma insulin concentration, in conjunction with an increase in counterregulating hormones, activates the hormone-sensitive lipase present in the cytoplasm of the adipocytes and of the muscle tissue. In the adipose tissue, the action of this enzyme releases FAs and glycerol from the deposit of triacylglycerol.[13,36]

The reserves of glycogen last approximately 24 h; therefore, the glucose has to be synthesized again, using protein as a substratum. The protein in the muscles and other sources is broken down, and amino acids (alanine and glutamine) are released and transported to the liver, where glyconeogenesis takes place. After 24 h of fasting, the oxidation of FAs becomes, progressively, the main source in the production of energy for the tissues; however, the nervous system and red blood cells continue to partially use glucose as an energetic fuel.

The oxidation of FAs produces an accumulation of acetyl-CoA that is then converted to ketone bodies (KBs) through the ketogenic pathway. The production of KB during fasting is regulated by the high ratio of plasma glucagon/insulin and also by the reduced concentration of malonyl-CoA of the hepatocyte (this metabolite has the function of inhibiting the activity of carnitine palmitoyl transferase [CPT], which is the key enzyme in the β-oxidation).[36]

The KB present in the circulation together with free FAs are used for production of ATP by the peripheral and principally muscular tissues.

During the first week of fasting, intense muscular catabolism occurs for glucose production by the liver. Following this, there is an adaptation response to the prolonged fasting, such that after about 4 weeks of fasting, the consumption of body protein is considerably reduced, mainly due to the adaptation for using KB as an alternative fuel in response to prolonged fasting.[13,36]

The use of KB during prolonged fasting and the consequent inhibition of the utilization of glucose occurs not only in the central nervous system but also in the muscles, renal cortex, mammary glands, and small intestine, thus enabling a normal adult to survive for up to 2 months of fasting.[13,36]

LIPID METABOLISM IN A STRESSED STATE

The term *stress* is frequently employed in the scientific literature in the area of nutrition to describe certain clinical situations. Physiological stress is characterized by neurological and endocrinological alterations that affect the normal physiological function of the organism. Pathological stress may be defined as that which emerges from prolonged physiological stress or an additional stress due to disease or trauma and is also denominated severe stress. In this chapter, we will consider stress as a pathological response to an illness or injury.

ALTERATIONS IN THE METABOLISM OF LIPIDS DURING STRESS

In critically ill patients, the ingestion of fats and other nutrients may be reduced or even completely absent in relation to the increased energy needs of the organism. This is due to the fact that individuals in a condition of stress frequently suffer a significant loss of appetite, a syndrome known as anorexia. Although the causes of anorexia are complex, there are indications that factors such as leptin and proinflammatory cytokines are involved.[37,38]

Leptin is a hormone that is synthesized and secreted by adipocytes, bound to receptors in the hypothalamus and other tissues. Leptin may act as a regulator of the mass of body fat. A decrease in the fat deposits reduces the production of leptin. In the hypothalamus, a low concentration of leptin leads to a greater expression of neuropeptide Y, which increases alimentary ingestion.[39] However, under stress there is an increase of leptin release, despite the reduction in fat reserves, with a consequent decrease in appetite.[37,38]

In situations of fasting, the organism resorts to compensatory mechanisms that protect it from the possible damage caused by the lack of nutrients. These mechanisms include a breaking down of protein and fat and a reduction in the use of energy. However, in the presence of stress, these mechanisms of adaptation to prolonged fasting do not occur. The presence of tissue damage leads to the installation of a catabolic picture in a desperate attempt to recover homeostasis in the organism. The magnitude of the catabolic reaction seems to be related more to the intensity of the tissular injury than to the type of stress.

During stress, the liberation of catabolic hormones leads to an increase in lipolytic activity. Paralleling this is a preferential oxidation of fat by various tissues, such as the muscles, where a resistance to insulin is developed.[40,41] However, nervous and immune cells continue to need glucose as an energy source, but this is supplied by neoglucogenesis.

Despite the intense lipolysis observed during the metabolic response to stress, there is not always an increase in the plasma concentrations of free FAs, suggesting that the clearance rate of free FAs in the plasma is increased.[42] On the other hand, under certain conditions, the activity of LPL is inhibited by the production of proinflammatory cytokines (such as INF-γ and IL-1), impairing the clearance of TGs from the circulation and installing a picture of hypertriglyceridemia.[43]

The increased rates of lipolysis previously described are so intense that they frequently exceed the energy requirements of the organism. The FAs that are not oxidized can be reesterified into TGs in the liver and inserted in the VLDLs. The hepatic production of TGs may be increased in stress situations, propitiating the development of hepatic steatosis. VLDLs, in turn, seem to have protective effects against endotoxemia through their capacity to bind with endotoxins and enable their degradation in hepatic parenchymal cells.[44,45]

In relation to the metabolic alterations of lipids in stress conditions, there is a decrease in the concentrations of plasma cholesterol, in spite of the increase in its hepatic production. Likewise, probably due to the increased catabolism, there is a decrease in the concentration of plasma LDLs together with HDLs. The decrease in HDLs seems to be related to the increase of its subendothelial uptake and retention.[44,45]

In addition, cytokines liberated during stress can modify the composition of HDLs and LDLs, influencing functional properties of these lipoproteins. In this way, alterations of proteins associated with HDLs, for instance, can lead to a reduced capacity for actuating in the reverse transport of cholesterol.[44,45]

Modulation of the Metabolism of Lipids Induced by Stress

Hormonal Response to Stress and the Metabolism of Lipids

The neuroendocrine alterations released in a stress situation are characterized by the high presence of neural stimuli as much from the central nervous system as from autonomous nerves that activate the endocrine system to liberate glucagon, cortisol, and catecholamines, thereby significantly increasing the plasmatic levels of these hormones. Consequently, there is an alteration of the balance between insulin, the principal anabolic hormone (the functions of which are outlined in Table 4.5),

TABLE 4.5
Main Functions of Insulin on Fat

Activity	Effect
Anticatabolic (to prevent degradation)	Inhibit lipolysis, prevent the excess of ketone and ketoacidosis production
Anabolic (to promote storage)	Facilitate the pyruvate reduction into free FA by stimulating the lipogenesis
Transport	Activate the lipoprotein lipase, facilitating the transport of TG to adipose tissue

and these important catabolic hormones, favoring catabolism. In burn patients, the amount of glucagon may double, cortisol may increase fourfold, and catecholamines may increase by eight and up to ten times compared with normal controls. These changes are related to the metabolic effects of the disease, which include a significant increase of lipolysis.[46]

There are indications that adipocytes may have direct contact with nerve endings that, when stimulated provoke an increase in lipolysis. Therefore, it is possible that the stimulation of these nerves does not alter the metabolism by the modulation of endocrine functions alone but also by direct effects on peripheral tissues.[47]

Cortisol

Cortisol produces important effects in the energy metabolism during sepsis and trauma. Its effects on the lipid metabolism, however, are not well understood. Hypercortisolemia increases the arterial concentration of nonesterified (free) FAs (NEFA) and of their organic turnover. However, arterial–venous studies have shown that hypercortisolemia reduces the efflux of NEFAs from some deposits of fatty tissue. This inhibition of lipid mobilization seems to be associated with a reduction in the rate of activity of the hormone-sensitive lipase in these deposits.[48] The increase in the arterial concentration of NEFAs may be explained by the higher rate of LPL activity, since the plasma concentrations of TGs are reduced. Another possible effect on the metabolism might be through specific sites of cortisol activity.

Catecholamines

The infusion of adrenaline in humans leads to an increase in the efflux of NEFAs from adipose tissue, due to the increase of its transcapillary efflux resulting from the increase of lipolysis in the adipose tissue.[49] Adrenaline also causes an important elevation in the blood flow in adipose tissues, which results in an increased presentation of the triacylglycerol lipoprotein, as a substratum for LPL, to be hydrolyzed in the vascular component.

The effect of noradrenaline on the lipid metabolism in adipose tissue is similar to that of adrenaline. The infusion of noradrenaline leads to an increased blood flow in the adipose tissue that in turn results in an increase in the efflux of NEFAs and glycerol from the adipose tissue, indicating intense activity of hormone-sensitive lipase.[50] Apparently, the blood flow in the adipose tissue, together with its catecholamines, is an important regulator of the metabolism.[50]

In the presence of severe injury, perfusion of the adipose tissue may be impaired; this can lead to a lower concentration of NEFAs and to their reduced turnover. One of the major differences between sepsis and trauma seems to be the hypertriglyceridemia induced by sepsis. This effect during sepsis seems to be mediated partially through the liver by the selective cleavage of NEFAs into TGs and an increased de novo synthesis of TGs. Additionally, the clearance of TGs from peripheral areas is reduced through a decrease in the levels of LPL.[51]

A schematic of the neuroendocrine response to stress is shown in Figure 4.7.

Cytokine Response to Stress and Lipid Metabolism

Injury to tissues interferes in the metabolism through the neuroendocrine nervous system and also by the induction of proinflammatory mediators. In sepsis and in trauma, the levels of plasmatic cytokines, which include TNF-α, IL-1β and IL-6, can increase rapidly.[52,53]

TNF-α seems to have an important effect in the induction of anorexia and in the loss of adipose tissue. The administration of TNF-α in laboratory animals induces cachexia with anorexia and a depletion of adipose tissue.[54] This cytokine is also involved in the genesis of a resistance to insulin by inhibiting the phosphorylase of receptors.[55] IL-1 presents the same effects as those of TNF-α by suppressing the activity of LPL and increasing intracellular lipolysis. IL-6 appears to have an important effect in the development of cachexia.[56] This cytokine is an important modulator in human metabolism, which is capable of stimulating lipolysis and fat oxidation without causing hypertriglyceridemia.

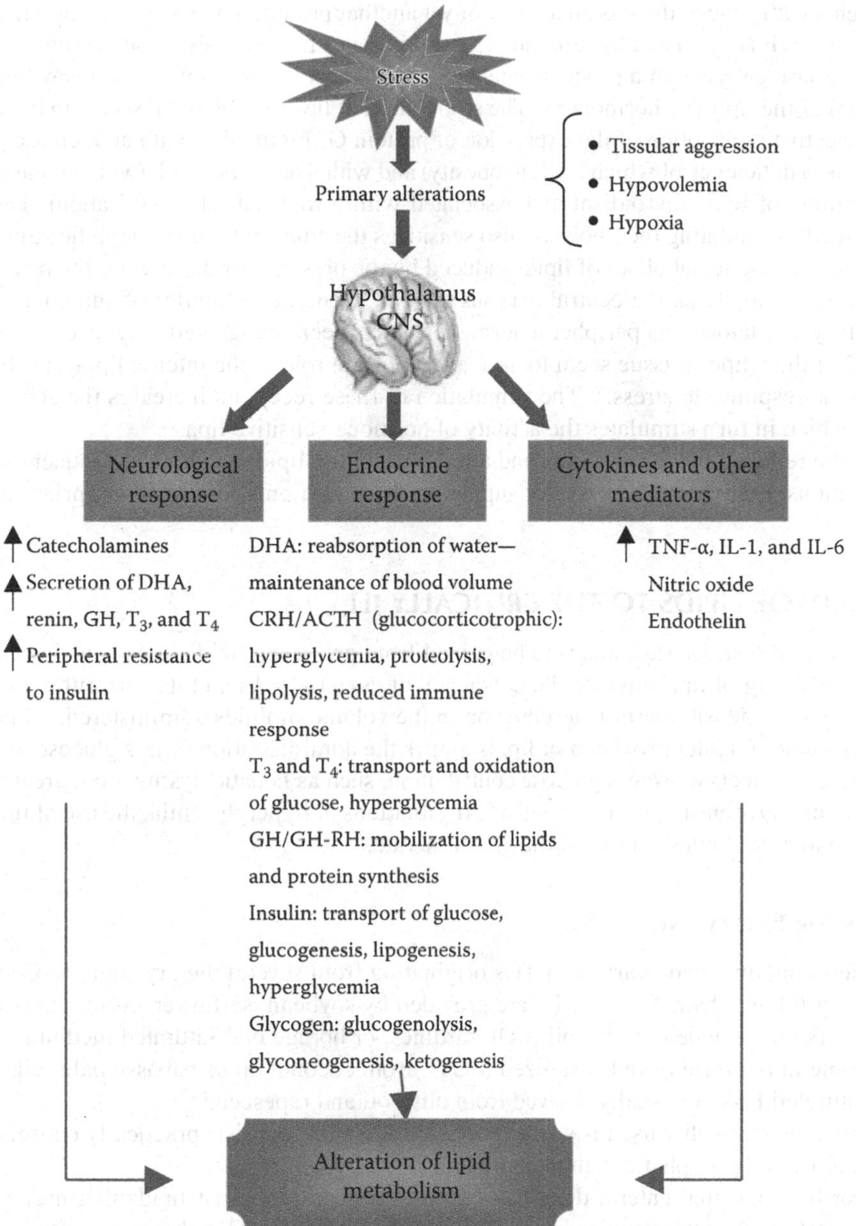

FIGURE 4.7 CNS, central nervous system; DHA, docosahexaenoic acid; GH, growth hormone; T, thyroxine hormone; CRH, corticotropin-releasing hormone; ACTH, adrenocorticotropic hormone; GH-RH, growth hormone-releasing hormone; TNF, tumor necrosis factor; and IL, interleukin.

The cytokine response to trauma or sepsis may vary according to the nature of the insult. These cytokines can affect directly the metabolism of the adipose tissue, and they can even influence indirectly the lipid metabolism through alterations of the counterregulatory hormone plasma concentrations. IL-6 and TNF-α, for example, induce important neuroendocrine alterations, by stimulating the secretion of corticotrophin, cortisol, noradrenaline, adrenaline, and glucagon.[57,58] In the last decade, it has been demonstrated that cytokines such as TNF-α, leptin, and plasminogen activator inhibitor-1, which are produced by adipose tissue, act in an endocrine and paracrine manner, thus allowing the adipose tissue to regulate the metabolism of its lipid content.[59]

In patients with cancer, there is an activity of yet another protein, known as lipid mobilization factor (LMF).[60] LMF is produced by tumoral cells and initiates the lipolysis through stimulation of the adenylate cyclase enzyme, in a process dependent on guanosine triphosphate, in a way homologous to the action of the lipolytic hormones.[61] The stimulation of lipolysis by LMF seems to be associated with the selective modulation of the expression of protein G (Figure 4.6) with an increase in protein G of type Gs (a deficiency of which leads to obesity) and with a decrease in Gi (with increased expression in pictures of hyperthyroidism and associated with a reduced fat mobilization). Thus, LMF, besides directly stimulating the lipolysis, also sensitizes the adipose tissue to lipolytic stimulation.[62]

Alterations in the metabolism of lipids induced by the presence of disease are the result of complex interactions involving the central nervous system, hormones, stimulus of autonomous nerves, inflammatory mediators, and peripheral hormones. It has been recognized only recently that receptors beta-2 of the adipose tissue seem to have an important role in the intense lipolysis observed in the metabolic response to stress.[63] The stimulation of these receptors increases the concentrations of cAMP, which in turn stimulates the activity of hormone-sensitive lipase.

Due to the reduced ingestion of fats and alterations in the lipid metabolism, frequently found in stress situations, there is a necessity for supplying these nutrients through appropriate nutritional therapy.

PROVISION OF LIPIDS TO THE CRITICALLY ILL

There are several distinct advantages to be gained from providing lipids to patients in critical condition. The offering of lipids avoids the deficiency of essential FAs and its harmful consequences. Their high-energy density permits a reduction in the volume of fluids administered, without a loss of energy content. Greater provision of lipids allows the administration of less glucose, thus reducing the negative effects of excess glucose contribution, such as hepatic dysfunction, greater production of CO_2, and O_2 consumption of oxygen.[64] In situations of hyperglycemia, the use of lipids offers a safe alternative for better control of the glycemic rate.

Formulas for Enteral Nutrition

Enteral diets contain a wide variety of TGs originating from several dietary sources. Generally, in these diets, n-6 long-chain TGs (LCTs) are provided by soybean, safflower, corn, or sunflower oil. The n-3 LCTs are provided by fish oil (FO), sardines, or borage oil. Saturated medium-chain TGs (MCTs) come in the form of industrialized MCTs, from coconut oil or babassu palm oil, while the monounsaturated FAs are usually derived from olive oil and rapeseed.[65]

Normally, the emulsifier used is soybean lecithin. Lecithin consists practically entirely of phosphatidylcholine and phosphatidylethanolamine.[65]

It is worth noting that enteral diets have distinct concentrations of lipids that may vary from 1.5 g/L in certain elementary diets, up to 93.7 g/240 mL in specialized formulas for seriously ill patients in the ICU with adult respiratory distress syndrome (ARDS).

Regarding critically ill patients, randomized studies, both prospective and controlled, have indicated that the provision of an enteral diet enriched with ω-3 FA, arginine, and derivatives of RNA, to elective surgical patients, was accompanied by a decrease in the rate of infection and a shorter hospital stay, without changes in mortality.[66–68] However, these effects cannot be attributed exclusively to the dietary content of ω-3 FAs, because these diets also provide other nutrients with immunomodulating properties, like arginine, nucleotides, and antioxidants. In these patients, it is important to determine the amount and the type of available fat in each product of the enteral diet offered.

In critically ill adult patients, suffering from acute lung injury (ALI) or ARDS, the administration of an enteral diet containing FO, borage oil, and antioxidants was associated to less morbidity.[69] The European Society for Parenteral and Enteral Nutrition (ESPEN) guideline for enteral nutrition was published in 2006.[70] It contains specific recommendations regarding

TABLE 4.6
Indications of Enteral Immunomodulating Formulae (Enriched with Arginine, Nucleotides, and ω-3 Fatty Acids)

Clinical Setting	Yes	No	Observations
Elective upper GI surgery	×		Formulae enriched with arginine, nucleotides, and ω-3 fatty acids.
Mild sepsis (APACHE II < 15)	×		Formulae enriched with arginine, nucleotides, and ω-3 fatty acids.
Trauma	×		Formulae enriched with arginine, nucleotides, and ω-3 fatty acids.
Acute respiratory distress syndrome	×		Formulae containing ω-3 fatty acids and antioxidants.
Severe sepsis (APACHE II > 25)		×	Immunomodulating formulae may be harmful.
Burn		×	Only trace elements (Cu, Se, and Zn) should be supplemented in a higher than standard dose.
ICU		×	Very severe illness that do not tolerate more than 700 mL enteral diet per day should not receive an immunomodulating formula.

immunomodulating formulae, provided in Table 4.6. The American Society of Parenteral and Enteral Nutrition (ASPEN) has reviewed their guidelines regarding the use of lipids and recommends that patients with ARDS and severe ALI should be placed on an enteral formulation characterized by an anti-inflammatory lipid profile (i.e., ω-3 FOs, borage oil) and antioxidants. Special high-lipid, low-carbohydrate enteral formulations designed to manipulate the respiratory quotient and reduce CO_2 production are not recommended for routine use in ICU patients with acute respiratory failure.[71] The Canadian guidelines are available at http://www.criticalcarenutrition.com/.[76]

Parenteral Formulas: Lipid Emulsions

Lipid emulsions (LEs) have been an integral part of parenteral nutritional therapy for more than 40 years and are composed of TGs that constitute the central part of exogenous chylomicrons, emulsified and covered by a layer of phospholipids, which helps to maintain the fats in an aqueous phase in the emulsion. Antioxidants such as liposoluble vitamins (vitamin E) and vegetable esters are also present. The chylomicrons diameter present in the LEs generally ranges from 200 to 350 nm.[65]

The clinical use of parenteral LEs gained momentum with the development of a safe and effective LE for clinical practice, consisting of a soybean oil derivative combined with egg phosphatide.[72]

The LE offer advantages in having a high-energy density, in having a neutral pH, and in being isosmotic with the plasma. They can be infused alone or associated to parenteral nutrition formulation, respecting its stability. For optimal use, some days of adaptation are necessary. Occasionally, patients may present episodes of fever. Anaphylactic reactions are very rare. It is advisable to measure the plasma TGs to verify that they are clearing adequately, especially in conditions in which the metabolism of fats might be impaired.[65]

The LEs available for clinical use are differentiated by the content of FAs, which should be determined and taken into consideration before indicating them to patients in critical condition.[65] Conventional LEs can be composed exclusively by soybean, sunflower, or cotton oils (10% or 20%), by physical or chemical (structured lipids) mixture of soybean oil and MCTs from coconut oil or by a mixture of soybean oil and olive oil (2:8).[73] Soybean LE has been contraindicated for critical patients because this LE is rich in ω-6 PUFAs and these types of FAs can impair the immune functions.[65]

Standard LEs containing MCTs or olive oil are commercially available in Europe, Asia, and South America and were designed to decrease the infusion of n-6 PUFAs.[73] Due to its easiest and fastest metabolism, the addition of MCTs provides biochemical and metabolic advantages upon soybean oil LEs. Since its development, LEs rich in MCTs are being indicated to critical patients, because they are less susceptible to lipid peroxidation, do not participate in eicosanoids synthesis, and have less impact under reticuloendothelial system and systemic inflammatory response than n-6 PUFAs.[73] Olive oil–based LEs have only 20% of n-6, an amount sufficient to prevent or to correct essential FAs deficiency.[73] In addition, olive oil LE is rich in vitamin E, important to the prevention of lipid peroxidation and cell damage.[73]

A weekly measurement of the TGs is recommended in order to monitor the supply of parenteral LE.

The ESPEN, in 2009, had published their guideline on parenteral nutrition.[74] It contains the following recommendations regarding lipids and LEs:

1. Lipids should be an integral part of parenteral nutrition for energy and to ensure essential FA provision in long-term ICU patients.
2. Intravenous LEs (LCT, MCT, or mixed emulsions) can be administered safely at a rate of 0.7 g/kg up to 1.5 g/kg over 12–24 h.
3. The tolerance of mixed LCT/MCT LEs in standard use is sufficiently documented. Several studies have shown specific clinical advantages over soybean LCT alone but require confirmation by prospective controlled studies.
4. Olive oil–based parenteral nutrition is well tolerated in critically ill patients.

Additionally, the ASPEN guidelines recommend that in the first week of hospitalization in the ICU, when parenteral nutrition is required and enteral nutrition is not feasible, patients should be given a parenteral formulation without soy-based lipids.[71]

ω-3 Lipid Emulsions

Parenteral supply of n-3 PUFAs occurs by the infusion of LEs composed by pure FO or by FO mixed with other oils, which are commercially available for clinical use in Europe, Asia, and South America.[5] They were designed to provide higher n-3 PUFAs and lower n-6:n-3 PUFA ratios than that provided by standard soybean oil LE, as one of the alternatives to minimize the risks associated with the infusion of high amount of the potentially inflammatory n-6 PUFAs.[28]

Only one LE contains only FO. Pure FO LE is traditionally infused as a supplement form physically mixed with standard LEs (based on soybean oil, 50% soybean oil and 50% MCTs or 80% olive oil and 20% soybean oil).[28] Pure FO LE should be given to make up between 10% and 20% of total fat, in order to attain a n-6: n-3 ratio within what is considered to be the ideal range by the current literature for treating severely ill patients (approximately 2.5:1) and providing approximately 1 g/100 mL of EPA plus DHA.[28]

Mixed FO LEs are recently commercially available for clinical use and their formulas seek to provide n-3 PUFAs using the recommended n-6:n-3 PUFA ratio for promoting immune modulation: One of them is composed by 50% MCT, 40% soybean oil, and 10% FO, providing approximately 0.6 g/100 mL of EPA plus DHA; the other one is composed by 30% soybean oil, 30% MCT, 25% olive oil, and 15% FO, providing approximately 0.4 g/100 mL of EPA plus DHA. Mixed FO LEs are infused as ready-to-use parenteral LEs and exclusive fat source.[28]

Because of the high number of double bonds in their carbon chain, n-3 PUFAs are susceptible to lipid peroxidation, but the risk of oxidation of LEs containing FO is efficiently counterbalanced by adding enough alpha-tocopherol in their formulas.[28]

In surgical patients, FO-containing LEs fast increased the incorporation of n-3 PUFAs in the phospholipids of cell membranes. In general, this LE seems to preserve immune functions and favorably modulate the inflammatory response in the postoperative period.[28] FO emulsions changed lipid mediator synthesis toward more n-3 FA-derivated eicosanoids (e.g., increased LTB5), which are less inflammatory, and downregulated postoperative inflammatory response (e.g., decreased postoperative IL-6 and TNF-α levels) and improved postoperative immune functions (e.g., maintained HLA-DR expression and increased CD4/CD8 lymphocyte populations). In patients with sepsis and other inflammatory conditions, the use of FO LE is associated with increased production of odd number series eicosanoids and decrease of proinflammatory cytokines.[28] However, a recent study did not find benefits in ICU patients treated with MCT/LCT LE and FO LE (n-3:n-6 ratio = 1:2), regardless of the presence or not of SIRS.[28] A recent meta-analysis has evaluated prospective, randomized trials studying FO LE in surgery and sepsis and concluded that against control LE as soy lipid or MCT/LCT and olive, parenteral LE with FO significantly decreased complications and length of hospital stay, without changing mortality.[75]

Regarding FO LE, the guideline published by ESPEN on parenteral nutrition considers that the addition of ω-3 FAs EPA and DHA to LEs has demonstrable effects on cell membranes and inflammatory processes, and therefore it specifically recommends FO-enriched LEs in preoperative and in critically ill patients, to probably decrease length of stay.[75]

Thus, modern nutritional planning should consider the provision of lipids as a source of energy and of essential FA and also as modulators of the immune-inflammatory response.

PERSPECTIVES

Lipids and their FAs are involved in a range of functions in the human body, in normal and stressed state. It cannot be considered as just another energy source. In accordance with their FA composition, such as ω-3 or ω-6, a different metabolism path is utilized with different immune mediators and pro- or anti-inflammatory end products.

As part of the nutrition therapy for the critically ill, the provision of lipids should be considered not only as source of energy and essential FAs but also as a potential modulator of the immune and inflammatory response.

Within the current literature available, it is possible to recognize that an excess of PUFA ω-6 promotes proinflammatory eicosanoids production. Therefore, in severely ill patients, particularly in surgery and ICU, the delivery of diet rich in this type of FAs should be carefully evaluated, as it could have a deleterious impact in the patient.

It is currently available for enteral and parenteral nutrition therapy, a range of diets containing different types, quantities, and proportion of FAs. FO, as a PUFA ω-3 source, has been accepted and recommended in recent nutrition therapy guidelines for their demonstrable positive effects on cell membranes and inflammatory processes.

PRACTICAL ACTIVITY

To answer the following questions, consider the following clinical findings:

> Critically ill surgical patient, hemodynamically stable, with indication for nutritional therapy, and contraindication of using enteral pathway.

1. Indicate the alternative that best meets the needs of the patient:
   A. The offer of parenteral LE is not recommended to critically ill patients.
   B. The patient should receive the isolated infusion of parenteral LE to prevent the deficiency of essential FAs and to provide nonglucidic energy source.
   C. The patient should receive the infusion of parenteral LE associated with glucose and amino acids to prevent deficiency of essential FAs and to provide nonglucidic energy source.

Answer: Alternative C—The patient needs to receive parenteral LE, to avoid deficiency of essential FAs, and to provide nonglucidic energy source. Considering the impossibility to use enteral path to provide nutrients, it should be opted to infuse parenteral LE mixed with glucose and amino acids (3:1 mixture).

2. How long should be the parenteral infusion of lipids?
   A. We can consider the maximum period of 24 h to infuse parenteral LE.
   B. For critically ill patients, the time of LE infusion cannot exceed the maximum period of 12 h.
   C. For critically ill patients, parenteral infusion of lipids should not be done.

Answer: Alternative A—Considering the infusion of LE associated with amino acids and glucose, it can be considered the maximum infusion time of 24 h, observing the criteria of stability of the parenteral nutrition formulation. Consider the possible suspension of the LE infusion when serum levels of TG are elevated (usually above 400 mg/dL).

3. What is the amount of fat that should be daily infused in patient?
   A. As in any parenteral regimen, the amount of fat infused must be included into 25%–35% of the total energy value of the diet and should be infused from 2 to 3 g/kg/day of lipid. It should not exceed 3.5 g/kg/day to minimize the risk of metabolic complications.
   B. There are no safe levels for parenteral infusion of LE in critically ill patients.
   C. In the case of critically ill patients, we should provide from 0.7 to 1.5 g/kg/day of fat.

Answer: Alternative C—In the critically ill patient, we should avoid excessive intake of fat, due to its possible association to immunosuppressive effects, which may increase the frequency of infections. The amount of fat to provide may be from 0.7 g/kg to 1.5 g/kg/day, not to exceed 1.5 g/kg/day.

4. What is the most indicated LE for this patient?
   A. Soybean oil–based LE
   B. Mixed LE containing FO

Answer: Alternative B—For critically ill patients, the total FA content must be well distributed because it can, among other conditions, influence eicosanoid synthesis pathways. According to the ESPEN guidelines, the addition of FO (rich in EPA and DHA) to LEs may be useful to decrease hospitalization length of stay. In this situation, we may prescribe FO LE supplementation. This can be done by adding the FO LE to the conventional LE at the concentration of 20% of the total fat offered (≅0.2 g/kg/day) or by using a mixed LE containing FO.

REFERENCES

1. Holum, R.J. Lipids, in *Fundamentals of General, Organic and Biological Chemistry*, Holum, R.J. (Ed.) John Wiley & Sons, Inc., pp. 566–582, 1994.
2. Gunstone, F. Fatty acids nomenclature, structure, isolation and structure determination, biosynthesis and chemical synthesis, in *Fatty Acid and Lipid Chemistry*, 1st edition, Black Academic & Professional, Springer Science+Business Media Dordrecht, Glasgow, U.K., pp. 1–33, 1996.
3. Borges, V. and Waitzberg, D.L. Gorduras, in *Nutrição enteral e parenteral na prática clínica*, Waitzberg, D.L., ed., Atheneu, São Paulo, Brazil, pp. 21–32, 1995.
4. Gunstone, F. Fatty acids—Nomenclature, structure, isolation and structure determination, biosynthesis and chemical synthesis, in *Fatty Acid and Lipid Chemistry*, 1st edition, Black Academic & Professional, Springer Science+Business Media Dordrecht, Glasgow, U.K., pp. 35–59, 1996.
5. Calder, P.C. Long-chain n-3 fatty acids and inflammation: Potential application in surgical and trauma patients, *Braz. J. Med. Biol. Res.*, 36, 433, 2003.
6. Liao, T.H., Hamosh, P., and Hamosh, M. Fat digestion by lingual lipase: Mechanism of lipolysis in the stomach and upper small intestine, *Pediatr. Res.*, 18, 402, 1984.
7. Corey, M.C., Small, D.M., and Bliss, C.M. Lipid digestion and absorption, *Annu. Rev. Physiol.*, 45, 651, 1983.
8. Livesey, G. and Elia, M. Short-chain fatty acids as an energy source in the colon: Metabolism and clinical applications, in *Physiological and Clinical Aspects of Short-Chain Fatty Acid*, Cumings, J.H., Rombeau, J.L., and Sakata, T., eds., Cambridge University Press, Cambridge, U.K., pp. 427–481, 1995.

9. Havel, R.J. and Kane, J.P. Introduction: Structure and metabolism of plasma proteins, in *The Metabolic and Molecular Bases of Inherited Disease*, 7th edn., Scriver, C.R., Beaudet, A.L., Sly, W.S., Valle, D., eds., McGraw-Hill, Inc., New York, Vol. II, pp. 1841–1851, 1995.
10. Dominiczak, M.H. Apolipoproteins and lipoproteins, in *Handbook of Lipoprotein Testing*, Rifai, N., Russel Warnick, G., Dominiczak, M.H., eds., AACC Press, Washington, DC, pp. 123–134, 1997.
11. Vilela, A.L.M. O Colesterol. http://www.afh.bio.br/digest/digest2.asp, (accessed January 14, 2015) (Portuguese).
12. Barter, P.J. and Rye, K.A. High-density lipoproteins and coronary artery disease, *Atherosclerosis*, 121, 1, 1996.
13. Mahan, L.K. and Escott-Stump, S. (Eds.), *Krause: Alimentos, Nutrição e Dietoterapia*, 10th edn., Roca, São Paulo, Brazil, 2002, (Portuguese version).
14. Glatz, J.F.C. and Van der Vusse, G.J. Cellular fatty acid binding protein: Their function and physiological significance, *Prog. Lipid Res.*, 35, 243, 1996.
15. Graber, R., Sumida, C., and Nunez, E.A., Fatty acids and cell signal transduction, *J. Lipid Mediat. Cell Signal*, 9, 91, 1994.
16. Sumida, C., Graber, R., and Nunez, E.A. Role of fatty acids in signal transduction: Modulators and messengers, *Prostaglandins Leukot. Essent. Fatty Acids*, 48, 117, 1993.
17. Alexander, J.W. Immunonutrition: The role of omega-3 fatty acids, *Nutrition*, 14, 627, 1998.
18. Sprecher, H. An update on the pathways of polyunsaturated fatty acid metabolism, *Curr. Opin. Clin. Nutr. Metab. Care*, 2, 135, 1999.
19. Calder, P.C. and Deckelbaum, R.J. Dietary lipids: More than just a source of calories, *Curr. Opin. Clin. Nutr. Metab. Care*, 2, 105, 1999.
20. Kinsella, J.E. Lipids, membrane receptors, and enzymes: Effects of dietary fatty acids, *JPEN*, 14(Suppl.), 200S, 1990.
21. Calder, P.C. and Grimble, R.F. Polyunsaturated fatty acids, inflammation and immunity, *Eur. J. Clin. Nutr.*, 56(Suppl.), S14, 2002.
22. Calder, P.C. Lipid metabolism in critically ill, in *Nutrition and Critical Care*, Cynober, C.L. and Moore, F.A., (eds.), Nestlé Nutrition Workshop Series Clinical & Performance Program, Southampton, UK, Vol. 8, p. 75, 2003.
23. James, M.J., Gibson, R.A., and Cleland, L.G. Dietary polyunsaturated fatty acids and inflammatory mediator production, *Am. J. Clin. Nutr.*, 71(Suppl.), S343, 2000.
24. Calder, P.C. N-3 polyunsaturated fatty acids and cytokine production in health and disease, *Ann. Nutr. Metab.*, 41, 203, 1997.
25. Endres, S. et al. The effect of dietary supplementation with n-3 polyunsaturated fatty acids on the synthesis of interleukin-1 and tumor necrosis factor by mononuclear cells, *N. Engl. J. Med.*, 320, 265, 1989.
26. Meydani, S.N. Oral (n-3) fatty acid supplementation suppresses cytokine production and lymphocyte proliferation: Comparison between young and older women, *J. Nutr.*, 121, 547, 1991.
27. Meydani, S.N. Modulation of cytokine production by dietary polyunsaturated fatty acids, *Proc. Soc. Exp. Biol. Med.*, 200, 189, 1992.
28. Waitzberg, D.L. and Torrinhas, R.S. Fish oil lipid emulsions and immune response: What clinicians need to know, *Nutr. Clin. Pract.*, 24, 487, 2009.
29. Poynter, M.E. and Daynes, R.A. Peroxisome proliferator-activated receptor alpha activation modulates cellular redox status, repress nuclear factor-kappa B signaling, and reduces inflammatory cytokine production in aging, *J. Biol. Chem.*, 273, 32833, 1998.
30. Mascaro, C. et al. Control of human muscle-type carnitine palmitoyltransferase I gene transcription by peroxisome proliferator-activated receptor, *J. Biol. Chem.*, 273, 8560, 1998.
31. Rodriguez, J.C. et al. Peroxisome proliferator-activated receptor mediates induction of the mitochondrial 3-hydroxy-3-methylglutaryl-CoA synthase gene by fatty acids, *J. Biol. Chem.*, 269, 18767, 1994.
32. Baillie, R.A. et al. Coordinate induction of peroxisomal acyl-CoA oxidase and UCP-3 by dietary fish oil: A mechanism for decreased body fat deposition, *Prostaglandins Leukot. Essent. Fatty Acids*, 60, 351, 1999.
33. Desvergne, B. and Wahli, W. Peroxissome proliferator-activated receptors: Nuclear control of metabolism, *Endocrinol. Rev.*, 20, 249, 1999.
34. Nichols, D.G. and Locke, L. Thermogenic mechanism in brown adipose tissue, *Pysiol. Rev.*, 64, 1, 1984.
35. Pénicaud, L. et al. The autonomic nervous system, adipose tissue plasticity, and energy balance, *Nutrition*, 16, 903, 2000.
36. Curi, R., Pompéia, C., Miyasaka, C.K., and Procópio, J. *Entendendo a gordura*, 1st edn., Manole, São Paulo, Brazil, 2002 (Portuguese).

37. Grunfeld, C. and Feingold, K.R., Regulation of lipid metabolism by cytokines during host defense, *Nutrition*, 12(Suppl.), S24, 1996.
38. Gaillard, R.C. et al. Cytokines, leptin, and the hypothalamo-pituitary-adrenal axis, *Ann. N. Y. Acad. Sci.*, 917, 647, 2000.
39. Inui, A. Cancer anorexia-cachexia syndrome: Current issues in research and management, *CA Cancer J. Clin.*, 52, 72, 2002.
40. Shaw, J.H.F. and Wolfe, R.R. Fatty acid and glycerol kinetics in septic patients and in patients with gastrointestinal cancer, *Ann. Surg.*, 205, 368, 1987.
41. Stoner, H.B. et al. The relationships between plasma substrates and hormones and the severity of injury in 277 recently injured patients, *Clin. Sci.*, 56, 563, 1979.
42. Martinez, A. et al. Assessment of adipose tissue metabolism by means of subcutaneous microdialysis in patients with sepsis or circulatory failure, *Clin. Physiol. Funct. Imaging*, 23, 286, 2003.
43. Hardardottir, I., Grunfeld, C., and Feingold, K.R. Effects of endotoxin and cytokines on lipid metabolism, *Curr. Opin. Lipidol.*, 5, 207, 1994.
44. Khovidhunkit, W. et al. Infection and inflammation-induced proatherogenic changes lipoproteins, *J. Infect. Dis.*, 181(Suppl.), S462, 2000.
45. Carpentier, Y.A. and Scruel, O. Changes in concentration and composition of plasma lipoproteins during the acute phase response, *Curr. Opin. Clin. Nutr. Metab. Care*, 5, 153, 2002.
46. Wolfe, R.R. et al. Regulation of lipolysis in severely burned children, *Ann. Surg.*, 206, 214, 1987.
47. Youngstrom, T.G. and Bartness, T.J. Catecholaminergic innervation of white adipose tissue in Siberian hamsters, *Am. J. Physiol.*, 268, 744, 1995.
48. Samra, J.S. et al. Effects of physiological hypercortisolemia on the regulation of lipolysis in subcutaneous adipose tissue, *J. Clin. Endocrinol. Metab.*, 83, 626, 1998.
49. Samra, J.S. et al. Effects of adrenaline infusion on the interstitial environment of subcutaneous adipose tissue as studied by microdialysis, *Clin. Sci.*, 91, 425, 1996.
50. Kurpad, A. et al. Effect of noradrenaline on glycerol turnover and lipolysis in the whole body and subcutaneous adipose tissue in humans in vivo, *Clin. Sci.*, 86, 177, 1994.
51. Feingold, K.R. et al. Endotoxin rapidly induces changes in lipid metabolism that produce hypertriglyceridemia: Low doses stimulate hepatic triglyceride production while high doses inhibit clearance, *J. Lipid Res.*, 33, 1765, 1992.
52. Michie, H.R. et al. Detection of circulating tumor necrosis factor after endotoxin administration, *N. Engl. J. Med.*, 318, 1481, 1988.
53. Maass, D.L., White, J., and Horton, J.W. IL-1beta and IL-6 act synergistically with TNF-alpha to alter cardiac contractile function after burn trauma, *Shock*, 18, 360, 2002.
54. Tisdale, M.J. Biology of cachexia, *J. Natl. Cancer Inst.*, 89, 1763, 1997.
55. Uysal, K.T. et al. Protection from obesity- induced insulin resistance in mice lacking TNF alfa function, *Nature*, 389, 610, 1997.
56. Barton, B.E. and Murphy, T.F. Cancer cachexia is mediated in part by the induction of IL-6-like cytokines from the spleen, *Cytokine*, 16, 251, 2001.
57. Vander Poll, T. et al. Tumor necrosis factor mimics the metabolic response to acute infection in healthy humans, *Am. J. Physiol.*, 261, 457, 1991.
58. Stouthard, J.M. et al. Endocrinologic and metabolic effects of interleukin-6 in humans, *Am. J. Physiol.*, 268, 813, 1995.
59. Ronti, T., Lupattelli, G., Mannarino, E. The endocrine function of adipose tissue: An update. *Clin Endocrinol (Oxf).*, 64, 355, 2006.
60. Todorov, P.T. et al. Purification and characterization of a tumor lipid-mobilizing factor, *Cancer Res.*, 58, 2353, 1998.
61. Tisdale, M.J. Biochemical mechanisms of cellular catabolism, *Curr. Opin. Clin. Nutr. Metab. Care*, 5, 401, 2002.
62. Islam-Ali, B. et al. Modulation of adipocyte G-protein expression in cancer cachexia by a lipid-mobilizing factor (LMF), *Br. J. Cancer*, 85, 758, 2001.
63. Herndon, D.N. et al. Lipolysis in burned patients is stimulated by the beta 2-receptor for catecholamines, *Arch. Surg.*, 129, 1301, 1994.
64. Ribeiro, P.C. Terapia Nutricional na Sepse. *RBTI Revista Brasileira Terapia Intensiva*, 16, 175, 2004, http://professor.ucg.br/SiteDocente/admin/arquivosUpload/7541/material/ARTIGO%20TERAPIA%20NUTRICIONAL%20NA%20SEPSE.pdf, (accessed January 14, 2015) (Portuguese).
65. Carpentier, Y.A. et al. Recent developments in lipid emulsions: Relevance to intensive care, *Nutrition*, 13(9 Suppl.), S73, 1997.

66. Heyland, D.K. et al. Should immunonutrition become routine in critically ill patients? A systematic review of the evidence, *JAMA*, 286, 944, 2001.
67. Gianotti, L. and Braga, M. Perioperative nutrition in cancer patients, *Nutr. Clin. Metab.*, 15, 298, 2001.
68. Gianotti, L. et al. A randomized controlled trial of preoperative oral supplementation with a specialized diet in patients with gastrointestinal cancer, *Gastroenterology*, 122, 1763, 2002.
69. Pontes-Arruda, A., Demichelem, S., Seth, A., and Singer, P. The use of an inflammation-modulating diet in patients with acute lung injury or acute respiratory distress syndrome: A meta-analysis of outcome data, *JPEN J. Parenter. Enteral Nutr.*, 32, 596, 2008.
70. Kreymann, K.G. et al. ESPEN guidelines on enteral nutrition: Intensive care. *Clin. Nutr.*, 25, 210, 2006.
71. McClave, S.A. et al. Guidelines for the provision and assessment of nutrition support therapy in the adult critically ill patient: Society of Critical Care Medicine (SCCM) and American Society for Parenteral and Enteral Nutrition (A.S.P.E.N.). *JPEN J. Parenter. Enteral Nutr.*, 33, 277, 2009.
72. Wretlind, A. Development of fat emulsions, *JPEN J. Parenter. Enteral Nutr.*, 5, 230, 1981.
73. Waitzberg, D.L., Torrinhas, R.S., and Jacintho, T.M. New parenteral lipid emulsions for clinical use, *JPEN J. Parent. Enteral Nutr.*, 30, 351, 2006.
74. Singer, P., Berger, M.M., Van den Berghe, G., Biolo, G., Calder, P., Forbes, A., Griffiths, R., Kreyman, G., Leverve, X., and Pichard, C., ESPEN. ESPEN guidelines on parenteral nutrition: Intensive care, *Clin. Nutr.*, 28, 387, 2009.
75. Pradelli, L., Mayer, K., Muscaritoli, M., and Heller, A.R. n-3 fatty acid-enriched parenteral nutrition regimens in elective surgical and ICU patients: A meta-analysis, *Crit Care*, 16, R184, October 4, 2012.
76. Critical Care Nutrition, Canadian Clinical Practice Guidelines, http://www.criticalcarenutrition.com/docs/cpgs2012/4.2a.pdf, (accessed January 13, 2014.)

Section II

Nutrients for the Critically Ill

5 Nutrition Assessment and Monitoring

Kavitha Krishnan and Michael D. Taylor

CONTENTS

Screening and assessing the nutritional status of a critically ill patient should involve a systematic approach to help implement appropriate interventions. Malnutrition remains a significant problem in the hospital setting despite the evidence describing both the clinical and economical consequences. Malnutrition increases the risk of adverse complications for the critically ill patient. In 2009, an International Consensus Guideline Committee developed an etiology-based approach for the diagnosis of adult malnutrition in the clinical setting, which was endorsed by the American Society for Parenteral and Enteral Nutrition (ASPEN) and the European Society for Parenteral and Enteral Nutrition (ESPEN). The committee proposed the following diagnosis [1]:

1. Starvation-related malnutrition
2. Chronic disease–related malnutrition
3. Acute disease–related or injury-related malnutrition

Nutrition care involves screening, assessment, and intervention in patients with malnutrition [2].

SCREENING

Nutrition screening has been defined by ASPEN as a "process to identify an individual who is malnourished or who is at risk for malnutrition to determine if a detailed nutrition assessment is indicated" [2]. In the United States, the Joint Commission mandates nutrition screening for every patient admitted within 24 h [3]. Nursing screening tools may include questions such as

1. Has the patient lost weight unintentionally?
2. Does the patient look poorly nourished?
3. Does the patient have a poor appetite?
4. Does the patient have any pressure ulcer stage 2 or greater?

An ideal screening tool is convenient, easy to use, less time consuming, and noninvasive. It also involves no calculations and laboratory data [4]. The screening tool selected should have been tested in patient populations similar to the ones where it will be utilized [5].

The commonly cited screening tools found in literature include Birmingham nutrition risk score, malnutrition screening tool (MST), malnutrition universal screening tool (MUST), nutrition risk index (NRI), prognostic inflammatory and nutritional index, prognostic nutritional index (PNI), and simple screening tool (see Table 5.1) [6]. The parameters used in these screening tools are related to anthropometry, diet, and severity of illness.

In 2006, a workgroup of dietitians proposed an evidence analysis project to identify reliable and valid screening tools [5]. In this project, the MST was the only tool shown to be both valid and reliable for identifying nutrition problems in the acute care and hospital-based ambulatory care settings. The MUST is another valid screening tool and has been recommended for use in inpatient care settings [7]. The MUST includes evaluation of weight loss and adequacy of intake with the calculation and evaluation of body mass index (BMI) and estimation of the severity of the medical condition [8].

TABLE 5.1
Criteria Used in Selected Screening Tools

Nutrition Screening Tools	Developed by	Criteria Used
Malnutrition screening tool (MST)	Ferguson M, Capra S, Bauer J, Banks M	Recent weight loss, appetite
Malnutrition universal screening tool (MUST)	Malnutrition Advisory Group, a standing committee of the British Association for Parenteral and Enteral Nutrition (BAPEN)	Body mass index (BMI), unintentional weight loss, and acute disease effect
Nutrition risk screening (NRS 2002)	Kondrup et al. and an ESPEN working group	Weight loss BMI, appetite and disease severity
Mini Nutritional Assessment® (MNA-SF)	Center for Internal Medicine and Clinical Gerontology of Toulouse (France), the Clinical Nutrition Program at the University of New Mexico (United States), and the Nestlé Research Center (Switzerland)	Recent weight loss, appetite, disease severity, housebound, dementia/depression, difficulty with eating
Simple two-part tool	Nursal TZ, Noyan T, Atalay BG, Koz N, Karakayali H	Unintentional weight loss and loss of subcutaneous fat
Tool #1	Laporte et al.	Recent weight loss, BMI
Nutritional risk index	Veterans Affairs Parenteral Nutrition Cooperative Study Group	Body weight, serum albumin

Sources: Anthony, P.S., *Nutr. Clin. Pract.*, 23, 373, 2008; Skipper, A. et al., *JPEN J. Parenter. Enteral. Nutr.*, 36, 293, 2012; Veterans affairs Total Parenteral Nutrition Cooperative Study Group, *N. Engl. J. Med.*, 324, 525, 1991; Laporte, M. et al., *Can. J. Diet. Pract. Res.*, 62, 26, 2001.

Screenings may be repeated at regular intervals of time as part of the continuous monitoring process. After the screening process is complete and the patient has been identified as being at nutritional risk, a thorough assessment should be completed. The data collected during the nutrition assessment process is similar to nutrition screening but it is more in depth and detail [10].

ASSESSMENT

Nutrition assessment has been defined by ASPEN as "a comprehensive approach to diagnosing nutrition problems that uses a combination of the following: medical, nutrition, and medication histories; physical examination; anthropometric measurements; and laboratory data" [12]. Clinical assessment is a continuous process. The specific methods used to perform a clinical nutrition assessment are determined by the clinical skill, resource availability, and the clinical setting [13,14].

Validated nutrition assessment tools include the subjective global assessment (SGA), patient-generated SGA, and Mini Nutritional Assessment [7]. SGA distinguishes between well-nourished and malnourished individuals without the use of anthropometric and laboratory methods [15].

A comprehensive nutrition assessment should include the following components [1]:

1. History and clinical diagnoses
2. Clinical signs and physical examination
3. Anthropometric data
4. Laboratory indicators of inflammation
5. Dietary data
6. Functional outcomes

History and Clinical Diagnoses

The medical, surgical, and psychosocial history as well as the clinical diagnosis may help in early identification of inflammation and malnutrition. Admitting diagnosis may be associated with an acute inflammatory response. Examples of these conditions include critical illness, major infection/sepsis, adult respiratory syndrome, severe burns, major abdominal surgeries, and trauma. Acute or chronic conditions may place a patient at greater risk for malnutrition. Weight loss may be one of the best validated nutrition assessment parameter [16,17]. The degree and duration of weight loss is important to determine the severity of weight loss. It is pertinent to take into account the factors that may influence existing or potential access sites for the delivery of nutrition support.

Knowledge of the medications prior to and during admission is important. Certain drugs may promote anorexia or interfere with the absorption and metabolism of nutrients [18]. Other drugs may increase appetite and cause weight gain.

Clinical Signs and Physical Examination

A comprehensive nutrition-focused physical examination (NFPE) is systematic from head to toe. This approach ensures an organized and competent approach to care [19]. Equipment required to perform the NFPE may include but not limited to a stethoscope, thermometer, penlight or flashlight, tongue depressor, tape measure, and reflex hammer.

A NFPE employs the technique of inspection, palpation, percussion, and auscultation. See Table 5.2 for techniques of a physical examination [20].

The following is an outline for NFPE. The table is intended to be a sample and may need modifications depending upon the patient population and clinical scenario [21].

Subcutaneous fat and muscle loss may also be observed during the physical examination and these are useful parameters in assessing the nutritional status of a patient (Tables 5.3 and 5.4).

TABLE 5.2
Four Techniques of Physical Assessment

Technique	Description
Inspection	Used throughout the exam using eyes for observation. Critically observe color, shape, size, and texture.
Palpation	Uses touch to examine location, texture size, tenderness, temperature, and mobility of the body. For texture and shape, use tips and pads of fingers. For temperature, use the back side (dorsal) of the hand and for vibrations, use the underside (ulnar) of the hand.
Percussion	Tapping of fingers to assess sounds of the body to determine the border, shape, and position of organs.
Auscultation	Listening with the ear or stethoscope to sounds produced by organs like the lungs, heart, abdomen, intestines, and also vasculature.

Source: Adapted from Hammond, K.A., *Nutrition*, 15, 411, 1999.

Anthropometric Data

Anthropometry is the measurement of the body composition. Anthropometric data include height, weight, muscle, and fat mass.

Height is usually measured to determine ideal body weight. Height should be measured in a consistent manner. A stadiometer can be used to measure the height of a patient in standing position without his or her shoes on. For adults who cannot stand safely, estimated height can be obtained by arm span or knee height measurements. Arm span measure involves the arms being extended straight out to the sides at a 90° angle from the body and measuring from the patient's sterna notch to the end of the longest finger [18,23].

The knee height is measured from under the heel of the foot to the anterior surface of the thigh, which is bent 90°. Height is then calculated from the following equations [23]:

$$\text{Men: Height (cm)} = 64.19 - [0.04 \times \text{age (year)}] + [2.02 \times \text{knee height (cm)}]$$
$$\text{Women: Height (cm)} = 84.88 - [0.24 \times \text{age (year)}] + [1.83 \times \text{knee height (cm)}]$$

Weight can be affected in the clinical setting by changes in fluid status. Careful review of fluid status from intravenous fluid administration, diuretic therapy, edema, and ascites is necessary [23].

Comparing actual body weight to ideal or desirable weight may help estimate adipose stores, but measuring unintentional weight loss may provide meaningful information on the patient's nutritional risk. Seltzer et al. [24] looked at the frequency of unintentional weight loss greater than 10 lb in 4382 elective surgery patients. Higher mortality rates were observed among patients with greater than 10 lb weight loss versus patients with less than 10 lb weight loss or no weight loss at all (see Table 5.5).

Body Mass Index

BMI is a gross estimate of body fat. BMI is calculated using the following formula (Table 5.6). BMI is not valid in pregnancy, in extremely muscular individuals, and in patients whose weight is altered by fluid status [21].

Skin folds and mid-arm circumferences are not used routinely in hospital settings due to the amount of training required and also the possibility of inter- and intraobserver error [21]. In the critically ill population, these measurements do not correlate well with lean body mass since the measurements are affected by the patient's fluid status [27].

TABLE 5.3
Components of Nutrition-Focused Physical Examination

System		What the examination may reveal in regard to nutritional status.
Vital signs	Temperature	Elevated temperature increases fluid and energy requirements.
	Respirations	Increased rate increases energy requirements.
	Pulse	Increases with anemia, hyperthyroidism, fever, anxiety, pain, exercise, and medications; decreases with sleep/rest, organic heart disease, hypothyroidism, and medications.
	Blood pressure	Decreases with dehydration, blood loss, heart attack, heart failure, irregular heart rate, and certain medications.
Skin	Color	Pallor—iron, folate, or B12 deficiency.
	Lesions, pigmentation	Dermatitis—essential fatty acid, zinc, niacin, or riboflavin deficiency. Pellagrous dermatitis—niacin or tryptophan deficiency. Flaky paint dermatitis—hyperpigmented areas on thighs; buttocks—protein deficiency.
	Wound healing, pressure ulcers	Poor wound healing—zinc, vitamin C, and/or protein deficiency.
	Moisture, turgor	Poor skin turgor—dehydration. Sweating increases fluid requirements. Edema—generalized (anasarca) with accumulation of serum in connective tissue.
	Texture	Scaly, dry—vitamin A or essential fatty acid deficiency. Small lumps or nodules on elbows or eyelids—hypercholesterolemia.
	Temperature	Increased ambient temperature increases fluid and energy requirements.
Nails	Shape, color, angle contour, lesions	Spoon shape (koilonychia)—iron deficiency; lackluster; dull—protein deficiency. Mottled, pale, poor blanching—vitamin A or C deficiency.
Scalp/hair	Shape and symmetry of scalp; masses; hair distribution, color, texture	Dull, lackluster, thin, sparse—protein, iron, zinc, or essential fatty acid deficiency. Easily pluckable—protein deficiency.
Face (general)	Shape and symmetry	Moon face, bilateral temporal wasting—protein-energy deficiency.
Eyes	Vision impairments	Night blindness—vitamin A deficiency.
	Skin color and texture, cracks	Cracked and reddened corners of eyes, brows, lids (angular palpebritis)—riboflavin or niacin deficiency.
	Sclera	Foamy spots on eyes (Bitot's spots) or dull, dry rough appearance—vitamin A deficiency; pallor—iron, folate, or B12 deficiency.
	Conjunctiva	Dull, dry rough appearance to inner lids (conjunctival xerosis)—vitamin A deficiency.
	Cornea	Dull, milky, or opaque (corneal xerosis) or softening (keratomalacia)—vitamin A deficiency.
Nose	Shape, septum, nares, mucosa, discharge	Skin scaly, greasy, with gray or yellowish material around nares (nasolabial seborrhea)—riboflavin or pyridoxine deficiency.
Lips	Color, temperature, cracking, lesions, symmetry	Bilateral cracks, redness of lips (angular stomatitis)—riboflavin, niacin, and/or pyridoxine deficiency.
Mucosa (mouth)	Color, texture, lesions, integrity, moisture	Pallor—iron, B12, or folate deficiency; dryness—dehydration; cracking—vitamin C deficiency; general inflammation—vitamin B complex, C, or iron deficiency.

(Continued)

TABLE 5.3 (*Continued*)
Components of Nutrition-Focused Physical Examination

Tongue	Color	Magenta color—riboflavin deficiency; beefy red color—niacin, folate, riboflavin, iron deficiency.
	Texture, moisture, lesions	Smooth, slick, loss of papillae—folate, niacin, iron, riboflavin, B12 deficiency.
	Distorted taste (dysgeusia), Diminished taste (hypogeusia)	Zinc deficiency.
Teeth	State of repair, missing dentures	Affects ability to chew; caries—tooth decay; enamel erosion associated with bulimia.
Gums	Lesions, integrity, moisture, color	Spongy, bleeding, receding—vitamin C deficiency; dry—dehydration; pale—iron deficiency.
Neck	Vasculature appearance	Distended neck veins—fluid overload.
	Symmetry, midline structures (trachea, thyroid)	Enlarged thyroid—iodine deficiency.
	Parotid glands	Bilateral enlargement—protein deficiency or bulimia.

Body composition may also be assessed by bioelectrical impedance analysis (BIA), dual-energy x-ray absorptiometry (DEXA), computed tomography (CT), and magnetic resonance imaging (MRI). Baracos et al. have shown that it is possible to evaluate musculature using CT scans being done for routine care [28]. Bemben [33] documented the reliability and cost effectiveness of using diagnostic ultrasound to assess muscle mass.

Laboratory Indicators of Inflammation

It has been common practice to utilize plasma proteins for the interpretation of biochemical assessment of protein status. However, these proteins are indicators of inflammation rather than malnutrition in the critically ill patient [18]. Albumin, prealbumin, transferrin, retinol-binding protein, C-reactive protein, and ceruloplasmin are affected by intercompartmental fluids shifts, the acute-phase response, and provision of exogenous blood products (Table 5.7). Hepatic acute-phase response is an orchestrated cascade of events initiated by proinflammatory cytokines that result in an increase in acute-phase protein production by the liver with a concomitant decrease in serum protein levels [34].

During metabolic stress, albumin synthesis is depressed and albumin degradation is increased. The degraded amino acids become part of the amino acid pool to be used for protein synthesis [35]. Half-life of albumin is 21 days. Significant losses of albumin occur with thermal injury, nephrotic syndrome, protein-losing enteropathy, cirrhosis, and chronic bronchitis [36,37]. Albumin is a poor indicator of nutritional status in the critically ill patient but is a sensitive indicator of morbidity, mortality, and length of hospitalization [38,39], and in the acute phase of inflammation, it can be used as a marker of injury and metabolic stress.

Prealbumin, also known as transthyretin or transthyretin-bound prealbumin, like albumin, is a visceral protein and a negative acute-phase reactant. It is also affected by many of the same factors that affect albumin. Prealbumin's advantage over albumin is its shorter half-life (2–3 days) and quick response to the onset of malnutrition and rapid rise with adequate protein and energy intake [40–42]. This is not the case in the presence of sepsis, acute respiratory distress syndrome, and similar clinical situations [43]. Only in the presence of normalized inflammatory parameters does prealbumin reflect adequacy of nutrition support [44].

Albumin, prealbumin, and other negative acute-phase reactants such as transferrin- and retinol-binding protein are expected to return to normal as the inflammatory process resolves.

TABLE 5.4
Assessment of Subcutaneous Fat and Muscle

	Tips	Severe Malnutrition	Mild–Moderate Malnutrition	Well Nourished
Exam areas—subcutaneous fat loss				
Orbital region—surrounding the eye	View patient when standing directly in front of them, touch above cheekbone.	Hollow look, depressions, dark circles, loose skin.	Slightly dark circles, somewhat hollow look.	Slightly bulged fat pads. Fluid retention may mask loss.
Upper arm region—triceps/biceps	Arm bent, roll skin between fingers, do not include muscle in pinch.	Very little space between folds, fingers touch.	Some dept pinch, but not ample.	Ample fat tissue obvious between folds of skin.
Thoracic and lumbar region—ribs, lower back, midaxillary line	Have patient press hands hard against a solid object.	Depression between the ribs very apparent. Iliac crest very prominent.	Ribs apparent, depressions between them less pronounced. Iliac crest somewhat prominent.	Chest is full, ribs do not show. Slight to no protrusion of the iliac crest.
Exam areas—muscle loss				
Temple region—temporalis muscle	View patient when standing directly in front of them, ask patient to turn head side to side.	Hollowing, scooping, depression.	Slight depression.	Can see/feel well-defined muscle.
Clavicle bone region—pectoralis major, deltoid, trapezius muscles	Look for prominent bone. Make sure patient is not hunched forward.	Protruding prominent bone.	Visible in male, some protrusion in female.	Not visible in male, visible but not prominent in female.
Clavicle and acromion bone region—deltoid muscle	Patient arms at side: observe shape.	Shoulder to arm joint looks square. Bones prominent. Acromion protrusion very prominent.	Acromion process may slightly protrude.	Rounded, curves at arm/shoulder/neck.
Scapular bone region—trapezius, supraspinatus, infraspinatus muscle	Ask patient to extend hands straight out, push against solid object.	Prominent, visible bones, depressions between ribs/scapula or shoulder/spine.	Mild depression or bone may show slightly.	Bones not prominent, no significant depressions.
Dorsal hand—interosseous muscle	Look at thumb side of hand; look at pads of thumb when tip of forefinger touching tip of thumb.	Depressed area between thumb–forefinger.	Slightly depressed.	Muscle bulges, could be flat in some well-nourished people.
Lower body less sensitive to change				
Patellar region—quadriceps muscle	Ask patient to sit with leg propped up, bent at knee.	Bones prominent, little sign of muscle around knee.	Kneecap less prominent, more rounded.	Muscles protrude, bones not prominent.
Anterior thigh region—quadriceps muscles	Ask patient to sit, prop leg up on low furniture. Grasp quads to differentiate amount of muscle tissue from fat tissue.	Depression/line on thigh, obviously thin.	Mild depression on inner thigh.	Well rounded, well developed.

(Continued)

TABLE 5.4 (*Continued*)
Assessment of Subcutaneous Fat and Muscle

	Tips	Severe Malnutrition	Mild–Moderate Malnutrition	Well Nourished
Posterior calf region—gastrocnemius muscle	Grasp the calf muscle to determine amount of tissue.	Thin, minimal to no muscle definition.	Not well developed.	Well-developed bulb of muscle.
Edema				
Rule out other causes of edema, patient at dry weight	View scrotum/vulva in activity-restricted patient: ankles in mobile patient.	Deep to very deep pitting, depression lasts a short to moderate time (31–60 s), extremity looks swollen (3–4+).	Mild to moderate pitting, slight swelling of the extremity, indentation subsides quickly (0–30 s).	No sign of fluid accumulation.

Source: Adapted from Nutrition Focused Physical Assessment Tables: Copyright-Cleveland Clinic.

TABLE 5.5
Evaluation of Percent Weight Loss

$$\text{Patient weight loss} = \frac{\text{usual body weight} - \text{actual body weight}}{\text{usual body weight}} \times 100$$

Time Frame	Significant Weight Loss (%)
1 Week	1–2
1 Month	5
3 Months	7.5
6 Months	10

TABLE 5.6
Interpretation of Body Mass Index

$$\text{Body mass index} = \frac{\text{weight (kg)}}{\text{height}^2\text{ (m)}}$$

Underweight	<18.5
Normal range	18.5–24.9
Overweight	25–29.9
Class I obesity	30–34.9
Class II obesity	35–39.9
Class III obesity	>40

Source: National Institutes of Health, *Obes. Res.*, 6, 51S, 1998.

C-reactive protein (CRP) is a positive acute-phase reactant whose levels are elevated with both acute and chronic inflammation. It has a short half-life of 19 h [45]. If CRP is elevated and serum albumin or prealbumin are decreased, then inflammation is likely to be a contributing factor. Monitoring the trends over the clinical course may be helpful. Research findings suggest that proinflammatory cytokines, particularly interleukin-6, may also offer promise as indicators of inflammatory status but may not be practical to monitor in all situations [46,47].

TABLE 5.7
Acute-Phase Reactants

Protein	Half-Life	Increased in	Decreased in
Albumin	20 days	Dehydration, blood transfusions, exogenous albumin infusions	Overhydration Liver failure Inflammation/metabolic stress/postsurgery Protein-losing enteropathy Cancer Corticosteroid use Zinc deficiency
Prealbumin (transthyretin)	2 days	Renal failure Corticosteroid use	Inflammation/metabolic stress/postsurgery Liver disease Infection/stress/inflammation Dialysis Hyperthyroidism Significant hyperglycemia
C-reactive protein	19 h	Acute inflammation Infection	Resolving acute inflammation and infection
Transferrin	8 days	Iron deficiency Blood loss Dehydration Hepatitis Chronic renal failure	Pernicious anemia (B12 deficiency) Folate-deficiency anemia Overhydration Chronic infection Iron overload Acute catabolic states Nephrotic syndrome Severe liver disease/hepatic congestion Zinc deficiency Corticosteroids Cancer

Source: Russell, M.K., Laboratory monitoring, in: Matarese, L.E. and Gottschlich, M.M., eds., *Contemporary Nutrition Support Practice*: *A Clinical Guide*, Saunders, St Louis, MO, 1998.

Nitrogen Balance Studies

Nitrogen balance reflects net protein synthesis, the difference between whole-body protein synthesis, and breakdown (Table 5.8). In the setting of severe acute systemic inflammatory response, negative nitrogen balance is expected [18]. Ideally, total urinary nitrogen measurements should be made; however, estimates of nitrogen loss can be obtained from urine urea nitrogen (UUN) and approximation of nonurinary nitrogen losses. The usual goal for nitrogen balance is 2–4 g/day.

In the critically ill patient, abnormal nitrogen losses may occur through burn exudates, fistula drainage, gastrointestinal fluid loss, diarrhea, or dialysis and positive nitrogen balance is difficult to achieve [21].

TABLE 5.8
Nitrogen Balance

Nitrogen Balance = Nitrogen in [protein intake/6.25] − Nitrogen out [urinary urea nitrogen ± 4 (insensible losses)]
Nitrogen balance, protein intake, and urinary urea nitrogen are expressed as grams/24 h

Glycemic Control

In critical illness, acute insults like the stress of surgery, trauma, or sepsis alter carbohydrate metabolism; cause excessive secretion of counterregulatory hormones like catecholamines, cortisol, glucagon, and growth hormone; promote insulin resistance; increase hepatic glucose production; and impair peripheral glucose utilization and insulin action [48]. Hyperglycemia is commonly observed in critically ill patients. ASPEN guidelines recommend a target blood glucose goal range of 140–180 mg/dL (7.8–10 mmol/L) in critically ill patients [49]. Routine monitoring of blood glucose levels and maintaining glycemic control will help prevent the adverse effects of hyperglycemia.

Electrolytes

Phosphate is essential for the synthesis of adenosine triphosphate (ATP) and 2,3-diphosphoglycerate, which are involved in optimal pulmonary function. Mechanically ventilated patients with hypophosphatemia are at greater risk for weaning failure [50]. The Society of Critical Care Medicine (SCCM) and ASPEN recommend monitoring serum phosphate levels and replacing phosphate when needed [51].

Monitoring phosphate, potassium, and magnesium levels in patients at risk for refeeding syndrome should also be considered. Refeeding syndrome is discussed in Chapter 14.

Dietary Data

Obtaining information on diet using 24 h recall or modified diet history is useful in detecting inadequate food or nutrient intakes. In the critically ill patient, diet history is usually obtained from medical records, family, and caregivers. The patient's intake during the hospital stay should also be monitored and assessed. If enteral and parenteral nutrition has been initiated, the clinician should monitor the amount of nutrition that the patient receives compared to the amount ordered.

Functional Outcomes

Impaired muscle strength is common in patients with disease-related malnutrition. Handgrip strength is a validated and most feasible method for clinical purposes [52]. Handgrip strength is measured using a handgrip dynamometer. In geriatric patients, timed gait, chair stands, and stair steps are used in the assessment of physical function and strength [18]. Lee et al. [53] showed that handgrip strength measurements did not predict length of stay in the surgical intensive care patients as well as manual muscle testing. In critically ill patients, grip strength measurements may not be feasible.

CRITICAL ILLNESS AND SARCOPENIA

Critically ill patients are predisposed to skeletal muscle weakness and wasting. Malnutrition is one of the factors contributing to muscle weakness and atrophy [29]. Sarcopenia is usually observed in the aging populations but it is also being identified in critical illness. Sarcopenia was originally described by Evans and Campbell [30] and was further defined by Evans [31] as age-related loss of muscle mass.

Cachexia has been defined by Evans et al. [32] as "a complex metabolic syndrome associated with underlying illness and characterized by loss of muscle with or without loss of fat mass."

It is worthwhile to mention the importance of identifying muscle loss/atrophy in the critically ill since ICU-acquired muscle weakness is an independent predictor of prolonged weaning from mechanical ventilation [29,54]. Muscle weakness can be manifested directly by critical illness or result from motor neuron dysfunction. Factors regulating muscle mass and function in critically ill patients include aging, nutritional status, immobility, sepsis, inflammation, and drugs [55]. Early identification and assessment of muscle loss and atrophy can facilitate early treatment and impact patient outcomes.

ASSESSING THE PRESENCE OF MALNUTRITION

Malnutrition negatively impacts the patient at a cellular, physical, and psychological level [57,58]. Malnutrition contributes to loss of muscle and fat mass as well as atrophy of visceral proteins.

Identification of malnutrition in the context of illness and injury or social/environmental circumstances followed by nutrition intervention may improve clinical outcomes.

The Academy/ASPEN clinical characteristics (Table 5.9) used to recommend the diagnosis of malnutrition [1] are

Insufficient food intake
Weight loss
Loss of muscle mass

TABLE 5.9
Malnutrition Assessment

Characteristics	Nonsevere/Moderate Malnutrition	Severe Malnutrition
Malnutrition in the context of acute illness or injury		
Energy intake	<75% of estimated requirements for >7 days	≤50% of estimated requirements for ≥5 days
Weight loss	1%–2% in 1 week	>2% in 1 week
	5% in 1 month	>5% in 1 month
	7.5% in 3 months	>7.5% in 3 months
Physical findings—loss of subcutaneous fat	Mild	Moderate
Loss of muscle mass	Mild	Moderate
Fluid accumulation	Mild	Moderate to severe
Reduced grip strength	Not applicable	Measurable reduced
Malnutrition in the context of chronic illness		
Energy intake	≤75% of estimated requirements for >1 month	≤75% of estimated requirements for ≥1 month
Weight loss	5% in 1 month	>5% in 1 month
	7.5% in 3 months	>7.5% in 3 months
	10% in 6 months	>10% in 6 months
	20% in 1 year	>20% in 1 year
Physical findings—loss of subcutaneous fat	Mild	Severe
Loss of muscle mass	Mild	Severe
Fluid accumulation	Mild	Severe
Reduced grip strength	Not applicable	Measurable reduced
Malnutrition in the context of social or environmental circumstances		
Energy intake	<75% of estimated requirements for ≥3 months	≤50% of estimated requirements for ≥1 month
Weight loss	5% in 1 month	>5% in 1 month
	7.5% in 3 months	>7.5% in 3 months
	10% in 6 months	>10% in 6 months
	20% in 1 year	>20% in 1 year
Physical findings—loss of subcutaneous fat	Mild	Severe
Loss of muscle mass	Mild	Severe
Fluid accumulation	Mild	Severe
Reduced grip strength	Not applicable	Measurable reduced

Source: Adapted from White, J.V. et al., *JPEN J. Parenter. Enteral. Nutr.*, 36(3), 277, 2012.

Loss of subcutaneous fat
Localized or generalized fluid accumulation
Diminished functional status

The presence of at least two or more of these characteristics is recommended for diagnosis. Specifications of these characteristics distinguish between severe and nonsevere malnutrition.

The academy and ASPEN experts agree that it is not possible to differentiate between mild and moderate malnutrition and have not developed definitions for mild malnutrition at this time [1].

Proper identification and treatment of malnutrition can help prevent its negative consequences for the patient. Malnutrition has an indirect effect on healthcare costs by influencing the case-mix index [57]. Malnutrition can have an impact on hospital reimbursement by influencing the DRG. Severity of illness and risk of mortality may be increased if malnutrition is appropriately diagnosed, documented, and coded.

CASE STUDIES

What classification of malnutrition would you recommend for the following patient?

CASE STUDY 1

A 44 year-old female with a past medical history significant for gastric adenocarcinoma stage 3 was diagnosed 6 months ago. Four months ago, she had a total gastrectomy, splenectomy, distal pancreatectomy, omentectomy, and small bowel resection. The patient has lost 60 lb in the last 6 months. The patient was in an outpatient visit today and was sent to the ER for severe weight loss, nausea, and vomiting. The patient admits to poor appetite and only has been able to eat crackers and mashed potatoes and drink one to two cups of apple juice per day for the past 1 month. She exhibited severe generalized loss of muscle in the temple, clavicle bone, and scapular bone region. Severe muscle loss was also noted in the anterior thigh region and posterior calf region.

Height, 5′5; admission weight, 29.4 kg (65 lb); BMI, 10.82

Vital signs:

Blood pressure, 104/73; temperature, 37.2°C; pulse, 84

Laboratory values:

White blood cell count, 7.8; C-reactive protein, 0.7 mg/dL; serum albumin, 4.2 g/dL; fasting blood glucose, 95 mg/dL; sodium, 150

Answer: The National Center for Health Statistics defines chronic as a disease/condition lasting 3 months or longer [59]. Gastric carcinoma was diagnosed in this patient 6 months ago and as such is consistent with the existence of a chronic illness.

Using Table 5.10 as a reference, patient exhibits four out of the six mentioned characteristics for severe malnutrition. Recommended diagnosis will be severe malnutrition in the context of chronic illness as a result of reduced dietary intake, unintended weight loss, physical exam with loss of muscle, and subcutaneous fat.

CASE STUDY 2

A 50 year-old male with history of alcoholism, pancreatitis, and diverticulitis lost his wife 3 months ago. He presented to the emergency department due to generalized weakness, abdominal pain, and respiratory distress, which developed over the past 10–12 days. The patient states he had not been eating well due to grief from his wife's death. He lost about 9 lb in the last month. NFPE revealed mild loss of muscle and subcutaneous fat.

Height, 6′0; admission weight, 71 kg; BMI, 21

Vital signs:

Blood pressure, 99/65; temperature, 36.3°C

TABLE 5.10
Case Study 1: Malnutrition in the Context of Chronic Illness

Characteristics	Nonsevere/Moderate Malnutrition	Severe Malnutrition
Energy intake	<75% of estimated requirements for >1 month	*≤75% of estimated requirements for ≥1 month*
Weight loss	5% in 1 month	>5% in 1 month
	7.5% in 3 months	>7.5% in 3 months
	10% in 6 months	*≥10% in 6 months*
	20% in 1 year	>20% in 1 year
Physical findings—loss of subcutaneous fat	Mild	*Severe*
Loss of muscle mass	Mild	*Severe*
Fluid accumulation	Mild	Severe
Reduced grip strength	Not applicable	Measurable reduced

TABLE 5.11
Case Study 2: Malnutrition in the Context of Social or Environmental Circumstances

Characteristics	Nonsevere/Moderate Malnutrition	Severe Malnutrition
Energy intake	*<75% of estimated requirements for ≥3 months*	≤50% of estimated requirements for ≥1 month
Weight loss	*5% in 1 month*	>5% in 1 month
	7.5% in 3 months	>7.5% in 3 months
	10% in 6 months	>10% in 6 months
	20% in 1 year	>20% in 1 year
Physical findings—loss of subcutaneous fat	*Mild*	Severe
Loss of muscle mass	*Mild*	Severe
Fluid accumulation	Mild	Severe
Reduced grip strength	Not applicable	Measurable reduced

Laboratory values:

White blood cell count, 13.88; serum albumin, 2.8 g/dL; fasting glucose, 79 mg/dL

Answer: Using Table 5.11 as reference, the recommended diagnosis will be moderate malnutrition in the context of social/environmental circumstances based on energy intake, 5% weight loss in 1 month, mild subcutaneous fat, and muscle loss.

REFERENCES

1. White JV, Guenter P, Jensen G, Malone A, Schfield M. Consensus Statement of the Academy of Nutrition and Dietetics/American Society for Parenteral and Enteral Nutrition: Characteristics recommended for the identification and documentation of adult malnutrition (undernutrition). *JPEN J Parenter Enteral Nutr* 2012; 36(3): 277.
2. Mueller C, Compher C, Druyan ME. A.S.P.E.N clinical guidelines: Nutrition screening, assessment and intervention. *JPEN J Parenter Enteral Nutr* 2011; 35(1): 16–24.
3. Joint Commission on Accreditation of Healthcare Organizations. *Comprehensive Accreditation Manual for Hospitals*. Chicago, IL: Joint Commission on Accreditation of Healthcare Organizations; 2007.

4. Anthony PS. Nutrition screening tools for hospitalized patients. *Nutr Clin Pract* 2008; 23: 373.
5. Skipper A, Ferguson M, Thompson K, Castellanos VH, Porcari J. Nutrition screening tools: An analysis of the evidence. *JPEN J Parenter Enteral Nutr* 2012; 36: 293.
6. Thomas DR. Nutrition assessment in long-term care. *Nutr Clin Pract* 2008; 23: 383–387.
7. Kondrup J, Allison SP, Elia M, Vellas B, Plauth M. ESPEN guidelines for nutrition screening. *Clin Nutr* 2003; 22(4): 415–421.
8. Stratton RJ, King CL, Stroud MA, Jackson AA, Elia M. "Malnutrition Universal Screening Tool" predicts mortality and length of hospital stay in acutely ill elderly. *Br J Nutr* 2006; 95(2): 325–330.
9. Veterans affairs Total Parenteral Nutrition Cooperative Study Group. Perioperative total parenteral nutrition in surgical patients. *N Engl J Med* 1991; 324: 525–532.
10. Charney P. Nutrition screening vs nutrition assessment: How do they differ? *Nutr Clin Pract* 2008; 23(4): 366–372.
11. Laporte M, Villalon L, Payette H. Simple nutrition screening tools for healthcare facilities: Development and validity assessment. *Can J Diet Pract Res* 2001; 62: 26–34.
12. Teitelbaum D, Guenter P, Howell WH, Kochevar ME, Roth J, Seidner DL. Definition of Terms, Style, and Conventions Used in A.S.P.E.N. Guidelines and Standards. *Nutr Clin Pract* 2005; 20(2): 281–285.
13. Pesce-Hammond K, Wesssel J. Nutrition assessment and decision making. In: Merrit R, ed. *The A.S.P.E.N Nutrition Support Practice Manual*. Silver Spring, MD: A.S.P.E.N; 2005, pp. 3–26.
14. Russel MK, Mueller C. Nutrition screening and assessment. In: Gottschlich M, ed. *The A.S.P.E.N Nutrition Support Core Curriculum: A Case-Based Approach—The Adult Patient*. Silver Spring, MD: A.S.P.E.N; 2007, pp. 163–186.
15. Baccaro F, Moreno JB, Borlenghi C, Aquino L, Armesto G, Plaza G, Zapata S. Subjective global assessment in the clinical setting. *JPEN J Parenter Enteral Nutr* 2007; 31(5): 406–409.
16. Jensen GL, Bistrian BM, Roubenoff R, Heimburger DC. Malnutrition syndromes: A conundrum vs continuum. *JPEN J Parenter Enteral Nutr* 2009; 33: 710–716.
17. Jensen GL, Mirtallo J, Compher C et al. Adult starvation and disease-related malnutrition: A rational approach for etiology-based diagnosis in the clinical practice setting from the International Consensus Guideline Committee. *JPEN J Parenter Enteral Nutr* 2010; 34: 156–159.
18. Jensen GL, Hsiao Y, Wheeler D. Adult nutrition assessment tutorial. *JPEN J Parenter Enteral Nutr* 2012; 36: 267–297.
19. Hammond K. History and physical examination. In: Matarese LE, Gottschlich MM, eds. *Contemporary Nutrition Support Practice: A Clinical Guide*, 2nd edn. St. Louis, MO: Saunders; 2003, pp. 14–30.
20. Hammond KA. The nutritional dimension of physical assessment. *Nutrition* 1990; 15(5): 411–419.
21. DeChicco R, Hamilton C. Nutrition assessment. In: Coughlin KL, DeChicco R, Hamilton C, eds. *Cleveland Clinic Nutrition Support Handbook*, 3rd edn. Cleveland, OH: The Cleveland Clinic Foundation; 2011, pp. 17–34.
22. Table Physical Exam-Parameters Useful in the Assessment of Nutritional Status, accessed at: www.eatright.org/search.aspx?search=physical+exam&type=Site (accessed February 17, 2014.)
23. Shopbell JM, Hopkins B, Shronts EP. Nutrition screening and assessment. In: Gottschlich M, ed. *The Science and Practice of Nutrition Support: A Case-Based Core Curriculum*. Kendall/Hunt Publishing Company; 2001, pp. 107–140.
24. Seltzer MH, Slocum BA, Cataldi-Betcher EL, Fileti C. Instant nutritional assessment: Absolute weight loss and surgical mortality. *JPEN J Parenter Enteral Nutr* 1985; 9: 239–241.
25. Blackburn GL, Bistrian BR, Maini BS et al. Nutritional and metabolic assessment of the hospitalized patient. *JPEN J Parenter Enteral Nutrition* 1977; 1: 11–22.
26. National Institutes of Health. Clinical guidelines on the identification and treatment of overweight and obesity in adults: The evidence report. *Obes Res* 1998; 6: 51S–209S.
27. Campbell IT, Watt T, Withers D, England R, Sukumar S, Keegan MA, Faragher B, Martin DF. Muscle weakness, measured with ultrasound, may be an indicator of lean tissue wasting in multiple organ failure in the presence of edema. *Am J Clin Nutr* September 1995; 62(3): 533–539.
28. Baracos VE, Reiman T, Mourtzakis M, Gioulbasanis I, Antoun S. Body composition in patients with non-small cell lung cancer: A contemporary view of cancer cachexia with the use of computed tomography image analysis. *Am J Clin Nutr* 2010; 91(suppl.): 1133S–1137S.
29. Supinsky G. Acquired weakness in critically ill patients. *110th Abott Nutrition Research Conference*. Downloaded at http://images.abbottnutrition.com/ANHI2010/MEDIA/20–110TH%20ANHI%20Conf%20Supinsk%20Final.pdf, (accessed March 15, 2014.)
30. Evans WJ, Campbell WW. Sarcopenia and age-related changes in body composition and functional capacity. *J Nutr* 1993; 123: 465–468.

31. Evans W. What is sarcopenia? *J Gerontol* 1995; 50A(special issue): 5–8.
32. Evans WJ, Morley JE, Argiles J et al. Cachexia: A new definition. *Clin Nutr* 2008; 27: 793–799.
33. Bemben MG. Use of diagnostic ultrasound for assessing muscle size. *J Strength Cond Res* 2002; 16(1): 103–108.
34. Cioffi WG. What's new in burns and metabolism. *J Am Coll Surg* 2001; 192–241.
35. Russell MK. Laboratory monitoring. In: Matarese LE, Gottschlich MM, eds. *Contemporary Nutrition Support Practice: A Clinical Guide*. St Louis, MO: Saunders; 2003, pp. 45–62.
36. Doweiko JP, Nompleggi DJ. The role of albumin in human physiology and pathophysiology. Part III. Albumin and disease states. *J Parenter Enteral Nutr* 1991; 15(4): 476–483.
37. Fleck A, Raines G, Hawker F et al. Increased vascular permeability: A major cause of hypoalbuminemia in disease and injury. *Lancet* 1985; 1(8432): 781–784.
38. Higgins PA, Daly J, Lipson AR, Guo SE. Assessing nutritional status in chronically ill patients. *Am J Crit Care* 2006; 15: 1–99.
39. Chan S, McCowen KC, Blackburn GL. Nutrition assessment in the ICU. *Chest* 1999; 115: 145S–148S.
40. Church M, Hill GL. Assessing the efficacy of intravenous nutrition in general surgical patients: Dynamic nutritional assessment with plasma proteins. *J Parenter Enteral Nutr* 1987; 11(2): 135–139.
41. Spiekerman AM. Nutritional assessment (protein nutriture). *Anal Chem* 1995; 67(12): 429R–436R.
42. Shetty PS, Watrasiewicz KE, Jung RT, James WP. Rapid- turnover proteins: An index of subclinical protein-energy malnutrition. *Lancet* 1979; 2(8136): 230–232.
43. Veldee M. Nutrition assessment, therapy and monitoring. In: Burtis C, Ashwood E, eds. *Tietz Textbook of Clinical Chemistry*. Philadelphia, PA: WB Saunders; 1999, pp. 1359–1394.
44. Lopez-Hellin J, Baena-Fustegueras JA, Schwartz-Riera S, Garcia-Arumi E. Usefulness of short lived proteins as nutritional indicators in surgical patients. *Clin Nutr* April 2002; 21(2): 119–125.
45. Vigushin DM, Pepys MB, Hawkins PN. Metabolic and scintigraphic studies of radioiodinated human C-reactive protein in health and disease. *J Clin Invest* 1993; 91: 1351–1357.
46. Ohzato H, Yoshizaki K, Nishimoto N et al. Interleukin-6 as a new indicator of inflammatory status: Detection of serum levels of interleukin-6 and C-reactive protein after surgery. *Surgery* 1992; 111(2): 201–209.
47. Clarke SJ, Chua W, Moore M et al. Use of inflammatory markers to guide cancer treatment. *Clin Pharmacol Ther* 2011; 90: 475–478.
48. Nomikos IN, Sidiropoulos A, Vamvakopoulou DN et al. Surgical complications of hyperglycemia. *Curr Diab Rev* 2009; 5(2): 145–150.
49. Molly McMahon M, Erin N, Carol B, John M, Charlene C. A.S.P.E.N Clinical Guidelines: Nutrition support of adult patients with hyperglycemia. *J Parenter Enteral Nutr* January 2013; 37(1): 23–26, first published on June 29, 2012.
50. Alsumrain MH, Jawad SA, Imran NB, Riar S, DeBari VA, Adelman M. Association of hypophosphatemia with failure to wean from mechanical ventilation. *Ann Clin Lab Sci Spring* 2010; 40(2): 144–148.
51. McClave SA, Martindale RG, Vanek VW, McCarthy M, Roberts P, Taylor B, Ochoa JB, Napolitano L, Cresci G. Guidelines for the provision and assessment of nutrition support therapy in the critically ill patient: Society of Critical Care Medicine (S.C.C.M) and American Society for Parenteral and Enteral Nutrition (A.S.P.E.N). *JPEN J Parenter Enteral Nutr* 2009; 33: 277.
52. Norman K, Stobaus N, Gonzales MC, Schulzke JD, Pirlich M. Hand grip strength: Outcome predictor and marker of nutritional status. *Clin Nutr* April 2011; 30(2): 135–142.
53. Lee JJ, Waak K, Grosse-Sundrup M, Xue F, Lee J, Chipman D, Ryan C, Bittner EA, Schmidt U, Eikermann M. Global muscle strength but not grip strength predicts mortality and length of stay in a general population in the surgical intensive care unit. *Phys Ther* 2012; 92(12): 1546–1555.
54. De Jonghe B, Bastuji-Garin S, Durand MC et al. Respiratory weakness is associated with limb weakness and delayed weaning in critical illness. *Crit Care Med* 2007; 35: 2007–2015.
55. Puthucheary Z, Montgomery H, Moxham J, Harridge S, Hart N. Structure to function: Muscle failure in critically ill patients. *J Physiol* 2010; 588(P23): 4641–4648.
56. Holmes S. The effects of undernutrition in hospitalized patients. *Nurs Stand* 2007; 22: 35–38.
57. Barker L, Gout BS, Crowe TC. Hospital malnutrition: Prevalence, identification and impact on patients and the healthcare system. *Int J Environ Res Public Health* 2011; 8: 514–527.
58. Chumlea WC, Roche AF, Steinbaugh ML. Estimating stature from knee height for persons 60 to 90 years of age. *J Am Geriatr Soc* 1985; 33: 116–120.
59. Hagan JC. Acute and chronic diseases. In: Mulner RM, ed. *Encyclopedia of Health Services Research*, Vol. 1. Thousand Oaks, CA: Sage; 2009, p. 25.

6 Energy Expenditure in the Critically Ill Patient

David Frankenfield

CONTENTS

Accurate determination of energy needs is an important part of the nutritional assessment of critically ill patients. Data are accumulating that early achievement of energy balance has important influence on outcome [1–5]. The goal of this chapter is to describe the energy requirements of the critically ill patient and to examine the methods for determining energy expenditure.

INFLAMMATORY RESPONSE IN CRITICALLY ILL PATIENTS

As a result of traumatic or surgical injury, infection, cancer, and other illnesses, the human body mounts an inflammatory response [6]. At the mediation level, several interacting systems are involved. The central nervous system, hormones, cytokines, eicosanoids, growth factors, and catabolic factors all play a role (see Chapter 1) [7]. Clinically apparent hallmarks of the response include fever, tachycardia, tachypnea, and leukocytosis [6]. These patients tend to be hyperdynamic. Blood chemistry hallmarks of the inflammatory response include fasting hyperglycemia, hypertriglyceridemia (but hypocholesterolemia), and hypoalbuminemia (but increased acute phase proteins) [8]. Metabolically, the patient undergoing an inflammatory response has an increase in resting metabolic rate, an increase in muscle catabolism and nitrogen loss, an enhanced gluconeogenesis that is resistant to feeding, a blunting of ketone production if the patient is starved, and increased peripheral glutamine production, but an even greater increase in glutamine consumption centrally. This chapter will emphasize the changes in resting metabolic rate brought about by the inflammatory response in critically ill patients.

IS HYPERMETABOLISM LINKED TO ILLNESS PER SE OR TO THE INFLAMMATORY RESPONSE TO ILLNESS?

Most research on resting metabolic rate in critically ill patients categorizes those patients based on their reason for being critically ill (trauma vs. surgery vs. pancreatitis, etc.). Long's seminal paper [9] is a good example of this, with division of subjects into elective surgery, blunt and penetrating trauma, trauma with steroids, sepsis, and burn groups. Typically burns and sepsis are found to be the most hypermetabolic condition, followed by blunt trauma, surgery, and medical conditions (Table 6.1). However, categorization by illness type alone does not explain all of the variability in the published research on resting metabolic rate in critically ill patients.

Frankenfield et al. [10] examined inflammatory response relative to injury type in a diverse group of nonburn trauma, surgery, and medical intensive care unit (ICU) patients. Patients were classified by these illness types as well as by the presence of systemic inflammatory response syndrome (SIRS) at the time of measurement. SIRS was defined as the presence of at least two of the following criteria: (1) body temperature greater than 38°C or less than 36°C; (2) white blood cell count greater than 12,000 cells/mL or less than 3,000 cells/mL; or (3) heart rate greater than 90 beats/min. Patients were also classified by whether they were febrile at any time during the 24 h prior to metabolic rate measurement (body temperature >38.0°C recorded at least once by nursing staff). The result was that neither illness type nor SIRS status was associated with higher level of hypermetabolism, but fever in the 24 h prior to measurement did increase the level of hypermetabolism no matter why the patient was admitted to the ICU or whether the patient had SIRS (Table 6.2). Although all groups had elevated resting metabolic rate, in afebrile subjects, hypermetabolism was less pronounced than in febrile subjects, and there was almost no difference by injury type (Table 6.2). There was more separation by illness type in febrile subjects (trauma being somewhat more hypermetabolic than either surgery or medicine), but when subjects' body temperature was controlled by covariate analysis, resting metabolic rates among the febrile subjects equalized (137% ± 21% of healthy resting metabolic rate for trauma, 135% ± 20% for surgery, and 135% ± 21% for medicine). In a similar study, Raurich et al. [11] controlled for body temperature

TABLE 6.1
Stress and Activity Multipliers for Injury and Illness Suggested by Long in 1979 (Multiply Basal Metabolic Rate by Harris–Benedict Equation by Activity Factor and by Injury Factor)

Activity factor	
Confined to bed	1.20
Out of bed	1.30
Injury factor	
Minor operation	1.20
Skeletal trauma[a]	1.35
Major sepsis (fever, hypotension, tachypnea, tachycardia, i.e., SIRS)	1.60
Severe thermal burn	2.10

[a] This appears to be an average of skeletal trauma (auto crashes without brain injury) at ×1.32, blunt trauma (gunshot wounds) at ×1.37, and trauma with steroids (brain injury) at ×1.61. It should also be pointed out that the major sepsis and severe thermal burn stress factors do not match the percent increase over basal measured in the study (1.32 for burns and 1.79 for sepsis).

TABLE 6.2
Influence of Injury/Disease Type, SIRS, and Fever as the Cause for Hypermetabolism in Critically Ill Patients (Percent of Calculated Basal Metabolic Rate by Harris–Benedict Equation)

	Maximum Body Temperature >38°C		
	Yes	No	All
Injury group			
Trauma	1.45 ± 0.22	1.23 ± 0.14	1.34 ± 0.23
Major surgery	1.38 ± 0.22	1.25 ± 0.14	1.32 ± 0.22
Medical	1.39 ± 0.20	1.25 ± 0.20	1.32 ± 0.20
All	1.41 ± 0.24	1.24 ± 0.17	
SIRS group			
SIRS	1.41 ± 0.23	1.23 ± 0.17	1.32 ± 0.26
Non-SIRS	1.49 ± 0.20	1.25 ± 0.24	1.37 ± 0.36
All	1.45 ± 0.34	1.24 ± 0.21	

by excluding febrile patients from examination and found no differences in resting metabolic rate between trauma, surgical, and medical ICU patients. Furthermore, the presence of infection did not change the resting metabolic rate among patients who did not develop fever.

Another way of examining the relation of resting metabolic rate and fever is to examine the change in resting metabolic rate as febrile patients are cooled [12–14]. Metabolic rate has been found to drop in sedated febrile patients treated with external cooling. A 10% decrease in resting metabolic rate occurred as body temperature was lowered from 39.2°C to 37.2°C [12]. In another study, body temperature was reduced 12% (to 33°C) resulting in a 25%–30% reduction in resting metabolic rate [13]. These patients were heavily sedated or medically paralyzed, which is critical because if not, shivering could have occurred, resulting in increased metabolic rate [15].

Thus, it seems that the presence of fever is a major factor in determining the degree of hypermetabolism in critically ill patients. Within any disease or SIRS category, fever denotes an increase in resting metabolic rate. This points out the importance of an evaluation of inflammatory state or perhaps specifically body temperature as a feature of clinical nutrition assessment/practice in the ICU.

WHAT IS THE IMPACT OF PHYSICAL ACTIVITY AND SEDATION ON METABOLIC RATE?

Intuitively, sedation and medical paralysis should be associated with a decrease in resting metabolic rate. Indeed, in a randomized trial on the effect of propofol versus midazolam on time to sedation and time to awaken, Kress et al. [16] used 33 medical ICU patients as their own controls to determine the change in oxygen consumption as subjects went from the awake to sedated state. Oxygen consumption dropped from 4.58 to 3.89 mL/min/kg body weight (equivalent to an 18% drop in metabolic rate from 32 to 27 kcal/kg body weight) with no difference noted between the propofol and the midazolam.

Similarly, Marik and Kaufman [17] used eight medical ICU patients as their own controls as medical paralysis was induced. In these subjects, oxygen consumption fell 34% from 200 ± 77 mL/min/m^2 body surface area to 149 ± 35 mL with no change in body temperature. Paradoxically, septic trauma patients in whom a clinical decision had been made to medically paralyze have been observed to have higher resting metabolic rates than septic trauma patients in whom medical paralysis was not clinically indicated (48 ± 16 vs. 42 ± 6 kcal/kg body weight) [18]. The most likely explanation of this observation is that the medically paralyzed patients were more seriously ill and therefore had more inflammatory injury and higher resting metabolic rate. Thus, it is safe to say that sedation and medical paralysis will decrease resting metabolic rate in an individual as he or she enters from a conscious to a drugged state, but it is not true to state that subjects requiring heavy sedation or paralysis are less hypermetabolic than those not requiring such drug therapy, because those requiring these medications are probably sicker.

Physical activity also contributes to the total metabolic rate of critically ill patients. Activities such as bathing, chest physiotherapy, and dressing changes may increase metabolic rate by 20%–45% [19,20]. However, because these activities are usually short-lived, the overall impact on daily metabolic rate is more on the order of about 5%–10% [18–20]. Shivering is another physical activity that if not prevented by medication can markedly increase metabolic rate [15].

WHAT IS THE THERMOGENIC EFFECT OF FEEDING ON RESTING METABOLIC RATE?

In healthy individuals, consumption of a meal increases metabolic rate for a short time afterward. The degree is variable, as is the duration of the effect, based on the size and composition of the meal [21]. For this reason, when resting metabolic rate is measured in healthy people, it is done so in a fasted state. On the other hand, resting metabolic rate measurements in the critically ill are typically conducted during feeding, and a thermogenic effect is presumed to be present. No attempt is made to measure in a fasted state because the thermic effect is expected to be constant, so measuring during a fast would be counterproductive. In actuality, there may be minimal thermogenic effect of feeding in critically ill patients, for several reasons. First, most critically ill patients are fed through feeding tubes and do not need to swallow. Swallowing seems to be part of the process of generating the thermogenic effect of feeding [22,23]. Second, most feedings are delivered continuously at a slow rate rather than in large amounts intermittently, and this act further minimizes the thermogenic effect of feeding [23]. In one study of critically ill brain-injured patients (stroke and traumatic brain injury), Frankenfield reported on 10 patients who by clinical happenstance had not received feeding in 24 h prior to being measured [24]. These patients had a resting metabolic rate of 2002 ± 425 kcal/day compared to 1982 ± 249 kcal/day for a group of 120 patients who were receiving continuous feeding during the measurement. These metabolic rates were normalized to body size and were not significantly different from one another, suggesting that thermogenic effect of feeding did not have a major role in increasing the metabolic rate of critically ill patients. In an unpublished analysis of data from Ref. [25], 16 patients unfed for 24 h prior to measurement had a resting metabolic rate of 2089 ± 558 versus 1993 ± 533 kcal/day in 186 patients who received continuous feeding prior and during the study. Controlling for body size, sex, and age reduced the difference to 2009 ± 334 versus 2000 ± 335 kcal/day. In a study of obese patients [26], there were no differences in resting metabolic rate in unfed versus fed patients being mechanically ventilated (1741 ± 502 vs. 1883 ± 550 kcal/day) or spontaneously breathing (2039 ± 405 vs. 1934 kcal/day). On the other hand, Miles [27] conducted a comprehensive review of resting metabolic rate papers published between 1980 and 2006. The mean resting metabolic rate in studies of fed patients (n = 11) was 117% ± 3% of Harris–Benedict value, whereas the increase in studies of unfed patients (n = 5) was only 105% ± 4% of Harris–Benedict ($p < 0.047$). However, the authors noted that overfeeding was likely a common occurrence in the fed studies, and overfeeding is known to stimulate the thermogenic effect of feeding [28]. It thus appears that thermogenic effect of feeding is not a prominent factor in the metabolic rate of critically ill patients.

HOW DOES BODY SIZE AND COMPOSITION AFFECT RESTING METABOLIC RATE?

All body sizes are encountered in the ICU, from the emaciated to the morbidly obese. Although obesity is common in the general population and underweight is a common feature of chronic illness, the metabolic rate of these body types has not been well-studied in critically ill patients. Metabolic assessments are therefore often extrapolated from data from normal weight patients or are based on conjecture and assumption.

Two studies of obese trauma patients have demonstrated that resting metabolic rate is similar to that of non-obese trauma patients if it is indexed to fat-free mass [29,30]. However, as obesity becomes more severe, the relationship changes. Obesity causes an increase in adipose tissue, extracellular mass, and muscle but little change in organ mass (brain, heart, liver, kidney) [31,32]. The tissues with expanding mass have metabolic rates that range from <1 kcal/kg (extracellular mass) to 15 kcal/kg (muscle), while the tissues with stable mass have very high metabolic rates, ranging from 202 kcal/kg for liver to 440 kcal/kg for heart and kidney. Therefore, as obesity worsens the overall mass of respiring, tissue increases, but the proportion of high metabolic rate tissue falls, while the proportion of low metabolic rate tissue increases, resulting in a nonlinear increase in resting metabolic rate among the classifications of obesity. However, since the overall mass of metabolically active tissue is higher in obese people than non-obese people, their overall resting metabolic rate is also higher (Figure 6.1) [25,33,34]. In these groups of patients, fat-free mass was calculated from the data presented in Ref. [35]:

Men: Fat-free mass (kg) = 33 + Wt(0.59) − BMI(0.73)
Women: Fat-free mass (kg) = 24 + Wt(0.57) − BMI(0.71)

The fat-free mass in Class I–II obesity was increased by 19% compared to non-obese patients, and resting metabolic rate followed suit with an 18% increase. In Class III obesity, however, the fat-free mass increased by 52%, but resting metabolic rate increased by only 36%, resulting in a downward deflection of the line relating metabolic rate to fat-free mass.

A similar but opposite situation occurs in underweight patients. As humans lose body weight during starvation, muscle and body fat are catabolized for fuel, while the mass of high metabolism tissues (the internal organs) is usually preserved until very late in the starvation process [36]. In an underweight person who has lost muscle and fat but preserved brain, heart, liver, and kidney, the proportion of total weight composed of high metabolic rate tissue is elevated, and so the

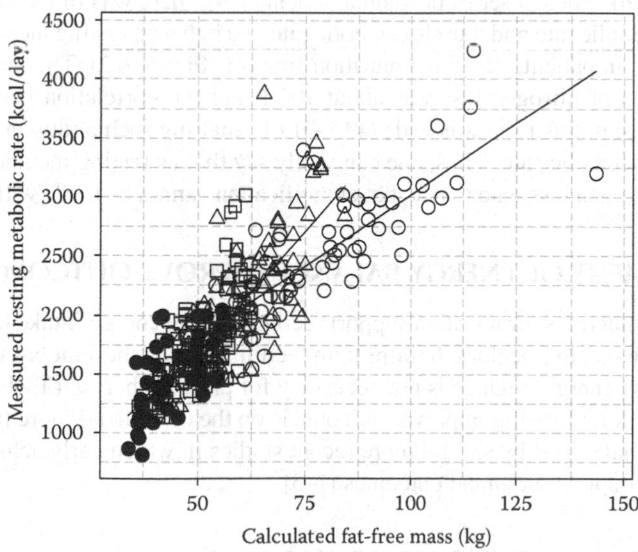

FIGURE 6.1 The resting metabolic rate of critically ill, mechanically ventilated patients plotted against estimated fat-free mass, subdivided by body mass index (closed circles, body mass index <20.0 kg/m^2; open squares, body mass index 20.0–29.9 kg/m^2; open triangles, body mass index 30.0–39.9 kg/m^2; open circles, body mass index ≥40.0 kg/m^2). In the highest body mass index group, the measured resting metabolic rate fails to increase at the same rate as the fat-free mass causing a change in the relationship between the two. This is presumably due to the expansion of low metabolic rate tissues (muscle and extracellular mass) with little change in high metabolic rate tissues (organ mass).

resting metabolic rate when indexed to body weight is elevated compared to normal weight people. In the data from Refs. [25,33,34], there are 42 patients with body mass index <20.0 kg/m^2. While the overall resting metabolic rate of these underweight patients was 20% lower than those with body mass index 20–30 kg/m^2 (1447 ± 331 vs. 1813 ± 391 kcal/day), the resting metabolic rate per kg body weight was 16% higher (29.1 ± 7.2 vs. 25.1 ± 4.1 kcal/kg), as Hoffer predicted [36]. However, there was no difference in resting metabolic rate per kg fat-free mass (34.0 ± 6.0 vs. 35.0 ± 5.3 kcal/kg).

DOES AGE AFFECT RESTING METABOLIC RATE IN THE CRITICALLY ILL?

Just as the general population is getting heavier, it is also growing older [37]. The elderly make up a substantial percentage of the population in a critical care unit. Typical aging is associated with a drop in fat-free mass (although those who maintain physical activity can minimize this change) [37]. Since fat-free mass is the *engine* of the body, burns all of the fuel, and performs all the work [38], it follows that resting metabolic rate decreases with typical aging. Indeed, most predictive equations for resting metabolic rate include a negative age multiplier to account for the attenuation in resting metabolic rate.

Changes in the metabolic response to critical illness in the elderly have not been extensively studied. In one investigation [30], elderly trauma patients were found to have a lower incidence of fever on day 5–7 post-injury. In young trauma patients, more than 80% were febrile, while in the elderly, fewer than 50% were. This was true despite higher infection rates in the elderly group. Resting metabolic rate was 12% lower in the elderly than in the young. Controlling for body compositional differences in the elderly only partly reduced the difference (an 8% difference remained).

WHAT IS THE LINK BETWEEN HYPERMETABOLISM AND HYPERCATABOLISM?

Increased muscle catabolism and nitrogen loss are hallmarks of critical illness [8]. Hypermetabolism is thought to go hand-in-hand with this catabolic state, as both are consequences of the inflammatory response. In Frankenfield's series of trauma patients [39], there was in fact a linear association between resting metabolic rate and muscle catabolic rate and between resting metabolic rate and total urinary nitrogen loss in patients receiving nutrition support (Figure 6.2). The mean ratio of energy expenditure per gram of nitrogen loss was about 100:1, but the correlation between the two was quite low, so the range in this ratio was wide (49:1–319:1), making such a ratio useless in estimating nitrogen loss from metabolic rate. Thus, one can safely say that as resting metabolic rate rises, then catabolic rate and nitrogen loss tend to rise, but quantification cannot be made without measurement.

DOES ACHIEVEMENT OF ENERGY BALANCE IMPROVE OUTCOME?

Many critical care guidelines for nutrition support recommend an energy intake target <100% in the first week and permissive hypocaloric high-protein feeding for the obese. It has been demonstrated in several studies that energy balance is not necessary for protein sparing (Table 6.3) [39–41]. The evidence that hypocaloric feeding improves outcome is on the other hand more limited [42,43], and that view has been challenged by several more recent studies in which early achievement of energy and protein balance improved clinical outcomes [1–5].

DETERMINATION OF RESTING METABOLIC RATE

If it is confirmed that achieving energy balance is important in improving clinical outcome [1–5], then accurate assessment of that demand becomes imperative. Energy demand can be assessed either by measurement or by calculation. The next sections of this chapter will review the factors involved in these methods.

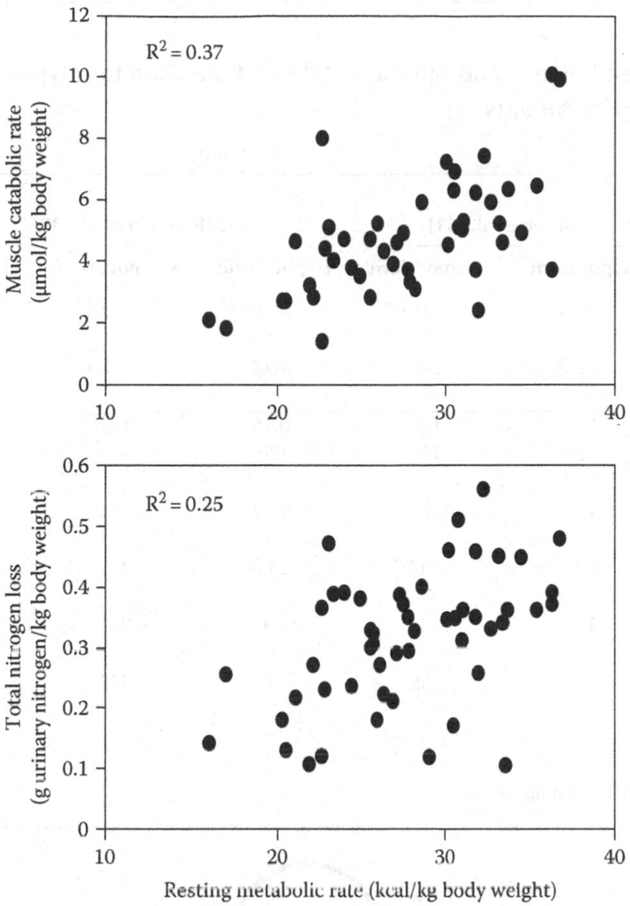

FIGURE 6.2 Relationship between muscle catabolic rate and resting metabolic rate and between urinary nitrogen loss and resting metabolic rate in critically ill trauma patients. (From data Frankenfield, D.C. et al., *J. Trauma*, 48, 49, 2000.)

HOW IS RESTING METABOLIC RATE MEASURED?

Indirect calorimetry is the measurement of respiratory gas exchange in order to make inference about cellular gas exchange (which equates to metabolic rate and substrate utilization). The measured parameters of indirect calorimetry are oxygen consumption (VO_2) and carbon dioxide production (VCO_2). From these measurements, respiratory quotient (RQ) and metabolic rate can be calculated. Indirect calorimetry is valid only when the respiratory gas exchange and the cellular gas exchange are equivalent. Equivalence is fairly easy to attain for oxygen consumption, since oxygen is not stored in the body and is not used for purposes other than metabolism. Thus, a change in cellular oxygen consumption is quickly detected as a change in respiratory VO_2. Carbon dioxide, on the other hand, is stored extensively in the body and participates in acid–base homeostasis. Therefore, a change in carbon dioxide production in the cells can take time to manifest as a change in respiratory VCO_2 [44], and a need to convert back and forth to bicarbonate or to ventilate carbon dioxide from the blood in order to normalize pH will result in an uncoupling of cellular and respiratory carbon dioxide (Figure 6.3).

TABLE 6.3
Energy and Nitrogen Balance and Muscle Catabolic Rate Data for Hypocaloric versus Full Feeding in Critically Ill Patients

	Study					
	Burge et al. [41]		Frankenfield et al. [39]			Dickerson et al. [40]
Parameter	**Hypocaloric**	**Normocaloric**	**Hypocaloric**	**Normocaloric**	**Overfed**	**Hypocaloric**
Resting metabolic rate (kcal/day)	1767	2199	2095	2175	2257	2205
Total calorie intake (kcal/day)	1285	2429	1600	2280	2815	1397
Intake/RMR	0.73	1.13	0.75	1.05	1.24	0.63
Protein intake (g/day)	111	130	120	120	124	129
Nitrogen intake (g/day)	17.8	20.8	19.2	19.2	19.8	20.6
Urea nitrogen output (g/day)	8.1[a]	10.7[a]	26.8	24.9	26.6	15.0
Nitrogen balance (g/day)	+1.3	+2.8	−7.9	−7.5	−8.3	+2.4
3-Methylhistidine excretion (μmol/day)	255	335	357	422	375	—

[a] Urine urea nitrogen value is fasting value.

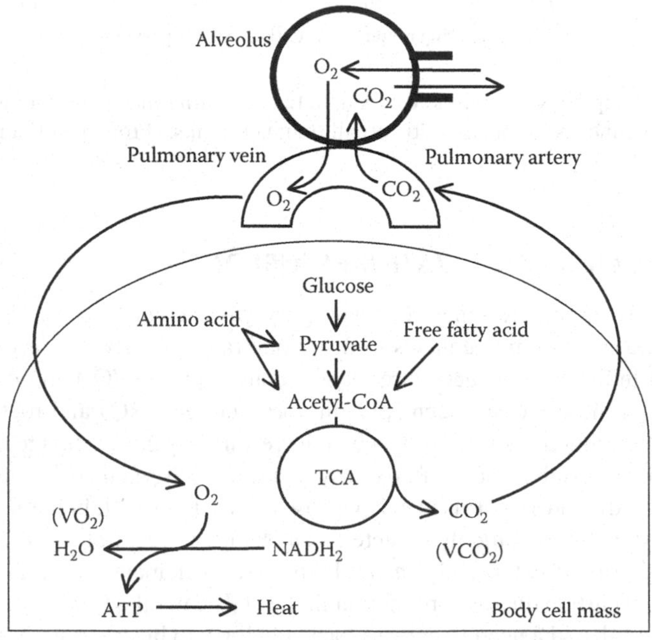

FIGURE 6.3 Diagram illustrating the relationship between pulmonary gas exchange and cellular metabolism. This relationship makes indirect calorimetry possible. For a given type of fuel being oxidized, a constant and known amount of oxygen is consumed, carbon dioxide produced, and heat released. Therefore, measurement of the oxygen and/or carbon dioxide volumes equates directly with energy expenditure.

Equipment

Most indirect calorimeters in use today are portable, open-circuit devices. Open circuit refers to the fact that while the entire expired air is captured and measured for gas concentration and volume by the calorimeter, the inspired air is only sampled. Total inspired volume is instead calculated from inspired and expired gas concentrations and expired volume. This puts an upper limit on the FIO_2 at which measurements can be conducted, but it makes the calorimetry device much easier to use because the inspired air does not need to pass through the indirect calorimeter on its way to the patient.

Calorimeters have five basic components. Two of the components relate to analysis of gas concentrations: separate sensors for analyzing carbon dioxide and oxygen consumption in the inspired and expired air. The calorimeter must also have a device for measuring expired air volume. A calibration system is included for the gas sensors and sometimes pressure or volume. Finally, a computer is used to calculate inspired volume, RQ, and metabolic rate, to run test algorithms, and to manage data output.

Measurement Protocols

In order for indirect calorimetry measurements to have meaning, they must be performed under known conditions. Ideally, all clinical indirect calorimetry measurements would be performed continuously, resulting in a value for total daily metabolic rate. Such a measurement would include the effect of physical activity, feeding state, and change in clinical condition on the patient's metabolic rate and would average out respiratory artifact (the times when the respiratory and cellular gas exchanges are not equivalent) or actively remove it based on data algorithms. Systems exist for continuous gas-exchange monitoring, some single unit [45], and some multiunit [46]. However, the most common indirect calorimetry measurement is one in which metabolic rate is measured over a short time period (less than 1 h), and in such cases, more attention must be paid to the clinical state of the patient at the time of the measurement, so that the result can be properly interpreted and acted upon. The most desired measurement condition for a short indirect calorimetry test is that of steady-state rest. Steady-state rest is desirable because it is reproducible, minimizes the chance of respiratory artifact, and in critical care represents >90% of the total metabolic rate unless the patient is agitated or otherwise physically active [15,18,19]. The resting state is one in which the patient has been left undisturbed and is lying nearly motionless in bed. It is generally proclaimed that this condition should be maintained for at least 30 min prior to measurement (less if the patient is deeply sedated or medically paralyzed) and continued through the duration of the measurement [21]. In healthy people undergoing indirect calorimetry, resting conditions require a fast, but in the ICU, with patients typically receiving continuous feeding, thermogenic effect of feeding is minimized (see the previous section "Equipment"), so feeding should not be stopped for indirect calorimeter measurements. Steady state refers to a condition in which the subject's gas-exchange measurements are varying from minute to minute within a tight range and is another way of assuring that respiratory and metabolic gas exchange are the same [21]. If a change in respiratory rate or tidal volume (the components of minute ventilation) [47] or FIO_2 has been made recently, the patient will be in a state of change, so indirect calorimetry should not be performed.

When resting conditions are known to exist, and it is also known that no ventilator changes have been recently made [47], an indirect calorimetry measurement can commence. The remaining criterion for steady state (tight variation in VO_2 and VCO_2) can only be determined after the measurement commences. Typical allowable coefficient of variation to define steady state is 5% in a 10 min test or 10% coefficient of variation in a 30 min test (discarding the first 5 min of data automatically). Either protocol has been shown to reflect 24 h resting metabolic rate [21,48,49].

If a resting steady state cannot be achieved, the indirect calorimetry measurement can be prolonged over several hours, while typical nursing activities are allowed to occur as usual. The resulting data do not require a minimum coefficient of variation on the gas-exchange parameters.

Interpretation

There are two aspects to the interpretation of indirect calorimetry studies. The first is an assessment of whether the results are technically acceptable, and the second is an integration of the results with clinical conditions at the time of the measurement. The points to note regarding technical acceptability are whether the device was calibrated, whether steady-state conditions were met, and whether the RQ was within the physiologic range (0.68–1.2) [21].

Integration of the measurement with clinical condition entails assessing whether the measurement was performed in a resting state or whether it was prolonged to capture physical activity, whether the patient was sedated or medically paralyzed during the measurement, and whether the patient was febrile or afebrile. These factors are important to note because if they change, it is likely that resting metabolic rate will change as well. In fact, one study indicates that measurement of resting metabolic rate results in no better accuracy over estimation methods unless the measurement is repeated every 3 or 4 days [50]. Strict interpretation of RQ as an indicator of substrate utilization is not feasible because of significant variability within the physiologic range [21,51,52]. If the patient was measured in the resting state, a factor of 5%–10% can be added to account for physical activity.

There are significant limitations to indirect calorimetry. First and foremost, the cost of the devices severely limits their availability, and the operational cost in terms of manpower and time can be significant. Even if indirect calorimetry is available, a number of conditions common to the critical care unit will limit the number of patients who can be measured. Such conditions include air leaks, extracorporeal membrane oxygenation, use of nitric oxide or other inhaled gasses, and high fraction of inspired oxygen. In one international study of energy balance in critically ill patients, fewer than 1% of all patients included in the study had their metabolic rate measured [4].

HOW IS RESTING METABOLIC RATE PREDICTED?

Given the obstacles to routine measurement of resting metabolic rate in critically ill patients, the clinician often has little choice but to determine metabolic needs by estimation. It is not possible to list or comment on all of the estimation methods, so in this chapter, only a few pertinent methods will be discussed.

Common practice for predicting resting metabolic rate in critically ill patients is to calculate resting metabolic rate on a kcal/kg basis, with little standardization in the amount of energy per kg or the weight to use in obesity. It also remains commonplace to calculate healthy resting metabolic rate (often using the Harris–Benedict equations [53]) and then to multiply this rate by a stress factor. Calvin Long's stress factors from 1979 are still sometimes used for this purpose [9]. In the 1990s, a different approach emerged that de-emphasized patient categorization into stress factors and instead used dynamic physiologic variables in regression equations to predict resting metabolic rate. Swinamer et al. [54] was one of the first to report such an equation, developed from 112 mechanically ventilated critical care patients (47% trauma):

$$\text{RMR} = \text{BSA}(941) - \text{age}(6.3) + \text{Temp}(104) + \text{RR}(24) + V_T(804) - 4243 \tag{6.1}$$

in which BSA was body surface area (m^2), age was in years, Temp was body temperature (degrees centigrade), RR was respiratory rate in breaths/minute, and V_T was tidal volume in liters/breath. This is the prototypical form of resting metabolic rate equations in critical care in that the body surface area and age terms reflect the classic determinants of healthy resting metabolic rate (i.e., metabolic body size) and that the Temp, RR, and V_T terms reflect the effect of inflammatory response on metabolic rate. Of note is the absence of a factor for type of injury even though a heterogeneous patient population was used to develop the equation. Soon after the release of the Swinamer equation, Ireton-Jones et al. [55] published an equation in regression form that also accounted for the typical predictors of healthy resting metabolism (body weight, age, sex) and added categories of illness (trauma, burn injury) but did not utilize clinical variables such as body temperature, respiratory rate, or tidal volume to account for degree of inflammation:

$$\text{RMR} = \text{wt}(5) - \text{age}(10) - \text{sex}(281) + \text{trauma}(292) + \text{burn}(851) + 1925 \quad (6.2)$$

This equation was developed from a group of 65 ventilator-dependent ICU patients. Fifty-two percent were burn victims. In 1997, an amended equation was published from the same data, but with corrections to the statistics [56]:

$$\text{RMR} = \text{wt}(5) - \text{age}(11) - \text{sex}(244) + \text{trauma}(239) + \text{burn}(804) + 1784 \quad (6.3)$$

In 1994, Frankenfield et al. [57] published an equation developed from 423 measurements in 56 mechanically ventilated trauma and septic trauma patients that again relied on a marker of healthy resting metabolic rate (RMR(healthy), in this case the Harris–Benedict equation), physiologic variables (V_E, minute ventilation in L/min), and disease category (septic multiple-organ failure [SMOF]):

$$\text{RMR} = \text{RMR(healthy)}(1.3) + V_E(100) + \text{SMOF}(300) - 1000 \quad (6.4)$$

A more recent equation published by Frankenfield was constructed retrospectively from the data in Ref. [10] and referred to as the Penn State equation. This equation was developed on a broad mix of trauma, surgical, and medical ICU patients [58]:

$$\text{RMR} = \text{RMR(healthy)}(1.1) + V_E(32) + \text{Tmax}(140) - 5340 \quad (6.5)$$

The RMR(healthy) term was the Harris–Benedict equation using actual weight for non-obese and adjusted weight for obese patients (25% of the excess weight added to the ideal body weight), V_E was minute ventilation in L/min, and Tmax was maximum body temperature in the previous 24 h (degrees centigrade). The investigators later found that the Mifflin–St. Jeor standard for resting metabolic rate was more accurate than the Harris–Benedict in healthy people and that use of adjusted body weight caused marked underestimation of resting metabolic rate in obese people [59]. Therefore, the Penn State ICU equation was recomputed from the original data using the Mifflin–St. Jeor equation actual body weight for obese as well as non-obese people [60]:

$$\text{RMR} = \text{RMR(healthy)}(0.96) + V_E(31) + \text{Tmax}(167) - 6212 \quad (6.6)$$

Faisy published another equation for predicting resting metabolic rate in mechanically ventilated critically ill patients [61]. The equation was calculated from resting metabolic rate measurements in 70 medical ICU patients. The format of the equation was similar to that used by Swinamer and Frankenfield:

$$\text{RMR} = \text{Wt}(8) + \text{Ht}(14) + V_E(32) + \text{Temp}(94) - 4834 \quad (6.7)$$

Validation

The number of calculation equations published over the years is legion. The number of validation studies of published equations is not. One of the first validation studies of any of the aforementioned equations was conducted by Flancbaum et al. [62] in which the 1992 Ireton-Jones and Frankenfield equations (Equations 6.2 and 6.4) were examined. Neither equation performed particularly well. Correlation coefficients between measured and predicted resting metabolic rate were low

($R^2 = 0.15$ for Frankenfield and 0.07 for Ireton-Jones). The Ireton-Jones equation was prone to underestimation (doing so in 89% of cases vs. 37% for Frankenfield). On the other hand, the Frankenfield equation could markedly overestimate true resting metabolic rate (by 1617 kcal in one case).

Similarly, MacDonald and Hildebrandt [63], using continuous gas-exchange technology (thus probably measuring total metabolic rate, which is greater than resting metabolic rate) in 76 critically ill patients with body mass index <30 kg/m², tested the validity of the Swinamer, 1992 Ireton-Jones, Frankenfield, and Penn State equations (Equations 6.1, 6.2, 6.4, and 6.5). The 1992 Ireton-Jones equation underestimated the measured metabolic rate (on average 85% ± 16% of the total metabolic rate) with low correlation ($R^2 = 0.23$), while the Frankenfield equation correlated with the total metabolic rate ($R^2 = 0.52$) and on average was 90% ± 20% of the measured. In both the Ireton-Jones and Frankenfield equations, only 63% of the subjects were predicted to be within 20% of the measured metabolic rate. The Penn State equation (Equation 6.4) correlated with the measured total metabolic rate ($R^2 = 0.66$) and on average calculated at 87% ± 11% of the measured total metabolic rate. Seventy-two percent of the subjects were estimated to be within 20% of the measured total metabolic rate. The Swinamer equation predicted the total metabolic rate to be within 20% of the measured in 88% of the subjects, and on average, metabolic rate was predicted at 93% ± 12% of the measured.

In another validation study, the Ireton-Jones and Penn State equations (Equations 6.2, 6.3, 6.5, and 6.6) were tested against the measured resting metabolic rate in 47 critically ill patients (trauma, surgical, and medical ICU, with no restriction on body mass index) [60]. Defining an accurate prediction of resting metabolic rate as one lying within 10% of the measured and defining a clinically important error as a prediction that was more than 15% above or below the measured resting metabolic rate, the modified Penn State equation (Equation 6.6) was accurate 72% of the time versus 60% of the time for the Ireton-Jones equation and made a clinically important error 11% of the time versus 28% of the time for the Ireton-Jones equation.

Savard conducted an analysis of the Faisy, Swinamer, and Ireton-Jones equations in 45 medical ICU patients, published in 2008 [64]. Accuracy rate was not included in the analysis, but Bland–Altman calculations indicated bias toward overestimation in all three equations. This bias was least pronounced for the Faisy equation (192 ± 277 kcal/day compared to 1172 ± 447 kcal/day for Swinamer and 339 ± 356 kcal/day for Ireton-Jones), and limit of agreement was narrowest.

The largest validation study yet published appeared in 2009. Frankenfield et al. [25] tested the Penn State, Faisy, ACCP, Brandi, and Ireton-Jones equations plus several variations of the Harris–Benedict and Mifflin equations in 202 critically ill patients (trauma, surgery, medical). The subject pool was large enough to allow subdivision by body mass index and age. The Penn State equation was found to be unbiased and to predict accurately in more patients than any of the other equations. However, a limitation was noted in patients 60 years old or older who had body mass index ≥30.0 kg/m². In this group, the equation was accurate only 53% of the time. A modification to the equation was proposed and subsequently validated [33]:

$$\text{RMR} = \text{Mifflin}(0.71) + \text{Tmax}(85) + V_E(64) - 3085 \tag{6.8}$$

The overall accuracy of the Penn State equation (combining Refs. [25,33]) and using the modified equation in older obese patients was 73%. Follow-up studies to this validation included a study emphasizing morbidly obese and underweight patients [34] and another testing validity over time [50]. The Penn State equation was accurate in 76%–80% of morbidly obese patients (body mass index ≥45.0 kg/m²) but in only 58% of patients with body mass index <20.5 kg/m². Another modification of the equation was proposed for these underweight patients but awaits validation:

$$\text{RMR} = \text{Mifflin}(0.78) + \text{Tmax}(50) + V_E(58) - 1762 \tag{6.9}$$

Longitudinal validation of the Penn State equation showed that over 7 days, daily recalculation of the Penn State equation was as accurate as weekly measurement of resting metabolic rate [50].

In order to be more accurate than daily estimation with the Penn State equation, resting metabolic rate must be measured every 3 or 4 days.

IS IT BETTER TO MEASURE OR ESTIMATE METABOLIC RATE IN CRITICALLY ILL PATIENTS?

As reviewed earlier, estimation of resting metabolic rate in critically ill patients has important limitations. Measurement of metabolic rate is possible clinically by the use of indirect calorimetry. However, the equipment is expensive, the technique can be time-consuming, and there are some patients who cannot be measured accurately. Furthermore, precise knowledge of resting metabolic rate has not been shown to improve clinical outcome. Measurement of metabolic rate may have a role in the clinical care of patients in whom a reasonable estimate of metabolic rate cannot be expected. Examples of this are significant changes in body shape or composition (amputation, spinal cord injury with quadriplegia, scoliosis, very small adults as occurs with some forms of retardation, prolonged bed rest with its attendant loss of muscle mass). Another instance in which measurement of metabolic rate may be desirable is when the patient is not progressing as expected (unexplained high minute ventilation, unexplained failure to wean from ventilator) or instances when hypometabolism is expected (high SvO_2, shock, hypothermia, spinal cord injury with quadriplegia).

CONCLUSION

The importance of achieving energy balance in critically ill patients is under active investigation. Early studies indicated that moderate underfeeding is associated with positive outcome, but more recent studies indicate the opposite, even if parenteral nutrition is necessary to meet the energy target. If it becomes clear that energy balance is beneficial, accurate determination of resting metabolic rate by measurement or prediction will be confirmed as an important component of nutrition assessment in the ICU patient. Measurement is presumed accurate 100% of the time if conducted according to protocol, but in a significant percentage of cases, patient condition or equipment availability limits the number of patients that can be measured. The best predictive equations are accurate about 75% of the time. It remains to be seen whether the accuracy rate of current equations is good enough to guide the setting of energy intake targets in the critically ill or whether frequent measurement is necessary.

CASE STUDY: Use of Indirect Calorimetry

FN is an 81-year-old female involved in a motor vehicle crash in which she sustained rib fractures, bilateral pneumothorax, pulmonary contusion, a skull fracture, and fractures of the second and fourth lumbar vertebrae. There was a distal femur and proximal open tibia fracture on the right side resulting in a floating knee. On the left was also a femur fracture. She had fractured her pelvis and distal radius, and there was a degloving injury to the hand. She arrived in the Emergency Room intubated and hypotensive. There was no reliable previous medical history. She was resuscitated and orthopedic repairs were made on the first, second, and fifth day post-injury. Tube feeding was initiated on the second day after injury but was interrupted frequently because of the surgeries. After the final orthopedic repair on day 5, her daily enteral feeding intake was noted to average 90% of target for the following week. At that point, having failed to be liberated from the ventilator due to high tidal volumes, a tracheostomy was performed in the hope that the reduced dead space would facilitate ventilator weaning. At the same time, an endoscopic gastrostomy tube placement was planned. During the procedure, it was revealed that the patient had in the past undergone a roux-en-y gastrojejunostomy. The surgery was therefore converted to an exploratory laparotomy, for placement of a jejunostomy tube, and she also underwent lysis of adhesions. She remained on mechanical ventilation for the next week, with enteral feeding continuing to reach 90% of daily target volume on average. Then on day 20 post-injury, she was noted to have fascial dehiscence and focal evisceration. Repeat laparotomy revealed that the sutures tacking her bowel to her abdominal wall had failed, creating an enterotomy that had been leaking. Her small bowel was resected, and she had debridement of her abdominal wall and removal of the jejunostomy tube. Her abdomen was left open, and a vacuum-assisted closure (VAC) dressing was applied. The next day, she returned to the operating room for further debridement and replacement of the jejunostomy tube. The abdomen was closed and a VAC dressing applied over the wound. Over the next 5 days, her enteral feeding intake was noted to be minimal, so parenteral nutrition was suggested if enteral feeding could not be advanced. This was initiated the next day. After 10 days of combined enteral and parenteral nutrition (on day 37 post-injury), an enterocutaneous fistula was noted. Her VAC output ranged from 400 to 2000 mL/day during this period. She continued receiving tube feeding, but the formula was changed to an elemental-type feeding with minimal fat. She received on average 1600 mL of tube feeding per day with a fistula output of 150–400 mL/day. The parenteral nutrition was stopped, but on day 56 post-injury, her fistula output was 700 mL, and her stool output was noted to look like the tube feeding. Reducing substances in the stool were +3 indicating carbohydrate malabsorption. The tube feeding rate was reduced but not stopped, and she was restarted on parenteral nutrition. Ventilator management also was not going as planned, with a high minute ventilation, and therefore, on day 61 post-injury, the critical care team ordered an indirect calorimetry study to help optimize feeding and ventilator management.

FN was evaluated by the dietitian for feasibility to have an indirect calorimetry measurement. There were no air leaks, the inspired oxygen concentration was acceptable, and her other ventilator settings were stable. She was not being sedated, so the dietitian decided to wait until the next morning to conduct the test as it was felt that FN would more likely be in a resting state, and the chance of interruption before obtaining a valid study was felt to be lower. At 0500 on day 62 post-injury, patient's conditions were rechecked and found to be in order. The indirect calorimeter was prepared for measurement following manufacturer guidelines and the evidence-based measurement protocol published by AND was used [21]. The intent was to measure the patient for 30 min. However, at the 22nd minute, a surgical resident entered the room. Visual inspection of the data suggested to the dietitian that steady-state conditions had already been achieved, so he offered to end the test so that the resident could conduct his examination of the patient. The results of the indirect calorimetry test and other pertinent clinical data are shown in the box.

From an arterial blood gas and CO_2 data from the indirect calorimeter, FN was found to have a compensated respiratory alkalosis and a high dead space ventilation fraction (Vd/Vt) (59%). Dead space ventilation was calculated with the modified Bohr equation using the expired CO_2 measured by the indirect calorimeter [65]. A predictive equation for Vd/Vt that relies on blood gas data but does not require the indirect calorimetry data [65] also predicted a high dead space fraction (60%). Ventilatory efficiency (Ve/VCO_2), which requires no blood gas data, likewise was consistent with high dead space ($Ve/VCO_2 = 72$).

The metabolic application of the indirect calorimetry data revealed a hypermetabolic state (35%–50% increase in metabolic rate above that predicted by the Mifflin–St. Jeor equation, depending upon which body weight was used to calculate the Mifflin value). The measured resting metabolic rate was similar to the value predicted by the Penn State equation (1455 or 1550 kcal/day, again depending on which body weight is used) despite the potential for dead space ventilation to disturb the accuracy of the equation (i.e., to cause overprediction of expenditure because the minute ventilation is so high). Notably, FN's RQ was elevated, though not high enough to suspect measurement error [21]. The measured RQ was 1.21. Against a measured resting metabolic rate of 1500 kcal/day and additional energy expended on movement probably not raising the total expenditure beyond 1800 kcal/day, FN was receiving a total of 3065 kcal from the combination of tube feeding and parenteral nutrition. Of this total, 2300 kcal was nonprotein energy. She was experiencing substrate loss through the fistula, through the stool, and through the VAC, so her effective nutrient intake was probably substantially less than 3065 kcal, but this loss could not be quantified. Nearly all the nonprotein energy intake was from carbohydrate (93%) because of the choice of tube feeding and because of a nationwide shortage of intravenous lipid for the parenteral nutrition. Therefore, although RQ alone is generally not a reliable indicator of substrate utilization because of variability [21], in this case, it was consistent with other data suggesting that FN was being overfed. One other note on RQ is that the respiratory alkalosis could potentially have contributed to her high RQ also (removal of CO_2 from the bloodstream in excess of true CO_2 production).

The overall interpretation of the indirect calorimetry study was that the patient was being overfed, though the degree could not be determined because of unmeasurable losses from the GI tract. She was hypermetabolic but not outside of the degree predicted by the Penn State equation, and her high minute ventilation was a result of high dead space ventilation along with some overventilation leading to respiratory alkalosis. The dietitian recommended a reduction in tube feeding rate (given the volume of fistula output) and dextrose load in the parenteral nutrition, although total substrate load remained greater than energy expenditure in recognition of the substrate loss from the GI tract (total energy intake was reduced to 2200 kcal/day). The day after the indirect calorimetry study, the radiologist read her chest radiograph as being consistent with ARDS.

DATA

Clinical: Fistula output 1450 mL, stool output 1375 mL, VAC output 1000 mL. Arterial blood gas 7.45/28.0/83.0/19.5, end tidal CO_2 24 mm Hg, maximum body temperature 37.3°C, minute ventilation from mechanical ventilator 15.1 L/min, heart rate 98 beats/min. Body weight: 65 kg on admission, ±80 over the first 14 days of hospitalization, +75 kg over the next 30 days, ±70 kg thereafter. Weight for calculations 55 kg (assuming a 15% loss of tissue mass since admission) and 65 kg (admission weight).

Calorimetry results: VCO_2 240 mL/min (coefficient of variation 3%), VO_2 199 mL/min (coefficient of variation 5%), minute ventilation 17.5 L/min.

Calculated results: RQ 1.21, resting metabolic rate 1500 kcal/day, Ve/VCO_2 72, Vd/Vt (measured) 59%, Vd/Vt (estimated) 60%; PSU equation using 55 kg estimated current dry wt. 1455 kcal/day, PSU equation using 65 kg admission body weight 1550 kcal/day.

REFERENCES

1. Weijs PJM, Stapel SN, de Groot SDW, Driessen RH, de Jong E, Girbes ARJ, Strack van Schijndel RJN, Beishuizen A. Optimal protein and energy nutrition decreases mortality in mechanically ventilated, critically ill patients: A prospective observational cohort study. *J Parenter Enteral Nutr* 2012; 36: 60–68.
2. Heidegger CP, Graf S, Thibault R, Darmon P, Berger M, Pichard C. Supplemental parenteral nutrition (SPN) in intensive care unit (ICU) patients for optimal energy coverage: Improved clinical outcome. *Clin Nutr* 2011; 1(S): 2–3.
3. Heyland DK, Cahill NE, Day AG. Optimal amount of calories for critically ill patients: Depends on how you slice the cake! *Crit Care Med* 2011; 39: 2619–2626.
4. Alberda C, Gramlich L, Jones N, Jeejeebhoy K, Day AG, Dhaliwal R, Heyland DK. The relationship between nutritional intake and clinical outcomes in critically ill patients: Results of an international multicenter observational study. *Intensive Care Med* 2009; 35: 1728–1737.
5. Singer P, Anbar R, Cohen J, Shapiro H, Salita-Chesner M, Lev S, Grozouski E, Theilla M, Frishman S, Madar Z. The tight calorie control study (TICACOS): A prospective randomized clinical pilot study of nutrition support in critically ill patients. *Intensive Care Med* 2011; 37: 601–609.

6. American College of Chest Physicians/Society of Critical Care Medicine Consensus Conference Committee: American College of Chest Physicians/Society of Critical Care Medicine Consensus Conference. Definitions for sepsis and organ failure and guidelines for the use of innovative therapies in sepsis. *Crit Care Med* 1992; 20: 864.
7. Chrousos GP. The hypothalamic-pituitary-adrenal axis and immune-mediated inflammation. *N Eng J Med* 1995; 332: 1351.
8. Chiolero R, Revelly JP, Tappy L. Energy metabolism in sepsis and injury. *Nutrition* 1997; 13: 45S.
9. Long CL, Schaffel N, Geiger JW et al. Metabolic response to injury and illness: Estimation of energy and protein needs from indirect calorimetry and nitrogen balance. *J Parenter Enteral Nutr* 1979; 3: 452.
10. Frankenfield DC, Smith JS, Cooney RN et al. Relative association of fever and injury with hypermetabolism in critically ill patients. *Injury* 1997; 28: 617.
11. Raurich JM, Ibanez J, Marse P, Riera M, Homar X. Resting energy expenditure during mechanical ventilation and its relationship with type of lesion. *J Parenter Enteral Nutr* 2007; 31: 58–62.
12. Problete B, Romand JA, Pichard C et al. Metabolic effects of i.v. propacetamol, metamizol or external cooling in critically ill febrile sedated patients. *Brit J Anaesth* 1997; 78: 123.
13. Bardutzky J, Gergiadis D, Kollmar R et al. Energy expenditure in ischemic stroke patients treated with moderate hypothermia. *Intensive Care Med* 2004; 30: 151.
14. Saur J, Leweling H, Trinkmann F et al. Modification of the Harris-Benedict equation to predict the energy requirements of critically ill patients during mild therapeutic hypothermia. *In Vivo* 2008; 22: 143.
15. Badjatia N, Strongilis E, Gordon E et al. Metabolic impact of shivering during therapeutic temperature modulation: The bedside shivering assessment scale. *Stroke* 2008; 38: 3242.
16. Kress JP, O'Connor MF, Pohlman AE et al. Sedation of critically ill patients during mechanical ventilation. *Am J Respir Crit Care Med* 1996; 153: 1012.
17. Marik P, Kaufman D. The effects of neuromuscular paralysis on systemic and splanchnic oxygen utilization in mechanically ventilated patients. *Chest* 1996; 109: 1038.
18. Frankenfield DC, Wiles CE, Bagley S et al. Relationship between resting and total energy expenditure in injured and septic patients. *Crit Care Med* 1994; 22: 1796.
19. Weissman C, Kemper M, Damask MC et al. Effect of routine intensive care interactions on metabolic rate. *Chest* 1984; 86: 815.
20. Swinamer DL, Phang PT, Jones RL et al. Twenty-four hour energy expenditure in critically ill patients. *Crit Care Med* 1987; 15: 637.
21. Compher C, Frankenfield DC, Keim N et al. Best practice methods to apply to measurement of resting metabolic rate in adults: A systematic review. *J Am Diet Assoc* 2006; 106: 881.
22. Garrel DR, de Jonge L. Intragastric vs. oral feeding: Effect on the thermogenic response to feeding in lean and obese subjects. *Am J Clin Nutr* 1994; 59: 971.
23. Heymsfield SB, Hill JO, Evert M et al. Energy expenditure during continuous intragastric infusion of fuel. *Am J Clin Nutr* 1987; 45: 526.
24. Frankenfield DC, Ashcraft CM. Description and prediction of resting metabolic rate after stroke and traumatic brain injury. *Nutrition* 2012; 28: 906.
25. Frankenfield DC, Schubert A, Alam S et al. Validation study of predictive equations for resting metabolic rate in critically ill patients. *J Parenter Enteral Nutr* 2009; 33: 27.
26. Alves VGF, da Rocha EEM, Gonzalez MC et al. Assessment of resting energy expenditure of obese patients: Comparison of indirect calorimetry with formulae. *Clin Nutr* 2009; 28: 299.
27. Miles JM. Energy expenditure in hospitalized patients: Implications for nutritional support. *Mayo Clin Proc* 2006; 81: 809.
28. Segal KR, Edano A, Blando L et al. Comparison of thermic effects of constant and relative caloric loads in lean and obese men. *Am J Clin Nutr* 1990; 51: 14.
29. Jeevanandam M, Young DH, Schiller WR. Obesity and the metabolic response to severe multiple trauma in man. *J Clin Invest* 1991; 87: 262.
30. Frankenfield DC, Cooney RN, Smith JS et al. Age-related differences in the metabolic response to injury. *J Trauma* 2000; 48: 49.
31. Muller MJ, Bosy-Westphal A, Kutzner D et al. Metabolically active components of fat-free mass and resting energy expenditure in humans: Recent lessons from imaging technologies. *Obes Rev* 2002; 3: 113.
32. Javed F, He Q, Davidson LE et al. Brain and high metabolic rate organ mass: Contributions to resting energy expenditure beyond fat-free mass. *Am J Clin Nutr* 2010; 91: 907.
33. Frankenfield DC. Validation of a metabolic rate equation in older obese critically ill people. *J Parenter Enteral Nutr* 2011; 35: 264.

34. Frankenfield DC, Ashcraft CM, Galvan DA. Prediction of resting metabolic rate in critically ill patients at the extremes of body mass index. *J Parenter Enteral Nutr*. 2013; 37: 361–367.
35. Frankenfield DC, Rowe WA, Cooney RN et al. Limits of body mass index to detect obesity and predict body composition. *Nutrition* 2001; 17: 26.
36. Hoffer LJ. Protein and energy provision in critical illness. *Am J Clin Nutr* 2003; 78: 906.
37. Johnson RE, Chernoff R. Geriatrics. In: Matarese LE, Gottschlich MM (eds.), *Contemporary Nutrition Support Practice: A Clinical Guide*, 2nd edn., Vol. 9. Philadelphia, PA: WB Saunders; 2002, p. 376.
38. Ravussin E, Lillioja S, Anderson TE et al. Determinants of 24-hour energy expenditure in man. *J Clin Invest* 1986; 78: 1568.
39. Frankenfield DC, Smith JS, Cooney RN. Accelerated nitrogen loss after traumatic injury is not attenuated by achievement of nitrogen balance. *J Parenter Enteral Nutr* 1997; 21: 324.
40. Dickerson RN, Rosato EF, Mullen JL. Net protein anabolism with hypocaloric parenteral nutrition in obese stressed patients. *Am J Clin Nutr* 1986; 44: 747.
41. Burge JC, Goon A, Choban PS et al. Efficacy of hypocaloric total parenteral nutrition in hospitalized obese patients: A prospective, double-blind randomized trial. *J Parenter Enteral Nutr* 1994; 18: 203.
42. Dickerson RN, Boschert KJ, Kudsk KA et al. Hypocaloric enteral tube feeding in critically ill obese patients. *Nutrition* 2002; 18: 241.
43. Kutsogiannis J, Alberda C, Gramlich L et al. Early use of supplemental parenteral nutrition in critically ill patients: Results of an international multicenter observational study. *Crit Care Med* 2011; 39: 2691.
44. Barstow TJ, Cooper DM, Sobel E et al. Influence of increased metabolic rate on ^{13}C bicarbonate washout kinetics. *Am J Physiol* 1990; 259: R163.
45. Headley JM. Indirect calorimetry: A trend toward continuous metabolic assessment. *AACN J* 2003; 14: 155.
46. Turney SZ, McCaslan TC, Cowley RA. The continuous measurement of pulmonary gas exchange and mechanics. *Ann Thorac Surg* 1972; 13: 229.
47. Brandi LS, Bertolini R, Santini L et al. Effects of ventilator resetting on indirect calorimeter measurement in the critically ill surgical patient. *Crit Care Med* 1999; 27: 531.
48. Frankenfield DC, Sarson GY, Cooney RN et al. Validation of a five minute steady state indirect calorimetry protocol for resting energy expenditure in critically ill patients. *J Am Coll Nutr* 1996; 15: 397.
49. Petros S, Engelmann L. Validity of an abbreviated indirect calorimetry protocol for measurement of resting energy expenditure in mechanically ventilated and spontaneously breathing critically ill patients. *Intensive Care Med* 2001; 27: 1164.
50. Frankenfield DC, Ashcraft CM, Galvan DA. Longitudinal prediction of metabolic rate in critically ill patients. *J Parenter Enteral Nutr*. 2012; 36: 700–712.
51. McClave SA, Lowen CC, Kleber MJ et al. Clinical use of the respiratory quotient obtained from indirect calorimetry. *J Parenter Enteral Nutr* 2003; 27: 21.
52. Liusuwan Monotak RA, Palmieri TL, Greenhalgh DG. The respiratory quotient has little value in evaluating the state of feeding in burn patients. *J Burn Care Res* 2008; 29: 655.
53. Harris JA, Benedict FG. *A Biometric Study of Basal Metabolism in Man*. Publication No. 279. Washington, DC: Carnegie Institute; 1919.
54. Swinamer DL, Grace MG, Hamilton SM et al. Predictive equation for assessing energy expenditure in mechanically ventilated critically ill patients. *Crit Care Med* 1990; 18: 657.
55. Ireton-Jones CS, Turner WW, Liepa GU et al. Equations for estimation of energy expenditures of patients with burns with special reference to ventilatory status. *J Burn Care Rehab* 1992; 13: 330.
56. Ireton-Jones CS, Jones JD. Why use predictive equations for energy expenditure assessment? *J Am Diet Assoc* 1997; 97: A-44.
57. Frankenfield DC, Omert LA, Badellino MM et al. Correlation between measured energy expenditure and clinically obtained variables in trauma and sepsis patients. *J Parenter Enteral Nutr* 1994; 18: 393.
58. Frankenfield DC. Energy dynamics. In: Matarese LE, Gottschlich MM (eds.), *Contemporary Nutrition Support Practice: A Clinical Guide*, 2nd edn. Philadelphia, PA: WB Saunders; 2003, p. 89.
59. Frankenfield DC, Rowe WA, Smith JS et al. Validation of several established equations for resting metabolic rate in obese and nonobese people. *J Am Diet Assoc* 2003; 103: 1152.
60. Frankenfield DC, Smith JS, Cooney RN. Validation of two approaches to predicting resting metabolic rate in critically ill patients. *J Parenter Enteral Nutr* 2004; 28: 259.
61. Faisy C, Guerot E, Diehl JL et al. Assessment of resting energy expenditure in mechanically ventilated patients. *Am J Clin Nutr* 2003; 78: 241.

62. Flancbaum L, Choban PS, Sambucco S et al. Comparison of indirect calorimetry, the Fick method, and prediction equations in estimating the energy requirements of critically ill patients. *Am J Clin Nutr* 1999; 69: 461.
63. MacDonald A, Hildebrandt L. Comparison of formulaic equations to determine energy expenditure in the critically ill patient. *Nutrition* 2003; 19: 233.
64. Savard JF, Faisy G, Lerolle N et al. Validation of a predictive method for assessment of resting energy expenditure in medical mechanically ventilated patients. *Crit Care Med* 2008; 36: 1175.
65. Frankenfield DC, Alam S, Bekteshi E, Vender RL. Predicting dead space ventilation in critically ill patients using clinically available data. *Crit Care Med* 2012; 38: 288–291.

7 Macronutrient Requirements
Carbohydrate, Protein, and Fat

Michael D. Taylor, Kavitha Krishnan, Jill Barsa, and Kendra Glassman Perkey

CONTENTS

INTRODUCTION

The metabolic response to critical illness is characterized by hypermetabolism, hyperglycemia, increased lipolysis, and net protein catabolism [1]. Skeletal muscle is broken down, and the amino acids are used for gluconeogenesis and protein synthesis. Reprioritization of hepatic protein synthesis occurs resulting in synthesis of positive acute phase proteins (e.g., C-reactive protein) and decreased synthesis of negative acute phase proteins (e.g., prealbumin, albumin) [2]. Additionally, bed rest and suboptimal nutrient intake contribute to depletion of lean body mass (see Chapter 1). Nutritional support in the critically ill should occur early, be tailored to the patient's medical condition, nutritional status, and available route of administration; provide nutrients compatible with current metabolism while avoiding complications; and improve patient outcomes [3]. This chapter reviews the suggested macronutrient (carbohydrates, protein, and lipids) composition of nutritional support provided to critically ill patients.

CARBOHYDRATES

Carbohydrates, organic compounds of carbon, hydrogen, and oxygen in the ratio of C:H:O as 1:2:1, should provide approximately 45%–65% of our daily energy [4]. Upon oxidation, carbohydrates yield 4 kilocalories per gram (kcal/g); intravenous (IV) dextrose monohydrate provides 3.4 kcal/g [4]. Carbohydrates are constituents of DNA and RNA, coenzymes, glycoproteins, and glycolipids. The brain and red and white blood cells, to a large extent, obligate glucose [4].

Carbohydrate Requirements

Approximately 120 g/day of exogenous glucose is necessary to maintain central nervous system function [5,6]. Optimal carbohydrate delivery should be at a level to allow maximal protein sparing while minimizing hyperglycemia [7]. The amount of carbohydrate that can be safely provided during critical illness is a direct function of the patient's oxidative capacity. The maximal glucose oxidation rate is 4–7 mg/kg/min, or roughly 400–700 g/day in a 70 kg person [4]. In a hypermetabolic patient, a large portion of oxidized glucose is derived from amino acid substrates via gluconeogenesis yielding up to 2–3 mg/kg/min of glucose. Exogenous insulin delivery can increase cellular glucose uptake in critically ill patients; however, it is relatively ineffective in improving glucose oxidation. Providing exogenous glucose does little to suppress this endogenous glucose production, therefore providing excessive exogenous glucose stimulates hyperglycemia and hyperinsulinemia. The maximum rate suggested for carbohydrate infusion in the critically ill patients is 4–5 mg/kg/min [8,9] and 2.5–4.0 mg/kg/min for patients with diabetes, with stress hyperglycemia, or receiving steroid therapy (Table 7.1) [9]. Providing glucose at a rate of 3–4 mg/kg/min or approximately 50%–60% of total energy requirements in critically ill patients as well as administering insulin to maintain normal glycemia is recommended [4]. For patients at risk for refeeding syndrome, it is a safe recommendation to provide 100–150 g dextrose/day [4,9]. Measurement of respiratory quotient (RQ) by indirect calorimetry can provide feedback on macronutrient utilization. RQ >1 reflects lipogenesis and excess carbohydrate administration.

During critical illness, underfeeding energy requirements leads to tissue catabolism (e.g., adipose, muscle) liberating carbon to enter into the gluconeogenic pathway to assist the body's need for glucose. Unlike adipose tissue, muscle tissue is not considered a stored body fuel, making protein catabolism detrimental leading to decreased skeletal muscle mass, visceral proteins, and structural and metabolically active proteins of the body [4]. This can lend to poor wound healing, impaired immune response, and physiologic exhaustion contributing to total body failure.

Overfeeding carbohydrates can result in hypercapnia, hyperglycemia, and fatty infiltration of the liver [8]. Hyperglycemia as a result of overfeeding carbohydrates may further result in electrolyte imbalances, mainly potassium, due to hyperinsulinemia that leads to a shift of this electrolyte intracellularly. Respiratory distress [10], hypercapnia during weaning [11], and respiratory failure [12] have been reported in patients receiving excessive carbohydrate loads in parenteral nutrition (PN). Carbon dioxide (CO_2) retention, increased minute ventilation, difficulty

TABLE 7.1
Calculating Dextrose Infusion Rates

To calculate the suggested maximum dextrose:
4 mg/kg/min × weight (kg) × 1440 (min/24 h) ÷ 1000
For example,
How many grams of dextrose should be infused over 24 h at a rate of 4 mg/kg/min for a 72 kg patient?
4 mg/kg/min × 72 kg × 1440 min ÷ 1000 = 414 g dextrose/day

To calculate the dextrose infusion rate:
g dextrose ÷ weight (kg) ÷ 1440 (min/24 h) × 1000 = dextrose mg/kg/min
For example,
What is the dextrose infusion rate for a 72 kg patient receiving 400 g dextrose daily?
400 g dextrose ÷ 72 kg ÷ 1440 × 1000 = 3.85 mg/kg/min

weaning from the ventilator, acute respiratory acidosis or metabolic alkalosis, and a RQ greater than 1 may indicate overfeeding of carbohydrate or total calories [8]. The reported low sensitivity and specificity of RQ may limit its use as an indicator of over- and underfeeding [13]. A thorough review of the patient's condition, nutritional regimen, and response to therapy must be performed frequently to assure appropriate feeding. When overfeeding is suspected, a reduction in carbohydrate or total caloric intake may prevent elevated CO_2 production and respiratory compromise [14]. Strategies to prevent and treat complications associated with overfeeding macronutrients are shown in Table 7.2.

While hyperglycemia may indicate overfeeding, critically ill patients may experience hyperglycemia as a result of factors other than nutrition [8]. Blood glucose should be monitored closely and controlled with exogenous insulin as needed. The presence of hyperglycemia may be an independent risk factor for the development of infection, and the use of intensive insulin therapy has been shown to reduce morbidity and mortality in surgical patients [15,16]. The amount of glucose control has been an area of interest as aggressive glycemic control (<110 mg/dL) leading to hypoglycemia is associated with adverse patient outcomes to include mortality. Maintaining blood glucose levels between 140 and 180 mg/dL is currently recommended based on the available research [17].

PROTEIN

Proteins are the most abundant organic molecules in cells and are fundamental to cell structure and function. Proteins serve many roles in the body including the maintenance and growth of body tissues, enzymes, hormones, and antibodies and the synthesis of nucleic acids and genetic material. Proteins are also used for transporting substances such as lipids, vitamins, minerals, albumin, and oxygen throughout the body. Blood proteins are essential in maintaining and regulating fluid balance between blood and tissues through oncotic pressure. Each gram of protein will produce 4 kcal of energy [18].

Protein Requirements

Protein needs are elevated in critical illness due to the increased protein loss associated with the stress response. Although providing optimal protein during critical illness cannot reverse the catabolic process, protein synthetic rate is responsive to amino acid provision [19]. In the 2009 Consensus statement issued jointly by the Society of Critical Care Medicine (SCCM) and the American Society for Parenteral and Enteral Nutrition (ASPEN) guidelines and recommendations for metabolically stressed patients with body mass index (BMI) <30, protein requirements should be in the range of 1.2–2.0 g/kg actual body weight per day [20]. Patients with severe sepsis and burns often require up to 2.5–3.0 g/kg protein per day [18,21]. Providing burn patients high-protein regimens improves nitrogen balance [22,23], restores body weight and muscle function [24], enhances immune function (fewer bacteremic and antibiotic days), and increases survival [25] (see Chapter 24). Evidence suggests that protein requirements in the critically ill obese patient are greater than in the nonobese. Protein requirements are estimated to be >2.0 g/kg ideal body weight (IBW)/day for classes I and II obesity and >2.5 g/kg/day for class III [26] (see Chapter 7).

Protein is necessary for the synthesis of enzymes involved in wound healing, proliferation of cells and collagen, and formation of connective tissue. Optimal wound healing requires increased energy and protein. Protein recommendations are 1.25–1.5 g/kg [27,28] for those with chronic wounds and for those with more than one wound or a stage III to IV pressure ulcer may require up to 2.0 g/kg/day [28,29]. Protein losses via open and draining wounds can add to the protein needs. Protein losses from large open wounds depend on the amount of drainage, and

TABLE 7.2
Indicators of Overfeeding, Characteristics of Patients at Risk, and Considerations for Monitoring and Intervention

Complication with Indicator	Patients at Risk	Monitoring and Intervention
Azotemia		
Progressively increasing blood urea nitrogen (BUN) level (30 mg/dL)	Patients ≥65 years old. Patients given >2 g protein/kg.	Check creatinine clearance; serum creatinine may be less than 2 mg/dL despite renal impairment. Ratio of BUN to creatinine greater than 15 suggests abnormal renal function and/or excessive protein intake, muscle catabolism, or dehydration. Provide adequate energy intake and monitor hydration. Readjust protein as needed.
Fat-overload syndrome		
Respiratory distress Sudden hypertriglyceridemia Prolonged prothrombin and partial thromboplastin times Bleeding from orifices Elevated bilirubin level	Patients receiving more than 3 g lipid/kg body weight/day. Account for lipid in medications. Patients with elevated C-reactive protein (acute phase response and heightened cytokine production).	Symptoms may arise within a few days of initiating IVLE or after months of tolerance. Monitor triglyceride level; hold lipids when triglyceride is >300–400 mg/dL. Monitor respiratory, hematologic, and hepatic systems. Symptoms abate as lipemia resolves.
Hepatic steatosis		
Hepatomegaly with/without right-upper quadrant pain or tenderness Abnormal, high-fat liver biopsy	Patients receiving high-carbohydrate, very-low-fat PN.	Liver function tests do not correlate well with hepatic steatosis. Monitor glucose and triglyceride levels and actual feeding. Adjust energy or carbohydrate intake as needed; use mixed fuel feedings that include fat daily. Hepatic steatosis is rarely confirmed.
Hypercapnia		
Elevated $PaCO_2$ Increased minute ventilation; difficulty in weaning from ventilator Acute respiratory acidosis: $PaCO_2 >$ 40 mm Hg and pH < 7.40 Acute metabolic alkalosis: $PaCO_2$ 50–60 mm Hg, serum bicarbonate > 24 mmol/L, and pH > 7.40	Patients with poor ventilatory status. Indirect calorimetry is preferred to estimate energy needs, especially for patients with unusual body sizes and for the elderly.	The RQ is an insensitive indicator of overfeeding, remaining less than 1.0 even with excessive respiratory workload and distress. Adjustments in ventilation may mask elevated CO_2 production. Decrease energy intake, particularly from dextrose; add lipid daily. Monitor the patient's response ($PaCO_2$, blood pH) to changes in feeding.
Hyperglycemia		
Glucose > 200 mg/dL Insulin administration	Patients with systemic inflammatory response syndrome, with pancreatitis, on steroids or peritoneal dialysis containing dextrose. Infusing more than 4 mg/kg/min.	Monitor hydration, blood glucose level, insulin administration, and actual dextrose feeding. Replace some energy from dextrose with energy from lipid.

(Continued)

TABLE 7.2 (*Continued*)
Indicators of Overfeeding, Characteristics of Patients at Risk, and Considerations for Monitoring and Intervention

Complication with Indicator	Patients at Risk	Monitoring and Intervention
Hyperglycemic hyperosmolar nonketotic syndrome		
Glucose level > 600 mg/dL Intravascular dehydration: that is, plasma level > 350 mOsm/L Fever Tachycardia, hypotension	Patients receiving high carbohydrate loads followed by prolonged osmotic diuresis; patients with severe burns, reduced renal function, or pancreatitis; or patients that underwent cardiopulmonary bypass or are elderly with type 2 diabetes.	Monitor central venous pressure or pulmonary capillary wedge pressure. Restore intravascular volume using 0.9% sodium chloride until vital signs stabilize, then 0.45% sodium chloride. Bolus of 10–15 U insulin, then 0.1 U/kg/h. When glucose level is <300 mg/dL, use 5% dextrose in water and 0.45% sodium chloride, and decrease insulin. Manage potassium and other electrolytes.
Hypertonic dehydration		
Hypernatremia Elevated hematocrit Azotemia	Tube-feeding with a high-protein formula, loss of large amounts of fluid, and elderly age increase risk.	Reduce sodium and protein intake; use isotonic feeding. Provide rehydration over 24–48 h or longer. Treatment may require IV solutions. Avoid water intoxication. Replete minerals as needed, especially after the extracellular space has expanded.
Hypertriglyceridemia		
Triglyceride > 300 mg/dL	Patients receiving lipid-based drugs (propofol > 6 mg/kg/h; lipid loads > 2 g/kg/day) or patients with infections, particularly gram-negative sepsis.	If triglyceride level rises over 300–400 mg/dL, then restrict lipids (e.g., provide 500 mL 10% emulsion at ≤21 mL/h once or twice per week). If triglyceride level rises over 500 mg/dL, then hold infusions and monitor essential fatty acid status. Avoid overfeeding energy, fat, and dextrose.
Metabolic acidosis		
Blood pH < 7.35 Bicarbonate < 21 mEq/L	Patients receiving formulas with low ratios of energy to nitrogen (90:1). Ability to deal with acid loads is diminished in the elderly.	Monitor hydration, renal function, pH, bicarbonate, potassium, and BUN. Reduce protein intake and follow the patient's response.
Refeeding syndrome		
Hypophosphatemia Acute respiratory failure Arterial hypotension Tachycardia	Patients with chronic malnutrition and/or extended nil per os without nutritional support are at risk.	Monitor cardiac function. Decrease total energy and dextrose; adjust fluids for appropriate hydration. Monitor minerals in blood and urine. Replete phosphorus, magnesium, and potassium as needed.

Source: Adapted from Klein, C.J. et al., *J. Am. Diet. Assoc.*, 98, 795, 1998.

protein content can be estimated as approximately 2.9 g protein/dL of exudate [30]. The open abdomen represents a significant source of protein/nitrogen loss in the critically ill, and failure to account for these additional losses may lead to underfeeding and inadequate nutrition support with a direct effect on patient outcome. An estimate of 2–4 g of nitrogen per liter of abdominal fluid output should be included in the nitrogen balance calculations of any patient with an open abdomen [31,32]. Mean total protein loss was 25 ± 17 g/day for open abdomens and 8 ± 5 g/day for soft tissue wounds [32]. The rate of protein loss from wounds is similar to the presently assumed insensible loss rate of 12–25 g/day [32]. Freise found that the single most reliable indicator of appropriate nutrition support for wound healing was timely and adequate wound closure [33].

Declining kidney function produces a buildup of nitrogenous waste, an imbalance of electrolytes, accumulation of extracellular fluid (ECF), and acid–base disturbances [34]. Acute kidney injury (AKI) affects approximately 10%–30% of critically ill patients [35] with 5%–10% requiring some form of renal replacement therapy. All methods of dialysis cause activation of protein catabolism through loss of amino acids in the effluent, release of cytokines causing a chronic inflammatory state, and chronic blood loss, but these losses are seen as negligible when compared with what is already altered in critical illness [36]. In addition to the hypercatabolic rate, methods of continuous renal replacement therapy (CRRT) that use convection show higher protein losses in the effluent when compared to those using diffusion. Approximately 10%–17% of centrally infused protein is lost and needs to be considered when calculating supplementation [34]. Ongoing assessment of adequacy of protein provision should be performed. One prospective trial suggested that intake up to 2.5 g/protein/kg may be needed to achieve positive nitrogen balance [37] (see Chapter 28).

Many clinicians believe that higher amounts of protein (2.0–2.5 g/kg/day) may be preferable for most critically ill patients; however, limited amount and poor quality of the evidence preclude such conclusions or clinical recommendations. At the present time, most critically ill adults receive less than half of the most common current recommendation, 1.5 g/kg/day, for the first week or longer of their stay in an intensive care unit [38]. Hoffer and Bistrian concluded, after their systematic and narrative review of appropriate protein in critical illness, that there is still need for well-designed clinical trials to identify appropriate levels of protein provision in critical illness [38] (Table 7.3).

Serum-negative acute phase proteins (e.g., albumin, prealbumin) can be difficult to interpret in the critically ill and may not be reflective of the adequacy of nutritional support [2,39]. Monitoring negative acute phase proteins during critical illness lends insight into the severity of illness, but not necessarily a good measure of nutrition support outcomes [39]. Nitrogen balance studies can be used to determine protein requirements or to assess the adequacy of current nutrient intake. A nitrogen balance that is positive 2–4 would indicate anabolism. Monitoring trends in nitrogen balance is more useful than a single measurement, and the trends should reflect improvement as the patient recovers from their illness. Other parameters that can be monitored to determine adequacy of protein provision is wound healing and functional status.

TABLE 7.3
Suggested Protein Guidelines in Adult Hospitalized Patients

Clinical Condition	Protein Requirement
Moderate stress (most ICU patients)	1.5–2.0 g/kg
Severe obesity	2.0–2.5 g/kg IBW
Severe stress, catabolic, burns	2.0–2.5 g/kg
Hemodialysis, CRRT	2.0–2.5 g/kg
Wounds	1.5–2.5 g/kg

LIPIDS

Fat serves as a source of calories (9 cal/g) and thus a major fuel source [40]. Intravenous lipid emulsions (IVLEs) contain an emulsifier that contributes additional calories and therefore provides 10 cal/g. Fatty acids perform a wide variety of functions in the body including providing insulation and cushion to organs and structure to cell membranes and function as a lubricant for body surfaces, joints, and mucous membranes [40]. Fat is also needed for fat-soluble vitamin digestion and absorption and provides essential fatty acids [40]. Fatty acid metabolites are important mediators for a variety of metabolic processes. Metabolism of membrane phospholipids produces some of the mediators of the systemic inflammatory response syndrome. Lipoproteins appear to play a role in the binding and processing of bacterial endotoxins [41–43]. In critical illness, alterations in lipid metabolism occur. Changes in serum lipid and lipoprotein concentration may have prognostic value in critically ill patients [44–46]. It is increasingly recognized that lipids are not merely a source of calories but that they play an important role in the pharmaconutritional support of the critically ill patient [47,48].

Fat Requirements

There is no defined level of adequate intake, recommended dietary allowance, or tolerable upper intake level; however, an acceptable macronutrient distribution range has been estimated for total fat—it is 20%–35% of total energy intake [49]. The minimum amount of fat needed is 2%–4% of total calories for the essential fatty acids, alpha-linolenic and linoleic acid [3]. When used as a source of calories, generally 15%–30% of total calories can be provided as fat [3,40]. The absolute maximum amount of fat is suggested to be no more than 2.5 g/kg/day [1] or less than 60% of total calories. Intravenous fat emulsions should not exceed 1 g/kg/day in critically ill patients [1,40]. The infusion rate for IVLEs is also important to consider and should not exceed 0.11 g/kg/h to avoid metabolic complications [1]. Contraindications to the use of IVLE include egg allergy and hypertriglyceridemia. Provision of IVLE is generally considered safe as long as triglyceride concentrations are less than 400 mg/dL [1]. There is no strong evidence to suggest a benefit in restricting IVLE for patients with low platelet counts.

Providing insufficient amounts of lipids over time can result in an essential fatty acid deficiency (EFAD). The timing of EFAD is variable and dependent on nutritional status, disease state, and age of the patient. In general, the majority of hospitalized patients who receive no dietary fat develop biochemical evidence of EFAD within 4 weeks. Physical signs and symptoms of an EFAD include alterations in platelet function, hair loss, poor wound healing, and dry, scaly skin unresponsive to water miscible creams. A suspected EFAD can be confirmed by obtaining a triene-to-tetraene ratio that is greater than 0.4. For prevention of EFAD, 2%–4% total daily calorie needs should come from fat (1%–2% from linoleic and 0.5% from alpha-linolenic acid) [50].

Provision of excessive amounts of fat can lead to hypertriglyceridemia and fat overload (Table 7.2). Manifestations of fat overload include respiratory distress, coagulopathies, abnormal liver function tests, and impaired reticuloendothelial system (RES) function [8]. Overfeeding of IVLE may also be associated with immunosuppression as a result of the breakdown of linoleic acid (an omega-6 polyunsaturated fatty acid) to pro-inflammatory eicosanoids [40]. Battistella et al. [51] found that IVLE provided in the early post injury period resulted in greater susceptibility to infection, prolonged pulmonary failure, and delayed recovery. However, patients receiving the lipid-free TPN regimen did not have the calories replaced with dextrose. Therefore, it was unclear if these results were related to the absence of IVLE or the hypocaloric regimen. Limiting total fat calories to 15%–30% should reduce complications related to overfeeding of fat, and monitoring triglyceride clearance is recommended.

TABLE 7.4
Macronutrient Requirements in the Critically Ill

Macronutrient	Minimum Requirement	Maximum Requirement	% of Total Calories
Carbohydrate	100–150 g/day	<4 mg/kg/min	30%–70%
Protein	1 g/kg body weight	2 g/kg body weight	20%–25%
Fat	2%–4% total calories	<1 g fat/kg/day	15%–30%

Further complicating nutrition regimens is the use of propofol (Diprivan™) for sedation in the critically ill population. Propofol is provided in a 10% lipid emulsion and is a calorie source providing 1.1 cal/mL. Calories delivered from propofol should be included in calculations of total nutrient and fat intake with adjustments to the nutrition regimen made if needed. Adjustments may include a reduction in the rate of total calories for tube-fed patients or a reduction in the amount of IVLE provided with TPN. In some cases, the high amounts of propofol given may negate the need for additional IVLE (Table 7.4) [52].

SUMMARY

Nutritional support in the critically ill is aimed at supporting the patient through recovery, providing macronutrient substrates appropriate for metabolic alterations, and reducing potential complications associated with nutritional support. Provision of macronutrients in the amounts suggested (Table 7.4) will help to achieve outcome goals and avoid complications of under- or overfeeding in critically ill patients.

CASE STUDIES

CASE STUDY 1

A 65-year-old man with short bowel syndrome (secondary to Crohn's disease) is admitted to the hospital for elective cardiac surgery. He uses a premixed parenteral formula containing 15% dextrose and 7.5% amino acids infusing at 70 mL/h plus 250 mL of 20% IVLE. The total amount of macronutrients is calculated as follows:

To calculate dextrose grams and carbohydrate calories:

70 mL/h × 24 h = 1680 mL
1680 mL × 0.15 = 252 g dextrose
252 g dextrose × 3.4 cal/g = 857 cal from dextrose

To calculate amino acid grams and protein calories:

1680 mL × 0.075 = 126 g amino acid
126 g amino acid × 4 cal/g = 504 cal from amino acid

To calculate lipid calories:

250 mL × 2 cal/mL = 500 cal
Total calories = 857 dextrose calories + 504 amino acid calories + 500 lipid calories = 1861 cal

CASE STUDY 2

A 40-year-old man is admitted with short bowel obstruction. He had a ventral hernia repair 3 weeks ago. Since then, he has been having poor appetite and 8 lb weight loss. His height is 5′8 and current weight 160 lb (72 kg). He continues to have high outputs from a nasogastric tube.

The surgical team plans to initiate PN and asks the nutrition support clinician to calculate a formula to meet the patient's needs, providing 2200 mL daily total (excluding the IV lipid volume).

The patient's nutritional needs were estimated:

25 cal/kg current weight = 1800 cal/day
1.5 g protein/kg current weight = 108 g protein/day

The following steps can be used to calculate TPN formulation to meet the patient's macronutrient needs:

1. Calculate the percentage of calories to be delivered as fat and determine the amount of IVLE needed:
   To provide 20% calories as fat:
   1800 cal × 0.20 fat = 360 cal as fat
   360 cal as fat/2 cal = 180 mL 20% IVLE
2. Calculate final concentration of amino acids:
   108 g protein ÷ 2200 mL = 0.04 or 4% amino acids
   108 g protein × 4 cal/g = 432 protein calories
3. Calculate calories left to provide as dextrose:
   360 fat calories + 432 protein calories = 792 cal
   1800 total calories – 792 cal = 1008 cal
4. Calculate final concentration of dextrose needed to meet calorie needs:
   1008 dextrose calories ÷ 3.4 cal/g = 296 g dextrose
   296 g dextrose ÷ 2200 mL = 0.134 or 13.4% dextrose
   The final TPN solution would be for 13.4% dextrose and 4% amino acids, with 180 mL 20% IVLE. This would be started at one-half of goal rate and advanced in increments toward the goal of 92 mL/h if serum glucose and electrolytes remain well controlled.

CASE STUDY 3

The patient described earlier is now intubated and receiving propofol at the rate of 20 mL/h for sedation. How would you reformulate a TPN solution to avoid overfeeding fat and total calories?

The following steps can be used to calculate a TPN formulation to meet the patient's calorie and macronutrient needs:

1. Calculate fat calories from propofol:
   20 mL/h × 24 h/day = 480 mL propofol
   480 mL propofol × 1.1 cal/mL = 528 cal from fat
2. Calculate the final concentration of amino acids:
   108 g protein ÷ 2200 mL = 0.04 or 4% amino acids
   108 g protein × 4 cal/g = 432 protein calories
3. Calculate calories left to provide as dextrose:
   528 fat calories + 432 protein calories = 960 cal
   1800 cal – 960 cal = 840 cal as dextrose
4. Calculate final concentration of dextrose needed to meet calorie needs:
   840 dextrose calories ÷ 3.4 cal/g = 247 g dextrose
   247 g ÷ 2200 mL = 0.11% or 11% dextrose
   The TPN solution could be changed to 92 mL/h with 11% dextrose and 4% amino acids. The IVLE will be held while propofol was being given to avoid providing excess lipid and calories.

CASE STUDY 4

A 60-year-old male is status post abdominal aortic aneurysm repair. He is currently intubated and not tolerating enteral feeds. He is 5′7 and weighs 260 lb. His BMI is 40.7 kg/m^2. The nutrition support clinician is asked to calculate a TPN formula to meet the patient's needs with 2000 mL daily.

The patient's nutritional needs were estimated:

14 cal/kg current weight = 14 cal/kg × 118 kg = 1652 cal/day
2 g protein/kg ideal body weight = 2 g protein × 67 kg = 134 g protein/day
(Calorie and protein requirements were based on 2009 Guidelines for the Provision and Assessment of Nutrition Support Therapy in the Adult Critically Ill Patient: Society of Critical Care Medicine and ASPEN [20].)

The following steps can be used to calculate TPN formulation to meet the patient's macronutrient needs:

1. Calculate the percentage of calories to be delivered as fat and determine the amount of IVLE needed:
   To provide 20% calories as fat:
   1652 cal × 0.20 fat = 330 cal as fat
   330 fat calories ÷ 2 cal/mL = 165 mL 20% IVLE
2. Calculate final concentration of amino acids:
   134 g protein ÷ 2000 mL = 0.067% or 6.7% amino acids
   134 g protein × 4 cal/g = 536 protein calories
3. Calculate calories left to provide as dextrose:
   330 fat calories + 536 protein calories = 866 cal
   1652 total calories – 866 cal = 786 cal
4. Calculate final concentration of dextrose needed to meet calorie needs:
   786 dextrose calories ÷ 3.4 cal/g = 231 g dextrose
   231 g dextrose ÷ 2000 mL = 0.115% or 11.5% dextrose
   The final TPN solution is 11.5% dextrose and 6.7% amino acids, with 165 mL 20% IVLE. This can be started at one-half of goal rate and advanced incrementally toward the goal of 83 mL/h if serum glucose and electrolytes remain well controlled.

REFERENCES

1. Mirtallo J, Canada T, Johnson D, Kumpf V, Petersen C, Sacks G, Seres D, Guenter P. Task force for the revision of safe practice for parenteral nutrition. *JPEN J Parenter Enteral Nutr.*, 2004; 28S: S52–S57.
2. Gabay C, Kushner I. Acute-phase proteins and other systemic responses to inflammation. *N Engl J Med.*, 1999; 340: 448–454.
3. Cerra FB, Benitez MR, Blackburn GL et al. Applied nutrition in ICU patients. A consensus statement of the American college of chest physicians. *Chest*, 1997; 111: 769–778.
4. Ling P, McCowen KC. Carbohydrates. In: Gottschlich MM (ed.), *The Science and Practice of Nutrition Support—A Case-Based Core Curriculum*. A.S.P.E.N, Silver Spring, MD, 2007, pp. 33–47.
5. Fredstrom S. Carbohydrate. In: Matarese LM, Gottschlich MM (eds.), *Contemporary Nutrition Support Practice—A Clinical Guide*. W.B. Saunders Company, Philadelphia, PA, 1998, pp. 110–116.
6. Skipper A. Principles of parenteral nutrition. In: Matarese LE, Gottschlich MM (eds.), *Contemporary Nutrition Support Practice—A Clinical Guide*. W.B. Saunders Company, Philadelphia, PA, 1998, pp. 227–242.
7. Wilmore DW. Postoperative protein sparing. *World J Surg.*, 1999; 23: 545–552.

8. Klein CJ, Stanek GS, Wiles CE. Overfeeding macronutrients to critically ill adults: Metabolic complications. *J Am Diet Assoc.*, 1998; 98: 795–806.
9. Kumpf VJ, Gervasio J. Complications of parenteral nutrition. In: Mueller CM (ed.), *The ASPEN Adult Nutrition Support Core Curriculum*, 2nd edn. A.S.P.E.N., Silver Spring, MD, 2012, pp. 284–295.
10. Askanazi J, Elwyn DH, Silverberg PA, Rosenbaum SH, Kinney JM. Respiratory distress secondary to a high carbohydrate load: A case report. *Surgery*, 1980; 87: 596–598.
11. Dark DS, Pingleton SK, Kerby GR. Hypercapnia during weaning: A complication of nutritional support. *Chest*, 1985; 88: 141–143.
12. Covelli HD, Black JW, Olsen MS, Beekman JF. Respiratory failure precipitated by high carbohydrate loads. *Ann Intern Med.*, 1981; 95: 579–581.
13. McClave SA, Lowen CC, Kleber MJ, McConnell JW, Jung LY, Goldsmith LJ. Clinical use of the respiratory quotient obtained from indirect calorimetry. *J Parenter Enteral Nutr.*, 2003; 27: 21–26.
14. Talpers SS, Romberger DJ, Bunce SB et al. Nutritionally associated increased carbon dioxide production. Excess total calories vs. high proportion of carbohydrate calories. *Chest*, 1992; 102: 551–555.
15. Pomposelli JJ, Baxter JK, Babineau TJ, Pomfret EA, Driscoll DF, Forse RA, Bistrian BR. Early postoperative glucose control predicts nosocomial infection rate in diabetic patients. *J Parenter Enteral Nutr.*, 1998; 22: 77–81.
16. Van den Berghe G, Wouters P et al. Intensive insulin therapy in critically ill patients. *N Engl J Med.*, 2001; 345: 1359–1367.
17. McMahon MM, Nystrom E, Braunschweig C et al. A.S.P.E.N. clinical guidelines: Nutrition support of adult patients with hyperglycemia. *JPEN J Parenter Enteral Nutr.*, 2012; 37(1): 23–36.
18. Young LS, Kearns LR, Schoepfel SL. Protein. In: Gottschlich MM (ed.), *The Science and Practice of Nutrition Support—A Case-Based Core Curriculum.* A.S.P.E.N., Silver Spring, MD, 2007, pp. 71–87.
19. Streat SJ, Beddore SH, Hill GL. Aggressive nutritional support does not prevent protein loss despite fat gain in septic intensive care patients. *J Trauma*, 1987; 27: 262–266.
20. McClave SA, Martindale RG, Vanek VW et al. Guidelines for the provision and assessment of nutrition support therapy in the adult critically ill patient: Society of critical care medicine (SCCM) and American Society for Parenteral and Enteral Nutrition (A.S.P.E.N.). *JPEN J Parenter Enteral Nutr.*, 2009; 33: 277–316.
21. Lawson CM, Miller KR, Smith VL. Appropriate protein and specific amino acid delivery can improve patient outcome: Fact or fantasy? *Curr Gastroenterol Rep.*, 2011; 13: 380–387.
22. Matsuda T, Kagan RJ, Hanumadass M, Jonasson O. The importance of burn wound size in determining the optimal calorie: Nitrogen ration. *Surgery*, 1983; 94: 562–568.
23. Kagan RJ, Matsuda T, Hanumadass M, Castillo B, Jonasson O. The effect of burn wound size on ureagenesis and nitrogen balance. *Ann Surg.*, 1982; 195: 70–74.
24. Demling RH, DeSanti L. Increased protein intake during the recovery phase after severe burns increases body weight gain and muscle function. *J Burn Care Rehabil.*, 1998; 19: 161–168.
25. Alexander JW, MacMillan BG, Stinnett JD, Ogle CK, Bosian RC, Fischer JE, Oakes JB, Morris MJ, Krummel R. Beneficial effects of aggressive protein feeding in severely burned children. *Ann Surg.*, 1980; 192: 505–517.
26. McClave SA, Kushner R, Van Way III CW. Nutrition therapy of the severely obese, critically ill patient: Summation of conclusions and recommendations. *JPEN J Parenter Enteral Nutr.*, 2011; 35: 88S–96S.
27. Stechmiller JK, Cowen L, Logan K. Nutrition support for wound healing. *Support Line*, 2009; 31: 2–8.
28. Campos ACL, Groth AK, Branco A. Assessment and nutritional aspects of wound healing. *Curr Opin Clin Nutr Metab Care*, 2008; 11: 281–288.
29. Dorner B, Posthauer ME, Thomas D; National Pressure Ulcer Advisory Panel. The role of nutrition in pressure ulcer prevention and treatment: National Pressure Ulcer Advisory Panel white paper. *Adv Skin Wound Care*, 2009; 22: 212–221.
30. Hourigan LA, Linfoot JA, Chung KK et al. Protein loss, immunoglobulins, and electrolytes in exudates from negative pressure wound therapy. *Nutr Clin Pract.*, 2010; 25: 510–516.
31. Cheatham ML, Safcsak K, Brzezinski SJ, Lube MW. Nitrogen balance, protein loss, and the open abdomen. *Crit Care Med.*, 2007; 35: 127–131.
32. Wade C, Wolf SE, Salinas R et al. Loss of protein, immunoglobulins, and electrolytes in exudates from negative pressure wound therapy. *Nutr Clin Pract.*, 2010; 25: 510–516.
33. Freise RS. The open abdomen: Definitions, management principals, and nutrition support considerations. *Nutr Clin Pract.*, 2012; 27: 492–498.

34. Wooley JA, Btaiche IF, Good KL. Metabolic and nutritional aspects of acute renal failure in critically ill patients requiring continuous renal replacement therapy. *Nutr Clin Pract.*, 2005; 20: 176–191.
35. Gervasio JM, Garmon WP, Holowatyj MR. Nutrition support in acute kidney injury. *Nutr Clin Pract.*, 2011; 26: 374–381.
36. Maursetter L, Kight CE, Mennig J, Hofmann M. Review of the mechanism and nutrition recommendations for patients undergoing continuous renal replacement therapy. *Nutr Clin Pract.*, 2011; 26: 382–390.
37. Scheinkestel CD, Kar L, Marshall K et al. Prospective randomized trial to assess caloric and protein needs of critically ill, anuric, ventilated patients during continuous renal replacement therapy. *Nutrition*, 2003; 19: 909–916.
38. Hoffer JL, Bistrian BR. Appropriate protein provision in critical illness: A systematic and narrative review. *Am J Clin Nutr.*, 2012; 96: 591–600.
39. Mueller C. True or false: Serum hepatic protein concentrations measure nutritional status. *Support Line*, 2004; 26(1): 8–16.
40. Hise ME, Brown JC. Lipids. In: Mueller C (ed.), *The ASPEN Adult Nutrition Support Core Curriculum*, 2nd edn. A.S.P.E.N., Silver Spring, MD, 20012, pp. 63–77.
41. Harris HW, Grunfeld C. Human very low density lipoproteins and chylomicrons can protect against endotoxin-induced death in mice. *J Clin Invest.*, 1990; 86: 696–702.
42. Harris HW, Grunfeld C. Chylomicrons alter the fate of endotoxin, decreasing tumor necrosis factor release and preventing death. *J Clin Invest.*, 1993; 91: 1028–1034.
43. Van Lenten BJ, Fogelman A. The role of lipoproteins and receptor-mediated endocytosis in the transport of bacterial lipopolysaccharide. *Proc Natl Acad Sci USA*, 1986; 83: 2704–2708.
44. Gordon BR, Parker TS. Low lipid concentrations in critical illness: Implications for preventing and treating endotoxemia. *Crit Care Med.*, 1996; 24: 584–589.
45. Chien JY, Jerng JS. Low serum level of high-density lipoprotein cholesterol is a poor prognostic factor for severe sepsis. *Crit Care Med.*, 2005; 33: 1688–1693.
46. Barlage S, Gnewuch C. Changes in HDL-associated apolipoproteins relate to mortality in human sepsis and correlate to monocyte and platelet activation. *Intensive Care Med.*, 2009; 35: 1877–1885.
47. Hasselmann M, Reimund JM. Lipids in the nutritional support of the critically ill patients. *Curr Opin Crit Care.*, 2004; 10: 449–455.
48. Calder PC, Jensen GL. Lipid emulsions in parenteral nutrition of intensive care patients: Current thinking and future directions. *Intensive Care Med.*, 2010: 36: 735–749.
49. Institute of Medicine of the National Academies. *Dietary Reference Intakes for Energy, Carbohydrate, Fiber, Fat, Fatty Acids, Cholesterol, Protein, and Amino Acids*. The National Academies Press, Washington, DC, 2005.
50. Barr LH, Dunn GD. Essential fatty acid deficiency during total parenteral nutrition. *Ann Surg.*, 1981; 193: 304–311.
51. Battistella FD, Widegreen JT, Anderson JT, Siepler JK, Weber JC, MacCall K. A prospective, randomized trial of intravenous fat emulsion administration in trauma victims requiring total parenteral nutrition. *J Trauma*, 1997; 43: 52–60.
52. Eddleston JM, Shelly MP. The effect on serum lipid concentrations of a prolonged infusion of propofol—Hypertriglyceridemia associated with propofol administration. *Intensive Care Med.*, 1991; 17: 424–426.

8 Micronutrient and Antioxidant Therapy in Adult Critically Ill Patients

Krishnan Sriram

CONTENTS

The term *micronutrient* includes vitamins and trace elements. Vitamins are substances not generally synthesized by the body and are cofactors for various enzymes. Trace elements are metals present in minute quantities that act as cofactors or as part of the structure of specific enzymes. Trace metals (selenium, zinc, manganese, iron, and copper) and 13 essential vitamins (4 fat soluble and 9 water soluble) are essential in stabilizing or catalyzing homeostatic reactions in the human organism.[1–4]

This chapter will discuss the role of micronutrients in critically ill patients, and trace element deficiency will be addressed individually, except in the tables listed. Otherwise, only the most crucial deficiency states dealing with critical illness will be discussed. The second half of this chapter will be dedicated to past and current studies highlighting the increasingly important role antioxidant therapy plays in critically ill patients during the acute inflammatory and oxidative stress states.

Micronutrient deficiencies in critically ill patients may occur as preexisting conditions in patients with poor nutritional status prior to hospitalization, as a result of severe illness with depletion of micronutrients, or iatrogenically, when the physician fails to recognize the nutrient-wasting illness or when there is a failure to institute replacement therapy early in the care of critically ill patients.[1,2] These deficient states can affect numerous biochemical processes and enzymatic functions, resulting in organ dysfunction, poor wound healing, and altered immune status, all with deleterious patient outcomes.

Literature on critical care nutrition often concentrates on macronutrients highlighting the optimal requirement of protein, carbohydrate, and lipid along with monitoring of the adequacy of these components of nutrition therapy. Clinicians may not realize that for the optimal functioning and utilization of macronutrients, it is imperative that adequate amounts of micronutrients, both vitamins and trace elements, are provided. The role of micronutrients is often neglected. This is especially true for obese patients who have macronutrient excess but may still be micronutrient deficient. Deficiencies of almost every micronutrient have been reported in bariatric surgery patients, both pre- and postoperatively.[5,6] It has been strongly suggested that micronutrient deficiency should also form an integral part of the malnutrition syndrome and should be included in the definition of malnutrition.[7]

Although the American Medical Association has established guidelines for the daily recommended intake of vitamins and trace elements, these have been formulated for a healthy population. The exact formulation of micronutrient replacement required for health maintenance or replacement is not well known in critically ill patients.[8–11] The FDA has recognized that parenteral vitamin requirements are increased in disease states and manufacturers have been instructed to modify their products accordingly,[12] but a similar recommendation for trace elements has not been initiated. The American Society for Parenteral and Enteral Nutrition (ASPEN) has taken the lead in establishing guidelines on the administration of parenteral trace element additives.[13] Table 8.1 summarizes the various actions of the essential vitamins and trace elements, the clinical sequelae of the deficient states for each, and the recommendations for replacement. Table 8.2 gives the suggested composition of parenteral micronutrients for adults.

ABSORPTION AND INTERACTIONS

VITAMINS

Most water-soluble vitamins are absorbed easily from the proximal gastrointestinal (GI) tract (see Figure 8.1). Fat-soluble vitamins are thought to be absorbed in the mid and distal ileum, due to the necessity of bile acid and pancreatic lipase to facilitate absorption. Absorptions of fat-soluble vitamins (such as vitamin B_{12}, which is absorbed in the terminal ileum) are affected by all conditions with fat malabsorption. Deficiencies will occur with excessive GI losses, such as high-output fistulas and prolonged diarrhea. Re-instillation of upper GI secretions into the jejunum via nasojejunal tube or jejunostomy will facilitate the absorption of fat-soluble vitamins that require bile and pancreatic secretions for optimal absorption. This will help to avoid the loss of micronutrients that will occur if the aspirated fluid is discarded. Differences between intragastric and intrajejunal administration have not been studied in depth. In the case of vitamin B_{12}, intrajejunal administration results in better absorption, even though the stomach (source of intrinsic factor) is bypassed.[14] This may be due to the increased binding of cobalamin to intrinsic factor at alkaline pH levels seen in the ileum.[15]

TABLE 8.1
Micronutrient Functions and Recommended Intakes

Nutrient	Role	Cause of Deficient State	Perifollicular Petechiae, Poor Wound Healing, and Gingivitis	Toxicity/Adverse Effects	Recommendations
Vitamin A	Maintains mucosal integrity and wound healing. Fatsoluble vitamin with antioxidant activity.	GI losses, use of steroids.	Poor wound healing, diarrhea, poor epithelial cell regeneration, factor in bacterial translocation, impairs neutrophil function.	Excess amounts can lead to liver dysfunction and failure.	1 mg/d or 3000 IU/d. Enteral nutrition formulas contain 2,600 to 5,200 IU/l, and enhanced formulas contain 4,500 to 12,000 IU/l. Amount needed to counteract steroid effects is 10,000 to 15,000 IU/d × 7 days.
Vitamin B_1	A cofactor for oxidation of pyruvate, alpha ketoacids, and branched-chain amino acids. Water soluble.	Alcoholism, high carbohydrate intake, as a component of refeeding syndrome, iatrogenic (when TPN is given without thiamine).	TPN given without thiamine results in refractory metabolic (lactic) acidosis. Mental changes, confabulation, confusion and congestive heart failure, socalled wet beri beri.	None known.	Give additional thiamine (100 mg/d) to patients at risk for deficiency, especially alcoholics and patients with preexisting malnutrition.
Vitamin B_6	Metabolism of amino acids and fatty acids, synthesis of heme and neurotransmitters. Water soluble.	Levels are decreased in renal failure.	Anemia, skin and mucosal changes, mental changes (depression, confusion).	Very high doses of over 2 g can cause convulsions.	RDA is 1.5 mg.
Vitamin B_{12}	Needed for the conversion of methyl folate to tetrahydrofolate, thus affecting DNA synthesis. Water soluble.	Due to adequate body reserves, a deficiency state in critically ill patients is unlikely. Exposure to nitrous oxide anesthesia can result in vitamin B12 deficiency.	Macrocytic anemia.	None known.	RDA is 2.4 μg. A single dose of 1 mg virtually saturates body stores for several months.
Vitamin C	A nonenzymatic antioxidant that is also needed for collagen synthesis and wound healing. It is required for the synthesis of carnitine. Water soluble.	Increased requirements in burns. Abrupt cessation can lead to rebound scurvy.	Perifollicular petechiae, poor wound healing, and gingivitis.	Increases free Fe, which promotes bacterial proliferation and decreases bacteriocidal activity. Known to produce hyperoxaluria and renal calculi.	75 to 90 mg/d. Standard PN recommendation is 20 mg/d. Standard EN solutions contain 125 to 250 mg/l. Supplementation recommendations are 500 to 3000 mg/d. Enhanced formulas have 80 to 850 mg/l.

(Continued)

TABLE 8.1 (*Continued*)
Micronutrient Functions and Recommended Intakes

Nutrient	Role	Cause of Deficient State	Perifollicular Petechiae, Poor Wound Healing, and Gingivitis	Toxicity/Adverse Effects	Recommendations
Vitamin D	Calcium and bone metabolism. Fat soluble.	Lack of sunlight, hepatic and renal insufficiency. Vitamin D levels decrease with stress, but the significance of this is not known.	Osteomalacia and osteoporosis are not relevant for critically ill patients. Prolonged inactivity can result in osteoporosis.	Paucity of data for recommending in critically ill patients. RDA is 5 μg (200 IU), present 1 l of EN formulas. Use active 1,25 dihydroxy form in renal or hepatic failure.	Hypercalcemia. Toxicity occurs only when intakes are in the range of 40,000 IU/d (1,000 μg/d), a situation unlikely to occur.
Vitamin E	Antioxidant, cofactor for selenium, membrane fluidity and integrity. Fat soluble.	Vitamin E levels decline with stress. The decrease seen when septic shock occurs in parallel with lipid peroxidation and may represent increased free radical activity.	None.	Excess antagonizes vitamin A. High doses may adversely affect wound healing and may contribute to platelet dysfunction. It may also upregulate proinflammatory cytokines. Doses as high as 3 g/d have been given without deleterious clinical effects.	RDA is 15 mg. Multivitamin preparations for PN contain 10 mg/dose. EN formulas have variable amounts: 25 to 50 mg/l. In critically ill patients, higher parenteral doses of 50 to 60 mg/d are recommended.
Vitamin K	Required in the hepatic production of serine proteases of the coagulation cascade. Fat soluble.	There are no storage forms. Alterations in microbiologic flora can diminish bacterial synthesis. Deficiencies occur rapidly in patients, especially when TPN void of vitamin K is administered.	Estimation of prothrombin time (PT) may not detect subclinical vitamin K deficiency states, which may become pronounced after surgery or resuscitation.	Rapid intravenous administration can result in hypotension. Excessive administration of vitamin K results in inability to anticoagulate patients adequately with warfarin.	RDA (150 μg) in enteral feeding. Multivitamin preparations have recently been reformulated to provide 150 μg/d.

(*Continued*)

TABLE 8.1 (*Continued*)
Micronutrient Functions and Recommended Intakes

Nutrient	Role	Cause of Deficient State	Perifollicular Petechiae, Poor Wound Healing, and Gingivitis	Toxicity/Adverse Effects	Recommendations
Folic acid	Homocysteine metabolism. Water soluble.	Alcoholism, nitrous oxide exposure, dialysis, antiepileptic drugs.	Macrocytic anemia, skin rash, increased serum homocysteine levels	None known.	RDA is 400 μg present in EN and PN. One mg/day is needed in deficiency states, including dialysis.
Niacin	An indirect role in oxidation through NAD^+. Water soluble.	Alcohol abuse produces niacin deficiency. Isonicotinic acid hydrazine (INH), an antituberculosis medication, and 6-mercaptopurine, an anticancer drug, also produce niacin deficiency.	Deficiency is a chronic problem with pellagra, or dry skin, and associated with diarrhea, dermatitis, and dementia.	None known.	RDA for niacin is 16 μg, adequate in most enteral formulas. Recommend 40 mg/d for PN. Some infused tryptophan gets converted to niacin. Niacin deficiency can also occur acutely in patients with severe GI problems. Supplemental niacin can rapidly reverse symptoms. No specific recommendations for critically ill patients.
Zinc	Zn content is the highest of any trace element except for Fe. Ninety-five percent of body Zn is intracellular. Functions in the formation of metalloenzymes, RNA conformation and membrane stabilization, and protein metabolism. Zn interacts with insulin and has important roles in the immune system.	Zn content is the highest of any trace element except for Fe. Ninety-five percent of body Zn is intracellular. Functions in the formation of metalloenzymes, RNA conformation and membrane stabilization, and protein metabolism. Zn interacts with insulin and has important roles in the immune system.	Skin rash involving elbows and knees, also called acrodermatitis enteropathica, characteristic rash around ala nasi, glucose intolerance, poor wound healing, abnormal hemostasis, immune dysfunction, loss of hair, altered taste (dysgeusia) and smell perception, diarrhea.	High doses of Zn result in immune dysfunction, as noted in text.	Parenteral, 2.5 to 4 mg/d. Additional amounts are as follows: 2 mg/d in acute catabolism, 12.2 mg/l of small bowel fluid losses, and 17.1 mg/kg of stool or ileostomy output. Enteral RDA is 15 mg. Additional doses are given when indicated.

(*Continued*)

TABLE 8.1 (*Continued*)
Micronutrient Functions and Recommended Intakes

Nutrient	Role	Cause of Deficient State	Perifollicular Petechiae, Poor Wound Healing, and Gingivitis	Toxicity/Adverse Effects	Recommendations
Selenium	Se has antioxidant functions. Its function is linked with that of vitamin E. Selenocysteine is in glutathione peroxidase. Se is also important for thyroid hormone production. Supplemental Se in trauma patients has been shown to normalize thyroxine (T4) and reverse T3 plasma levels. Se inhibits nuclear transcription factor κB expression, a key step in the development of inflammation.	Administration of Se-free TPN or EN, history of alcoholism, surgical resection of duodenum and proximal jejunum, especially when EN formulas deficient in Se are used.	Se deficiency manifests as congestive heart failure and arrhythmias. Involvement of peripheral muscles is manifested as myositis, with weakness and muscle cramps.	No report of Se toxicity due to nutritional support.	PN intake of 30 to 100 µg/d. The recommended enteral intake is 55 to 70 µg/d. Enteral formulas may also be deficient in bioavailable forms of Se. Se levels should be monitored in renal insufficiency and intake decreased if indicated. GI excretion of Se offers some protection against Se toxicity.
Iron	In association with hemoglobin, Fe is an oxygen carrier.	Fe deficiency is seen in critical illness as part of anemia, blood loss with microcytic anemia.	Low hemoglobin production, with possible hypoxia at the tissue level.	Free Fe is released in critical illness. Free Fe interferes with the reticuloendothelial system (RES), decreases macrophage activity, and promotes bacterial growth.	IV supplementation is not recommended in acute phase of illness, but enteral is recommended during recovery phase to support production of red cells. Diminished in renal failure, and IV supplementation may be useful.

(*Continued*)

TABLE 8.1 (*Continued*)
Micronutrient Functions and Recommended Intakes

Nutrient	Role	Cause of Deficient State	Perifollicular Petechiae, Poor Wound Healing, and Gingivitis	Toxicity/Adverse Effects	Recommendations
Copper	Part of proteins; ferroxidase and ceruloplasmin. Component of metalloenzymes (SOD, cytochrome oxidase).	Seen most often in malnourished young children, in patients with disrupted gastric and small bowel anatomy.	Neutropenia, anemia, arrested maturation of myeloid cell line in bone marrow with megaloblastic changes. Bone spur formation, osteoporosis, and long bone fractures.	Red cell toxin, damages cell membranes and inhibits red cell enzymes. Manifests as hemolysis and GI disturbances. Accumulation of metal in liver and other organs, leading to death of hepatocytes.	RDA is for 1.0 to 1.5 mg for adolescents and adults and about 50 mcg/kg body weight in infants.
Manganese	Involved in sustaining several enzyme systems, most notably that of SOD.	Lack of proper diet, mostly seen in vegan and similar diets.	Impaired insulin production, altered lipid profile, deficient oxidant defense, and abnormal growth factor metabolism.	Decreased appetite and growth, reproductive failure. CNS abnormalities with inhaled form in miners.	RDA about 2 to 5 mg. Rarely of concern because EN and PN formulas with trace metals supply sufficient amounts.

TABLE 8.2
Suggested Composition of Parenteral Multivitamin and Trace Element Products for Adults

Vitamin/Trace Element	Unit of Measurement	Amount
A	mg (IU)	1.0 (~3000)
B_1 (thiamine)	mg	3
B_6 (pyridoxine)	mg	3.6
B_{12} (cyanocobalamin)	μg	5
C (ascorbic acid)	mg	100
D	μg[a] (IU)	5 (200)
E	mg[b] (IU)	6.7 (10)
Folic acid	μg	400
K	μg	150
Niacin	mg	40
Copper	mg	0.3–0.5
Manganese	μg	60–100
Selenium	μg	20–60
Zinc	mg	2.5–5.0

Sources: Mirtallo, J.M., Parenteral formulas, in *Patenteral Nutrition*, 3rd ed., Rombeiau, J.L., Rolandelli, R.H., Eds. W.B. Saunders, Philadelphia, 2001, 124; American Medical Association, *JAMA*, 241, 2051, 1979; ASPEN Board of Directors and Clinical Guidelines Task Force, *J. Parenter. Enteral Nutr.*, 26, 1, Supplement, 1SA, 2002; and Fuhrman, P.M. and Herrmann, V.M., in *Nutritional Considerations in the Intensive Care Unit*, American Society for Parenteral and Enteral Nutrition, Silver Springs, MD, 2002, 51–60.

Note: IU = international units.

[a] As cholecalciferol.

[b] As di-alpha tocopherol.

Interactions between various vitamins are very complex and not well understood.[16] For example, vitamins E and C are synergistic. Vitamin C recycles vitamin E; thus, vitamin C deficiency decreases the function of the latter. Excess of vitamin E antagonizes vitamin A function. Pyridoxine (vitamin B_6) and riboflavin (vitamin B_2) deficiencies increase requirements for niacin. Therefore, single vitamin supplementation can counteract the action of other vitamins. See Table 8.2 for suggested composition of parenteral multivitamin and trace element products for adults.

Trace Elements

There is a paucity of information about the exact location in the GI tract where specific trace elements are absorbed. However, certain generalizations can be made. Zinc and selenium are absorbed mainly in the duodenum and also in the ileum. The latter location is especially important when food requires digestion before the zinc is bioavailable. Iron is also absorbed in the duodenum (see Figure 8.1). Numerous interactions exist between trace elements affecting absorption via the GI tract. Factors affecting bioavailability of trace elements are numerous:[17]

- Dietary factors including chemical form of the nutrient (e.g., the organic form of chromium is better absorbed than the ionized form).
- Antagonistic ligands (e.g., phytate decreases zinc absorption, fiber decreases zinc and iron absorption, vitamin C decreases copper absorption but increases iron absorption).
- Facilitating ligands (e.g., picolinic acid and citric acid aid zinc absorption).
- Competitive interactions (e.g., iron depresses the absorption of copper and zinc; zinc depresses copper absorption and vice versa).

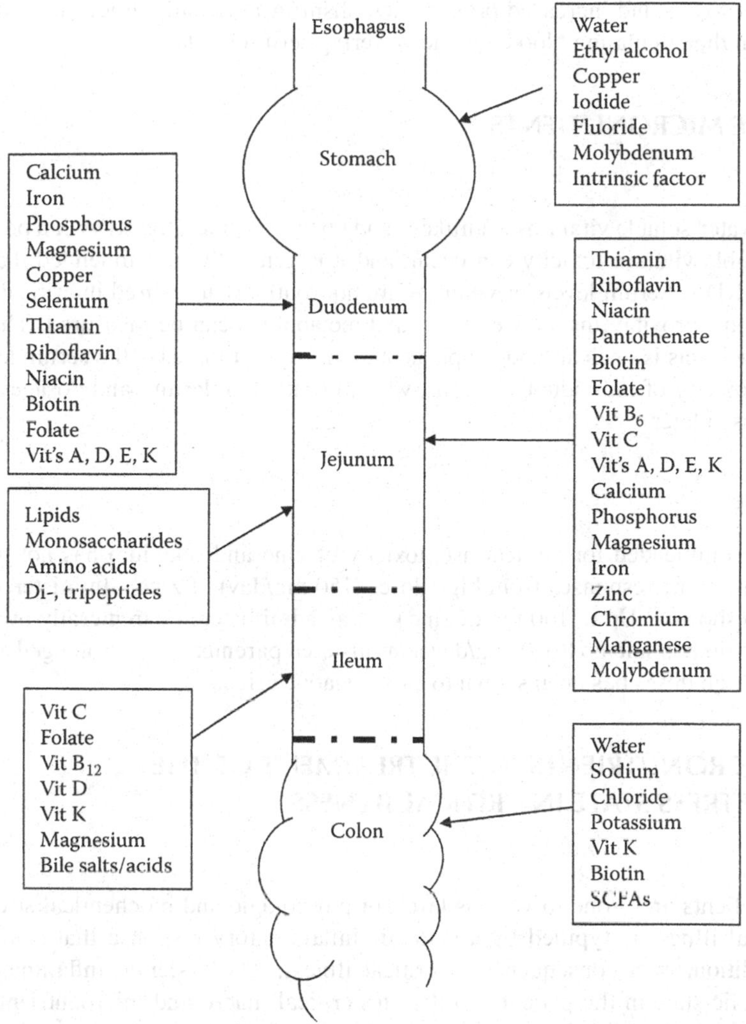

FIGURE 8.1 Sites of absorption of micronutrients.

EFFECT OF THE INFLAMMATORY RESPONSE ON MICRONUTRIENT STATUS

Vitamins

Serum levels of various vitamins decrease with the inflammatory response although the specific clinical consequences are unclear.[18] It is hypothesized that decreased levels of antioxidant vitamins may inhibit the body's ability to fight oxidative stress.[9,19] It is well known that vitamin C levels are decreased in severe illness.[11] However, other vitamin levels are not affected and if low may represent a true deficiency. Vitamin levels may be decreased for various reasons, losses in body fluids and drains, dilution, renal replacement therapy, or true deficiency. However, there is no conclusive proof to indicate that additional supplementation is needed when the serum level of a specific vitamin declines.

Trace Elements

Serum levels of various trace elements decrease in critical illness, as is well summarized by Berger.[9,20] Serum levels of selenium, copper, and zinc are decreased. This may be due to increased urinary or other losses and increased protein catabolism. Additionally, trace elements are sequestered away from the circulating blood volume, lowering serum levels.

TOXICITY OF MICRONUTIENTS

VITAMINS

Toxicity from water-soluble vitamins is unlikely, and up to 100 times, the RDA can be safely administered. Fat-soluble vitamin toxicity can occur, and it is generally recommended that a safe limit is 10 times the RDA. Serum levels of vitamins are not routinely measured in critical care. Several forms of vitamins, provitamins, active forms, and metabolites can be measured. The clinical significance of low levels is unclear, and supplementation may not increase the serum levels. Adverse reactions and toxicity of individual vitamins, where clinically relevant, and dosage recommendations are discussed later.

TRACE ELEMENTS

In the doses recommended for clinical use, toxicity of zinc and selenium has not been reported. Depression of immune responses from high doses (150 mg/day) of zinc administered for 6 weeks orally has been shown.[21] Up to 100 mg of zinc per day administered parenterally over 24 h is well tolerated.[22] Selenium is safe up to 400 μg/day administered parenterally.[23] Prolonged administration of selenium in high doses has been shown to have negative effects.[9]

ROLE OF MICRONUTRIENTS IN THE TREATMENT OF THE OXIDATIVE STRESS STATE IN CRITICAL ILLNESS

INTRODUCTION

Critically ill patients are prone to various levels of physiologic and biochemical stress. The acute phase of critical illness is typified by a systemic inflammatory response that can be a cause, a comorbid condition, or a consequence of critical illness. The systemic inflammatory response causes a catabolic state in the patient that depletes critical macro and micronutrients. It has been emphasized throughout this book that an essential tool in our armamentarium to care for critically ill patients includes providing the appropriate combination of macronutrients in an attempt to reverse the catabolic process in critical illness. Micronutrient replacement also plays a significant role in the nutritional management of critical illness. Micronutrients act to stabilize many of the homeostatic processes and enzymatic reactions required to sustain life.

In the prolonged inflammatory response, there has been an increasing recognition that critically ill patients have an imbalance between prooxidant and antioxidant mechanisms. This imbalance can lead to the production of large quantities of reactive oxygen species (ROS). The effects of this oxidative stress state have been shown to respond to antioxidant treatment, many of which are the very same micronutrients that are essential in the daily care of the critically ill patient.

OXIDATIVE STRESS STATE

In critically ill patients, the systemic inflammatory response syndrome (SIRS) leads to the release of numerous pro- and anti-inflammatory cytokines. In the initial phase of the inflammatory response is a local activation of lymphocytes at the site of injury.[24] ROS act to facilitate and induce the production of cytokines that activate the immune system, as well as acting to promote cell damage locally. This initial response is then amplified systemically via cytokines and other signaling mechanisms, which leads to further production of ROS. ROS interact with cell membranes, protein, DNA, and lipids causing oxidative damage from free radical electrons leading to mitochondrial dysfunction, cell death, tissue injury, and ultimately organ failure.[25] This excessive SIRS response then leads to the commonly encountered syndromes of organ dysfunction seen in the ICU (adult respiratory distress syndrome, septic shock, disseminated intravascular coagulation, and multi-organ dysfunction syndrome).[24]

Endogenous Antioxidant Activity

Endogenous mechanisms act in a network-like fashion to neutralize the production of ROS in an attempt to ablate the deleterious effects of these agents. Intracellular glutathione acts as one of the major antioxidant buffers. Nonenzymatic ROS scavengers also include commonly occurring molecules such as utate, ubiquinone, bilirubin, and vitamins such as ascorbic acid (vitamin C), β-carotene, and α-tocopherol (vitamin E). Once vitamin E is oxidized, vitamin C and glutathione play a role in reducing the vitamin E back to its active form.

Enzymatic systems then act in concert to detoxify ROS further. Thus, superoxide dismutase (SOD) converts O_2 to H_2O_2; catalase and glutathione peroxide convert H_2O_2 to water and alcohols. These enzyme systems are inducible and dependent on minerals such as selenium, copper, zinc, and manganese as important cofactors in these enzymatic reactions.

There has been an abundance of research in the last decade showing that these critical micronutrient stores are depleted in critically ill patients. These deficits may be due to increased loss, decreased nutritional intake, and redistribution from blood to tissue. The result is a decrease in the antioxidant potential and increased cellular damage from oxidative stress.[24,25] Currently, recommendations exist for the supplementation of micronutrients, parenteral or enteral, in the nutritional support of critically ill patients. This list is constantly undergoing modification as new data becomes available.[9,24]

Micronutrient Replacement in Critical Illness

The previous sections discussed the etiology of an oxidative stress state in the critically ill patient and how data have demonstrated an increase in oxidative stress in critically ill patients. It has also been shown that there is a decline in endogenous micronutrients in the critically ill. This situation clearly lends itself to directed therapy to replace depleted micronutrients where beneficial effects may be demonstrated.

The goal of this therapy would be to provide the necessary factors to replenish the endogenous antioxidants at appropriate levels to counteract the toxic effects of ROS and to supply these factors through the most appropriate route. Numerous studies have shown that supplementation of antioxidants in critically ill patients have demonstrated measurable benefits for the patients.

Summary of Recent Recommendations and Review of Data

There have been numerous studies examining micronutrient therapy in critically ill patients. It has been established that in critically ill patients, levels of selenium, zinc, vitamin C and other antioxidant micronutrients are depleted for various reasons.[9–11] While there are no universally agreed-upon replacement protocols, there is a growing body of evidence advocating replacement of micronutrients in critically ill patients, especially those most at risk for oxidative stress.

Many of the earliest studies on micronutrient and antioxidant replacement have dealt with premedication in surgical patients. Over the last 10 years, there have been numerous studies looking specifically at micronutrient replacement in critically ill patients. These studies have focused primarily on vitamins C and E, selenium, and zinc, either alone or in combination therapy.

Vitamin C has been shown in numerous studies to be beneficial in patients with severe burn injury. Patients who received parenteral vitamin C in doses of 1000–3000 mg have been shown to have decreased infectious complications and lower fluid requirements with no complications or side effect of vitamin C administration.[26,27]

Selenium replacement in doses of 200–1000 mcg/day has also been studied individually and has been shown in critically ill patients and has been associated with improvement in mortality and other secondary indicators of oxidative stress, as well as fewer infections.[26,28] However, other studies of selenium have shown no improvement in mortality.[29]

While the replacement of individual micronutrients has provided interesting data, it has been well established that levels of selenium, zinc, vitamin C, and vitamin E are all decreased in critically ill patients in the oxidative stress state.[24,25] There have been numerous studies that have examined replacement of multiple micronutrients in various protocols. Multiple prospective randomized control studies have shown that combination antioxidant replacement can improve mortality, morbidity, degree of organ failure, and length of ICU stay.[30–33] The findings of these and other studies have been confirmed by meta-analysis showing that there is a measurable clinical benefit in antioxidant replacement. Manzanares et al. in a 2012 meta-analysis were able to show that antioxidant therapy especially those protocols containing selenium in doses of 500 μg or more appears to confer the greatest benefit.[34] They were also able to show that antioxidant therapy did decrease mortality and shorten ventilator days as well as trend toward fewer infectious complications. In this study, the sickest patients were shown to derive the greatest benefit.

SUMMARY

Nutritional support of the critically ill patient is a key component of therapy. Although great pains are taken to provide adequate carbohydrate, lipid, and protein combinations, the role of micronutrients must not be overlooked.

A growing body of literature indicates that critical illness provides a setting for the formation of ROS as a result of the activation of various mechanisms. At the same time, this overproduction of ROS overwhelms endogenous mechanisms, leading to depletion in nonenzymatic and enzymatic antioxidant activity. This situation leads to an oxidative stress state that will ultimately cause damage to cellular molecules and structural proteins, resulting in cell death, organ dysfunction, and organ failure, with prolongation of critical illness and diminished survival.

Clinical evidence has defined a role for the use of antioxidant vitamins and trace minerals to improve ICU mortality, ventilator times, and ICU length of stay and reduce organ failure and infectious complications. There is evidence that clearly shows that replacement of micronutrients is safe, effective, and low in cost.[26] While intravenous replacement is advocated in the critically ill due to unpredictable absorption,[34] there are still several questions that need to be answered about the amount and timing of replacement: Is early in the course of ICU admission good enough, or is this too late, and should timing of replacement be considered at admission? Further research continues in this field.

RECOMMENDATIONS FOR SUPPLEMENTATION

Who Needs Supplementation

All critically ill patients need micronutrient supplementation. Parenteral supplementation can be given with or without parenteral nutrition. Enteral supplementation should be instituted once enteral feeding has begun.

We recommend a practical approach to micronutrient supplementation based on clinical signs and symptoms, without depending on laboratory confirmation, as shown in Refs. 6, 36.

Timing

The largest increase in ROS production occurs early in the course of acute illness. Likewise, decreased serum levels of micronutrients are seen in this period. In burns, early administration of micronutrients has been shown to be beneficial.[24–26] Recent randomized studies and meta-analyses

TABLE 8.3
Micronutrients in Critical Illness

		Standard Dose			
Micronutrient	**RDA**	**Recommended PN**	**Recommended PN**	**Supplementation (per day)**	**Enhanced EN Formulas**
Vitamin A	1 mg	1.0 mg	0.9–1.0 mg	PN: 3.5 mg EN: 8.6 mg	1.5–4.0 mg/l
Vitamin C	75–90 mg	200 mg	125–250 mg/l	500–3000 mg	80–844 mg/l
Vitamin E (α-tocopherol)	15 mg	10 mg	25–50 mg/l	PN: 400 mg EN: 40–1000 mg	40–212 mg/l
Vitamin K	150 μg	150 μg	40–135 μg		
Iron	10–15 mg	0 mg	12–20 mg/l		
Selenium	50–100 μg	20–60 μg	20–70 μg/l	100–400 μg	77–100 μg/l
Zinc	15 mg	2.5–5.0 mg	11–19 mg/l	10–30 mg	15–24 mg/l

Sources: From Fuhrman, P.M. and Herrmann, V.M., in *Nutritional Considerations in the Intensive Care Unit*, Shikora, S.A., Martindale, R.G., Schwartberg, S.D., Eds., American Society for Parenteral and Enteral Nutrition, Silver Springs, MD, 2002, 51–60.

Note: EN: enteral nutrition; PN: parenteral nutrition. 1 IU of vitamin A = 0.344 μg.

have recommended that supplementation begin early and continue for 1–2 weeks. Once enteral or parenteral nutrition therapy is established and has reached goal therapy routine supplementation can begin.

Route

In critically ill patients, the intravenous route is the only reliable method by which micronutrients can be administered. Very few clinical trials have used the enteral route for supplementation in critically ill patients. Absorption by the enteral route in critically ill patients is unpredictable, due to hemodynamic instability, bowel edema, and alterations in blood supply.[37] Thus, micronutrients are initially administered intravenously, either as a component of total parenteral nutrition or separately. If and when enteral feeding is initiated and tolerated, micronutrient supplementation can be provided enterally.

Dose

There are currently no universal recommendations for routine micronutrient supplementation in critically ill patients. Based on the evidence available, selenium supplementation at doses between 500 and 1000 μg has been shown to be of benefit. Vitamin C in doses of 1000–3000 mg has been proven to be beneficial and of no harm in critically ill burn patients.[9,26] Current ASPEN guidelines advocate replacement of micronutrients but acknowledges that optimal dosing ranges have yet to be established.[38]

Monitoring

Though serum levels can be used to detect deficiencies, they are not easy to obtain in most hospitals and may not reflect a true deficiency. There are no reliable laboratory indicators for vitamins and trace elements to determine adequacy of supplementation. Functional end points, such as using enzyme assays (alkaline phosphatase for zinc and glutathione peroxidase for selenium), are also not reliable.

CONCLUSION

We have attempted to provide some general and safe guidelines for the use of vitamins in critically ill patients. The information available is, at best, incomplete. However, this discussion should assist the clinician to make individual choices in the management of critically ill patients, specifically regarding the use of micronutrients.

The routine inclusion or supplementation of standard doses of vitamins and trace elements with enteral and parenteral nutritional support is accepted. The data on antioxidant supplementation in critically ill patients are evolving, but supplementation is considered safe.

REFERENCES

1. Vrees, M.D. and Albina, J.E. Metabolic response to illness and its mediators, in *Clinical Nutrition: Parenteral Nutrition*, Rombeau, J.L. and Rolandelli, R.H., eds., W.B. Saunders, Philadelphia, PA, 2000.
2. Solomons, N.W. and Ruz, M. Trace element requirements in humans: An update. *J. Trace Elem. Exp. Med.*, 11, 177, 1998.
3. Kelly DG. Guideline and available products for parenteral and vitamin and trace elements. *J Parenter Enteral Nutr.*, 26(5), S34, 2002.
4. American Medical Association, Department of Foods and Nutrition. Guidelines for essential trace element preparations for parenteral use: A statement by and expert panel. *JAMA*, 241, 2051, 1979.
5. Shankar, P., Boylan, M., and Sriram, K. Micronutrient deficiencies after bariatric surgery. *Nutrition*, 26, 1031, 2010.
6. Valentino, D., Sriram, K., and Shankar, P. Micronutrient supplementation in bariatric surgery. *Curr. Opin. Clin. Nutr. Metab. Care*, 14, 635, 2011.
7. Correira, M.I.T.D., Hegazi, R., Llido, L., Rugeles, S., and Sriram, K. (in alphabetic order). *TNT 3.0, Total Nutrition Therapy: An Integral Approach to Patient Care*, Abbott Health Nutrition Institute, Chicago, IL, 2011.
8. Elia, M. Changing concepts for nutrient requirements in disease: Implications for artificial nutritional support. *Lancet*, 5, 1279, 1995.
9. Berger, M. and Shenkin, A. Updated on clinical micronutrient supplementation studies in the critically ill. *Curr. Opin. Clin. Nutr. Metab. Care*, 9, 711, 2006.
10. Marik, P.E. and Hooper, M. Immunonutrition in the critically ill. *ImmunoGastroenterology*, 1(1), 0–1, 2012.
11. Weitzel, L.B., Mayles, W.J., Sandoval, P.A., and Wishmeyer, P.E. Effects of pharmaconutrients of cellular dysfunction and the microcirculation in critical illness. *Curr. Opin. Anaesthesiol.*, 22, 177, 2009.
12. Food and Drug Administration (FDA). Parenteral multivitamin products: Drugs for human use: Drug efficacy study implementation. *Federal Register*, 65(77), 21200–21201, 2000.
13. ASPEN Board of Directors and Clinical Guidelines Task Force. Guidelines for the use of parenteral and enteral nutrition in adult and pediatric patients. *J. Parenter. Enteral Nutr.*, 261(supp. 1), 1Sa, 2002.
14. Sriram, K., Gergans, G., and Badger, H. Vitamin B12 (cobalamin) absorption via feeding jejunostomy. *J. Am. Coll. Nutr.*, 8(1), 75, 1989.
15. Goldberg, L.S. and Fundenberg, H.H. Effect of pH on the vitamin B12-bining capacity of intrinsic factor. *J. Lab. Clin. Med.*, 73, 469, 1969.
16. Demling, R.H. and De Biasse, M.A. Micronutrients in critical illness. *Crit. Care Clin.*, 11, 651, 1995.
17. Kenny, F., Sriram, K., and Hammond, J. Clinical zinc deficiency during adequate enteral nutrition. *J. Am. Coll. Nutr.*, 8(1), 75, 1989.
18. Galloway, P., McMillan, D.C., and Sattar, N. Effect of the inflammatory response on trace element and vitamin status. *Ann. Clin. Biochem.*, 37, 289, 2000.
19. Mechanick, J.I. and Berger, M.M. Convergent evidence and opinion on intensive metabolic support. *Curr. Opin. Clin. Nutr. Metab. Care*, 15, 144, 2012.
20. Berger, M.M. and Chiolero, R.L. Key vitamins and trace elements in the critically ill, in *Nutrition and Critical Care*, Cynober, L. and Moore, F.A., eds., Nestle Nutrition Workshop Series Clinical & Performance Program, 2003, pp. 8–9, 1999.
21. Chandra, R.K. Excessive intake of zinc impairs immune responses. *JAMA*, 252, 1443, 1984.
22. Baumgartner, T.G., ed. *Clinical Guide to Parenteral Micronutrition*, 3rd edn., Fujisawa, Chicago, IL, 1997.

23. Bielsalki, H.K. The role of antioxidants in nutritional support. *Nutrition*, 16, 578, 2000.
24. Mizock, B.A. Immunonutrition and critical illness: An update. *Nutrition*, 26, 701, 2010.
25. Berger, M.M. and Cholero, R.L. Antioxidant supplementation in sepsis and systemic inflammatory response syndrome. *Crit. Care Med.*, 35(9), S584, 2007.
26. Reddell, L. and Cotton, B.A. Antioxidants and micronutrient supplementation in trauma patients. *Curr. Opin. Clin. Nutr. Metab. Care*, 15, 181, 2012.
27. Berger, M.M., Soguel, L., Pinget, C. et al. Antioxidant supplements modulate clinical course after complex cardiac surgery and major trauma. *Intensive Care Med.*, 31(supp. 1), S32, 2005.
28. Angstwurm, M.W., Engelmann, L., Zimmerman, T. et al. Selenium in intensive care (SIC): Results of a prospective randomized, placebo-controlled, multiple-center study in patients with severe systemic inflammatory response syndrome, sepsis, and septic shock. *Crit. Care Med.*, 35, 118, 2007.
29. Valenta, J., Brodska, H., Drabek, T. et al. High dose selenium substitution in sepsis: A prospective randomized clinical trial. *Intensive Care Med.*, 37, 808, 2011.
30. Nathens, A.B., Neff, M.J., Jurkovich, G.J. et al. Randomized, prospective trial of antioxidant supplementation in critically ill surgical patients. *Ann. Surg.*, 236, 814, 2002.
31. Collier, B.R., Giladi, A., Dossett, L.A. et al. Impact of high-dose antioxidants on outcomes in acutely injured patients. *J. Parenter. Enteral Nutr.*, 32, 384, 2008.
32. Giladi, A.M., Dossett, L.A., Fleming, S.B. et al. High-dose antioxidant administration is associated with a reduction in post injury complications in critically ill trauma patients. *Injury*, 48, 78, 2010.
33. Berger, M.M., Soguel, L., Shenkin, A. et al. Influence of early antioxidant supplements on clinical evolution and organ function in critically ill cardiac surgery, major trauma, and subarachnoid hemorrhage patients. *Crit. Care*, 12, R101, 2008.
34. Manzanares, W., Dhaliwal, R., Jiang, X. et al. Antioxidant micronutrients in the critically ill: A systematic review and meta-analysis. *Crit. Care*, 16, R66, 2012.
35. Sriram K. and Lonchyna, V.A. Micronutrient supplementation in adult nutrition therapy: Practical considerations. *J Parenter Enteral Nutr.*, 33(5), 548, 2009.
36. Sriram, K., Mazanares, W., and Joseph, K. Thiamine supplementation in nutrition support. *Nutr. Clin. Pract.*, 27, 50, 2012.
37. Berger, M.M., Berger-Gryllaki, M., Wiesel, P.H. et al. Gastrointestinal absorption after cardiac surgery. *Crit. Care Med.*, 28, 2217, 2000.
38. McClave, S.A., Martindale, R.G. et al. Guidelines for the provision and assessment of nutrition support therapy in the adult critically ill patient. *J. Parenter. Enteral Nutr.*, 33, 277, 2009.

9 Fluid, Electrolyte, and Acid–Base Requirements in the Critically Ill Patient

Maria R. Lucarelli, Lindsay Pell Ryder, Mary Beth Shirk, and Jay M. Mirtallo

CONTENTS

INTRODUCTION

Critically ill patients manifest a multitude of fluid, electrolyte, and acid–base disturbances. Nutrition support in the form of enteral tube feeding or parenteral nutrition (PN) may be associated with these disorders either by being a primary cause or by being the major mode of treatment. As such, the clinician providing nutrition support must know basic and advanced concepts of fluid, electrolyte, and acid–base balance. The purpose of this chapter is to summarize the etiology, symptoms, and treatments of fluid, electrolyte, and acid–base disorders commonly observed in the intensive care patient receiving nutrition support.

BODY FLUID COMPARTMENTS

Maintenance of fluid and electrolyte homeostasis is necessary for normal cell function, and the human body has an incredible ability to compensate for excessive fluid and electrolyte losses and intake. Figure 9.1 illustrates the distribution of fluid and electrolytes of the body. In the critically ill patient, the balance may be challenged, at times to such an extreme that the body is unable to compensate. Early recognition and treatment of such abnormalities by critical care practitioners can avoid morbidity and mortality.

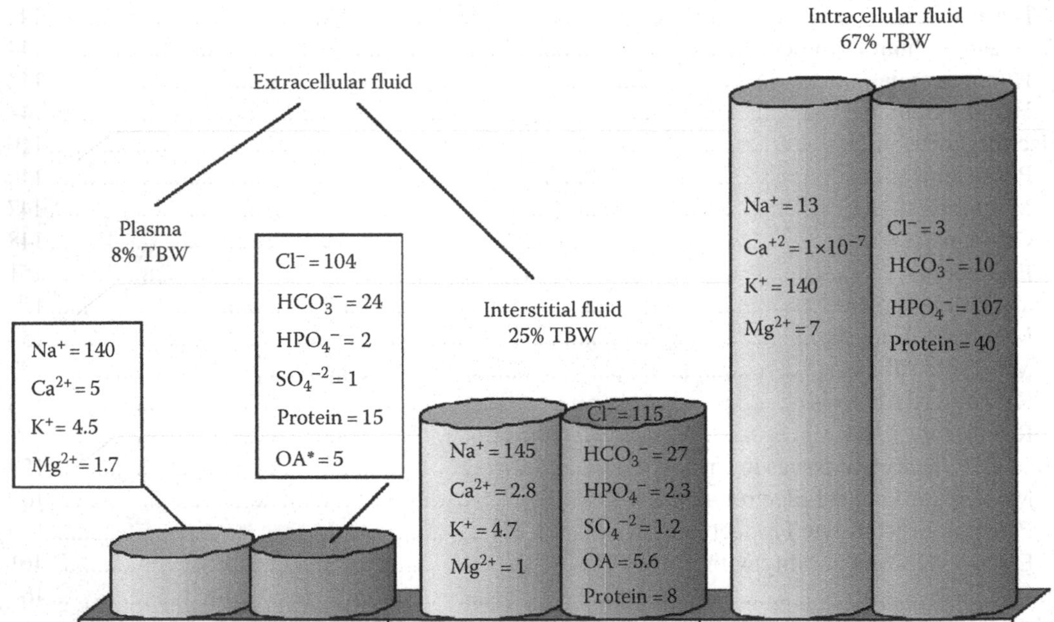

FIGURE 9.1 Distribution and composition of body fluids. TBW, total body water; OA, organic acids. (Adapted with permission from Whitmire, S.J., Fluid and electrolytes, in: Matarese, L.E. and Gottschlich, M.M. (eds.), *Contemporary Nutrition Support Practice: A Clinical Guide*, WB Saunders, Philadelphia, PA, 1998, p. 128; Ohs, M.S. and Uribarri, J., Electrolytes, water, and acid–base balance, in: Shils, M.E., Olson, J.A., and Shike, M., and Ross, A.C. (eds.), *Modern Nutrition in Health and Disease*, 9th edn., Williams & Wilkins, Baltimore, MD, 1999, p. 107; Shapiro, J. and Kaehny, W., Pathogenesis and management of metabolic acidosis and alkalosis, in: Schrier, R.W. (ed.), *Renal and Electrolyte Disorders*, 6th edn., Lippincott Williams & Wilkins, Philadelphia, PA, 2003, pp. 115–153; Lumpkin, M.M., *Am. J. Hosp. Pharm.*, 51, 1427, 1994.)

EFFECTS OF STARVATION AND CRITICAL ILLNESS ON FLUID/ELECTROLYTE STATUS

During periods of prolonged starvation, there is a loss of lean tissue mass, water, and minerals. Up to 150 g of lean muscle is lost daily during simple starvation resulting in the release of 15–20 mmol of potassium and 110 mL of water from the intracellular to the extracellular fluid.[1] Stress or injury increases the lysis of lean tissue and may result in as much as 1.2 g of phosphorus, 60 mmol of potassium, and 450 mL of water loss per day.[1] These deficits predispose the patient to acute electrolyte abnormalities, fluid retention, and dysfunction of various organ systems. As such, nutrition support in the presence of severe malnutrition may lead to acute electrolyte shifts and fluid retention, which are well-known symptoms of the refeeding syndrome (RFS).[2] For PN patients, the RFS has been associated with severe complications of hypophosphatemia in patients being refed after severe weight loss.[3] The effects of the RFS on fluid/electrolytes and organ function however are much more comprehensive than those of hypophosphatemia. Solomon and Kirby proposed a definition/components of the *RFS* as the metabolic and physiologic consequences of the depletion, repletion, and compartmental shifts and interrelationships of the following: phosphorus, potassium, magnesium, glucose metabolism, vitamin deficiency, and fluid resuscitation.[3] As such, the nutritional status of the patient must be considered when determining fluid/electrolyte requirements and then diagnosing and managing electrolyte disorders.

REQUIREMENTS FOR FLUID AND ELECTROLYTES

When providing nutrition support, the enteral nutrition (EN) or PN fluid becomes a major, if not the primary, source of fluid and electrolytes for the patient. The critically ill patient may have conditions that alter the tolerance to fluid and electrolytes so these parameters are frequently monitored. During patient assessment, adjustment of the electrolyte content of PN or the fluid content of EN or PN is often considered. Therefore, the fluid volume and electrolyte composition of nutrition support are based on normal nutritional requirements, and adjustments are based on patient clinical condition and overall response to the fluids and electrolytes being administered.

FLUID

Normal requirements for water are 30–40 mL/kg or 1–1.5 mL/kcal provided in nutrition support. Adjustments are usually required for those patients with cardiac, renal, and hepatic dysfunction. Critically ill patients need fluid in adequate amounts to maintain blood pressure, urine output, and perfusion to vital organs. Nutrition support fluids are only one of many sources of fluids infused in these patients. Other sources include parenteral maintenance fluids (Table 9.1), parenteral medications, blood products, or fluids from renal replacement therapy. These fluids are important to

TABLE 9.1
Electrolyte Composition and Osmolality of Common IV Fluids

IV Fluid	Glucose (G/L)	Osmolality (mOsm/L)	Sodium (mEq/L)	Chloride (mEq/L)	Potassium (mEq/L)	Lactate (mEq/L)	Calcium (mEq/L)
Dextrose 5% in water (D5W)	50	252	0	0	0	0	0
Lactated Ringer's solution (LR)	0	273	130	109	4	28	2.7
0.9% sodium chloride (NS)	0	308	154	154	0	0	0
0.45% sodium chloride (1/2 NS)	0	154	77	77	0	0	0

consider when the need for fluid restriction is present. Where appropriate, fluid restriction may be accomplished by limiting the volume of drug infusions and maintenance IV solutions so that the fluid for nutrition support may be spared. In some cases, the electrolyte content of PN can be adjusted to include the electrolytes previously provided by IV fluids so that the IV fluid may be discontinued.

Electrolytes

Electrolyte requirements are based on three conditions: (1) replacement of a deficit, (2) normal nutritional needs, and (3) recognition and appropriate replacement of extraneous fluid losses.

1. Conditions that predispose to electrolyte deficiency are listed in Table 9.2. With severe malnutrition, the deficits may be intracellular and may not be apparent from serum chemistries. If renal function is adequate, normal serum levels may be maintained even though significant cellular deficits are developing. For example, there may be as much as a 40% total body deficit of magnesium before it is demonstrated as a low serum level.[4] Therefore, patients with severe malnutrition are at high risk of electrolyte deficiencies, some of which only become manifest or symptomatic when nutrition support is initiated. Since nutrition support increases the demand of these electrolytes, there are some circumstances in which the electrolyte disorder should be corrected prior to initiating the nutrient infusion, for example, hypokalemia (serum K < 2.7 mEq/L), hypophosphatemia (serum phosphorus < 2 mg/dL), and hypochloremic metabolic alkalosis (serum carbon dioxide content > 50 mEq/L or arterial blood gas [ABG] pH > 7.50).
2. Rudman et al.[5] demonstrated that a proper proportion of electrolytes per gram of nitrogen administered was required to promote repletion of lean body mass. In this investigation, a ratio of phosphorus 0.8 g, sodium 3.9 mEq, potassium 3 mEq, chloride 2.5 mEq, and calcium of 1.2 mEq per gram of nitrogen was required to achieve positive nitrogen balance and improve lean body mass rather than fat or water mass. These data support the concept that electrolytes are required for nutritional purposes irrespective of renal, liver, or cardiac function and serve as the basis for the normal requirements for EN and PN (Table 9.3).[6,7]
3. Deficits in fluid, electrolyte, and acid or base may occur in critically ill patients resulting from large amounts of extraneous fluid outputs. Extraneous fluid outputs are those that are not normally present (e.g., ostomy, fistula, or nasogastric drainage, high urine output or diarrhea) and are in volumes in excess of that which can be managed without some form of intravenous replacement fluid. Generally, volume losses <600 mL/day in patients with normal renal function can be tolerated with minimal adjustments in intravenous fluid content

TABLE 9.2
Etiology of Common Electrolyte Deficiencies

Electrolyte	Cause of Deficiency
Sodium	Loss from skin, GI system, lungs Kidney: diuretic use, renal damage, adrenal insufficiency
Potassium	Starvation, loss from skin, bile, lower GI, or fistula Kidney: diuretic use, alkalosis, amphotericin
Bicarbonate	Diarrhea, pancreas, or small bowel loss, mineralocorticoid deficiency Kidney: renal tubular acidosis
Chloride	Loop diuretics, gastric loss, intestinal loss
Magnesium	Starvation, intestinal loss due to malabsorption or diarrhea, alcoholism, laxative abuse, diuretics, cyclosporine
Phosphorus	Starvation, alkalosis, glucose administration, diabetic ketoacidosis, gastrointestinal losses, use of Al-containing antacids

TABLE 9.3
Daily Electrolyte Requirements

Electrolyte	Enteral RDA/AI Reference Value	Parenteral
Sodium	500 mg (22 mEq/kg)	1–2 mEq/kg
Potassium	2 g (51 mEq/kg)	1–2 mEq/kg
Chloride	750 mg (21 mEq/kg)	As needed to maintain acid–base balance with acetate
Magnesium	420 mg (17 mEq/kg)	8–20 mEq
Calcium	1200 mg (30 mEq/kg)	10–15 mEq
Phosphorus	700 mg (23 mg/kg)	20–40 mmol

(e.g., addition of potassium or magnesium to a maintenance IV solution or adjustment of the sodium, potassium chloride, or acetate content of PN). When this volume is exceeded, a parenteral replacement fluid is required to be administered such that the fluid and electrolytes in the extraneous output are replaced. To assure proper replacement, the electrolyte content of the fluid being lost should be known (Table 9.4), and a replacement fluid should be selected that is similar in electrolyte content (Table 9.5). Lactated Ringer's solution should be used with caution in critically ill patients with low perfusion states. These patients may be prone to a lactic acidosis due to anaerobic glucose oxidation and the lactate dose provided by the IV solution. Other fluids such as 0.45% sodium chloride may need to be modified by adding sodium or potassium acetate in order to provide a source of bicarbonate.

TABLE 9.4
Electrolyte Content of Extraneous Fluid Loss

	Electrolyte Content of Fluid Loss (mEq/L)				
Source	Sodium	Hydrogen	Potassium	Chloride	Bicarbonate
Gastric	40–65	90	10	100–140	—
Pancreatic	135–150		5–10	60–75	70–90
Bile	128–160		4–12	90–120	30
Intestinal (jejunum)	95–120		5–15	80–130	10–20
Intestinal (ileum)	110–130		10–20	90–110	20–30
Diarrhea	90–120		5–10	75–120	5–40

TABLE 9.5
Electrolyte Replacement for Extraneous Fluid Loss

Source	Major Electrolyte Lost	Parenteral Replacement Fluid
Gastric	Hydrogen (acid), chloride	0.9% sodium chloride 0.45% sodium chloride if receiving acid suppression therapy
Pancreatic	Sodium, bicarbonate	Lactated Ringer's solution with added bicarbonate
Biliary and small bowel syndrome	Sodium, chloride, bicarbonate	Lactated Ringer's solution
Diarrhea	Sodium, potassium, chloride, bicarbonate	Lactated Ringer's solution or lactated Ringer's solution with added bicarbonate

FLUID AND SODIUM DISORDERS

Hyponatremia

Abnormally low sodium values are commonly encountered with an estimated incidence of 1% in all hospitalized patients and an incidence of 14% in the critically ill.[8,9] Hyponatremia is defined as serum sodium levels <135 mmol/L, though clinically significant hyponatremia usually occurs at levels <130 mmol/L. In evaluating patients with hyponatremia, it is important to assess tonicity. Hyponatremia may occur in hypotonic, normotonic, and hypertonic states. Pseudohyponatremia seen in patients with hyperlipidemia or hyperproteinemia reflects a decreased sodium in whole plasma, while the sodium concentration in plasma water remains constant. Hyperglycemia is the most common setting of hypertonic hyponatremia as increased plasma glucose results in a shift of water from the intracellular to extracellular space in response to the osmolar effect of glucose. In hyperglycemic states, the serum sodium is expected to decrease 1.6 mmol/L for every 100 mg/dL rise in serum glucose.[10]

Patients with hypotonic hyponatremia are often seen in the critical care setting. Attention to volume status is important in determining an etiology. Isovolemic hypotonic hyponatremia encompasses common conditions associated with hyponatremia in the hospitalized patient. The syndrome of inappropriate antidiuretic hormone (SIADH) is the most common cause of hyponatremia.[11] Clinically, the patient appears euvolemic, but is total body water overloaded as there is inappropriate concentration of the urine. Spot urine sodium values are elevated (>20 mmol/L) with a corresponding elevated urine osmolality (>100 mOsm/L).[12] This results in hypotonic hyponatremia. SIADH can be seen in patients with central nervous system (CNS) disease, malignancy, and lung disease and with the administration of some drugs including diuretics, antidepressants, and analgesics. This is a diagnosis of exclusion as normal thyroid, adrenal, and renal functions need to be confirmed.

Other causes of hypotonic hyponatremia (Figure 9.2) need to be considered in the critically ill patient. In patients who are volume depleted, one must consider both renal and extrarenal salt wasting. Most commonly, this occurs in the setting of dehydration, diuretic use, vomiting, or diarrhea. Hyponatremia can also occur in edematous patients, such as those with heart failure or liver failure as a result of increased extracellular water.

Clinical manifestations of hyponatremia include malaise, headache, seizures, coma, and even death. The rate at which the decreased sodium develops contributes to the degree of signs and symptoms a patient will demonstrate. That is, the more rapid the decline in serum levels, the more symptomatic a patient may become. Acute decline in serum sodium levels (<48 h) can lead to cerebral edema resulting in severe neurologic findings and potentially terminating in brain herniation. Correction of the serum sodium should be <10–12 mmol/L in the first 24 h and <18 mmol/L in 48 h to avoid the potential complication of the osmotic demyelination syndrome.[13] In patients with high risk for osmotic demyelination, efforts should be made to remain well below these limits.[13] In situations with acute declines in serum sodium and neurologic findings suggestive of edema, a quick increase in serum sodium of 2–4 mmol/L is effective in reducing intracranial pressure.[13] Treatment is aimed at the underlying mechanism. Hypovolemic patients can usually be treated with isotonic saline. In the settings of symptomatic normovolemic or hypervolemic hyponatremia, hypertonic saline infusions in conjunction with furosemide-induced diuresis can be attempted. This must be performed under close monitoring of the serum sodium levels. In all patients with hyponatremia, access to free water should be limited.

Hypernatremia

Hypernatremia, defined as a serum sodium of >145 mmol/L, has been estimated to occur at a frequency of 6% in the intensive care unit (ICU).[14] This is despite the often daily monitoring of

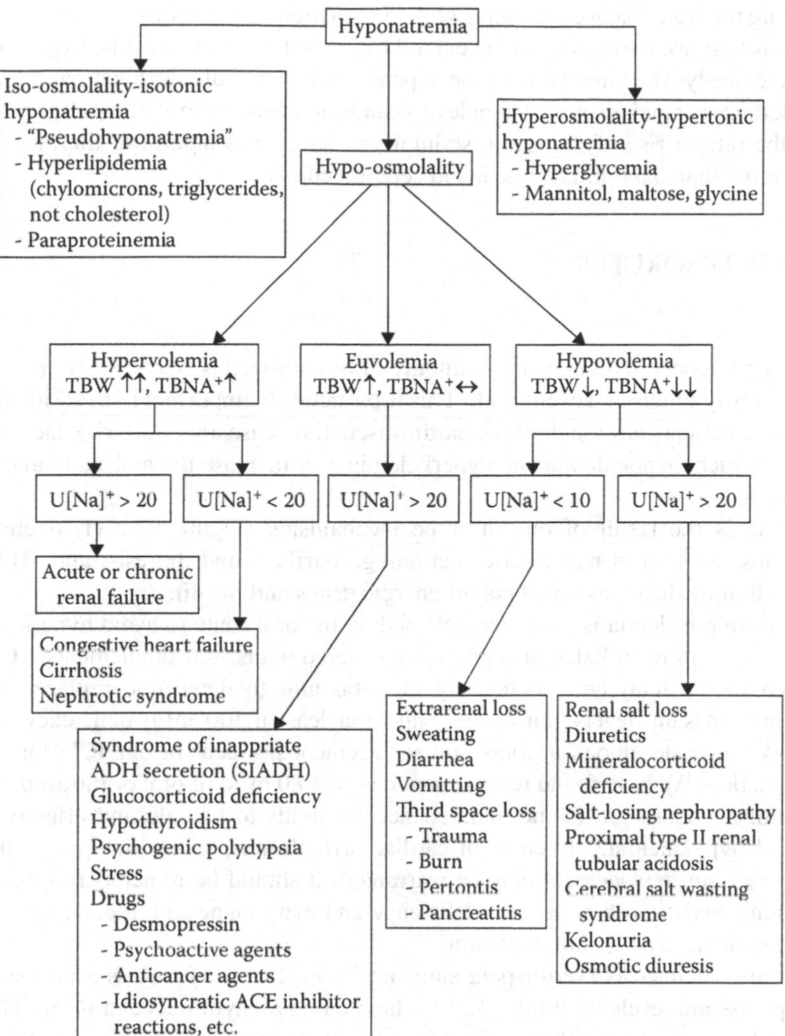

FIGURE 9.2 Etiology of hyponatremia. (Reprinted from *Best Pract. Res. Clin. Endocrinol. Metab.*, 17, Weiss-Guillet, E.M., Takala, J., and Jakob, S.M., Diagnosis and management of electrolyte emergencies, 623–651, Copyright 2003, with permission from Elseveir.)

fluid and electrolytes. Hypernatremia that develops during a patient's ICU stay has been linked to an increase in overall mortality compared to patients that present with elevated serum sodium levels.[14] Hypernatremia denotes an imbalance between body water and sodium in the body. In the hospital setting, this is usually a combination of patient's lack of access to free water and excessive loss of hypotonic fluids (i.e., gastrointestinal and respiratory fluid loss). This is compounded by inappropriate fluid prescriptions, sodium bicarbonate administration, medications, and hypertonic PN.

Clinical manifestations include lethargy, altered mental status, irritability, hyperreflexia, and spasticity. If the rise in serum sodium occurs rapidly, it can lead to rapid brain shrinkage and intracranial hemorrhage. Management of hypernatremia involves addressing the underlying cause as well as restoring the water balance. Patients with hypernatremia will require hypotonic fluid administration. This is best accomplished via the enteral route. If this is not possible, hypotonic fluids can be given intravenously. The rate of correction depends on how rapidly the hypernatremia developed. If the rise in sodium is rapid, serum sodium levels can be returned to normal rapidly without sequela. However, if the rate of rise of the serum sodium was slow or is unknown, the rate of correction should be no more than 0.5 mmol/L/h to avoid cerebral edema.[15]

ELECTROLYTE DISORDERS

POTASSIUM

Hypokalemia and hyperkalemia occur commonly in hospitalized patients.[16,17] Both conditions can lead to cardiac arrhythmias and even death. This is particularly important in the critically ill patient as many of these patients have underlying cardiovascular disease and other risk factors for cardiac arrhythmias. As such, hypokalemia and hyperkalemia may increase the morbidity and mortality of these patients.

Hypokalemia is the result of one of three mechanisms (Figure 9.3): (1) decreased intake; (2) increased loss as seen in nasogastric suctioning, diarrhea, and diuresis; and (3) transcellular shifts as a result of medications (i.e., beta-adrenergic drugs and insulin).

Treatment of hypokalemia is best accomplished by the oral route to avoid hyperkalemia, as the most common cause of hyperkalemia is physician-ordered potassium supplements.[17] Consideration must be given to the total body deficiency of potassium to determine replacement. Changes of 0.3 mEq in potassium levels can correspond to at least a 100 mEq deficiency in total body potassium.[18] We have developed a potassium replacement protocol in our ICU for patients with intact renal function. We have found replacement doses of 80 mEq of oral or intravenous potassium in patients with no potassium in the maintenance IV fluids to be safe and effective in correcting episodes of hypokalemia.[19] In cases of cardiac arrhythmias, severe myopathy, and paralysis, intravenous potassium replacement may be warranted. It should be remembered that magnesium deficiency often coexists with potassium deficiency and that magnesium replacement is necessary in this setting to achieve potassium repletion.

Hyperkalemia is defined as a serum potassium of >5 mEq/L and is seen less commonly than hypokalemia. At potassium levels >6.0 mEq/L, life-threatening arrhythmias can occur. Hyperkalemia results from either impaired renal excretion, drug effect, or impaired potassium entry into the cell or can be factitious (i.e., hemolysis, severe leukocytosis/thrombocytosis, fist clenching during venipuncture). Renal insufficiency is present in 80% of clinical episodes of hyperkalemia.[17]

Clinically, hyperkalemia is usually silent but can result in cardiac conduction abnormalities. The earliest sign is peaking of the T waves followed by widening of the QRS. Slow idioventricular rhythms, ventricular fibrillation, or cardiac standstill can occur.

Treatment to lower serum potassium levels should be initiated when serum levels are >6.0 mEq/L or cardiac conduction abnormalities are present.[17] Intravenous calcium in the form of either calcium gluconate or calcium chloride can be given with continuous ECG monitoring to reverse these abnormalities and should be given in this setting. Glucose and insulin, administered intravenously usually as 10 units of insulin and 25 g of dextrose to prevent hypoglycemia, can be used to encourage transcellular shift in the potassium. High-dose beta-2 agonists such as albuterol can be given 10–20 mg in 4 cc by nebulizer over 10 min, which will also result in transcellular potassium shifts. These are temporizing measures that can be used until therapy to remove potassium from the body is initiated. Sodium polystyrene (Kayexalate®) can be given to bind potassium in the colon. Hemodialysis can be undertaken for rapid removal of potassium. Sodium bicarbonate should be reserved for patients with coexisting acidosis and should not be used as a single agent. Any offending agents should be removed. The mainstay of management is to reduce dietary potassium intake.

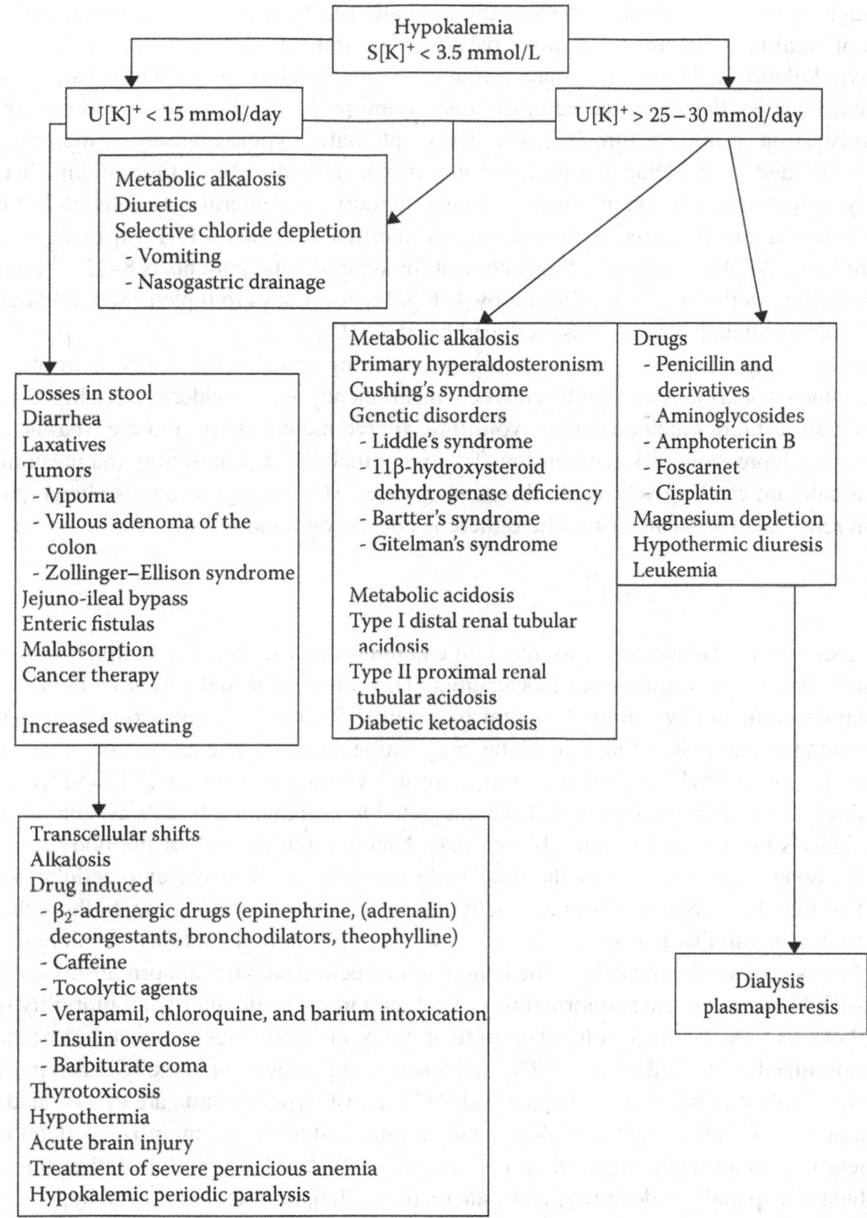

FIGURE 9.3 Etiology of hypokalemia. (Reprinted from *Best Pract. Res. Clin. Endocrinol. Metab.*, 17, Weiss-Guillet, E.M., Takala, J., and Jakob, S.M., Diagnosis and management of electrolyte emergencies, 623–651, Copyright 2003, with permission from Elseveir.)

Magnesium

Many of the conditions associated with hypokalemia can result in decreased serum magnesium levels. Magnesium is affected by dietary intake, gastrointestinal absorption, and renal loss. Magnesium wasting can occur with volume expansion or diuresis, as magnesium reabsorption by the kidneys is dependent on urine volume. Renal tubular damage and many drugs can contribute to magnesium wasting. The most common drugs to cause hypomagnesemia include ethanol, diuretics, aminoglycosides, amphotericin, and foscarnet. Proton pump inhibitors have also been implicated. It is often accompanied by hypocalcemia, hypokalemia, and metabolic alkalosis.

Hypomagnesemia occurs in 60%–65% of the critically ill.[20] Clinically, patients can present with symptoms of weakness, dizziness, tremors, paresthesias, and seizures as well as cardiac arrhythmias. As hypokalemia and hypocalcemia are often present, the clinical symptoms can overlap.

Treatment includes therapy directed at the underlying problem, if possible, and oral or parenteral administration of magnesium. In cases of asymptomatic hypomagnesemia, the oral route is preferred in divided doses. Diarrhea may become problematic and limit the amount that can be given orally. In patients with symptomatic hypomagnesemia, parenteral infusions of 1–2 mEq/kg body weight (a parenteral source is magnesium sulfate that provides 8.12 mEq mg/g of salt) are administered over 8–24 h.[21] Suggested replacement for symptomatic patients is 8–12 g of parenteral magnesium sulfate in the first 24 h followed by 4–6 g/day for 3 days to replete stores. Patients with renal insufficiency should have the dose reduced by 25%–50%.[22]

Hypermagnesemia is rare and usually iatrogenic resulting from intake in PN or in magnesium-containing antacids or laxatives. Patients with renal insufficiency and the elderly are at highest risk.[23,24]

Clinical manifestations include nausea, vomiting, altered mental status, muscle weakness, paralysis, respiratory depression, and hypotension. Treatment includes discontinuing magnesium intake. Intravenous calcium can be given in life-threatening cases. Hemodialysis can also be employed for magnesium removal, usually in cases where there is coexisting renal failure.

Calcium

The body goes to extreme measures to maintain calcium homeostasis. It is willing to sacrifice its skeleton and dentition to maintain normocalcemia. This alone is an indication of the critical role calcium plays in human physiology. Calcium is essential for muscle contraction, neural conduction, bone strength, and proper function of the coagulation cascade. The actions of three hormones (parathyroid hormone [PTH], calcitonin, and activated vitamin D or $1,25(OH)_2VitD_3$) and three organs (kidney, bone, and small intestine) are integrated to regulate the body's content of calcium, one of the body's most abundant ions (Figure 9.4). Ninety-eight percent of the body's calcium is stored in the bone. Less than 1% of the total body calcium exists in the extracellular fluid, and nearly half of that 1% exists in a bound, inactive form. It is the remaining 0.5%, the unbound, or ionized, serum calcium that is responsible for most of the physiologic actions of calcium. Despite the integral physiologic role of calcium, the benefit of correcting calcium abnormalities is unknown. An association between extreme abnormalities of calcium in the critically ill and mortality has been identified, but recommendations as to when to treat hypo- or hypercalcemia have not been defined through randomized controlled trials.[25,26] The incidence of hypocalcemia in the ICU is reported to be up to 90% for total calcium and 50% for ionized.[27] Causes of hypocalcemia are diverse and include insufficient action of PTH or $1,25(OH)_2VitD_3$ and an impaired ability to mobilize skeletal calcium; hypomagnesemia, as adequate magnesium is required for PTH release and its action; increases in calcium chelation; parathyroidectomy; and pancreatitis. Chelation as a cause of hypocalcemia is common in the ICU because of the greater frequency of citrated packed red blood cell transfusions. Citrate, which is also used as an anticoagulant for continuous renal replacement therapies in the ICU, binds calcium and results in a decrease in effective serum levels.[28] Other causes of hypocalcemia specific to the critically ill are not well understood. In a study evaluating hypocalcemia in septic ICU patients, Lind et al. found that bone resorption was not attenuated nor was there an increase in urinary excretion of calcium; the authors proposed that hypocalcemia in septic patients is related to the inflammatory response.[29]

Hypocalcemia is more likely to be symptomatic if it develops acutely. Tetany, paresthesias, circumoral numbness, decreased myocardial contractility, bradycardia, hypotension, psychosis, and confusion are a few of the common symptoms of hypocalcemia. Most of these symptoms have multifactorial causes, particularly in the critically ill patient, and a thorough assessment should include a calcium level (Figure 9.5). When interpreting low serum calcium levels, one must first ask, "Is it real?" Recall that slightly less than half of the serum calcium is protein bound and that it

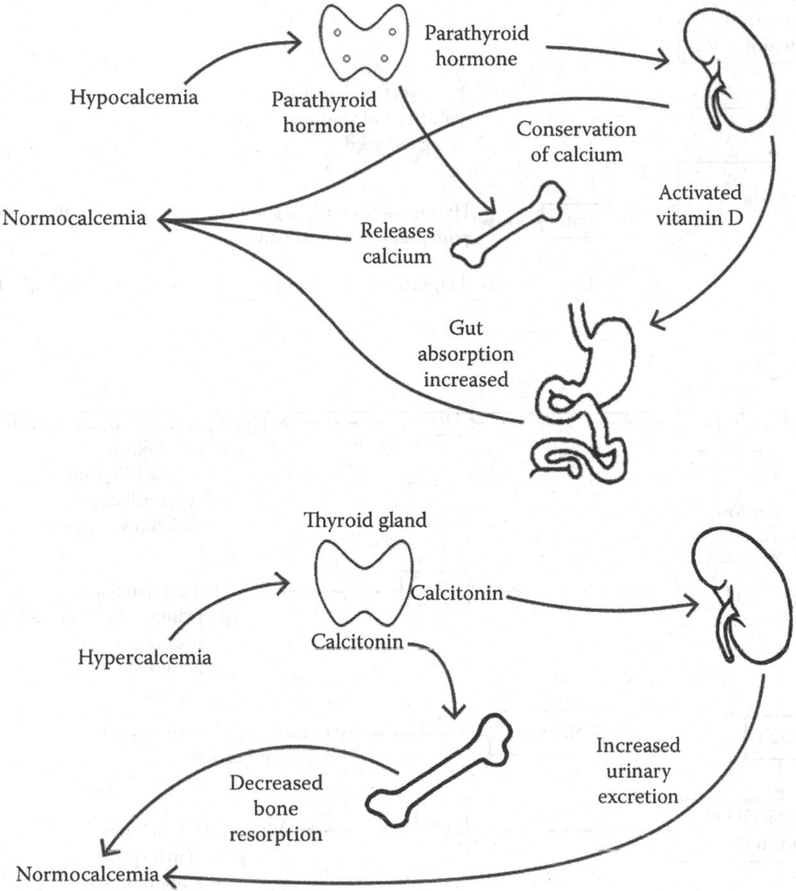

FIGURE 9.4 Regulation of calcium homeostasis.

is the unbound form of calcium that is active. Low total serum calcium levels need not be treated if the unbound or ionized portion is within the normal range. But often it is the total, not the unbound, calcium measurement that is available. Factors affecting the ionized fraction include albumin available for binding (each 1 g/dL decrease of serum albumin results in a decrease of total serum calcium by 0.8 mg/dL)[30] and serum pH (alkalosis decreases ionized calcium by increasing the protein binding of calcium; acidosis increases available ionized calcium). For critically ill patients, these factors are highly variable. While ionized calcium can be predicted from a total calcium when all other factors affecting its binding are considered, in the critically ill patient, this method has not been shown to be reliable; therefore, the most accurate method for measuring calcium in this setting is the ionized calcium.[31]

As with all electrolyte abnormalities, the cause of hypocalcemia should be identified and corrected. For example, if hypocalcemia is accompanied by hypomagnesemia, treatment of hypomagnesemia must be initiated; otherwise, attempts to correct the calcium will be unsuccessful. If hypocalcemia is a result of hyperphosphatemia, attempts to correct the hyperphosphatemia should be undertaken prior to replacing with calcium, and replacement delayed until serum phosphate has fallen below 6 mg/dL.[32]

Hypocalcemia is typically symptomatic if total calcium is <7–8 mg/dL or if the ionized calcium is <2.8 mg/dL (0.7 mmol/L).[33,34] A replacement threshold of 3.2 mg/dL (0.8 mmol/L) in the critically ill patient has been proposed; mild degrees of hypocalcemia (ionized calcium <>0.8 mmol/L) are typically well tolerated and often not acutely replaced.[31] Patients with symptomatic hypocalcemia

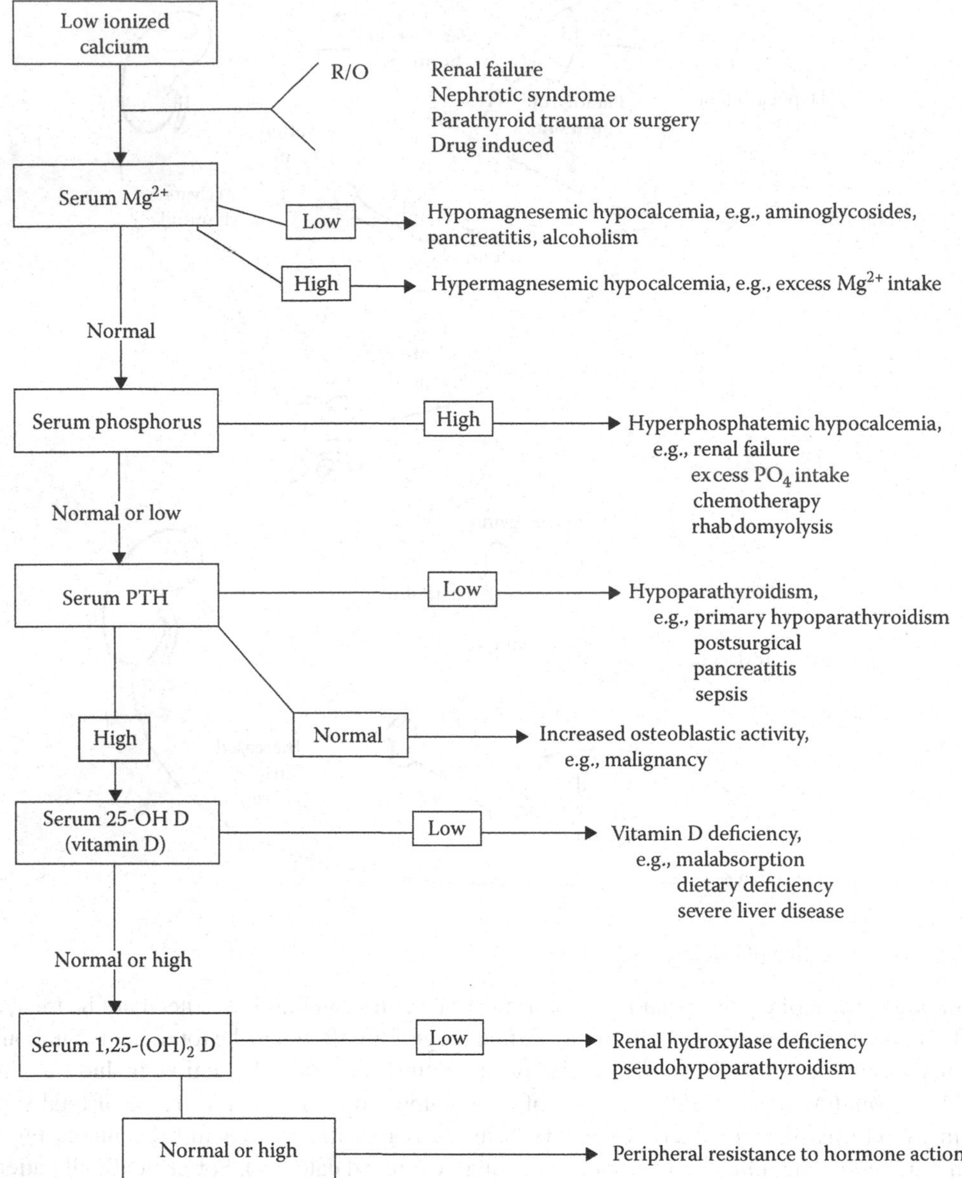

FIGURE 9.5 Evaluation of hypocalcemia. (Reprinted with permission from Zaloga, G.P. and Chernow, B., Divalent ions: Calcium, magnesium, and phosphorus, in: Chernow, B. (ed.), *Pharmacologic Approach to the Critically Ill Patient*, 3rd edn., Lippincott, Williams & Wilkins, Baltimore, MD, 1994, p. 784, Chapter 46.)

and those with corrected serum levels of 7.5 mg/dL (1.875 mmol/L) or less should be treated with parenteral calcium until the symptoms cease.

Calcium gluconate is the preferred injectable product, as calcium chloride is extremely hyperosmolar and irritating to the veins. Calcium chloride 10%, however, provides more elemental calcium per volume than does calcium gluconate 10% injectable solution (27.2 vs. 9.4 mg/mL). Chronic, asymptomatic, mild hypocalcemia should be treated enterally.[32] Available calcium products are listed in Table 9.6.

At our institution, the ICU replacement protocol includes an IV dose of 4 g calcium gluconate followed by six doses of enteral calcium citrate over 72 h for values 3.5 mg/dL and below. This was

TABLE 9.6
Agents for Calcium Replacement

Product	Dose Form	Elemental Calcium Content
Calcium acetate	667 mg tablet/capsule	8.5 mEq or 169 mg
(Phos-Lo®)	333.5 mg capsule	4.2 mEq or 84.5 mg
Calcium carbonate tablets	500 mg tablets, chewable	10 mEq or 200 mg
(Tums®, various)	650 mg tablet	13 mEq or 260 mg
	1000 mg tablet	20 mEq or 400 mg
	1250 mg tablet	25 mEq or 500 mg
	1.25 g/5 mL	25 mEq or 500 mg/5 mL
Calcium citrate	950 mg chewable tablet	10.6 mEq or 211 mg
(Citracal®, various)		
Calcium gluconate	500 mg tablet	2.25 mEq or 45 mg
Calcium chloride for injection	10% solution, 1 g/10 mL	13.6 mEq or 273 mg
Calcium gluconate for injection	10% solution, 1 g/10 mL	4.65 mEq or 93 mg

found to be effective unless patients were receiving multiple blood transfusions. Implementation of protocol-driven calcium replacement decreased the frequency of unnecessary IV calcium replacement and blood draws.[35]

Hypercalcemia does not occur as frequently as hypocalcemia in the critically ill patient. The primary causes of hypercalcemia include malignancy, hyperparathyroidism, and increased calcium intake. Mild hypercalcemia is generally asymptomatic (up to 12 mg/dL or 3 mmol/L). Initial symptoms may include fatigue, weakness, anorexia, constipation, or depression. Levels >12 mg/dL can result in confusion, hallucinations, and somnolence. High calcium levels can cause acute pancreatitis, and levels of 16 mg/dL or greater can result in stupor or coma. The therapeutic intervention undertaken should reflect the severity of the clinical manifestation. Treatment includes aggressive hydration, a loop diuretic such as furosemide to increase urinary excretion, and agents directed at bone resorption such as calcitonin and bisphosphonates.

Phosphorus

Phosphorous is a vital electrolyte, particularly in the ICU patient. It is the source for the high-energy bonds of adenosine triphosphate, which supplies energy for all physiologic functions. In addition, it is required for the proper synthesis of 2,3-diphosphoglycerate in red blood cells, a substance required for normal oxygen delivery to tissues. Phosphorous thus facilitates electrolyte transport, muscle contractibility, and the metabolism of protein, carbohydrates, and fat.

Phosphate is the body's most abundant intracellular anion. Almost all plasma phosphorous exists as either free or protein-bound phosphate. Approximately 85% of phosphorous is in the bones, about 14% in the body's soft tissues, leaving only 1% of total body phosphorous in the extracellular fluid (ECF). Homeostasis is maintained via interactions of hormones and organs, as with calcium. The exchange between the ECF and other forms of phosphorus is relatively slow.

Hypophosphatemia results from poor gastrointestinal absorption, significant intracellular shifts, or excessive loss of phosphate via the kidneys. True hypophosphatemia takes 4–8 weeks to develop. Patients particularly at risk for severe hypophosphatemia include chronic alcoholics and patients with diabetic ketoacidosis.

Seizures, chest and muscle pain, red blood cell hemolysis, and numbness and tingling occur with acute hypophosphatemia. Chronic depletion can result in bone stiffness, lethargy, memory loss, bruising, and bleeding. In critical illness, shifts in the oxygen dissociation curve resulting from hypophosphatemia can result in significant pulmonary compromise. As with calcium, an association between increased mortality and hypophosphatemia is known to exist. It remains unclear whether hypophosphatemia is merely a marker or an abnormality that, when corrected, lowers mortality. Prospective trials are needed.[36]

Current protocols for phosphate supplementation provide a weight-based replacement for phosphorus levels of <2[37] or <3 mg/dL.[38] It has been suggested to adjust the dose for renal function and to replace phosphorus until a level above 2 mg/dL is achieved.[37] Phosphate maintenance replacement following initiation of the protocol is recommended although it is for a brief period of time.

A point of debate is the recommended infusion time for phosphate-containing products. Recommendations range from at a rate of 7.5 mmol/h[37] to 0.64 mM/kg over up to 12 h, which equates to a rate of 3.7 mmol/h for a 70 kg patient.[38] Our preference is to infuse 15 mmol of phosphate over 2 h.

Potassium phosphate injection is included in the Institute for Safe Medication Practices (ISMP) list of high-alert medications. Confusion surrounds the injectable phosphate products due to the dose terminology—mmoles and mEqs for the products. One of ISMP's safety recommendations is to always order phosphate products in both millimoles of phosphate and mEqs of potassium (or sodium). ISMP also featured two oral phosphate products K-Phos Neutral® and Neutra-Phos-K® on the *Look-Alike/Sound-Alike Drug Names* list. Neutra-Phos-K contains a significant amount of potassium, and K-Phos Neutral does not. The report included a case in which a patient received the incorrect product following hospital discharge and later required readmission to the hospital as a result of the error.[39,40] Despite this and other highly publicized cases, ISMP later reported that just one in three computer systems provided alerts when Neutra-Phos-K was prescribed for a patient with an elevated potassium.[41] Caution should be exercised when prescribing, dispensing, or administering any phosphate product (Table 9.7).

Hyperphosphatemia in the ICU is most often the result of renal insufficiency but can also be due to its release from intracellular fluid following the lysis of red blood cells or injury to skeletal muscle. Symptoms of hyperphosphatemia are commonly associated with the resultant hypocalcemia; the primary complication of hyperphosphatemia is metastatic calcification of calcium phosphate in soft tissues, blood vessels, and organ parenchyma. The risk of metastatic calcification is increased when the phosphorus and calcium product exceeds 70, that is, inorganic phosphorus (mg/dL) × total calcium (mg/dL) exceeds 70.[42]

If hyperphosphatemia is acute and life threatening, hemodialysis should be considered. Dextrose and insulin cause an intracellular shift of phosphate into cells and can be administered for an immediate response. Phosphate excretion can be increased with a saline infusion. In the more chronic setting, phosphate-binding salts can be used. Agents such as calcium carbonate, calcium acetate, sevelamer, and aluminum hydroxide are effective.

TABLE 9.7
Agents for Phosphorous Replacement

	Phosphorus		Potassium		Sodium	
Product	**(mg)**	**(mmol)**	**(mg)**	**(mEq)**	**(mg)**	**(mEq)**
K-Phos Neutral Tablet	250	8	45	1.1	298	13
Neutra-Phos Powder® (75 mL reconstituted)	250	8	278	7.125	164	7.125
Neutra-Phos-K Powder (75 mL reconstituted)	250	8	556	14.25	0	0
Uro-KP-Neutral Tablet®	250	8	49.4	1.27	250.5	10.9
Fleet Phospho-Soda® (per 5 mL)	640	20.5	0	0	552	24
Skim milk (per quart)	1000	32	1600	40	552	24
Sodium phosphate for injection	3 mmol phosphate and 4 mEq sodium/mL					
Potassium phosphate for injection	3 mmol phosphate and 4.4 mEq potassium/mL					

ACID–BASE DISORDERS

Acid–base disorders are common in critically ill patients and can cause alterations in physiologic function that have a deleterious effect on a patient's medical condition. Prompt identification and appropriate management of these disorders are essential to patient care. The following sections will discuss the principles of acid–base regulation, pathophysiology of the common acid–base disorders, and treatment strategies in the critically ill patient.

An acid is a substance that donates hydrogen ions, while a base is a substance that accepts hydrogen ions. The balance between acid and base determines the pH, which is representative of the hydrogen ion concentration. The normal pH of blood is 7.35–7.45. Lower pH values indicate acidemia, while higher values are indicative of an alkalemic state.

Acidosis is defined as a process that decreases the pH of the blood, and alkalosis is a process that increases the pH. There are three processes that occur within the body to regulate acid–base balance in an attempt to maintain the pH within or close to its normal range. The first is chemical buffering. A buffer is a substance that can both accept and donate hydrogen ions. When a buffer is present in a solution, addition of acid or base to a solution will have a blunted effect on the pH. There are three buffers that serve to regulate acid–base balance: carbonic acid/bicarbonate, protein, and inorganic phosphate. Of these three, the carbonic acid/bicarbonate buffer is the most important. Buffering acts very quickly and its effects are immediate.[43]

The other two physiologic mechanisms for acid–base balance are compensatory responses. Compensation is defined as the physiologic changes that occur within the body to shift the pH toward a normal value in response to a primary acidosis or alkalosis. Respiratory compensation involves changes in the depth and rate of ventilation to control CO_2 excretion. This type of compensation is rapid and takes place within minutes of onset of the disorder. Metabolic or renal compensation is a much slower process than respiratory compensation because it involves alterations in renal acid excretion, bicarbonate reabsorption, and bicarbonate generation. These changes can take 6–24 h to take effect.[43]

Acid–base disorders can be divided into simple and mixed disorders. In a simple disturbance, there is only a single acid–base process and its expected compensation. Mixed disturbances consist of more than one primary acid–base disorder. The pH is determined by the magnitude of each of the individual disturbances. There are four types of simple acid–base disorders. These are defined by the direction of the pH deviation from normal (acidosis vs. alkalosis) and the primary abnormality that exists (metabolic vs. respiratory). Hence, the four disorders are referred to as metabolic acidosis, metabolic alkalosis, respiratory acidosis, and respiratory alkalosis.

The assessment and diagnosis of acid–base disorders involves ABGs, serum electrolytes, history and clinical signs and symptoms, and a review of the patient's medications and nutrition. The ABG is used to determine both oxygenation status and acid–base condition. The components of an ABG report are pH, partial pressure of oxygen (PaO_2), oxygen saturation (SaO_2), partial pressure of carbon dioxide ($PaCO_2$), and bicarbonate (HCO_3^-). Normal ABG values are found in Table 9.8.

TABLE 9.8
Normal ABG Values

pH	7.40 (7.35–7.45)
pO_2	80–100 mmHg
SaO_2	95%
pCO_2	35–45 mmHg
HCO_3^-	22–26 mEq/L

Source: Devlin, J.W. and Matzke, G.R., Acid–base disorders, in: DiPiro, J.T., Talbert, R.L., Yee, G.C., Matzke, G.R., Wells, B.G., and Posey, L.M. (eds.), *Pharmacotherapy: A Pathophysiologic Approach*, 8th edn., McGraw-Hill, New York, 2008.

TABLE 9.9
ABG Interpretation

Disorder	pH	Primary Change	Compensatory Response	Expected Compensation
Metabolic acidosis	Decreased	↓ HCO_3^-	↓ pCO_2	pCO_2 decreases by 10–13 mmHg for each 10 mEq/L decrease in HCO_3^-.
Metabolic alkalosis	Increased	↑ HCO_3^-	↑ pCO_2	pCO_2 increases by 6–7 mmHg for each 10 mEq/L increase in HCO_3^-.
Respiratory acidosis	Decreased	↑ pCO_2	↑ HCO_3^-	Acute: HCO_3^- increases by 1 mEq/L for each 10 mmHg increase in pCO_2. Chronic: HCO_3^- increases by 3–4 mEq/L for each 10 mmHg increase in HCO_3^-.
Respiratory alkalosis	Increased	↓ pCO_2	↓ HCO_3^-	Acute: HCO_3^- decreases by 2 mEq/L for each 10 mmHg decrease of pCO_2. Chronic: HCO_3^- decreases by 5 mEq/L for each 10 mmHg decrease in pCO_2.

Source: Adapted from Shapiro, J. and Kaehny, W., Pathogenesis and management of metabolic acidosis and alkalosis, in: Schrier, R. (ed.), *Renal and Electrolyte Disorders*, 6th edn., Lippincott Williams & Wilkins, Philadelphia, PA, 2003, pp. 115–153.

The components of the ABG can be assessed one at a time in a stepwise fashion starting with the pH, followed by the $PaCO_2$ and HCO_3^-. Table 9.9 provides the values that would be expected in each of the four types of simple acid–base disorders. It also indicates the expected compensation for each of the disorders. If the actual compensation is greater or less than expected, a mixed acid–base abnormality exists.[44]

The consequences of acidosis involve numerous organ systems. The cardiovascular system may undergo arteriolar dilatation, decreased cardiac contractility and cardiac output, and predisposition to arrhythmias. In addition, patients can experience CNS depression, hyperventilation, and GI symptoms such as nausea and vomiting. Hyperglycemia can result from insulin resistance and hyperkalemia often occurs secondary to a shift in intracellular potassium to the extracellular fluid.[45]

Like acidosis, alkalosis has detrimental physiologic effects. These include arteriolar vasoconstriction, decreased myocardial and cerebral perfusion, arrhythmias, hypoventilation, and low serum concentrations of potassium, magnesium, phosphorus, and ionized calcium.[46]

Metabolic Acidosis

Metabolic acidosis occurs when serum pH is decreased secondary to a decrease in the serum bicarbonate concentration. Metabolic acidosis can be classified as either anion gap or nonanion gap acidosis. The anion gap measures the difference between the unmeasured anions (proteins, sulfates, phosphates, organic anions) and the unmeasured cations (magnesium, calcium, potassium) in the serum and can be determined using the following equation:

$$\text{Anion gap} = [Na^+] - ([Cl^-] + [HCO_3^-])$$

Because the total concentration of cations and anions must be equal in the serum, increases in the anion gap indicate accumulation of unmeasured anions in the serum. The normal value for anion gap is 9 mEq/L (range of 3–11 mEq/L), and a value of 17–20 mEq/L or greater reflects an increase in unmeasured serum anions. The presence or absence of an increased anion gap can assist in determining the cause of a metabolic acidosis. Increased anion gap acidosis is seen when bicarbonate losses are replaced by an anion other than chloride (i.e., phosphates, sulfates, or organic anions such as lactate and ketones). This occurs in conditions such as lactic acidosis, ketoacidosis, renal failure, excessive electrolyte administration, dehydration, and toxic ingestion of methanol, ethylene glycol, and salicylates. Additionally, administration of some ICU-specific drugs may result in an anion gap metabolic acidosis. The intravenous formulation of lorazepam contains propylene glycol, which is metabolized to lactic acid and can cause lactic acidosis.[47–52] Propofol has a rare adverse effect known as propofol-related infusion syndrome, which is characterized by lactic acidosis, elevated serum triglyceride levels, cardiac dysrhythmias, and hypotension.[49,53–55] Normal anion gap acidosis is also referred to as hyperchloremic acidosis because of its association with increased serum chloride that has replaced depleted bicarbonate. This type of acidosis is seen with diarrhea, renal tubular acidosis with renal wasting of bicarbonate, and excessive exogenous chloride administration. The latter may be observed in the ICU setting when large volumes of chloride-rich fluids (sodium chloride 0.9% and hydroxyethyl starches) are administered to patients with shock.[49] Several studies have demonstrated a correlation between intravenous chloride load and the development of hyperchloremia and metabolic acidosis.[56,57] Although intravenous fluids such as lactated Ringer's solution and Plasma-Lyte A contain physiologic concentrations of chloride, the use of such fluids in critically ill patients has been demonstrated to increase the incidence of metabolic alkalosis.[57] Thus, the ideal strategy for fluid resuscitation in regard to maintaining acid–base balance is still under investigation.

The anion gap has some limitations when employed in critically ill patients. First, administration of large volumes of chloride-rich fluids (such as is seen in patients with septic shock) complicates diagnosis as the presence of excess chloride ions can mask a coexisting anion gap metabolic acidosis.[58] Hypoalbuminemia, which is common in critically ill patients, may also confound interpretation of the anion gap. Because albumin is one of the unmeasured anions, hypoalbuminemia decreases the anion gap and may cause an organic metabolic acidosis to exhibit the laboratory criteria for a nonanion gap acidosis.[44,58]

When metabolic acidosis is present, the body compensates by increasing its respiratory rate, which in turn increases CO_2 excretion. The result is a decrease in $PaCO_2$. Respiratory compensation typically starts within 15–30 min of the onset of metabolic acidosis, but its full compensatory effects are not seen for 12–24 h. This compensation occurs such that for every 1 mEq/L decrease of bicarbonate, the $PaCO_2$ decreases by 1–1.5 mmHg (Table 9.9).[59]

Treatment of metabolic acidosis should first be aimed at correcting the underlying cause (Table 9.10). In addition, resuscitation and adequate ventilation are of immediate concern. Pharmacologic alkali therapy can be used to moderate the acidosis until the underlying cause is adequately treated or endogenously corrected. The available alkalinizing agents include sodium bicarbonate, sodium acetate, sodium citrate, sodium lactate, and tromethamine (THAM). Sodium bicarbonate is the most commonly used alkali therapy in critically ill patients.[58] However, controlled clinical studies have not shown a benefit of sodium bicarbonate over general supportive care.[43] In addition, sodium bicarbonate should be avoided in lactic acidosis and other acidotic conditions associated with tissue hypoxia due to its propensity to increase CO_2 production.[43] Other risks associated with intravenous sodium bicarbonate include overshoot alkalosis, hypernatremia, and pulmonary edema.[43,49] The sodium salts of acetate, citrate, and lactate all require metabolism to sodium bicarbonate and have not been studied widely in this setting. Tromethamine is a sodium-free buffer that accepts hydrogen ions from both dissolved carbon dioxide and conventional acid solutions.[49] Its place in therapy is not clear as it has not demonstrated significant benefit over sodium bicarbonate.[60,61] For patients with metabolic acidosis receiving PN, the acetate content in the formulation should be increased and the chloride content decreased (particularly in hyperchloremic patients).[44]

TABLE 9.10
Etiology-Specific Treatment of Acid–Base Disorders

Disorder	Etiology	Treatment
Metabolic acidosis	Methanol or ethylene glycol ingestion	• Forced diuresis. • Alkali replacement. • Thiamine and pyridoxine supplementation. • Ethanol or fomepizole administration. • Hemodialysis.

	Lactic acidosis	• Correct underlying cause.
		• Ensure adequate tissue oxygenation.
		  • Mechanical ventilation.
		  • Fluid repletion.
		  • Inotropic drugs.
		  • Avoid vasoconstricting agents.

	Diabetic ketoacidosis	• Insulin. • Fluid, sodium, and potassium replacement. • Alkali therapy not advisable unless pH < 7.10 or hypotension is refractory to fluid repletion.
	Alcoholic ketoacidosis	• Fluid repletion with 5% dextrose in 0.9% sodium chloride. • Replace phosphorus, magnesium, and potassium as needed. • Benzodiazepines may be required for prevention of delirium tremens.
	Administration of non-alkali-containing IV fluids	• Add bicarbonate to the IV fluid.
	GI bicarbonate losses	• Correct GI pathology. • Oral or IV alkali replacement. • Correct associated losses of fluid and electrolytes (sodium and potassium).
	Renal failure	• Increase bicarbonate or acetate in dialysate. • Oral alkali replacement over several days, followed by maintenance alkali regimen.
	Type I RTA (distal)	• Alkali therapy. • Potassium replacement usually not necessary if alkali therapy is effective.
	Type II RTA (proximal)	• Large doses of alkali. • Potassium replacement. • Vitamin D for prevention of bone disorders.
	Type IV RTA (hyperkalemia)	• Treat hyperkalemia. • Low dose alkali therapy may be necessary.
Metabolic alkalosis	GI acid losses	• Administer H2-blocker or proton pump inhibitor to reduce gastric acid secretion. • Administer antiemetics for vomiting.
	Villous adenomas	• Surgical removal.
	Chloride responsive with volume depletion	• Administer IV normal saline. • Potassium replacement to correct concomitant hypokalemia.

(Continued)

TABLE 9.10 (*Continued*)
Etiology-Specific Treatment of Acid–Base Disorders

Disorder	Etiology	Treatment
	Chloride responsive with volume overload	• Administer potassium chloride. • Administer acetazolamide or a potassium-sparing diuretic (spironolactone, triamterene, amiloride) if diuresis is indicated.
	Chloride resistant due to primary hyperaldosteronism or Cushing's syndrome	• Administer a potassium-sparing diuretic. • Surgical removal of adrenal tumor if present.
	Excessive black licorice ingestion	• Discontinue licorice ingestion. • May administer potassium-sparing diuretics until alkalosis corrects.
Respiratory acidosis	Upper airway obstruction	• Immediate oxygenation. • Airway suctioning for secretion removal.
	Impaired alveolar gas exchange	• Immediate oxygenation. • Antibiotic therapy for pneumonia. • Diuresis for pulmonary edema.
	Obstructive airway disease	• Immediate oxygenation. • Inhaled bronchodilator for bronchospasm.
	Disorders of the respiratory muscles and chest wall	• Immediate oxygenation. • Consider inspiratory aids or assisted ventilation.
	Inhibition of central respiratory control	• Immediate oxygenation. • Reversal of narcotic agents with naloxone.
	Chronic obstructive pulmonary disease	• Smoking cessation. • Bronchodilators. • Inhaled or oral corticosteroids.
Respiratory alkalosis	Anxiety/pain	• Provide reassurance and nonpharmacologic pain control. • Treat with appropriate pain and antianxiety medication.
	Mechanical hyperventilation	• Decrease tidal volume. • Decrease respiratory rate.

	Voluntary hyperventilation	• Reassurance.
		• Rebreathing into paper bag.
		• Treat underlying psychological stress.
		  • Consider sedative agents.
		  • Consider beta-adrenergic antagonists.

	Salicylate toxicity	• Provide airway protection and stabilization. • Contact poison control center for information about gastric lavage or activated charcoal administration. • Fluid replacement. • Potassium repletion. • Consider hemodialysis in severe cases.

METABOLIC ALKALOSIS

Metabolic alkalosis presents as increased arterial pH associated with elevated serum bicarbonate. Metabolic alkalosis can be caused by excessive loss of hydrogen ions via the GI tract (nasogastric suctioning, vomiting, secretory diarrhea) or kidneys (diuretic use). Other causes include volume depletion, high-dose penicillin therapy, excess mineralocorticoid activity, and organic anion administration (lactate from lactated Ringer's solution, acetate from PN, and citrate from blood transfusion). Inappropriate alkali therapy for respiratory acidosis can also lead to metabolic alkalosis.

Furthermore, restricting the use of chloride-rich fluids in an attempt to avoid metabolic acidosis has been shown to increase the incidence of metabolic alkalosis.[57] Finally, in critically ill patients with chronic respiratory acidosis, a posthypercapnic metabolic alkalosis can occur when mechanical ventilation is employed and the respiratory acidosis is rapidly corrected. The compensatory elevated plasma sodium bicarbonate persists after correction of the hypercapnia if chloride replacement is inadequate.[62–64]

Patients with normal kidney function are able to maintain acid–base balance, even in the presence of factors that are known to cause metabolic alkalosis. However, there are two renal mechanisms that result in maintenance of metabolic alkalosis. The first occurs with diuretic use and GI losses and is characterized by volume depletion and chloride loss. Metabolic alkalosis of this type is referred to as sodium chloride-responsive alkalosis and is characterized by a low urine chloride (<10 mEq/L).[62] The second metabolic alkalosis is sodium chloride resistant and is most often associated with excess mineralocorticoid activity and associated hypokalemia secondary to renal loss of potassium. This subset of metabolic alkalosis manifests with both elevated urine chloride (>10 mEq/L) and urine potassium (>30 mEq/L).[62]

The body's compensation for metabolic alkalosis is hypoventilation, which leads to an increase in $PaCO_2$ within hours. For every 10 mEq/L increase in bicarbonate, the $PaCO_2$ increases by 6–7 mmHg (Table 9.9).[59]

The treatment of sodium chloride-responsive metabolic alkalosis should first be directed at correcting the factor that is maintaining the alkalosis, followed by a correction of the causative factors (Table 9.10). Administration of sodium chloride and potassium chloride-containing IV fluids will replenish both chloride and fluid. As chloride is repleted and sodium and/or potassium are excreted, bicarbonate will also be renally eliminated.[63] Patients with volume overload or an inability to tolerate a volume load may receive the carbonic anhydrase inhibitor acetazolamide that inhibits the reabsorption of bicarbonate by the kidneys. Acetazolamide also causes increased potassium and phosphorus excretion so these electrolytes will need to be monitored and replaced as necessary.[63] In severe or refractory cases of metabolic alkalosis, acidifying agents may be considered. These include hydrochloric acid, arginine monohydrochloride, and ammonium chloride.[43,63] Hemodialysis using a low-bicarbonate dialysate can also expedite correction of metabolic alkalosis.[63]

Sodium chloride-resistant metabolic alkalosis is rarely life threatening and can often be managed by reducing or eliminating the cause of mineralocorticoid excess. Approaches to achieve this goal include decreasing corticosteroid dosages or changing to a corticosteroid with less mineralocorticoid activity in patients receiving these agents. For those individuals with an endogenous source of mineralocorticoid excess, a potassium-sparing diuretic (spironolactone, triamterene, amiloride) may be administered or aggressive potassium repletion may be undertaken.[62,63]

Respiratory Acidosis

Respiratory acidosis is primary CO_2 retention that decreases the serum pH and results from the pulmonary system's failure to excrete CO_2 normally. Because metabolic compensation is slow and does not occur for at least 12–24 h after the onset of the disturbance, respiratory acidosis can be divided into two categories: acute and chronic. Acute respiratory acidosis occurs over minutes to hours and does not allow enough time for metabolic compensation. Causes of this type of disturbance include severe pulmonary disease, neuromuscular conditions that affect control of ventilation, and incorrect mechanical ventilator settings. Critically ill patients with acute respiratory distress syndrome are managed with a low-tidal volume strategy of mechanical ventilation in order to prevent alveolar overdistension.[65] The resulting mild hypercapnia has become acceptable to clinicians treating this disease state.[62] Finally, the administration of PN with greater than 50% of nonprotein calories provided by glucose can result in drastic increases in CO_2 production and consequently lead to respiratory acidosis. Chronic respiratory acidosis is seen when the increase in $PaCO_2$ and hypoxia occur to a non-life-threatening degree, allowing time for metabolic compensation to occur. Conditions that are often associated with chronic respiratory acidosis include chronic obstructive pulmonary disease and disorders involving restriction of the chest wall or lung.

The body's immediate response to acute respiratory acidosis is chemical buffering via the carbonic acid/bicarbonate mechanism. As a result of this buffering, the serum bicarbonate increases by 1 mEq/L for each 10 mmHg increase in $PaCO_2$. When respiratory acidosis persists beyond 12–24 h, metabolic compensation occurs in the form of increased renal bicarbonate reabsorption, increased hydrogen ion secretion, and ammoniagenesis. This compensation causes an increase of serum bicarbonate of 4 mEq/L for every 10 mmHg rise in $PaCO_2$ (Table 9.9).[59]

The treatment of acute respiratory acidosis consists of providing immediate adequate oxygenation, which may require intubation and mechanical ventilation. In addition, airway secretions should be adequately removed. The underlying cause must then be addressed. Specifically, patients receiving nutrition support should be assessed for overfeeding as this can cause excess CO_2 production (Table 9.10). Alkali therapy is rarely necessary and may in fact decrease the patient's respiratory drive or cause a metabolic alkalosis. Patients with a severe respiratory acidosis with hemodynamic compromise may require careful administration of sodium bicarbonate or tromethamine.

Patients with chronic respiratory acidosis may experience respiratory decompensation with precipitating conditions such as infection, oxygen therapy, or narcotic use. As with acute respiratory acidosis, the primary intervention is provision of adequate oxygenation. However, it is imperative to recognize that at baseline, these patients have a lower PaO_2 and higher $PaCO_2$ than patients without chronic lung disease. Therefore, the respiratory drive is dependent upon hypoxemia, not hypercarbia, and oxygen administration can eliminate the drive to breathe.

Respiratory Alkalosis

Respiratory alkalosis is a primary decrease in $PaCO_2$ caused by increased excretion of CO_2 by the lungs. This may occur via central or peripheral stimulation of respiration, mechanical ventilation, or voluntary hyperventilation.

The body's most rapid response to acute respiratory alkalosis occurs through the carbonic acid/bicarbonate buffer system, which takes only minutes to exert its full effect. For each 10 mmHg drop in $PaCO_2$, the serum bicarbonate concentration decreases by 3 mEq/L. If the respiratory alkalosis is still present 6 h after its onset, subsequent metabolic compensation will begin. The renal response is to increase bicarbonate elimination and decrease bicarbonate production. This compensation leads to a decrease in bicarbonate by 4 mEq/L per 10 mmHg decrease in $PaCO_2$ (Table 9.9).[59]

Identification and correction of the underlying cause are the initial steps in treatment of respiratory alkalosis (Table 9.10). Patients who are awake and alert can breathe into a paper bag to increase the pCO_2 in inspired air. If severe hypoxemia occurs, oxygen therapy should be initiated. In more severe cases ($pH > 7.60$), complications such as seizures and arrhythmias may be seen. If this is the case, mechanical ventilation, accompanied by sedation and possible neuromuscular blockade, may be necessary. For patients who are already undergoing mechanical ventilation, consider the possibility that the ventilator settings are the cause of the alkalosis and need to be adjusted.

FLUID AND ELECTROLYTE ISSUES IN CRITICAL CARE

The system of care for critically ill patients is important to consider when dealing with fluid and electrolyte problems in these patients. Areas that require attention are as follows: electrolyte disorders associated with medications[66] and parenteral electrolyte shortages and electrolyte compatibilities with EN and PN.

Medication-Induced Electrolyte Disorders

Buckley et al. identified and summarized the potential mechanisms of drug-induced electrolyte disorders that are likely in critically ill patients.[66] Most mechanisms are related to excess or too little intake and/or alterations in renal regulation of losses due to abnormal physiology. A list of agents associated with electrolyte disorders is provided in Table 9.11. The medications may be primarily involved with the disorder or may contribute to or exacerbate the disorder arising from other causes.

Parenteral Electrolyte Product Shortages

Since 2011 there has been a continuous or intermittent shortage of commercially available parenteral electrolyte products.[67] Historically, shortages of drugs have occurred intermittently but

TABLE 9.11
Medication-Induced Electrolyte Disturbances

Electrolyte Disturbance (Criteria)	Medications
Hyponatremia (Na_s < 135 mmol/L)	Thiazide and loop diuretics, mannitol, ACE inhibitors, trimethoprim–sulfamethoxazole
SIADH secretion	Proton pump inhibitors, nicotine, chlorpropamide, tolbutamide, clofibrate, cyclophosphamide, morphine, barbiturates, vincristine, acetaminophen, NSAIDs, antipsychotics, desmopressin, oxytocin, antidepressants (SSRIs, TCAs)
Hypernatremia (Na_s > 145 mmol/L)	Loop diuretics, mannitol, amphotericin B, demeclocycline, dexamethasone, dopamine, ifosfamide, lithium, ofloxacin, orlistat, foscarnet, hypertonic 3% saline or normal (0.9%) saline, antibiotics containing sodium, hypertonic sodium bicarbonate infusion Osmotic cathartic agents (lactulose, sorbitol)
Hypokalemia (K_s < 3.6 mmol/L)	Sympathomimetics (epinephrine, terbutaline, fenoterol, albuterol) Insulin, methylxanthines (theophylline, aminophylline), dobutamine Loop, thiazide and osmotic diuretics, carbonic anhydrase inhibitors Adrenocorticoid steroids, penicillin, aminopenicillins, aminoglycosides, amphotericin
Hyperkalemia (K_s > 5.3 mEq/L)	Citrate, penicillin G, EN and PN, spironolactone/amiloride, triamterene, trimethoprim, metoprolol, propranolol, labetalol, digoxin, ACE/ARB, heparin, LMWH, succinylcholine
Hypocalcemia	Fluoride poisoning, chemotherapeutic agents (cisplatin, carboplatin, 5-fluorouracil with leucovorin, dactinomycin, cyclophosphamide, ifosfamide, doxorubicin with cytarabine), bisphosphonates, calcitonin, amphotericin B, cimetidine, ethanol
Hypercalcemia	Vitamin D, vitamin A, estrogen, tamoxifen, diuretics, lithium
Hypophosphatemia (0.32–0.65 mmol/L)	Antacids (aluminum or magnesium containing), sucralfate, phosphate binders (calcium-containing products), aspirin (overdose), albuterol, catecholamines (epinephrine, dopamine), insulin (exogenous), sodium bicarbonate, acetaminophen (overdose), chemotherapeutic agents (ifosfamide, cisplatin, cyclophosphamide, doxorubicin), diuretics (thiazides, loop, osmotic, carbonic anhydrase inhibitors), glucocorticoids, theophylline (overdose), low or no-phosphate PN or EN
Hyperphosphatemia	Phosphate-containing enema/laxative, phosphate (exogenous intravenous or oral sources)
Hypomagnesemia	Aminoglycosides, amphotericin B, cisplatin, cyclosporine, colony-stimulating factors, digoxin, diuretics (thiazides, loop, osmotic, carbonic anhydrase inhibitors), foscarnet, methotrexate, pentamidine, polymyxin B, ticarcillin
Hypermagnesemia	Catecholamines (exogenous), insulin (exogenous), lithium intoxication, magnesium-containing enema/laxatives/antacids, magnesium (exogenous) administration (intravenous or oral)

Source: Buckley, M.S.et al., *Crit. Care. Med.*, 38(6 Suppl.), S253, 2010.

are resolved with time. However, commercial shortages of electrolytes do seem to occur periodically and have prompted professional societies to make recommendations for conserving product for those patients in most need. The following is an adaptation of recommendations made by the Shortage Subcommittee of the American Society for Parenteral and Enteral Nutrition for electrolyte replacement during product shortages[67]:

- Consider providing medications via the oral or enteral route when possible.
- Consider prioritizing patients, saving supply for those vulnerable populations such as neonatal, pediatric, or short bowel or malabsorption syndrome PN patients.
- Minimize use of electrolyte/mineral additives to parenteral fluids or as a supplement to EN.
- Revise electrolyte replacement algorithms based on serum electrolytes prioritizing symptomatic or at-risk patients.
- Use oral or enteral electrolyte product replacement whenever possible.
- Use premixed, parenteral electrolyte replacement products.
- Identify national availability of alternate salt forms or package volumes.
- Consider a standardized, commercial PN product with standard electrolytes for a portion of your patient population.
- Modify routine electrolyte monitoring for the patient population and the current ability to access sufficient quantities of electrolyte products.
- Realize the likelihood of an inferior outcome due to prioritizing use of electrolytes to at-risk patients, thereby denying access to others.

Electrolyte Compatibility with EN or PN

Electrolyte disorders are common in nutrition support patients. As such, electrolyte replacement is considered via nutrition support fluids and access devices. This coadministration with nutritional fluids creates issues of compatibility and sterility.

For EN, most organizations use a closed system to avoid inadvertent contamination that may result in clinical infections if infused into the patient. With a closed EN delivery system, electrolytes may not be added to the formula without opening the system and creating the possibility of contamination. Compatibility of oral liquid electrolyte products with EN fluids must also be considered. Liquid formulations of potassium chloride, magnesium, and phosphorus are not compatible with EN products.[68] These medications should not be infused with EN. If compatibility of the electrolyte product is not known, in general, syrups cause coagulation of EN products and should be avoided. The best practice of administering electrolytes via enteral feeding tubes should be to turn off the tube feeding, flush the catheter with 10–30 mL of fluid, administer the electrolyte, flush the catheter, and then resume the tube feeding. Another concern of electrolyte replacement is with gastrointestinal tolerance. Potassium chloride is very hyperosmolar (3000–3500 mOsm/kg) and may cause abdominal discomfort and diarrhea if administered in an undiluted form. Magnesium citrate and milk of magnesia are 1000 and 1250 mOsm/kg, respectively, and sodium phosphate (Fleet Phospho-Soda) is 2250 mOsm/kg. It is recommended that these formulations be diluted prior to administration.[67] Other formulations contain sorbitol, which may also cause GI distress.

Compatibility of electrolyte additives in PN is a continual concern. Some of the additives are conditionally compatible (interactions and precipitation are dependent on electrolyte concentration, final PN pH, order of admixture into PN, and environmental temperature and light during dispensing, distribution, and storage). Calcium salts are reactive compounds and readily form insoluble products with phosphorus, oxalate, and bicarbonate. The formation of the insoluble product dibasic calcium phosphate is an incompatibility of calcium and phosphorus in PN. Many factors influence the solubility of calcium and phosphorus including high concentrations of calcium and phosphorus, decreased amino acid concentrations, increased environmental temperature, increased PN formulation pH, or hang time prolonged beyond 24 h.[69] In 1994, a FDA Safety Alert addressed two

TABLE 9.12
Electrolyte Compatibility with PN

PN Type	2-in-1	3-in-1
Calcium gluconate	C	C
Hydrochloric acid	C	I
Magnesium sulfate	C	I
Potassium chloride	C	C
Potassium/sodium phosphate	I	I

C, compatible; I, incompatible.

deaths and two near fatal injuries associated with the infusion of an incompatible mixture of calcium phosphate.[70] To avoid problems with calcium phosphate compatibility, it is recommended to only use the gluconate salt for PN admixture, follow the proper sequence for electrolyte addition to PN during compounding, and not to exceed maximal compatible doses of calcium and phosphorus. Also, *borderline* doses should be avoided by considering separate infusions of calcium and/or phosphorus when higher-than-normal doses are required. Calcium may also react with bicarbonate in PN formulations. As such, bicarbonate is contraindicated, especially since acetate salts of potassium and sodium are effective sources of bicarbonate that are compatible in PN. Electrolytes administered separate from PN may be coinfused if compatible (Table 9.12).

PATIENT CASE

A 40-year-old female with metastatic ovarian cancer is admitted via the emergency room following a 2-week history of abdominal pain, persistent nausea, vomiting, and constipation. Her vital signs are as follows: SBP 96, DBP 69, HR 120, RR 16, T 97.5°F, and SpO_2 95%. On a physical exam, she appears thin, with no acute distress. Her lungs are clear bilaterally without wheezes, rhonchi, or rales. Cardiac assessment is normal. She has well-healed midline incisions and is distended but compressible with no tenderness to palpation. Her past medical history is significant for multiple surgeries, chemotherapy, and radiation complicated with deep vein thrombosis and pulmonary embolus. Most recently, she has developed abdominal ascites that requires frequent palliative paracentesis. Her current medications include paclitaxel (Taxol®) and bevacizumab (Avastin®). Her nutritional status as follows: height = 5′4″, weight = 60 kg, ideal body weight = 54.5 kg, and weight loss = 6 kg (10%) over the past 30 days diagnosed with acute starvation-related malnutrition. The patient is admitted with initial diagnosis of bowel obstruction and malnutrition. The plan is for operative repair of the bowel obstruction and PN. After successful repair of her bowel obstruction, she continues to remain in the ICU for inability to be weaned from mechanical ventilation and is to be initiated on PN. Parameters assessed at that time are provided in the following table:

WBC—9.6 × 109/L	Na—130 mmol/L	K—2.6 mmol/L	Cl—76 mmol/L	CO_2—44 mmol/L
BUN—20 mg/dL	Cr—1.26 mg/dL	Gluc—91 mg/dL	Mg—1.8 mmol/L	Ca—9.8 mg/dL
Phosphorus—1.9 mg/dL	Prealbumin—8 mg/dL	Osm—278 mOsm/kg	ABG	
pH, 7.59; pCO_2, 47; HCO_3, 45; pO_2, 97%; O_2 Sat, 97%; Base excess, 20.3				

WBC, white blood cell; Na, sodium; K, potassium; Cl, chloride; CO_2, bicarbonate; BUN, blood urea nitrogen; Cr, creatinine; Gluc, glucose; Mg, magnesium; Ca, calcium; Osm, osmolality, pCO_2, arterial carbon dioxide; pO_2 arterial oxygen; HCO_3, arterial bicarbonate (calculated); O_2 Sat, oxygen saturation.

WHAT APPROACH SHOULD BE TAKEN FOR PROPER FLUID/ELECTROLYTE MANAGEMENT WHEN INITIATING PARENTERAL NUTRITION?

On assessment, the patient has a hypochloremic metabolic alkalosis due to excess loss of stomach acid (nasogastric drainage over the past 24 h = 1670 mL). Hypokalemia and hypophosphatemia are also present. Since the patient is malnourished, they are at risk of the RFS on initiation of PN. It is recommended to replace the chloride (acid) deficit as well as correct the potassium and phosphorus levels prior to initiating PN. When initiating PN, use chloride salts of potassium and sodium and normal dose of phosphorus as the potassium salt (monitor renal function; the estimated creatinine clearance is 31 mL/min). Some who may argue would consider a pH < 7.50 to be a life-threatening condition. As such, the PN should be withheld PN until since it is likely to adversely affect correction of the alkalosis, with pH < 7.50. Once started, no more than 1 L/day of PN should be administered until it is assured that potassium and phosphorus levels are acceptable and the risk of RFS is resolved.

DEVELOP A PLAN FOR INITIATION, MONITORING, AND MANAGEMENT OF PN

Fluid and electrolyte management of a critically ill patient should be based on their initial status, ongoing needs, and alterations caused by critical illness. Table 9.13 provides a suggested monitoring protocol for critically ill patients receiving PN. On an acute basis, electrolyte deficiencies should be made immediately with either oral or intravenous replacements. Adjustments may be made to the PN but no more frequently than every 24 h. Once electrolyte derangements are corrected, the electrolyte composition of the PN needs to be reassessed in order to prevent high serum levels caused by amounts needed to correct deficits that no longer exist.

SUMMARY

Fluid, electrolyte, and acid–base disorders are a frequent concern to the clinician providing nutrition support to the intensive care patient. The underlying condition of the patient along with its treatment often results in derangements in fluid, electrolyte, and acid–base status. The clinical significance and management of these disorders (Table 9.14) is important to providing optimal nutrition support. The principles and concepts addressed in this chapter are commonly used by the clinician providing nutrition support to the critically ill patient.

TABLE 9.13
Monitoring Fluid and Electrolyte Status in a Critically Ill Malnourished Patient on PN

Parameter	Baseline	Initiation (Days 1–7)	Stable Patients
Electrolytes—Na, K, Cl, CO_2, Mg, Ca, phosphorus, BUN, Cr	Yes	Daily	1–2 times per week
ABG	Yes	As needed based on baseline and subsequent respiratory and metabolic assessment	
Serum glucose	Yes		1–2 times per week
Weight	Yes	Daily	2–3 times per week
Intake and output	Yes	Daily unless fluid status assessed by physical exam	
Individual electrolyte or ABG	Yes	At least 1 h after intravenous replacement dose administered	

Na, sodium; K, potassium; Cl, chloride; CO_2, bicarbonate; Mg, magnesium; Ca, calcium, BUN, blood urea nitrogen; Cr, serum creatinine.

TABLE 9.14
Clinical Significance and Management of Electrolyte Disorders

Electrolyte Disorder	Threshold of Clinical Significance	Treatment Approach
Hyponatremia	• Clinical symptoms • Usually sodium <130	• Treat underlying disorder • Water restriction (<1–2 L/day) • Saline infusion with goal 8 mmol/L/day correction[71] • Diuretics can increase free water excretion but should be used cautiously • In hypertonic hyponatremia treat increased glucose • Can consider 3% saline in cases of severe hyponatremia (<110) and CNS symptoms • Careful monitoring of sodium
Hypernatremia	• Clinical symptoms • Serum sodium >158	• Correction should be <0.5 mmol/L/h[15] • Hypotonic saline infusion • Hypovolemic patients should be given saline to stabilize hemodynamics, then proceed with hypotonic saline solutions • In central diabetes insipidus desmopressin 2–4 mcg IV • Careful monitoring of sodium
Hypokalemia	• Clinical symptoms • Serum K^+ <3.5 mEq/L in patient with cardiovascular disease	ECG monitoring Oral potassium replacement preferred Intravenous potassium rate should not exceed 20 mEq/h and serum potassium rechecked after 60 mEq[17]

Hyperkalemia	• Clinical symptoms
	• Serum K^+ >6.5 mEq/L
		• Confirm laboratory finding
		• Discontinue any potassium or potassium-containing agents
		• Nonemergent
		  • Loop diuretic increases renal excretion; its effects last up to 2 h
		  • Sodium polystyrene sulfonate (Kayexalate) ion-exchange resin; its effects last 1–3 h
		  • Hemodialysis/peritoneal dialysis; its effects last 48 h
		• Emergent
		  • Calcium antagonizes cardiac conduction abnormalities; onset 5 min; duration 1 h
		  • Bicarbonate causes transcellular shift; onset 15–30 min; duration 1–2 h
		  • Insulin causes transcellular shift; onset 15–60 min; duration 4–6 h
		  • Albuterol causes transcellular shift; onset 15–30 min; duration 2–4 h

Hypomagnesemia	• Clinical symptoms • Magnesium <1.0 mg/dL	• Oral replacement preferred in asymptomatic individuals • Symptomatic patients consider parenteral administration 1–2 mEq/kg of magnesium over 8–24 h Rapid infusion can lead to renal magnesium wasting
Hypermagnesemia	Clinical symptoms	• Discontinuing magnesium intake • Intravenous calcium for life-threatening circumstances • Hemodialysis

(Continued)

TABLE 9.14 (*Continued*)
Clinical Significance and Management of Electrolyte Disorders

Electrolyte Disorder	Threshold of Clinical Significance	Treatment Approach
Hypocalcemia[31]	Clinical symptoms 3.2 mg/dL (0.8 mmol/L)	• Symptomatic patient parenteral administration of 1–2 g calcium gluconate IVPB over 10 min, then 1–2 mg/kg/h of elemental calcium until serum calcium normalizes; then decrease rate based on patient response
	Ionized calcium <2.5 mg/dL urgently	• Replace serum magnesium and phosphorus • Oral calcium replacement when stable • Consider addition of vitamin D (calcitriol) 0.25 mcg po daily
Hypercalcemia[31]	Clinical symptoms Calcium >12 mg/dL Ionized calcium >mg/dL	• Discontinue calcium intake • Correct underlying cause • Aggressive hydration (approximately 200 mL/h, 0.9% sodium chloride) • Loop diuretic (e.g., furosemide 20–40 mg IVP) • Calcitonin 1–2 units/kg IV, SC every 12 h up to 8 units/kg every 6 h. • (onset in 6–10 h; unreliable response) • Bisphosphonates (e.g., pamidronate 60–90 mg IV infusion over 2–24 h; onset 4–7 days) • Hemodialysis with low calcium bath for life-threatening cases
Hypophosphatemia[27]	Clinical symptoms iPhos <2.5 mg/dL iPhos <1 mg/dL urgently	• IV if symptomatic • IV administration rates are highly variable (0.3–4 mg/kg/h) • Evaluate need for magnesium replacement • Oral route causes diarrhea in large doses • Administer for 5–7 days to replace stores, then maintain dose of 1200 mg/day orally or 1000 mg/day intravenously
Hyperphosphatemia[31]	Laboratory evidence Symptomatic from hypocalcemia	• Discontinue phosphate intake • Correct underlying cause • 0.9% sodium chloride infusion (250–500 mL/h) • Acetazolamide (500 mg every 6 h) • Enteral phosphate binders (e.g., aluminum hydroxide, calcium acetate, or sevelamer) • Hemodialysis for life-threatening cases

REFERENCES

1. Moore FD, Brennan MF, Ballinger WF et al. Surgical injury: Body composition, protein metabolism and neuroendocrinology. In: *Manual of Surgical Nutrition*. Philadelphia, PA: WB Saunders; 1975, pp. 169–222.
2. Kraft MD, Btaiche IF, Sacks GS. Review of the refeeding syndrome. *Nutr Clin Pract* 2005;20:625–633.
3. Solomon SM, Kirby DF. The refeeding syndrome: A review. *JPEN J Parenter Enteral Nutr* 1990;14:90–97.
4. Juan D. Clinical review: The clinical importance of hypomagnesemia. *Surgery* 1982;91:510–517.
5. Rudman D, Millikan WJ, Richardson TJ, Bixler TJ, Stackhouse J, McGarrity WC. Elemental balances during intravenous hyperalimentation of underweight adult subjects. *J Clin Invest* 1975;55:94–104.

6. Guidelines for the use of parenteral and enteral nutrition in adult and pediatric patients. *JPEN J Parenter Enteral Nutr* 2002;26:1SA–138SA.
7. National Advisory Group on Standards and Practice Guidelines for Parenteral Nutrition. Safe practices for parenteral nutrition formulations. *JPEN J Parenter Enteral Nutr* 1998;22:49–66.
8. Al Salman J, Kemp D, Randall D. Hyponatremia. *West J Med* 2002;176:173–176.
9. Bennani SL, Abouqal R, Zeggwagh AA et al. Incidence, causes and prognostic factors of hyponatremia in intensive care. *Rev Med Interne* 2003;24:224–229.
10. Katz MA. Hyperglycemia-induced hyponatremia—Calculation of expected serum sodium depression. *N Engl J Med* 1973;289:843–844.
11. Peixoto AJ. Critical issues in nephrology. *Clin Chest Med* 2003;24:561–581.
12. Fried LF, Palevsky PM. Hyponatremia and hypernatremia. *Med Clin North Am* 1997;81:585–609.
13. Verbalis JG, Goldsmith SR, Greenberg A, Schrier RW, Sterns RH. Hyponatremia treatment guidelines 2007: Expert panel recommendations. *Am J Med* 2007;120:S1–S21.
14. Polderman KH, Schreuder WO, Strack van Schijndel RJ, Thijs LG. Hypernatremia in the intensive care unit: An indicator of quality of care? *Crit Care Med* 1999;27:1105–1108.
15. Kahn A, Brachet E, Blum D. Controlled fall in natremia and risk of seizures in hypertonic dehydration. *Intens Care Med* 1979;5:27–31.
16. Gennari FJ. Hypokalemia. *N Engl J Med* 1998;339:451–458.
17. Gennari FJ. Disorders of potassium homeostasis. Hypokalemia and hyperkalemia. *Crit Care Clin* 2002;18:273–288, vi.
18. Asmar A, Mohandas R, Wingo CS. A physiologic-based approach to the treatment of a patient with hypokalemia. *Am J Kidney Dis* 2012;60:492–497.
19. Pell L, Shirk MB, Hoffmann S. Evaluation of a potassium replacement protocol in the medical intensive care unit. *Crit Care Med* 2003;31:A107.
20. Wong ET, Rude RK, Singer FR, Shaw ST Jr. A high prevalence of hypomagnesemia and hypermagnesemia in hospitalized patients. *Am J Clin Pathol* 1983;79:348–352.
21. Agus ZS, Wasserstein A, Goldfarb S. Disorders of calcium and magnesium homeostasis. *Am J Med* 1982;72:473–488.
22. Ayuk J, Gittoes NJL. How should hypomagnesaemia be investigated and treated? *Clin Endocrinol* 2011;75:743–746.
23. Clark BA, Brown RS. Unsuspected morbid hypermagnesemia in elderly patients. *Am J Nephrol* 1992;12:336–343.
24. Schelling JR. Fatal hypermagnesemia. *Clin Nephrol* 2000;53:61–65.
25. Egi M, Kim I, Nichol A et al. Ionized calcium concentration and outcome in critical illness. *Crit Care Med* 2011;39:314–321. doi: 10.1097/CCM.0b013e3181ffe23e.
26. Forsythe RM, Wessel CB, Billiar TR, Angus DC, Rosengart MR. Parenteral calcium for intensive care unit patients. *Cochrane Database Syst Rev* 2008:CD006163.
27. Zaloga GP. Hypocalcemia in critically ill patients. *Crit Care Med* 1992;20:251–262.
28. Morgera S, Schneider M, Slowinski T et al. A safe citrate anticoagulation protocol with variable treatment efficacy and excellent control of the acid-base status. *Crit Care Med* 2009;37:2018–2024. doi: 10.1097/CCM.0b013e3181a00a92.
29. Lind L, Carlstedt F, Rastad J et al. Hypocalcemia and parathyroid hormone secretion in critically ill patients. *Crit Care Med* 2000;28:93–99.
30. Whitmire S, Gottschlich MM. Fluids and electrolytes. In: *The Science and Practice of Nutrition Support: A Case Based Core-Curriculum*. Dubuque, IA: American Society of Parenteral and Enteral Nutrition; 2001.
31. Zaloga GP, Chernow B. Divalent ions: Calcium, magnesium, and phosphorus. In: *Pharmacologic Approach to the Critically Ill Patient*. Baltimore, MD: Lippincott, Williams & Wilkins.
32. Bushinsky DA, Monk RD. Electrolyte quintet: Calcium. *Lancet* 1998;352:306–311.
33. Weiss-Guillet EM, Takala J, Jakob SM. Diagnosis and management of electrolyte emergencies. *Best Pract Res Clin Endocrinol Metab* 2003;17:623–651.
34. Vanek VW, Shikora SA, Martindale RG, Schwaitzberg SD. Assessment and management of fluid and electrolyte abnormalities. In: *Nutritional Considerations in the Intensive Care Unit*. Dubuque, IA: Kendall/Hunt Publishing Company; 2002.
35. Shirk MB, Donahue K, Reilly K. Evaluation of an ICU calcium replacement protocol. *Pharmacotherapy* 2007;27:e33, A138.
36. Geerse DA, Bindels AJ, Kuiper MA, Roos AN, Spronk PE, Schultz MJ. Treatment of hypophosphatemia in the intensive care unit: A review. *Crit Care* 14:R147.

37. Guidelines for phosphorus supplementation in adults. *Formulary* 1998;33:263.
38. Clark CL, Sacks GS, Dickerson RN, Kudsk KA, Brown RO. Treatment of hypophosphatemia in patients receiving specialized nutrition support using a graduated dosing scheme: Results from a prospective clinical trial. *Crit Care Med* 1995;23:1504–1511.
39. Look-alike/sound-alike drug names and other product related issues. *ISMP Medication Safety Alert* 2002.
40. ISMP's list of high-alert medications. *ISMP Medication Safety Alert* 2003.
41. Safety still compromised by computer weaknesses: Comparing 1999 and 2005 pharmacy computer field test results. *ISMP Medication Safety Alert* 2005.
42. Brenner R, Brenner BM, Braunwald E et al. Disorders of the kidney and urinary tract. In: *Harrison's Principle's of Internal Medicine*. New York: McGraw-Hill Professional; 2001.
43. Devlin JW, Matzke GR. Acid–base disorders. In: DiPiro JT, Talbert RL, Yee GC, Matzke GR, Wells BG, Posey LM, eds. *Pharmacotherapy: A Pathophysiologic Approach*, 8th edn. New York: McGraw-Hill; 2008.
44. Vanek V. Assessment and management of acid–base abnormalities. In: Shikora SA, Martindale RG, Schwaitzberg SD, eds. *Nutritional Considerations in the Intensive Care Unit*. Dubuque, IA: Kendall/Hunt; 2002, pp. 101–109.
45. Adrogue HJ, Madias NE. Management of life-threatening acid–base disorders. Part 1. *N Engl J Med* 1998;338:26–34.
46. Adrogue HJ, Madias NE. Management of life-threatening acid-base disorders. Part 2. *N Engl J Med* 1998;338:107–111.
47. Arroliga AC, Shehab N, McCarthy K, Gonzales JP. Relationship of continuous infusion lorazepam to serum propylene glycol concentration in critically ill adults. *Crit Care Med* 2004;32:1709–1714.
48. Cate JCt, Hedrick R. Propylene glycol intoxication and lactic acidosis. *N Engl J Med* 1980;303:1237.
49. Morris CG, Low J. Metabolic acidosis in the critically ill: Part 2. Causes and treatment. *Anaesthesia* 2008;63:396–411.
50. Reynolds HN, Teiken P, Regan ME et al. Hyperlactatemia, increased osmolar gap, and renal dysfunction during continuous lorazepam infusion. *Crit Care Med* 2000;28:1631–1634.
51. Wilson KC, Farber HW. Propylene glycol accumulation during continuous-infusion lorazepam in critically ill patients. *J Intens Care Med* 2008;23:413; author reply 4–5.
52. Yaucher NE, Fish JT, Smith HW, Wells JA. Propylene glycol-associated renal toxicity from lorazepam infusion. *Pharmacotherapy* 2003;23:1094–1099.
53. Diedrich DA, Brown DR. Analytic reviews: Propofol infusion syndrome in the ICU. *J Intens Care Med* 2011;26:59–72.
54. Kam PC, Cardone D. Propofol infusion syndrome. *Anaesthesia* 2007;62:690–701.
55. Roberts RJ, Barletta JF, Fong JJ et al. Incidence of propofol-related infusion syndrome in critically ill adults: A prospective, multicenter study. *Crit Care* 2009;13:R169.
56. Klemz K, Ho L, Bellomo R. Daily intravenous chloride load and the acid–base and biochemical status of intensive care unit patients. *J Pharm Pract Res* 2008;38:296–299.
57. Yunos NM, Kim IB, Bellomo R et al. The biochemical effects of restricting chloride-rich fluids in intensive care. *Crit Care Med* 2011;39:2419–2424.
58. Morris CG, Low J. Metabolic acidosis in the critically ill: Part 1. Classification and pathophysiology. *Anaesthesia* 2008;63:294–301.
59. Shapiro J, Kaehny W. Pathogenesis and management of metabolic acidosis and alkalosis. In: Schrier RW, ed. *Renal and Electrolyte Disorders*, 6th edn. Philadelphia, PA: Lippincott Williams & Wilkins; 2003, pp. 115–153.
60. Hoste EA, Colpaert K, Vanholder RC et al. Sodium bicarbonate versus THAM in ICU patients with mild metabolic acidosis. *J Nephrol* 2005;18:303–307.
61. Rehm M, Finsterer U. Treating intraoperative hyperchloremic acidosis with sodium bicarbonate or tris-hydroxymethyl aminomethane: A randomized prospective study. *Anesth Analg* 2003;96:1201–1208, table of contents.
62. Dzierba AL, Abraham P. A practical approach to understanding acid–base abnormalities in critical illness. *J Pharm Pract* 2011;24:17–26.
63. Galla JH. Metabolic alkalosis. *J Am Soc Nephrol* 2000;11:369–375.
64. Webster NR, Kulkarni V. Metabolic alkalosis in the critically ill. *Crit Rev Clin Lab Sci* 1999;36:497–510.
65. The Acute Respiratory Distress Syndrome Network. Ventilation with lower tidal volumes as compared with traditional tidal volumes for acute lung injury and the acute respiratory distress syndrome. *N Engl J Med* 2000;342:1301–1308.
66. Buckley MS, Leblanc JM, Cawley MJ. Electrolyte disturbances associated with commonly prescribed medications in the intensive care unit. *Crit Care Med* 2010;38(6 Suppl.):S253–S264.

67. Holcombe B, Andris DA, Brooks G, Houston DR, Plogsted SW. Parenteral nutrition electrolyte/mineral product shortage considerations. *JPEN J Parenter Enteral Nutr* 35:434–436.
68. Dickerson RN, Melnik G. Osmolality of oral drug solutions and suspensions. *Am J Hosp Pharm* 1988;45:832–834.
69. Niemiec PW Jr., Vanderveen TW. Compatibility considerations in parenteral nutrient solutions. *Am J Hosp Pharm* 1984;41:893–911.
70. Lumpkin MM. Safety alert: Hazards of precipitation associated with parenteral nutrition. *Am J Hosp Pharm* 1994;51:1427–1428.
71. Whitmire SJ. Fluids and electrolytes. In: *Contemporary Nutrition Support Practice: A Clinical Guide*. Gottschlich MM, Matarese LE (eds.), Philadelphia, PA: WB Saunders; 1998, p. 128.
72. Ohs MS, Uribarri J, Shils ME, Olson JA, Shike M, Ross AC. Electrolytes, water, and acid–base balance. In: *Modern Nutrition in Health and Disease*. Baltimore, MD: Williams & Wilkins; 1999, p. 107.

10 Gut Microbiome in the Critically Ill

Gail A. Cresci

CONTENTS

Although a healthy human fetus develops in a sterile environment, the human host's bacterial cells outnumber its eukaryotic cells 10-fold (Hooper et al., 2002). Newborns are first colonized based upon their mode of delivery. Heavily colonized by microbes, the mammalian birth canal provides the initial inoculum for all mammals delivered vaginally. At time of delivery, the vaginal ecosystem is typically comprised of *Lactobacillus*, >50% of all bacteria present, and *Prevotella* spp. (Dominguez-Bello et al., 2010). It appears that the vaginal community changes to provide newborns with beneficial bacteria (Dominguez-Bello et al., 2011). Bacteria identified on newborn's skin and mouth and present in the first meconium are noted to be the same as the mother's vaginal bacteria in vaginally delivered newborns (Dominguez-Bello et al., 2011). In contrast, babies birthed by cesarean section (C-section) harbor bacterial communities that resemble those of the skin, comprising *Staphylococcus*, *Corynebacterium*, and *Propionibacterium* spp. (Dominguez-Bello et al., 2010; Mackie et al., 1999). Because C-section babies do not receive that first vaginal maternal inoculum, it may not only influence the gut microbiota development but also contribute to the vulnerability they have to certain pathogens (Dominguez-Bello et al., 2011). C-section-delivered babies have a higher incidence of atopic disease (Penders et al., 2007), allergies, and asthma (Bager, 2008; Negele, 2004), and 64%–82% of cases of skin infection with methicillin-resistant *Staphylococcus aureus* in newborns occurs in C-section babies (Watson et al., 2004).

The gut is home to approximately 100 trillion predominantly anaerobic bacteria comprised of approximately 800 different bacterial species and over 7000 strains (Ley et al., 2006). The proximal gastrointestinal tract (GIT) (stomach, duodenum, jejunum) houses relatively low densities of bacteria, 10^2 colony-forming units (CFU/mL of luminal contents) due to an acidic gastric pH, bile, and peristalsis. Bacterial counts markedly increase in the distal ileum (10^8 CFU/mL) and colon

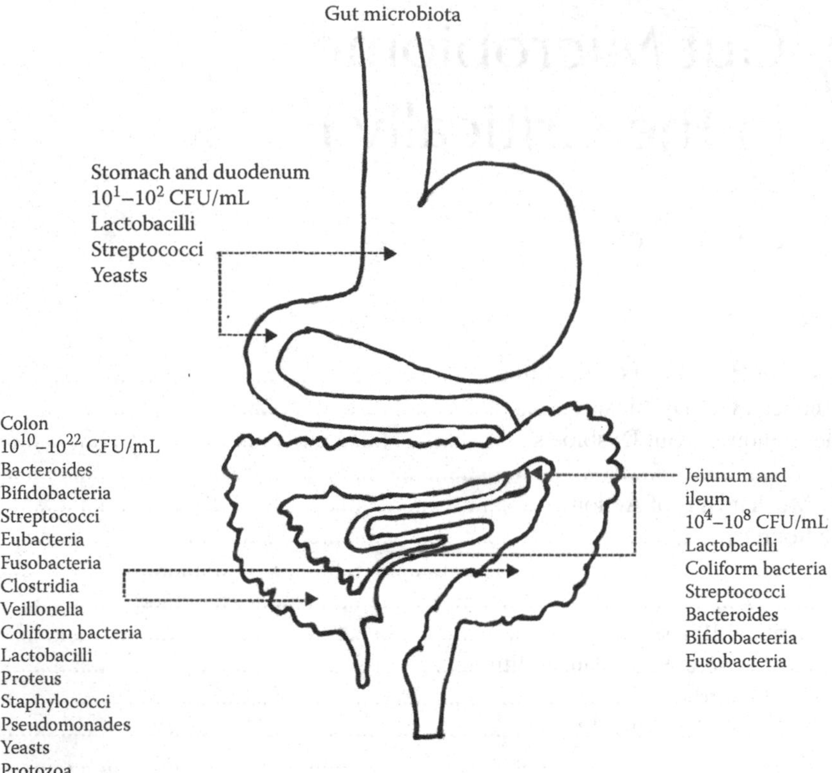

FIGURE 10.1 Gut microbiota.

(10^{11}–10^{12} CFU/mL) (Figure 10.1) (Savage, 1977). Diversity in the gut microbiome rapidly increases after the first few years of life (Koenig et al., 2011). This may be due in part to an enlarging intestinal tract that provides a larger habitat for more bacteria, increased exposure to environmental bacteria, and/or dietary changes (Dominguez-Bello et al., 2011). Breast milk contains bifidobacteria, with *Bifidobacterium longum* the most widely found species followed by *Bifidobacterium animalis*, *Bifidobacterium bifidum*, and *Bifidobacterium catenulatum*; all are *Bifidobacterium* species that may promote healthy microbiota development (Cani and Delzenne, 2009). A change in the relative ratio of bacterial phyla in the GIT, from an unstable community dominated by *Actinobacteria* and *Proteobacteria*, to a stable mixture dominated by *Firmicutes* and *Bacteroidetes*, was found when diet was advanced from simple solid foods (rice cereal) to a more complex plant polysaccharide-containing (peas) diet (Koenig et al., 2011). Discovering that African children had an increased abundance and diversity of *Bacteroidetes* compared to Italian children opened up the possibility that gut microbiota are influenced by local diet and can adapt via genomic changes to changes in the host's diet (De Filippo et al., 2010).

There seems to be interfamily member influences on the composition of the gut microbiota as similarities are noted between family members compared to unrelated people with sharing of the same bacterial strains (Falush et al., 2003; Moodley et al., 2009; Turnbaugh et al., 2009; Vaishampayan et al. 2010). There are also geographical variances in the gut microbiota pattern within the host (De Filippo et al., 2010), as well as with age, noting gut microbiome variance between the elderly and younger adults (Biagi et al., 2010; Claesson et al., 2011; Rajilic-Stojanovic et al., 2009). Organisms have defined life spans, playing different roles throughout the life span. Nature has created biologic clocks to monitor the position of an individual in the aging matrix; these clocks are phylogenetically deep and well conserved (Harley, 1991). One type of clock includes bifunctional genes, which are genes beneficial to young individuals but costly in aging individuals (Williams, 1957). Subsets of endogenous microbiota may have bifunctional genes (Dominguez-Bello et al., 2011) with evidence for selection of microbes that coevolve with their host (Ley et al., 2008). This could impact drug and nutrient metabolism, making it even more important to perform drug and nutrition trials in age- and location-matched populations to avoid the effects of differences in the metabolic capabilities of the human gut microbiota (Rajilic-Stojanovic et al., 2009). This could influence the outcome after provision of probiotic supplements. Particular species that are beneficial to younger age groups (e.g., *Lactobacillus* and *Bifidobacterium*) might actually be harmful if provided to the elderly population. These are important topics for study. In addition to diet, age, and geographical residence of the host, the gut microbiota can be altered by other factors such as medications and both physiological and psychological stress (Ley et al., 2008).

GUT MICROBIOTA IN HEALTH AND CRITICAL ILLNESS

Humans have a mutualistic relationship with their gut microbiota, one which both benefit from coexistence. As hosts, we provide a safe niche and food supply, and in return, the gut microbiota synthesize enzymes, vitamins, and beneficial fermentation by-products, provide protection against pathogenic bacteria and their by-products, influence gene expression, and are involved with host and immune interactions within the intestine (Backhed et al., 2005; Hooper et al., 2002). However, altered gut microbiota, or dysbiosis, is involved with the pathogenesis of a wide variety of diseases, including metabolic syndrome, obesity, congestive heart failure, pancreatitis, inflammatory bowel disease, and critical illness (Cani et al., 2009; Othman et al., 2008; Sandek et al., 2008; Shimizu et al., 2010).

ANTIBIOTIC-INDUCED GUT DYSBIOSIS

When discussing gut dysbiosis in hospitalized patients the use of antibiotics must be considered. Nearly every hospitalized patient receives one or more doses of antibiotics during their hospital stay (World Health Organization, 2011). The elimination of anaerobic gut microbiota with broad-spectrum antibiotics, particularly the fluoroquinolones, not only causes antibiotic-associated diarrhea (AAD) but also predisposes to colonization and overgrowth of pathogens, such as *Clostridium difficile* (Marra et al., 2007). It is estimated that approximately 25%–30% of cases of AAD in hospitalized patients involve *C. difficile* (Mehmet et al., 2006). *C. difficile* can be debilitating with a high recurrence rate; it can cause pseudomembranous lesions in the colonic mucosa, causing severe inflammation (Asha et al., 2006; Rohde et al., 2009). The associated diarrhea typically begins 4–9 days following antibiotic cessation, but can occur up to 8 weeks later. Other risk factors include severe illness, advanced age, presence of a nasogastric tube, provision of medications that raise gastric pH, GI surgery or manipulation, immunocompromise, and extended hospital stay (Rohde et al., 2009). The most effective treatment of AAD/CDAD is to stop the inciting antibiotic. Identification of *C. difficile* with a positive stool culture is typically treated with metronidazole initially with correction of fluid and electrolyte imbalance as needed. Treatment failures are then treated with oral vancomycin. Relapses may occur within 1–2 weeks of discontinuing antibiotic treatment. Relapse is believed to be caused by the survival of *C. difficile* spores that later germinate producing vegetative forms and critical illness (Rohde et al., 2009).

Critically ill high-risk patients, otherwise assumed to have healthy microbiota prior to admission, who were receiving systemic antibiotics per ICU protocol, were evaluated for changes in their gut microbiota (Iapichino et al., 2008). Patients were fed with a fiber-free enteral formula and were receiving insulin, vasoactive drugs, or stress ulcer prophylaxis as needed. Patients sustained an overall alteration in gut microbiota within 1 week of ICU stay, which was amplified in patients requiring greater than 2 weeks of ICU stay. A decrease in anaerobes and an overgrowth of *Enterococcus* were found; this was associated with organ failure, ICU duration, and incidence of diarrhea.

CRITICAL ILLNESS–INDUCED GUT DYSBIOSIS

In addition to receiving antibiotics, critically ill patients are recipients of multiple therapies and metabolic conditions that can alter the gut microbiota in a negative manner. Most studies investigating gut microbiota in critical illness have examined hospitalized patients receiving intensive care (Shimizu et al., 2006, 2010). The gut has been described as the *motor* of multiple organ dysfunction syndrome (MODS) and is now considered a crucial target organ after severe insults such as trauma and sepsis. The gut has an important role in promoting infectious complications and MODS. This is due to deteriorated intestinal epithelia, gut immune system, and commensal bacteria (Mittal, 2014). The gut microbiota and the gut environment (fecal pH and presence of organic acids) of patients with systemic inflammatory response syndrome (SIRS) were evaluated (Shimizu et al., 2006). In comparison to healthy controls, patients with severe SIRS had significantly lower total anaerobic bacterial counts (especially 2–4 log fewer commensal *Bifidobacterium* and *Lactobacillus*) and 2 log higher potentially pathogenic *Staphylococcus* and *Pseudomonas* group counts. Concentrations of total organic acids, in particular the short-chain fatty acids (SCFAs) acetate, propionate and butyrate, were significantly decreased in the patients, whereas pH was markedly increased. This group of researchers further investigated the impact of fecal pH in critical illness in 138 trauma patients (Osuka, 2012). Patients with acidic or alkaline feces were noted to have decreased *Bacteroides* and *Bifidobacterium* spp. The incidence of bacteremia in patients with an acidic or alkaline fecal pH was significantly higher than those with a fecal pH in the normal range ($p < 0.05$ vs. normal range). The incidence of both bacteremia and mortality was associated with an increased pH of 6.6 and that, when the pH level was increased or decreased by one, the incidence of bacteremia more than tripled and mortality more than doubled. Total SCFA concentrations decreased with pH > 6.6 (propionate, butyrate); lactic, succinic, and formic acids were increased in acidic feces, which is notable as these are produced by *Enterobacteriaceae* (Junko, 2005). Whether these changes are a cause or consequence of SIRS is yet to be determined. While this study lends potential that fecal pH could be a risk factor marker, it does have limitations as these data were made with the use of culture-based interrogation of the microbiota and because the pH was not specified by GIT region.

While a change in gut microbiota balance is now recognized in critically ill patients, the timing of when alterations occur was just recently investigated. Fifteen critically ill patients were followed from the admission to the emergency department after sustaining a sudden and severe metabolic insult (e.g., trauma, cardiac arrest, cerebral vascular accident) through 2 weeks in their ICU stay and were compared to health controls (Hayakawa et al., 2011). Prior to any antibiotic administration, a fecal swab was obtained, followed by serial sampling (days 1, 2, 5, 7, 10, 14). At baseline time point, a 1000-fold reduction in commensal gut microbiota was noted in patients with acute trauma/critical illness compared to healthy controls, with obligate anaerobes being most affected. Within 2 weeks, overgrowth of pathogenic bacteria occurred, while commensal bacteria did not recover. Additionally, there was a reduction in SCFA. Causes of this rapid depletion of commensal microbiota and their fermentation by-products are unknown. But to speculate, it could be related to hypotension, reduced mesenteric blood flow, provision of supplemental oxygen, or systemic inflammation. These potential contributors deserve further study.

Gut dysmotility is frequently encountered in critically ill patients, complicating delivery of enteral nutrition. Therefore, it is of interest to identify a cause and resolve gut dysmotility so that enteral feeding can proceed. Recently, an association between the gut microbiota and gut dysmotility in critically ill patients was made (Shimizu et al., 2011). Sixty-three ICU patients with severe SIRS were evaluated, based upon their feeding tolerance, for gut microbiota composition, incidences of bacteremia, and mortality. Patients with feeding intolerance, defined as >300 mL reflux from nasal gastric feeding tube in 24 h, had significantly lower numbers of obligate anaerobes including *Bacteroidaceae* and *Bifidobacterium*, higher numbers of *Staphylococcus*, lower concentrations of acetic acid and propionic acid, and higher concentrations of succinic acid and

TABLE 10.1
Biological Roles of SCFAs

- Involved with ion transport (Na^+, HCO_3^-)
- Metabolic fuel source for colonic epithelium
- Modulate intracellular pH and cell volume
- Regulators of
  - Proliferation
  - Differentiation
  - Gene expression

Butyrate

- Contributes to differentiation of epithelial cells
- Enhancement of electrolyte and water absorption
- Promotes angiogenesis
- Modulates immune function
- Associated with decreased incidence of colorectal cancer and inflammatory bowel disease
- Inhibitor of HDAC

lactic acid than those patients without feeding intolerance ($p < 0.05$). Patients with feeding intolerance also had higher incidences of bacteremia (86% vs. 18%) and mortality (64% vs. 20%).

This same group of researchers further characterized patterns of SCFAs in critically ill ICU patients (n = 141) who fulfilled the criteria of SIRS and had a serum C-reactive protein level of >10 mg/dL comparing results with healthy volunteers (Yamada et al., in press). Fecal samples were collected and analyzed weekly for 6 weeks after admission. SCFA concentrations (butyrate, propionate, and acetate) were decreased significantly compared to healthy volunteers throughout the 6-week time period ($p < 0.001$). SCFAs are fermentation by-products of fermentable fiber by commensal gut microbiota. Gut dysbiosis occurring during critical illness and feedings that lack fermentable fibers lend to a decrease in luminal SCFA concentrations. Because SCFAs, particularly butyrate, serve multiple biological roles in the gut (Table 10.1), these data indicating depletion during critical illness could help explain many gut-related phenomena that critically ill patients experience.

PROBIOTICS

A probiotic is defined by the World Health Organization as "a live microbial feed that when consumed in adequate amounts confers a health benefit on the host" (Schlundt, 2012). In order to be a probiotic, meaning "for life," a live microbial strain must meet very stringent criteria. These include, being of human origin, resistant to acid and bile; able to survive the upper intestinal tract environment and reach the distal gut (ileum and colon), attach to the intestinal epithelium, colonize the distal intestine, and confer health benefit to the host; and having scientifically proven health benefits (Cresci, 2012). Because of these strict criteria, most supplements termed *probiotics* are not truly probiotics, and their use may be misleading to clinicians and consumers. To appropriately identify a probiotic, one should look at the genus, species, and strain designations, for example, *Bifidobacterium* (genus) *lactis* (species) Bb-12 (strain). Most manufacturers do not include this information in their product labeling such as yogurts or other fermented milk products. Oftentimes, manufacturers have not conducted research on the particular probiotic strain used in their fermented milk product or supplement and typically generalize health claims from the other research sources for the genus and/or species included in the product. This poses a challenge for the clinician and the consumer regarding whether the product actually confers a health benefit.

Probiotic Mechanisms of Action

Not all probiotic strains exert the same mechanisms of action possessing considerable interstrain diversity. *Therefore, properties of one probiotic should not be extrapolated to another.* Additionally, it should not be assumed that probiotic actions in vitro reflect mechanisms of action in vivo. Another issue is whether the same probiotic strain exerts the same mechanism of action in different metabolic environments of the host, such as a patient in the ambulatory care setting versus an intensive care setting.

Probiotic strains may have multiple activities (Table 10.2) and therefore may be influential at various stages (Sherman, 2009). Different probiotics exert their predominant action either in the lumen, at the mucosal surface, by engagement with the mucosal innate immune response, or by action beyond the gut with stimulation of the acquired immune response (Shanahan, 2010). An example of a protective luminal action against *Listeria monocytogenes* is via the production of an antimicrobial bacteriocin by the probiotic *Lactobacillus salivarius UCC118* (Corr et al., 2007). The same probiotic was effective in protecting against salmonella infection, but by a different mechanism. Another luminal action of a probiotic is via metabolic alterations of the commensal resident microbiota. Inoculation of germ-free mice with probiotic bacteria results in marked changes in gene expression within the resident commensal microbiome (Sonneburg et al., 2006).

Probiotics have been shown to have action at the mucosal surface by inducing mucins (MUC2 and MUC3) (Mack et al., 1999). An enhanced mucus layer overlying the gut epithelial lining then serves as an antibacterial shield that prevents the binding of enteric pathogens to mucosal surfaces and increases the clearance of pathogens from the gut (Linden et al., 2008). Additionally, mucin-producing cells secrete trefoil factors in response to microbial pathogens that act together with mucins to prevent their binding to mucosal surfaces (Clyne et al., 2004). Probiotics also have a direct effect on enhancing gut integrity and its barrier function by preventing changes in tight junction proteins (e.g., occludins, claudins) and enhancing the tight junction electrical resistance (Cresci et al., 2013;

TABLE 10.2
Probiotic Potential Mechanisms of Action

- Beneficially alter gut microbiota pattern
    - Restore gut microbiota homeostasis correcting dysbiosis
- Competitively inhibit adherence of potentially pathogenic microorganisms (PPMs)
    - Secrete proteins that affect PPM adherence
- Antimicrobial factors
    - Host cell
        - Commensal microbiota upregulate expression and secretion of defensins and cathelicidins
    - Probiotic factors
        - Produce antimicrobial molecules (SCFA, bacteriocins, microcins)
        - Reduce intraluminal pH (secretin, acetic acid, lactic acid)
- Secrete proteins that alter apoptosis and inflammation
- Maintain intestinal barrier function
- Immunologic effects
    - Upregulate mucin encoding genes to increase mucus production
        - Prevent *E. coli* adherence/invasion
    - Increase IL-10—anti-inflammatory
    - Regulate toll-like receptor signaling
    - Increase immunoglobulin (IgA, IgG, IgM) production
- Metabolic effects
    - Nutrient metabolism
    - Quorum sensing

TABLE 10.3
Some Commercially Available Probiotics

Strain	Initial Product	Supplier
L. casei strain Shirota	Yakult	Yakult
B. longum BBS36	Bifidus milk	Morinaga Milk Products
B. breve strain Yakult	Mil-Mil (Bifiene)	Yakult
B. lactis BB-12	Yogurt	Chr. Hansen
L. rhamnosus GG	Gefilus	Valio
L. casei DN-114-001 (*L. casei* Immunitas)	Actimel (DanActive)	Danone
L. johnsonii La-1	LC1	Nestle
L. plantarum 299v	ProViva	Probi
B. animalis DN-173-010 (*Bifidus regularis*)	BIO (Activia)	Danone
L. gasseri LG21	LG21	Meiji Milk Products
B. lactis HN-019	Supplement	Danisco
L. casei KW2110	Yogurt	Kirin Holdings
L. casei F19	Cultura	Arla Foods
Bifidobacterium breve, B. longum, B. infantis, L. acidophilus, L. plantarum, Lactobacillus paracasei, Lactobacillus bulgaricus, and Streptococcus thermophiles	VSL#3	Sigma Tau
L. salivarius UCC118	Supplement	Metagenics

Lebeer et al., 2010). Probiotics express microorganism-associated molecular patterns (MAMPs) capable of engaging with the same pattern recognition receptors as do pathogens and thus have the means to protect the mucosal surface by competitive exclusion (Lebeer et al., 2010).

The ability to stimulate the innate and acquired immune system via induction of regulatory T-cell function has been exhibited by some probiotics (O'Mahony et al., 2008). The secretion of anti-inflammatory (e.g., IL-10) and pro-inflammatory (e.g., IL-12) cytokines by immune cells can be affected in a strain-specific manner by some probiotic strains (Sherman, 2009). Some probiotics activate specific gut opioid and cannabinoid receptors, thus having the potential to modulate visceral pain (Rousseaux et al., 2007).

Probiotic Sources

A challenge to clinicians is finding a commercially available probiotic product that has scientific evidence demonstrating benefit to patients. Many probiotic strains reported in the literature are not commercially available limiting the ability to readily translate scientific evidence into clinical practice. Additionally, most manufacturers lack disclosure of strain specificity or quantity of viable organisms (CFU) on products, thus further confusing the clinical application. Table 10.3 lists a select number of commercially available probiotic products.

PREBIOTICS

The gut microbiota ferment undigested polysaccharides and proteins. A prebiotic is defined as "a selectively fermented ingredient that allows specific changes, both in the composition and/or activity in the gut microbiota, which confer benefits upon host well-being and health" (Gibson et al., 2004). An ingredient must exhibit necessary criteria to be considered a prebiotic. In order to selectively stimulate the growth and/or activity of the gut microbiota in a beneficial manner, a prebiotic must be resistant to the host's gastric acidity and digestive enzymes and must be fermented in the distal intestine (ileum and colon) by the commensal anaerobic gut microbiota. Demonstration of prebiotic activity of an ingredient is very difficult; therefore, it's likely an ingredient may have prebiotic effects, but not yet be called a prebiotic because the necessary criteria have not yet been proven. Prebiotics are simple, naturally occurring, or synthetic sugars that vary with their degree of polymerization (DP). A prebiotic is not available to all bacterial species that inhabit GIT ecosystem, and currently *Lactobacillus* and *Bifidobacterium* are considered indicator organisms.

Upon reaching the distal intestine (ileum and colon), prebiotics are fermented by endogenous anaerobic bacteria producing SCFA and gases (CO_2 and H_2). Prebiotic fermentation increases bacterial cell mass and alters bacterial enzyme activities. This has been shown to cause a drop in intraluminal pH, thus favoring an increase of *Bifidobacteria*, *Lactobacilli*, and nonpathogenic *Escherichia coli* and decreasing *Bacteroidaceae* (Damaskos, 2008). As with a high-fiber diet, with wide individual variation in consumption of prebiotics (5–20 g/day), a prebiotic can produce several unwanted symptoms such as flatulence, bloating, abdominal pain, eructation, and borborygmi (Cummings and Macfarlane, 2002). The stoichiometry of fermentation differs for carbohydrates of differing chain lengths and monosaccharide composition, DP, and branching, with slower fermentation associated with longer chain length. Prebiotics can also affect bowel habits resulting in a laxative effect through stimulation of microbial growth and increased bacterial cell mass leading to stimulation of peristalsis by increased bowel content (Cummings and Macfarlane, 2002). However, the effect is small and there is a need for well-controlled studies to detect. The type of prebiotic influences fecal stool weight with inulin and fructooligosaccharide increasing stool weight by 1.3–2 g and wheat bran, fruits, and vegetables increasing stool weight by 5.4–4.7 g (Cummings and Macfarlane, 2002).

Prebiotics are fermented by endogenous commensal gut microbiota producing SCFA, predominantly acetate, propionate, and butyrate, but not all prebiotics yield equal amounts and types of SCFA (Cummings et al., 2001). SCFAs are known to serve several biological functions to include ion transport (e.g., Na^+, HCO_3^-), modulate intracellular pH and cell volume, serve as metabolic cellular fuel source, and regulate proliferation, differentiation, and gene expression (Topping and Clifton, 2001). Butyrate in particular is known to contribute to differentiation of epithelial cells, enhance water and electrolyte absorption, modulate immune function, exert anti-inflammatory effects, and possess tumor suppressor effects in the colon through its role as an inhibitor of histone deacetylases (HDACs) and serving as a ligand for a butyrate transporter and receptor (Thangaraju et al., 2008, 2009).

SYNBIOTIC

A synbiotic is a physical combination of prebiotics and probiotics. A synbiotic could then beneficially affect the host by improving the survival and implantation of live microbial dietary supplements in the gut as the fermentable substrate for the probiotic is packaged together and readily available (Lolida and Gibson, 2011). Oftentimes, candidates for probiotic therapy may not have adequate dietary intake of prebiotics, and/or they may have gut dysbiosis. Therefore, providing only one substrate, a prebiotic or a probiotic, may not exhibit a beneficial effect. Provision of a synbiotic could assist in maintaining/stimulating the viability and growth of the probiotic, outside and inside the recipient (Bengmark, 2000).

PROBIOTICS IN CRITICAL ILLNESS

Due to physiologic complexity (e.g., hypotension, decreased intestinal motility, increased levels of stress hormones, medications, and altered nutrient intake), illness severity, and simultaneously occurring gut dysbiosis in critically ill patients, knowing potential mechanisms of certain probiotics makes probiotic therapy a potentially attractive intervention in this setting. Probiotic supplementation has been studied in multiple types of critically ill patients. These include acute pancreatitis, trauma, major abdominal surgery, liver transplantation, and medical intensive care. These studies vary not only in patient population and underlying disease but also in probiotic strains and combinations, dosage, duration, delivery method, supplemental feeding, concomitant therapies, and outcome measurements. A narrative review of 10 randomized controlled trials (RCTs) in which probiotics and/or prebiotics were provided to critically ill patients was performed (Alberda et al., 2007; Falcao de Arruda et al., 2004; Jain et al., 2004; Klarin et al., 2005; Koretz, 2009; Kotzampassi et al., 2006; McNaught et al., 2005; Rayes et al., 2002, 2005, 2007; Spindler-Vesel et al., 2007). Combined outcomes of the trials were mortality, infections, length of intensive care unit stay, and length of hospital stay. Combining the data from these trials showed no effect of probiotics on mortality. A decrease incidence of infections with probiotic provision was found in nine of the studies; however, methodological bias is suspected to lead to this conclusion as when separated by risk of bias scores, the effect was diminished. No significant differences were seen in length of stay.

Evaluating single studies implementing the use of probiotics or synbiotics in critically ill patients is challenging. In addition to study heterogeneity, most of the studies also have included small numbers of subjects and therefore lack both study rigor and power to make a conclusion or recommendation. In the past few years, several systematic reviews have been performed with varying conclusions largely due to study heterogeneity and variability in the definitions used to define outcomes (Gu et al., 2012; Petrof et al., 2012; Siempos et al., 2010; Sun et al., 2009; Watkinson et al., 2007; Zhang et al., 2010). In attempts to reduce study heterogeneity, more recent systematic reviews have narrowed their focus and thus limited the studies included in the analysis, resulting in reviews analyzing similar outcomes (e.g., ventilator-associated pneumonia [VAP], infection, mortality) with varying conclusions. For example, in the analysis by Petrof et al., studies were included if they met the following criteria: (1) study design was an RCT; (2) studied adult patient populations (>18 years of age) are critically ill patients; (3) intervention was probiotics compared to a placebo; and (4) outcomes included infectious complications (primary) and other clinical outcomes such as diarrhea, mortality, and ICU and hospital length of stay. Critically ill patients were defined as those cared for in an ICU environment and had an urgent or life-threatening complication (high baseline mortality rate ≥5%) to distinguish them from patients with elective surgery who are also cared for in some ICUs but have a low baseline mortality rate (<5%). Sixty-one studies were identified, but only twenty-three were included in the analysis. Realizing the likelihood of significant heterogeneity in the primary outcome, an a priori analysis consisting of five subgroups was performed to examine the possible causes of heterogeneity. These subgroups included dosing of probiotics (high vs. low dose), use of *Lactobacillus plantarum* versus other probiotic, use of *Lactobacillus rhamnosus* GG versus other probiotic, higher versus lower mortality, and higher methodological quality versus lower methodological quality trials. The initial publication of this study found probiotics were associated with lower rates of infections, including VAP, and a trend toward reduced ICU mortality. Probiotics had no effect on hospital mortality, ICU or hospital length of stay, or diarrhea. Results of the subgroup analysis did not show a difference between which probiotic was provided and its dosage. Also notable is that subgroup analysis suggested that low-quality trials reported larger treatment effects than higher quality trials. Interestingly, the majority of the included trials did not confirm viability of the probiotic supplement prior to administering it, rendering one to consider the lack of response may be due to nonviable supplements being provided. As a follow-up to this meta-analysis and in response to a letter to the editor from Gu et al. critiquing these results stating incorrect data were entered into analysis evaluating probiotics and VAP and that an included study should be omitted, Petrof et al. reanalyzed their data. Interestingly, upon reanalysis, they report that a revised effect of probiotics on VAP, as reflected in a pooled risk ratio of 0.74 (95% confidence interval [CI] 0.55, 1.01; $p = 0.06$, test for heterogeneity $p = 0.11$, $I^2 = 45\%$) (Heyland, 2013). Despite a nonsignificant result ($p = 0.06$), the authors still conclude that that probiotics are associated with lower VAP rates in critically ill patients based upon a trend toward lower VAP rates.

Gu et al. (2012) also performed a meta-analysis for the use of probiotics in preventing VAP in critically ill patients. Studies were included in this analysis if they were RCTs with the following inclusion criteria: adult patients undergoing mechanical ventilation, probiotics compared with a control (placebo or another active agent), VAP specifically defined, and data available on the incidence of VAP. The primary outcome was the incidence of VAP. The definition of VAP varied across studies; no standard definition was used in all studies. Secondary outcomes included ICU mortality, hospital mortality, urinary tract infection, catheter-related bloodstream infection, diarrhea, length of stay (ICU and hospital), and duration of mechanical ventilation. Of the 51 RCTs identified, only 7 were included in this analysis; studies were evaluated for methodological quality. In this review, probiotics were not associated with a significant reduction in the incidence of VAP (OR, 0.82; 95% CI, 0.55–1.24; $P = 0.35$), with low heterogeneity among the studies ($I^2 = 36.5\%$, $P = 0.15$). Likewise, probiotics had no effect on any of the secondary outcomes (ICU mortality, hospital mortality, urinary tract infection, catheter-related blood stream infection, diarrhea, ICU length of stay, or duration of mechanical ventilation).

This issue of heterogeneity and lack of good quality studies is a highlight of systematic reviews of probiotic use in critically ill patients. With the combined knowledge that gut dysbiosis occurs early after metabolic insult and does not recover and the potential mechanisms of action of certain probiotic strains, further rigorous study on probiotic provision in the critically ill deserves attention. Future studies should focus on (1) clarification of viable probiotic strain(s) provided and their dosage, route, and timing of delivery, (2) clear definitions for the outcomes attempting to modify (VAP, diarrhea), and (3) focus effect of probiotic supplementation on meaningful clinical endpoints (mortality, duration of mechanical ventilation, other infections, length of stay).

Probiotics and Severe Acute Pancreatitis

Acute pancreatitis is an acute inflammatory process with mild to severe forms. High mortality rates are frequent particularly with necrosis and infection of the gland. Prophylactic antibiotic therapy is widely used but with variable benefits. With a need for new anti-infectious strategies, several researchers have investigated the provision of probiotics, prebiotics, or synbiotics to reduce the severity and improve the outcomes of acute pancreatitis. As with probiotic studies in general critically ill patients, those with patients with pancreatitis also have much heterogeneity and a small number of patients included. Early studies in patients with severe acute pancreatitis show benefit when providing a symbiotic containing four strains of *Lactobacillus* bacteria and four prebiotic fibers (Olah et al., 2002). However, a large multicenter study conducted in Europe was stopped early because patients receiving probiotics had higher mortality (16% vs. 6%, $p < 0.05$) than those receiving a placebo (Besselink et al., 2008). This study involved 296 patients with predicted severe acute pancreatitis that were randomized to receive a probiotic supplement containing 6 strains of viable probiotics (*Lactobacillus acidophilus*, *Lactobacillus casei*, *L. salivarius*, *Lactococcus lactis*, *B. bifidum*, and *B. lactis* [10^{10} CFU/day] + cornstarch and maltodextrin) or placebo (cornstarch and maltodextrin). In addition to enteral feeding, these supplements were provided through the nasojejunal feeding tube. The authors concluded that probiotics, particularly this combination, should not be provided routinely in patients with predicted severe acute pancreatitis.

In attempts to assimilate several trials of probiotics, prebiotics, or synbiotics in patients with acute pancreatitis, a meta-analysis was performed (Zhang et al., 2010). Studies were included if they were RCTs evaluating the use of prebiotics, probiotics, or synbiotics with at least one of the following as a primary outcome variable: number of infections and pancreatic infectious complications, incidence of multiple organ failure (MOF) and SIRS, surgical interventions, length of hospital stay, and mortality. Studies were scored on their methodological quality. Of the 48 papers available for review, only 7 RCTs involving 559 patients met the inclusion criteria and were included in the meta-analysis. Most of the analyzed studies were small in size (<100 patients) and had moderate to high methodological scores. Overall, there were no significant differences of incidence of total infections in pancreatic patients between the probiotics/synbiotics group and the control group and no significant differences in the incidence of MOF and SIRS between the probiotics/synbiotics group and the control group; combination analysis of MOF and SIRS also showed no significant differences between the two groups; there was no significant difference in the mortality between the probiotics/synbiotics group and the control group. The use of prebiotics, probiotics, or synbiotics had no significant influence on the main surgical outcomes including septic morbidity, pancreatic infections, surgical intervention, mortality, MOF, and SIRS in severe acute pancreatitis. Four studies reported length of hospital stay which was significantly shorter in the probiotics/synbiotics group. The authors concluded that few recommendations for use of probiotics, prebiotics, or synbiotics can be made at this time.

Probiotics and Diarrhea

Diarrhea in the ICU patient is common with most episodes being mild and self-limiting. Multiple factors may contribute to acute diarrhea including enteral feeding (type and dosage of fiber in enteral formula, osmolarity of formula, delivery mode, enteral feeding contamination), medications (antibiotics, proton pump inhibitors, prokinctics, glucose-lowering agents, selective serotonin reuptake inhibitors, laxatives, and sorbitol-containing preparations), and infectious etiologies including *C. difficile* (Chang and Huang, 2013). Fermentable oligosaccharides, disaccharides, and monosaccharides and polyols (FODMAPS) are highly osmotic and rapidly fermented by gut bacteria. Enteral formulas with a high content of FODMAPS may play a role in diarrhea, especially if the patient is also receiving antibiotics that have a detrimental effect on intestinal microbiota (Halmos, 2013). An attempt should be made to distinguish infectious diarrhea from osmotic diarrhea. Assessment should include an abdominal exam, fecal leukocyte test, quantification of stool, stool culture for *C. difficile* (and/or toxin assay), serum electrolyte panel (to evaluate for excessive electrolyte losses or dehydration), and review of medications (Maroo and Lamont, 2006).

There have been attempts made to modify the gut microbiota in critically ill patients to mitigate diarrhea. A few studies have investigated the use of probiotics on reducing incidence of diarrhea in critically ill patients. A meta-analysis (Petrof et al., 2012) included a subanalysis for probiotics and diarrhea. None of the probiotics studied had an effect on incidence of diarrhea.

Provision of soluble fiber (prebiotics) has been evaluated and appears more consistent in reducing diarrhea than enteral formulas containing a mixture of fibers (soluble and insoluble) in ICU patients. Use of a soluble fiber additive theoretically may pose lower risk of intestinal obstruction than use of a mixed fiber formula. Five small RCTs have evaluated the use of a commercial soluble fiber-containing supplement added to a standard enteral formula (Hart and Dobb, 1988; Heather et al., 1991; Karakan et al., 2007; Rushdi et al., 2004; Spapen et al., 2001). Of the trials that included diarrhea as a study endpoint, three showed significant reductions in diarrhea in critically ill patients (Heather et al., 1991; Rushdi et al., 2004; Spapen et al., 2001).

Probiotic Safety in the Critically Ill

Several *Bifidobacteria* (e.g., *B. bifidum*, *B. longum*, and *Bifidobacterium infantis*) are common safe species as are many lactic acid bacteria (LAB). While considered harmless for their use for years in foods, these particular bacteria fall under the Medical Food and Supplement Act and are afforded GRAS status. LAB that grow as adventitious microbiota or that are added to foods as cultures do not pose a health risk to healthy humans. Several strains of LAB species have been isolated from the human GIT and administered to humans without reported adverse effects. These include *L. reuteri*, *L. plantarum*, and *L. casei* (ssp. *rhamnosus*). However, although probiotics are normal commensals of mammalian microbiota and are generally thought to be without pathologic potential, individual patients may be susceptible to opportunistic infections via normal gut microbiota. There have been case reports of adverse effects, including sepsis (bacteremia, fungemia), bowel ischemia, and mortality, when probiotics were administered, most of which occurred in patients who had underlying medical conditions (Besselink et al., 2008; Boyle et al., 2006; Enache-Angoulvant et al., 2005). Other potential theoretical risks are deleterious metabolic activities related to altered polysaccharide fermentation, lipid metabolism, and glucose homeostasis, immune deviation or excessive immune stimulation, and microbial resistance (Boyle et al., 2006).

In review of 92 cases of invasive *Saccharomyces* infections, treatment with antibiotic therapy and existing intravenous catheters were identified as the most frequent predisposing factors (Enache-Angoulvant et al., 2005). *Lactobacillus* has been isolated in the blood from patients with short-gut syndrome, leukemia, mitral regurgitation, and cardiac surgery (Boyle et al., 2006). Risk factors for developing infectious complications associated with probiotic provision include presence of a central venous catheter, immunocompromise, administration of the probiotic directly into the small intestine, concomitant administration of broad-spectrum antibiotics in which the probiotic is resistant, cardiac valvular disease, and compromised intestinal barrier (Boyle et al., 2006).

SUMMARY

The gut microbiota are complex and known to be altered negatively during critical illness. Current research indicates a potential for modifying the gut microbiota to improve clinical outcomes in critically ill. However, exactly how that modification should be provided is unknown. Well-designed RCTs are needed to further explore the mechanistic issues and probiotic interactions and assess the effect and safety of prebiotics, probiotics, or synbiotics in the critically ill population.

REFERENCES

Alberda C, Gramlich L, Meddings J et al. Effect of probiotic therapy in critically ill patients: A randomized, double-blind, placebo-controlled trial. *Am J Clin Nutr.* 2007;85:816–823.

Asha N, Tompkins D, Wolcox MH. Comparative analysis of prevalence, risk factors, and molecular epidemiology of antibiotic-associated diarrhea due to *Clostridium difficile, Clostridium perfringens,* and *Staphylococcus aureus. J Clin Microbiol.* 2006;44:2785–2791.

Backhed F, Ley R, Sonnenburg JL, Peterson DA, Gordon JI. Host–bacterial mutualism in the human intestine. *Science* 2005;307:1915–1920.

Bager P, Wohlfahrt J, Westergaard T. Caesarean delivery and risk of atopy and allergic disease: Meta-analyses. *Clinical & Experimental Allergy*. 2008;38:634–642.

Bengmark S. Bacteria for optimal health. *Nutrition* 2000;16:611–615.

Besselink MG, van Santvoort HC, Buskens E et al. Probiotic prophylaxis in predicted severe acute pancreatitis: A randomized, double-blind, placebo-controlled trial. *Lancet* 2008;371:651–659.

Biagi E, Nylund L, Candela M et al. Through ageing, and beyond: Gut microbiota and inflammatory status in seniors and centenarians. *PLoS One* 2010;5:e10667.

Boyle R, Robins-Browne R, Tang M. Probiotic use in clinical practice: What are the risks? *Am J Clin Nutr.* 2006;83:1256–1264.

Cani P, Lecuort E, Dewulf EM et al. Gut microbiota fermentation of prebiotics increases satietogenic and incretin gut peptide production with consequences for appetite sensation and glucose response after a meal. *Am J Clin Nutr.* 2009;90:1236–1243.

Cani PD, Delzenne NM. Interplay between obesity and associated metabolic disorders: New insights into the gut microbiota. *Curr Opin Pharmacol.* 2009;9:737–743.

Chang SJ, Huang HH. Diarrhea in enterally fed patients: Blame the diet? *Curr Opin Clin Nutr Metab Care.* 2013;16:588–594.

Claesson MJ, Cusack S, O'Sullivan O et al. Composition, variability, and temporal stability of the intestinal microbiota of the elderly. *Proc Natl Acad Sci USA.* 2011;108(Suppl. 1):4680–4687.

Clyne M, Dillon P, Daly S et al. *Helicobacter pylori* interacts with the human single-domain trefoil protein TFF1. *Proc Natl Acad Sci USA.* 2004;101:7409–7414.

Corr S, Li Y, Riedel CU et al. Bacteriocin production as a mechanism for the antiinfective activity of *Lactobacillus salivarius UCC118. Proc Natl Acad Sci USA.* 2007;104:7617–7621.

Cresci G. Probiotics and prebiotics. In: *ASPEN Adult Nutrition Support Core Curriculum.* Mueller CM (ed.) ASPEN, Silver Spring, MD, 2012; pp. 51–62.

Cresci G, Nagy LE, Ganapathy V. *Lactobacillus GG* and tributyrin supplementation reduce antibiotic-induced intestinal injury. *JPEN J Parenter Enteral Nutr.* 2013;37:763–774.

Cummings J, Macfarlane GT. Gastrointestinal effects of prebiotics. *Br J Nutr*. 2002;87(Suppl. 2):S145–S151.

Cummings JH, Macfarlane GT, Englyst HN. Prebiotic digestion and fermentation. *Am J Clin Nutr.* 2001;73:415S–420S.

Damaskos D, Kolios G. Probiotics and prebiotics in inflammatory bowel disease: Microflora "on the scope". *BJCP British J Clin Pharm.* 2008;65:453–467.

De Filippo C, Cavalieri D, Di Paola M et al. Impact of diet in shaping gut microbiota revealed by a comparative study in children from Europe and rural Africa. *Proc Natl Acad Sci USA*. 2010;107:14691–14696.

Dominguez-Bello M, Costtello EK, Contreras M et al. Delivery mode shapes the acquisition and structure of the initial microbiota across multiple body habitats in newborns. *Proc Natl Acad Sci USA.* 2010;107:11971–11975.

Dominguez-Bello MG, Blaser M, Ley R, Knight R. Development of the human gastrointestinal microbiota and insights from high throughput sequencing. *Gastroenterology*. 2011;140:1713–1719.

Enache-Angoulvant A, Hennequin C. Invasive saccharomyces infection: A comprehensive review. *Clin Infect Dis*. 2005;41:1559–1568.

Falcao de Arruda I, de Aguilar-Nascimento JE. Benefits of early enteral nutrition with glutamine and probiotics in brain injury patients. *Clin Sci.* 2004;106:287–292.

Falush D, Wirth T, Linz B et al. Traces of human migrations in *Helicobacter pylori* populations. *Science* 2003;299:1582–1585.

Gibson GR, Probert HM, Van Loo J et al. Dietary modulation of the human colonic microbiota: Updating the concept of prebiotics. *Nutr Res Rev*. 2004;17:259–275.

Gu WJ, Wei CY, Yin RX. Lack of efficacy of probiotics in preventing ventilator-associated pneumonia: A systematic review and meta-analysis of randomized controlled trials. *Chest* 2012;142(4):859–868.

Halmos EP. Role of FODMAP content in enteral nutrition-associated diarrhea. *J Gastroenterol Hepatol.* 2013;28(Suppl. 4):25–28.

Harley C. Telomere loss: Mitotic clock or genetic time bomb? *Mutat Res*. 1991;256:271–282.

Hart GK, Dobb GJ. Effect of a fecal bulking agent on diarrhea during enteral feeding in the critically ill. *JPEN J Parenter Enteral Nutr*. 1988;12(5):465–468.

Hayakawa M, Asahara T, Henzan N et al. Dramatic changes of the gut flora immediately after severe and sudden insults. *Dig Dis Sci.* 2011;56:2361–2365.

Heather DJ, Howell L, Montana M, Howell M, Hill R. Effect of a bulk-forming cathartic on diarrhea in tube-fed patients. *Heart Lung*. 1991;20(4):409–413.

Heyland D. Do probiotics decrease the incidence of ventilator-associated pneumonia in critically ill patients? *Crit Care Med.* 2013;41:e28–e29.

Hooper L, Midtvedt T, Gordon JI. How host-microbial interactions shape the nutrient environment of the mammalian intestine. *Annu Rev Nutr*. 2002;22:283–307.

Iapichino G, Callegari ML, Marzorati S et al. Impact of antibiotics on the gut microbiota of critically ill patients. *J Med Microbiol.* 2008;57:1007–1014.

Jain P, McNaught CE, Anderson ADG, MacFie J, Mitchell CJ. Influence of synbiotic containing *Lactobacillus acidophilus* La5, *Bifidobacterium lactis* Bb 12, *Streptococcus thermophilus*, *Lactobacillus bulgaricus* and oligofructose on gut barrier function and sepsis in critically ill patients: A randomized controlled trial. *Clin Nutr*. 2004;23:467–475.

Junko W. Carbohydrate fermentation in the colon. *J Intest Microbiol*. 2005;19:169–177.

Karakan T, Ergun M, Dogan I, Cindoruk M, Unal S. Comparison of early enteral nutrition in severe acute pancreatitis with prebiotic fiber supplementation versus standard enteral solution: A prospective randomized double-blind study. *World J Gastroenterol*. 2007;13(Suppl. 19):2733–2737.

Klarin B, Johansson ML, Molin G, Larsson A, Jeppsson B. Adhesion of the probiotic bacterium *Lactobacillus plantarum* 299v onto the gut mucosa in critically ill patients: A randomised open trial. *Crit Care.* 2005;9:R285–R293.

Koenig J, Spor A, Scalfone N et al. Microbes and health sackler colloquium: Succession of microbial consortia in the developing infant gut microbiome. *Proc Natl Acad Sci USA*. 2011;108(Suppl. 1):4578–4585.

Koretz R. Probiotics, critical illness, and methodologic bias. *Nutr Clin Pract*. 2009;24:45–49.

Kotzampassi K, Giamarellos-Bourboulis EJ, Voudouris A, Kazamias P, Eleftheriadis E. Benefits of a synbiotic formula (Synbiotic 2000Forte) in critically ill trauma patients: Early results of a randomized controlled trial. *W J Surg*. 2006;30:1848–1855.

Lebeer S, Vanderleyden J, De Keersmaecker SCJ. Host interactions of probiotic bacterial surface molecules: Comparison with commensals and pathogens. *Nat Rev Microbiol*. 2010;8:171–184.

Ley R, Lozupone CA, Hamady M et al. Worlds within worlds: Evolution of the vertebrate gut microbiota. *Nat Rev Microbiol.* 2008;6:776–788.

Ley R, Peterson DA, Gordon JI. Ecological and evolutionary forces shaping microbial diversity in the human intestine. *Cell* 2006;124:837–848.

Linden S, Sutten P, Karlsson NG, Korolik V, McGuckin MA. Mucins in the mucosal barrier to infection. *Nat Mucosal Immunol.* 2008;1:183–197.

Lolida S, Gibson GR. Synbiotics in health and disease. *Annu Rev Food Sci Technol.* 2011;2:373–393.

Mack D, Michail S, Wei S, McDougall L, Hollingsworth MA. Probiotics inhibit enteropathogenic *E. coli* adherence in vitro by inducing intestinal mucin gene expression. *Am J Physiol.* 1999;276:G941–G950.

Mackie RI, Sighir A, Gaskins HR. Developmental microbial ecology of the neonatal gastrointestinal tract. *Am J Clin Nutr.* 1999;69:S1035–S1045.

Maroo S, Lamont JT. Recurrent *Clostridium difficile*. *Gastroenterology* 2006;130(Suppl. 4):1311–1316.

Marra AR, Edmond MB, Wenzel RP, Bearman GM. Hospital-acquired *Clostridium difficile*-associated disease in the intensive care unit setting: Epidemiology, clinical course and outcome. *BMC Infect Dis.* 2007;7:42.

McNaught C, Woodcock NP, Anderson ADG, MacFie J. A prospective randomized trial of probiotics in critically ill patients. *Clin Nutr.* 2005;24:211–219.

Mehmet C, Bulent B, Ismail A et al. Prophylactic *Saccharomyces boulardii* in the prevention of antibiotic-associated diarrhea: A prospective study. *Med Sci Monit.* 2006;12:119–122.

Mittal R, Coopersmith CM. Redefining the gut as the motor of critical illness. *Trends Mol Med.* 2014;20:214–223.

Moodley Y, Linz B, Yamaoka Y et al. The peopling of the Pacific from a bacterial perspective. *Science* 2009;323:527–530.

Negele K, Heinrish J, Borte M et al. Mode of delivery and development of atopic disease during the first 2 years of life. *Pediatr Allergy Immunol.* 2004;15:48–54.

Oláh A, Belágyi T, Issekutz A et al. Randomized clinical trial of specific lactobacillus and fibre supplement to early enteral nutrition in patients with acute pancreatitis. *Br J Surg.* 2002;89:1103–1107.

Oláh A, Belágyi T, Pótó L et al. Synbiotic control of inflammation and infection in severe acute pancreatitis: A prospective, randomized, double blind study. *Hepatogastroenterology.* 2007;54:590–594.

O'Mahony C, Scully P, O'Mahony D et al. Commensal-induced regulatory T cells mediate protection against pathogen-stimulated NF-kB activation. *PLoS Pathogens.* 2008;4:e1000112.

Osuka A, Shimizu K, Ogura H et al. Prognostic impact of fecal pH in critically ill patients. *Crit Care.* 2012;16:R119.

Othman M, Aguero R, Lin HC. Alterations in intestinal microbial flora and human disease. *Curr Opin Gastroenterol.* 2008;24:11–16.

Penders J, Thijs C, van den Brandt PA et al. Gut microbiota composition and development of atopic manifestations in infancy: The KOALA Birth Cohort Study. *Gut.* 2007;56:661–667.

Rajilic-Stojanovic M, Heilig HG, Molenaar D et al. Development and application of the human intestinal tract chip, a phylogenetic microarray: Analysis of universally conserved phylotypes in the abundant microbiota of young and elderly adults. *Environ Microbiol.* 2009;11:1736–1751.

Rayes N, Seehofer D, Hansen S et al. Early enteral supply of lactobacillus and fiber versus selective bowel decontamination: A controlled trial in liver transplant recipients. *Transplantation* 2002;74:123–128.

Rayes N, Seehofer D, Theruvath T et al. Supply of pre- and probiotics reduces bacterial infection rates after liver transplantation—A randomized, double-blind trial. *Am J Transplant.* 2005;5:125–130.

Rayes N, Seehofer D, Theruvath T et al. Effect of enteral nutrition and synbiotics on bacterial infection rates after pylorus-preserving pancreatoduodenectomy. *Ann Surg.* 2007;246:36–41.

Rohde C, Bartolini V, Jones N. The use of probiotics in the prevention and treatment of antibiotic-associated diarrhea with special interest in *Clostridium difficile*-associated diarrhea. *Nutr Clin Pract.* 2009;24:33–40.

Rousseaux C, Thuru X, Gelot A et al. *Lactobacillus acidophilus* modulates intestinal pain and induces opioid and cannabinoid receptors. *Nat Med.* 2007;13:35–37.

Rushdi TA, Pichard C, Khater YH. Control of diarrhea by fiber-enriched diet in ICU patients on enteral nutrition: A prospective randomized controlled trial. *Clin Nutr.* 2004;23(Suppl. 6):1344–1352.

Sandek A, Rauchhaus M, Anker SD, von Haehling S. The emerging role of the gut in chronic heart failure. *Curr Opin Clin Nutr Metab Care.* 2008;11632–11639.

Savage D. Microbial ecology of the gastrointestinal tract. *Ann Rev Microbiol.* 1977;31:107–133.

Schlundt, J. Evaluation of health and nutritional properties of probiotics in food including powder milk with live lactic acid bacteria. Report of a joint FAO/WHO expert consultation. FAO/WHO, 2012. http://www.who.int/foodsafety/publications/fs_management/en/probiotics.pdf (retrieved December 17, 2012).

Shanahan F. Probiotics in perspective. *Gastroenterology* 2010;139:1808–1812.

Sherman P, Ossa JC, Johnson-Henry K. Unraveling mechanisms of action of probiotics. *Nutr Clin Pract.* 2009;24:10–14.

Shimizu K, Ogura H, Asahara T et al. Gastrointestinal dysmotility is associated with altered gut flora and septic mortality in patients with severe systemic inflammatory response syndrome: A preliminary study. *Neurogastroenterol Motil.* 2011;23:330–335.

Shimizu K, Ogura H, Goto M et al. Altered gut flora and environment in patients with severe SIRS. *J Trauma.* 2006;60:126–133.

Shimizu K, Ogura H, Hamasaki T et al. Altered gut flora are associated with septic complications and death in critically ill patients with systemic inflammatory response syndrome. *Dig Dis Sci.* 2010;56:1171–1177.

Siempos II, Ntaidou TK, Falagas ME. Impact of the administration of probiotics on the incidence of ventilator-associated pneumonia: A meta-analysis of randomized controlled trials. *Crit Care Med.* 2010;38:954–962.

Sonnenburg J, Chen CTL, Gordon JI. Genomic and metabolic studies of the impact of probiotics on a model gut symbiont and host. *PLoS Biol.* 2006;4:2213–2226.

Spapen H, Diltoer M, Van Malderen C, Opdenacker G, Suys E, Huyghens L. Soluble fiber reduces the incidence of diarrhea in septic patients receiving total enteral nutrition: A prospective, double-blind, randomized, and controlled trial. *Clin Nutr.* 2001;20(Suppl. 4):301–305.

Spindler-Vesel A, Bengmark S, Vovk I, Cerovic O, Kompan L. Synbiotics, prebiotics, glutamine, or peptide in early enteral nutrition: A randomized study in trauma patients. *JPEN J Parenter Enteral Nutr.* 2007;31:119–126.

Sun S, Yang K, He X et al. Probiotics in patients with severe acute pancreatitis: A meta-analysis. *Langenbecks Arch Surg.* 2009;394:171–177.

Thangaraju M, Cresci G, Itagaki S, Mellinger J, Browning D, Berger F, Prasad P, Ganapathy V. Sodium-coupled transport of the short-chain fatty acid butyrate by SLC5A8 and its relevance to colon cancer. *J Gastrointest Surg.* 2008;12:1773–1782.

Thangaraju M, Cresci G, Liu K et al. GPR109A is a G-protein-coupled receptor for the bacterial fermentation product butyrate and functions as a tumor suppressor in colon. *Cancer Res.* 2009;69:2826–2832.

Topping D, Clifton PM. Short-chain fatty acids and human colonic function: Roles of resistant starch and non-starch polysaccharides. *Physiol Rev.* 2001;81:1031–1064.

Turnbaugh P, Hamady M, Yatsunenko T et al. A core gut microbiome in obese and lean twins. *Nature.* 2009;457:480–484.

Vaishampayan P, Kuehl JV, Froula JL et al. Comparative metagenomics and population dynamics of the gut microbiota in mother and infant. *Genome Biol Evol.* 2010;6:53–66.

Watkinson PJ, Barber VS, Dark P et al. The use of pre-pro-and synbiotics in adult intensive care unit patients: Systematic review. *Clin Nutr.* 2007;26:182–192.

Watson J, Jones R, Cortes C et al. Community-associated methicillin-resistant *Staphylococcus aureus* infection among healthy newborns—Chicago and Los Angeles County, 2004. *JAMA.* 2004;296:36–38.

Williams G. Pleiotropy, natural selection and the evolution of senescence. *Evolution.* 1957;11:398–411.

World Health Organization. Obesity and Overweight. Fact Sheet Number 311. Geneva, Switzerland: World Health Organization; 2011.

Yamada T, Shimizu K, Ogura H et al. Rapid and sustained long-term decrease of fecal short-chain fatty acids in critically Ill patients with systemic inflammatory response syndrome. *J Parenter Enteral Nutr.* in press. http://www.ncbi.nlm.nih.gov/pubmed/24711120.

Zhang MM, Cheng JQ, Lu YR et al. Use of pre-, pro- and synbiotics in patients with acute pancreatitis: A meta-analysis. *World J Gastroenterol.* 2010;16:3970–3978.

Section III

Delivery of Nutrition Therapy in the Critically Ill

11 Parenteral versus Enteral Nutrition

Gail A. Cresci

CONTENTS

INTRODUCTION

Nutritional support has progressed tremendously since 1678, when Sir Christopher Wren used a quill and a pig bladder to inject wine and ale into dogs. However, specialized nutrition support showed little real progress until the 1950s, when the concept of intensive care units was conceived. With the development of these areas of *intensive* care came the inception of nutritional support of the ICU patient. In 1967, Dudrick et al. [1] demonstrated that a central venous cannula could be used to deliver a concentrated mixture of protein hydrolysate and glucose. Parenteral nutrition was refined and found extensive clinical use in the 1970s. Clinicians were enamored by total parenteral nutrition (TPN) until the 1980s and 1990s, when its disadvantages became apparent. At the same time, the benefits of using the enteral route to provide nutrition were being reported [2–5].

The 1990s saw an increasing utilization of enteral nutrition (EN) as literature supported its numerous benefits over TPN. The purported role of EN in modulating the immune system continues to occupy a central place in comparisons between EN and TPN. Indeed, leaders in the field consider the immunologic benefits of EN more important than delivering calories or improving the nitrogen balance [6].

The proposed advantages of EN in surgical and critically ill patients are now well described. They include attenuation of the metabolic response to stress [7–9], improved nitrogen balance [10–13], better glycemic control [14–17], increased visceral protein synthesis [18,19], increased gastrointestinal (GI) anastomotic strength [20], and increased collagen deposition [21]. Other benefits of EN include decreased nosocomial infections [22], enhanced visceral blood flow [9,23–25], increased variety of nutrients available for delivery, and decreased risk of GI bleeding [26–28]. The cost–benefit analysis has also shown EN to be superior to TPN [13,17,29], though in the light of more aggressive enteral access techniques, this may have to be reevaluated. Many of the proposed physiologic benefits of EN are based on animal studies with limited corroborating human data. The advantages of EN have been largely supported by prospective randomized trials [30,31], though conflicting data exist [17,32–37].

TPN offers the obvious advantage that a functional GI tract is not required. The parenteral route provides considerable ease in nutrient delivery, and, as shown in recent large series, the nutritional requirements are met more consistently [17,38]. These *ease of delivery* advantages may be overshadowed by TPN's alleged disadvantages. The adverse effect of TPN on the mucosal barrier and gut-associated lymphoid tissue (GALT) [39–41] has been extensively investigated.

Other adverse effects often associated with TPN are hepatic impairment including steatosis, cholestasis, and cholelithiasis [42,43]; systemic immunosuppression [44–46] or, conversely, a proinflammatory condition [47]; venous thrombosis [48]; and local complications at the venous access site [49].

There is little doubt that EN is the preferred method of nutrient delivery in patients with functioning GI tracts. However, despite heroic attempts, the GI tract may be insufficient for adequate nutrient delivery. Access difficulties remain [37], there is difficulty in achieving nutritional delivery goals, and up to 50% of patients are intolerant to enteral feeds [50,51]. Complications of EN include jejunal necrosis [51–54], aspiration [55,56], and respiratory compromise [57]. High gastric residuals, constipation, diarrhea, abdominal distension, vomiting, and the risk of gut ischemia have been described as additional limitations to EN [58–62].

It must be kept in mind that nutritional support is just one of the many treatment variables affecting outcome. Timely and appropriate resuscitation, wound care, respiratory support, and infection control all have an important impact on outcome. These factors should be taken into account when formulating an optimal nutrition plan. Recommendations for nutritional support should include not only the quantity of nutrient and its composition but also the timing of its institution and the route of delivery.

ROLE OF EN IN MAINTAINING STRUCTURE AND FUNCTION OF THE GI TRACT

Lack of luminal nutrients and ischemia both result in an alteration of intestinal barrier function. Rats maintained on TPN alone show as much as 50% loss in the mass of their proximal small bowel mucosa within a week, accompanied by an increase in permeability [63–65]. Intestinal mucosal epithelial cells provide a mechanical barrier to pathogen entry and are an important part of the body's innate immune system. Increased permeability due to intravenous feeding is associated with increased bacterial translocation to the mesenteric lymph nodes in animals [66,67]. Changes in interferon-gamma expression [68] and keratinocyte growth factor levels [69] may be some of the mechanisms responsible for the loss of the epithelial barrier associated with TPN. Another mechanism may be abnormalities of the *tight junctions*, which in the fed state prevent small molecules and pathogens from penetrating through the intercellular spaces between adjoining intestinal epithelial cells [70]. There are several contributing factors that drive this diminished epithelial barrier function with TPN, such as loss of local growth factors, increased levels of proinflammatory mucosal cytokines, and alterations in intraluminal microbiota [71]. These TPN-induced changes result in a proinflammatory state within the intestinal mucosa, leading to villous atrophy, an increase in epithelial cell apoptosis, and a decrease in epithelial cell proliferation, as also demonstrated by the reduction in overall length of the small and large bowels.

The lack of enteral nutrient delivery to the gut mucosa during TPN also deprives the gut microbiota putting it in a state of nutrient deprivation. This corresponds with alterations in gut microbiota composition (see Chapter 10 for further discussion). Typically comprised of predominantly Gram-positive Firmicutes, TPN shifts the gut microbiota to a Gram-negative Proteobacteria-dominated population. Additional phylum-level changes include increases in Bacteroidetes and Verrucomicrobia (predominantly *Akkermansia*). This shift is associated with increased toll-like receptor (TLR) signaling with upregulation of TLRs 2,4,7, and 9 [72].

Partial confirmation of these animal studies came from Buchman et al. [73], who showed 10%–15% reductions in small bowel mucosal thickness occur in healthy humans receiving TPN, as well as increased villus cell count and an increase in the urinary lactulose–mannitol ratio (indicating an increase in intestinal permeability). However, mitotic index was not significantly diminished. Other investigators have shown a decrease in villous height, as well as an increase in intestinal permeability in nutritionally depleted patients [74,75]. TPN is associated with greater jejunal mucosal atrophy in patients of chronic pancreatitis than is seen in those who are maintained on enteral feeds [76]. After an injury, gut disuse and TPN are particularly liable to increase intestinal mucosal permeability. Increased gut permeability due to TPN has been shown to increase systemic endotoxemia in humans [77]. However, these small studies do not conclusively show that increased permeability and mucosal atrophy predispose humans to bacterial translocation, and bacterial translocation was not increased with TPN when compared to EN in a well-designed study by Sedman et al. [78]. The clinical significance of bacterial translocation itself is very controversial [79]. Some argue that translocation occurs and is responsible for septic complications [77]. Others propose that translocation increases septic complications, but not mortality [80].

A recent study has begun to elucidate whether a similarly significant change in gut microbial diversity occurs with enteral deprivation in humans [72]. Human intestinal mucosa-associated microbiota diversity was noted in 12 patients undergoing intestinal resection, as noted in other studies of human intestinal microbiota [81]. While an accurate characterization of the typical makeup of intestinal microbiota with TPN in humans was not possible, an interesting finding was that the level of microbial diversity appeared to be closely related to clinical outcome. Patients with low enteric bacterial diversity were significantly more likely to develop postoperative infection or intestinal anastomotic disruption [72].

EN is proposed to maintain the immune function of the gut better than TPN does. Two-thirds of the mammalian immune cells reside in the GI tract. With 8.5×10^{10} Ig producing cells (compared to 2.5×10^{10} for bone marrow, spleen, and lymph nodes combined), GALT is the largest lymphoid organ in the body. There are four configurations of GALT: single cells close to the epithelium (IELs), collections in the lamina propria, aggregates in the form of Peyer's patches, and finally mesenteric lymph nodes. By a process of continual sampling of intestinal contents and sensitization of inflammatory cells in Peyer's patches, GALT is constantly exposed to inflammatory stimuli from intestinal contents yet maintains a level of tolerance to normal bacterial flora and antigens. The lamina propria is a unique constituent of the GALT because it is continually in a state of physiologic inflammation, populated by activated lymphocytes and plasma cells. This is important for the sustained production of secretory IgA (sIgA), which inhibits bacterial attachment to the mucosa and is a vital component of the local immune response. Gut disuse results in a decrease in sIgA secretion within 5 days [82], accompanied by an increased susceptibility to infections normally controlled by sIgA in mice [83].

GALT is important for systemic immunity as well, since sensitized immune cells sourced from the GALT migrate to and maintain other mucosal-associated lymphoid tissues (MALT), specifically those associated with the bronchial tree. Loss of GALT mass due to gut disuse adversely affects the entire MALT system. Gut disuse combined with TPN in mice decreases immunity against respiratory viruses. Refeeding the gut restores the protection and improves viral clearance [84]. Mice fed on TPN alone have persistent respiratory viral infections, compared to enterally fed animals [85]. Trauma patients receiving EN have significantly less intra-abdominal abscesses and pneumonia than those receiving TPN.

In animal studies, TPN shrinks Peyer's patches and decreases the CD4–CD8 cell ratio in the lamina propria. It diminishes extraintestinal cellular immune mechanisms as well [44] and is associated with defective pulmonary macrophage function in rats [86]. Defective cellular immunity reverses when the animals are subsequently fed enterally.

Infants receiving long-term TPN have impaired bacteriocidal activity against coagulase-negative staphylococcus [87]. Excessive caloric intake, with resultant hyperglycemia and hepatic steatosis, may contribute to TPN-induced systemic immune suppression. Excessive long-chain triglycerides in TPN cause reticuloendothelial system dysfunction, excess PGE_2, and altered macrophage function. In addition, TPN formulas lack glutamine, an important immunonutrient. EN improves the host's ability to kill bacteria that do translocate [88]. A reversal of some of these detrimental effects occurs when the neuropeptide bombesin is given intravenously along with parenteral nutrition [89,90]. Possibly, enteroendocrine mechanisms that are affected by luminal nutrition play a role in maintaining the immune function of the GI mucosa by increasing mucin and IgA production and stimulating GALT function.

A TPN-induced decrease in mucosal immunity could increase the susceptibility to virulent pathogens, increasing bacterial adherence to mucosa and subsequent inflammation. This may also serve to prime neutrophils, promoting a systemic proinflammatory condition [47]. Preinjury priming of neutrophils plays an important role in systemic inflammatory response syndrome and multiple organ dysfunction syndrome by augmenting the inflammatory response to a subsequent insult. Feeding the gut improves survival and decreases lung and liver damage after ischemia/reperfusion injury in mice [69]. Administration of EN improves gut function and improves the global immunosuppressive and inflammatory response compared to TPN in patients with acute pancreatitis and in postsurgical patients [75,91]. However, this association of TPN with intestinal immune dysfunction in humans is not universally accepted [92]. Cerra et al. [93] showed no difference in either the mortality or incidence of multiorgan failure syndrome in 66 septic patients prospectively randomized to isocaloric, isonitrogenous EN or TPN.

Diminished visceral blood flow due to any global insult results in intestinal ileus. Ileus promotes microbial overgrowth and disturbs the normal gut ecology, which increases microbial translocation in humans [94]. Ischemia-induced dysmotility can be prevented by providing nutrients intraluminally [95]. Enteral feeding stimulates peristalsis and biliary secretion, which is rich in sIgA, which assists with bacterial movement downstream and decreases bacterial adhesiveness. Early oral feeding within 4 h after colorectal resection and anastomosis is associated with earlier flatus, bowel movements, and tolerance of diet than observed in traditionally managed patients [96]. It is hypothesized that by maintaining or improving intestinal motility in the critical care or postoperative setting, EN will help maintain the relative sterility of the proximal gut. Burn patients fed enterally within 24 h of injury show less endotoxin absorption from the gut than patients who are fed after 48 h [97]. EN prevents the increase in IgM endotoxin antibodies seen in patients of acute pancreatitis receiving TPN [75].

EN has also been shown to protect against hypoperfusion by increasing visceral and mucosal blood flow. In postoperative cardiac patients with hemodynamic compromise, the introduction of postpyloric EN increases cardiac index and splanchnic blood flow, without any adverse affects on the myocardium or systemic hemodynamics. At the same time, there is an increased absorption and utilization of nutrients [98]. Early EN has recently been reported to preserve mucosal ATP levels and gut absorptive capacity [24]. There may be a hyperemic response to the presence of luminal nutrients, which actually improves blood flow and oxygen delivery to all layers of the gut following EN compared to a fasting gut in the presence of shock. In animal models and human studies of burns, hemorrhagic shock, and septic shock, EN improves gut blood flow [99,100], gut motility [95], and outcomes [101,102].

Delivery of nutrients to the lumen may offer other benefits. Human intestinal cell cultures exposed to nutrients on the luminal surface as well as the vascular side show increased cell proliferation, motility, and enzyme production [103] when compared to cells exposed to nutrition only on the vascular side. Following major upper GI surgery, there is an improvement of peripheral protein kinetics and utilization of nutrients when they are provided enterally, compared to isonitrogenous, isocaloric TPN [104]. However, in some studies, this did not translate into actual improvement in visceral protein markers [11], postoperative muscle function, fatigue, weight loss, or body composition [21]. In fact, enteral carbohydrate administration, which normally promotes hepatic glucose uptake, actually failed to do so in a small number of critically ill patients [105]. Enteral delivery of nutrients may also fail to suppress endogenous glucose production and gluconeogenesis in this patient population [106].

EN's proposed benefits appear to extend to other organ systems. By maintaining renal blood flow, EN decreases renal injury resulting from rhabdomyolysis [107] and improves recovery in a rodent model of ischemia-induced acute renal failure when compared with isocaloric, isonitrogenous TPN [108]. EN has also been reported to minimize liver injury and improve survival after hemorrhagic shock [109].

The etiology of feeding-associated nonobstructed bowel necrosis (NOBN) during EN is unclear, but is probably multifactorial. Underlying bowel injury, hyperosmolar feeds, poor splanchnic perfusion secondary to excessive vasoconstriction, poor local bowel perfusion due to bowel dilatation, aggressive advancement of feeds, bacterial toxins, the use of tube instead of needle jejunostomies, and even flushing the jejunostomy tube with tap water [54] have been implicated. There is no clear association between NOBN and EN use in the presence of hemodynamic instability; in fact, enteral feeds may be beneficial after hemorrhagic shock [109]. In patients requiring inotropic support after cardiac surgery, EN is well tolerated and may even increase cardiac output and splanchnic blood flow [98,110]. Neither is there an association with early EN and NOBN: several studies have pointed out the benefits of early EN without any reported episodes of NOBN [111–114].

There are no prospective, randomized studies to accurately determine the risk of NOBN due to EN. In trauma patients, retrospective data would suggest that the incidence of NOBN is 0.3% of all critically ill trauma patients receiving EN by any route [115] and 0.29% of all feeding jejunostomies [52]. In a retrospective analysis of 2022 consecutive needle catheter jejunostomies for early EN, only 0.15% developed NOBN [116]. Witzel tube jejunostomies may be associated with higher necrosis rates (1%–2%) [117]. NOBN seems to occur more in patients undergoing abdominal surgery. A retrospective review of 524 consecutive patients who underwent elective upper GI operations with insertion of a feeding jejunostomy (needle catheter jejunostomy (NCJ) and tube jejunostomy (TJ)) for benign or malignant disease was conducted [118]. Six cases of NOBN were identified (1.15%) with no difference in incidence between routine NCJ ($n = 5$; 1.16%) and selective TJ ($n = 1$; 1.06%). The median rate of feeding at time of diagnosis was 105 mL/h (range, 75–125 mL/h), and the diagnosis was made at a median of 6 days (range, 4–18 days) postoperatively. All patients developed abdominal distension, hypotension, and tachycardia in 24 h before reexploratory laparotomy. Five patients died and one patient survived.

In nonsurgical patients, high-dose clonidine has been implicated. NOBN has even been reported with gastric tube feeding [119]. Additionally, the type of enteral formula has been implicated. A case report of two patients with no previous history of vascular problems experienced septic shock due to bowel ischemia [120]. Both were fed a fiber-rich enteral formula. Surgical finding showed hemorrhagic ischemia in the bowel. Pathologic finding suggests these changes may have been due to inspissations of bowel contents, which may put direct pressure on the mucosa of the bowel wall, leading to local impairment of mucosal and submucosal blood flow with subsequent bowel necrosis. Bowel ischemia may have been precipitated by an increased mesenteric blood flow requirement in combination with a metabolically stressed bowel.

Though it is a rare event, bowel perforation during EN has a mortality of over 85% [52], and therefore any signs of intolerance to feeds, emesis, diarrhea, cramp-like abdominal pain, abdominal distension, fever, tachycardia, and especially hypotension and hypovolemia during EN must be viewed with due suspicion. The risk of NOBN seems greatest during the first 24 h of starting feeds, but anecdotal evidence points to onset even after several days of successful enteral feeds. Daily abdominal exams prior to advancing feeds are strongly encouraged. Timely operative intervention can significantly improve outcome [121,122]. Overall, up to 92% of patients are successfully fed through needle jejunostomies after major abdominal operations [123].

HUMAN STUDIES: ENTERAL VERSUS PARENTERAL

In 1984, Bauer et al. showed that nutritional parameters increased faster with EN than with TPN in 60 prospectively randomized postoperative patients [4]. A study soon after showed that EN was associated with faster resolution of malabsorption than TPN in a small, prospective randomized study of infants with intractable diarrhea [124]. However, several prospective randomized studies are published at that time [32,125–127] and more recently [128] have shown no significant nutritional advantage of EN over isonitrogenous, isocaloric TPN. Kotler et al. looked at the effect of EN and TPN on 23 AIDS patients suffering from malabsorption [129]. There were no differences in intestinal function or CD4+ lymphocyte numbers in the peripheral blood, though the TPN group consumed more total calories, and this correlated with better weight gain.

In 1991, a large VA study [130] showed that preoperative TPN administered to surgical patients increased infectious morbidities compared to patients randomized to standard preoperative care.

However, this trial has been criticized for a poorly selected patient population. Patients at low risk of malnutrition will show minimal benefit from any nutrition plan. In fact, in a post hoc analysis of the 50 malnourished patients in this trial, TPN actually showed some benefit in reducing the non-infectious complication rate. The TPN group was clearly given excessive calories (3300 kcal/day). The resultant hyperglycemia and other complications of overfeeding are potential confounding variables [131].

Brennan et al. [132] showed a significant increase in complications after major pancreatic resection for cancer in patients randomized to TPN, compared to standard care. A meta-analysis by Heyland et al. [133] of 26 trials with a total of 2211 critically ill and surgical patients compared TPN to standard care (intravenous hydration and oral feeds when tolerated). Though TPN had no overall affect on mortality and malnourished patients benefited with a lower complication rate, the subset of critically ill patients and studies of a higher methodological quality showed an increase in mortality and complication rates with TPN. However, the adverse effects of TPN could have been exaggerated by the fact that several studies included patients who were accepting oral diets, and some studies provided inadequate TPN calories. Koretz et al. [134] reported a meta-analysis of 82 randomized, controlled trials that compared postoperative TPN with standard care and found that the TPN-fed patients had significantly more infectious complications. However, this meta-analysis included very few studies that looked specifically at malnourished patients, raising the question of whether nutritional support was justified at all in most of these studies.

In contrast, EN decreased complications in trials comparing it to standard postoperative care. Beier-Holgersen et al. [135] showed a significant decrease in postoperative infective complications with EN compared to placebo in a randomized, double-blind trial of 60 patients undergoing major abdominal surgery. In a meta-analysis of 11 prospective randomized trials with a total of 837 patients [136], there was a significant decrease in infectious complications and postoperative hospital stay in the early EN group (within 24 h of surgery) compared to those receiving standard care: nil by mouth. The only adverse effect was an increase in vomiting. Singh et al. [137] showed a similar significant reduction in septic morbidity with EN compared to standard care in a prospective, randomized study of 43 patients with nontraumatic perforative peritonitis.

Studies showing that, compared to TPN, EN improves resistance to infection in humans came from Moore et al. in 1986 and 1989. Data from two prospective, randomized studies of patients (n = 75 and 59) with an abdominal trauma index greater than 15 and less than 40 showed that patients randomized to EN had reduced major septic complications (abdominal abscesses and pneumonia) compared to those randomized to no supplemental nutrition [11] or TPN [30]. A study by the same author in a similar patient population showed a blunting of the hepatic stress response, with higher constitutive proteins and lower acute-phase proteins in the EN-fed patients than in the TPN fed [138]. In a subsequent meta-analysis of 8 prospective randomized trials comparing EN to TPN in a total of 230 high-risk surgical patients, Moore et al. found that EN-fed trauma patients had significantly fewer septic complications [22].

A report of findings from a prospective study of 98 patients of blunt and penetrating trauma with an abdominal trauma index of at least 15, randomized to either enteral or parenteral feeding within 24 h of injury, was published in 1992 [31]. Patients were fed formulas with almost identical amounts of fat, carbohydrate, and protein, though the TPN patients received 19.1 kcal/kg/day compared to 15.7 kcal/kg/day in the EN group. The enteral group sustained significantly fewer pneumonias, intra-abdominal abscesses, and line sepsis and sustained significantly fewer infections per patient, as well as significantly fewer infections per infected patient. The beneficial effects were more in severely injured patients and in patients with penetrating injuries. There was no significant benefit in the less severely injured subgroup.

An Italian group of surgical oncologists and nutritionists led by Bozzetti et al. studied 317 malnourished GI cancer patients in a multicenter prospective randomized trial of early EN or isonitrogenous, isocaloric TPN after elective surgery [139]. There was a significant decrease in infectious complications (27% with TPN, 16% with EN) and hospital stay, as well as a tendency toward decreased mortality with EN-treated patients. This suggested a decrease in the deleterious systemic inflammatory and metabolic responses associated with TPN. However, there were more therapy-associated adverse effects attributable to EN. Significantly more EN patients could not tolerate treatment due to GI adverse effects and were switched to TPN. This study was criticized for not including a control arm with no nutritional support (standard care), but the authors' rebuttal was that in this study of malnourished patients, not providing any nutritional support would be unjust in the face of established recommendations for postoperative care [140,141]. A meta-analysis of RCTs comparing EN, TPN, and standard care (no nutritional therapy) did in fact show that in malnourished patients, standard care had a worse outcome than TPN [37].

A study by Baïgrie et al. [142] also found a trend of reduction in postoperative septic complications with EN compared to TPN in 97 patients prospectively randomized after major surgery. Braga et al. [17] was unable to show any overall difference in complication rates or mortality with EN in 257 GI patients prospectively randomized to postoperative isonitrogenous, isocaloric EN or TPN. However, less than 80% of the EN patients reached nutritional goals within 4 days, significantly less than the TPN group. GI adverse effects to EN contributed to this difference, as well as to the eventual crossover of patients from the EN to the TPN groups. Interestingly, the EN arm had significantly better intestinal oxygenation, earlier flatus, and earlier bowel movements than the TPN arm did. Subset analysis of malnourished patients showed that EN was beneficial, but not significantly better than TPN.

Significant nutritional and immune benefits of EN over TPN have been shown in randomized controlled trials in the setting of severe acute ulcerative colitis [143], liver transplantation [12], neurosurgery [19], and acute pancreatitis [16,144]. In acute pancreatitis, the concept of early enteral feeds went against the established, if arbitrary dictum of NPO for 10 days and TPN [145]. However, early EN has been shown to decrease the rate of septic complications compared to TPN in these patients [146]. In the presence of necrosis, EN combined with prophylactic antibiotics decreased the rates of septic complications, multiorgan failure, and mortality compared to TPN and antibiotics [147]. Windsor et al. [75] also showed that early EN reduced the systemic inflammatory response syndrome, sepsis, and organ failure compared to TPN in acute pancreatitis.

Recently, several large meta-analyses of randomized controlled trials comparing enteral to parenteral nutrition have been published. Lipman et al. [35] found that the only benefit of EN was lower cost and probably reduced septic morbidity in acute abdominal trauma. However, this meta-analysis did not examine the quality of the studies it included, nor did it attempt to comprehensively evaluate the methodology of each study.

Subsequently, a more vigorous meta-analysis by Braunschweig et al. [37] included 27 prospective randomized studies comparing TPN versus EN or TPN versus standard care in a total of 1829 patients with compromised GI function. Aggregate results showed that TPN was associated with a higher relative risk of infection, even accounting for catheter sepsis, than either the EN or standard care groups, especially in normally nourished populations. Hyperglycemia in the TPN-fed patients was reported in several of the studies that showed a benefit of EN over TPN, and this could have played a confounding role. In a subset analysis of studies with more malnourished patients, TPN showed significantly less mortality than standard care did. In that same subset, enteral feeding significantly increased the risk of mortality. Of note, several studies delivered inadequate nutrition to the EN patients because of tolerance issues. The authors hypothesized that inadequate nutritional delivery by EN caused the increased mortality in malnourished populations. Nutritional support complications were more in the EN group, unless catheter sepsis was included, in which case they were no significant differences.

A meta-analysis of trials comparing EN to TPN in patients with acute pancreatitis by Al-Omran et al. [148] showed a trend toward improved outcomes with EN but suffered from the usual failings of this genre: heterogeneity of inclusion criterion, therapeutic parameters, and study quality.

The evidence from the last 20 years of prospective randomized trials is seemingly contradictory. Many studies have been criticized for including patient populations who were at low risk of malnutrition with normal GI function and therefore not expected to show much benefit from any nutritional intervention. At the same time, several studies randomized patients to EN or aggressive advancement of feeds, despite known GI dysfunction, and that could have led to a higher rate of nutritional support complications. Earlier studies delivered excessive calories to their TPN patients, causing hyperglycemia. Conversely, underfeeding with EN due to intolerance was frequently reported, and the resultant persistent calorie debt probably clouded the outcome [149].

In a study that attempted to determine the effect of underfeeding due to inadequate EN, Bauer et al. [150] prospectively randomized 120 patients to early EN plus placebo or early EN plus TPN. Retinol-binding protein and prealbumin increased significantly in the treatment group, and there was a reduction in hospital stay, though there was no difference in morbidity. The study failed to address the core issue of long-term underfeeding due to GI dysfunction or intolerance to EN, since patients in both groups tolerated similar mean amounts of EN and treatment extended for 7 days or less though outcome was measured till 2 years. Moreover, the majority (59%) of patients in the study were not malnourished and included patients who were anticipated to have only 2 or more days of inadequate oral intake.

A well-designed randomized prospective trial by Woodcock et al. [151] addressed some of the criticisms of patient selection in previous trials of EN versus TPN and attempted to provide answers that could be used in a clinical setting. In this study, the clinical assessment of GI function determined route of delivery in 562 patients who had at least 7 days of inadequate oral intake, actual or anticipated. Patients assessed to have inadequate GI function were given TPN, those assessed as having functional GI tracts were given EN, and the 64 patients in which there was a reasonable doubt were randomized equally to TPN or EN. The study had few well-nourished patients (11.2%). Invasive techniques of EN were not routinely initially employed. Clinical judgment of GI function was accurate across all groups, though poorest in randomized EN patients. Significantly more patients on TPN got their target intake than patients on EN, in both the nonrandomized and the randomized groups, and significantly fewer randomized than nonrandomized EN patients got their target caloric intake. There was no significant difference in the incidence of septic complications between EN and TPN in either the randomized or the nonrandomized groups or in malnourished and well-nourished subsets. Significantly more nonseptic delivery-related complications occurred with both EN groups than in the TPN groups. This study showed more mortality in the EN groups than in the TPN groups, reaching statistical significance in the nonrandomized groups. The authors attributed this to differences in patient populations between these two nonrandomized groups.

The beneficial effects of EN when compared to TPN in critical illness are well documented in numerous randomized controlled trials involving a variety of patient populations (e.g., trauma, burns, head injury, major surgery, acute pancreatitis). Few studies have been designed and powered to exhibit a differential effect on mortality; the most consistent outcome effect for EN is a reduction in infectious morbidity and ICU length of stay. Infectious morbidity includes general pneumonia and central line infections in most patients and abdominal abscess formation in trauma patients [22,30,31]. In the absence of those data, meta-analyses are the best available evidence, despite the inherent shortcoming of study heterogeneity. Overall, EN does have metabolic and immune benefits over TPN, as reflected by a reduction in hyperglycemia and infectious complications in most studies. This may not translate into a reduction in mortality but is probably accompanied by a significant cost savings.

CLINICAL APPROACH

The literature reviewed earlier clearly shows that both parenteral nutrition and EN have specific detrimental and beneficial effects. The question is, How should we use each method to minimize the disadvantages and maximize the advantages of nutritional therapy in our most gravely ill patients? In patients with a functional GI tract, the enteral route is undoubtedly superior because of its ability to maintain the immune system. In critically ill patients, greater success in achieving enteral tolerance has been reported by implementing a standardized protocol and may be further improved by feeding beyond the ligament of Treitz [152]—see Chapter 39 for further discussion. Gastric feeding, however, has the advantage of earlier institution than small bowel feeding [153]. Determining tolerance to EN is not always an easy task, especially in the ICU patient where the abdominal exam may be confounded by paralysis, mechanical ventilation, bulky dressings, and the occasional open abdomen. However, abdominal distension, pain, increased gastric residuals and nasogastric output, diarrhea, and pneumatosis are all signs of intolerance.

Critically ill patients often suffer from GI dysmotility, which is an important cause of intolerance to EN [154]. Contributing factors include electrolyte imbalances, mechanical ventilation [155], burns, extensive abdominal trauma, spinal cord injury, and pancreatitis [156], as well as increased intracranial pressure following a head injury [157]. Surgical trauma activates resident macrophages within the intestinal muscularis, which release several proinflammatory cytokines, contributing to postoperative ileus [158]. Other risk factors include medications (opiates, antidepressants, calcium channel blockers, ganglion-blocking agents, sedatives, dopamine, clonidine, and anticholinergics), sepsis, abdominal compartment syndrome, hypovolemia, hyperglycemia, previous vagotomy, systemic sclerosis, and muscular disease [159]. Patient overhydration, hemodynamic instability, inadequate gastric decompression, and overly aggressive feeding are all important contributing factors. To restore normal GI motility, it is important to correct these, as well as any electrolyte imbalances, establish strict glucose control, and discontinue drugs that decrease motility, especially opiate narcotics. Prokinetic agents like erythromycin, neostigmine, metoclopramide, and octreotide may all be considered, though they each have disadvantages. Since high-fat formulas with long-chain triglycerides increase dysmotility, tolerance can be improved with the use of relatively low-fat formulas or some of the newer enteral formulas, which contain medium-chain triglycerides.

A key factor in successful EN is to start conservatively and advance only as tolerated. Critically ill patients require fewer calories than was previously believed. It is now apparent that 20–30 kcal/kg/day is adequate in the ICU setting, a marked decrease from the past goals of 40–50 kcal/kg/day. In fact, enteral delivery of only 15%–30% of the usual caloric intake is believed to be enough to maintain both the GALT and the gut barrier function, with the consequent local and systemic immunologic benefits [44,160,161]. In a prospective randomized trial in which 53 patients with acute pancreatitis required nutritional support, the jejunal fed patients had shorter hospital stays, significantly faster progression to oral diets, and significantly fewer complications (hyperglycemia, septic complications, catheter related infections) than those receiving TPN, despite getting fewer calories (49% compared to 85% of the goal 25–30 kcal/kg/day) [29]. Initial trophic feedings (defined as 10–20 mL/h) for up to 6 days resulted in a lower incidence of GI intolerance over the first week of ICU stay than full feeding in one randomized single center study of a heterogeneous population of patients with acute respiratory failure and another larger randomized multicenter trial enrolling patients with acute lung injury and adult respiratory distress syndrome [162,163]. Compared to full feeding, initial trophic feedings resulted in similar clinical outcomes, including ventilator-free days, ICU-free days, 60-day mortality, and development of nosocomial infections. While trophic feeding seems appropriate for low-nutrition-risk patients to enhance gut immune function and improve GI tolerance, efforts should be made to reach at least 60%–70% goal nutrition requirements within 48–72 h in those patients at nutrition risk in order to achieve clinical benefit of EN over the first week of hospitalization (see Chapter 5). Contraindications to enteral feeding include continuing emesis, intestinal obstruction, major upper GI bleeds, inaccessibility, and hemodynamic instability. A dietitian with the experience and patience to place the tube in the small intestine may better address accessibility issues than the use of expensive fluoroscopic equipment [164].

Guidelines for nutritional support in critically ill patients have been formulated based on an analysis of the existing data [165]. Nutritional support should be initiated within 24–48 h, using a standard, polymeric enteric formula fed either gastrically or postpylorically, based on patient risk factors and local expertise in gaining postpyloric access. Aspiration precautions, including feeding in a semirecumbent posture and elevation of the head of the bed at least 30°, should be observed.

Using an algorithmic approach optimizes success with EN. This includes starting at a target rate of 10–15 mL/h, advancing feeds based on clinical exam, and taking the steps outlined earlier to optimize GI motility. EN should progress to 80% of target caloric intake (25–30 kcal/kg/day) within 72 h and to 100% soon after. If after 7 days EN cannot be advanced to meet these goals, the balance of the target should be supplemented with TPN. The patient should receive EN challenges every 12 h in an effort to increase the enteral delivery and wean off TPN. If the gut is not available or EN is not tolerated, nutritional support should be instituted with TPN in malnourished patients or be delayed for 7 days in patients not malnourished, while continuing EN challenges every 12 h wherever appropriate. Hypocaloric dosing, using less long-chain triglycerides, and maintaining optimal glycemic control (blood glucose <180 mg%) will help minimize the adverse metabolic effects of TPN. The implementation of such an evidence-based algorithm has been shown to improve patient outcomes in the intensive care setting [166].

REFERENCES

1. Dudrick S J, Wilmore D W, Vars H M, Rhoads J E. Long-term total parenteral nutrition with growth, development, and positive nitrogen balance. *Surgery* 1968; 64: 134–142.
2. Chrysomilides S A, Kaminski M V Jr. Home enteral and parenteral nutritional support: A comparison. *Am J Clin Nutr* 1981; 34: 2271–2275.
3. Kudsk K A, Stone J M, Carpenter G, Sheldon G F. Enteral and parenteral feeding influences mortality after hemoglobin–*E. coli* peritonitis in normal rats. *J Trauma* 1983; 23: 605–609.
4. Bauer E, Graber R, Brodtke R, Lunstedt B, Seifert J. Nutrition physiologic, immunologic and clinical parameters in prospective randomized patients by enteral or parenteral nutrition therapy following large intestine operations. *Infusionsther Klin Ernahr* 1984; 11: 165–167.
5. Hull S. Enteral versus parenteral nutrition support-rationale for increased use of enteral feeding. *Zeitschrift fur Gastroenterologie* 1985; 23: 55–63.
6. Bengmark S. Enteral nutrition in HPB surgery: Past and future. *J Hepatobiliary Pancreat Surg* 2002; 9: 448–458.
7. Taylor S J, Fettes S B, Jewkes C, Nelson R J. Prospective, randomized, controlled trial to determine the effect of early enhanced enteral nutrition on clinical outcome in mechanically ventilated patients suffering head injury. *Crit Care Med* 1999; 27: 2525–2531.
8. Fong Y M, Marano M A, Barber A et al. Total parenteral nutrition and bowel rest modify the metabolic response to endotoxin in humans. *Ann Surg* 1989; 210: 449–456; discussion 456–457.
9. Gianotti L, Nelson J L, Alexander J W, Chalk C L, Pyles T. Post injury hypermetabolic response and magnitude of translocation: Prevention by early enteral nutrition. *Nutrition* 1994; 10: 225–231.
10. Chiarelli A, Enzi G, Casadei A, Baggio B, Valerio A, Mazzoleni F. Very early nutrition supplementation in burned patients. *Am J Clin Nutr* 1990; 51: 1035–1039.
11. Moore E E, Jones T N. Benefits of immediate jejunostomy feeding after major abdominal trauma—A prospective, randomized study. *J Trauma* 1986; 26: 874–881.
12. Hasse J M, Blue L S, Liepa G U et al. Early enteral nutrition support in patients undergoing liver transplantation. *JPEN J Parenter Enteral Nutr* 1995; 19: 437–443.
13. Carr C S, Ling K D, Boulos P, Singer M. Randomised trial of safety and efficacy of immediate postoperative enteral feeding in patients undergoing gastrointestinal resection. *Bmj* 1996; 312: 869–871.
14. Vernet O, Christin L, Schutz Y, Danforth E Jr., Jequier E. Enteral versus parenteral nutrition: Comparison of energy metabolism in healthy subjects. *Am J Physiol* 1986; 250: E47–E54.
15. Magnusson J, Tranberg K G, Jeppsson B, Lunderquist A. Enteral versus parenteral glucose as the sole nutritional support after colorectal resection. A prospective, randomized comparison. *Scand J Gastroenterol* 1989; 24: 539–549.
16. McClave S A, Greene L M, Snider H L et al. Comparison of the safety of early enteral vs parenteral nutrition in mild acute pancreatitis. *JPEN J Parenter Enteral Nutr* 1997; 21: 14–20.
17. Braga M, Gianotti L, Gentilini O, Parisi V, Salis C, Di Carlo V. Early postoperative enteral nutrition improves gut oxygenation and reduces costs compared with total parenteral nutrition. *Crit Care Med* 2001; 29: 242–248.
18. Kudsk K A, Minard G, Wojtysiak S L, Croce M, Fabian T, Brown R O. Visceral protein response to enteral versus parenteral nutrition and sepsis in patients with trauma. *Surgery* 1994; 116: 516–523.

19. Suchner U, Senftleben U, Eckart T et al. Enteral versus parenteral nutrition: Effects on gastrointestinal function and metabolism. *Nutrition* 1996; 12: 13–22.
20. Moss G, Greenstein A, Levy S, Bierenbaum A. Maintenance of GI function after bowel surgery and immediate enteral full nutrition. I. Doubling of canine colorectal anastomotic bursting pressure and intestinal wound mature collagen content. *JPEN J Parenter Enteral Nutr* 1980; 4: 535–538.
21. Schroeder D, Gillanders L, Mahr K, Hill G L. Effects of immediate postoperative enteral nutrition on body composition, muscle function, and wound healing. *JPEN J Parenter Enteral Nutr* 1991; 15: 376–383.
22. Moore F A, Feliciano D V, Andrassy R J et al. Early enteral feeding, compared with parenteral, reduces postoperative septic complications. The results of a meta-analysis. *Ann Surg* 1992; 216: 172–183.
23. Bengmark S, Gianotti L. Nutritional support to prevent and treat multiple organ failure. *World J Surg* 1996; 20: 474–481.
24. Kozar R A, Hu S, Hassoun H T, DeSoignie R, Moore F A. Specific intraluminal nutrients alter mucosal blood flow during gut ischemia/reperfusion. *JPEN J Parenter Enteral Nutr* 2002; 26: 226–229.
25. Gosche J R, Garrison R N, Harris P D, Cryer H G. Absorptive hyperemia restores intestinal blood flow during *Escherichia coli* sepsis in the rat. *Arch Surg* 1990; 125: 1573–1576.
26. Cook D, Heyland D, Griffith L, Cook R, Marshall J, Pagliarello J. Risk factors for clinically important upper gastrointestinal bleeding in patients requiring mechanical ventilation. Canadian Critical Care Trials Group. *Crit Care Med* 1999; 27: 2812–2817.
27. Raff T, Germann G, Hartmann B. The value of early enteral nutrition in the prophylaxis of stress ulceration in the severely burned patient. *Burns* 1997; 23: 313–318.
28. Laggner A N, Lenz K. Prevention of stress ulcer in intensive care patients. *Wien Med Wochenschr* 1986; 136: 596–599.
29. Abou-Assi S, Craig K, O'Keefe S J. Hypocaloric jejunal feeding is better than total parenteral nutrition in acute pancreatitis: Results of a randomized comparative study. *Am J Gastroenterol* 2002; 97: 2255–2262.
30. Moore F A, Moore E E, Jones T N, McCroskey B L, Peterson V M. TEN versus TPN following major abdominal trauma—Reduced septic morbidity. *J Trauma* 1989; 29: 916–922; discussion 922–923.
31. Kudsk K A, Croce M A, Fabian T C et al. Enteral versus parenteral feeding. Effects on septic morbidity after blunt and penetrating abdominal trauma. *Ann Surg* 1992; 215: 503–511; discussion 511–513.
32. Burt M E, Stein T P, Brennan M F. A controlled, randomized trial evaluating the effects of enteral and parenteral nutrition on protein metabolism in cancer-bearing man. *J Surg Res* 1983; 34: 303–314.
33. Merkle N M, Wiedeck H, Herfarth C, Grunert A. Immediate postoperative enteral tube feeding following resection of the large intestine. Experiences with a controlled clinical study. *Chirurg* 1984; 55: 267–274.
34. Hausmann D, Mosebach K O, Caspari R, Rommelsheim K. Combined enteral-parenteral nutrition versus total parenteral nutrition in brain-injured patients. A comparative study. *Intensive Care Med* 1985; 11: 80–84.
35. Lipman T O. Grains or veins: Is enteral nutrition really better than parenteral nutrition? A look at the evidence. *JPEN J Parenter Enteral Nutr* 1998; 22: 167–182.
36. Heyland D K, MacDonald S, Keefe L, Drover J W. Total parenteral nutrition in the critically ill patient: A meta-analysis. *JAMA* 1998; 280: 2013–2019.
37. Braunschweig C L, Levy P, Sheean P M, Wang X. Enteral compared with parenteral nutrition: A meta-analysis. *Am J Clin Nutr* 2001; 74: 534–542.
38. Gianotti L, Braga M, Gentilini O, Balzano G, Zerbi A, Di Carlo V. Artificial nutrition after pancreaticoduodenectomy. *Pancreas* 2000; 21: 344–351.
39. Tanaka S, Miura S, Tashiro H et al. Morphological alteration of gut-associated lymphoid tissue after long-term total parenteral nutrition in rats. *Cell Tissue Res* 1991; 266: 29–36.
40. Khan J, Iiboshi Y, Nezu R et al. Total parenteral nutrition increases uptake of latex beads by Peyer's patches. *JPEN J Parenter Enteral Nutr* 1997; 21: 31–35.
41. Janu P, Li J, Renegar K B, Kudsk K A. Recovery of gut-associated lymphoid tissue and upper respiratory tract immunity after parenteral nutrition. *Ann Surg* 1997; 225: 707–715; discussion 715–717.
42. Quigley E M, Marsh M N, Shaffer J L, Markin R S. Hepatobiliary complications of total parenteral nutrition. *Gastroenterology* 1993; 104: 286–301.
43. Kaufman S S. Prevention of parenteral nutrition-associated liver disease in children. *Pediatr Transplant* 2002; 6: 37–42.
44. Shou J, Lappin J, Minnard E A, Daly J M. Total parenteral nutrition, bacterial translocation, and host immune function. *Am J Surg* 1994; 167: 145–150.

45. Kudsk K A, Li J, Renegar K B. Loss of upper respiratory tract immunity with parenteral feeding. *Ann Surg* 1996; 223: 629–635; discussion 635–638.
46. King B K, Kudsk K A, Li J, Wu Y, Renegar K B. Route and type of nutrition influence mucosal immunity to bacterial pneumonia. *Ann Surg* 1999; 229: 272–278.
47. Fukatsu K, Lundberg A H, Hanna M K et al. Route of nutrition influences intercellular adhesion molecule-1 expression and neutrophil accumulation in intestine. *Arch Surg* 1999; 134: 1055–1060.
48. Lokich J J, Bothe A Jr., Benotti P, Moore C. Complications and management of implanted venous access catheters. *J Clin Oncol* 1985; 3: 710–717.
49. Reimund J M, Arondel Y, Finck G, Zimmermann F, Duclos B, Baumann R. Catheter-related infection in patients on home parenteral nutrition: Results of a prospective survey. *Clin Nutr* 2002; 21: 33–38.
50. Jones T N, Moore F A, Moore E E, McCroskey B L. Gastrointestinal symptoms attributed to jejunostomy feeding after major abdominal trauma—A critical analysis. *Crit Care Med* 1989; 17: 1146–1150.
51. Heyland D, Cook D J, Winder B, Brylowski L, Van deMark H, Guyatt G. Enteral nutrition in the critically ill patient: A prospective survey. *Crit Care Med* 1995; 23: 1055–1060.
52. Schunn C D, Daly J M. Small bowel necrosis associated with postoperative jejunal tube feeding. *J Am Coll Surg* 1995; 180: 410–416.
53. Zetti G, Tagliabue F, Barabino M, Fontana S, Ceppi M, Samori G. Small bowel necrosis associated with postoperative enteral feeding. *Chir Ital* 2002; 54: 555–558.
54. Schloerb P R, Wood J G, Casillan A J, Tawfik O, Udobi K. Bowel necrosis caused by water in jejunal feeding. *JPEN J Parenter Enteral Nutr* 2004; 28: 27–29.
55. Heyland D K, Drover J W, MacDonald S, Novak F, Lam M. Effect of postpyloric feeding on gastroesophageal regurgitation and pulmonary microaspiration: Results of a randomized controlled trial. *Crit Care Med* 2001; 29: 1495–1501.
56. McClave S A, DeMeo M T, DeLegge M H et al. North American Summit on Aspiration in the Critically Ill Patient: Consensus statement. *JPEN J Parenter Enteral Nutr* 2002; 26: S80–S85.
57. Watters J M, Kirkpatrick S M, Norris S B, Shamji F M, Wells G A. Immediate postoperative enteral feeding results in impaired respiratory mechanics and decreased mobility. *Ann Surg* 1997; 226: 369–377; discussion 377–380.
58. Seron Arbeloa C, Avellanas Chavala M, Homs Gimeno C, Larraz Vileta A, Laplaza Marin J. Descriptive analysis of the nutritional support in a polyvalent intensive care unit. Complications of enteral nutrition. *Nutr Hosp* 1999; 14: 217–222.
59. Montejo J C. Enteral nutrition-related gastrointestinal complications in critically ill patients: A multicenter study. The Nutritional and Metabolic Working Group of the Spanish Society of Intensive Care Medicine and Coronary Units. *Crit Care Med* 1999; 27: 1447–1453.
60. Jorba R, Fabregat J, Borobia F G, Torras J, Poves I, Jaurrieta E. Small bowel necrosis in association with early postoperative enteral feeding after pancreatic resection. *Surgery* 2000; 128: 111–112.
61. Mentec H, Dupont H, Bocchetti M, Cani P, Ponche F, Bleichner G. Upper digestive intolerance during enteral nutrition in critically ill patients: Frequency, risk factors, and complications. *Crit Care Med* 2001; 29: 1955–1961.
62. Braga M, Gianotti L, Gentilini O, Liotta S, Di Carlo V. Feeding the gut early after digestive surgery: Results of a nine-year experience. *Clin Nutr* 2002; 21: 59–65.
63. Johnson L R, Copeland E M, Dudrick S J, Lichtenberger L M, Castro G A. Structural and hormonal alterations in the gastrointestinal tract of parenterally fed rats. *Gastroenterology* 1975; 68: 1177–1183.
64. Levine G M, Deren J J, Steiger E, Zinno R. Role of oral intake in maintenance of gut mass and disaccharide activity. *Gastroenterology* 1974; 67: 975–982.
65. Saito H, Trocki O, Alexander J W, Kopcha R, Heyd T, Joffe S N. The effect of route of nutrient administration on the nutritional state, catabolic hormone secretion, and gut mucosal integrity after burn injury. *JPEN J Parenter Enteral Nutr* 1987; 11: 1–7.
66. Alverdy J C, Aoys E, Moss G S. Total parenteral nutrition promotes bacterial translocation from the gut. *Surgery* 1988; 104: 185–190.
67. Deitch E A, Xu D, Naruhn M B, Deitch D C, Lu Q, Marino A A. Elemental diet and IV-TPN-induced bacterial translocation is associated with loss of intestinal mucosal barrier function against bacteria. *Ann Surg* 1995; 221: 299–307.
68. Yang H, Kiristioglu I, Fan Y et al. Interferon-gamma expression by intraepithelial lymphocytes results in a loss of epithelial barrier function in a mouse model of total parenteral nutrition. *Ann Surg* 2002; 236: 226–234.

69. Yang H, Wildhaber B, Tazuke Y, Teitelbaum D H. 2002 Harry M. Vars Research Award. Keratinocyte growth factor stimulates the recovery of epithelial structure and function in a mouse model of total parenteral nutrition. *JPEN J Parenter Enteral Nutr* 2002; 26: 333–340; discussion 340–341.
70. Yang H, Feng Y, Teitelbaum D. Enteral versus parenteral nutrition: Effect on intestinal barrier function. *Ann N Y Acad Sci* 2009; 1165: 338–346.
71. Demehri F R, Barrett M, Ralls M W et al. Intestinal epithelial cell apoptosis and loss of barrier function in the setting of altered microbiota with enteral nutrient deprivation. *Front Cell Infect Microbiol* 2013; 3: 105.
72. Ralls M W, Miyasaka E, Teitelbaum D H. Intestinal microbial diversity and perioperative complications. *JPEN J Parenter Enteral Nutr* 2014; 38(3): 392–399.
73. Buchman A L, Moukarzel A A, Bhuta S et al. Parenteral nutrition is associated with intestinal morphologic and functional changes in humans. *JPEN J Parenter Enteral Nutr* 1995; 19: 453–460.
74. Hadfield R J, Sinclair D G, Houldsworth P E, Evans T W. Effects of enteral and parenteral nutrition on gut mucosal permeability in the critically ill. *Am J Respir Crit Care Med* 1995; 152: 1545–1548.
75. Groos S, Hunefeld G, Luciano L. Parenteral versus enteral nutrition: Morphological changes in human adult intestinal mucosa. *J Submicrosc Cytol Pathol* 1996; 28: 61–74.
76. Windsor A C, Kanwar S, Li A G et al. Compared with parenteral nutrition, enteral feeding attenuates the acute phase response and improves disease severity in acute pancreatitis. *Gut* 1998; 42: 431–435.
77. O'Boyle C J, MacFie J, Dave K, Sagar P S, Poon P, Mitchell C J. Alterations in intestinal barrier function do not predispose to translocation of enteric bacteria in gastroenterologic patients. *Nutrition* 1998; 14: 358–362.
78. Sedman P C, MacFie J, Palmer M D, Mitchell C J, Sagar P M. Preoperative total parenteral nutrition is not associated with mucosal atrophy or bacterial translocation in humans. *Br J Surg* 1995; 82: 1663–1667.
79. Van Leeuwen P A, Boermeester M A, Houdijk A P et al. Clinical significance of translocation. *Gut* 1994; 35: S28–S34.
80. MacFie J. Enteral versus parenteral nutrition: The significance of bacterial translocation and gut-barrier function. *Nutrition* 2000; 16: 606–611.
81. Costello E K, Stagaman K, Dethlefsen L, Bohannan B J, Relman D A. The application of ecological theory toward an understanding of the human microbiome. *Science* 2012; 336: 1255–1262.
82. Li J, Kudsk K A, Gocinski B, Dent D, Glezer J, Langkamp-Henken B. Effects of parenteral and enteral nutrition on gut-associated lymphoid tissue. *J Trauma* 1995; 39: 44–51; discussion 51–52.
83. Kudsk K A. Current aspects of mucosal immunology and its influence by nutrition. *Am J Surg* 2002; 183: 390–398.
84. Renegar K B, Small P A Jr. Immunoglobulin A mediation of murine nasal anti-influenza virus immunity. *J Virol* 1991; 65: 2146–2148.
85. Johnson C D, Kudsk K A, Fukatsu K, Renegar K B, Zarzaur B L. Route of nutrition influences generation of antibody-forming cells and initial defense to an active viral infection in the upper respiratory tract. *Ann Surg* 2003; 237: 565–573.
86. Shou J, Lappin J, Daly J M. Impairment of pulmonary macrophage function with total parenteral nutrition. *Ann Surg* 1994; 219: 291–297.
87. Okada Y, Klein N J, van Saene H K, Webb G, Holzel H, Pierro A. Bactericidal activity against coagulase-negative staphylococci is impaired in infants receiving long-term parenteral nutrition. *Ann Surg* 2000; 231: 276–281.
88. Gianotti L, Alexander J W, Nelson J L, Fukushima R, Pyles T, Chalk C L. Role of early enteral feeding and acute starvation on postburn bacterial translocation and host defense: Prospective, randomized trials. *Crit Care Med* 1994; 22: 265–272.
89. Zarzaur B L, Wu Y, Fukatsu K, Johnson C D, Kudsk K A. The neuropeptide bombesin improves IgA-mediated mucosal immunity with preservation of gut interleukin-4 in total parenteral nutrition-fed mice. *Surgery* 2002; 131: 59–65.
90. Li J, Kudsk K A, Hamidian M, Gocinski B L. Bombesin affects mucosal immunity and gut-associated lymphoid tissue in intravenously fed mice. *Arch Surg* 1995; 130: 1164–1169; discussion 1169–1170.
91. Braga M, Vignali A, Gianotti L, Cestari A, Profili M, Carlo V D. Immune and nutritional effects of early enteral nutrition after major abdominal operations. *Eur J Surg* 1996; 162: 105–112.
92. Buchman A L, Mestecky J, Moukarzel A, Ament M E. Intestinal immune function is unaffected by parenteral nutrition in man. *J Am Coll Nutr* 1995; 14: 656–661.
93. Cerra F B, McPherson J P, Konstantinides F N, Konstantinides N N, Teasley K M. Enteral nutrition does not prevent multiple organ failure syndrome (MOFS) after sepsis. *Surgery* 1988; 104: 727–733.

94. MacFie J, O'Boyle C, Mitchell C J, Buckley P M, Johnstone D, Sudworth P. Gut origin of sepsis: A prospective study investigating associations between bacterial translocation, gastric microflora, and septic morbidity. *Gut* 1999; 45: 223–228.
95. Grossie V B, Jr., Weisbrodt N W, Moore F A, Moody F. Ischemia/reperfusion-induced disruption of rat small intestine transit is reversed by total enteral nutrition. *Nutrition* 2001; 17: 939–943.
96. Stewart B T, Woods R J, Collopy B T, Fink R J, Mackay J R, Keck J O. Early feeding after elective open colorectal resections: A prospective randomized trial. *Aust N Z J Surg* 1998; 68: 125–128.
97. Peng Y Z, Yuan Z Q, Xiao G X. Effects of early enteral feeding on the prevention of enterogenic infection in severely burned patients. *Burns* 2001; 27: 145–149.
98. Revelly J P, Tappy L, Berger M M, Gersbach P, Cayeux C, Chiolero R. Early metabolic and splanchnic responses to enteral nutrition in postoperative cardiac surgery patients with circulatory compromise. *Intensive Care Med* 2001; 27: 540–547.
99. Kazamias P, Kotzampassi K, Koufogiannis D, Eleftheriadis E. Influence of enteral nutrition-induced splanchnic hyperemia on the septic origin of splanchnic ischemia. *World J Surg* 1998; 22: 6–11.
100. Purcell P N, Davis K Jr., Branson R D, Johnson D J. Continuous duodenal feeding restores gut blood flow and increases gut oxygen utilization during PEEP ventilation for lung injury. *Am J Surg* 1993; 165: 188–193; discussion 193–194.
101. Gianotti L, Alexander J W, Gennari R, Pyles T, Babcock G F. Oral glutamine decreases bacterial translocation and improves survival in experimental gut-origin sepsis. *JPEN J Parenter Enteral Nutr* 1995; 19: 69–74.
102. Zaloga G P, Roberts P, Black K W, Prielipp R. Gut bacterial translocation/dissemination explains the increased mortality produced by parenteral nutrition following methotrexate. *Circ Shock* 1993; 39: 263–268.
103. Perdikis D A, Basson M D. Basal nutrition promotes human intestinal epithelial (Caco-2) proliferation, brush border enzyme activity, and motility. *Crit Care Med* 1997; 25: 159–165.
104. Harrison L E, Hochwald S N, Heslin M J, Berman R, Burt M, Brennan M F. Early postoperative enteral nutrition improves peripheral protein kinetics in upper gastrointestinal cancer patients undergoing complete resection: A randomized trial. *JPEN J Parenter Enteral Nutr* 1997; 21: 202–207.
105. Tappy L, Berger M, Schwarz J M et al. Hepatic and peripheral glucose metabolism in intensive care patients receiving continuous high- or low-carbohydrate enteral nutrition. *JPEN J Parenter Enteral Nutr* 1999; 23: 260–267; discussion 267–268.
106. Schwarz J M, Chiolero R, Revelly J P et al. Effects of enteral carbohydrates on de novo lipogenesis in critically ill patients. *Am J Clin Nutr* 2000; 72: 940–945.
107. Roberts P R, Black K W, Zaloga G P. Enteral feeding improves outcome and protects against glycerol-induced acute renal failure in the rat. *Am J Respir Crit Care Med* 1997; 156: 1265–1269.
108. Mouser J F, Hak E B, Kuhl D A, Dickerson R N, Gaber L W, Hak L J. Recovery from ischemic acute renal failure is improved with enteral compared with parenteral nutrition. *Crit Care Med* 1997; 25: 1748–1754.
109. Bortenschlager L, Roberts P R, Black K W, Zaloga G P. Enteral feeding minimizes liver injury during hemorrhagic shock. *Shock* 1994; 2: 351–354.
110. Berger M M, Berger-Gryllaki M, Wiesel P H et al. Intestinal absorption in patients after cardiac surgery. *Crit Care Med* 2000; 28: 2217–2223.
111. Galban C, Montejo J C, Mesejo A et al. An immune-enhancing enteral diet reduces mortality rate and episodes of bacteremia in septic intensive care unit patients. *Crit Care Med* 2000; 28: 643–648.
112. Gadek J E, DeMichele S J, Karlstad M D et al. Effect of enteral feeding with eicosapentaenoic acid, gamma-linolenic acid, and antioxidants in patients with acute respiratory distress syndrome. Enteral Nutrition in ARDS Study Group. *Crit Care Med* 1999; 27: 1409–1420.
113. Caparros T, Lopez J, Grau T. Early enteral nutrition in critically ill patients with a high-protein diet enriched with arginine, fiber, and antioxidants compared with a standard high-protein diet. The effect on nosocomial infections and outcome. *JPEN J Parenter Enteral Nutr* 2001; 25: 299–308; discussion 308–309.
114. Atkinson S, Sieffert E, Bihari D. A prospective, randomized, double-blind, controlled clinical trial of enteral immunonutrition in the critically ill. Guy's Hospital Intensive Care Group. *Crit Care Med* 1998; 26: 1164–1172.
115. Marvin R G, McKinley B A, McQuiggan M, Cocanour C S, Moore F A. Nonocclusive bowel necrosis occurring in critically ill trauma patients receiving enteral nutrition manifests no reliable clinical signs for early detection. *Am J Surg* 2000; 179: 7–12.

116. Myers J G, Page C P, Stewart R M, Schwesinger W H, Sirinek K R, Aust J B. Complications of needle catheter jejunostomy in 2,022 consecutive applications. *Am J Surg* 1995; 170: 547–550; discussion 550–551.
117. Holmes J H t, Brundage S I, Yuen P, Hall R A, Maier R V, Jurkovich G J. Complications of surgical feeding jejunostomy in trauma patients. *J Trauma* 1999; 47: 1009–1012.
118. Spalding D R C, Behranwala K A, Straker P et al. Non-occlusive small bowel necrosis in association with feeding jejunostomy after elective upper gastrointestinal surgery. *Ann R Coll Surg Engl* 2009; 9: 477–482.
119. Frey C, Takala J, Krahenbuhl L. Non-occlusive small bowel necrosis during gastric tube feeding: A case report. *Intensive Care Med* 2001; 27: 1422–1425.
120. Gwon J G, Lee Y J, Kyoung K H et al. Enteral nutrition associated non-occlusive bowel ischemia. *J Korean Surg Soc* 2012; 83: 171–174.
121. Lawlor D K, Inculet R I, Malthaner R A. Small-bowel necrosis associated with jejunal tube feeding. *Can J Surg* 1998; 41: 459–462.
122. Andersen D R, Christensen L T. Small bowel necrosis associated with postoperative percutaneous jejunal tube feeding. *Ugeskr Laeger* 2003; 165: 2750–2751.
123. De Gottardi A, Krahenbuhl L, Farhadi J, Gernhardt S, Schafer M, Buchler M W. Clinical experience of feeding through a needle catheter jejunostomy after major abdominal operations. *Eur J Surg* 1999; 165: 1055–1060.
124. Orenstein S R. Enteral versus parenteral therapy for intractable diarrhea of infancy: A prospective, randomized trial. *J Pediatr* 1986; 109: 277–286.
125. Muggia-Sullam M, Bower R H, Murphy R F, Joffe S N, Fischer J E. Postoperative enteral versus parenteral nutritional support in gastrointestinal surgery. A matched prospective study. *Am J Surg* 1985; 149: 106–112.
126. Fletcher J P, Little J M. A comparison of parenteral nutrition and early postoperative enteral feeding on the nitrogen balance after major surgery. *Surgery* 1986; 100: 21–24.
127. Adams S, Dellinger E P, Wertz M J, Oreskovich M R, Simonowitz D, Johansen K. Enteral versus parenteral nutritional support following laparotomy for trauma: A randomized prospective trial. *J Trauma* 1986; 26: 882–891.
128. Borzotta A P, Pennings J, Papasadero B et al. Enteral versus parenteral nutrition after severe closed head injury. *J Trauma* 1994; 37: 459–468.
129. Kotler D P, Fogleman L, Tierney A R. Comparison of total parenteral nutrition and an oral, semielemental diet on body composition, physical function, and nutrition-related costs in patients with malabsorption due to acquired immunodeficiency syndrome. *JPEN J Parenter Enteral Nutr* 1998; 22: 120–126.
130. The Veterans Affairs Total Parenteral Nutrition Cooperative Study Group. Perioperative total parenteral nutrition in surgical patients. *N Engl J Med* 1991; 325: 525–532.
131. Nordenstrom J, Thorne A. Benefits and complications of parenteral nutritional support. *Eur J Clin Nutr* 1994; 48: 531–537.
132. Brennan M F, Pisters P W, Posner M, Quesada O, Shike M. A prospective randomized trial of total parenteral nutrition after major pancreatic resection for malignancy. *Ann Surg* 1994; 220: 436–441; discussion 441–444.
133. Heyland D K, Montalvo M, MacDonald S, Keefe L, Su X Y, Drover J W. Total parenteral nutrition in the surgical patient: A meta-analysis. *Can J Surg* 2001; 44: 102–111.
134. Koretz R L, Lipman T O, Klein S. AGA technical review on parenteral nutrition. *Gastroenterology* 2001; 121: 970–1001.
135. Beier-Holgersen R, Boesby S. Effect of early postoperative enteral nutrition on postoperative infections. *Ugeskr Laeger* 1998; 160: 3223–3226.
136. Lewis S J, Egger M, Sylvester P A, Thomas S. Early enteral feeding versus "nil by mouth" after gastrointestinal surgery: Systematic review and meta-analysis of controlled trials. *BMJ* 2001; 323: 773–776.
137. Singh G, Ram R P, Khanna S K. Early postoperative enteral feeding in patients with nontraumatic intestinal perforation and peritonitis. *J Am Coll Surg* 1998; 187: 142–146.
138. Moore E E, Moore F A. Immediate enteral nutrition following multisystem trauma: A decade perspective. *J Am Coll Nutr* 1991; 10: 633–648.
139. Bozzetti F, Braga M, Gianotti L, Gavazzi C, Mariani L. Postoperative enteral versus parenteral nutrition in malnourished patients with gastrointestinal cancer: A randomised multicentre trial. *Lancet* 2001; 358: 1487–1492.
140. Koretz R L. Enteral nutrition led to fewer postoperative complications than did parenteral feeding in gastrointestinal cancer. *ACP J Club* 2002; 136: 93.

141. Koretz R L. One if by gut and two if iv. *Gastroenterology* 2002; 122: 1537–1538; discussion 1538.
142. Baigrie R J, Devitt P G, Watkin D S. Enteral versus parenteral nutrition after oesophagogastric surgery: A prospective randomized comparison. *Aust N Z J Surg* 1996; 66: 668–670.
143. Gonzalez-Huix F, Fernandez-Banares F, Esteve-Comas M et al. Enteral versus parenteral nutrition as adjunct therapy in acute ulcerative colitis. *Am J Gastroenterol* 1993; 88: 227–232.
144. Kalfarentzos F, Kehagias J, Mead N, Kokkinis K, Gogos C A. Enteral nutrition is superior to parenteral nutrition in severe acute pancreatitis: Results of a randomized prospective trial. *Br J Surg* 1997; 84: 1665–1669.
145. Bank S, Singh P, Pooran N, Stark B. Evaluation of factors that have reduced mortality from acute pancreatitis over the past 20 years. *J Clin Gastroenterol* 2002; 35: 50–60.
146. Olah A, Pardavi G, Belagyi T, Nagy A, Issekutz A, Mohamed G E. Early nasojejunal feeding in acute pancreatitis is associated with a lower complication rate. *Nutrition* 2002; 18: 259–262.
147. Olah A, Pardavi G, Belagyi T. Early jejunal feeding in acute pancreatitis: Prevention of septic complications and multiorgan failure. *Magy Seb* 2000; 53: 7–12.
148. Al-Omran M, Groof A, Wilke D. Enteral versus parenteral nutrition for acute pancreatitis. *Cochrane Database Syst Rev* 2003: CD002837.
149. Griffiths R D. Nutrition in intensive care: Give enough but choose the route wisely? *Nutrition* 2001; 17: 53–55.
150. Bauer P, Charpentier C, Bouchet C, Nace L, Raffy F, Gaconnet N. Parenteral with enteral nutrition in the critically ill. *Intensive Care Med* 2000; 26: 893–900.
151. Woodcock N P, Zeigler D, Palmer M D, Buckley P, Mitchell C J, MacFie J. Enteral versus parenteral nutrition: A pragmatic study. *Nutrition* 2001; 17: 1–12.
152. Kozar R A, McQuiggan M M, Moore E E, Kudsk K A, Jurkovich G J, Moore F A. Postinjury enteral tolerance is reliably achieved by a standardized protocol. *J Surg Res* 2002; 104: 70–75.
153. Neumann D A, DeLegge M H. Gastric versus small-bowel tube feeding in the intensive care unit: A prospective comparison of efficacy. *Crit Care Med* 2002; 30: 1436–1438.
154. Adam S, Batson S. A study of problems associated with the delivery of enteral feed in critically ill patients in five ICUs in the UK. *Intensive Care Med* 1997; 23: 261–266.
155. Mutlu G M, Mutlu E A, Factor P. GI complications in patients receiving mechanical ventilation. *Chest* 2001; 119: 1222–1241.
156. Ritz M A, Fraser R, Tam W, Dent J. Impacts and patterns of disturbed gastrointestinal function in critically ill patients. *Am J Gastroenterol* 2000; 95: 3044–3052.
157. Kao C H, ChangLai S P, Chieng P U, Yen T C. Gastric emptying in head-injured patients. *Am J Gastroenterol* 1998; 93: 1108–1112.
158. Kalff J C, Turler A, Schwarz N T et al. Intra-abdominal activation of a local inflammatory response within the human muscularis externa during laparotomy. *Ann Surg* 2003; 237: 301–315.
159. DeMeo M T, Mutlu E A, Keshavarzian A, Tobin M C. Intestinal permeation and gastrointestinal disease. *J Clin Gastroenterol* 2002; 34: 385–396.
160. Okada Y, Klein N, van Saene H K, Pierro A. Small volumes of enteral feedings normalise immune function in infants receiving parenteral nutrition. *J Pediatr Surg* 1998; 33: 16–19.
161. Sax H C, Illig K A, Ryan C K, Hardy D J. Low-dose enteral feeding is beneficial during total parenteral nutrition. *Am J Surg* 1996; 171: 587–590.
162. Rice T W, Wheeler A P, Thompson B T et al. Enteral omega-3 fatty acid, gamma-linolenic acid, and antioxidant supplementation in acute lung injury. *JAMA* 2011; 306: 1574–1581.
163. National Heart, Lung, and Blood Institute Acute Respiratory Distress Syndrome (ARDS) Clinical Trials Network, Rice T W, Wheeler A P et al. Initial trophic vs full enteral feeding in patients with acute lung injury: The EDEN randomized trial. *JAMA* 2012; 307: 795–803.
164. Cresci G, Martindale R. Bedside placement of small bowel feeding tubes in hospitalized patients: A new role for the dietitian. *Nutrition* 2003; 19: 843–846.
165. McClave S, Martindale R, Vanek V et al., Guidelines for the provision and assessment of nutrition support therapy in the adult critically ill patient. Society of Critical Care Medicine and the American Society for Parenteral and Enteral Nutrition. *J Parenter Enteral Nutr* 2009; 33: 277.
166. Martin C M, Doig G S, Heyland D K, Morrison T, Sibbald W J. Multicentre, cluster-randomized clinical trial of algorithms for critical-care enteral and parenteral therapy (ACCEPT). *CMAJ* 2004; 170: 197–204.

12 Vascular Access in the Critically Ill Patient

Lindsay M. Dowhan, Jesse Gutnick, and Ezra Steiger

CONTENTS

INTRODUCTION

Central venous catheters (CVCs) are critical devices needed for patient care during intensive care unit (ICU) hospitalization. They are used to administer many therapies including parenteral nutrition (PN), chemotherapy, IV medications and fluid resuscitation, hemodialysis, and hemodynamic monitoring. This chapter will focus on CVC use for PN in the critically ill patient.

HISTORY

Central venous access was first performed through insertion of a glass tube into the left jugular vein of a horse in order to measure central venous pressure (CVP) by Stephen Hales in 1733 (Kalso 1985). It was not until 1929 that Werner Forssmann accomplished central access in a human when he inserted a urethral catheter into his own arm vein and advanced it to his right ventricle from which he, along with André Cournand and Dickenson Richards, was awarded the Nobel Prize in 1956 (Meyer 1990). Aubaniac described the infraclavicular route of catheterization in 1952 and was the first to use percutaneous access of the subclavian vein in order to achieve rapid transfusion. Rhoad and colleagues (Dudrick 2006) introduced peripherally inserted CVCs via the lower extremity veins for nutrition support of cancer patients in 1952; however, this technique was aborted due to thrombosis of the cannulated peripheral veins. The Seldinger technique, introduced in 1953, revolutionized vascular access by allowing nonsurgeons to access the vascular system safely (Varon and Nyman 2007). Wilson used peripherally inserted CVCs to monitor CVP in critically ill patients in 1960 (Dudrick 2006), while Dudrick pioneered research in the development of successful prolonged central venous feeding of Beagle puppies and humans via the superior vena cava (SVC) in 1966 (Dudrick 2009) laying the foundation for the development of PN that we know today.

TYPES OF CENTRAL ACCESS IN THE ICU

There are several CVCs that can be used for access in the ICU. They may have one, two, or multiple lumens depending on the goals of therapy.

Short-term access CVCs typically include peripherally inserted central catheters (PICCs); internal jugular (IJ) and external jugular, subclavian, and femoral CVCs; and pulmonary artery catheters (PACs) (also called the Swan–Ganz catheters). If the only concern is providing PN support, the subclavian vein is preferred over IJ or femoral sites, due to lower infectious complications (van der Kooi et al. 2012) and catheter-associated deep venous thrombosis (Malinoski et al. 2013). Patients with renal failure are best served by IJ lines to avoid long-term arteriovenous (AV) fistula outflow obstruction due to subclavian stenosis, making dialysis catheter placement difficult.

Long-term CVC access typically involves catheters used for dialysis and long-term PN patients. Historically, AV fistulas have been used for vascular access in the Netherlands for long-term PN patients and have proven to be a safe alternative with low rates of infection (Versleijen et al. 2009). Tunneled cuffed catheters (such as Hickman, Leonard, Groshong, and Broviac) are used for long-term PN patients. The Dacron velour cuff adheres to the tissue in the subcutaneous tunnel to prevent displacement and infection (Galloway and Bodenham 2004). Previously implanted ports may be used in the ICU for the administration of chemotherapeutic agents (Figures 12.1 through 12.4).

When determining what access is best for PN in a particular patient, it is important to consider the duration of therapy. PAC and midline catheters are not appropriate for PN administration; PACs

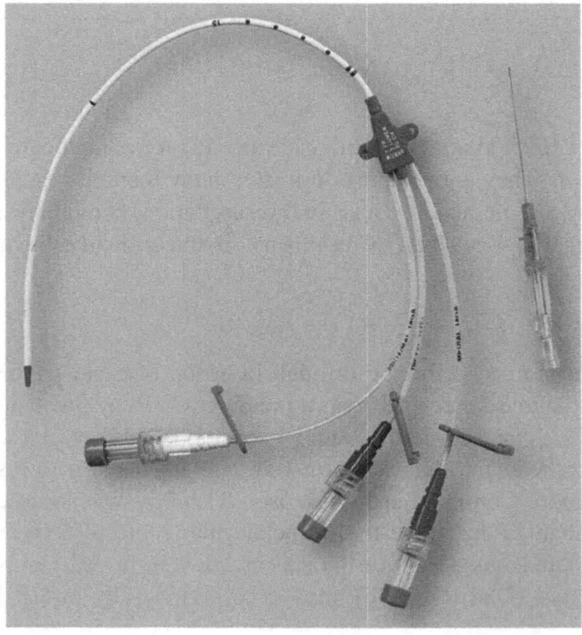

FIGURE 12.1 Triple-lumen CVC on the left. Peripheral vein catheter on the right.

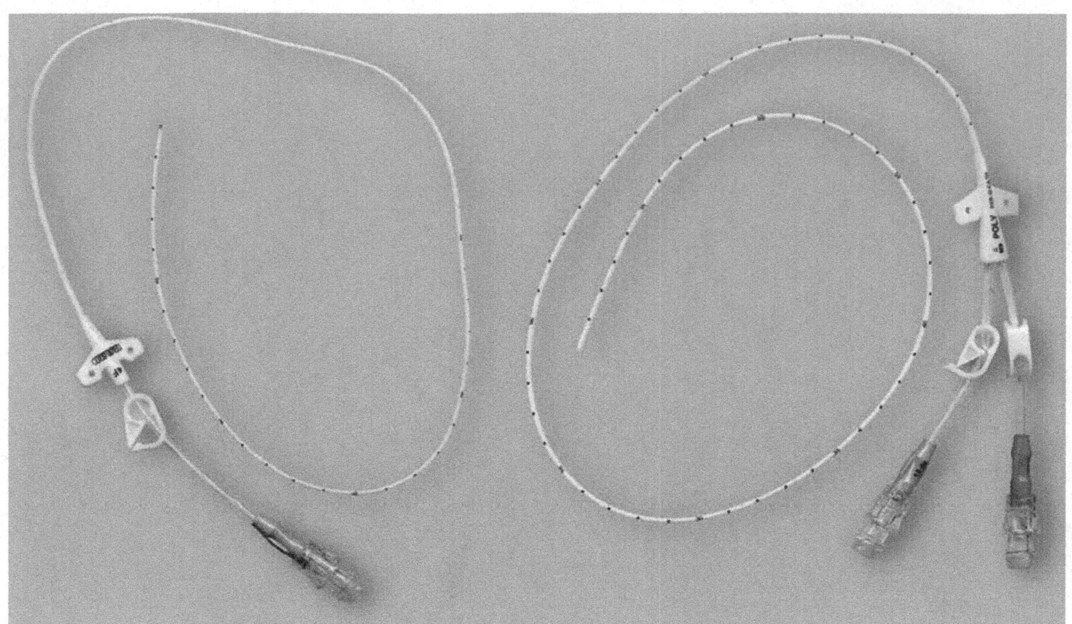

FIGURE 12.2 Single- and double-lumen PICCs.

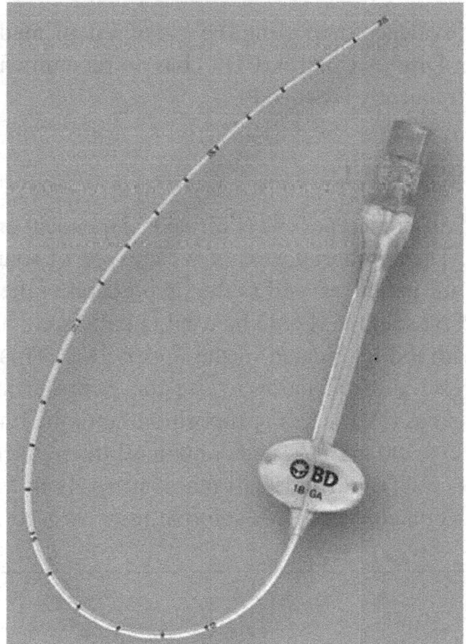

FIGURE 12.3 Midline catheter.

are only used for hemodynamic monitoring, and the high osmolarity of PN may cause peripheral veins to sclerose or thrombose. Due to the tip position of midline catheters, which are located deep in a peripheral vein, it has been proven difficult to determine the formation of thrombus, therefore challenging for the clinician to monitor the status of the line. If PN is expected to exceed more than 6 days, the use of a central line via tunneled CVC (subclavian, IJ, femoral) or nontunneled CVC (PICC, Hohn) is suitable.

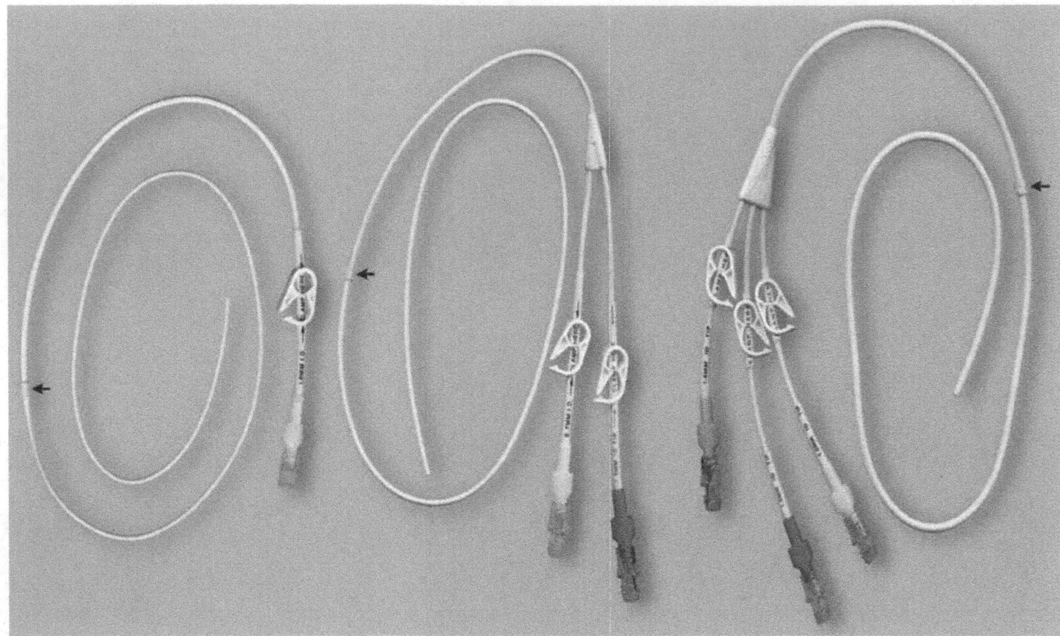

FIGURE 12.4 Single-, double-, and triple-lumen Hickman catheters. Arrow points to the Dacron cuff.

Although there is no clear evidence supporting the use of a dedicated lumen for the administration of PN and the Centers for Disease Control (CDC) has no recommendation regarding this issue (O'Grady et al. 2011), this is frequently practiced.

PN INFUSIONS USED IN THE ICU

The pharmacy can compound different types of PN infusion dependent on the type of central venous access and location of its tip. The appropriateness of which type of solution to choose depends on the clinical characteristics of the patient as well as the tip position of the central line (Table 12.1).

A 3-in-1 peripheral PN (PPN) solution should be used in patients that do not have central access or in patients with a CVC with the tip located in the upper SVC. This may include patients that receive short-term PN and have an expectation to use the gastrointestinal tract within the next 14 days; hence, central intravenous (IV) access or repositioning of the line has been deferred. These solutions have an osmolarity of <900 mmol/L and contain all three macronutrients in the infusion.

A 3-in-1 central PN (CPN) solution includes all macronutrients in the admixture; however, the osmolarity of the solution is not a concern. This solution may be used in patients with central IV

TABLE 12.1
Types of PN Infusions

	3-in-1 PPN	3-in-1 CPN	2-in-1 CPN
IV access	Peripheral IV or central IV with a tip located outside of a high flow area of circulation	Central IV with a tip located in a high flow area of circulation	Central IV with a tip located in a high flow area of circulation
PN constituents	Dextrose, amino acids, lipids	Dextrose, amino acids, lipids	Dextrose, amino acids
Osmolarity	<900 mmol/L	>900 mmol/L	>900 mmol/L
Duration of therapy	Short term (<14 days)	Short term or long term	Long term

access whose tip is located in the mid-to-lower portion of the SVC, considered a high flow area of circulation. These patients typically have blood sugar levels that may be difficult to control; therefore, the addition of lipids will help to decrease the dextrose load to aid in optimal blood sugar maintenance.

A 2-in-1 CPN solution is reserved for patients that have central IV access with the tip of the line positioned in the mid-to-lower portion of the SVC. These solutions contain higher dextrose kilocalories along with amino acids while the IV lipid emulsion is administered separately.

INSERTION TECHNIQUES

A complete focused preprocedural evaluation, a thorough knowledge of 3D vascular anatomy, familiarity with the catheter and imaging technology, meticulous technique, and prudent postprocedural evaluation provide the best chance for a complication-free insertion, a functional catheter, and minimal long-term morbidity. Although case volume is an imprecise surrogate for these attributes, insertion of a CVC by an operator who has performed more than 50 catheterizations is half as likely to result in a mechanical complication as insertion by a physician who has performed fewer than 50 catheterizations (Sznajder et al. 1986).

OPTIMAL SITE SELECTION

The patient's past history, current condition, and anatomy must be considered when choosing the best site for CVC placement (Figure 12.5).

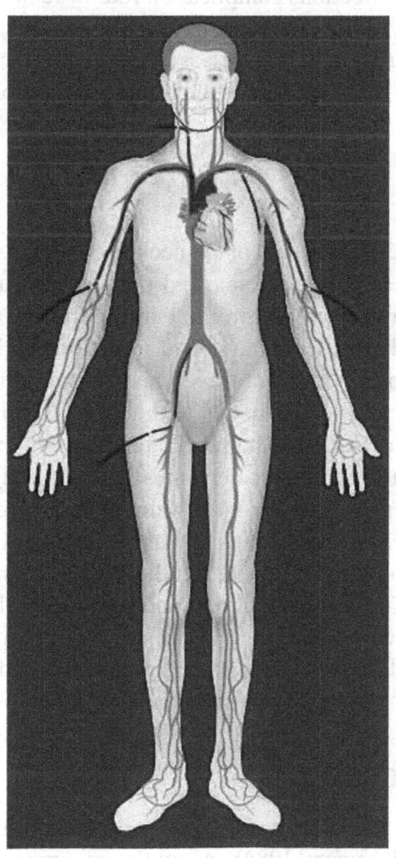

FIGURE 12.5 Vascular access sites.

Selecting the best site for central venous access begins with a focused history. The site and duration of all prior central lines (including PICCs) should be assessed, and a history of upper extremity or IJ deep venous thrombosis should be investigated, as these may result in venous stenosis and a technically difficult catheterization. Similarly, if a patient is at risk for renal failure, subclavian catheterization may worsen the venous outflow of a future AV fistula and should be avoided; catheterization ipsilateral to a current AV fistula should also be avoided. Prior neck or chest surgery should be assessed as the natural tissue planes and the vascular anatomy of the neck and chest may have been disrupted. If the anatomy or patency of the neck and chest vessels is unclear, a preprocedural vascular ultrasound study can delineate the anatomy and flow. The presence of intravascular devices (such as cardiac pacers or inferior vena cava filters) should be assessed as these may tangle with the wires and catheters used during insertion.

The presence of a coagulopathy should be assessed. Common coagulopathies in the ICU include liver failure, uremia, thrombocytopenia, heparinization, warfarinization (or the presence of other oral anticoagulants, such as dabigatran), and antiplatelet agents (such as plavix). Nonemergent central venous access should be deferred until as many of these can be safely normalized within the overall medical status of the patient. The subclavian approach should be avoided in patients with a coagulopathy, as the clavicle precludes compression of the vein. The subclavian approach should also be avoided in patients with hypoxemia, as pneumothorax or hemothorax is more likely to occur at this site and these complications are less likely to be well tolerated. Catheterization should not be attempted through an active infection or malignancy of the skin.

All other factors being equal, catheterization of the right neck or chest is preferred, as it is technically easier for right-handed operators, it has the shortest, most direct route for the catheter, the right-sided pleural apex is lower than the left, and the thoracic duct is avoided. Because of the extremely high mechanical and infectious complication rate of femoral venous catheterization, it is appropriate only for emergency resuscitation, rather than the medium- to long-term PN use. In the unfortunate patient whose venous system is so diseased that femoral catheterization is being considered for PN access, vascular surgery or interventional/vascular radiology consultation is suggested to assess for other options.

ANATOMY

A thorough understanding of the 3D anatomy of the neck and chest is necessary for safe CVC placement. The IJ vein is deep to the sternocleidomastoid muscle and runs from the superior anterior margin to the inferior posterior margin within the carotid sheath, anterior–lateral to the carotid artery. When the head is rotated away from the side of insertion, the IJ vein is immediately deep to the apex of the triangle formed by the heads of the sternocleidomastoid muscle and the clavicle. The axillary vein crosses under the clavicle just medial to the midclavicular point and becomes the subclavian vein as it crosses over the first rib. The subclavian vein reliably runs anterior to the subclavian artery and is separated by the anterior scalene muscle. On the right side, the IJ and subclavian veins join as the right brachiocephalic (innominate) vein, which travels nearly directly inferiorly to the SVC. On the left, the IJ and subclavian veins join as the left brachiocephalic (innominate) vein, which traverses laterally and gently inferiorly within the mediastinum, anterior to the left common carotid and the brachiocephalic (innominate) artery and superior to the aortic arch, to join the right brachiocephalic as it becomes the SVC. The SVC descends directly into the right atrium of the heart. The apical pleura of the lung is slightly lower on the right side, and the main thoracic duct enters the innominate vein on the left side (Valentine and Wind 2003).

ULTRASOUND ASSISTANCE TECHNIQUE

Ultrasound is a useful adjunct to the anatomic approach to central venous catheterization, first described in 1984 (Legler and Nugent 1984). As with any image guidance technique, a complete understanding of 3D anatomy, 2D cross-sectional projections, and expertise in utilizing the technology is necessary for correct image interpretation (and safe utilization). We emphasize that prior to utilizing this technique, operators undergo didactic and proctored training. When appropriately applied, ultrasound guidance decreases the number of unsuccessful needle passes and decreases the number of mechanical complications during IJ vein cannulation and may decrease complications during subclavian vein cannulation (Randolph et al. 1996).

To utilize the ultrasound, position the patient appropriately and position the ultrasound monitor directly in view of the operator. No compromises in patient or operator positioning should be made. Set the frequency to the highest frequency that penetrates deep enough to visualize the target vein. Using the nondominant hand to manipulate the ultrasound probe, perform a survey of the anatomy, identifying the veins, arteries, muscles, and bones along their course from the head or arm to the chest. Identify the correct image window for the ideal access site. For IJ vein cannulation, the probe position is just superior to the clavicle at the insertion of the heads of the sternocleidomastoid muscle, oriented perpendicular to the vein. For subclavian vein cannulation, the probe position is just inferior to the clavicle. Prep and drape the patient with the anatomic landmarks visible and the ultrasound probe in a sterile sleeve. The needle is passed in the same orientation as for the anatomic approach when using ultrasound guidance. The needle appears hyperechoic and may be followed as it passes into the vein. Blood return should occur at the moment the needle enters the vein. After the wire is placed, its course should be followed from the skin into the vein and along the vein lumen until the vein is too deep in the chest to visualize. From this point, the catheterization continues as usual.

MAINTAINING SAFE TECHNIQUE

Specific techniques are used during central venous catheterization to prevent technical complications. The patient should be on a cardiac and oxygen saturation monitor, which should be easily visible to the operator, to assist in the early detection of rapidly fatal complications. Air embolism is prevented by maintaining the Trendelenburg (head down) position during insertion and occluding catheter hubs during the procedure. Arterial injury is avoided by recognition of arterial puncture prior to dilating the vessel. If ultrasound is used, the course of the needle should be visualized into the vein. In the critical care setting, venous (dark, nonpulsatile) blood may be difficult to distinguish from arterial blood in a patient in shock. If there is any suspicion of arterial puncture, pressure transduction and/or blood gas sampling should be performed prior to passing dilators. A single lumen catheter may be advanced over the wire and attached via flushed pressure tubing to the bedside monitor to evaluate for venous pressures and waveforms. A venous blood gas should be significantly different from an arterial blood gas even in a patient in shock. Pneumothorax is prevented by minimizing the number of needle passes (Mansfield et al. 1994). Guidewire embolism is prevented by keeping one hand on the guidewire at all times. Cardiac perforation is prevented by only using the wire included in the kit and by only inserting the floppy or j-tipped end of the wire into the vein.

INTERNAL JUGULAR VEIN ACCESS

The IJ vein may be approached from the anterior, central, or posterior route. The most common approach is the central route, which will be described. The landmarks are the apex of the inverted triangle of the heads of the sternocleidomastoid, the clavicle, the ipsilateral nipple, and the carotid pulse. The head is rotated away from the side of cannulation, the ipsilateral arm is tucked at the patient's side, and the patient is placed in a 15° Trendelenburg position, and the bedside monitor is positioned facing the operator. The operator stands at the head of the bed and palpates the carotid pulse with the nondominant hand. If ultrasound is used, the ultrasound anatomic survey is completed with the probe in the nondominant hand. The neck and chest is prepped with skin antiseptic, a full body drape is placed, and the operator uses full sterile barrier precautions. Local anesthetic is applied to the apex of the triangle. The access needle with a syringe is used to access the vein. With the nondominant hand on the carotid or holding the ultrasound probe, the access needle pierces the skin at apex of the triangle and is advanced at a 45° angle from the skin from the apex of the triangle toward the ipsilateral nipple, while maintaining negative pressure on the syringe. The vein is typically encountered before 3 cm of the needle has been inserted. After venous cannulation is confirmed, the operation proceeds using the Seldinger technique. To minimize the risk complications of accidental arterial puncture, using a micropuncture needle/catheter/wire kit or a small gauge finder needle should be considered for the initial access, particularly if ultrasound guidance is not utilized.

SUBCLAVIAN VEIN ACCESS

The subclavian vein is accessed in a standard fashion. The landmarks are the clavicle, the sternal notch, and the deltopectoral groove. A small towel roll is placed between the shoulder blades, the ipsilateral arm is tucked at the side, and the patient is placed in a 15° Trendelenburg position, and the bedside monitor is positioned facing the operator. The operator stands at the side of the bed and places the index finger of the nondominant hand in the sternal notch and the thumb of the same hand at the junction of the medial and middle third of the clavicle, which is at the junction of the clavicle and the deltopectoral groove. Alternatively, the nondominant hand holds the ultrasound probe just inferior to the clavicle. If ultrasound is used, the ultrasound anatomic survey is completed with the probe in the nondominant hand. The lower neck and chest is prepped with skin antiseptic, a full body drape is placed, and the operator uses full sterile barrier precautions. Local anesthetic is applied to the skin and clavicular periosteum. The needle is inserted just lateral and inferior to the operator's thumb and advanced parallel to the clavicle, aiming to the sternal notch, maintaining negative pressure on the syringe. The needle is advanced just under the clavicle toward the suprasternal notch. After venous cannulation is confirmed, the operation proceeds using the Seldinger technique.

COMPLETION OF CATHETERIZATION

After venous access is achieved and confirmed, the soft tip of the included guidewire is passed through the needle (or catheter) into the vein, and the needle is removed. During passage of the guidewire, the operator should observe the bedside monitor for arrhythmias caused by passing the wire too far into the atrium or ventricle; if these occur, the wire is pulled back. If fluoroscopy is available, this is done under radiographic visualization. If ultrasound is used, the course of the wire can be traced for a distance within the lumen of the vein. The skin is nicked with the included scalpel, the dilator is passed over the wire, the catheter is passed over the wire, and the wire is removed. Each port is aspirated and flushed, the catheter is secured to the skin, and a sterile dressing is applied. If the catheterization was not performed under fluoroscopy, upright chest radiography (CXR) should be obtained. The course of the catheter should follow the expected path of the vein, and the tip should be at the cavoatrial junction, which is at the level of the carina. The angle of the catheter tip compared to the vein wall should be near parallel. Any deviation from this should raise a suspicion for arterial placement of the line or cardiac puncture. The apices, paramediastinal area, and costophrenic angle should be inspected for pneumothorax or hemothorax. The rest of the CXR should be inspected in a routine manner to assess for incidental findings.

COMPLICATIONS OF CENTRAL IV ACCESS

Complications occur both with CVC insertion and with catheter extraction. Complications of IV access insertion are defined by the Food and Drug Administration as either short term, characterized as less than 4 weeks, or long term, occurring more than 4 weeks after CVC placement (Ge et al. 2012). Acute complications arise with less experienced practitioners and increase with multiple venipuncture attempts and more failures to catheterize, as well as with patients whose body mass index is greater than 30 kg/m^2 and less than 20 kg/m^2. Uncorrected coagulopathies and the use of larger bore catheters increase complications (Kusminsky 2007).

INSERTION COMPLICATIONS

We emphasize that operative technique is the most modifiable risk factor for preventing CVC complications and early recognition is important to mitigate the effects of complications.

Pneumothorax comprises 30% of all mechanical adverse events. Risk factors for pneumothorax include the number of venipuncture attempts (much higher after >3), emergency situations, and the use of larger bore catheters. Subclavian venipuncture is associated with an increased incidence of pneumothorax in comparison to IJ venipuncture. Delayed pneumothorax occurs in approximately 0.5%–4% of insertions (Kusminsky 2007).

Arterial punctures (subclavian, carotid, aorta) are critical to recognize early to avoid major complications. Risk factors for arterial puncture is more commonly seen with IJ and femoral cannulation (in comparison to subclavian access) and with cannulation of the right side due to the sharper angle of the subclavian vein when entering the innominate vein (Kusminsky 2007). Hemothorax is commonly seen in arterial injuries. Carotid punctures are most often seen with cannulation of the IJ and are associated with hematoma. Perforation of the aorta is associated with cardiac tamponade, and if the perforation occurs within the pericardial reflection, mortality increases to 90% (Kusminsky 2007). The use of larger catheters, increased number of insertion attempts, and right-sided cannulation with straight-tipped guidewires are associated with greater chance for perforation to occur. AV fistulas may occur immediately or can develop years after catheter attempts.

Brachial plexus and lymphatic injuries, such as chylothorax and chylopericardium, can be seen after IJ and subclavian vein cannulation.

The use of a guidewire may also cause complications. Guidewires can loop and become entrapped within the catheter, knot, or fracture. Guidewires increase the risk of cardiac ectopy, specifically with the use of a straight-tipped guidewire (Kusminsky 2007). The occurrence of cardiac ectopy reaches 75% when the wire is advanced between 25 and 32 cm from the IJ entry site, and signs of premature atrial contractions may occur; symptoms subside once the guidewire is withdrawn.

INDWELLING COMPLICATIONS

The most common complication that develops after insertion is infection, either from the catheter hub, skin insertion site, or hematogenous seeding of the catheter (McGee and Gould 2003). Catheter days are defined as the total number of days of exposure to CVCs, and it has been estimated that there are approximately 15 million CVC days each year in the ICU alone (Mermel et al. 2009). The CDC estimates that there is a 12%–25% rate of mortality among the critically ill population that is attributed to CVC-related infections (O'Grady et al. 2011). This has initiated evidence-based guidelines to help in the prevention of catheter-related bloodstream infection (CRBSI).

The administration of PN increases CRBSI risk (Elke et al. 2008), and a recent study by Walshe et al. (2012) found that 25% of nontunneled catheters used for PN were culture positive and were associated with the development of CRBSI in an ICU population.

Organisms most frequently associated with CRBSI include *Staphylococcus epidermidis*, *Staphylococcus aureus*, and *Candida* species (O'Grady et al. 2011).

The factors that may attribute to higher infection rates include femoral access and use of a multiple lumen catheter and material of the IV catheter.

Femoral lines are associated with higher risk of infection when compared to subclavian and IJ access, and this may be due to the proximity of the catheter to the perineal region of the patient. Femoral sites are typically used in emergency situations due to ease of insertion in comparison to the IJ and subclavian vein; however, femoral lines should be removed once a more permanent line is established, optimally within 24 h.

Some studies have shown that infectious complications increase as the number of lumens and/or ports from the catheter increases (Tan et al. 2007), while some studies have not observed a difference in infection rates (McGee and Gould 2003). It has been recognized by the CDC that the choice of lumen number should be based on the management of the patient and what is necessary for treatment (O'Grady et al. 2011).

To help in the reduction of line-associated infections, the CDC has recommended the use of standardized protocols when caring for central lines. This includes using the subclavian vein when possible, removing central lines when they are no longer needed, proper hand hygiene and use of sterile barriers during insertion, and the use of chlorhexidine gluconate prep solution (O'Grady et al. 2011).

The formation of biofilm, which can occur within 24 h of insertion, has also been implicated in the development of CRBSI. Development of a fibrin sheath is more prevalent on silicone catheters, therefore enhancing the adherence of Gram-positive and Gram-negative bacteria (Mehall et al. 2002). *Candida albicans* species adhere to the biofilm present on silicone elastomer when compared to polyurethane and 100% silicone (Hawser and Douglas 1994). The nonalbican species have been shown to increase mortality in the nonimmunosuppressed, nonneutropenic ICU population (Dimopoulos et al. 2008).

If CRBSI is suspected, verification is achieved through obtaining cultures peripherally and through all lumens of the vascular access device (Guembe et al. 2010) prior to the initiation of antibiotic therapy. Quantitative blood cultures are the most accurate test for diagnosing CRBSI, and a diagnosis can be made if the culture taken from the catheter is greater than threefold higher than that of the sample taken peripherally (Safdar et al. 2005).

Complications arising from CRBSI include septic thrombosis, endocarditis, and metastatic septic foci, and the risk of infection has been shown to increase with the presence of thrombosis (Timsit et al. 1998). Crowley et al. (2008) also found that the rate of thrombosis increases with the presence of CRBSI, specifically *S. aureus* bacteremia, with an incidence rate of 71% in patients studied using ultrasonography.

Thrombosis occurs in 33%–59% indwelling catheters and clinical symptoms are present in only a small percentage of patients (Kusminsky 2007). Factors that increase the risk include endothelial injury, venous flow turbulence, catheter thrombogenicity, and composition of infusate. The femoral and IJ sites are more susceptible to thrombus formation in comparison to cannulation of the subclavian vein, in which the rate of thrombosis is reported to be 1.9% with subclavian vein and up to 29% with femoral cannulation. The location of the catheter within an inlet vein will also increase the incidence of thrombus formation (Cadman et al. 2004).

Occlusion and stenosis occur more readily with longer catheter dwell times, with larger bore catheters, with previously infected catheters within the CVC, and with previously catheterized CVCs (especially through the subclavian vein).

Catheter fractures and embolization are delayed complications of indwelling catheters. They can lead to arrhythmia, cardiac arrest, pulmonary emboli and hemoptysis, cardiac perforation, thrombosis, and infection. The overall morbidity and mortality rates are 71% and 30%–38%, respectively (Kusminsky 2007). Fractures and embolization may occur from mechanical shearing of the catheter often seen with pinch-off syndrome. This is characterized by compression of the CVC between the clavicle and first rib, creating a functional occlusion with postural changes, which can be visualized via CXR (McMenamin 1993).

Symptoms associated with fracture include pain and swelling during infusion, resistance of infusion, withdrawal occlusion, shoulder or chest pain, and palpitations.

EXTRACTION COMPLICATIONS

Several noninsertion complications may develop during intentional or accidental CVC removal. Air embolism is seen in 0.13%–0.5% patients, with fatality observed at rates of 23%–50% (Kusminsky 2007). This is more common with tunneled catheters inserted through a pull-away sheath. Air emboli may occur with accidental hub disconnection or through inadvertent arterial cannulation. It may also be seen during accidental removal, demonstrated by hemorrhage. Breakage can be resultant from excessive traction force and may be due to the material of the catheter.

VERIFICATION OF CATHETER TIP POSITION

After placement of a CVC, tip verification should be done via CXR in order to visualize the tip of the catheter. Verification is important and can be used to determine the presence of local toxicity, perforation, and venous thrombosis. Optimal location of a CVC is within the long axis of the SVC just outside the right atrium (Schummer et al. 2004). When the catheter tip is located in smaller-diameter vessels, the risk of catheter wedging, endothelial injury, thrombus and vascular stenosis, or perforation increases.

During visualization of the CVC on CXR, the clinician should follow the line from its origin to the tip of the catheter. The tip of the CVC should be positioned in the mid-to-lower portion of the SVC in order to deliver CPN as shown in Figure 12.1. CPN solutions have a higher osmolarity in comparison to PPN solutions and need to be delivered in a high flow area of circulation. Studies have shown a higher incidence of thrombus formation, specifically 41.7%, in patients whose CVC tip lies in the upper portion of the SVC and coordinate veins (Cadman et al. 2004) in comparison to those in which the tip lies in the mid-to-lower SVC.

The lower SVC can be identified using several landmarks visible on the CXR since the pericardial reflection cannot be visualized. Use of the carina as a landmark has proven valuable in the identification of CVC tip (Stonelake and Bodenham 2006).

Obstructive complications have been observed in patients whose CVC tip is not located near the cavoatrial junction, thereby increasing the risk for venous thrombus and SVC syndrome, resulting in permanent loss of upper torso vascular access. Those CVCs where the catheter tip is within the right atrium have increased incidence of heart arrhythmias and risk for perforation of the heart wall (Askegard-Giesmann et al. 2009). PICC lines have been associated commonly with malposition (DeChicco et al. 2007), mostly related to left-side insertions. The left subclavian vein has a more horizontal approach; and as it enters the SVC, the tip of the catheter may abut the wall of the SVC if the catheter length is of insufficient length. Steady pressure and friction applied to the vessel wall by the catheter tip has the potential to lead to vessel wall erosion, increasing the risk of perforation. If the tip of the catheter is in direct contact with the vessel wall, thrombus formation may develop, and catheter dysfunction ensues. During visualization of the CXR, the catheter tip should lie parallel to the SVC and remain above the pericardial reflection.

Several case reports have also shown that PICC lines placed within the right atrium have increased risk of cardiac tamponade (Booth et al. 2001). PICC lines and central catheters have the ability to move significantly with postural changes in comparison to tunneled catheters, thereby increasing the risk of possible perforation and extravasation of infusate into the pericardial cavity (Orme et al. 2007). It is important to visualize the central line on a daily basis in order to observe changes in the length of the catheter and catheter tip position, specifically with PICC lines. Cardiac tamponade symptoms include dyspnea, chest pain, tachycardia, hypotension, and pulsus paradoxus and are associated with a mortality rate of 65%–100% (Shamir and Bruce 2011). Symptoms of malpositioned central lines may include complaints of pain and/or discomfort in the neck, shoulder, or chest regions during PN infusion (Figures 12.6 and 12.7)

CATHETER MAINTENANCE

In order to prevent the occurrence of infections, high-dose concentrations of lock solutions have been infused directly in the catheter and allowed to dwell after cyclic PN administration. Antibiotic locks have been used for the prevention of CRBSI but have since been implicated in increasing antibiotic resistance with methicillin-resistant *S. aureus* infection. A recent study by

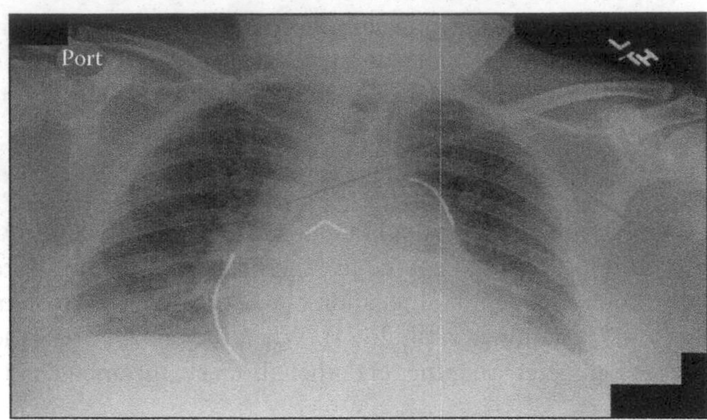

FIGURE 12.6 CXR showing left-sided PICC line in the upper SVC.

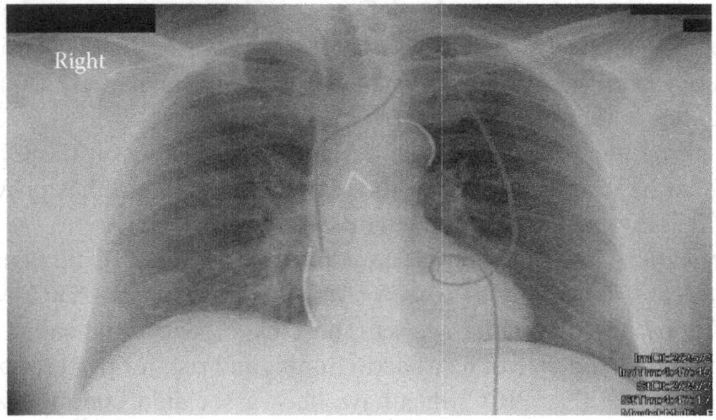

FIGURE 12.7 CXR showing right-sided IJ Hickman in the SVC/RA junction.

Ramos et al. (2011) showed that CVCs coated with minocycline and rifampin helped to decrease catheter line–associated bloodstream infection (CLABSI) rates with their prolonged use in comparison to noncoated catheters. Taurolidine lock has been shown to be highly effective in preventing CRBSI in patients on home PN. One such study by Bisseling et al. (2010) showed a decrease from 71% to 6% by using a catheter lock with taurolidine as compared to using a heparin lock after cyclic PN administration. Ethanol lock solutions, consisting of 70% ethanol, have been shown to be an effective means of reducing the rate of CVC infections in PN-dependent children (Jones et al. 2010) and have been shown to be superior in comparison to antibiotic solutions in decreasing the amount of biofilm development in concentrations of 20% (Ou et al. 2009; Chaudhury et al. 2012). However, new case reports have emerged implicating ethanol lock as contributing to the development of thrombosis or occlusion in long-term CVCs (Wong et al. 2011). Ethanol lock solutions are typically used in tunneled catheters for use in patients that need long-term IV access (John et al. 2012); however, these solutions are only used with catheters made of silicone.

Needleless valve connectors were introduced in order to decrease the incidence of needle stick injuries and exposure of blood-borne viruses to health-care professionals. This increased the incidence of CRBSI due to the introduction of microorganisms to the connector and fluid path, as well as facilitating biofilm formation on the interior surface of the valved connectors (Jarvis et al. 2009). A nanosilver-impregnated polycarbonate-valved needleless connector was used to help decrease biofilm formation, thus decreasing the incidence of CLABSI. This connector has the ability to release minute quantities of bactericidal ionic silver off the surface of the polycarbonate matrix into the fluid path (Maki 2010).

Exposure of mechanical valve needleless connectors to nutritional fluids and blood enables biofilm development, thus enhancing bacterial growth. Because of their more complex design, negative or positive pressure mechanical valve needleless connectors may be more prone to inadvertent contamination and inadequate disinfection contributing to increased incidence of bloodstream infection (Jarvis et al. 2009).

Disinfecting caps have recently been introduced to help prevent infection. They protect the needleless connector and can be used on any swabable luer access valve and contain 70% isopropyl alcohol in a saturated sponge. This ultimately protects the connector from airborne contamination and provides a physical barrier for up to 7 days if not removed (Menyhay and Maki 2008).

CASE STUDY

E. F. is a 31-year-old female with a history of end-stage renal disease and multiple deep vein thromboses due to antithrombin III deficiency, factor V Leiden, and antiphospholipid syndrome. She has failed warfarin, unfractionated heparin, enoxaparin, and fondaparinux therapies. She has also failed peritoneal dialysis and is admitted for IV access for intermittent hemodialysis. Vascular surgery was consulted for creation of an AV fistula; however, it was deemed not to remain patent, and subsequently a hepatic vein tunneled catheter was placed with its tip located in the right atrium. She developed gallstone pancreatitis during her admission and underwent a cholecystectomy, which was complicated by postoperative ileus. On postoperative day 7, PN was started for nutrition support. A left-sided single lumen IJ CVC was placed for PN access. A CXR was completed, which showed the tip overlying the lower left IJ vein.

- Which catheter would you use for IV access, and why?
- Would you prescribe a central PN formula or a peripheral PN formula?
- Why would you recommend this formula?

REFERENCES

Askegard-Giesmann, JR., Caniano, DA., Kenney, BD. Rare but serious complications of central line insertion. *Seminars in Pediatric Surgery* 2009; 18: 73–83.

Aubaniac, R. L'injection intraveineuse sous-claviculaire. *La Presse médicale* October 25, 1952; 60(68): 1456.

Bisseling, TA., Willems, MC., Versleijen, MW. et al. Taurolidine lock is highly effective in preventing catheter-related bloodstream infections in patients on home parenteral nutrition: A heparin-controlled prospective trial. *Clinical Nutrition* 2010; 29(4): 464–468.

Booth, SA., Norton, B., Mulvey, A. Central venous catheterization and fatal cardiac tamponade. *British Journal of Anaesthesia* 2001; 87 (2): 298–302.

Cadman, A., Lawrance, JAL., Fitzsimmons, L., Spencer-Shaw, A., Swindell, R. To clot or not to clot? That is the question in central venous catheters. *Clinical Radiology* 2004; 59: 349–355.

Chaudhury, A., Rangineni, J., Venkatramana, B. Catheter lock technique: In vitro efficacy of ethanol for eradication of methicillin-resistant staphylococcal biofilm compared with other agents. *FEMS Immunology and Medical Microbiology* 2012; 65: 305–308.

Crowley, AL., Peterson, GE., Benjamin, DK. et al. Venous thrombosis in patients with short- and long-term central venous catheter-associated Staphylococcus aureus bacteremia. *Critical Care Medicine* 2008; 36(2): 385–390.

DeChicco, R., Seidner, DL., Brun, C. et al. Tip position of long-term central venous access devices used for parenteral nutrition. *Journal of Parenteral and Enteral Nutrition* 2007; 31(5): 383–387.

Dimopoulos, G., Ntziora, F., Rachiotis, G. et al. Candida albicans versus non-albicans intensive care unit-acquired bloodstream infections: Differences in risk factors and outcome. *Critical Care and Trauma* 2008; 106(2): 523–529.

Dudrick, SJ. History of vascular access. *Journal of Parenteral and Enteral Nutrition* 2006; 30(1): S47–S56.

Dudrick, SJ. History of parenteral nutrition. *Journal of the American College of Nutrition* 2009; 28(3): 243–251.

Elke, G., Schadler, D., Engel, C. et al. Current practice in nutritional support and its association with mortality in septic patients—Results from a national, prospective, multicenter study. *Critical Care Medicine* 2008; 36(6): 1762–1767.

Galloway, S., Bodenham, A. Long-term central venous access. *British Journal of Anaesthesia* 2004; 92(5): 722–734.

Ge, X., Cavallazzi, R., Li, C. et al. Central venous access sites for the prevention of venous thrombosis, stenosis and infection. *Cochrane Database of Systematic Reviews* 2012; 3: CD004084.

Guembe, M., Rodriguez-Creixems, M., Sanchez-Carrillo, C. How many lumens should be cultured in the conservative diagnosis of catheter-related bloodstream infections? *Clinical Infectious Diseases* 2010; 50: 1575–1579.

Hawser, AP, Douglas, LJ. Biofilm formation by Candida species on the surface of catheter materials in vitro. *Infection and Immunology* 1994; 62(3): 915–921.

Jarvis, WR., Murphy, C., Hall, KK. et al. Health care-associated bloodstream infections associated with negative or positive-pressure or displacement mechanical valve needleless connectors. *Clinical Infectious Diseases* 2009; 49: 1821–1827.

John, BK., Khan, MA., Speerhas, R. et al. Ethanol lock therapy in reducing catheter-related bloodstream infections in adult home parenteral nutrition patients: Results of a retrospective study. *Journal of Parenteral and Enteral Nutrition* 2012; 36(5): 603–610.

Jones, BA., Hull, MA., Richardson, DS. et al. Efficacy of ethanol locks in reducing central venous catheter infections in pediatric patients with intestinal failure. *Journal of Pediatric Surgery* 2010; 45: 1287–1293.

Kalso, E. A short history of central venous catheterization. *Acta Anaesthesiologica Scandinavica* 1985; 81: 7–10.

Kusminsky, RE. Complications of central venous catheterization. *Journal of the American College of Surgeons* 2007; 204(4): 681–696.

Legler, D., Nugent, M. Doppler localization of the internal jugular vein facilitates central venous catheterization. *Anesthesiology* 1984; 60: 481–482.

Maki, DG. In vitro studies of a novel antimicrobial luer-activated needleless connector for prevention of catheter-related bloodstream infection. *Clinical Infectious Diseases* 2010; 50(12): 1580–1587.

Malinoski, D., Ewing, T., Bhakta, A. et al. Which central venous catheters have the highest rate of catheter-associated deep venous thrombosis: A prospective analysis of 2,128 catheter days in the surgical intensive care unit. *Trauma Acute Care Surgery* 2013; 74(2): 454–462.

Mansfield, PF., Hohn, DC., Fornage, BD., Gregurich, MA., Ota, DM. Complications and failures of subclavian-vein catheterization. *The New England Journal of Medicine* 1994; 331: 1735–1738.

McGee, DC., Gould, M. Preventing complications of central venous catheterization. *The New England Journal of Medicine* 2003; 348(12): 1123–1133.

McMenamin, EM. Catheter fracture: A complication in venous access devices. *Cancer Nursing* 1993; 16(6): 464–467.

Mehall, JR., Saltzman, DA., Jacksom, RJ. et al. Fibrin sheath enhances central venous catheter infection. *Critical Care Medicine* 2002; 30(4): 908–912.

Menyhay, SZ., Maki, DG. Preventing central venous catheter-associated bloodstream infections: Development of an antiseptic barrier cap for needleless connectors. *American Journal of Infection Control* 2008; 36(10): S174.e1–S174.e5

Mermel, LA., Allon, M., Bouza, E. et al. Clinical practice guidelines for the diagnosis and management of intravascular catheter-related infection: 2009 update by the Infectious diseases society of America. Guideline Summary NGC-7382.

Meyer, JA. Werner Forssmann and catheterization of the heart, 1929. *The Annals of Thoracic Surgery* 1990; 49(3): 497–499.

O'Grady, N., Alexander, M., Burns, L. et al. Guidelines for the prevention of intravascular catheter-related infections. *Clinical Infectious Diseases* 2011; May 1; 52(9): e162–e193.

Orme, RML'E., SmSwiney, MM., Chamberlain-Webber, RFO. Fatal cardiac tamponade as a result of a peripherally inserted central venous catheter: A case report and review of the literature. *British Journal of Anaesthesia* 2007; 99(3): 384–388.

Ou, Y., Istivan, TS., Daley, AJ. et al. Comparison of various antimicrobial agents as catheter lock solutions: Preference for ethanol in eradication of coagulase-negative staphylococcal biofilms. *Journal of Medical Microbiology* 2009; 58: 442–450.

Ramos, ER., Reitzel, R., Jiang, Y. et al. Clinical effectiveness and risk of emerging resistance associated with prolonged use of antibiotic-impregnated catheters: More than 0.5 million catheter days and 7 years of clinical experience. *Critical Care Medicine* 2011; 39(2): 245–251.

Randolph, AG., Cook, DJ., Gonzales, CA., Pribble, CG. Ultrasound guidance for placement of central venous catheters: A meta-analysis of the literature. *Critical Care Medicine* 1996; 24: 2053–2058.

Safdar, N., Fine, JP, Maki, DG. Meta-analysis: Methods for diagnosing intravascular device-related bloodstream infection. *Annals of Internal Medicine* 2005; 142(6): 451.

Schummer, W., Schummer C., Bredle, D. et al. The anterior jugular venous system: Variability and clinical impact. *International Anesthesia Research Society* 2004; 99: 1625–1629.

Shamir, M., Bruce, LJ. Central venous catheter-induced cardiac tamponade: A preventable complication. *Anesthesia and Analgesia* 2011; 112(6): 1280–1282.

Stonelake, PA., Bodenham, AR. The carina as a radiological landmark for central venous catheter tip position. *British Journal of Anaesthesia* 2006; 96(3): 335–340.

Sznajder, JI., Zveibil, FR., Bitterman, H., Weiner, P., Bursztein, S. Central vein catheterization: Failure and complication rates by three percutaneous approaches. *Archives of Internal Medicine* 1986; 146: 259–261.

Tan, CC., Zanariah, Y., Lim, KI. et al. Central venous catheter-related blood stream infections: Incidence and an analysis of risk factors. *Medical Journal of Malaysia* 2007 December; 62(5): 370–374.

Timsit, JF., Farkas, JC., Boyer, JM. et al. Central vein catheter-related thrombosis in intensive care unit patients. *Chest* 1998; 114(1): 207–213.

Valentine, RJ., Wind, GG. *Anatomic Exposures in Vascular Surgery*, 2nd edn. Philadelphia, PA: Lippincott Williams & Wilkins, 2003.

Van Der Kooi, T III., Wille, JC., Van Benthem, BHB. Catheter application, insertion vein and length of ICU stay prior to insertion affect the risk of catheter-related bloodstream infection. *Journal of Hospital Infection* 2012; 80: 238–244.

Varon, J., Nyman, U. Sven-Ivar Seldinger: The revolution of radiology and acute intravascular access. *Resuscitation* 2007; 75: 7–11.

Versleijen, MWJ., Huisman-De Waal, GJ., Kock, MC. et al. Arteriovenous fistulae as an alternative to central venous catheters for delivery of long-term home parenteral nutrition. *Gastroenterology* 2009; 136: 1577–1584.

Walshe, C., Bourke, J., Lynch, M. et al. Culture positivity of CVC's used in TPN: Investigation of an association with catheter-related infection and comparison of causative organisms between ICU and non-ICU CVC's. *Journal of Nutrition and Metabolism* 2012; 2012: 1–7.

Wong, T., Clifford, V., McCallum, Z. et al. Central venous catheter thrombosis associated with 70% ethanol locks in pediatric intestinal failure patients on home parenteral nutrition: A case series. *Journal of Parenteral and Enteral Nutrition* 2011; 36(3): 358–360.

13 Enteral Feeding Access in the Critically Ill Patient

Beth Taylor and John E. Mazuski

CONTENTS

ENTERAL ACCESS DEVICES

The usefulness of enteral feeding for critically ill patients has been well documented [1–7]. Although there is debate over the type and amount of enteral feeding that is most beneficial, there is a consensus that critically ill patients with a functioning gastrointestinal (GI) tract should be fed enterally if specialized nutritional support is thought to be warranted [2,8]. There is considerable debate, however, with regard to the techniques that should be used for enteral feeding in the critically ill patient and, specifically, what enteral access device is most appropriate for this patient. In order to answer these questions, a clear understanding of the enteral access devices presently available is needed. The selection of a specific device will be based, in part, on whether the patient will be fed into the stomach (prepyloric feeding) or the small bowel (postpyloric feeding) and whether the patient is likely to need short-term (<4 weeks) or long-term (≥4 weeks) enteral access.

In this overview, we will first discuss the general characteristics of feeding devices and the methods of using them and then review the specific issues related to feeding device selection, based on duration of use and where the patient will be fed.

GENERAL CHARACTERISTICS OF ENTERAL ACCESS DEVICES

Enteral access devices vary markedly in the type of material used for their construction, their length and diameter, the presence of a stylet or guidewire, weighting of the tube, the presence of a Y-port, and the presence of more than one lumen.

CONSTRUCTION

Currently available adult feeding tubes are made of polyvinyl chloride, polyurethane, silicone, or polyurethane–silicone mix material (see Table 13.1). Polyurethane, silicone, and the combination tubes are soft and made of nonreactive materials. Silicone tubes are the softest and may collapse when aspirating. Polyvinyl chloride is an inexpensive material, but in the presence of acid, it may stiffen over time, leading to increased risks of naris irritation, cracking or breaking of the tube, or possible gastric perforation as the distal tip hardens. Foley catheters are made of latex, which may be irritating to the skin of some patients and dangerous to those with latex allergies [9]. Tubes designed for bedside, surgical, endoscopic, or fluoroscopic placement usually are completely radiopaque or have a radiopaque stripe to facilitate radiographic confirmation of their location.

TUBE SIZE: LENGTH AND DIAMETER

The length of the feeding tube is dictated both by the site of its insertion and by the desired site of feeding (see Table 13.1). Lengths can range from 6 in. for a gastrostomy tube to 60 in. for a nasojejunal tube. The shortest surgically implanted tubes are called *button* or *skin-level* tubes, but these are rarely placed acutely in the critically ill patient. Some surgically placed devices are combination tubes that have a shorter gastric lumen for decompression and medication administration and a longer jejunal limb for feeding purposes. Other gastrostomy tubes, especially those implanted endoscopically, can accommodate a second jejunal tube inserted through the gastrostomy and thereby function as a combination tube.

Besides having different lengths, tubes also differ with regard to diameter (see Table 13.1). Usually the tube diameter is measured in French units, where 1 Fr unit equals 0.33 mm. In general, for nasoenteric tubes, the smallest-diameter tube that allows optimal delivery of the nutritional formula should be used. Smaller-diameter tubes are more comfortable for the patient and less likely to produce sinusitis but are also more susceptible to clogging.

TABLE 13.1
Properties of Enteral Access Devices

Tube Type	Material	Length (in.)	French Size (Fr)	Stylet or Guidewire	Y-Port
Nasogastric/Salem sump	Polyvinyl chloride or silicone	36–48	12–20	No	No
Nasoenteric feeding tube	Polyurethane, silicone, or mixture	36–60	8–14	Yes/No	Yes/No
PEG	Silicone or polyurethane	Cut to fit	14–24	No	Yes
Gastrostomy	Silicone or polyurethane	4–6	12–24	No	Yes
Jejunostomy	Silicone or polyurethane	6–10	8–14	No	Yes/No
Jejunostomy via PEG	Silicone or polyurethane	35–45	8–10	Yes	Yes/No
Needle jejunostomy	Silicone or polyurethane	6–10	8–10	Yes	No
Gastrojejunostomy	Silicone or polyurethane	Jejunal length, 35–45	G-port, 22–24; J-port, 8–10	Yes	Yes
MOSS gastrostomy	Silicone	18 to feeding tip	18	Yes	Yes

Stylets

Stylets are often used to stiffen softer feeding tubes made of polyurethane or silicone to facilitate insertion (see Table 13.1). Most stylets end in a blunt loop or a spring tip to decrease the risk of tube puncture during placement. In addition, they do not extend completely to the end of the tube. Most stylets have a flow-through design that allows air or water to be flushed through the tube ports while the stylet is in place. In most tubes with stylets, the inner lumen is coated with a water-soluble lubricant for ease of stylet removal.

Y-Ports

Most nasoenteric feeding tubes have a Y-port on the end to facilitate flushing of the tube and medication administration without having to disconnect the feeding administration set (see Table 13.1). Some feeding tubes have only a single port. In this case, a Y extension set can be added to the end of the tube. The port may be designed to accommodate a feeding set, a syringe, or both. The use of the Y-port is effective in minimizing contamination of the nutritional formulation. The use of Y-ports occasionally causes some confusion with gastrostomy tubes, because a gastrostomy tube with a Y-port might be misinterpreted as a gastrojejunal combination tube. To avoid this misinterpretation, ports should be labeled as clearly as possible with respect to the purpose (e.g., gastrostomy port, for flushing only).

Weighted versus Nonweighted Feeding Tips

Nasoenteric feeding tubes are available on the market with or without a tungsten weight (see Table 13.1). Initially, it was thought that the weight would facilitate tube placement. However, clinical trials have not clearly identified an advantage to the use of weighted tubes, and some studies suggest that placement of a nasoenteric feeding tube into the small bowel is easier with nonweighted tubes [10–12]. Ultimately, the decision whether to use a weighted or a nonweighted tube is a matter of personal preference and should be based on the experience of those performing the procedure on a routine basis. Choosing a feeding tube strictly based on cost or facility contract without considering the clinicians' expertise is unlikely to result in any cost savings, because of increased device wastage after unsuccessful deployments.

FEEDING METHODS AND EQUIPMENT

Feeding Methods

Enteral feedings can be infused either continuously or intermittently by two different methods. In critically ill patients, feeding pumps should be used for all continuous feedings, so that the rate of feeding can be adequately regulated. Intermittent feedings may be administered either by gravity, using a gravity drip bag, or via a syringe to provide a bolus feeding. Critically ill patients rarely tolerate large volumes via the syringe or bolus feeding method, but these patients will often tolerate a gravity feeding delivered over 20–40 min several times a day.

Feeding Sets and Pumps

Feeding sets are designed for either gravity or pump feeding. Feeding sets are often preattached to the gravity or pump feeding bags and cannot be separated. The gravity feeding delivery sets have a roller clamp to help control the flow rate. Generally, the feeding sets designed for the continuous method are pump specific, which must be taken into consideration when contracting for these items. Most of the connectors on a feeding set will not attach to an intravenous (IV) needle or a luer connector, making it impossible to administer enteral feeding inadvertently into an IV line.

Enteral feeding containers come in different sizes and hold different volumes. In the hospital setting, they are generally changed every 24 h. Closed-system containers are available that are prefilled with a specific volume. Theoretically, these should decrease the risk of contamination. However, use of these closed systems in the critically ill patient population may lead to increased wastage of enteral formulas. Enteral feedings are often withheld in the critically ill patient because of a change in the patient's clinical status or the need for the patient to undergo an invasive procedure. As for other hospitalized patients, any product that remains in the container after 24 h should be discarded.

Several factors should be considered when selecting a pump for use in the intensive care setting. Most importantly, the pump should come with clear instructions and be simple to use. The pump should be quiet but have both audio and visual alarms to protect against overinfusion. The pump should provide accurate volumetric delivery and offer the ability to preset an intermittent dose or a continuous flow rate. Given space limitations in an ICU, a 24 h battery and built-in IV pole clamp are also highly desirable.

INSERTION AND CARE OF FEEDING TUBES

The major differences between various types of enteral access devices are the following:

- Where the tip of the tube is located (stomach vs. small bowel)
- Whether the tube is inserted via the nasal or oral cavity directly into the GI tract (for short-term access) or is surgically placed through the skin of the abdomen into the stomach or small bowel (for longer-term access)
- Whether the tube has different lumens and can be used to decompress the stomach while allowing feeding into the small bowel

Each tube type has potential advantages and disadvantages for the critically ill patient (see Table 13.2).

SHORT-TERM FEEDING TUBES

As previously mentioned, many critically ill patients will have a large-bore tube inserted nasally or orally for gastric decompression [13]. When the patient no longer requires gastric decompression, these tubes may be used for medication administration and enteral feeding. The disadvantage of these tubes is that they are uncomfortable and may become even more irritating to the patient over time as they harden. In addition, these larger, stiffer tubes are more likely to cause sinusitis or nasal necrosis [14,15]. Therefore, if a patient no longer requires gastric decompression, the larger-bore nasogastric tube should be replaced with a smaller-bore, more flexible nasoenteric tube for patient comfort and safety. These tubes can usually be successfully placed at the bedside by the staff nurse. If a patient's condition precludes gastric feeding and only short-term access is needed, a nasoduodenal or nasojejunal tube can be utilized. Although usually placed transnasally, these tubes can be inserted transorally in patients with facial or sinus fractures. In general, the goal is to place the feeding tip at or beyond the ligament of Treitz, in order to decrease the risk of reflux of feedings into the stomach. Placement of these tubes by any method (endoscopic, fluoroscopic, or at the bedside) requires trained personnel.

Confirmation of Placement and Monitoring of Short-Term Feeding Access

Prior to utilization of any feeding tube placed at the bedside, radiographic confirmation of its location remains the gold standard. This virtually eliminates the risk of inadvertent administration of enteral feedings into the lungs, although it does not eliminate the initial risk of misplacement of the tube down the tracheobronchial tree [16–20]. In many mechanically ventilated, critically ill patients, the use of sedative and paralytic medications or the patient's underlying disease process itself impairs the normal reflexes protecting the airway and allows a nasoenteric tube to be inserted

TABLE 13.2
Advantages and Disadvantages

Tube Type	Access Duration	Placement Technique and Expertise Level	Advantages	Disadvantages and Risks	Patient Types
Nasogastric/Salem sump	Short term	Bedside/RN	Large bore; less clogging; nasal or oral route; staff RN can replace if needed; used for decompression	Aspiration risk; patient discomfort; sinusitis; nasal necrosis.	Normal gastric emptying; low risk of aspiration
Nasoenteric feeding tube—gastric or small bowel placement	Short term	Bedside gastric placement/RN bedside small bowel placement/trained RN, RD, MD endoscopy, fluoroscopy/MD	Softer more flexible material for improved patient comfort; nasal or oral placement; patient can swallow *around* tube; if larger than 8 Fr, unlikely to clog with good flushing techniques; available for immediate use after placement verification	Cannot be used for decompression; sinusitis. If placed in stomach, may migrate easily into the small bowel; aspiration risk. If placed in small bowel, tube may *flip* back to stomach; may not be able to be placed in patients with altered anatomy.	Gastric—low risk of aspiration Small bowel—delayed gastric emptying, increased risk of aspiration secondary to condition or positioning
PEG or fluoroscopically placed gastrostomy	Long term	Endoscopy, fluoroscopy/MD	Large bore; low risk of clogging; may feed via intermittent or syringe method; may accommodate an SBFT, if necessary	Hemorrhage; infection at insertion site; risk of peritonitis; may have to wait 24 h to use; persistent gastrocutaneous fistula if tract does not close when removed. Cannot be placed if endoscopy is unable to be done.	Normal gastric emptying, low risk of aspiration; need for long-term enteral feeding
Surgical gastrostomy	Long term	Surgical/MD	Large bore; low risk of clogging; may feed via intermittent or syringe method	Requires surgical placement; hemorrhage; infection at incision or insertion site; anesthetic complications; may have to wait 24 h to use; persistent gastrocutaneous fistula if tract does not close when removed.	Normal gastric emptying, low risk of aspiration; need for long-term enteral feeding; unable to place gastrostomy via endoscopic or fluoroscopic techniques
PEJ	Long term	Endoscopy/MD	Decreased risk of aspiration; can provide supplemental feeds at night; may use immediately post placement; bypasses the stomach if decreased gastric motility is a problem	Hemorrhage; infection at insertion site; risk of peritonitis; may *flip* back into stomach; difficult to replace; cannot check residuals; requires continuous infusion; smaller bore; may occlude easily; persistent gastrocutaneous fistula if tract does not close when removed; cannot be placed if endoscopy is unable to be done.	Increased risk of aspiration, gastric motility disorders

(*Continued*)

TABLE 13.2 (*Continued*)
Advantages and Disadvantages

Tube Type	Access Duration	Placement Technique and Expertise Level	Advantages	Disadvantages and Risks	Patient Types
Jejunostomy via PEG	Long term	Endoscopy, fluoroscopy/MD	Decreased risk of aspiration; can provide supplemental feeds at night; may use immediately post placement; simultaneous gastric decompression and small bowel feeding possible	May be difficult to get tube in position; jejunal extension may *flip* back into stomach; requires continuous infusion; smaller bore; may occlude easily.	Increased risk of aspiration, gastric motility disorders
Double-lumen gastrojejunostomy	Long term	Surgical/MD	Decreased risk of aspiration; can provide supplemental feeds at night; may use immediately post placement; simultaneous gastric decompression and small bowel feeding possible	Requires surgical placement; hemorrhage; infection at incision or insertion site; anesthetic complications; jejunal extension may *flip* back into stomach; small-bore tube; may clog easily; unable to be replaced if inadvertently pulled; persistent gastrocutaneous fistula if tract does not close when removed.	Increased risk of aspiration, motility disorders; endoscopic placement not feasible
Surgical jejunostomy	Long term	Surgical/MD	Decreased risk of aspiration; can provide supplemental feeds at night; may use immediately post placement; bypasses the stomach if decreased gastric motility is a problem	Requires surgical placement; hemorrhage; infection at incision or insertion site; anesthetic complications; small-bore tube may clog easily, unable to easily replace if inadvertently pulled.	Increased risk of aspiration, motility disorders, gastric outlet obstruction or other anatomy precluding gastric placement

past the balloon of an endotracheal or tracheostomy tube without detection. Oral placement of the feeding tube is recommended in patients who have sustained craniofacial trauma, to reduce the risk of intracranial placement [21].

During blind bedside placement, several tools exist that can be utilized to aid in the correct placement of a nasoenteric tube into the GI tract and its correct positioning into the stomach or small bowel. These tools include capnography, electromagnetic device, auscultation, and comparison of gastric and small bowel aspirates.

Capnography

Capnography is a common noninvasive technique used in critically ill patients to determine the adequacy of ventilation by measuring end-tidal carbon dioxide (CO_2). To use this technique for nasoenteric or nasogastric tube placement, it is only necessary to distinguish the presence or absence of a CO_2 waveform. An end-tidal CO_2 detector is attached to the end of the feeding tube for continuous monitoring during placement. Theoretically, the presence of an end-tidal CO_2 >15 mm Hg, a respiratory waveform, or both implies inadvertent placement of the tube into the airway. The absence of these two findings suggests that the tube has been placed correctly and is not in the respiratory tract.

Some authors have found this technique to be highly sensitive. This finding was replicated in our institution, when the technique was used with placements of larger-bore nasogastric tubes [22,23]. However, we did have inadvertent placement of a nasojejunal tube into the airway, despite the fact that end-tidal CO_2 monitoring did not identify detectable CO_2 or a respiratory waveform. We hypothesize that this failure may have been due in part to the small diameter of the tube (10 Fr) or the total length of the nasoenteric tube and end-tidal CO_2 detector tubing combined. We presently do not advocate using this technique for nasoenteric tube placement.

Electromagnetic Device

An electromagnetic tube placement device (ETPD) (Corpak MedSystems, Wheeling, IL) provides real-time imaging of FT tip position during bedside placement. The tip of the stylet is a transmitter. The signal is picked up by an external receiver unit placed on the patient's chest. The signal is fed to an attached monitor unit. One group found a 66.1% agreement between the abdominal radiographs of the reading of ETPD, with the strongest agreement when the tubes were determined to be in the second portion of the duodenum or beyond by the ETPD [24]. We currently utilize this device in our own institution and have found a decrease in placement time and decreased learning curve for professionals training in tube placement. The decision to replace the abdominal radiograph for tube placement confirmation will need to be made at each individual institution.

Auscultation

Auscultation of air over the stomach and small bowel is a commonly used method for detecting placement of the feeding tube [25–27]. Sounds of air injected into the stomach are heard best in the midline or left upper quadrant regions. In the small bowel, these sounds are best heard in the right upper quadrant for the proximal duodenum and in the left flank area for the distal duodenum or proximal jejunum. Unfortunately, air injection in the thoracic cavity may be auscultated in the abdomen and misinterpreted as indicating correct placement of the tube into the stomach. A more sensitive technique of auscultation is to determine whether the location of the sound changes during tube advancement. Such a finding makes it unlikely that the tube has been inadvertently placed into the tracheobronchial tree.

Aspiration

Aspiration of gastric and small bowel contents for color and pH testing is also used to determine tube placement [28–31]. Gastric fluid typically has a lower pH (3–4) than respiratory (6–8) and small bowel fluid (>6). However, because many critically ill patients receive H_2 blockers or proton pump inhibitors to protect against bleeding from stress ulceration, they may have a higher gastric pH (5–7).

Therefore, color and appearance of the aspirate may be more important than pH in determining placement. A small bowel aspirate is generally a clear, golden, syrupy fluid. If the stomach and small bowel aspirates are different in appearance and pH, the tip of the feeding tube is usually found to be within the small bowel.

Because nasogastric tubes may migrate into the small bowel, rechecking for correct tube placement should be performed on a routine basis. Inadvertent bolus feeding into the intestine instead of the stomach may result in diarrhea. A gastric pH should be rechecked prior to each bolus or intermittent feed. If the color or pH changes, an abdominal radiograph is ordered to determine where the tip of the tube is located. In patients with nasoenteric tubes, it is also advisable to check color and pH of small bowel aspirate at least one time per day in continuously fed patients, because the tip of the feeding tube can migrate back into the stomach.

Bilirubin concentrations of enteral aspirates have been evaluated as a method by which to monitor feeding tube location [32,33]. The bilirubin content of the small bowel should be higher than that of the stomach or lung. However, because commercially available bedside methods for measuring bilirubin are not yet available, this technique is not yet in common practice.

In order to compare gastric and small bowel aspirates, it must be possible to sample them. In our experience, aspirates can be obtained approximately 70% of the time. The success of obtaining an aspirate may depend on the number of exit holes at the end of the tube; successful aspiration of GI contents is more likely using tubes that have more than one exit hole.

Long-Term Feeding Tubes

A surgically implanted feeding tube should be considered if feeding will be required for longer than 4 weeks. In general, these tubes are less disturbing to the patient than are tubes placed via the nasal or oral route. The risks of sinusitis and nasal or pharyngeal injuries are also eliminated. Implanted tubes transverse two epithelial barriers: the skin and the mucosa of the GI tract. Because these barriers are the primary defenses against bacterial invasion, there is a significant risk of infection at the tube site [34,35]. Also, if the patient or caregiver inadvertently removes the tube, particularly soon after it has been placed, an operative procedure of the stomach or intestine may be needed to prevent ongoing peritoneal soilage [36]. As with all surgical procedures, placement of enteral access devices entails risks of anesthetic complications and hemorrhage, in addition to infection.

Several options are available for the placement of gastrostomy tubes. Currently, the most common technique is percutaneous endoscopic gastrostomy (PEG) [37–39]. Placement of a PEG requires that an endoscope be passed into the stomach for visualization and manipulation of the insertion site. After placement, an external bolster holds the tube in position and keeps the stomach up against the abdominal wall to prevent leakage of feedings or gastric contents. This procedure can usually be performed under local anesthesia with conscious sedation and is done with an either *push* or *pull* technique [40]. Besides infection and hemorrhage, uncommon complications include inadvertent placement of the tube through the colon or another intra-abdominal viscus and erosion or extrusion of the tube, with resultant leakage of gastric contents and tube feedings into the abdominal cavity [41–44]. Within 1–2 weeks of placement, significant adhesions form between the stomach and the abdominal wall, and the leakage of material into the peritoneal cavity is unlikely, even when the tube is removed. The general practice is to wait 24 h after PEG tube insertion to initiate feedings; however, there is evidence that feeding can begin as soon as 4–6 h after placement [45].

Fluoroscopically guided percutaneous gastrostomy is an alternative to the PEG technique, although it is done less often [46]. This technique requires the introduction of a tube into the stomach for the delivery of contrast and air for dilation of the stomach, after which the stomach is punctured percutaneously. For patients with pharyngeal or esophageal abnormalities that preclude endoscopic or fluoroscopic placement of a tube, a surgical gastrostomy may be placed. The surgical gastrostomy tube can be implanted using either an open technique (with laparotomy) or a laparoscopic approach [47–49]. Both methods generally require general anesthesia to be administered. Because of its more invasive nature, surgical placement of a gastrostomy tube is generally associated with a higher complication rate than is endoscopic or fluoroscopic placement. However, because the stomach is secured to the abdominal wall directly, there is usually a lower risk of gastric leakage than with the other techniques [34].

The small bowel can be accessed through the abdominal wall using several different methods. A percutaneous endoscopic jejunostomy (PEJ) tube can be placed, using a technique similar to that for a PEG tube, except that the tube is endoscopically positioned beyond the pylorus into the jejunum. Alternatively, if the patient already has a gastrostomy tube in place or is having one inserted, a small bowel feeding tube (SBFT) may be inserted through the gastrostomy tube and into the duodenum or jejunum. In addition, a SBFT can be inserted through a preexisting gastrostomy fluoroscopically [50,51]. Also available are combination tubes that have dual ports: one for drainage of the stomach and one for delivery of nutritional formulas into the small bowel. These can be inserted via an endoscopic technique or, more commonly, during an open operative procedure [52–54]. With all SBFTs placed transgastrically, there is a risk that the distally placed small bowel tube will migrate back into the stomach; thus, the tube may have to be repositioned endoscopically or fluoroscopically in order for the patient to be fed into the small bowel [55].

A feeding jejunostomy implanted directly into the small bowel provides the most secure means of accessing the small bowel [56]. Placement of a feeding jejunostomy almost always requires an operative procedure, via either an open or a laparoscopic approach [51,57,58]. Many times, these tubes are implanted during laparotomy for another reason, such as abdominal trauma or resection of a major neoplasm. Occasionally, they are placed during a primary procedure for a patient who will require long-term enteral feeding and has contraindications to gastric feeding. Generally, jejunostomy tubes are of a smaller caliber than gastrostomy tube and thus more susceptible to clogging, particularly a needle catheter jejunostomy tube [59]. They are frequently placed through a serosal (Witzel) tunnel, which makes it unlikely that an enterocutaneous fistula will persist when the tube is discontinued but also makes it difficult to restore access if the tube is inadvertently removed [60].

Care of the Insertion Site

Care of the insertion site for various tube types should begin as soon as the tube is placed and continue until the tube is removed and the exit site is healed (Table 13.3). The loss of any permanent feeding tube should be considered a medical emergency. If the tube is inadvertently removed before the tract has had time to mature, the viscus into which the tube was inserted may fall away from the abdominal wall, with leakage of GI contents into the peritoneal cavity [36]. However, the loss of a tube from a mature site requires early reinsertion if the feeding device is to be maintained. The failure to recannulate the tube tract within a few hours may result in permanent closure of the tract, with the need to perform another procedure to gain access for a new tube.

Maintaining Tube Patency

Several considerations are important in maintaining patency of all types of feeding tubes. The smaller-bore (14 Fr or less) polyurethane, silicone, or polyurethane–silicone combination tubes are more prone to clogging than are larger-bore or stiffer tubes. Regular flushing with water or normal saline has been shown to be the best way to prevent clogging. The tube should be flushed with a minimum of 30 mL of water or saline solution before and after each intermittent feeding or every 3–4 h during continuous feeding [61]. Medications administered via feeding tubes should be in a liquid form or crushable [62]. Tablets should be crushed finely and dissolved in water prior to administration. The tube should be flushed with 30 mL of water before and after administering medications. Medications should not be mixed with the nutritional product, because formula–medication interactions may result in coagulation of the formula and clogging of the tube or in precipitation of the medication and loss of its effectiveness. If enteral feedings are held for any reason, the tube should continue to be flushed every 3–4 h to maintain patency. If the feeding tube does become clogged, several maneuvers can be attempted, as outlined in Figure 13.1 [63–65].

TABLE 13.3
Care of Insertion

Type of Placement	Evaluate	Assessment	Care	Precautions
Nasal or oral	Daily	Redness, dryness, or fissures noted around nose or mouth.	Lubricate nares with water-soluble lubricant. Change anchoring method.	If condition worsens, it may need to change site of insertion.
Nasal or oral	Twice daily	Decreased oral hygiene.	Mouth care.	
Nasal	Daily	Sores or increased nasal drainage.	Replace via the oral route, it may require antibiotics.	May indicate sinusitis; report to MD.
Gastrostomy or jejunostomy	Daily—start 24 h post placement	Check exit site.	Clean tube site twice daily with soap and water and the area immediately around the skin opening. If site is covered by a bolster, use cotton swab for cleaning.	
	Immediately post placement, then daily	Increased bleeding or drainage at exit site.	Place additional gauze dressing around the site and the tube.	Do not place dressings directly under the external bolster—it may dislodge tube. Report to MD.
	Daily	Increased tenderness, swelling, or redness.	More frequent cleaning; cap feeding ports when not in use; possibly antibiotics or tube removal.	Report immediately to MD—may be sign of an infection.
	Daily	Inadvertent tube removal.	Contact MD—may be able to reinsert through established tract if done quickly.	If tract is not mature, this should be considered a medical emergency.

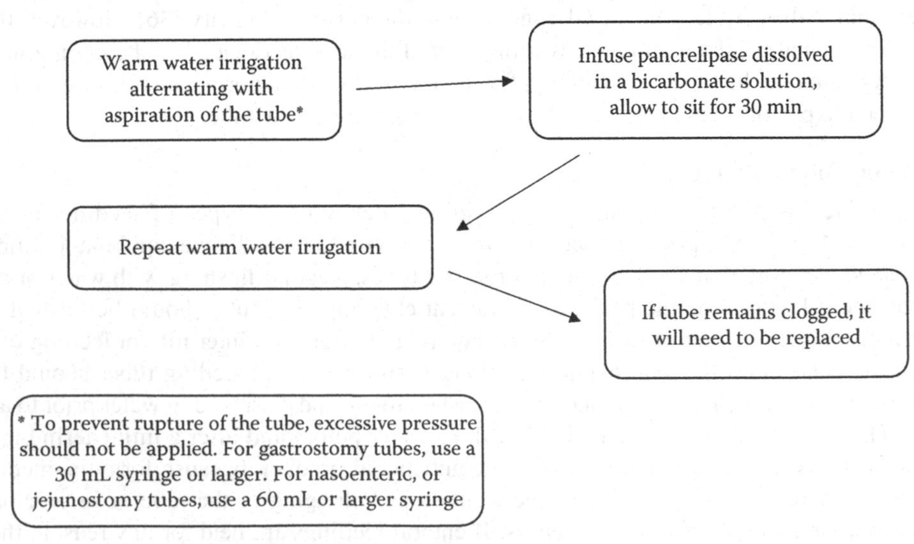

FIGURE 13.1 Steps for unclogging enteral feeding tubes.

GASTRIC VERSUS SMALL BOWEL ACCESS

Enteral nutritional support has become standard for many patients admitted to an intensive care unit, and the use of early enteral support has gained popularity over the past decade in many institutions [6,66–68]. There is considerable debate regarding the best site for feeding the ICU patient: prepyloric or postpyloric [69,70]. Ultimately, this decision will be based on the perceived advantages and disadvantages of either site, as well as the physician's assessment of the specific needs of the particular patient.

The advantages of gastric (prepyloric) feedings include preservation of the reservoir function of the stomach, the allowance for bolus feedings, the ease of tube placement for short-term access, the need for less equipment (such as a feeding pump), and decreased costs, because specifically trained personnel are not needed for tube placement. The disadvantages of gastric feeding relate to prolonged retention of formula in the stomach as a result of decreased gastric motility, leading to regurgitation and possible tracheobronchial aspiration, and the frequent development of high gastric residuals or feeding intolerance, which leads to a delay in achieving caloric goals [71,72].

The advantages of small bowel (postpyloric) feeding include bypassing the pylorus if gastric emptying is a problem and a theoretical decreased risk of aspiration [73–78]. It should be pointed out, however, that this latter issue remains an area of marked controversy and a decreased risk of aspiration pneumonia with use of postpyloric feedings has not been clearly established. The disadvantages of small bowel feedings relate to the greater difficulty in placing postpyloric feeding tubes, which may necessitate transport of a critically ill patient for fluoroscopy or endoscopically guided placement, and the greater costs associated with having experienced personnel available for tube placement, the tube itself, and the use of additional equipment, particularly a pump for delivery of the formula [79–83].

Placement of SBFTs has been reported to be highly successful with the use of endoscopic and fluoroscopic guidance [82–84]. However, the initial placement of the tube into the small bowel may give the clinician a false sense of security, because the tube may migrate out of position and back into the stomach. If this occurs, repeat endoscopy or fluoroscopy is generally required to reposition the tube, increasing costs further.

Placement of SBFTs at the bedside obviates some of the risks and costs associated with small bowel feedings and eliminates the need for patient transport. Several methods for blind bedside placement of postpyloric feeding tubes have been described [10,25,79,85–88]. Earlier techniques required long periods for *tube migration* (4–72 h) prior to obtaining an abdominal radiograph to confirm correct placement [77]. Salasidis et al. [89] described a technique utilizing air insufflation and reported a 78% success rate in achieving small bowel placement; however, the authors waited 2 h prior in obtaining an abdominal radiograph to allow time for tube migration. Thurlow [85] utilized a corkscrew technique and reported an 87% success rate at time of placement. Zaloga [86] reported a 92% success rate with this method using trained personnel; however, when the task was given to untrained residents, the success rate dropped to 70%. Recently, the use of a magnetic device has been described; however, the success rate with this technique was lower than that reported with other techniques [90].

Promotility agents (see Table 13.4) have been used in an effort to facilitate SBFT placements. There have been mixed reports on their efficacy in improving success rates, and the utility of these agents remains uncertain [85,91–93].

Several studies have shown that consistently higher success rates can be achieved when specifically trained personnel are designated for feeding tube placements [79,86,87]. The type of professional appears to be immaterial, with successful tube placements being achieved by physicians, nurses, and dietitians [87].

The practice at our institution is based on the technique described by Lord et al. [10], which is outlined in Table 13.5. Nasoduodenal or nasojejunal feeding tubes are placed at the bedside in most ICU patients. We have recently reported the results of blind bedside placement of SBFTs in 1220 critically ill patients [94]. Trained professionals from the nutrition support service, including one physician, four nurses, and three dietitians, were responsible for SBFT placements in all patients in the surgical trauma, medical, cardiothoracic, and cardiac units;

TABLE 13.4
Motility Agents

Trade Name	Metoclopramide Reglan	Erythromycin E-mycin
Effect on GI tract	Increases resting esophageal sphincter tone, improves gastric tone and peristalsis, relaxes pyloric sphincter, and augments duodenal peristalsis.	Increases gastric emptying and improves intestinal motility (not presently FDA approved for this function).
Contraindications	Do not use in patients with seizure disorder.	Do not use in patients with preexisting liver disease or hepatic impairment.
Most common adverse reactions	Restlessness, drowsiness, diarrhea, weakness.	Abdominal pain, cramping, nausea, and vomiting.
Form	Available in oral or IV.	Available in oral or IV (shortages of IV form have occurred).

TABLE 13.5
Sample Placement Protocol
Bedside SBFT Placement
Variation of the "10–10–10" Protocol

Policy statement: A Nutrition Support Service member or APN who has shown clinical competency with insertion will place a SBFT at the bedside, with verification of placement by KUB prior to initiation of feeding.

Description: A protocol involving the insertion of all but **10** cm of a nonweighted 43 in. or 55 in. Corpak® feeding tube with a stylet **10** min after IV metoclopramide **10** mg in order to obtain small bowel placement.

Procedure:

1. Administer 10 mg IV metoclopramide (5 mg if patient in renal failure) over 1–2 min approximately 10 min prior to tube insertion.
2. Put on gloves.
3. If NGT or OGT is in place, obtain aspirate, noting color and pH, clamp NGT/OGT for SBFT insertion.
4. Set the hub of the stylet firmly into the main port of feeding tube; close the medication port with cap.
5. Flush tube with approximately 10 cc tap water to check for patency or leaks, and activate lubricant.
6. Elevate patient's HOB as tolerated.
7. Insert SBFT into nostril and advance to nasopharynx and into esophagus. Flexion of patient's neck or having patient swallow will facilitate passage of tube into esophagus.
8. Advance tube to 55–60 cm and auscultate over the epigastric area and attempt to aspirate gastric contents, comparing aspirate with previous NGT aspirate if available. Gastric aspirate is bilious in appearance. The pH may range from 1 to 7, depending on the use of gastric prophylaxis medication.
9. Continue to advance SBFT slowly with a gentle touch. Infuse approximately 60 cc air slowly, starting at 70–75 cm, to help open the pylorus. Never force the tube; if resistance is met, pull back and attempt to readvance. Continue to advance to the 100 cm mark. There should be a vacuum present on the syringe when the tube is in the small bowel.
10. Aspirate and check pH and color of output when tube is at 100 cm mark. The color of small bowel aspirate is generally yellow in appearance with a pH of 7+.
11. Remove stylet and check for kinks or loops, then attempt to reinsert. The stylet should be easy to insert. Upon reinsertion of stylet, if any resistance is met, pull tube back until stylet is easily inserted. After stylet is in place, readvance tube.
12. When tube is in position, remove stylet and secure tube with tape to nose. Place stylet in plastic bag to use in future if SBFT needs to be repositioned.
13. Return NGT to suction, if this was on prior to procedure.
14. Order KUB to verify placement.
15. If SBFT pulled back from original insertion cm marking, reinsert stylet and advance SBFT per preceding procedure. Obtain KUB to verify position.

neurologic ICUs; and the ICU step-down unit. The overall success rate of this team in achieving postpyloric placement was 86% (1045/1220), with 72% of the feeding tips delivered distal to the second portion of the duodenum and 57% at or beyond the ligament of Treitz. We did note a learning curve with each newly trained practitioner. The individual with the most experience was a dietitian, who achieved a 93% success rate (401/432). Our results are consistent with the evidence indicating that designating and training specific personnel for SBFT placement will lead to improved success with the procedure.

CONCLUSION

The clinician has a wide variety of enteral access devices and equipment from which to choose. The specific choice will be influenced by the desired site for feeding, the duration of enteral feeding needed, and the availability of trained staff for feeding tube placement. Once the enteral access device is in position, care should be taken to maintain the integrity of the site and the patency of the tube, to ensure the provision of effective enteral nutritional support.

CASE STUDY

K.D. is a 53-year-old male involved in a motor vehicle collision. A head and abdominal CT scans were both negative. The patient sustained a T7 vertebral body fracture, a right femur fracture, a left distal femur fracture, bilateral postacetabular fractures, multiple rib fractures, and a pneumothorax. A chest tube was placed. The patient was intubated and placed on mechanical ventilation. The patient has a history of atrial fibrillation and chronic pancreatitis. The patient was sent to the trauma intensive care unit.

On postadmission day 3, the patient remains intubated and the decision is made to begin enteral feeds. The plan for the next several days is for the patient to undergo several orthopedic procedures. The patient is expected to be weaned from the ventilator in approximately 7–10 days.

Anthropometrics: height 5 ft 11 in., weight 86 kg, IBW 81 kg, BMI 26

Inputs/outputs:

IVFs, D51/2NS with 20 mEq KCL at 100 mL/h
Nasogastric tube (Salem sump—16 Fr), 2200 mL
Urine output, 2500 mL
Chest tube, 150 mL
The patient has had two bowel movements.

Question: What are the possible causes of the high gastric output?
Answer: The possible causes of the high output are decreased gastric motility, gastric outlet obstruction, and migration of the nasogastric tube tip into the duodenum. An abdominal radiograph should be done to check for obstruction or migration of the tube.

Question: The abdominal radiograph demonstrated the nasogastric tube to be in good position. There was no evidence of an obstruction. It was determined the patient has decreased gastric motility. Where should the patient be fed (stomach or small bowel), and what is the appropriate enteral access device to use in this patient?
Answer: To reduce the risk of aspiration, the patient should be continued on low-intermittent gastric suction. Therefore, a nasoenteric feeding tube at or beyond the ligament of Treitz would be preferred. The patient's injuries will not affect his swallowing function. Given the short period of time (7–10 days) anticipated that the patient will require tube feeds, a permanent

enteral access is not warranted. Because the Salem sump nasogastric tube is in the left naris, the nasoenteric tube is placed through the right naris.

Question: The patient was started on IV metoclopramide 10 mg q 6 h, and his gastric output decreased to 300 mL in 24 h. He has developed pneumonia and is not expected to wean from the ventilator for another 7 days. He is presently tolerating his feeds at goal via a 10 Fr nasoenteric tube. The RN notes he is developing a sore on his left naris. The patient is receiving several medications via his nasogastric tube. The patient's weight has increased 12 kg since admission. Should any changes be made?

Answer: The patient's poor gastric motility has resolved. Because he no longer requires gastric decompression, the stiff Salem sump can be removed and his ulceration treated. His enteral medications should be in liquid or crushable form. Because the medications are to be given into the small bowel, they need to be diluted with 10–30 mL of water; in addition, adequate flushing between administrations of medications needs to be continued.

Question: The patient's SBFT is pulled accidentally when the patient is being turned. What type of tube should be placed?

Answer: Because the patient's decreased gastric motility has resolved, a small bowel tube may no longer be necessary. At many institutions, a specially trained professional is needed to place the small bowel tube; the bedside nurse can place a nasogastric tube. Therefore, a 12 Fr nasoenteric tube placed into the stomach would be appropriate.

REFERENCES

1. Heyland, D.K., Cook, D.J., and Guyatt, G.H., Enteral nutrition in the critically ill patient: A critical review of the evidence, *Intens. Care Med.*, 19, 435, 1993.
2. Kudsk, K.A., Croce, M.A., Fabian, T.C. et al., Enteral versus parenteral feeding: Effects on septic morbidity after blunt and penetrating abdominal trauma, *Ann. Surg.*, 215, 503, 1992.
3. McMahon, M.M., Farnell, M.B., and Murray, M.J., Nutritional support of critically ill patients, *Mayo Clin. Proc.*, 68, 911, 1993.
4. Moore, E.E. and Jones, T.N., Benefits of immediate jejunostomy feeding after major abdominal trauma: A prospective, randomized study, *J. Trauma*, 26, 874, 1986.
5. Moore, F.A. and Moore, E.E., The benefits of enteric feeding, *Adv. Surg.*, 30, 141, 1996.
6. Zaloga, G.P., Bortenschlager, L., Black, K.W. et al., Immediate postoperative enteral feeding decreases weight loss and improves wound healing after abdominal surgery in rats, *Crit. Care Med.*, 20, 115, 1992.
7. Heyland, D., Cook, D.J., Winder, B. et al., Enteral nutrition in the critically ill patient: A prospective survey, *Crit. Care Med.*, 23, 1055, 1995.
8. Meyer, N.A. and Kudsk, K.A., Enteral versus parenteral nutrition: Alterations in mechanisms of function in mucosal host defenses, *Nestle Nutr. Workshop Ser. Clin. Perform. Programme*, 8, 133, 2003.
9. Ciaccia, D., Quigley, R.L., Shami, P.J. et al., A case of retrograde jejunoduodenal intussusception caused by a feeding gastrostomy tube, *Nutr. Clin. Pract.*, 9, 18, 1994.
10. Lord, L.M., Weiser-Maimone, A., Pulhamus, M. et al., Comparison of weighted vs. unweighted enteral feeding tubes for efficacy of transpyloric intubation, *J. Parenter. Enteral Nutr.*, 17, 271, 1993.
11. Levenson, R., Turner, W.W. Jr., Dyson, A. et al., Do weighted nasoenteric feeding tubes facilitate duodenal intubations? *J. Parenter. Enteral Nutr.*, 12, 135, 1988.
12. Ugo, P.J., Mohler, P.A., and Wilson, G.L., Bedside postpyloric placement of weighted feeding tubes, *Nutr. Clin. Pract.*, 7, 284, 1992.
13. Montgomery R.C., Bar-Natan, M.F., and Thomas S.E., Postoperative nasogastric decompression: A prospective randomized trial, *South. Med. J.*, 89, 1063, 1996.
14. Caplan, E.S. and Hoyt, N.J., Nosocomial sinusitis, *JAMA*, 247, 639, 1982.
15. Landis, E.E. Jr., Hoffman, H.T., and Koconis, C.A., Upper airway obstruction associated with large bore nasogastric tubes, *South. Med. J.*, 81, 1333, 1988.
16. Biggart, M., McQuillan, P.J., Choudhry, A.K. et al., Dangers of placement of narrow bore nasogastric feeding tubes, *Ann. R. Coll. Surg. Engl.*, 69, 119, 1987.

17. McWey, R.E., Curry, N.S., Schabel, S.I. et al., Complications of nasoenteric feeding tubes, *Am. J. Surg.*, 155, 253, 1988.
18. Bankier, A.A., Wiesmayr, M.N., Henk, C. et al., Radiographic detection of intrabronchial malpositions of nasogastric tubes and subsequent complications in intensive care unit patients, *Intens. Care Med.*, 23, 406, 1997.
19. Rolfe, I. and Nair, B., Complications associated with the insertion of narrow-bore feeding-tubes, *Med. J. Aust.*, 152, 108, 1990.
20. Alessi, D.M. and Berci, G., Aspiration and nasogastric intubation, *Otolaryngol. Head Neck Surg.*, 94, 486, 1986.
21. Ferreras, J., Junquera, L.M., and Garcia-Consuegra, L., Intracranial placement of a nasogastric tube after severe craniofacial trauma, *Oral Surg. Oral Med. Oral Pathol. Oral Radiol. Endod.*, 90, 564, 2000.
22. Burns, S.M., Carpenter, R., and Truwit, J.D., Report on the development of a procedure to prevent placement of feeding tubes into the lungs using end-tidal CO_2 measurements, *Crit. Care Med.*, 29, 936, 2001.
23. Araujo-Preza, C.E., Melhado, M.E., Gutierrez, F.J. et al., Use of capnometry to verify feeding tube placement, *Crit. Care Med.*, 30, 2255, 2002.
24. Rivera, R., Campana, J., Hamilton, C. et al. Small bowel feeding tube placement using an electromagnetic tube placement device: Accuracy of tip location. *J. Parenter. Enteral Nutr.*, 35, 636, 2011.
25. Metheny, N., McSweeney, M., Wehrle, M.A. et al., Effectiveness of the auscultatory method in predicting feeding tube location, *Nurs. Res.*, 39, 262, 1990.
26. Stone, S.J., Pickett, J.D., and Jesurum, J.T., Bedside placement of postpyloric feeding tubes, *AACN Clin. Issues*, 11, 517, 2000.
27. Neumann, M.J., Meyer, C.T., Dutton, J.L. et al., Hold that x-ray: Aspirate pH and auscultation prove enteral tube placement, *J. Clin. Gastroenterol.*, 20, 293, 1995.
28. Metheny, N., Williams, P., Wiersema, L. et al., Effectiveness of pH measurements in predicting feeding tube placement, *Nurs. Res.*, 38, 280, 1989.
29. Metheny, N., Reed, L., Wiersema, L. et al., Effectiveness of pH measurements in predicting feeding tube placement: An update, *Nurs. Res.*, 42, 324, 1993.
30. Metheny, N.A., Clouse, R.E., Clark, J.M. et al., pH testing of feeding-tube aspirates to determine placement, *Nutr. Clin. Pract.*, 9, 185, 1994.
31. Metheny, N., Reed, L., Berglund, B. et al., Visual characteristics of aspirates from feeding tubes as a method for predicting tube location, *Nurs. Res.*, 43, 282, 1994.
32. Metheny, N.A., Stewart, B.J., Smith, L. et al., pH and concentration of bilirubin in feeding tube aspirates as predictors of tube placement, *Nurs. Res.*, 48, 189, 1999.
33. Metheny, N.A., Smith, L., and Stewart, B.J., Development of a reliable and valid bedside test for bilirubin and its utility for improving prediction of feeding tube location, *Nurs. Res.*, 49, 302, 2000.
34. Shellito, P.C. and Malt, R.A., Tube gastrostomy: Techniques and complications, *Ann. Surg.*, 201, 180, 1985.
35. Ephgrave, K.S., Buchmiller, C., Jones, M.P. et al., The cup is half full, *Am. J. Surg.*, 178, 406, 1999.
36. Holmes, J.H., Brundage, S.I., Yuen, P. et al., Complications of surgical feeding jejunostomy in trauma patients, *J. Trauma*, 47, 1009, 1999.
37. Gauderer, M.W., Ponsky, J.L., and Izant, R.J. Jr., Gastrostomy without laparotomy: A percutaneous endoscopic technique, *J. Pediatr. Surg.*, 15, 872, 1980.
38. Grant, J.P., Comparison of percutaneous endoscopic gastrostomy with Stamm gastrostomy, *Ann. Surg.*, 207, 598, 1988.
39. Gauderer, M.W., Percutaneous endoscopic gastrostomy and the evolution of contemporary long-term enteral access, *Clin. Nutr.*, 21, 103, 2002.
40. Hogan, R.B., DeMarco, D.C., Hamilton, J.K. et al., Percutaneous endoscopic gastrostomy: To push or pull. A prospective randomized trial, *Gastrointest. Endosc.*, 32, 253, 1986.
41. Larson, D.E., Burton, D.D., Schroeder, K.W. et al., Percutaneous endoscopic gastrostomy: Indications, success, complications, and mortality in 314 consecutive patients, *Gastroenterology*, 93, 48, 1987.
42. DeLegge, M.H., Effect of external bolster tension on PEG tube tract formation, *Gastrointest. Endosc.*, 43, 349, 1996.
43. Grant, J.P., Mortality with percutaneous endoscopic gastrostomy, *Am. J. Gastroenterol.*, 95, 3, 2000.
44. Stefan, M.M., Holcomb, G.W. 3rd, and Ross, A.J. 3rd, Cologastric fistula as a complication of percutaneous endoscopic gastrostomy, *J. Parenter. Enteral Nutr.*, 13, 554, 1989.

45. Ho, C.S., Yee, A.C., and McPherson, R., Complications of surgical and percutaneous nonendoscopic gastrostomy: Review of 233 patients, *Gastroenterology*, 95, 1206, 1988.
46. McLoughlin, R.F., So, B., and Gray, R.R., Fluoroscopically guided percutaneous gastrostomy: Current status, *Can. Assoc. Radiol. J.*, 47, 10, 1996.
47. Peitgen, K., von Ostau, C., and Walz, M.K., Laparoscopic gastrostomy: Results of 121 patients over 7 years, *Surg. Laparosc. Endosc. Percutan. Tech.*, 11, 76, 2001.
48. Murayama, K.M., Schneider, P.D., and Thompson, J.S., Laparoscopic gastrostomy: A safe method for obtaining enteral access, *J. Surg. Res.*, 58, 1, 1995.
49. Rosser, J.C. Jr., Rodas, E.B., Blancaflor, J. et al., A simplified technique for laparoscopic jejunostomy and gastrostomy tube placement, *Am. J. Surg.*, 177, 61, 1999.
50. Baskin, W. and Johanson, J.F., Trans-PEG ultra thin endoscopy for PEG/J placement, *Gastrointest. Endosc.*, 57, 146; author reply 146, 2003.
51. Bell, S.D., Carmody, E.A., Yeung, E.Y. et al., Percutaneous gastrostomy and gastrojejunostomy: Additional experience in 519 procedures, *Radiology*, 194, 817, 1995.
52. Parasher, V.K., Abramowicz, C.J., Bell, C. et al., Successful placement of percutaneous gastrojejunostomy using steerable guidewire: A modified controlled push technique, *Gastrointest. Endosc.*, 41, 52, 1995.
53. Duckworth, P.F. Jr., Kirby, D.F., McHenry, L. et al., Percutaneous endoscopic gastrojejunostomy made easy: A new over-the-wire technique, *Gastrointest. Endosc.*, 40, 350, 1994.
54. DeLegge, M.H., Patrick, P., and Gibbs, R., Percutaneous endoscopic gastrojejunostomy with a tapered tip, non-weighted jejunal feeding tube: Improved placement success, *Am. J. Gastroenterol.*, 91, 1130, 1996.
55. DeLegge, M.H., Duckworth, P.F. Jr., McHenry, L. Jr. et al., Percutaneous endoscopic gastrojejunostomy: A dual center safety and efficacy trial, *J. Parenter. Enteral Nutr.*, 19, 239, 1995.
56. McGonigal, M.D., Lucas, C.E., and Ledgerwood, A.M., Feeding jejunostomy in patients who are critically ill, *Surg. Gynecol. Obstet.*, 168, 275, 1989.
57. Duh, Q.Y., Senokozlieff-Englehart, A.L., Choe, Y.S. et al., Laparoscopic gastrostomy and jejunostomy: Safety and cost with local vs general anesthesia, *Arch. Surg.*, 134, 151, 1999.
58. Henderson, J.M., Strodel, W.E., and Gilinsky, N.H., Limitations of percutaneous endoscopic jejunostomy, *J. Parenter. Enteral Nutr.*, 17, 546, 1993.
59. Myers, J.G., Page, C.P., Stewart, R.M. et al., Complications of needle catheter jejunostomy in 2,022 consecutive applications, *Am. J. Surg.*, 170, 547, 1995.
60. Cogen, R., Weinryb, J., Pomerantz, C. et al., Complications of jejunostomy tube feeding in nursing facility patients, *Am. J. Gastroenterol.*, 86, 1610, 1991.
61. Massoni, M., *Gastrointestinal Care*, Springhouse Corporation, Ambler, PA, 1993.
62. Williams, N.T., Medication administration through enteral feeding tubes. *Am J Health Syst Pharm*, 65(24) 2347, 2008.
63. Tinckler, L., Nasogastric tube management, *Br. J. Surg.*, 59, 637, 1970.
64. Marcuard, S.P., Stegall, K.L., and Trogdon, S., Clearing obstructed feeding tubes, *J. Parenter. Enteral Nutr.*, 13, 81, 1989.
65. Marcuard, S.P. and Stegall, K.S., Unclogging feeding tubes with pancreatic enzyme, *J. Parenter. Enteral Nutr.*, 14, 198, 1990.
66. Inoue, S., Epstein, M.D., Alexander, J.W. et al., Prevention of yeast translocation across the gut by a single enteral feeding after burn injury, *J. Parenter. Enteral Nutr.*, 13, 565, 1989.
67. Moore, F.A., Moore, E.E., and Haenel, J.B., Clinical benefits of early post-injury enteral feeding, *Clin. Intens. Care*, 6, 21, 1995.
68. Carr, C.S., Ling, K.D., Boulous, P., and Singer M., Randomized trial of safety and efficacy of immediate postoperative enteral feeding in patients undergoing gastrointestinal resection, *BMJ*, 312, 869, 1996.
69. Hiyama, D.T. and Zinner, M.J., *Principles of Surgery*, McGraw-Hill, New York, 1994.
70. Marik, P.E. and Zaloga, G.P., Gastric versus post-pyloric feeding: A systematic review, *Crit. Care*, 7, R46, 2003.
71. Montecalvo, M.A., Steger, K.A., Farber, H.W. et al., Nutritional outcome and pneumonia in critical care patients randomized to gastric versus jejunal tube feedings. The Critical Care Research Team, *Crit. Care Med.*, 20, 1377, 1992.
72. Neumann, D.A. and DeLegge, M.H., Gastric versus small-bowel tube feeding in the intensive care unit: A prospective comparison of efficacy, *Crit. Care Med.*, 30, 1436, 2002.
73. Lazarus, B.A., Murphy, J.B., and Culpepper, L., Aspiration associated with long-term gastric versus jejunal feeding: A critical analysis of the literature, *Arch. Phys. Med. Rehabil.*, 71, 46, 1990.

74. Mullan, H., Roubenoff, R.A., and Roubenoff, R., Risk of pulmonary aspiration among patients receiving enteral nutrition support, *J. Parenter. Enteral Nutr.*, 16, 160, 1992.
75. Cataldi-Betcher, E.L., Seltzer, M.H., Slocum, B.A. et al., Complications occurring during enteral nutrition support: A prospective study, *J. Parenter. Enteral Nutr.*, 7, 546, 1983.
76. Botoman, V.A., Kirtland, S.H., and Moss, L.A., A randomized study of a pH sensor feeding tube vs a standard feeding tube in patients requiring enteral nutrition, *J. Parenter. Enteral Nutr.*, 18, 154, 1994.
77. Rees, R.G., Payne-James, J.J., King, C., and Silk, D.B.A., Spontaneous transpyloric passage and performance of "fine bore" polyurethane feeding tubes: A controlled clinical trial, *J. Parenter. Enteral Nutr.*, 12, 462, 1988.
78. Strong, R.M., Condon, S.C., Solinger, M.R. et al., Equal aspiration rates from postpylorus and intragastric-placed small-bore nasoenteric feeding tubes: A randomized, prospective study, *J. Parenter. Enteral Nutr.*, 16, 59, 1992.
79. Powers, J., Chance, R., Bortenschlager, L. et al., Bedside placement of small-bowel feeding tubes in the intensive care unit, *Crit. Care Nurse*, 23, 16, 2003.
80. Ott, D.J., Mattox, H.E., Gelfand, D.W. et al., Enteral feeding tubes: Placement by using fluoroscopy and endoscopy, *Am. J. Roentgenol.*, 157, 769, 1991.
81. Hillard, A.E., Waddell, J.J., Metzler, M.H. et al., Fluoroscopically guided nasoenteric feeding tube placement versus bedside placement, *South. Med. J.*, 88, 425, 1995.
82. Patrick, P.G., Marulendra, S., Kirby, D.F. et al., Endoscopic nasogastric-jejunal feeding tube placement in critically ill patients, *Gastrointest. Endosc.*, 45, 72, 1997.
83. Prager, R., Laboy, V., Venus, B. et al., Value of fluoroscopic assistance during transpyloric intubation, *Crit. Care Med.*, 14, 151, 1986.
84. Rives, D.A., LeRoy, J.L., Hawkins, M.L. et al., Endoscopically assisted nasojejunal feeding tube placement, *Am. Surg.*, 55, 88, 1989.
85. Thurlow, P.M., Bedside enteral feeding tube placement into duodenum and jejunum, *J. Parenter. Enteral Nutr.*, 10, 104, 1986.
86. Zaloga, G.P., Bedside method for placing small bowel feeding tubes in critically ill patients: A prospective study, *Chest*, 100, 1643, 1991.
87. Taylor, B. and Schallom, L., Bedside small bowel feeding tube placement in critically ill patients using a dietitian/nurse team approach, *Nutr. Clin. Pract.*, 16, 258, 2001.
88. Lenart, S. and Polissar, N.L., Comparison of 2 methods for postpyloric placement of enteral feeding tubes, *Am. J. Crit. Care*, 12, 357, 2003.
89. Salasidis, R., Fleiszer, T., and Johnston, R., Air insufflation technique of enteral tube insertion: A randomized, controlled trial, *Crit. Care Med.*, 26, 1036, 1998.
90. Boivin, M., Levy, H., and Hayes, J., A multicenter, prospective study of the placement of transpyloric feeding tubes with assistance of a magnetic device. The Magnet-Guided Enteral Feeding Tube Study Group, *J. Parenter. Enteral Nutr.*, 24, 304, 2000.
91. Heiselman, D.E., Hofer, T., and Vidovich, R.R., Enteral feeding tube placement success with intravenous metoclopramide administration in ICU patients, *Chest*, 107, 1686, 1995.
92. Kittinger, J.W., Sandler, R.S., and Heizer, W.D., Efficacy of metoclopramide as an adjunct to duodenal placement of small-bore feeding tubes: A randomized, placebo-controlled, double-blind study, *J. Parenter. Enteral Nutr.*, 11, 33, 1987.
93. Kalliafas, S., Choban, P.S., Ziegler, D. et al., Erythromycin facilitates postpyloric placement of nasoduodenal feeding tubes in intensive care unit patients: Randomized, double-blinded, placebo-controlled trial, *J. Parenter. Enteral Nutr.*, 20, 385, 1996.
94. Taylor, B., Everett, S., and Muckova, N., Bedside small bowel placement in over 1200 critically ill patients: A success story, *Crit. Care Med. (Suppl.)*, 31, A85, 2003.

14 Parenteral Formulations

Michael Christensen

CONTENTS

INTRODUCTION

Parenteral nutrition (PN) has been a lifesaving procedure for patients with short gut syndrome, very-low-birth-weight infants, and certain other patients with gut failure. The modern era of PN began in the 1960s with the development of a technique to catheterize the central venous circulation and the demonstration that normal growth and development could be achieved in immature dogs fed exclusively with PN (Dudrick et al., 1968; Wilmore and Dudrick, 1968). The placement of a central venous catheter allowed the provision of hypertonic PN formulas that were rapidly diluted in the high-flow central vein. Prior to this time, the provision of PN was limited to isotonic formulas or modestly hypertonic formulas that could be infused through a peripheral vein. The principle limitations were the large fluid volumes necessary to meet the nutritional needs of the patients leading to fluid overload and the loss of peripheral venous access in patients who required prolonged support with PN. Considerable knowledge about the provision of PN has evolved over the past 50 years. There is now a multitude of commercial products, amino acids, carbohydrates, fat emulsions, electrolytes, minerals, vitamins, and trace elements, available for inclusion in PN formulations. Unfortunately, one of the greatest challenges in the provision of PN has been the growing drug shortage crisis that has affected nearly every component of the PN formulation (Holcombe, 2012).

PN is indicated when the enteral route is inadequate, when the enteral route should be avoided, or when the enteral route may be harmful. A number of meta-analyses of the use of PN in different patient populations including intensive care, oncology, liver disease, and surgery have not shown a benefit and have generally reported increased complications; therefore, careful selection of patients for PN is necessary (Heyland et al., 1998, 2001; Koretz et al., 2001; McGeer et al., 1990; Torosian, 1999). Nutrition societies have published guidelines for the use of PN in various adult and pediatric patients (2009, 2011; Bozzetti and Forbes, 2009).

WATER

Water is the most abundant constituent of the human body accounting for approximately 60% of total body weight in the adult and 70%–75% in the infant. Water balance depends on fluid intake, urine and stool output, metabolic and respiratory rates, evaporative losses from skin, and body temperature. Fluid requirements vary depending on the age of the patient and concurrent disease. Normal fluid requirements are summarized in Table 14.1, which range from 150 mL/kg in preterm neonates to 30 mL/kg in normal adults (Holliday and Segar, 1957). Factors that increase fluid requirement included elevated body temperature, burn injury, fistula drainage, nasogastric losses, and diarrhea. In infants, radiant warmers and phototherapy increase evaporative losses. Factors that decrease fluid requirements include renal failure, congenital or congestive heart failure, and respiratory disorders. In evaluating fluid amounts in PN, it is important to consider fluids administered with parenteral drug administration, other intravenous fluids, and enteral feedings or oral intake.

ENERGY SOURCES

Intravenous sources of energy include carbohydrates, protein, and fat. The dietary reference intake in the adult diet is 45%–65% carbohydrate, 20%–35% fat, and 10%–35% protein (Dietary Reference Intake, 2005). The provision of optimal nutrition support to hospitalized patients is necessary to maintain or improve nutritional status while at the same time preventing complications associated with overfeeding or underfeeding. Measurement of energy expenditure using direct or indirect calorimetry or the double-labeled water method provides the most accurate method for determining energy requirements. These methods are expensive, time consuming, and require trained personnel. A number of predictive equations have been developed as more practical means for estimating energy requirements. The accuracy and applicability of these equations have been questioned (Elizabeth Weekes, 2007; Flancbaum et al., 1999; MacDonald and Hildebrandt, 2003; Reeves and Capra, 2003). Clinicians must carefully choose the method used for estimating energy requirement, understanding the degree of accuracy that is acceptable and the limitations in their application.

TABLE 14.1
Normal Fluid Requirements

<2.5 kg	150 mL/kg
2.5–10 kg	100 mL/kg
10–20 kg	1000 mL + 50 mL/kg (for each kg >10 kg)
≥20 kg	1500 mL ± 20 mL/kg (for each kg ≥20 kg)

Dextrose

Dextrose is the most common energy source used in PN. Anhydrous dextrose provides 4 kcal/g, whereas dextrose in aqueous solution is hydrated lowering the caloric content to 3.4 kcal/g. Commercial dextrose solution concentrations are available from 2.5% to 70%. Many institutions have the availability of an automated compounding system and predominately use 70% dextrose that can be admixed with sterile water to create a wide range of lower final dextrose concentrations. Dextrose solutions have an acidic pH of 3.5–5.5.

PN solutions with final dextrose concentrations less than 12.5% usually can be infused into a peripheral vein. The use of peripheral PN depends on having suitable veins that can tolerate high volume rates and modestly hyperosmolar solutions. In general, peripheral PN should be limited to a short period of time, usually less than 1 week. The osmolality of peripheral PN solutions can reach 800–900 mOsm/L, making these solutions relatively hypertonic. Coadministration of fat emulsion with the peripheral PN solution or the addition of heparin to the peripheral PN solution may increase the duration of the peripheral catheter (Barrington, 2000; Kamala et al., 2002; Phelps and Cochran, 1989; Phelps and Helms, 1987; Randolph et al., 1998; Shah and Shah, 2001). Dextrose concentration exceeding 12.5% or a total osmolality exceeding 900 mOsm/L should be infused into a central vein.

Lipids

Intravenous fat emulsions are used widely in PN as a source of energy and essential fatty acids (Dupont and Carpentier, 1999). The first fat emulsion introduced into the United States that contained cottonseed oil was withdrawn from the market soon after its introduction due to severe adverse reactions. Subsequently, a fat emulsion derived from soybean oil, which is high in long-chain triglycerides (LCTs), notably linolenic acid, was introduced and has been the principal fat emulsion in the United States. A safflower oil–based fat emulsion followed the soybean oil fat emulsion, but was withdrawn from the market in 2009. The most recent fat emulsion released in the United States is a combination of soybean and olive oil. Its approval and release were in response to recurring shortages of intravenous fat emulsions in the United States. Interestingly, this product was initially approved in 1975, but was never released in the United States until several decades later.

Fat emulsions are available in 10% (1.1 kcal/mL), 20% (2.0 kcal/mL), and 30% (3.0 kcal/mL). These products contain egg phospholipid as an emulsifying agent and glycerol to make the product isotonic. Outside the United States, there are a greater variety of fat sources included in the fat emulsion including olive oil (monounsaturated fatty acids), fish oil (n-3 polyunsaturated fatty acids [PUFAs]), and coconut oil (medium-chain triglycerides [MCTs]), as well as structured lipids. Representative fat emulsions are listed in Table 14.2. Structured lipid emulsions are manufactured triglycerides where medium-chain and long-chain fatty acids are esterified on the same glycerol backbone.

Fat emulsions are generally given continuously to infants, may be given intermittently to older children and adults, or included in a total nutrient admixture. To meet essential fatty acid requirements, only 2%–4% of the nonprotein calories need to be provided as essential fatty acid or about 10% as total fat. Adults usually receive 0.5–1.0 g/kg up to a maximum dose of 2.5 g/kg. Infants usually receive 2–3 g/kg up to a maximum dose of 4 g/kg (1981). In infants, lipids are usually started at 0.5–1.0 g/kg and advanced to 0.5–1 g/kg as tolerated. Slower titration schedules in preterm infants are often required because of the immaturity in clearance and metabolism pathways.

The currently available fat emulsions have a very different composition compared to lipids normally found in regular diet, infant formulas, or human milk (Uauy and Castillo, 2003). The 10% fat emulsion product provides twice the amount of phospholipid as the 20% when given in a gram equivalent amount. The excessive amount of phospholipid administered with the 10% fat emulsion has been associated with abnormal plasma lipid profile in infants (Haumont et al., 1989, 1992).

TABLE 14.2
Fatty Acid Composition of Intravenous Fat Emulsions

Fatty Acid Content % (Manufacturer)	Intralipid® 10%, 20%, 30% (Kabi Vitrum)	Liposyn III® 10%, 20%, 30% (Abbott)	Clinolipid® 20% (Baxter Healthcare)	Lipofundin® 10%, 20% (B. Braun)	ClinOleic® 20% (Baxter)	Omegaven® 10% (Fresenius Kabi)
Oil source	Soybean	Soybean	Soybean, olive	Soybean, coconut	Soybean, olive	Soybean, fish
Caprylic (C8:0)	—	—	—	27	—	—
Capric (C10:0)	—	—	—	18	—	—
Lauric (C12:0)	—	—	—	1	—	—
Myristic (C14:0)	—	—	—	—	—	4.9
Palmitic (C16:0)	10	10	13.4	16	13	10.7
Palmitoleic (C16:1n-7)	—	—	—	—	1	8.2
Stearic (C18:0)	4	4	2.8	3	3	2.4
Oleic (C18:1n-9)	21	21	61.9	12.5	60	12.3
Linoleic (C18:2n-6)	56	55	17.9	27	18	3.7
Linolenic (C18:3n-3)	8	8	2.4	3.5	2	1.3
Arachidonic (C20:4n-6)	1	—	—	0.5	0.3	2.6
Eicosapentaenoic (C20:5n-3)	—	—	—	—	—	18.8
Docosapentaenoic (C22:5n-3)	—	—	—	—	—	2.8
Docosahexaenoic (C22:6n-3)	—	—	—	—	—	16.5

Fat emulsions are prone to the formation of hydroperoxides on exposure to light, and phototherapy may enhance the formation of hydroperoxides (Helbock et al., 1993; Neuzil et al., 1995; Silvers et al., 2001; Torosian, 1999). Preterm infants have limited antioxidant reserves and may be at increased risk for oxidative damage. Protecting the fat emulsion from light has been advocated as a method to limit hydroperoxide formation (Baird, 2001). Current standards do not address the need for protecting the fat emulsion from light (Mirtallo et al., 2004).

The other major concerns with the administration of fat emulsion are the infection risk and the effect on immune function. Infection risk with the fungal organisms *Malassezia furfur* and *Staphylococcus epidermidis* has been reported with the use of fat emulsion (Avila-Figueroa et al., 1998; Freeman et al., 1990). There remains controversy regarding the modulation of immune function from the different oil sources (soy, fish, and olive oils and structured lipids) in lipid emulsions (Cury-Boaventura et al., 2008; Garnacho Montero et al., 1996; Guillou, 1993; Pomposelli and Bistrian, 1994; Suchner and Senftleben, 1994; Wanten, 2006a; Yaqoob, 1998). The content of PUFAs in fat emulsions, primarily the n-6 and n-3 series (precursors to different eicosanoids [leukotrienes, prostaglandins, and thromboxanes]), may alter the immune system, inflammation, and oxidant stress levels (Carpentier and Dupont, 2000; Wanten, 2006a,b).

Glycerol

Glycerol, a sugar alcohol that provides 4.3 cal/g, is a nonprotein caloric source in the PN product ProcalAmine® (B. Braun, Irvine, CA). ProcalAmine contains 3% amino acids and 3% glycerol premixed in 1 L containers (Table 14.3). This product is intended for short-term administration to postsurgical patients. ProcalAmine contains standard electrolytes that may not be appropriate for all patients. Glycerol as a nonprotein caloric source does offer an advantage over dextrose in that it does not require insulin for uptake into the cell. Postsurgical insulin-dependent patients had lower insulin requirements when given PN with glycerol as compared to glucose as the nonprotein caloric source (Freeman et al., 1983; Lev-Ran et al., 1987; Waxman et al., 1992). The potential benefits of short-term administration of the premixed solution must be weighed against the infusion of standard intravenous fluids or peripheral PN. Although the premixed solution is convenient, it likely does not offer a significant advantage (Sun et al., 2006).

Energy Utilization of Parenteral Carbohydrate Source

The maximum infusion of dextrose in patients receiving PN depends on the age of the patient and the underlying clinical condition. Net fat synthesis occurred when parenteral glucose intake exceeded 12.5 mg/kg/min in postsurgical newborns and 12.6 mg/kg/min in stable infants (Bresson et al., 1989; Jones et al., 1993). In critically ill children, maximal glucose oxidation occurred at glucose intakes of 5 mg/kg/min (Coss-Bu et al., 2001; Sheridan et al., 1998). The fraction of exogenous glucose that was oxidized decreased as glucose infusion rates increased up to an infusion rate of 8 mg/kg/min. Children with lipogenesis had an average glucose intake of 8.5 mg/kg/min (Coss-Bu et al., 2001). These results in critically ill children are similar to the glucose oxidation rates reported in critically ill adults. In adults, increasing glucose infusion rates from 4 to 8 mg/kg/min is associated with increased glucose oxidation rates, although efficiency of oxidation decreases (Burke et al., 1979; Wolfe et al., 1980). When glucose infusion rates exceed 9 mg/kg/min, there was no significant increase in glucose oxidation (Wolfe et al., 1980). Glucose infusion rates in excess of the oxidative capacity will enter nonoxidative metabolic pathways including glycolysis, glycogenesis, and lipogenesis. Alternately, excessive glucose infusion rates can lead to hyperglycemia and glycosuria, which has been associated with higher morbidity and mortality rates in critically ill adults (Finney et al., 2003; Kumar et al., 2011; van den Berghe et al., 2001, 2003).

TABLE 14.3
Glycerol-Containing Amino Acid Solution

Preparation	**ProcalAmine 3% (3% Amino Acid and 3% Glycerin with Electrolytes)**
Manufacturer	**B. Braun**
Nitrogen g/100 mL	0.46
Essential amino acids (mg/100 mL)	
Histidine	85
Isoleucine	210
Leucine	270
Lysine	220
Methionine	160
Phenylalanine	170
Threonine	120
Tryptophan	46
Valine	200
Nonessential amino acids (mg/100 mL)	
Alanine	210
Arginine	290
Proline	340
Serine	180
Taurine	—
Tyrosine	—
N-acetyl-L-tyrosine	—
Glycine	420
Cysteine	<20
Glutamic acid	—
Aspartic acid	—
Electrolytes (mEq/L)	
Calcium	3
Sodium	35
Potassium	24
Magnesium	5
Chloride	41
Acetate	47
Phosphate (mmol/L)	3.5
mOsm/L	735
pH	6.5–7

PROTEIN SOURCES

Parenteral protein products have undergone considerable change during the past 50 years. The initial protein sources were hydrolysates of casein and fibrin. They could be produced in large quantities at reasonable cost and met most of the essential amino acid requirements of adults. Deficiencies of hydrolysates included the uncertain metabolic fate of peptides, the uncontrollable batch-to-batch variation in the hydrolysate composition, the occurrence of hyperammonemia (especially in infants, likely due to low arginine rather than preformed ammonia), and the occasional severe allergic-type reaction. Early crystalline amino acid formulations resulted in a profound hyperchloremic metabolic acidosis in infants that was less severe in older children and adults. This chapter will focus on standard and modified disease-specific amino acid products available in the United States; there are similar products by different manufacturers available outside the United States. Although there is widespread use of PN, there is little comparative efficacy research to guide the selection of standard and specialty amino acid solutions or their appropriate dosing (Yarandi et al., 2011).

Standard Adult

The amino acid composition of standard amino acid solutions have been based on high-quality dietary proteins such as egg white, but modified to replace glutamine and asparagine with glycine (Table 14.4). Standard amino acid solutions are intended to meet the protein needs of the stable adult. Standard amino acid solutions are available in concentrations ranging from 3.5% to 20% and are available with and without added electrolytes. More concentrated amino acid solutions are often used in pharmacies that have automated formulators and may be used in fluid-restricted patients. Amino acid solutions that contain electrolytes are best used in stable patients who do not have unusual electrolyte requirements. The standard amino acid solutions may be inadequate in certain disease states and during infancy. This has led to the development of modified disease-specific amino acid solutions as well as amino acid solutions for use in infants.

Renal Failure

Modified amino acid solutions have been formulated for patients with renal failure (Table 14.5). These products contain predominately essential amino acids as well as histidine. One product also contains arginine, which is important in the urea cycle. The essential amino acid solutions for renal failure were based on the principles established for treating patients with chronic renal failure with a low-protein diet and an essential amino acid supplement. Because of underlying differences in the metabolic response between chronic and acute renal failures, essential-only amino acid solutions may not meet protein needs. The benefits of modified amino acid solutions for renal failure over standard amino acids in acute renal failure remain controversial (Abel et al., 1973; Feinstein et al., 1981; Mirtallo et al., 1982). Patients with acute renal failure are highly variable in terms of hypermetabolism and hypercatabolism as well as renal function. Protein and energy requirements will depend on their underlying disease state, rather than their renal failure. Nutrition therapy will need to be individualized given the degree of critical illness, use of renal replacement therapy, and nutritional status.

Hepatic Failure

There is only one modified amino acid solution approved for use in patients with hepatic failure (Table 14.5). The hepatic failure amino acid solution (HepatAmine®, B. Braun, Irvine, CA) contains high amounts of branched-chain amino acids (BCAAs) and low amounts of aromatic amino acid (AAA) solutions. The basis for the formulation of the hepatic failure amino solution emerges from the false neurotransmitter and unified theories of hepatic encephalopathy (Fischer and Baldessarini, 1971; James et al., 1979b). Patients with hepatic encephalopathy have elevated plasma AAAs because of decreased liver metabolism and decreased plasma BCAAs because of peripheral metabolism (Campollo et al., 1992; Cascino et al., 1978; Ferenci and Wewalka, 1978; James et al., 1979a; Watanabe et al., 1982). The reduction in the BCAA/AAA ratio favors brain uptake of AAA because they compete with BCAA to cross the blood–brain barrier. The AAA-derived neuroamines (phenylethylamine, tyramine, phenylethanolamine, octopamine, serotonin, and tryptamine) are elevated in the blood and in the CNS and have been associated with hepatic encephalopathy. The traditional approach to nutritional intervention in patients with hepatic encephalopathy was protein restriction. Patients with hepatic encephalopathy often have protein–calorie malnutrition. When the diet is restrictive, undernutrition and its associated complications further compromise patients with liver failure. Most patients can be supported with standard amino acid formulation with careful attention to protein intake. For patients who decompensate while receiving modest doses of standard amino

TABLE 14.4
Representative Standard Amino Acid Solutions

Preparation	Aminosyn® 10%	Aminosyn II® 10%	Aminosyn II 15%	FreAmine III® 10%	Clinisol® 15%	Travasol® 10%	Prosol® 20%
Manufacturer	Hospira	Hospira	Hospira	B. Braun	B. Braun	Baxter	Baxter
Essential amino acids (mg/100 mL)							
Histidine	300	300	450	280	894	480	1180
Isoleucine	720	660	990	690	749	600	1080
Leucine	940	1000	1500	910	1040	730	1080
Lysine	720	1050	1575	730	1180	580	1350
Methionine	400	172	258	530	749	400	760
Phenylalanine	440	298	447	400	1040	560	1000
Threonine	520	400	600	150	749	420	980
Tryptophan	160	200	300	660	250	180	320
Valine	800	500	750		960	580	1440
Nonessential amino acids (mg/100 mL)							
Alanine	1280	993	1490	710	2170	2070	2760
Arginine	980	1018	1527	950	1470	1150	19360
Proline	860	722	1083	1120	894	680	1340
Serine	420	530	795	590	592	500	1020
Taurine	—	—	—	—	—	—	50
Tyrosine	44	—	—	—	39	40	—
N-acetyl-L-tyrosine	—	270	405	—	—	—	—
Glycine	1280	500	750	—	1040	1030	2060
Glutamic acid	—	738	1107	—	749	—	1020
Aspartic acid	—	700	1050	—	434	—	600
Electrolytes mEq/L							
Sodium	—	38	50	10	—	—	—
Potassium	5.4	—	—	—	—	—	—
Chloride	—	—	—	—	—	40	—
Acetate	147	71.8	107.6	89	127	88	140
Phosphate (mmol/L)	—	—	—	10	—	—	—
mOsm/L	932	840	1270	950	1357	1000	1835
pH	5.2	5.8	5.8	6.5	6	6	6

TABLE 14.5
Representative Modified Amino Acid Solutions

Preparation	FreAmine HBC® 6.9%	Aminosyn HBC® 7%	HepatAmine 8%	Aminosyn RF® 5.2%	NephrAmine® 5.4%
Manufacturer	B. Braun	Hospira	B. Braun	Hospira	B. Braun
Essential amino acids (mg/100 mL)					
Histidine	160	154	240	429	250
Isoleucine	760	789	900	462	560
Leucine	1370	1576	1100	726	880
Lysine	410	265	610	535	640
Methionine	250	206	100	726	880
Phenylalanine	320	228	100	726	880
Threonine	200	272	450	330	400
Tryptophan	90	88	66	165	200
Valine	880	789	840	528	640
Nonessential amino acids (mg/100 mL)					
Alanine	400	660	770	—	—
Arginine	580	507	600	600	—
Proline	630	448	800	—	—
Serine	330	221	500	—	—
Taurine	—	—	—	—	—
Tyrosine	—	33	—	—	—
N-acetyl-L-tyrosine	—	—	—	—	—
Glycine	330	660	900	—	—
Glutamic acid	—	—	—	—	—
Aspartic acid	—	—	—	—	—
Electrolytes mEq/L					
Sodium	10	—	10	—	5
Potassium	—	—	—	—	—
Chloride	≤3	—	<3	—	<3
Acetate	57	71	62	113	44
Phosphate (mmol/L)	—	—	10	—	—
mOsm/L	620	623	785	427	435
pH	5.5	5.2	6.5	5.2	6.5

acids, use of the hepatic failure amino acid solution may be considered. Clinical studies support that the hepatic failure amino acid formulation improved hepatic encephalopathy (Cerra et al., 1985; Egberts et al., 1985; Marchesini et al., 2003; Michel et al., 1985; Naylor et al., 1989; Rocchi et al., 1985; Vilstrup et al., 1990). A Cochrane review found a 1.3-fold improvement in hepatic encephalopathy, but no significant difference in time to improvement or survival (Als-Nielsen et al., 2003). Because the hepatic failure amino acid solution is more costly than standard amino acid solutions, strict criteria should be implemented to prevent inappropriate use.

Trauma/Stress

Trauma, sepsis, or major surgery results in profound hypercatabolism. During the catabolic state, there is a significant breakdown of skeletal muscles resulting in increased release of amino acids to meet the increased demand for hepatic protein synthesis and increased metabolism of BCAAs as a preferred local energy source. Providing BCAAs, notably leucine, reduced skeletal muscle catabolism and increased skeletal muscle and hepatic protein synthesis

(Buse and Reid, 1975). Two modified amino acid products have been formulated with a high content of BCAAs (Table 14.5). Studies of BCAA-enriched PN solutions have not demonstrated a decreased catabolic rate or a reduction in morbidity or mortality (Bower et al., 1986; Cerra et al., 1985, 1987; Kuhl et al., 1990; von Meyenfeldt et al., 1990). Although there are theoretical reasons for the use of BCAA-enriched solutions, they have not been shown to be superior to standard amino acid solutions.

Pediatric

Infants have a number of immature enzymatic metabolic pathways making certain amino acids considered nonessential for adults essential in infants. The most notable inactive amino acid metabolic pathways are the conversion of phenylalanine to tyrosine and the transsulfuration pathway. When standard amino acid solutions are administered to infants, aberrant plasma amino acids have been observed including elevated plasma concentrations of methionine and phenylalanine and low concentrations of tyrosine, cysteine, and taurine (Winters et al., 1977). Three pediatric amino acid solutions are available in the United States (Table 14.6). One pediatric amino acid solution

TABLE 14.6
Representative Pediatric Amino Acid Solutions

Preparation	**Aminosyn-PF 10%**	**TrophAmine 10%**	**Premasol 10%**
Manufacturer	**Hospira**	**B. Braun**	**Baxter**
Essential amino acids (mg/100 mL)			
Histidine	312	480	480
Isoleucine	760	820	820
Leucine	1200	1400	1400
Lysine	677	820	820
Methionine	180	340	340
Phenylalanine	427	480	0.48
Threonine	512	420	420
Tryptophan	180	200	200
Valine	673	780	780
Nonessential amino acids (mg/100 mL)			
Alanine	698	540	540
Arginine	1227	1200	1200
Proline	812	680	680
Serine	495	380	380
Taurine	70	25	25
Tyrosine	44	24	24
N-acetyl-L-tyrosine	—	240	240
Glycine	385	360	360
Glutamic acid	820	500	500
Aspartic acid	527	320	320
Electrolytes (mEq/L)			
Sodium	—	5	0
Potassium	—	—	
Chloride	—	<3	<3
Acetate	46	97	94
Phosphate (mmol/L)	—	—	
mOsm/L	788	788	865
pH	5.5	5.5	5.5

(TrophAmine®, B. Braun, Irvine, CA) was designed to normalize plasma amino acids to a postprandial reference range developed in healthy 1-month-old breastfed infants (Heird et al., 1987, 1988; Winters et al., 1977; Wu et al., 1986). This product compared to a standard amino acid solution was associated with higher weight gain and nitrogen balance in postsurgical infants (Helms et al., 1987). A generic version (Premasol®, Baxter, Deerfield, IL) has been introduced. Another pediatric amino acid solution (Aminosyn-PF®, Abbott, Abbott Park, IL) is a modification of their standard amino acid solution, incorporating additional amino acids thought to be essential in infants, including glutamic acid, aspartic acid, and taurine; reducing alanine, glycine, methionine, and valine; and increasing leucine and arginine.

Cysteine

Preterm and newborn infants have a functional immaturity in the transsulfuration pathway leading to impairment in the metabolism of sulfur-containing amino acids. Low cysteine concentrations have been reported in infants receiving PN containing minimal amounts of cysteine. The initial pediatric amino acid solution released in the United States was designed to have cysteine added to the PN solution at the time of preparation. Cysteine is not included in the pediatric amino acid solution because it is not stable in solution for prolonged periods of time. When cysteine is included in the amino acid solution, it forms the dimer cystine, which has limited solubility in solution and precipitates out of solution. Cysteine HCl is available as a 50 mg/mL solution and is added to the PN solution at a dose of 40 mg/g of amino acids. Cysteine addition to a pediatric amino acid solution resulted in higher taurine levels and was necessary to achieve plasma taurine concentration within the normal reference range for infants (Helms et al., 1999). Short-term cysteine supplementation improves nitrogen balance, but the long-term effect on growth is not known (Soghier and Brion, 2006).

Glutamine

Glutamine is a nonessential amino acid but may be essential in certain clinical settings (i.e., critical illness) because the body is unable to synthesize sufficient amounts (Buchman, 2001; Weitzel and Wischmeyer, 2010b). Glutamine is not included in parenteral amino acid solutions because of limited solubility (3.5 g/dL), limited final concentration (1.5 g/dL), and instability (degradation with heat sterilization and prolonged storage), and it must be extemporaneously compounded and added to the PN solution (Vanek et al., 2011). The dose of parenteral glutamine has ranged from 0.26 to 0.57 g/kg per day with higher dosing appearing to be more effective (Novak et al., 2002). Recent meta-analysis has supported the beneficial effect of parenteral glutamine supplementation in critically ill postsurgical and ventilator-dependent patients on mortality, length of stay, and infectious morbidity (Weitzel and Wischmeyer, 2010a). Glutamine supplementation of PN has not been shown to be of benefit in other critically ill patients: bone marrow transplant, acute pancreatitis, burns, and preterm infants (Moe-Byrne et al., 2012; Tubman et al., 2008). The use of parenteral glutamine in the United States is limited because of the lack of availability of commercial glutamine products.

Dipeptides

The problem of free glutamine has been overcome by the synthesis of glutamine-containing dipeptides, alanyl-glutamine and glycyl-glutamine, which are available outside the United States. After the initial studies of compounded free glutamine solutions, most clinical studies have utilized one of the glutamine dipeptides (Çekmen et al., 2011; Grau et al., 2011; Tzaneva and Ajderian, 2009; Wang et al., 2010). One professional organization has encouraged the approval of commercial glutamine dipeptides in the United States (Vanek et al., 2011).

TABLE 14.7
Normal Daily Electrolyte and Mineral Requirements

	Adults	Infants and Children
Sodium	50–250 mEq	2–4 mEq/kg
Potassium	30–200 mEq	2–3 mEq/kg
Chloride	50–250 mEq	2–3 mEq/kg
Phosphate	10–40 mmole	0.5–2 mmol/kg
Calcium	10–20 mEq	1–3 mEq/kg
Magnesium	10–30 mEq	0.25–0.5 mEq/kg

ELECTROLYTES AND MINERALS

The management of electrolyte and mineral status in acutely ill patients receiving PN remains the most challenging aspect of providing PN. Once a patient's estimated caloric and protein needs have been met through the titration of the PN solution, most of the clinician's effort is focused on maintaining electrolyte and mineral status. Electrolytes may be added to PN solutions using single or multiple electrolyte formulations. Multiple electrolyte formulations are most appropriately used in patients who have normal organ function and normal serum electrolytes. The usual requirements of electrolytes and minerals are listed in Table 14.7. Sodium and potassium are available as chloride, acetate, and phosphate salts and magnesium is available as a sulfate salt. Calcium gluconate is the preferred salt for PN, but is also available as calcium chloride. The concern for calcium phosphate precipitation limits the amount of calcium and phosphate that can be added to PN solutions. This potential problem is even greater if calcium chloride is substituted for calcium gluconate. Therefore, preterm neonates, who have the highest requirements for both calcium and phosphate, have the greatest risk of calcium phosphate precipitation in PN solutions. Outside the United States, organic phosphates are available that have a much greater compatibly with calcium.

VITAMINS

Parenteral multivitamin products (Table 14.8) have been formulated according to the recommendations of the American Medical Association National Advisory Group (AMA-NAG) in adult and pediatric patients (1979b; Greene et al., 1988). The Food and Drug Administration (FDA) Division of Metabolic and Endocrine Drug Products and the AMA's Division of Personal and Public Health Policy sponsored a workshop in 1985 that led to recommended changes to adult multivitamin products. These included an increase in the dosage of vitamins B1, B6, C, and folic acid as well as the addition of vitamin K (2000b). The importance of the addition of parenteral vitamins to PN solutions has been highlighted by a number of national shortages of parenteral adult and pediatric multivitamins. The most serious consequence of the shortage was the development of refractory lactic acidosis due to thiamine deficiency resulting in significant morbidity and mortality (1997). Notably, there continues to be a lack of parenteral multivitamin products formulated to meet the unique needs of preterm neonates. One concern with the current multiple vitamin preparations is vitamin D deficiency in patients receiving long-term PN (Thomson and Duerksen, 2011). One recommendation is for the availability of a parenteral vitamin D product for use in PN-dependent patients who do not respond to oral vitamin D (Vanek et al., 2012).

TRACE ELEMENTS

Trace elements are essential micronutrients that are necessary cofactors for the function of a number of enzymatic systems. These are available as single entity and multiple trace element products. The AMA-NAG has published guidelines for four trace elements known to be important

TABLE 14.8
Multivitamin Preparations

	Current Adult Formulation	Pediatric Formulation
Fat-soluble vitamins		
Vitamin A	3300 IU	2300 IU
Vitamin D	200 IU	400 IU
Vitamin E	10 IU	7 IU
Vitamin K	150	200 mcg
Water-soluble vitamins		
Thiamine (B1)	6 mg	1.2 mg
Riboflavin (B2)	3.6 mg	1.4 mg
Pyridoxine (B6)	6 mg	1 mg
Cyanocobalamin	5 mcg	1 mcg
Ascorbic acid (C)	200 mg	80 mg
Niacin (B3)	40 mg	17 mg
Biotin	60 mg	20 mg
Folic acid	600 mcg	140 mcg
Pantothenic acid (B5)	15 mg	5 mg

to human nutrition (1979a, Greene et al., 1988). The recommended amounts for zinc, copper, manganese, and chromium are listed in Table 14.9. Selenium may also be an important trace element that should be considered for addition to PN solutions (Baptista et al., 1984; Hunt et al., 1984). Guidelines for the supplementation of molybdenum and iodine have not been established. Iron is an important element that is not routinely added to PN solutions, but should be considered in patients who are receiving long-term parental nutrition and unable to take oral iron supplementation.

Zinc requirements are increased in metabolic stress secondary to increased urinary excretion and in gastrointestinal diseases secondary to increased ostomy, fistula, or diarrheal losses. Manganese and copper are excreted via the biliary tract and should be restricted or withheld in patients with cholestatic liver disease. Zinc, chromium, and selenium are renally excreted and restriction or elimination may be needed with impaired renal function. Evidence is accumulating that the amount of contamination of chromium in PN solutions makes addition to PN unnecessary or the dose should be dramatically reduced (Moukarzel et al., 1992; Mouser et al., 1999). Recommended changes in commercially multiple trace element products have been made by the American Society for Parenteral and Enteral Nutrition (ASPEN) (Vanek et al., 2012).

TABLE 14.9
Guidelines for Daily Trace Elements

	Adults	Infants/Children
Zinc	2.5–4.0 mg	50–500 mcg/kg[a] (max 5000 mcg)
Copper	0.5–1.5 mg	20 mcg/kg
Manganese	0.15–0.8 mg	2–10 mcg/kg
Chromium	10–15 mcg	0.2 mcg/kg (max 5 mcg)
Selenium	40–80 mcg	1–3 mcg/kg

[a] Premature, 450–500 mcg/kg; infants < 3 months, 250 mcg/kg; infants > 3 months, 50 mcg/kg.

Aluminum

Aluminum is the most abundant metal in the earth's crust and is ubiquitous in its distribution, but has no known biological function. It is nearly impossible to completely prevent exposure because it is a contaminant in most parenteral products administered to patients. The accumulation of aluminum in human tissue is well recognized in certain patient populations. Aluminum contamination is associated with osteomalacia, encephalopathy, and microcytic anemia and may contribute to cholestasis in infants. Patients with impaired renal function and neonates are at the greatest risk for exposure to unsafe amounts of aluminum. Aluminum toxicity was first reported as an encephalopathy in adult patients on dialysis and subsequently in children with renal disease not on dialysis but receiving aluminum-containing phosphate binders (Baluarte et al., 1977; Foley et al., 1981; Polinsky and Gruskin, 1984; Sedman et al., 1984). High concentrations of aluminum were found in the gray matter of dialysis patients (Alfrey et al., 1976). Subsequently high concentrations of aluminum have been found in the bone, urine, and plasma of adults and infants receiving PN (Koo et al., 1986a,b; Ott et al., 1983).

Manufacturers must include information regarding aluminum content present in large and small volume parenterals. The aluminum content of all large volume parenterals should not exceed 25 mcg/L, which must be stated on the product label (1998a, 2000b). There is no limit to the aluminum content in small volume parenteral, but the label must include a statement of the maximum aluminum content. The aluminum contamination of small volume parenterals is highly variable ranging up to 28,000 mcg/L (Driscoll and Driscoll, 2005). The maximum intake of aluminum that has been deemed safe is 5 mcg/kg/day. Unfortunately, the estimated aluminum exposure from PN solutions basing from the aluminum content from the product label will exceed this safe limit in adults two- to threefold and more than 20-fold in infants (Driscoll and Driscoll, 2005). Using the product label to estimate aluminum content may significantly overestimate the amount of aluminum in PN solutions; however, the lower measured aluminum content still exceeded the safe recommended amount of <5 mcg/kg/day (Poole et al., 2010, 2011; Speerhas and Seidner, 2007).

PARENTERAL NUTRITION SOLUTION ORDER

PN is one of the most complicated pharmaceutical products administered to patients. The complexity of this solution makes it prone to errors, both in the prescribing as well as in the preparation (Mirtallo, 2012). Safe practices emphasize the use of standardized processes including standard order forms for PN to reduce potential errors (Kochevar et al., 2007; Mirtallo et al., 2004). Examples of PN order forms are provided in the safe practices for PN guidelines (Mirtallo et al., 2004). The order form should be designed to meet the unique needs of the practitioners and patient population of the institution. It can be fairly rigid in allowing the prescription of a few standardized PN solutions with only minimal additions allowed or a flexible order form that identifies the major components of the PN solution with the daily amounts written in by the practitioner. A number of institutions use the back of the PN order form to provide specific instructions and general guidelines for writing PN orders. Institutions must have written policies and procedures for the ordering and preparing of PN solutions and monitoring patients requiring PN. Prior to initiating PN, it is important to confirm the location of the venous access device. The order form must indicate if the PN solution is to be administered via a central or peripheral catheter. PN solution orders must be written or reviewed on a daily basis.

PREPARATION OF PARENTERAL NUTRITION SOLUTIONS

Typically, PN solutions contain 2.5%–5% amino acids and 10%–25% dextrose, plus electrolytes, minerals, vitamins, and trace elements sufficient to meet the patient's estimated daily requirements. Intravenous fat emulsions offer a concentrated source of calories and can be used as a source of essential fatty acids. In some medical centers and in home PN programs, the fat emulsion is added directly to the PN solution (Brown et al., 1986). Manual or automated methods of PN preparation are available. The manual method allows the pharmacist to decide the order of mixing and must be carefully undertaken to avoid potential incompatibilities. Manufacturers of automated compounders should provide the compounding sequence to ensure safety and compatibility.

PN solutions should be prepared in the pharmacy by appropriately trained staff using strict aseptic procedures and a laminar airflow hood. Although the hypertonicity of the solutions is not ideal for growth of many bacterial organisms, some pathogens such as *Candida albicans* can readily proliferate in these solutions at room temperature (Brennan et al., 1971; Goldmann et al., 1973). The total 24 h requirements for fluids and nutrients are generally prepared in a single container or occasionally in multiple containers depending on the volume of infusate. PN solutions should be refrigerated immediately if not administered to a patient soon after preparation.

The complex nature of PN solutions including the amino acid–dextrose solutions (two in one) and total nutrient admixtures (three in one) containing the intravenous fat emulsion requires careful attention to stability and compatibility issues. Total nutrient admixtures add an additional level of complexity. Acid pH, di- and trivalent cations, and trace elements can be disruptive to the emulsion. Only total nutrition admixture formulations that have been well documented should be used exactly as described. Proper preparation instructions should be obtained directly from the manufacturer of the amino acids and fat emulsion.

The American Society of Health-System Pharmacists (ASHP) and ASPEN have published quality assurance guidelines on the preparation of sterile products and safe practices related to PN (1998b; 2000a; Mirtallo et al., 2004). These guidelines emphasize policies and procedures for all personnel involved in the preparation of PN, appropriate training and education, facilities and equipment requirements, process validation, expiration dating, and labeling requirements. Observing the physical appearance of the final admixture for gross particulate contamination is one of the most fundamental quality assurance measures that pharmacists routinely apply. For total nutrient admixtures, the products should be inspected for any visual signs of phase separation. When possible, quantitative end-product testing of the accuracy of all additives to the PN solution should be done on a routine basis.

COMPOUNDED VERSUS STANDARDIZED COMMERCIAL FORMULATIONS

The Joint Commission's National Patient Safety Goals in 2007 focused on using standard drug concentrations and limiting the number in use. The commission went on further to state that drugs should be dispensed in the most ready-to-use commercial formulation. There were concerns about the standardization of PN solutions and the use of commercial premixed solutions. A task force at ASPEN worked with the commission to clarify this issue, and the commission released an answer in its frequently asked questions that this recommendation may apply to PN, but PN is more complex than the drug solutions for which the goal was intended and that standardized PN solutions were not required under the goal (Kochevar et al., 2007).

Prior to the widespread implementation of automated compounding devices, most patients received standardized PN (1983, Seltzer et al., 1978). A standardized process is advocated including the consideration of standardized commercial products because PN is a complex solution that is prone to errors in the process of prescribing, compounding, labeling, and administering (Kochevar et al., 2007). The process of individualized PN, even using standardized process, is far more complicated than ordering a commercial premixed solution (Figures 14.1 and 14.2).

In the United States, there is one commercial source of premixed PN solutions in a two-compartment product with one compartment as amino acids and the second compartment as dextrose. There is a total of 32 products available with dextrose content from 5% to 25% (5%, 10%, 15%, 20%, and 25%) and amino acid content from 2.75% to 5% (2.75%, 4.25%, and 5%), with or without electrolytes in 1 and 2 L containers. A challenge to the use of premixed solutions is selecting which products to inventory since it will likely not be practical to inventory all products, and it is

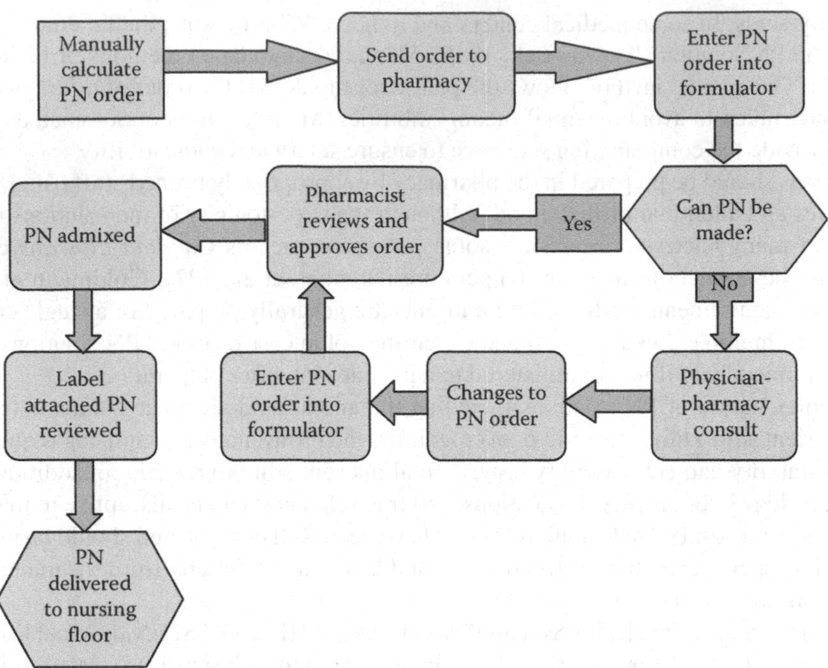

FIGURE 14.1 Process for ordering and preparing individualized PN solutions.

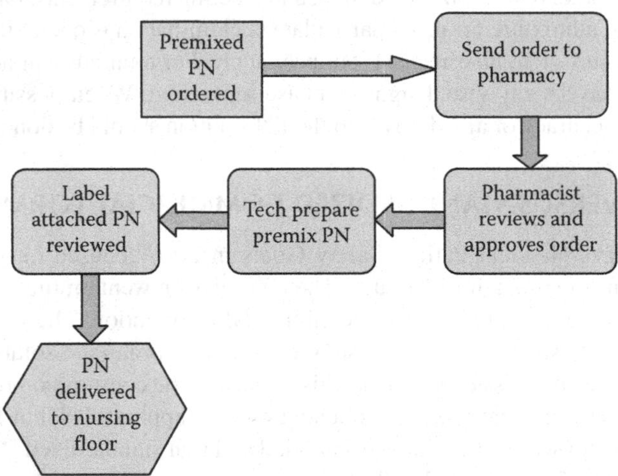

FIGURE 14.2 Process for ordering and preparing premixed PN solutions.

likely that some patients will have unique requirements that do not fit one of the available products. Outside the United States, three-compartment premixed products are available with the third compartment as lipid emulsion.

DRUG SHORTAGES

The growing drug shortage crisis threatens many aspects of patient care. The shortages have impacted every component of PN except dextrose and sterile water. Shortages have occurred for amino acids, electrolytes, minerals, multivitamins, trace elements (individual and combination), and lipid emulsion. These shortages have resulted in harm to patients; severe lactic acidosis from thiamine deficiency during multivitamin shortages has recurred over the past 30 years, and death from *Serratia*-contaminated extemporaneously compounded parenteral amino acids (1997; Cho et al., 2004; Cohen, 2012; Velez et al., 1985). The continually changing component shortages have put a great strain on the safe practice of providing PN, potentially leading to suboptimal care for some patients and the risk of harm to others. These shortages have led in multiple changes in the source or concentration of PN components (i.e., 3% saline in place of 23.4% saline) that could lead to errors in the configuration of the automated compounder (Holcombe, 2012). The current drug shortage crisis poses a significant risk to the entire PN process, from the procurement of high-quality products to the ordering of PN solution to the frequent changing in products used in the compounding of the PN formulation. This necessitates close communications, vigilance, and continuous assessment of procedures to ensure the safe delivery of PN to patients.

REFERENCES

Abel, R. M., Beck, C. H. Jr., Abbott, W. M., Ryan, J. A. Jr., Barnett, G. O., and Fischer, J. E. 1973. Improved survival from acute renal failure after treatment with intravenous essential L-amino acids and glucose. Results of a prospective, double-blind study. *N Engl J Med*, 288, 695–699.

Alfrey, A. C., Legendre, G. R., and Kaehny, W. D. 1976. The dialysis encephalopathy syndrome. Possible aluminum intoxication. *N Engl J Med*, 294, 184–188.

Als-Nielsen, B., Koretz, R. L., Kjaergard, L. L., and Gluud, C. 2003. Branched-chain amino acids for hepatic encephalopathy. *Cochrane Database Syst Rev*, CD001939.

AMA Department of Foods and Nutrition. 1979a. Guidelines for essential trace element preparations for parenteral use. A statement by an expert panel. *JAMA*, 241, 2051–2054.

American Medical Association Department of Foods and Nutrition. 1979b. Multivitamin preparations for parenteral use. A statement by the Nutrition Advisory Group. *JPEN J Parenter Enteral Nutr*, 3, 258–262.

American Academy of Pediatrics. Committee on Nutrition. 1981. Use of Intravenous fat emulsions in pediatric patients. *Pediatrics*, 68, 738–743.

American Society of Health System Pharmacists. 2000a. ASHP guidelines on quality assurance for pharmacy-prepared sterile products. *Am J Health Syst Pharm*, 57, 1150–1169.

American Society for Parenteral and Enteral Nutrition (ASPEN). 2009. Clinical guidelines for the use of parenteral and enteral nutrition in adult and pediatric patients. *J Parenter Enteral Nutr*, 33, 255–259.

A.S.P.E.N. 2011. Guidelines and Standards Library.

Avila-Figueroa, C., Goldmann, D. A., Richardson, D. K., Gray, J. E., Ferrari, A., and Freeman, J. 1998. Intravenous lipid emulsions are the major determinant of coagulase-negative staphylococcal bacteremia in very low birth weight newborns. *Pediatr Infect Dis J*, 17, 10–17.

Baird, L. L. 2001. Protecting TPN and lipid infusions from light: Reducing hydroperoxides in NICU patients. *Neonatal Netw*, 20, 17–22.

Baluarte, H. J., Gruskin, A. B., Hiner, L. B., Foley, C. M., and Grover, W. D. 1977. Encephalopathy in children with chronic renal failure. *Proc Clin Dial Transplant Forum*, 7, 95–98.

Baptista, R. J., Bistrian, B. R., Blackburn, G. L., Miller, D. G., Champagne, C. D., and Buchanan, L. 1984. Utilizing selenious acid to reverse selenium deficiency in total parenteral nutrition patients. *Am J Clin Nutr*, 39, 816–820.

Barrington, K. J. 2000. Umbilical artery catheters in the newborn: Effects of heparin. *Cochrane Database Syst Rev*, CD000507.

Bower, R. H., Muggia-Sullam, M., Vallgren, S., Hurst, J. M., Kern, K. A., Lafrance, R., and Fischer, J. E. 1986. Branched chain amino acid-enriched solutions in the septic patient. A randomized, prospective trial. *Ann Surg*, 203, 13–20.

Bozzetti, F. and Forbes, A. 2009. The ESPEN clinical practice Guidelines on Parenteral Nutrition: Present status and perspectives for future research. *Clin Nutr*, 28, 359–364.

Brennan, M. F., O'connell, R. C., Rosol, J. A., and Kundsin, R. 1971. The growth of Candida albicans in nutritive solutions given parenterally. *Arch Surg*, 103, 705–708.

Bresson, J. L., Narcy, P., Putet, G., Ricour, C., Sachs, C., and Rey, J. 1989. Energy substrate utilization in infants receiving total parenteral nutrition with different glucose to fat ratios. *Pediatr Res*, 25, 645–648.

Brown, R., Quercia, R. A., and Sigman, R. 1986. Total nutrient admixture: A review. *JPEN J Parenter Enteral Nutr*, 10, 650–658.

Buchman, A. L. 2001. Glutamine: Commercially essential or conditionally essential? A critical appraisal of the human data. *Am J Clin Nutr*, 74, 25–32.

Burke, J. F., Wolfe, R. R., Mullany, C. J., Mathews, D. E., and Bier, D. M. 1979. Glucose requirements following burn injury. Parameters of optimal glucose infusion and possible hepatic and respiratory abnormalities following excessive glucose intake. *Ann Surg*, 190, 274–285.

Buse, M. G. and Reid, S. S. 1975. Leucine. A possible regulator of protein turnover in muscle. *J Clin Invest*, 56, 1250–1261.

Campollo, O., Sprengers, D., and Mcintyre, N. 1992. The BCAA/AAA ratio of plasma amino acids in three different groups of cirrhotics. *Rev Invest Clin*, 44, 513–518.

Centers for Disease Control and Prevention (CDC). 1997. Lactic acidosis traced to thiamine deficiency related to nationwide shortage of multivitamins for total parenteral nutrition—United States. *MMWR Morb Mortal Wkly Rep*, 46, 523–528.

Carpentier, Y. A. and Dupont, I. E. 2000. Advances in intravenous lipid emulsions. *World J Surg*, 24, 1493–1497.

Cascino, A., Cangiano, C., Calcaterra, V., Rossi-Fanelli, F., and Capocaccia, L. 1978. Plasma amino acids imbalance in patients with liver disease. *Am J Dig Dis*, 23, 591–598.

Çekmen, N., Aydimathn, A., and Erdemli, Ö. 2011. The impact of L-alanyl-L-glutamine dipeptide supplemented total parenteral nutrition on clinical outcome in critically patients. *e-SPEN*, 6, e64–e67.

Cerra, F., Blackburn, G., Hirsch, J., Mullen, K., and Luther, W. 1987. The effect of stress level, amino acid formula, and nitrogen dose on nitrogen retention in traumatic and septic stress. *Ann Surg*, 205, 282–287.

Cerra, F. B., Cheung, N. K., Fischer, J. E., Kaplowitz, N., Schiff, E. R., Dienstag, J. L., Bower, R. H., Mabry, C. D., Leevy, C. M., and Kiernan, T. 1985. Disease-specific amino acid infusion (F080) in hepatic encephalopathy: A prospective, randomized, double-blind, controlled trial. *JPEN J Parenter Enteral Nutr*, 9, 288–295.

Cho, Y. P., Kim, K., Han, M. S., Jang, H. J., Kim, J. S., Kim, Y. H., and Lee, S. G. 2004. Severe lactic acidosis and thiamine deficiency during total parenteral nutrition—Case report. *Hepatogastroenterology*, 51, 253–255.

Cohen, M. R. 2012. Safe practices for compounding of parenteral nutrition. *J Parenter Enteral Nutr*, 36, 14S–19S.

Coss-Bu, J. A., Klish, W. J., Walding, D., Stein, F., Smith, E. O., and Jefferson, L. S. 2001. Energy metabolism, nitrogen balance, and substrate utilization in critically ill children. *Am J Clin Nutr*, 74, 664–669.

Cury-Boaventura, M. F., Gorjao, R., De Lima, T. M., Fiamoncini, J., Torres, R. P., Mancini-Filho, J., Soriano, F. G., and Curi, R. 2008. Effect of olive oil-based emulsion on human lymphocyte and neutrophil death. *JPEN J Parenter Enteral Nutr*, 32, 81–87.

Driscoll, M. and Driscoll, D. F. 2005. Calculating aluminum content in total parenteral nutrition admixtures. *Am J Health Syst Pharm*, 62, 312–315.

Dudrick, S. J., Wilmore, D. W., Vars, H. M., and Rhoads, J. E. 1968. Long-term total parenteral nutrition with growth, development, and positive nitrogen balance. *Surgery*, 64, 134–142.

Dupont, I. E. and Carpentier, Y. A. 1999. Clinical use of lipid emulsions. *Curr Opin Clin Nutr Metab Care*, 2, 139–145.

Egberts, E. H., Schomerus, H., Hamster, W., and Jurgens, P. 1985. Branched chain amino acids in the treatment of latent portosystemic encephalopathy. A double-blind placebo-controlled crossover study. *Gastroenterology*, 88, 887–895.

Elizabeth Weekes, C. 2007. Controversies in the determination of energy requirements. *Proc Nutr Soc*, 66, 367–377.

Feinstein, E. I., Blumenkrantz, M. J., Healy, M., Koffler, A., Silberman, H., Massry, S. G., and Kopple, J. D. 1981. Clinical and metabolic responses to parenteral nutrition in acute renal failure. A controlled double-blind study. *Medicine (Baltimore)*, 60, 124–137.

Ferenci, P. and Wewalka, F. 1978. Plasma amino acids in hepatic encephalopathy. *J Neural Transm Suppl*, 87–94.

Finney, S. J., Zekveld, C., Elia, A., and Evans, T. W. 2003. Glucose control and mortality in critically ill patients. *JAMA*, 290, 2041–2047.

Fischer, J. E. and Baldessarini, R. J. 1971. False neurotransmitters and hepatic failure. *Lancet*, 2, 75–80.

Flancbaum, L., Choban, P. S., Sambucco, S., Verducci, J., and Burge, J. C. 1999. Comparison of indirect calorimetry, the Fick method, and prediction equations in estimating the energy requirements of critically ill patients. *Am J Clin Nutr*, 69, 461–466.

Foley, C. M., Polinsky, M. S., Gruskin, A. B., Baluarte, H. J., and Grover, W. D. 1981. Encephalopathy in infants and children with chronic renal disease. *Arch Neurol*, 38, 656–658.

Food and Drug Administration (FDA). 1998a. Aluminum in large and small volume parenterals used in total parenteral nutrition—Food and Drug Administration (FDA). Proposed rule. *Fed Regist*, 63, 176–185.

Food and Drug Administration (FDA). 2000b. Parenteral multivitamin products; drugs for human use; drug efficacy study implementation; amendment. *Fed Regist*, 65, 21200–21201.

Freeman, J., Goldmann, D. A., Smith, N. E., Sidebottom, D. G., Epstein, M. F., and Platt, R. 1990. Association of intravenous lipid emulsion and coagulase-negative staphylococcal bacteremia in neonatal intensive care units. *N Engl J Med*, 323, 301–308.

Freeman, J. B., Fairfull-Smith, R., Rodman, G. H. Jr., Bernstein, D. M., Gazzaniga, A. B., and Gersovitz, M. 1983. Safety and efficacy of a new peripheral intravenously administered amino acid solution containing glycerol and electrolytes. *Surg Gynecol Obstet*, 156, 625–631.

Garnacho Montero, J., Shou, J., Ortiz Leyba, C., Jimenez Jimenez, F. J., and Daly, J. M. 1996. Lipids and immune function. *Nutr Hosp*, 11, 230–237.

Goldmann, D. A., Martin, W. T., and Worthington, J. W. 1973. Growth of bacteria and fungi in total parenteral nutrition solutions. *Am J Surg*, 126, 314–318.

Grau, T., Bonet, A., Minambres, E., Pineiro, L., Irles, J. A., Robles, A., Acosta, J. et al. 2011. The effect of L-alanyl-L-glutamine dipeptide supplemented total parenteral nutrition on infectious morbidity and insulin sensitivity in critically ill patients. *Crit Care Med*, 39, 1263–1268.

Greene, H. L., Hambidge, K. M., Schanler, R., and Tsang, R. C. 1988. Guidelines for the use of vitamins, trace elements, calcium, magnesium, and phosphorus in infants and children receiving total parenteral nutrition: Report of the Subcommittee on Pediatric Parenteral Nutrient Requirements from the Committee on Clinical Practice Issues of the American Society for Clinical Nutrition. *Am J Clin Nutr*, 48, 1324–1342.

Guillou, P. J. 1993. The effects of lipids on some aspects of the cellular immune response. *Proc Nutr Soc*, 52, 91–100.

Haumont, D., Deckelbaum, R. J., Richelle, M., Dahlan, W., Coussaert, E., Bihain, B. E., and Carpentier, Y. A. 1989. Plasma lipid and plasma lipoprotein concentrations in low birth weight infants given parenteral nutrition with twenty or ten percent lipid emulsion. *J Pediatr*, 115, 787–793.

Haumont, D., Richelle, M., Deckelbaum, R. J., Coussaert, E., and Carpentier, Y. A. 1992. Effect of liposomal content of lipid emulsions on plasma lipid concentrations in low birth weight infants receiving parenteral nutrition. *J Pediatr*, 121, 759–763.

Heird, W. C., Dell, R. B., Helms, R. A., Greene, H. L., Ament, M. E., Karna, P., and Storm, M. C. 1987. Amino acid mixture designed to maintain normal plasma amino acid patterns in infants and children requiring parenteral nutrition. *Pediatrics*, 80, 401–408.

Heird, W. C., Hay, W., Helms, R. A., Storm, M. C., Kashyap, S., and Dell, R. B. 1988. Pediatric parenteral amino acid mixture in low birth weight infants. *Pediatrics*, 81, 41–50.

Helbock, H. J., Motchnik, P. A., and Ames, B. N. 1993. Toxic hydroperoxides in intravenous lipid emulsions used in preterm infants. *Pediatrics*, 91, 83–87.

Helms, R. A., Christensen, M. L., Mauer, E. C., and Storm, M. C. 1987. Comparison of a pediatric versus standard amino acid formulation in preterm neonates requiring parenteral nutrition. *J Pediatr*, 110, 466–470.

Helms, R. A., Storm, M. C., Christensen, M. L., Hak, E. B., and Chesney, R. W. 1999. Cysteine supplementation results in normalization of plasma taurine concentrations in children receiving home parenteral nutrition. *J Pediatr*, 134, 358–361.

Heyland, D. K., Macdonald, S., Keefe, L., and Drover, J. W. 1998. Total parenteral nutrition in the critically ill patient: A meta-analysis. *JAMA*, 280, 2013–2019.

Heyland, D. K., Montalvo, M., Macdonald, S., Keefe, L., Su, X. Y., and Drover, J. W. 2001. Total parenteral nutrition in the surgical patient: A meta-analysis. *Can J Surg*, 44, 102–111.

Holcombe, B. 2012. Parenteral nutrition product shortages: Impact on safety. *JPEN J Parenter Enteral Nutr*, 36, 44S–47S.

Holliday, M. A. and Segar, W. E. 1957. The maintenance need for water in parenteral fluid therapy. *Pediatrics*, 19, 823–832.

Hunt, D. R., Lane, H. W., Beesinger, D., Gallagher, K., Halligan, R., Johnston, D., and Rowlands, B. J. 1984. Selenium depletion in burn patients. *JPEN J Parenter Enteral Nutr*, 8, 695–699.

James, J. H., Freund, H., and Fischer, J. E. 1979a. Amino acids in hepatic encephalopathy. *Gastroenterology*, 77, 421–423.

James, J. H., Ziparo, V., Jeppsson, B., and Fischer, J. E. 1979b. Hyperammonaemia, plasma aminoacid imbalance, and blood-brain aminoacid transport: A unified theory of portal-systemic encephalopathy. *Lancet*, 2, 772–775.

Jones, M. O., Pierro, A., Hammond, P., Nunn, A., and Lloyd, D. A. 1993. Glucose utilization in the surgical newborn infant receiving total parenteral nutrition. *J Pediatr Surg*, 28, 1121–1125.

Kamala, F., Boo, N. Y., Cheah, F. C., and Birinder, K. 2002. Randomized controlled trial of heparin for prevention of blockage of peripherally inserted central catheters in neonates. *Acta Paediatr*, 91, 1350–1356.

Kochevar, M., Guenter, P., Holcombe, B., Malone, A., and Mirtallo, J. 2007. ASPEN statement on parenteral nutrition standardization. *J Parenter Enteral Nutr*, 31, 441–448.

Koo, W. W., Kaplan, L. A., Bendon, R., Succop, P., Tsang, R. C., Horn, J., and Steichen, J. J. 1986a. Response to aluminum in parenteral nutrition during infancy. *J Pediatr*, 109, 877–883.

Koo, W. W., Kaplan, L. A., Horn, J., Tsang, R. C., and Steichen, J. J. 1986b. Aluminum in parenteral nutrition solution—Sources and possible alternatives. *JPEN J Parenter Enteral Nutr*, 10, 591–595.

Koretz, R. L., Lipman, T. O., and Klein, S. 2001. AGA technical review on parenteral nutrition. *Gastroenterology*, 121, 970–1001.

Kuhl, D. A., Brown, R. O., Vehe, K. L., Boucher, B. A., Luther, R. W., and Kudsk, K. A. 1990. Use of selected visceral protein measurements in the comparison of branched-chain amino acids with standard amino acids in parenteral nutrition support of injured patients. *Surgery*, 107, 503–510.

Kumar, P. R., Crotty, P., and Raman, M. 2011. Hyperglycemia in hospitalized patients receiving parental nutrition is associated with increased morbidity and mortality: A review. *Gastroenterol Res Pract*, pii 760720, 2011.

Lev-Ran, A., Johnson, M., Hwang, D. L., Askanazi, J., Weissman, C., and Gersovitz, M. 1987. Double-blind study of glycerol vs glucose in parenteral nutrition of postsurgical insulin-treated diabetic patients. *JPEN J Parenter Enteral Nutr*, 11, 271–274.

Macdonald, A. and Hildebrandt, L. 2003. Comparison of formulaic equations to determine energy expenditure in the critically ill patient. *Nutrition*, 19, 233–239.

Marchesini, G., Bianchi, G., Merli, M., Amodio, P., Panella, C., Loguercio, C., Rossi Fanelli, F., and Abbiati, R. 2003. Nutritional supplementation with branched-chain amino acids in advanced cirrhosis: A double-blind, randomized trial. *Gastroenterology*, 124, 1792–1801.

Mcgeer, A. J., Detsky, A. S., and O'rourke, K. 1990. Parenteral nutrition in cancer patients undergoing chemotherapy: A meta-analysis. *Nutrition*, 6, 233–240.

Michel, H., Bories, P., Aubin, J. P., Pomier-Layrargues, G., Bauret, P., and Bellet-Herman, H. 1985. Treatment of acute hepatic encephalopathy in cirrhotics with a branched-chain amino acids enriched versus a conventional amino acids mixture. A controlled study of 70 patients. *Liver*, 5, 282–289.

Mirtallo, J., Canada, T., Johnson, D., Kumpf, V., Petersen, C., Sacks, G., Seres, D., and Guenter, P. 2004. Safe practices for parenteral nutrition. *JPEN J Parenter Enteral Nutr*, 28, S39–S70.

Mirtallo, J. M. 2012. Parenteral nutrition ordering processes. *JPEN J Parenter Enteral Nutr*, 36, 29S–31S.

Mirtallo, J. M., Schneider, P. J., Mavko, K., Ruberg, R. L., and Fabri, P. J. 1982. A comparison of essential and general amino acid infusions in the nutritional support of patients with compromised renal function. *JPEN J Parenter Enteral Nutr*, 6, 109–113.

Moe-Byrne, T., Wagner, J. V., and Mcguire, W. 2012. Glutamine supplementation to prevent morbidity and mortality in preterm infants. *Cochrane Database of Systematic Reviews*, 3, CD001457.

Moukarzel, A. A., Song, M. K., Buchman, A. L., Vargas, J., Guss, W., Mcdiarmid, S., Reyen, L., and Ament, M. E. 1992. Excessive chromium intake in children receiving total parenteral nutrition. *Lancet*, 339, 385–388.

Mouser, J. F., Hak, E. B., Helms, R. A., Christensen, M. L., and Storm, M. C. 1999. Chromium and zinc concentrations in pediatric patients receiving long-term parenteral nutrition. *Am J Health Syst Pharm*, 56, 1950–1956.

National Advisory Group (NAG) 1998b. Safe practices for parenteral nutrition formulations. On standards and practice guidelines for parenteral nutrition. *J Parenter Enteral Nutr*, 22, 49–66.

Naylor, C. D., O'rourke, K., Detsky, A. S., and Baker, J. P. 1989. Parenteral nutrition with branched-chain amino acids in hepatic encephalopathy. A meta-analysis. *Gastroenterology*, 97, 1033–1042.

Neuzil, J., Darlow, B. A., Inder, T. E., Sluis, K. B., Winterbourn, C. C., and Stocker, R. 1995. Oxidation of parenteral lipid emulsion by ambient and phototherapy lights: Potential toxicity of routine parenteral feeding. *J Pediatr*, 126, 785–790.

Novak, F., Heyland, D. K., Avenell, A., Drover, J. W., and Su, X. 2002. Glutamine supplementation in serious illness: A systematic review of the evidence. *Crit Care Med*, 30, 2022–2029.

Ott, S. M., Maloney, N. A., Klein, G. L., Alfrey, A. C., Ament, M. E., Coburn, J. W., and Sherrard, D. J. 1983. Aluminum is associated with low bone formation in patients receiving chronic parenteral nutrition. *Ann Intern Med*, 98, 910–914.

Oxford Parenteral Nutrition Team. 1983. Total parenteral nutrition: Value of a standard feeding regimen. *Br Med J (Clin Res Ed)*, 286, 1323–1327.

Phelps, S. J. and Cochran, E. B. 1989. Effect of the continuous administration of fat emulsion on the infiltration of intravenous lines in infants receiving peripheral parenteral nutrition solutions. *JPEN J Parenter Enteral Nutr*, 13, 628–632.

Phelps, S. J. and Helms, R. A. 1987. Risk factors affecting infiltration of peripheral venous lines in infants. *J Pediatr*, 111, 384–389.

Polinsky, M. S. and Gruskin, A. B. 1984. Aluminum toxicity in children with chronic renal failure. *J Pediatr*, 105, 758–761.

Pomposelli, J. J. and Bistrian, B. R. 1994. Is total parenteral nutrition immunosuppressive? *New Horiz*, 2, 224–229.

Poole, R. L., Pieroni, K. P., Gaskari, S., Dixon, T. K., Park, K., and Kerner, J. A. Jr. 2011. Aluminum in pediatric parenteral nutrition products: Measured versus labeled content. *J Pediatr Pharmacol Ther*, 16, 92–97.

Poole, R. L., Schiff, L., Hintz, S. R., Wong, A., Mackenzie, N., and Kerner, J. A. Jr. 2010. Aluminum content of parenteral nutrition in neonates: Measured versus calculated levels. *J Pediatr Gastroenterol Nutr*, 50, 208–211.

Randolph, A. G., Cook, D. J., Gonzales, C. A., and Andrew, M. 1998. Benefit of heparin in central venous and pulmonary artery catheters: A meta-analysis of randomized controlled trials. *Chest*, 113, 165–171.

Reeves, M. M. and Capra, S. 2003. Predicting energy requirements in the clinical setting: Are current methods evidence based? *Nutr Rev*, 61, 143–151.

Rocchi, E., Cassanelli, M., Gibertini, P., Pietrangelo, A., Casalgrandi, G., and Ventura, E. 1985. Standard or branched-chain amino acid infusions as short-term nutritional support in liver cirrhosis? *JPEN J Parenter Enteral Nutr*, 9, 447–451.

Sedman, A. B., Wilkening, G. N., Warady, B. A., Lum, G. M., and Alfrey, A. C. 1984. Encephalopathy in childhood secondary to aluminum toxicity. *J Pediatr*, 105, 836–838.

Seltzer, M. H., Asaadi, M., Coco, A., Lucchino, E. T., and Catena, A. L. 1978. The use of a simplified standardized hyperalimentation formula. *JPEN J Parenter Enteral Nutr*, 2, 28–30.

Shah, P. and Shah, V. 2001. Continuous heparin infusion to prevent thrombosis and catheter occlusion in neonates with peripherally placed percutaneous central venous catheters. *Cochrane Database Syst Rev*, CD002772.

Sheridan, R. L., Yu, Y. M., Prelack, K., Young, V. R., Burke, J. F., and Tompkins, R. G. 1998. Maximal parenteral glucose oxidation in hypermetabolic young children: A stable isotope study. *JPEN J Parenter Enteral Nutr*, 22, 212–216.

Silvers, K. M., Darlow, B. A., and Winterbourn, C. C. 2001. Lipid peroxide and hydrogen peroxide formation in parenteral nutrition solutions containing multivitamins. *JPEN J Parenter Enteral Nutr*, 25, 14–17.

Soghier, L. M., and Brion, L. P. 2006. Cysteine, cystine or N-acetylcysteine supplementation in parenterally fed neonates. *Cochrane Database Syst Rev*, CD004869.

Speerhas, R. A. and Seidner, D. L. 2007. Measured versus estimated aluminum content of parenteral nutrient solutions. *Am J Health Syst Pharm*, 64, 740–746.

Suchner, U. and Senftleben, U. 1994. Immune modulation by polyunsaturated fatty acids during nutritional therapy: Interactions with synthesis and effects of eicosanoids. *Infusionsther Transfusionsmed*, 21, 167–182.

Sun, L. C., Shih, Y. L., Lu, C. Y., Chen, F. M., Hsieh, J. S., Chuang, J. F., and Wang, J. Y. 2006. Randomized controlled study of glycerol versus dextrose in postoperative hypocaloric peripheral parenteral nutrition. *J Invest Surg*, 19, 381–385.

Thomson, P. and Duerksen, D. R. 2011. Vitamin D deficiency in patients receiving home parenteral nutrition. *JPEN J Parenter Enteral Nutr*, 35, 499–504.

Torosian, M. H. 1999. Perioperative nutrition support for patients undergoing gastrointestinal surgery: Critical analysis and recommendations. *World J Surg*, 23, 565–569.

Tubman, T. R., Thompson, S. W., and Mcguire, W. 2008. Glutamine supplementation to prevent morbidity and mortality in preterm infants. *Cochrane Database Syst Rev*, CD001457.

Tzaneva, P. and Ajderian, S. 2009. Glutamine dipeptides in intensive therapy. *Anaesthesiol Intensive Care*, 39, 30–38.

Uauy, R. and Castillo, C. 2003. Lipid requirements of infants: Implications for nutrient composition of fortified complementary foods. *J Nutr*, 133, 2962S–2972S.

Van Den Berghe, G., Wouters, P., Weekers, F., Verwaest, C., Bruyninckx, F., Schetz, M., Vlasselaers, D., Ferdinande, P., Lauwers, P., and Bouillon, R. 2001. Intensive insulin therapy in critically ill patients. *N Engl J Med*, 345, 1359–1367.

Van Den Berghe, G., Wouters, P. J., Bouillon, R., Weekers, F., Verwaest, C., Schetz, M., Vlasselaers, D., Ferdinande, P., and Lauwers, P. 2003. Outcome benefit of intensive insulin therapy in the critically ill: Insulin dose versus glycemic control. *Crit Care Med*, 31, 359–366.

Vanek, V. W., Borum, P., Buchman, A., Fessler, T. A., Howard, L., Jeejeebhoy, K., Kochevar, M., Shenkin, A., and Valentine, C. J. 2012. A.S.P.E.N. Position paper: Recommendations for changes in commercially available parenteral multivitamin and multi-trace element products. *Nutr Clin Pract*, 27, 440–491.

Vanek, V. W., Matarese, L. E., Robinson, M., Sacks, G. S., Young, L. S., and Kochevar, M. 2011. A.S.P.E.N. position paper: Parenteral nutrition glutamine supplementation. *Nutr Clin Pract*, 26, 479–494.

Velez, R. J., Myers, B., and Guber, M. S. 1985. Severe acute metabolic acidosis (acute beriberi): An avoidable complication of total parenteral nutrition. *JPEN J Parenter Enteral Nutr*, 9, 216–219.

Vilstrup, H., Gluud, C., Hardt, F., Kristensen, M., Kohler, O., Melgaard, B., Dejgaard, A. et al. 1990. Branched chain enriched amino acid versus glucose treatment of hepatic encephalopathy. A double-blind study of 65 patients with cirrhosis. *J Hepatol*, 10, 291–296.

Von Meyenfeldt, M. F., Soeters, P. B., Vente, J. P., Van Berlo, C. L., Rouflart, M. M., De Jong, K. P., Van Der Linden, C. J., and Gouma, D. J. 1990. Effect of branched chain amino acid enrichment of total parenteral nutrition on nitrogen sparing and clinical outcome of sepsis and trauma: A prospective randomized double blind trial. *Br J Surg*, 77, 924–929.

Wang, Y., Jiang, Z. M., Nolan, M. T., Jiang, H., Han, H. R., Yu, K., Li, H. L., Jie, B., and Liang, X. K. 2010. The impact of glutamine dipeptide-supplemented parenteral nutrition on outcomes of surgical patients: A meta-analysis of randomized clinical trials. *JPEN J Parenter Enteral Nutr*, 34, 521–529.

Wanten, G. 2006a. An update on parenteral lipids and immune function: Only smoke, or is there any fire? *Curr Opin Clin Nutr Metab Care*, 9, 79–83.

Wanten, G. J. 2006b. Suppressive effect of a selective increase in plasma linoleic acid concentration and intravascular lipolysis on peripheral T cell activation. *Am J Clin Nutr*, 83, 918; author reply 918–919.

Watanabe, A., Hayashi, S., Higashi, T., Obata, T., Sakata, T., Takei, N., Shiota, T., and Nagashima, H. 1982. Characteristics change in serum amino acid levels in different types of hepatic encephalopathy. *Gastroenterol Jpn*, 17, 218–223.

Waxman, K., Day, A. T., Stellin, G. P., Tominaga, G. T., Gazzaniga, A. B., and Bradford, R. R. 1992. Safety and efficacy of glycerol and amino acids in combination with lipid emulsion for peripheral parenteral nutrition support. *JPEN J Parenter Enteral Nutr*, 16, 374–378.

Weitzel, L. R. and Wischmeyer, P. E. 2010a. Glutamine in critical illness: The time has come, the time is now. *Crit Care Clin*, 26, 515–525, ix–x.

Weitzel, L. R. B. and Wischmeyer, P. E. 2010b. Glutamine in critical illness: The time has come, the time is now. *Crit Care Clin*, 26, 515–525.

Wilmore, D. W. and Dudrick, S. J. 1968. Growth and development of an infant receiving all nutrients exclusively by vein. *JAMA*, 203, 860–864.

Winters, R. W., Heird, W. C., and Dell, R. B. 1977. Plasma amino acids in infants receiving parenteral nutrition. In: Greene, H. L., Holliday, M. A., and Munro, H. N. (eds.) *Clinical Nutrition Update: Amino Acids [proceedings]*. Chicago, IL: AMA.

Wolfe, R. R., O'donnell, T. F. Jr., Stone, M. D., Richmand, D. A., and Burke, J. F. 1980. Investigation of factors determining the optimal glucose infusion rate in total parenteral nutrition. *Metabolism*, 29, 892–900.

Wu, P. Y., Edwards, N., and Storm, M. C. 1986. Plasma amino acid pattern in normal term breast-fed infants. *J Pediatr*, 109, 347–349.

Yarandi, S. S., Zhao, V. M., Hebbar, G., and Ziegler, T. R. 2011. Amino acid composition in parenteral nutrition: What is the evidence? *Curr Opin Clin Nutr Metab Care*, 14, 75–82.

Yaqoob, P. 1998. Lipids and the immune response. *Curr Opin Clin Nutr Metab Care*, 1, 153–161.

15 Enteral Formulations

Ainsley M. Malone

CONTENTS

INTRODUCTION

Over the past several decades, the availability of enteral formulas for use in hospitalized patients has dramatically increased. In the late 1970s, when enteral nutrition support was in its infancy, approximately 16 enteral formulas were available for use [1]. Present-day marketplace offers well over 100 enteral formulas, many of which can be considered for use in the critically ill patient. Choosing an appropriate formula can present a challenge given the multiple formula variations that exist. Energy and protein requirements and fluid status are important considerations when choosing an appropriate formula. Promoting positive outcomes through the use of modified enteral formulas is a key component in formula decision making. Does the use of an immune-modulating formula (IMF) reduce infectious complications? Does a formula for acute respiratory distress syndrome (ARDS) result in a reduction in the need for ventilatory support? Many of these questions have been addressed via systematic reviews of existing research and via evidence-based guideline recommendations. It should be pointed out that enteral formulas are considered food supplements by the Food and Drug Association and therefore are not under regulatory control. With some formulations, there is a lack of prospective, randomized, controlled clinical trials supporting their proposed indications, while for others the data are conflicting. This chapter will focus on several areas: (1) the individual components of enteral formulas, their functions, and characteristics; (2) the categories of enteral formulas including formula types within each category; (3) a review of the available evidence evaluating the use of specialized formulas; and (4) guideline recommendations for use of specific types of enteral formulas.

NUTRIENT COMPONENTS OF ENTERAL FORMULAS

CARBOHYDRATE

Carbohydrates represent the primary macronutrient in most enteral formulas and range from 28% to 82% of total calories. It is the formula component that influences overall sweetness, with the simpler form yielding a sweeter product. Table 15.1 outlines the sources of carbohydrate available in enteral formulas. Generally, the shorter the carbohydrate molecule, the greater the osmolality and the sweeter the product requiring the least digestive capacity [2]. Most enteral formulas contain either oligosaccharides containing 3–10 glucose units or polysaccharides, polymers containing more than 10 glucose units. Polymeric formulas provide carbohydrate primarily in the form of corn syrup solids, while hydrolyzed formulas offer hydrolyzed cornstarch or maltodextrin as their source of carbohydrate. The majority of enteral formulas do not contain lactose, a disaccharide many individuals are unable to adequately digest due to insufficient quantities of the enzyme lactase [3]. Some products offer variations of total carbohydrate content to assist in management

TABLE 15.1
Macronutrient Sources in Enteral Formulas

Enteral Formula Type	Carbohydrate	Protein	Fat
Polymeric formulas	Corn syrup solids	Casein	Borage oil
	Hydrolyzed cornstarch	Sodium, calcium, magnesium, and potassium caseinates	Canola oil
	Maltodextrin		Corn oil
	Sucrose	Soy protein isolate	Fish oil
	Fructose	Whey protein concentrate	High-oleic sunflower oil
	Sugar alcohols	Lactalbumin	MCTs
		Milk protein concentrate	Menhaden oil
			Monoglycerides and diglycerides
			Palm kernel oil
			Safflower oil
			Soybean oil
			Soy lecithin
Hydrolyzed formulas	Cornstarch	Hydrolyzed casein	Fatty acid esters
	Hydrolyzed	Hydrolyzed whey protein	Fish oil
	Cornstarch	Crystalline L-amino acids	MCTs
	Maltodextrin	Hydrolyzed lactalbumin	Safflower oil
	Fructose	Soy protein isolate	Sardine oil
			Soybean oil
			Soy lecithin
			Structured lipids

of metabolic states such as hyperglycemia and hypercapnia. See the section "Disease Specific Formulas" for further discussion. See Chapter 2 for a thorough review of carbohydrate metabolism in the critically ill patient.

Protein

Proteins are the source of amino acids necessary for synthesis of structural proteins, enzymes, antibodies, and other vital functional components. In addition, in the critically ill patient, amino acids are often metabolized for use as energy substrates [4]. The content of protein in enteral formulas ranges from approximately 6% to 37%. A patient's protein requirements and underlying disease state are primary determinants for product selection. Both the protein quantity and quality provided in an enteral formula are important considerations when choosing a product [3]. Table 15.1 outlines various protein sources available in enteral formulas. One of the most common methods for assessing protein quality is the determination of the protein's biological value (BV). Proteins with a high BV offer a higher percent of absorbed nitrogen required for growth and maintenance [5]. The lower the protein's BV, the greater percentage of nonessential amino acids is present in the protein with a greater amount of total protein required to achieve nitrogen balance. A newer concept of protein quality assessment has been suggested when evaluating protein from a variety of sources. The Protein Digestibility Corrected Amino Acid Score (PDCAAS) is a method of evaluating protein quality based on both the amino acid requirements of humans and their ability to digest it. A PDCAAS value of 1 is the highest and 0 is the lowest. A score of 1 indicates that after digestion the protein provides 100% or more of the required indispensable amino acids [6].

The form of protein available in enteral formulations can vary from intact proteins, hydrolyzed proteins, or crystalline amino acids (see Table 15.1). In addition, some formulas offer increased doses of specific amino acids added primarily for pharmacologic function, amounts that should not be factored into a formula's total protein content. The protein form best suited for the critically ill patient has frequently been a source of controversy [3]. It has often been thought that the digestive and absorptive abilities of the small intestine in critical illness are impaired, a reason supporting the use of more chemically defined formulas. Whether this impairment exists is not well defined [3]. See Chapter 3 for an extensive review of protein metabolism.

Amino Acids

The term *elemental* formula became well accepted in the early days of enteral nutrition. The concept that free amino acids were better absorbed by the functionally impaired gut was commonly accepted, especially as it applied to the critically ill patient [7]. It is well known that di- and tripeptides are absorbed from the intestinal lumen without hydrolysis [8]. The use of peptide-based enteral formulas has been shown to be superior to free amino acids in promoting greater nitrogen absorption in both the healthy and diseased guts [9,10]. In addition, the use of intact protein may be as effective as amino acid use in promoting intestinal integrity. One study comparing the use of amino acids versus intact protein in patients with Crohn's disease found that the use of intact protein was equally as effective in promoting disease remission as were free amino acids [11]. The use of free amino acids in enteral formulas may be necessary in those who are intolerant to peptide-based formulas.

Peptides

Peptides are hydrolyzed proteins containing varying chain lengths with most peptide formulas containing a mixture of di- and tripeptides. These formulas have been suggested for use in critically ill patients as well as in those with impaired gastrointestinal function, that is, pancreatitis or short bowel syndrome [2,12,13]. Whether there is a benefit in using peptide-based formulas rather than intact protein formulas in the critically ill patient is unclear.

One study in critically ill patients demonstrated improvement in serum proteins in those who received a peptide-based versus an intact protein formula [14]. Whether a difference in formula tolerance or in intensive care unit (ICU) length of stay occurred with the use of a peptide formula was not evaluated. Other studies have documented a reduced incidence of hypoalbuminemia-related diarrhea with the use of peptide-based formulas [12,13].

Existing data support the use of intact protein formulas in critically ill patients. Heimburger et al. [15] demonstrated no difference in diarrhea incidence between a peptide-based and a whole protein formula in critically ill patients. Moreover, Dietscher et al. [16] compared a combined peptide and free amino acid formula with a whole protein formula in ICU patients and found no difference in diarrhea incidence. The Canadian Clinical Practice Guidelines group, in their 2012 systematic review, found no evidence that peptide use results in decreased diarrhea incidence and therefore recommend the use of a polymeric whole protein formulas [17]. It appears the primary issue regarding peptide-based formula usage relates to the presence of gastrointestinal dysfunction. Clearly in those patients with malabsorption, pancreatic dysfunction, short bowel syndrome, or other evidence of gastrointestinal disease, peptide-based enteral formulas should be considered for initial use. In those with normal gastrointestinal function, however, enteral formulas with an intact protein source should be routinely utilized as the first choice in enteral product selection.

Glutamine

Glutamine, a nonessential amino acid, is a contributor to multiple metabolic functions and is considered a *conditionally essential* amino acid in periods of metabolic stress including sepsis, trauma, burns, and critical illness. Glutamine is the most abundant amino acid in skeletal muscles and plasma and is the primary carrier of nitrogen from the skeletal muscles to the viscera due to its two amino groups. Glutamine has multiple functions, all of which are important in the critically ill patient. It assists in the regulation of acid–base balance through ammonia synthesis, is essential for the synthesis of nucleotides and nucleic acids, and is the preferred primary energy source for rapidly proliferating cells such as enterocytes, lymphocytes, and macrophages. It is known that glutamine levels in both the blood and muscle are reduced in injury, trauma, and critical illness [18]. It is glutamine's function with rapidly dividing cells, especially those of the intestinal mucosa, that has generated the most interest [19]. Glutamine has been shown to increase nutrient absorption, reduce bacterial translocation, and exert trophic effects on the small bowel mucosa [19].

The inclusion of free glutamine in enteral products is an advancement initiated in the mid-1990s. Previously, glutamine was available either as a component of a free amino acid formula or as a protein-bound form. With the protein-bound form, the actual glutamine content is estimated and will vary with the protein source as well as the amount and degree of processing. It is known that hydrolyzed formulas will have less glutamine than their constituent protein due to losses that occur during hydrolysis [20]. In addition to glutamine provided from a product's inherent protein, some enteral products contain added glutamine, in the free amino acid form.

Whether providing a formula with enhanced glutamine will benefit the critically ill patient is not entirely known. Glutamine's suggested role in maintenance of gut permeability was evaluated by Velasco and colleagues [21]. They compared the effects of a standard and a glutamine-supplemented enteral formula on improvement of gut permeability in critically ill patients and found no difference. Two studies specifically evaluating glutamine in critically ill patients have yielded positive results. Houdijk and colleagues [22] demonstrated a significant reduction in pneumonia, bacteremia, and sepsis in critically ill multiple trauma patients receiving a glutamine-supplemented enteral formula. Jones et al. [23] evaluated a glutamine-supplemented enteral formula and found a significant reduction in intensive care and hospital lengths of stay as well as in total patient costs in those who received the glutamine-supplemented formula.

Two recent systematic reviews of the available data evaluating enteral glutamine in critically ill patients have concluded that the use of glutamine-supplemented formulas has not shown benefit. Both the Academy of Nutrition and Dietetics (AND) Evidence Analysis Library (2012) and the Canadian Clinical Practice Guidelines (2013) do not recommend the routine use of enteral glutamine [24,25]. The Canadian guidelines suggest enteral glutamine may be beneficial in the burn and trauma patients [24]. However, based upon their REDOXS trial results in which severely ill patients receiving combined enteral and parenteral glutamine demonstrated increased mortality, they strongly recommend avoidance of all glutamine sources in patients with shock or multiorgan failure [24]. Further study evaluating glutamine is necessary to identify the population in whom enteral glutamine may be beneficial [25].

Arginine

Arginine is considered an essential amino acid during periods of stress due mainly to its increased requirements in tissue repair. Arginine serves a number of biochemical and functional roles within the body. Arginine is a precursor for the synthesis of important proteins including proline, glutamate, and polyamine. As an intermediate in the urea cycle, arginine is important for ammonia detoxification. In addition, arginine plays a role in cell signaling and in the regulation of key cellular processes [26]. It has been suggested that arginine enhances immune function through lymphocyte proliferation [27]. Arginine's role in the production of nitric oxide has generated the most interest in critically ill patients. Nitric oxide is an antimicrobial agent, a neurotransmitter, and a vasodilator. Its production is regulated by nitric oxide synthase induced by increasing arginine levels [4,27]. Increased nitric oxide levels have been associated with improvements in immune function in the critically ill patient [28].

The role of arginine in immune function has led to the inclusion of supplemental arginine in enteral formulas designed for the critically ill patient. Arginine content varies as there is some arginine that is a component of the primary protein source. Unfortunately, other constituents have also been included in these *immune-modulating* formulas so it is difficult to ascertain arginine's specific benefits. A review of recent data evaluating these types of formulas is outlined in the section "Immune-Modulating Formulas and Critical Illness."

Lipid

Lipids in enteral formulas serve as both a concentrated source of energy and a source of essential fatty acids. Due to their isotonicity, lipids exert no influence on formula osmolality. Fat sources vary among formulas. The percentage of total calories provided by fat in available enteral formulas ranges from 1% to 55%. Essential fatty acids (linoleic and linolenic acids) should comprise a minimum of 4% of total calories to meet absolute essential fatty acid requirements [29]. Standard enteral formulas contain 15%–30% of total calories from fat. Formulas with higher amounts have been developed for use with specific disease states such as pulmonary disease or diabetes (see section on formula category for a more thorough review).

Long-Chain Fatty Acids

Fats in enteral formulas are included as triglycerides, with constituent long-chain or medium-chain fatty acids. Recent interest has been generated in the structure of the available long-chain fat source. Initially, fatty acids in enteral formulas were predominately of the omega-6 family. In more recent years, the omega-3 family of fatty acids has been added in combination with omega-6 fatty acids. The class of fatty acids is defined by the position of the first double bond from the terminal methyl end on the carbon chain [32]. Omega-3 fats include alpha-linolenic acid, eicosapentaenoic acid (EPA), and docosahexaenoic acid (DHA). These fatty acids follow a differing metabolic pathway than do omega-6 fatty acids with regard to eicosanoid synthesis. Omega-3 fatty acids are precursors to the 3 series of prostaglandins and the 5 series of leukotrienes, compounds shown to have anti-inflammatory properties [29–31]. Conversely, omega-6 fats are metabolized to arachidonic acid, a precursor to the 2 series of prostaglandins and 4 series of leukotrienes, known proinflammatory and immunosuppressants [31]. These metabolic variations form an important foundation for the alterations in fat sources utilized in some enteral formulas.

Medium-Chain Triglycerides

Triglycerides esterified with fatty acids of medium-chain length (6–12 carbon chains) are classified as medium-chain triglycerides (MCTs) and offer unique advantages for use in enteral formulas [30,32]. MCTs do not require bile salts or pancreatic lipase for digestion and can be directly absorbed by the intestinal epithelial cells, a benefit to the patient with impaired fat digestion, such as in pancreatitis or short bowel syndrome. In addition, MCTs are absorbed directly into the portal circulation and are metabolized at the cellular level without the assistance of carnitine. MCTs, unlike LCTs, are not stored and are almost completely metabolized to CO_2 and H_2O [32]. Enteral formulas contain MCT amounts ranging from 0% to 85% of the total fat content. It is important to remember that MCTs do not offer a source of the essential fatty acids, linoleic and linolenic acids, and therefore must always be provided in combination with a source of long-chain fatty acids. In high quantities, MCTs are metabolized to ketones in the liver, a disadvantage to those at risk of ketosis (i.e., diabetic patients or those who are acidotic) [33].

Structured Lipids

A more recent form of lipid included in selected enteral formulas is a chemically synthesized lipid comprised of both long- and medium-chain fatty acids. These *structured* lipids are designed to house individual fatty acids on a single glycerol backbone, thereby providing the benefits of both long and medium fats, namely, ease of absorption, peripheral tissue metabolism, and a source of essential fats [33].

FIBER

The addition of fiber in enteral formulas was introduced in the 1980s when its beneficial role in gastrointestinal health was recognized [29]. Dietary fiber is defined as structural and storage polysaccharides in plants that are not digested by human enzymes [34]. Sources of fiber in enteral formulas include soy polysaccharide, hydrolyzed guar gum, and oat fiber, among others [3,34]. A newer form of fiber added to many enteral formulas is the prebiotic fructooligosaccharides (FOSs), short-chain oligosaccharides that are rapidly fermented by the colonic bacteria to short-chain fatty acids (SCFAs), which may aid in the management of diarrhea and contribute to overall gastrointestinal tract health [34]. SCFAs are used as an energy source by colonic bacteria, a potential benefit in maintaining healthy gut microbiota [35]. Fibers can be classified by their solubility in water. Soluble fibers, such as pectin and guar, are fermented by colonic bacteria and have been shown to prevent colonic mucosal atrophy, stimulate mucosal proliferation, and provide fuel for the colonocyte [3]. In addition, increased colonic sodium and water absorption has been demonstrated with soluble fiber use, a potential benefit in the treatment of diarrhea associated with tube feeding use [36]. Insoluble fiber, such as soy polysaccharide, increases fecal weight leading to increased peristalsis and decreased stool transit time [36].

The use of fiber-fortified enteral formulas in the critically ill patient is controversial mainly due to the paucity of data demonstrating benefit [37–40]. The reported incidence of diarrhea in patients receiving tube feedings ranges from 2% to 63% with the higher incidence reported in the critically ill patient population [40]. Variations in reported incidence are a result of a variety of factors including population studied, definition of diarrhea used, and whether reports accounted for other causes of diarrhea.

Both soluble and insoluble fibers have been studied in the management of diarrhea. Insoluble fibers such as soy polysaccharide have not been shown to conclusively improve diarrhea, especially in the acutely ill patient [38,39]. Soy polysaccharide-containing enteral formulas may be more beneficial in chronic long-term enteral feeding patients. Bass et al. demonstrated a significant reduction in diarrhea in chronically ill patients requiring tube feedings for greater than 25 days who received a soy polysaccharide-containing enteral formula compared with a fiber-free formula [38]. In an evaluation using soluble fiber, Schultz et al. demonstrated a trend toward diarrhea reduction when pectin was combined with an insoluble fiber formula compared with an insoluble fiber formula alone [41]. In 2004, Rushdi and colleagues evaluated the addition of soluble guar gum to an enteral regimen in a mixed ICU population. The mean number of liquid stools was lower for the guar group compared to the group who did not receive additional soluble fiber [42]. The AND Evidence Analysis Library's systematic review in 2011 on the use of fiber in critically ill patients concluded that "diarrhea may be reduced when guar gum is included in an enteral nutrition regimen. The impact of other types of fiber on reducing diarrhea is unclear due to variations in the fiber combinations and amounts used in the studies" (Grade II, fair evidence) [43].

The routine use of a fiber-supplemented enteral formula in critically ill patients has come into question. Several cases of bowel obstruction caused by the use of insoluble fiber-containing formulas have been reported in the surgical and burn population [44,45]. The 2009 Guidelines for the Provision and Assessment of Nutrition Support Therapy in the Adult Critically Ill Patient: Society of Critical Care Medicine and the American Society for Parenteral and Enteral Nutrition (SCCM/A.S.P.E.N.) suggest "mixed fiber formulas, both soluble and insoluble fiber, should not be used routinely in adult critically ill patients to promote bowel regularity or prevent diarrhea and recommend that mixed fiber formulas should be avoided in patients at high risk for bowel ischemia or severe dysmotility" [46]. This recommendation is supported by smaller, randomized trials without clear-cut results and therefore offers an opportunity for cautious use of fiber in patients who have demonstrated improving GI function.

FORMULA CATEGORIES

Enteral formulas for use in the critically ill patient can be classified as standard, chemically defined, or specialized. Many formulas are available within each category, some of which may be significantly different from one another. For example, standard enteral formulas will include formulas with varying nutrient density, inclusion or exclusion of fiber, and various macronutrient distributions. The decision regarding which formula to utilize in the critically ill patient will be based upon a number of factors, both patient and formula related, including, among others, gastrointestinal function, fluid status, and organ function (Table 15.2 outlines factors to consider in enteral formula selection). Formula selection frequently requires adjustment throughout the patient's hospital course as clinical status changes.

TABLE 15.2
Factors to Consider in Enteral Formula Selection

Assessment of Patient	Assessment of Formula
Past medical history and present problems	Composition of carbohydrate, protein, and fat
Age	Calorie/nitrogen ratio
Calorie and nutrient requirements	Osmolality
Gastrointestinal function	Renal solute load
Hepatic function	pH
Renal function	Residue/fiber content
Pulmonary status	Viscosity
	Caloric density
	Convenience of administration
	Bacteriologic safety
	Cost

Source: Gottschlich M.M. et al., Defined formula diets, in: Rombeau, J.L. and Rolandelli, R.H. (eds.), *Clinical Nutrition: Enteral and Tube Feeding*, 3rd edn., W.B. Saunders, Philadelphia, PA, 1997, pp. 207–239. With permission.

Disease-Specific Formulas

Specialized formulas encompass a wide range of formulas and are designed for a variety of clinical scenarios. Some are intended for patients with specific disease states such as pulmonary disease, acute kidney injury, and diabetes. Others are recommended for use in hypermetabolic and/or inflammatory states such as that common in the critically ill patient. A review of currently available formulas from the two national manufacturers indicates there are over 35 enteral formulas designed for a particular *condition* or *disease state.*

Specialized formulas may or may not result in improved outcomes for critically ill patients and their use is controversial [3,4,47–50]. It is essential that clinicians evaluate specialized enteral formulas prior to their use. Manufacturers market their products for a variety of disease states or conditions, which may not be supported by scientific evidence. It is important to remember that nutrition is only one aspect of a critically ill patient's treatment, and therefore, it is necessary to ask, "What possible difference in outcome will this enteral formula offer to the patient?" Additionally, the concept of benefit versus harm needs to be considered. Does the risk of harm outweigh the potential benefit that this type of product may offer? Figure 15.1 outlines other important considerations when evaluating specialized formulas. The following formulas for specific disease states or conditions will be reviewed: diabetes mellitus and/or hyperglycemia, hepatic disease, hypermetabolism (immune enhancing), pulmonary disease (ARDS and chronic obstructive pulmonary disease [COPD]), and acute kidney injury.

Diabetes Mellitus/Hyperglycemia

Hyperglycemia is a common metabolic disturbance found in both diabetic and nondiabetic critically ill patients. It has been associated with worse outcomes in both adults and children [51,52]. Maintenance of normal blood glucose levels in the critically ill patient is often difficult secondary to the hypermetabolic stress response [53]. The presence of counterregulatory hormones and increased reliance on fatty acid oxidation by the skeletal muscles result in reduced glucose uptake and resultant hyperglycemia [4]. Good glycemic control (140–180 mg/dL) has been widely accepted into clinical practice [54] and is routinely cited in international treatment guidelines [55]. Control of blood glucose levels has demonstrated both a reduced incidence of complications and improved outcomes [56–58]. Several diabetic formulas are currently available with similar characteristics. Carbohydrate sources vary but generally consist of oligosaccharides, fructose, cornstarch, and fiber. The use of more complex carbohydrates, such as fructose, cornstarch, and fiber, has been shown to improve glycemic control primarily from delayed gastric emptying and reduced intestinal transit [59]. Types of fiber and total fiber content vary among diabetic enteral formulas. Soluble fiber such as guar and pectin has been associated with improved glucose control [60]. Due to the inherent viscosity of soluble fiber, most enteral diabetic formulas contain both soluble and insoluble fiber sources. Total fat content ranges from 40% to 49%, raising the concern of impaired gastric emptying with the use of a formula with increased fat content [61].

- Is the nutrient profile appropriate based on known metabolic abnormalities and nutrient requirements of the specified condition?
- Has the product testing been limited to animal research only?
- Have prospective, controlled, randomized clinical trials evaluating the product been conducted?
- Is the research only product-specific?
- Can the study results be generalized to other populations or only that in which the product was studied?
- Has objective criteria been developed to evaluate the specific formula?
- Are recommendations for product use confined only to the population(s) studied or for use with additional population(s)?

FIGURE 15.1 Considerations in evaluation of specialized enteral formulas. (Adapted from Malone, A.M., *Support Line*, 24(1), 3, 2002.)

There are few randomized controlled trials (RCTs) evaluating diabetic formulas. In a series of two studies, Peters et al. demonstrated that the use of a diabetic formula results in a reduced glucose response compared to standard enteral formulas [62,63]. It should be noted that these studies were conducted in healthy volunteers using a study protocol that attempted to mimic continuous tube feeding administration. Results of these studies cannot be generalized to hospitalized patients. Craig et al. [64] compared a diabetic with a standard formula in type 2 diabetics residing in a long-term care facility. There were no significant differences in fasting serum glucose levels at baseline, monthly, or at the study completion. Finger-stick glucose checks were not significantly different over the entire course of the study period but were significantly lower in the diabetic formula group in weeks 1, 5, and 7. The overall clinical significance of these results is unknown. Selected clinical outcomes, such as fever, pneumonia, and pressure ulcers, were noted to be higher in the standard formula group but these differences were not significant. In one of two evaluations of a diabetic formula in hospitalized patients, Beyers et al. [65] compared the efficacy of blood glucose control using a standard enteral formula and a diabetic formula. In this small study, blood glucose levels were significantly higher when the standard enteral formula was provided. Both formulas required the use of supplemental insulin for blood glucose control. The nutrient cost of the diabetic formula was significantly higher than that of the standard formula. It is interesting to note that the amount of intravenous dextrose received when the standard formula was provided was three times that received during infusion of the diabetic formula. While the results were not statistically significant, a larger sample size may have yielded different results. Overall, despite the small study size, the results confirm that glucose control is variable in a hospital setting and that, while the use of a diabetic formula can affect blood glucose levels, the effect may not be clinically significant, irrespective of all other methods utilized for controlling blood glucose.

In a more recent study, Mesejo and colleagues compared a high-protein diabetic formula to a standard formula over a 14-day period in 61 critically ill diabetic and/or hyperglycemic patients [66]. Significant improvements were seen in the diabetic group, in both plasma glucose and capillary glucose levels as well in the amount of insulin use per day. However, outcome measures such as infection rate, ICU length of stay, and mortality were not significantly different between the two groups [66].

The routine use of a diabetic formula does not appear warranted [49,50]. A recommendation from the Canadian Clinical Practice Guidelines does not support the use of a diabetic or high-fat/low-carbohydrate formula [67] in critically ill patients. However, when blood glucose control becomes problematic, despite appropriate pharmacologic intervention and the avoidance of overfeeding, the use of a diabetic formula may offer an advantage in facilitating improved glucose control.

Hepatic Disease

In the late 1970s, research began to appear demonstrating the beneficial use of high branched-chain amino acid (BCAA) (valine, leucine, and isoleucine) parenteral formulations for the patient with advanced liver disease. Patients with liver disease are often malnourished and require increased amounts of protein to maintain nitrogen equilibrium [68,69]. These formulas provided increased amounts of BCAA and reduced amounts of the aromatic amino acids (AAAs), phenylalanine, tyrosine, and tryptophan. These alterations have been thought to promote a reduced uptake of AAA at the blood–brain barrier, reducing the synthesis of false neurotransmitters and thereby ameliorating the neurological symptoms that occur with hepatic encephalopathy (HE) [69].

Parenteral and enteral BCAA formulas have been studied in patients with both acute and chronic HEs and have yielded conflicting results [70–74]. These studies are difficult to evaluate due to patient heterogeneity, differences in secondary therapies, and differences in nutritional regimens. Some studies evaluated BCAA without providing a nitrogen source for the control group [75]. A meta-analysis conducted by Naylor et al. [76] reviewed nine RCTs evaluating parenteral BCAA. Five of the studies showed a highly significant improvement in mental recovery from acute encephalopathy and a significant reduction in mortality. The authors concluded that, due to short-term follow-up times and mortality discrepancy across the trials, recommendation of parenteral BCAA over conventional therapy is not indicated.

Several trials evaluating BCAA in chronic encephalopathy have been conducted in an attempt to determine whether BCAA improves neurological outcome or improves tolerance to dietary protein. In a multicenter trial, Horst et al. [72] compared a BCAA-enriched versus a mixed protein enteral supplement. The BCAA-supplemented group achieved nitrogen balance equal to that of the control group without precipitation of HE. Additional studies in which patients were randomized to receive either oral diets enriched with BCAA or control failed to demonstrate clinical benefits of the BCAA-enriched diet [19]. In a 2003 evaluation, Marchesini and colleagues [77] compared the use of oral BCAA supplementation versus standard protein or carbohydrate without protein on death, disease deterioration, and the need for hospital admission in ambulatory patients with advanced cirrhosis. BCAA supplementation resulted in a significant decrease in the primary occurrence events, death, and disease deterioration. The authors concluded that there are benefits to routinely supplementing BCAA in patients with advanced cirrhosis. While this study offers a possible benefit to routine BCAA supplementation, generalizing these results to the critically ill patient with HE is not recommended. A 2009 Cochrane review demonstrated that BCAA may have a modest effect in improving encephalopathy. However, this effect was not seen when only trials of high quality were included [78]. The review concluded there is no convincing evidence to support the use of BCAA for patients with HE.

The routine use of BCAA-enriched enteral formulas does not appear to be clinically beneficial in patients with advanced liver disease and/or HE. Standard enteral formulas can successfully be used with most patients. However, in those patients who are unable to tolerate standard protein intakes without precipitation of HE, the use of BCAA-enriched enteral formulas may be better tolerated, thus permitting achievement of desired protein intakes [48,50,79]. Evidence-based guideline recommendations favor this approach. The 2009 SCCM/A.S.P.E.N. guidelines recommend that "standard enteral formulations should be used in ICU patients with acute and chronic liver disease. Branched chain amino acid formulations (BCAA) should be reserved for the rare encephalopathic patient who is refractory to standard treatment with luminal acting antibiotics and lactulose" [46].

Immune-Modulating Formulas and Critical Illness

The availability of formulas with added nutrient components to potentially improve outcome began to appear in the 1990s [4]. Specific nutrients such as arginine, nucleotides, and n-3 fatty acids were added to enteral formulas to enhance the immune system. The underlying rationale for these formula modifications was that by providing immune enhancement, the immune suppression common in critical illness and other disease states such as trauma and surgery could be altered resulting in improved patient outcome [80]. There are multiple enteral formulas marketed for immune modulation with a variety of *IMFs*. These IMFs provide varying amounts of some or all of these nutrients; this variability by nature makes it difficult when evaluating the evidence for use of a specific formulation.

Of all the specialized enteral products available, IMFs have been studied the most. A decade of research evaluating these formulas has demonstrated potential benefits in selected populations but has also raised concern regarding potential detriment [81]. Early studies evaluating IMFs were harshly criticized for flaws in both study design and statistical analysis. Others included small sample sizes that failed to yield significant results [82]. Three meta-analyses [83–85] and an industry-sponsored review in the critically ill population [83–88] have been published with variable results. More recently, the focus of evaluating the efficacy of IMFs has centered around surgical and trauma patients, populations thought to be at greater risk for arginine deficiency [89].

Beale and colleagues [90] conducted a meta-analysis in critically ill patients following trauma, sepsis, or major injury. No effect on mortality was demonstrated with immunonutrition. There were, however, significant reductions in infection rate, ventilator days, and hospital length of stay, most notably in surgical patients who received IMFs. The authors recommended the use of IMFs in the surgical population and that further study is necessary before recommendations can be made to use these formulas in all critically ill patients.

Heys et al. [91] conducted a meta-analysis of eleven trials evaluating immunonutrition in 1009 critically ill surgery and trauma patients. The use of IMFs was associated with a significant decrease in the incidence of wound complications and in hospital length of stay in patients undergoing gastrointestinal surgery and in those with critical illness. There were no differences, however, in death rate or in incidence of pneumonia in those who received the immune-modulating enteral nutrition.

Focusing on a more mixed ICU population, Heyland et al. [92] reviewed 22 randomized trials including 2419 patients comparing immunonutrition with standard enteral formulas in both surgical and critically ill patients. The overall results demonstrated no benefit of immunonutrition on mortality; however, immunonutrition was associated with a shorter hospital stay and a reduced incidence of infectious complications. In a subgroup analysis, the authors found that infectious complications and hospital length of stay were significantly lower in patients receiving formulas higher in arginine content. Elective surgical patients, compared to critically ill patients, demonstrated a reduced incidence of infectious complications when fed an immune-enhancing formula. The authors concluded that immunonutrition may decrease rates of infectious complications; however, this effect varies with patient population. Elective surgical patients may benefit from an immune-enhancing formula. Due to the potential for harm in selected critically ill patients, the authors recommended against routine use of IMFs in all critically ill patients.

The use of IMFs in all critically ill patients remains controversial. Some have suggested that positive effects on outcome have been realized only in those patients *less sick*, that is, those with lower APACHE scores [93]. These investigators have raised concern that the use of IMFs in sicker patients, such as those with severe sepsis, may lead to a worsening of the inflammatory process, an effect that could explain a higher mortality rate in this patient subgroup [82,94]. As a result of this concern, Bertolini et al. [95] reported an interim analysis of a multicenter trial evaluating an IMF and parenteral nutrition on mortality in critically ill patients. Subgroup analysis distinguished patients with and without severe sepsis and septic shock. Results demonstrated that those severely septic patients who received the immune-modulated enteral nutrition had a significantly higher mortality in the ICU compared to those who received parenteral nutrition. The investigators altered their study protocol based upon their results and discontinued recruiting patients with severe sepsis. They agree with recommendations by other investigators that the use of IMFs in severe sepsis is contraindicated.

As previously described, surgical and trauma patient populations are at risk of becoming arginine deficient. This is a result of a number of different mechanisms, the most predominant being an increased induction of arginase 1 by myeloid cells, T helper cells, and specific cytokines common in the patient experiencing trauma and complicated surgery [96]. Two large meta-analyses including studies in these specific populations have demonstrated positive results compared to Heyland's 2001 evaluation of mixed ICU patients. Marik and Zaloga [97] evaluated high-quality randomized trials comparing an IMF with a standard control formula in patients undergoing complicated surgical procedures. Some of these studies included critically ill patients but not exclusively. The use of an IMF significantly reduced the risk of acquired infections, wound complications, and LOS. Mortality was not different between the groups. The authors concluded that IMFs have important beneficial effects on clinical outcomes in high-risk surgical patients. They further suggest that arginine and ω-3 PUFAs may act synergistically to improve outcomes in noninfected surgical patients.

When should IMFs be utilized? Several clinical guidelines provide recommendations for the use of IMFs. SCCM/A.S.P.E.N guidelines recommend that IMFs should be used for the appropriate patient population. Specific populations include major elective surgery, trauma, burns, and head and neck cancers. The recommendation goes on to suggest that these formulas be used with caution in patients with severe sepsis [46]. The Canadian Clinical Practice Guidelines differ in their recommendation and advise that "diets supplemented with arginine and other select nutrients not be used for critically ill patients [98]." It is important to keep in mind that this recommendation applies to all critically ill patients. It appears these formulas are beneficial in selected patients and may not be appropriate for all ICU patients. It is important to remember that the decision to use an IMF should be based upon each patient's clinical status at the time of evaluation. As clinical condition changes, further decision making regarding formula usage will ultimately be required.

Pulmonary Disease

Specialized enteral formulas have been developed for two types of pulmonary disease: COPD and ARDS.

COPD Formulas

In the 1980s, reports began to appear in the literature describing adverse ventilatory effects when large amounts of dextrose-based parenteral nutrition solutions were provided to patients with and without COPD [99–101]. It was felt that the high amounts of dextrose provided in standard parenteral nutrition formulas was the primary causative factor in the reported adverse effects [99]. This concept was carried over into enteral nutrition via the introduction of a modified macronutrient formula designed for the COPD patient. Substituting a portion of carbohydrate calories with those provided from fat would limit carbon dioxide production resulting in improved ventilatory status. Two pulmonary formulas are currently available.

Multiple studies exist comparing the effects of macronutrient metabolism on respiratory function and status. Most have studied ambulatory patients making it difficult to generalize to patients in the ICU setting, but selected details can be highlighted. In 1985, Angelillo et al. [102] studied the effect of fat and carbohydrate contents on carbon dioxide (CO_2) production in ambulatory COPD patients with hypercapnia. The authors found that use of a high-fat formula reduced CO_2 production and respiratory quotient (RQ) compared to those receiving a lower-fat formula. In a subsequent study, Akrabawi et al. [103] evaluated pulmonary function and gas exchange in ambulatory COPD patients. Patients received both a high-fat and a moderate-fat formula *meal* on two separate days. No significant differences in RQ were demonstrated between the moderate- and high-fat meals.

Two studies have been conducted evaluating the role of high-fat formulas in weaning patients from mechanical ventilation. Al-Saady et al. [104] studied the effects of a modified enteral formula on 20 ventilated patients in an ICU. Patients were randomized to receive either a high-fat formula or a standard formula in amounts equal to their estimated energy requirements. Significant decreases in $PaCO_2$ tidal volume and peak inspiratory pressure were observed in the high-fat group, whereas these parameters all increased in the group receiving the standard formula. Time spent on artificial ventilation was 42% less in the high-fat group compared to the standard formula group and was statistically significant. Van den Berg et al. [105] conducted a similar study with slightly differing results. Their unblinded study compared a high-fat formula with a standard formula in 32 medical patients in the ICU. The RQ during weaning was significantly lower in the high-fat formula. There were, however, no significant differences in VCO_2 during weaning, and both groups had similar successful weaning episodes.

It is important to note that in most of the early reports citing adverse respiratory effects, patients received excessive calories (1.7–2.25 times the measured energy expenditure) [99–101]. A classic study by Talpers et al. [106] demonstrated no significant change in CO_2 production with increasing carbohydrate intake; however, with increasing caloric intake, CO_2 production was significantly increased. The authors concluded that avoidance of overfeeding is of greater significance than carbohydrate intake in avoiding nutritionally related hypercapnia. An additional study comparing calorie versus CHO intake conducted by Vemereen in an ambulatory COPD patient population showed similar results. In 2001, Vermeeren et al. evaluated both high-fat and high-CHO nutritional supplements and higher versus lower calories on metabolism and exercise capacity in stable COPD patients [107]. Significant increases in VCO_2, VO_2, and RQ were observed when the higher-calorie load was consumed, while there were no significant differences in these parameters between high-CHO and high-fat supplement consumption. While these studies were conducted in different patient populations, collectively, they demonstrate it is likely avoidance of overfeeding will have a greater impact in preventing adverse ventilator effects rather than reducing CHO intake.

Current guideline recommendations do not support the use of an altered macronutrient enteral formula in critically ill patients on mechanical ventilation [46]. The SCCM/A.S.P.E.N. guidelines suggest that "efforts should be made to avoid total caloric provision that exceeds energy requirements, as CO2 production increases significantly with lipogenesis and may be tolerated poorly in the patient prone to CO2 retention [46]." As with most nutrition support practices, patient monitoring is essential. If challenges in ventilatory status occur resulting in difficult management with the use of a standard enteral formula, offering an altered macronutrient formula is a potential option.

ARDS Formula

ARDS is a clinical illness characterized by hypoxemia ultimately resulting in respiratory failure [108]. The cascade of events that occurs in ARDS is thought to involve alveolar macrophages and their release of proinflammatory eicosanoids derived from the metabolism of arachidonic acid. Several of these metabolites, thromboxane A_2, leukotrienes, and prostaglandin E_2, have been implicated in the development of acute lung injury (ALI) [109,110]. A specialized enteral formula is available offering a modified lipid component specifically designed to potentially modulate the inflammatory cascade in ARDS. This formula contains fish and borage oils, sources of EPA and γ-linolenic acid (GLA). These fatty acids, in conjunction with metabolic alterations known to occur in ARDS, lead to an increased production of prostaglandins of the 1 series and leukotrienes of the 5 series, metabolites associated with anti-inflammatory and vasodilatory states. Vasoconstriction, platelet aggregation, and neutrophil accumulation are reduced when the eicosanoid balance favors anti-inflammatory rather than proinflammatory mediators [111].

Early evidence has shown support for the use of a specialized enteral formula with EPA/GLA in patients with ARDS. A 1999 multicenter trial conducted by Gadek et al. evaluating the use of a EPA/GLA formula in patients with evidence of either ARDS or ALI demonstrated significant improvement in gas exchange, fewer days of mechanical ventilatory support, and a decreased ICU length of stay in those who received the specialized formula [112]. A subsequent study by Singer et al. demonstrated similar results. Fifty-two ventilated patients with $PaO_2/FiO_2 \leq 250$ mmHg were randomized to receive either an EPA/GLA or control formula [113]. Patients who received the study formula had a significantly shorter length of ventilator time as well as a reduced ICU length of stay compared to the control patients. In an effort to pool the cumulative evidence comparing EPA/GLA formula versus control, in 2009, Pontes-Arruda et al. published a meta-analysis [114]. Three RCTs were included providing a total sample size of 411 patients, of which 296 were evaluable. The use of an EPA/GLA formula was associated with a 60% reduction in the risk of a 28-day mortality (OR = 0.040; 95% confidence interval (CI) = 0.24–0.68; p = 0.001). With aggregation via intent to treat, a significant reduction in a 28-day mortality was still evident with the use of an EPA/GLA formula (49% reduction) (OR = 0.51; 95% CI = 0.33–0.79; p = 0.002). Other positive clinical outcomes including increased 28 ventilator-free days and improved oxygenation were also demonstrated.

More recent studies evaluating the use of EPA/GLA in ARDS patients have demonstrated results conflicting with earlier studies. The largest to date is the ARDSnet OMEGA trial (2011), a multicenter randomized controlled clinical trial whose aim was to compare a bolus of EPA/GLA and antioxidants to placebo in 273 adults with ALI requiring mechanical ventilation [115]. This was a two-part trial that also included comparison between early and late enteral feeding initiation, a component managed through an enteral feeding protocol. Patients receiving the EPA/GLA bolus had significantly fewer ventilator- and ICU-free days. Patients receiving EPA/GLA also had significantly fewer nonpulmonary organ failure–free days. Hospital mortality was not significantly different between the groups. The study was terminated for futility (OMEGA). An additional single RCT evaluating an EPA/GLA formula was reported by Grau-Carmona et al. [116]. This trial compared an EPA/GLA formula to a control in 132 patients with ARDS or ALI. The EPA–GLA group showed a trend toward a decreased SOFA score (primary outcome), which was not significant. No differences were observed in the PaO_2/FiO_2 ratio or the days on mechanical ventilation between the groups. The control group stayed longer in the ICU than the EPA–GLA group [116].

Several potential reasons may help to explain the conflicting evidence observed with EPA/GLA formula use. In the ARDSnet OMEGA trial, patients were given a bolus dose of EPA/GLA twice a day rather than via a continuously provided enteral formula. In addition, the placebo used in this study contained protein, whereas the EPA/GLA bolus did not. Lastly, the OMEGA evaluation was part of the early versus later enteral feeding initiation study. Some of the EPA/GLA bolus patients received minimal enteral nutrients. In the Grau-Carmona study, enteral feeding was initiated within 1–3 days of ICU admission and was different than the start of feedings within 24 h in the Gadek and Singer trials. Could these significant differences in study design have led to the differing results compared to earlier studies?

Should an EPA/GLA formula be used in patients with ALI or ARDS? Guideline recommendations advise the use of this type of formula; however, due to the conflicting data observed with the OMEGA trial and lack of clear-cut effect in the Grau-Carmona trial, the most recent Canadian guideline recommendation suggests the use of EPA/GLA formula *be considered* [117], whereas the SCCM/A.S.P.E.N. guidelines do not make a recommendation due to conflicting data [46]. Additional research is needed that mimics early study design and formula administration to clarify existing and future guideline recommendations.

Acute Kidney Injury

Patients with acute kidney injury are typically hypercatabolic and hypermetabolic, due to their underlying disease state in addition to the derangements related to key impairments in renal function. This, in addition to the type of renal replacement therapy (RRT) utilized, greatly influences the patient's energy and protein requirements [118]. Up to 73% of ICU patients with AKI will require RRT during the course of their ICU stay and therefore is an important consideration in nutrition care decision making [119]. Protein requirements in these patients may be significantly higher than the general recommendation of 1.5–2 g/kg body weight [46]. In an evaluation of patients undergoing continuous venovenous hemodiafiltration, Bellomo and colleagues reported that a high protein intake of 2.5 g/kg/day of parenteral amino acids resulted in a slightly negative overall nitrogen balance. The authors attributed this high requirement to losses during the filtration process [120]. Similar results were obtained by Scheinkestel and colleagues in 2003, thus confirming the need for high protein intakes in patients undergoing this type of RRT [121].

Standard calorically dense enteral formulas are frequently appropriate for patients with acute kidney injury, although, to achieve higher protein requirements, supplemental protein may often be required. Ongoing laboratory monitoring of renal excreted electrolytes, potassium, phosphorus, and magnesium, is essential when using standard enteral formulas. In patients undergoing continuous venovenous hemodialysis (CVVHD), renal formulas may not be the most appropriate formula choice. These patients may not require a significant fluid restriction and have higher protein requirements as noted earlier. In addition, losses of electrolytes, specifically phosphorous [122], during CVVHD coupled with very low intakes provided by renal formulations often result in the need for significant electrolyte supplementations. A standard high-protein formula may be best suited for this type of patient.

In patients in whom RRT is delayed or unintended, a calorically dense, reduced protein formula is indicated [49]. Protein requirements for the nondialyzed patient with chronic renal failure range from 0.55 to 1.0 gm/kg/day [118] and can be achieved with reduced protein formulas. In addition to modified protein levels, renal formulas offer alterations in electrolytes. This variation may offer benefits to those patients who are not in an RRT or in whom the therapy is not achieving its desired results.

CONCLUSION

Enteral formula selection in the critically ill patient can be a challenging process. Underlying clinical state, nutritional requirements, and gastrointestinal function are all key components in deciding which formula to utilize. Understanding the individual formula components as well as the specific product variations is essential in formula selection. The growth of formula availability has resulted in a large number of specialized products marketed for improving specific disease-related outcomes. It is important that the practitioner carefully evaluates these products in conjunction with available scientific evidence prior to routine use.

REFERENCES

1. Griggs B.A., Chernoff R., Hoppe M.C., and Wade J.E. *Enteral Alimentation*. American Society for Parenteral and Enteral Nutrition, Rockville, MD, 1979.
2. Fussell ST. Enteral nutrition: A comprehensive overview. In: Matarese L.E. and Gottschlich M.M. (eds.), *Contemporary Nutrition Support Practice: A Clinical Guide*, 2nd edn. W.B. Saunders, Philadelphia, PA, 2003, pp. 188–200.
3. Gottschlich M.M., Shronts E.P., and Hutchins A.M. Defined formula diets. In: Rombeau JL, Rolandelli RH (eds.), *Clinical Nutrition: Enteral and Tube Feeding*, 3rd edn. W.B. Saunders, Philadelphia, PA, 1997, pp. 207–239.
4. Marks D.B., Marks A.D., and Smith CM. Intertissue relationships in the metabolism of amino acids. In: Velker J., (ed.), *Basic Medical Biochemistry*. William & Wilkins, Baltimore, MD, 1996, pp. 647–665.
5. Bell S.J., Bistrian BR., Wade JE. et al. Modular enteral diets: Cost and nutritional value comparisons. *J Am Diet Assoc* 1987; 87: 1526–1530.
6. Schaafsma G. The protein digestibility-corrected amino acid score. *J Nutr* 2000; 130: 1865S–1867S.
7. Keohane P.P. and Silk D.B. Peptides and free amino acids. In: Rombeau JL, Caldwell MD (eds.), *Clinical Nutrition: Enteral and Tube Feeding*, 1st edn. W.B. Saunders, Philadelphia, PA, 1984, pp. 44–59.
8. Reeds P.J. and Beckett P.R. Protein and amino acids. In: Ziegler E.E., Filer L.J. (eds.), *Present Knowledge of Nutrition*, 7th edn. ISLI Press, Washington DC, 1996, pp. 67–86.
9. Silk D.B., Fairclough P.D., Clar ML. et al. Use of peptide rather than free amino acid nitrogen source in chemically defined enteral diet. *J Parent Ent Nutr* 1980; 4: 548–553.
10. Craft I.L, Geddes D., Hyde C.W. et al. Absorption and malabsorption of glycine and glycine peptides in man. *Gut* 1968; 9: 425–437.
11. Verma S., Brown S., Kirkwood B., and Giaffer M.H. Polymeric versus elemental diet as primary treatment in active Crohn's disease: A randomized, double-blind trial. *Am J Gastroenterol* 2000; 95: 735–739.
12. Brinson R.R. and Kolts B.E. Hypoalbuminemia as an indicator of diarrheal incidence in critically ill patients. *Crit Care Med* 1987; 15: 506–509.
13. Brinson RR. Enteral nutrition in the critically ill patient: Role of hypoalbuminemia. *Crit Care Med* 1989; 17: 367–370.
14. Ziegler F., Ollivier J.M., Cynober L. et al. Efficiency of enteral nitrogen support in surgical patients: Small peptides versus non-degraded proteins. *Gut* 1990; 31: 1277–1283.
15. Heimburger D.C., Geels W.J., Bilbrey J. et al. Effects of small peptide and whole protein enteral feedings on serum proteins and diarrhea in critically ill patients: A randomized trial. *J Parenter Ent Nutr* 1997; 21: 162–167.
16. Dietscher J.E., Foulks C.J., and Smith R.W. Nutritional response of patients in an intensive care unit to an elemental formula vs a standard enteral formula. *J Amer Diet Assoc* 1998; 98: 335–336.
17. Canadian Critical Care Practice Guidelines 2012. Strategies for optimizing and minimizing risks of EN: Whole Protein vs. Peptides. http://www.criticalcarenutrition.com/docs/cpgs2012/4.3.pdf. Accessed April 30, 2014.
18. Souba W., Smith R.J., and Wilmore D.W. Glutamine metabolism by the intestinal tract. *J Parenter Ent Nutr* 1985; 9: 609–617.
19. Smith R.J. Glutamine metabolism and its physiological importance. *J Parenter Ent Nutr* 1990; 14(Suppl): 40S–44S.
20. Swails W.S., Bell S.J., Borlase B.C. et al. Glutamine content of whole proteins; implications for enteral formulas. *Nutr Clin Pract* 1992; 7: 77–80.
21. Velasco N., Hernandez G., Wainstain C. et al. Influence of polymeric enteral nutrition supplemented with different doses of glutamine on gut permeability in critically ill patients. *Nutrition* 2001; 17: 907–911.

22. Houdijk A.P., Rijnsburger E.R., Jansen J. et al. Randomised trial of glutamine-enriched enteral nutrition on infectious morbidity in patients with multiple trauma. *Lancet* 1998; 352: 772–776.
23. Jones C., Palmer T.E., and Griffiths R.D. Randomized clinical outcome study of critically ill patients given glutamine-supplemented enteral nutrition. *Nutrition* 1999; 15: 108–115.
24. Canadian Critical Care Practice Guidelines 2013. Composition of EN: Glutamine. http://www.criticalcarenutrition.com/docs/cpgs2012/4.1c.pdf. Accessed May1, 2014.
25. Academy of Nutrition and Dietetics Evidence Analysis Library. Supplemental Glutamine. http://andevidencelibrary.com/template.cfm?template=guide_summary&key=3201. Accessed May 1, 2014.
26. Basu H.N. Arginine: A clinical perspective. *Nutr Clin Pract* 2002; 17: 218–225.
27. Nieves C. and Langkamp-Henken B. Arginine and immunity: A unique perspective. *Biomed Pharmacother* 2002; 56: 471–482.
28. Suchner U., Heyland D.K., and Peter K. Immune-modulating actions of arginine in the critically ill. *Br J Nutr* 2002; 87(Suppl): S121–S132.
29. Gottschlich M.M. Selection of optimal lipid sources in enteral and parenteral nutrition. *Nutr Clin Pract* 1992; 7: 152–156.
30. Mayes P.A. Lipids of physiologic significance. In: Murray RK, Granner DK, Mayes PA, Rodwell VW (eds.), *Harper's Biochemistry*, 24th edn. Appleton & Lange, Stamford, CT, 1996, pp. 146–157.
31. Kinsella J.E. and Lokesh B. Dietary lipids, eicosanoids and the immune system. *Crit Care Med* 1990; 18: S94–S113.
32. Marks D.B., Marks A.D., and Smith C.M. Digestion and transport of dietary lipids. In: Velker J., (ed.), *Basic Medical Biochemistry*. William & Wilkins, Baltimore, MD, 1996, pp. 491–500.
33. Phan T.C. and Tsao P. Intestinal lipid absorption and transport. *Front Biosci* 2001; 6: 299–319.
34. Position of the American Dietetic Association. Health implications of dietary fiber. *J Am Diet Assoc* 2008; 108: 1716–1731.
35. Scheppach W. Effects of short chain fatty acids on gut morphology and function. *Gut* 1994; 35(Suppl): S35–S38.
36. Compher C., Seto R.W. Lew J.I., and Rombeau J.L. Dietary fiber and its clinical applications to enteral nutrition. In: Rombeau JL, Rolandelli RH (eds.), *Clinical Nutrition: Enteral and Tube Feeding*, 3rd edn. W.B. Saunders, Philadelphia, PA, 1997, pp. 81–95.
37. Dobb G.J. and Towler S.C. Diarrhea during enteral feeding in the critically ill: A comparison of feeds with and without fiber. *Intens Care Med* 1990; 16: 252–255.
38. Bass D.J., Forman L.P., Abrams S.E. et al. The effect of dietary fiber in tube-fed elderly patients. *J Gerontol Nurs* 1996; 22(10): 37–44.
39. Belknap D., Davidson L.J., and Smith C.R. The effects of psyllium hydrophilic mucilloid on diarrhea in enterally fed patients. *Heart Lung* 1997; 26: 229–237.
40. Bliss D.Z., Guenter P.A., and Settle R.G. Defining and reporting diarrhea in tube-fed patients—What a mess! *Am J Clin Nutr* 1992; 16(5): 488–489.
41. Schultz A.A., Ashby-Hughes B., Taylor R. et al. Effects of pectin on diarrhea in critically ill tube-fed patients receiving antibiotics. *Amer J Crit Care* 2000; 9: 403–411.
42. Rushdi T.A., Pichard C., and Khater Y.H. Control of diarrhea by fiber-enriched diet in ICU patients on enteral nutrition: A prospective randomized controlled trial. *Clin Nutr* 2004; 23: 1344–1352.
43. Academy of Nutrition and Dietetics Evidence Analysis Library. Enteral nutrition and fiber. http://www.andeal.org/topic.cfm?menu=5302&cat=4725. Accessed June 29, 2014.
44. Scaife C.L., Saffle J.R., and Morris S.E. Intestinal obstruction secondary to enteral feedings in burn trauma patients. *J Trauma* 1999; 47: 859–863.
45. McIvor A.C., Meguid M.M., Curtas S., and Kaplan D.S. Intestinal obstruction from cecal bezoar; a complication of fiber-containing tube feedings. *Nutrition* 1990; 6: 115–117.
46. McClave S., Martindale R., Vanek V. et al. Guidelines for the provision and assessment of nutrition support therapy in the adult critically Ill patient: Society of critical care medicine and the American society for parenteral and enteral nutrition. *J Parenter Enteral Nutr* 2009; 33: 277.
47. A.S.P.E.N. Board of Directors and Clinical Guidelines Task Force. Guidelines for the use of parenteral and enteral nutrition in adult and pediatric patients. *J Parent Ent Nutr* 2002; 26: 1SA–138SA.
48. Matarese L.E. Rationale and efficacy of specialized enteral and parenteral formulas. In: Matarese LE, Gottschlich MM (eds.), *Contemporary Nutrition Support Practice: A Clinical Guide*, 2nd edn. W.B. Saunders, Philadelphia, PA, 1998, pp. 263–275.
49. Malone A.M. The clinical benefits and efficacy in using specialized enteral feeding formulas. *Support Line* 2002; 24(1): 3–11.

50. Russell M.K. and Charney P. Is there a role for specialized enteral nutrition in the intensive care unit? *Nutr Clin Pract* 2002; 17: 156–168.
51. Ulate K.P., Lima Falcao G.C., Bielefeld M.R., Morales J.M., and Rotta A.T. Strict glycemic targets need not be so strict: A more permissive glycemic range for critically ill children. *Pediatrics* 2008; 122(4): e898–e904.
52. Kong M.Y., Alten J., and Tofil N. Is hyperglycemia really harmful? A critical appraisal of "Persistent hyperglycemia in critically ill children" by Faustino and Apkon. *J Pediatr* 2005; 146: 30–34; Fischer J.E. Branched-chain enriched amino acid solutions in patients with liver failure: An early example of nutritional pharmacology. *J Par Ent Nutr* 1990; 14: 249S–256S.
53. Martindale R.G., Shikora S.A., Nishikawa R., and Siepler J.K. The metabolic response to stress and alterations in nutrient metabolism. In: Shikora S.A., Martindale R.G., Schwaitzberg S.D. (eds.), *Nutritional Considerations in the Intensive Care Unit: Science, Rationale and Practice*. Kendall-Hunt Publishing, Dubuque, IA, 2002, pp. 11–20.
54. Brunkhorst F.M., Engel C., Ragaller M. et al. German Sepsis Competence Network (SepNet) practice and perception–A nationwide survey of therapy habits in sepsis. *Crit Care Med* 2008; 36(10): 2719–2725.
55. Dellinger R.P., Levy M.M., Carlet J.M. et al. Surviving Sepsis Campaign: International guidelines for management of severe sepsis and septic shock: 2008. *Crit Care Med* 2008; 36(1): 296–327.
56. Zerr K.J., Furnary A.P., Grunkemeier G.L. et al. Glucose control lowers the risk of wound infections in diabetics after open heart surgery. *Ann Thorac Surg* February 1997; 63(2): 356–361.
57. Trick W.E., Scheckler W.E., Tokars J.I. et al. Modifiable risk factors associated with deep sternal site infection after coronary artery bypass grafting. *J Thorac Cardiovasc Surg* 2000; 119: 108–114.
58. van den Berghe G., Wouters P., Weekers F. et al. Intensive insulin therapy in the critically ill patients. *N Engl J Med* 2001; 345(19): 1359–1367.
59. Charney P. Diabetes mellitus. In: Matarese LE, Gottschlich MM (eds.), *Contemporary Nutrition Support Practice: A Clinical Guide*, 2nd edn. W.B. Saunders, Philadelphia, PA, 2003, pp. 33–545.
60. Jenkins D.J.A., Leeds A.R., and Gassull M.A. Unabsorbable carbohydrate and diabetes: Decreased postprandial hyperglycemia. *Lancet* 1976; 2: 172.
61. Kollef M.H. and Schuster D.P. The acute respiratory distress syndrome. *N Eng J Med* 1995; 332: 27–37.
62. Peters A.L. and Davidson M.B. Lack of glucose elevation after simulated tube feeding with a low-carbohydrate, high fat enteral formula in patients with type 1 diabetes. *Am J Med* 1989; 87: 178–181.
63. Peters A.L. and Davidson M.B. Effects of various enteral feeding products on postprandial blood glucose response in patients with type I diabetes. *J Parent Ent Nutr* 1992; 16: 69–74.
64. Craig L.D., Nicholson S., Silverstone F.A., and Kennedy R.D. Use of a reduced carbohydrate, modified-fat enteral formula for improving metabolic control and clinical outcomes in long-term care residents with type 2 diabetes: Results of a pilot trial. *Nutrition* 1998; 14: 529–534.
65. Beyers P., Silver H., and Restler C. Hyperglycemia: Is a disease specific enteral formula indicated? *A.S.P.E.N. 19th Clinical Congress*, Miami Beach, FL, 1996, p. 592.
66. Mesejo A., Acosta J.A., Ortega C. et al. Comparison of a high-protein disease-specific enteral formula with a high-protein enteral formula in hyperglycemic critically ill patients. *Clin Nutr* 2003; 22: 295–305.
67. Canadian Clinical Practice Guidelines 2013. Composition of enteral nutrition: (Carbohydrate/fat): High fat/low CHO. http://www.criticalcarenutrition.com/docs/cpgs2012/4.2a.pdf. Accessed June 30, 2014.
68. Raup S.M. and Kaproth P. Hepatic failure. In: Matarese LE, Gottschlich MM (eds.), *Contemporary Nutrition Support Practice: A Clinical Guide*, 2nd edn. W.B. Saunders, Philadelphia, PA,, 1998, pp. 445–459.
69. Fischer J.E. The role of plasma amino acids in hepatic encephalopathy. *Surgery* 1975; 78: 276–290.
70. Cerra F.B., Cheung N.K., and Fischer JF. Disease specific amino acid infusion in hepatic encephalopathy: A prospective, randomized, double-blinded controlled trial. *J Par Ent Nutr* 1985; 9: 288–295.
71. Michel H., Bories P., Aubin J.P. et al. Treatment of acute hepatic encephalopathy in cirrhotics with branched-chain amino acid enriched versus a conventional amino acid mixture. *Liver* 1985; 5: 282–289.
72. Horst D., Grace N.D., Conn H.O. et al. Comparison of dietary protein with an oral, branched chain enriched amino acid supplement in chronic portal-systemic encephalopathy: A randomized controlled trial. *Hepatology* 1984; 4: 279–287.
73. Cerra F.B., Cheung N.K., Fischer J.E. et al. Disease-specific amino acid infusion (F080) in hepatic encephalopathy: A prospective, randomized, double-blind, controlled trial. *J Parenter Ent Nutr* 1985; 9: 288–295.
74. Rossi-Fanelli F., Riggio O., Cangiano C. et al. Branched-chain amino acids vs lactulose in the treatment of hepatic coma: A controlled study. *Dig Dis Sci* 1982; 27: 929–935.
75. Zaloga G. and Ackerman M.H. A review of disease specific formulas. *AACN* 1994; 5: 421–435.

76. Naylor C.D., O'Rourke K., Detsky A.S., and Baker J.P. Parenteral nutrition with branched-chain amino acids in hepatic encephalopathy. *Gastroenterology* 1989; 97: 1033–1042.
77. Marchesini G., Bianchi G., Merli M. et al. Nutritional supplementation with branched-chain amino acids in advanced cirrhosis: A double-blind, randomized trial. *Gastroenterol*ogy 2003; 124: 1792–1801.
78. Als-Nielsen B., Koretz R., Gluud L., and Gluud C. Branched-chain amino acids for hepatic encephalopathy. *The Cochrane Review*. John Wiley & Sons, Chichester, U.K., 2009.
79. Mizok B.A. Nutritional support in hepatic encephalopathy. *Nutrition* 1999; 15: 220–228.
80. Gottschlich M.M., Jenkins M., Warden G.D. et al. Differential effects of three dietary regimens on selected outcome variables in burn patients. *J Parenter Ent Nutr* 1990; 14: 225–236.
81. McClave S. The effects of immune-enhancing diets (IEDs) on mortality, hospital length of stay, duration of mechanical ventilation and other parameters. *J Parent Ent Nutr* 2001; 25: S44–S50.
82. Heyland D.K., Dhaliwal R., Drover J.W. et al. Canadian clinical practice guidelines for nutrition support in mechanically, ventilated, critically ill adult patients. *J Parent Ent Nutr* 2003; 27: 355–373.
83. Schloerb P.R. Immune-enhancing diets: Products, components and their rationales. *J Parent Ent Nutr* 2001; 25: S3–S7.
84. Jurkovich G. Outcome studies using immune-enhancing diets: Blunt and penetrating torso trauma patients. *J Parent Ent Nutr* 2001; 25: S14–S18.
85. Sax H. Effect of immune-enhancing formulas in general surgery patients. *J Parent Ent Nutr* 2001; 25: S19–S23.
86. Oltermann M. and Rasses T. Immunonutrition in a multidisciplinary ICU population: A review of the literature. *J Parent Ent Nutr* 2001; 25: S30–S35.
87. Moore F. Effects of immune-enhancing diets on infectious morbidity and multiple organ failure. *J Parent Ent Nutr* 2001; 25: S36–S43.
88. Kudsk K.A., Schloerb P.R., DeLegge M.H. et al. Consensus recommendations from the U.S. summit on immune-enhancing enteral therapy. *J Parent Ent Nutr* 2001; 25: S61–S62.
89. Pribis J.P., Zhu X., Vodovotz Y., and Ochoa J.B. Systemic arginine depletion after a murine model of surgery or trauma. *J Parenter Enteral Nutr* 2012; 36: 53–59.
90. Beale R.J., Bryg D.J., and Bihari D.J. Immunonutrition in the critically ill: A systematic review of clinical outcome. *Crit Care Med* 1999; 27: 2799–2805.
91. Heys S.D., Wlker L.G., Smith I., and Eremin O. Enteral nutritional supplementation with key nutrients in patients with critical illness and cancer. *Ann Surg* 1999; 329: 467–477.
92. Heyland D.K., Novak F., Drover J.W. et al. Should immunonutrition become routine in critically ill patients? A systematic review of the evidence. *JAMA* 2001; 286: 944–953.
93. Heyland D.K. and Novak F. Immunonutrition in the critically ill patient: More harm than good? *J Parenter Ent Nutr* 2001; 25: S51–S55.
94. Heyland D.K. Immunonutrition in the critically ill patient: Putting the cart before the horse? *Nutr Clin Pract* 2002; 17: 267–272.
95. Bertolini G., Iapichino G., Radrizzani D. et al. Early enteral immunonutrition in patients with severe sepsis: Results of an interim analysis of a randomized multicentre clinical trial. *Intensive Care Med* 2003; 29: 834–840.
96. Popovic P.J., Zeh H.J., and Ochoa J.B. Arginine and immunity. *J Nutr* 2007; 137: 1681S–1686S.
97. Marik P. and Zaloga G. Immunonutrition in high-risk surgical patients: A systematic review and analysis of the literature. *J Parent Ent Nutr* 2010; 34: 378–386.
98. Canadian Clinical Practice Guidelines 2013. EN composition: Diets supplemented with arginine and select other nutrients. http://www.criticalcarenutrition.com/docs/cpgs2012/4.1a.pdf. Accessed July 10, 2014.
99. Askanasi J., Rosenbaum S.H., Hyman A.I. et al. Respiratory changes induced by the large glucose loads of total parenteral nutrition. *JAMA* 1980; 243: 1444–1447.
100. Covelli H.D., Black J.W., Olsen M.S., and Beekman J.F. Respiratory failure precipitated by high carbohydrate loads. *Ann Int Med* 1981; 95: 579–581.
101. Delafosse B., Bouffard Y., Viale J.P. et al. Respiratory changes induced by parenteral nutrition in postoperative patients undergoing inspiratory pressure support ventilation. *Anesthesiology* 1987; 66: 393–396.
102. Angelillo V.A., Sukhdarshan B., Durfee B. et al. Effects of low and high carbohydrate feedings in ambulatory patients with chronic obstructive pulmonary disease and chronic hypercapnia. *Ann Intern Med* 1985; 103: 883–885.
103. Akrabawi S.S., Mobarhan S., Stoltz R., Stoltz R., and Ferguson P.W. Gastric emptying, pulmonary function, gas exchange, and respiratory quotient after feeding a moderate versus high fat enteral formula meal in chronic obstructive pulmonary disease patients. *Nutrition* 1996; 12: 260–265.

104. Al-Saady N.M., Blackmore C.M., and Bennett E.D. High fat, low carbohydrate, enteral feeding lowers PaCO2 and reduces the period of ventilation in artificially ventilated patients. *Intensive Care Med* 1989; 15: 290–295.
105. Van den Berg B. and Stam H. Metabolic and respiratory effects of enteral nutrition in patients during mechanical ventilation. *Intens Care Med* 1988; 14: 206–211.
106. Talpers S.S., Romberger D.J., Bunce S.B. et al. Nutritionally associated increased carbon dioxide production: Excess total calories vs high proportion of carbohydrate calories. *Chest* 1992; 102: 551–555.
107. Vermeeren M.A., Wouters E.F., Nelissen L.H., van Lier A., Hofman Z., and Schols A.M. Acute effects of different nutritional supplements on symptoms and functional capacity in patients with chronic obstructive pulmonary disease. *Am J Clin Nutr* 2001; 73: 295–301.
108. Hudson L.D. and Steinberg K.P. Acute respiratory distress syndrome: Clinical features, management and outcome. In: Fishman A.P. (ed.), *Pulmonary Diseases and Disorders*. McGraw-Hill, New York, 1998, pp. 2549–2565.
109. Mancuso P., Whelan J., DeMichele S.J. et al. Dietary fish oil and fish and borage oil suppress intrapulmonary proinflammatory eicosanoid biosynthesis and attenuate pulmonary neutrophil accumulation in endotoxic rats. *Crit Care Med* 1997; 25: 1198–1206.
110. Karlstad M.D., Palombo J.D., Murray M., and DeMichele S.J. The anti-inflammatory role of γ-linolenic and eicosapentaenoic acids in acute lung injury. In: Haung Y.S., Mills D.E. (eds.), *Gamma Linolenic Acid: Metabolism and Its Roles in Nutrition and Medicine*. AOCS Press, Champaign, IL, 1996, pp. 137–167.
111. Wennberg A.K., Nelson J.L., DeMichele S.J., and Campbell A.M. Affecting clinical outcome in acute respiratory distress syndrome with enteral nutrition. Ross Products Division, Abbott Laboratories, North Chicago, IL, 1997.
112. Gadek J., DeMichele S., Karlstad M. et al. Effect of enteral with eicosapentaenoic acid, γ-linolenic acid, and antioxidants in patients with acute respiratory distress syndrome. *Crit Care Med* 1999; 27: 1409–1420.
113. Singer P., Theilla M., Fisher H., Gibstein L., Grozovski E., and Cohen J. Benefit of an enteral diet enriched with eicosapentaenoic acid and gamma-linolenic acid in ventilated patients with acute lung injury. *Crit Care Med* 2006; 34: 1033–1038.
114. Pontes-Arruda A., Demichele S., Seth A., and Singer P. The use of an inflammation-modulating diet in patients with acute lung injury or acute respiratory distress syndrome: A meta-analysis of outcome data. *JPEN J Parenter Enteral Nutr* 2008; 32: 596–605.
115. Rice T.W., Wheeler A.P., Thompson B.T., et al. Enteral omega-3 fatty acid, -linolenic acid, and antioxidant supplementation in acute lung injury. *JAMA* 2011; 3061574–3061581.
116. Grau-Carmona T., Moran-Garcia V., Garcia-de-Lorenzo A. et al. Effect of an enteral diet enriched with eicosapentaenoic acid, gamma-linolenic acid and anti-oxidants on the outcome of mechanically ventilated, critically ill, septic patients. *Clin Nutr* 2011; 30: 578–581.
117. Canadian Clinical Practice Guidelines 2013. Composition of enteral nutrition: Fish oils, borage oils and antioxidants. http://www.criticalcarenutrition.com/docs/cpgs2012/4.1b(i).pdf. Accessed July 10, 2014.
118. Goldstein D.J. and Abrahamian-Gebeshian C. Nutrition support in renal failure. In: Matarese L.E., Gottschlich M.M. (eds.), *Contemporary Nutrition Support Practice: A Clinical Guide*, 2nd edn. W.B. Saunders, Philadelphia, PA, 1998, pp. 447–471.
119. Uchino S. Outcome prediction for patients with acute kidney injury. *Nephron Clin Pract* 2008; 109: 217–223.
120. Bellomo R., Tan H., Bhonagiri S. et al. High protein intake during continuous hemodiafiltration: Impact on amino acids and nitrogen balance. *Int J Artif Organs* 2002; 25: 261–268.
121. Scheinkestel C., Adams F., Mahony L. et al. Impact of increasing parenteral protein loads on amino acid levels and balance in critically ill anuric patients on continuous renal replacement therapy. *Nutrition* September 2003; 19: 733–740.
122. Wilkens K.G., Jenja V., and Shanaman E. Medical nutrition therapy for renal disorders. In: Mahan K.E., Escott-Stump S., Raymond J.L. (eds.), *Krause's Food and the Nutrition Care Process*, 13th edn. Elsevier, St. Louis, MO, 2012, pp. 799–831.

16 Complications of Parenteral Nutrition

Mandy L. Corrigan

CONTENTS

INTRODUCTION

Parenteral nutrition (PN) is an important therapy to deliver nutritional requirements when enteral nutrition is contraindicated or when there is prolonged inability to gain access to the gastrointestinal tract. The use of PN is not without risk or potential for complications. Safe and reliable venous access is a key component in the management of patients requiring PN in the hospital setting. Clinicians caring for patients requiring PN should be well versed with the potential complications associated with the use of PN and vascular access devices in order to provide safe and effective monitoring of this complex therapy. Management of PN within the intensive care unit (ICU) can be further complicated by the lack of hemodynamic stability and alterations in metabolism in the presence of stress. This chapter intends to review the short-term metabolic complications associated with PN use in the ICU, catheter-associated complications associated with PN delivery, and successful monitoring and management of these potential complications.

CATHETER-ASSOCIATED COMPLICATIONS

Placement-Associated Complications

Placement-associated catheter complications include pneumothorax, lacerations, air embolism, thrombosis, hemothorax, hemopericardium, or malposition. Skilled personnel placing temporary central lines should be present to avoid these potential complications.

After placement of a catheter, a chest x-ray should be taken to verify the catheter is safe to use and the position of the catheter tip. The American Society for Parenteral and Enteral Nutrition (A.S.P.E.N.) Safe Practices recommends the tip of central vascular access devices to terminate in the lower third of the superior vena cava (SVC) or the right atrium to reduce the risk of thrombosis (Mirtallo, 2004). Every step should be taken to reposition or replace the catheter if the tip does not fall within this range, especially for ICU patients where anticoagulation may be contraindicated (e.g., neurology ICU). Ruesch and colleagues found that central catheters placed using the internal jugular veins were less likely to be malpositioned compared to subclavian vein–placed catheters (Ruesch et al., 2002). Currently, the Centers for Disease Control and Prevention recommend the subclavian site for temporary central catheters over the jugular or femoral vein due to decreased risk of infection (O'Grady et al., 2011).

Virchow's triad describes the predisposing factors for central vein thrombosis, which include stasis, altered coagulation, and local trauma (Krzywda et al., 2007; Steiger, 2006). Signs of catheter-associated upper extremity venous thrombosis include swelling of the arms or neck, tenderness of the axilla, warmth, shoulder pain, jaw pain, and discoloration of the arm, or patients can be asymptomatic. Risk factors for thrombosis include older age, cancer, underlying hypercoagulable state, *Staphylococcus aureus* catheter-related blood stream infection (CRBSI), immobility, traumatic catheter insertion, dehydration, malposition of the catheter, catheter size (larger French or multiple lumens), and catheter composition (less thrombosis with silicone or polyurethane compared to other materials) (Crowley, 2008; Dechicco et al., 2007; Steiger, 2006).

Noninfectious Catheter Complications

PN solutions should be visually inspected to ensure no destabilization has occurred. Many precipitates are too small to be seen and providers ordering PN solutions should follow institution or manufacturer compounding guidelines (Table 16.1). A pharmacist can assist with compatibility and determining which medications can safely be added to PN solutions. Medication precipitates, calcium–phosphorus precipitates, lipids, or other incompatibilities typically cause occlusions. The cause of an occlusion (fibrin sleeve, blood, drug or lipid precipitate) dictates the treatment (Table 16.2). Thrombolytic agents should not be used in the presence of fever based on the potential for septic emboli to be spread within the bloodstream. The Infectious Disease Society of America does not recommend thrombolytic agents in the presence of catheter sepsis.

TABLE 16.1
Compatibility Guidelines for Cleveland Clinic Nutrition Support Team and Pharmacy

Component	Acceptable Compounding Range
Protein	20–60 g/L
Dextrose	40–250 g/L
Lipid	20–60 g/L
Divalent cations (magnesium + calcium)	≤20 mEq/L
Calcium phosphate product (calcium/L × phosphorus/L)	<200

TABLE 16.2
Placement-Associated and Noninfectious Catheter Complications

Complication	Signs and Symptoms	Treatment
Occlusion	Inability to withdraw fluid from the catheter, may or may not have resistance infusing via the catheter	• Determine the cause of occlusion and treat accordingly Precipitate • Lipid, ethanol • Drug, 0.1 normal hydrogen chloride or sodium bicarbonate Fibrin sheath or blood • Thrombolytic agent
Air embolism	Sudden-onset chest pain, cough, dyspnea, breathlessness Causes: Air entering the bloodstream due to unclamped catheter and end cap disconnected, tubing not primed, catheter integrity compromised (i.e., hole in catheter)	• Lay patient on the left side; lower head of bed
Catheter-associated deep vein thrombosis	Asymptomatic or swelling of the arms and/or neck (same side as catheter), tenderness of the axilla, warmth, shoulder pain, jaw pain, and discoloration of the arm	• Anticoagulation (if not contraindicated)
SVC syndrome	Swelling (shoulder, neck, or face) on same side as the catheter, dyspnea, prominent/enlarged veins on the chest wall, distended temporal or jugular veins, sore throat, cough, excessive tearing, or rhinorrhea	• Dependent on cause • Usually ultrasonography of neck, subclavian, brachial veins, chest computed tomography, thrombolytics, and/or anticoagulation • Vascular surgery or endovascular intervention may be indicated
Pneumothorax (associated with catheter placement)	Air in the pleural space on CXR, shortness of breath	• If large, chest tube placement may be required
Malposition of catheter tip (Mirtallo safe practices)	Tip of the catheter outside of lower third of the SVC adjacent to the right atrium on radiology studies	• Catheter repositioning or replacement

Sources: Krzywda, E.A. et al., Parenteral access devices, in: Gottschlich, M.M., DeLegge, M.H., Mattox, T., Mueller, C., and Worthington, P. (eds.), *The A.S.P.E.N. Nutrition Support Core Curriculum: A Case Based Approach—The Adult Patient*, American Society for Parenteral and Enteral Nutrition, Silver Spring, MD, 2007, pp. 300–322; Steiger, E., *J. Parenter. Enteral Nutr.* (*JPEN*), 30, S70, 2006; Pittiruti, M. et al., *Clin. Nutr.*, 28, 365, 2009; Cheng, S., *Cardiol. Rev.*, 17, 16, 2009; Johnson, D.H. et al., Superior vena cava syndrome, in: Abeloff, M.D., Armitage, J.O., Niederhuber, J.E., Kastan, M.B., and McKenna, W.G. (eds.), *Abeloff's Clinical Oncology*, 4th edn., Churchill Livingstone, Philadelphia, PA, 2008, pp. 803–814; Emery, M. et al., Vascular access and catheter care, in: Logan Couglin, K., DeChicco, R., and Hamilton, C. (eds.), *Cleveland Clinic Nutrition Support Handbook*, 3rd edn., Cleveland Clinic, Cleveland, OH, 2010, pp. 121–142; Potter, P.A., Parenteral nutrition, in: Perry, A.G. and Potter, P.A. (eds.), *Clinical Nursing Skills and Techniques*, 5th edn., Mosby, St Louis, MO, 2002, pp. 683–699; Fuhrman, M.P., Complication management in parenteral nutrition, in: Matarese, L.E. and Gottschlich, M.M. (eds.), *Contemporary Nutrition Support Practice: A Clinical Guide*, 2nd edn., Saunders Co, St Louis, MO, 2003, pp. 242–262.

Other contraindications to thrombolytic agents include active bleeding, recent stroke, intracranial surgery in the last 2 months, recent trauma, intracranial neoplasm, aneurysm, and severe uncontrolled arterial hypertension (Szeszycki and Benjamin, 2005).

When thrombolytic agents, ethanol or N hydrogen chloride, are not successful in restoring catheter patency, exchange of the catheter over a guide wire may be required. Other noninfectious catheter complications are listed in Table 16.2.

Mechanical Complications of PN Catheters

Among the mechanical complications that can occur with catheters for PN are breaks and ruptures that leave the catheter nonfunctional. In these cases, the catheter should be clamped with a blunt-tipped clamp between the catheter exit site and the damaged site to prevent air from entering and causing an air embolism. Affected catheters should be promptly exchanged or repaired if the need for venous access is ongoing.

Infectious Complications

One of the greatest risks with use of PN is the requirement of a central catheter placing the patient at risk for CRBSI. For patients receiving long-term PN, CRBSI is the most common infectious complication of PN therapy, often leading to a general hospital or ICU admission. Patients may also develop CRBSI while hospitalized. CRBSI is a significant contributor to health-care costs, with the average cost of CRBSI ranging from $33,000 to $65,000 per occurrence (Orsi et al., 2002; Pittet et al., 1994). Prevention methods for avoiding CRBSI are listed in Table 16.3.

Signs of CRBSI include fever (especially greater than 101°F), rigors, increased white blood cell count, and positive blood cultures, or quantitative blood cultures confirm the diagnosis in the absence of another source of infection.

Determining whether to remove the line or treat the infection with antibiotics while salvaging the catheter is based on clinical factors (i.e., hemodynamic stability, vital signs, causative pathogens, presence of fungemia) as well as the type of catheter (e.g., short- or long-term device) (Mermel, 2009). After the pathogen has been identified from blood cultures, infectious disease specialists should be consulted for recommendations on whether a long-term catheter (Hickman, Broviac, Groshong, implanted mediport) can be salvaged and specific antibiotic treatment regimens should be initiated.

TABLE 16.3
Prevention of CRBSIs

Use the CVC with the fewest number of lumens to manage the patient
Promptly remove any catheter that is no longer essential
Assess the need for the CVC daily
Antimicrobial coated catheters (for short-term use)
Maximal barrier precautions during insertion or guide wire
Staff education and training for insertion, maintenance, and infection control measures
Hand washing policy
2% chlorhexidine as skin antiseptic
Adequate RN staffing in the ICU
Use of a subclavian site rather than jugular or femoral sites for nontunneled CVCs
Do not routinely replace catheters to prevent infection

Sources: O'Grady, N.P. et al., *Am. J. Infect. Control*, 39, S1, 2011; Pittiruti, M. et al., *Clin. Nutr.*, 28, 365, 2009.

Short-term catheters (temporary central venous catheters, peripherally inserted central catheters, Hohn catheters) are easily placed and removed and therefore do not require salvaging should they become infected. Long-term tunneled catheters are often salvaged when possible due to the level of care required for placement and the potential for long-term PN patients having limited sites for IV access to lost sites for venous access due to other complications.

Catheter salvage is contraindicated when the CRBSI is caused by *S. aureus,* mycobacteria, *Pseudomonas aeruginosa,* or a fungemia (Mermel, 2009). Withholding delivery of parenteral IVFE during fungemia seems prudent because fungi are lipophilic (Schleman et al., 2000). CRBSI caused by *S. aureus* places the patient at risk for septic thrombophlebitis, endocarditis, and venous thrombosis (Mermel et al., 2009; Steiger 2006). Infectious disease specialists routinely recommend ruling out endocarditis in the presence of *S. aureus* bacteremia (Mermel et al., 2009). Thrombosis is also associated with *S. aureus* CRBSI, although patients may not always present with signs of venous thrombosis on physical examination. Routine internal jugular and subclavian ultrasonography should be obtained within 48 h of a positive blood culture for *S. aureus* (Crowley et al., 2008). In one study, 71% of patients who had *S. aureus* CRBSI had no physical signs of thrombosis, but thrombosis was confirmed by ultrasound (Crowley et al., 2008).

METABOLIC COMPLICATIONS

Hyperglycemia

Hyperglycemia is the most common short-term complication of PN. Often, critically ill patients have some degree of glucose intolerance due to the inflammatory response mediated by the cytokine and interleukin cascade. In addition to this temporary glucose intolerance due to stress, large amounts of parenteral dextrose may further exacerbate the inability to achieve adequate glycemic control. Other factors that contribute to hyperglycemia are the concomitant use of steroids, overfeeding, history of diabetes, other sources of intravenous dextrose provided separately from PN solutions, pancreatitis, and presence of an underlying infection. Excess of glucose through PN can lead to hypertriglyceridemia, hepatic steatosis, and adverse outcomes (Van der Bergh et al., 2006).

The parenteral dextrose load should be gradually increased during the first few days of therapy, with simultaneous increase in the insulin dosage if needed. Often, 150 g of dextrose is a starting point for the initiation of PN with no more than 200 g of dextrose in the first PN bag (McMahon, 2004). Blood glucose levels require monitoring at frequent intervals (usually every 4–6 h until goal calories or euglycemia is achieved concurrently). Regular human insulin can be added into the PN solution. A common rule of thumb when there is mild hyperglycemia before starting PN is to add 0.1 units of regular human insulin per gram of dextrose to the first PN bag and then increase by 0.05 units of regular human insulin per gram of dextrose to subsequent bags (McManon et al., 2006) until blood sugars are controlled. Other sources of dextrose outside the PN bag should be identified and removed from the regimen in the presence of hyperglycemia.

There is some debate on what is the ideal level of glycemic control. In 2001, Van den Berghe instituted the idea of intensive insulin therapy within the surgical ICU (Van den Berghe et al., 2001). Van den Berghe targeted blood sugars between 80 and 110 mg/dL in the intensive group and between 180 and 200 mg/dL in the conventional insulin group. After this study with 1548 patients showing a decreased mortality in the intensive insulin group, a shift moved toward tighter glycemic control within ICUs. Unfortunately, these results could not be reproduced with other ICU patient populations.

A follow-up study by Van den Berghe and colleagues in 2006 expanded the patient population beyond the surgical patient and now focused on the medical ICU patient population (Van den Berghe et al., 2006). Patients were enrolled into the intensive or the conventional insulin group with the same target parameters as the 2001 study. Morbidity was reduced significantly in the intensive insulin group, but mortality was not. Of note, the studies differed slightly in the severity of illness (with the medical ICU patients having a higher severity of illness).

The Normoglycemia in Intensive Care Evaluation and Survival Using Glucose Algorithm Regulation (NICE-SUGAR) study was composed of 6104 patients randomized into 2 groups. The intensive glucose control group targeted blood sugars to a range of 81–108 mg/dL, and the conventional glucose control group had a target blood sugar range of 180 mg/dL or less. Severe hypoglycemia was defined at less than 40 mg/dL and occurred in 0.5% of the conventional group and 6.8% of the intensive group ($p < 0.001$) (NICE-SUGAR). The main conclusion of the study was that intensive glucose control increased mortality among ICU patients and a blood sugar target below 180 mg/dL was associated with a lower mortality. Based on the results of the NICE-SUGAR study, many institutions have moved away from intensive therapy to prevent hypoglycemia. Current clinical guidelines from A.S.P.E.N. suggest a target blood glucose range of 140–180 mg/dL (McMahon et al., 2012).

Hypoglycemia

Hypoglycemia is associated with sudden interruption in PN infusion or loss of central access, excess insulin in the PN formula, or too tight insulin control outside the PN bag. If hypoglycemia continues, the PN bag should be held and a 10% dextrose intravenous fluid should be initiated at the same rate until a new PN formula can be compounded with less insulin.

Electrolyte Imbalances

Frequently, critically ill patients will have electrolyte imbalances due to a variety of etiologies. Critically ill patients may experience dysnatremias, hypocalcemia, hypokalemia, hyperkalemia, hyperphosphatemia, hypophosphatemia, hypermagnesemia, or hypomagnesemia, which can be associated with the use of PN. Signs, symptoms, and treatment of these electrolyte imbalances have been discussed elsewhere in this text and elsewhere in depth (Baumgartner, 2001; Piazza-Barnett and Matarese, 1999; Whitmire, 2003, 2008).

Electrolyte abnormalities should be corrected before PN is initiated. In the presence of hypocalcemia, an ionized calcium level should be checked since serum calcium is protein bound before considering intravenous calcium supplementation. Refeeding syndrome, characterized by electrolyte abnormalities (such as hypophosphatemia, hypokalemia, hypomagnesemia, hyperglycemia), weakness, arrhythmias, dysoxia, cardiac dysfunction, and respiratory failure, can occur when malnourished patients are reintroduced to overzealous nutrition regimens after periods of starvation (Byrnes and Strangenes, 2011). See the section "Vitamin and Mineral Status in the ICU" for further discussion on prevention of refeeding syndrome.

Fluid Imbalances

Regulating fluid status can be tedious in the ICU. When patients are volume restricted, the clinician has a few tools to deliver the greatest nutrient content in a low fluid volume. The PN solution can be concentrated by utilizing 15% amino acid solutions or, if the patient is receiving a three-in-one PN solution, 30% intravenous fat emulsion (IVFE) can be suggested. PN calories may be temporarily limited by fluid restraints until fluids may be liberalized.

Overfeeding

Overfeeding of any macronutrient or the combination can negatively impact multiple organ systems within the body. The consequences of overfeeding are listed in Table 16.4. Non-PN sources of calories should be identified and the PN regimen should be adjusted to account for these calories. Patients receiving propofol receive 1.1 cal/mL as lipid. When propofol use is prolonged or at high doses, IVFEs are not necessary. Of note, the Society for Critical Care Medicine and A.S.P.E.N. guidelines for ICU patients suggest withholding IVFE for the first week in the ICU (McClave et al., 2009).

TABLE 16.4
Consequences of Overfeeding

Organ	Consequence
Lung	Hypercapnia (total calorie excess)
	Respiratory insufficiency (excess fluid, fat, or dextrose, or calories)
Liver	Elevated LFTs
	Hepatic steatosis (increased dextrose or fat)
	Increased blood ammonia (increased protein)
	Hypertriglyceridemia (dextrose overfeeding or rapid infusion IV fat emulsion)
Pancreas	Hyperinsulinemia (due to excess dextrose)
Kidney	Azotemia
	Fluid retention
	Sodium retention
Heart	Altered electrolytes leading to arrhythmias
	Heart failure with excess fluid

Although this is a controversial recommendation with low levels of evidence, it is clinically relevant in the United States where the only IVFE options for use are omega-6 soy-based IVFE that are immunosuppressive in nature.

Hypertriglyceridemia is another potential adverse effect associated with overfeeding that can be caused by excess dextrose calories or rapid infusion of IVFE. If serum triglycerides exceed 400 mg/dL, IVFEs should be withheld (Mirtallo et al., 2004). IVFE should be infused over 8–12 h as a preventative measure. When IVFs are omitted due to hypertriglyceridemia for prolonged periods of time (>14 days), the patient is at risk for developing essential fatty acid deficiency. Typically, patients can receive fat free PN solutions for 2–3 weeks without a concern for essential fatty acid deficiencies. If there is an enteral source of fat being delivered with adequate absorption, the concern for essential fatty acid deficiency is alleviated.

A final potential complication associated with IVFE includes an allergy interaction for patients with existing allergies to the egg phospholipid that is used to emulsify the solution.

Underfeeding

Underfeeding patients in the ICU may not be intentional, but rather from inadequate delivery of the prescribed quantity of nutrition support. In 2006, Jain and colleagues surveyed 66 Canadian ICUs and found that patients only received 58% of their recommended caloric requirements (Jain et al., 2006). In the critically ill obese patient, some research shows there may be some benefits of intentional underfeeding for patients with a body mass index greater than 30. In these obese patients, protein should not be restricted, but restrict total calories to 60%–70% of target energy requirements to offer better metabolic outcomes and a shorter length of stay (Choban et al., 1997; Dickerson et al., 2002). When underfeeding is utilized, the goal is for short-term underfeeding for 3–5 days and then advancing to target energy requirements over the next 3–5 days as hypermetabolism subsides.

Hepatic Abnormalities

Minor increases in liver function tests (LFTs) are common with initiation of PN and usually return to normal after a few weeks of therapy without intervention and continued PN infusion (Jeejeehboy, 2005). When LFTs suddenly increase or remain persistently elevated, the ICU team must investigate the underlying cause. Steatosis (fat accumulation in the liver), cholestasis (impaired bile secretion/biliary

TABLE 16.5
Monitoring and Treating Hepatic Complications

Assess indication for PN	Discontinue PN if able Start enteral nutrition
Assess for overfeeding of macronutrients	Decrease dextrose or lipid calories if overfeeding is present Limit IV fat emulsion to lowest dose to prevent essential fatty acid deficiency (500 mL of 20% lipid once weekly) Limit IV fat emulsion to less than 1 g/kg/day if patient requires three-in-one PN solution to achieve adequate glycemic control Investigate and account for other sources of calories (i.e., propofol, dextrose contacting intravenous fluids, dextrose containing medication drips, and dialysate solutions)
Assess indication for IV fat emulsion	• Discontinue IV fat emulsion if patient is tolerating adequate amount of fat from enteral nutrition
Assess medications or herbal supplements (promoting cholestasis or hepatotoxicity)	• Review current medications • Discontinue antisecretory agents and histamine-2 blockers in PN solutions that can cause cholestasis • Review any herbal supplements
Rule out sepsis/infection	• Review for signs of sepsis, including catheter-related sepsis
Assess for bacterial overgrowth	• Assess for signs of small bowel bacterial overgrowth in patients with short bowel syndrome or blind loops, and treat with a trial of oral cyclic antibiotics because released endotoxin reduces bile flow (Fuhrman)

Sources: Corrigan, M.L. et al., Parenteral nutrition, in: Mullen, G.E., Matarese, L.E., and Palmer, M. (eds.), *The Gastrointestinal and Liver Disease Nutrition Desk Reference*, CRC Press, Boca Raton, FL, 2011, pp. 343–358; Jeejeehboy, K.N., *Pract. Gastroenterol.*, 24, 62, 2005; Fuhrman, M.P., Complication management in parenteral nutrition, in: Matarese, L.E. and Gottschlich, M.M. (eds.), *Contemporary Nutrition Support Practice: A Clinical Guide*, 2nd edn., Saunders Co, St Louis, MO, 2003, pp. 242–262.

obstruction), and gallstones/gallbladder sludge (due to impaired bile flow and gallbladder contractility) are common causes (Jeejeehboy, 2005; Krzywda, 2007; Ulkeja and Romano, 2007). Frequently, PN solution components are the suggested contributors to liver-related complications, although sepsis, bacterial overgrowth, or lack of enteral stimulation can contribute and must be investigated (Jeejeehboy, 2005; Krzywda, 2007). Proinflammatory cytokines are released during infection and are activated by endotoxins, which may impact the liver. See Table 16.5 for suggestions on monitoring and treating hepatic complications.

When triglyceride levels exceed 400 mg/dL, IVFEs should be withheld. Hypertriglyceridemia may negatively impact the immune response and pulmonary hemodynamics and increase the risk of pancreatitis (Seidner et al., 1989).

Vitamin and Mineral Status in the ICU

When relying on biochemical markers of vitamin, mineral, or trace element levels while in the ICU setting, the clinician must acknowledge a few factors. Micronutrients exist in pools, micronutrients are protein bound whose carriers may decrease in the presence of inflammation despite adequate total body or tissue stores, and there is an altered distribution of micronutrients during the acute phase response (Prelack and Sheridan, 2001). Therefore, conducting a nutrition-focused physical examination, assessing nutrient laboratory values, and being aware of disease states that may cause increased requirements or losses of specific nutrients can aid the clinician in recognizing and treating true deficiencies or toxicities.

Use of a standard intravenous multivitamin (MVI) in PN solutions is prudent. Some MVI products contain 150 mcg of vitamin K, but this should not interfere with anticoagulation regimens since it is a small dose and is a consistent amount delivered daily. Lipid emulsion may also contribute to vitamin K delivery in PN solutions. There are 0.6–0.7 µg of vitamin K per milliliter of Intralipid (150–175 mg in 250 mL of 20% Intralipid) (Drittij-Reiinders et al., 1994).

Additional vitamins or trace elements can be supplemented via PN solutions, but caution should be taken to just relying on biochemical markers during the presence of inflammation. Frequently in clinical practice, 100 mg of thiamin is added to prevent refeeding syndrome for the first 3–5 days along with slow advancement of dextrose calories (starting at 150 g dextrose, increasing by 150–300 g daily to goal based on laboratory studies and glycemic control). Iron should not be added to IVFE contacting PN solutions due to the risk of destabilizing the IVFE (Kumpf, 2003). Routine supplementation of iron via PN solutions is not recommended in the critically ill due to controversy between iron supplementation in the presence of active infection or stress (Prelack and Sheridan, 2001).

CASE STUDY

TN is a 45-year-old male with a past medical history significant for Crohn's disease, deep venous thrombosis, and type 2 diabetes mellitus. He underwent multiple small bowel resections due to enterocutaneous fistulae resulting in short bowel syndrome and PN dependency for the last 6 years. He currently has 100 cm end jejunostomy and a Hartman's stump out of continuity.

TN presents to the emergency department feeling weak, new onset lower back pain, and a temperature of 101.3°F. He also exhibits abnormal hyperglycemia compared to baseline.

His home medications are

- 10 units of Lantus
- 50,000 IUs of vitamin D three times weekly
- Imodium two caps 30 min before meals and bedtime (eight caps daily)
- Lomotil two caps 30 min before meals and bedtime (eight caps daily)
- Codeine 15 mg cap 30 min before meals and bedtime (four caps daily)

Lab	Two Weeks Ago	ER Labs
White blood cell	6,000	**18,000**
Sodium	138	141
Potassium	4.2	3.5
Blood urea nitrogen	35	38
Creatinine	0.8	1
Glucose	220	**381**
AST	45	**136**
ALT	25	**224**
Total bilirubin	0.3	1

Note: Bold values mean the lab is abnormal.

His home diet regimen includes low simple sugar and high complex carbohydrate in three small meals and three small snacks daily.

His home PN formula contains 80 g amino acids, 2100 kcal total, 50 units of insulin, and IVFE of 500 mL of 20% once weekly.

He is 5′11″, weighs 68 kg, and has a BMI of 20.9, which is normal.
He has a single lumen right internal jugular Hickman catheter.
His home intake and output (preillness) data are

- Oral intake, 1000 mL oral rehydration solution
- PN volume, 4200 mL cycled over 12 h
- Urine output, 1200 mL
- Jejunostomy output, 4000 mL

TN was admitted directly from the ER to the ICU due to significant hypotension and started on pressors (Levophed) along with broad-spectrum antibiotics. The Hickman catheter was removed due to worsening hemodynamic instability and persistent fevers despite an antibiotic regimen. Blood cultures grew *Candida albicans*. TN was hydrated with intravenous fluids and PN was withheld due to instability and the patient was well nourished. Once repeated, blood cultures showed clearance of the fungus; PN was resumed with acceptable glycemic control and a lower volume since TN was not eating well and his ostomy output was below 2 L. Fungal endophthalmitis was ruled out before discharge with the assistance of an ophthalmologist. TN lost 4 kg and required physical therapy due to a 10-day hospital stay (6 ICU days).

REFERENCES

Baumgartner TG. Enteral and parenteral electrolyte therapeutics. *Nutr Clin Pract*. 2001;16:233–235.

Byrnes MC, Strangenes J. Refeeding in the ICU: An adult and pediatric problem. *Curr Opin Nutr Metab Care*. 2011;14:186–192.

Cheng S. Superior vena cava syndrome. A contemporary review of a historic disease. *Cardiol Rev*. 2009;17:16–23.

Choban PS, Burge JC, Scales D, Flanchbaum L. Hypoenergetic nutrition support in hospitalized obese patients: A simplified method for clinical application. *Am J Clin Nutr*. 1997;66:546–550.

Corrigan ML, John BK, Steiger E. Parenteral nutrition. In: Mullen GE, Matarese LE, Palmer M, eds. *The Gastrointestinal and Liver Disease Nutrition Desk Reference*. Boca Raton, FL: CRC Press;2011, pp. 343–358.

Crowley AL, Peterson GE, Benjamin DK Jr et al. Venous thrombosis in patients with short- and long-term central venous catheter-associated *Staphylococcus aureus* bacteremia. *Crit Care Med*. 2008;36:385–390.

DeChicco R, Seidner DL, Brun C, Steiger E, Stafford J, Lopez R. Tip position of long-term central venous access devices used for parenteral nutrition. *J Parenter Enteral Nutr* (*JPEN*). 2007;31:382–387.

Dickerson RN, Boschert KJ, Kudsk KA, Brown RO. Hypocaloric enteral tube feeding in critically ill obese patients. *Nutrition*. 2002;18(3):241–246.

Drittij-Reiinders MJ, Sels JP, Rouflart M, Thijssen HH. Vitamin K status and parenteral nutrition; the effect of Intralipid on plasma vitamin K1 levels. *Eur J Clin Nutr.* 1994;48(7):525–527.

Emery M, Stafford J, Pearson A, Steiger E. Vascular access and catheter care. In: Logan Couglin K, DeChicco R, Hamilton C, eds. *Cleveland Clinic Nutrition Support Handbook*, 3rd edn. Cleveland, OH: Cleveland Clinic;2010, pp. 121–142.

Fuhrman MP. Complication management in parenteral nutrition. In: Matarese LE, Gottschlich MM, eds. *Contemporary Nutrition Support Practice: A Clinical Guide*, 2nd edn. St Louis, MO: Saunders Co;2003, pp. 242–262.

Jain MK, Heyland D, Dhaliwal R. Dissemination of the Canadian clinical practice guidelines for nutrition support: Results of a cluster randomized controlled trial. *Crit Care Med*. 2006;34(9):2362–2369.

Jeejeehboy KN. Management of PN-induced cholestasis. *Pract Gastroenterol*. 2005;24:62–68.

Johnson DH, Laskin J, Cmelak A, Meranze S, Roberts JR. Superior vena cava syndrome. In: Abeloff MD, Armitage JO, Niederhuber JE, Kastan MB, McKenna WG, eds. *Abeloff's Clinical Oncology*, 4th edn. Philadelphia, PA: Churchill Livingstone;2008, pp. 803–814.

Krzywda EA, Andris DA, Edmiston CE, Wallace JR. Parenteral access devices. In: Gottschlich MM, DeLegge MH, Mattox T, Mueller C, Worthington P, eds. *The A.S.P.E.N. Nutrition Support Core Curriculum: A Case Based Approach—The Adult Patient*. Silver Spring, MD: American Society for Parenteral and Enteral Nutrition;2007, pp. 300–322.

Kumpf VJ. Update on parenteral iron therapy. *Nutr Clin Pract*. 2003;18:318–326.

McClave SA, Martindale RG, Vanek VW et al. Guidelines for the provision and assessment of nutrition support therapy in the adult critically ill patient. *J Parenter Enteral Nutr* (*JPEN*). 2009;33:277–316.

McMahon M. Management of parenteral nutrition in acutely ill patients with hyperglycemia. *Nutr Clin Pract*. 2004;19:120–128.

McMahon MM, Nystrom E, Braunschweig C, Miles J, Compher C. A.S.P.E.N. clinical guidelines: Nutrition support of the adult patient with hyperglycemia. *J Parenter Enteral Nutr* (*JPEN*) 2013;37(1):23–36.

Mermel LA, Allon M, Bouza E et al. Clinical practice guidelines for the diagnosis and management of intravascular catheter-related infection: 2009 update by the Infectious Diseases Society of America. *Clin Infect Dis*. 2009;49:1–45.

Mirtallo J, Canada T, Johnson D. Safe practices for parenteral nutrition. *J Parenter Enteral Nutr* (*JPEN*). 2004;28(6):S39–S70.

NICE-SUGAR Study investigators, Finfer S, Chittock DR et al. Intensive versus conventional glucose in critically ill patients. *N Engl J Med*. March 26, 2009;360(13):1283–1297.

O'Grady NP, Alexander M, Burns LA et al. Guidelines for the prevention of intravascular catheter-related infections. *Am J Infect Control*. 2011;39:S1–S34.

Orsi GB, Di Stefano L, Noah N. Hospital acquired, laboratory confirmed bloodstream infection: Increased hospital stay and direct costs. *Infect Control Hosp Epidemiol*. 2002;23:190–197.

Piazza-Barnett R, Matarese LE. Electrolyte management in total parenteral nutrition. *Support Line*. 1999;21(2):2–8.

Pittet D, Tarara D, Wenzel RP. Nosocomial blood stream infection in critically ill patients: Excess length of stay, extra costs, and attributable mortality. *JAMA*. 1994;271:1598–1601.

Pittiruti M, Hamilton H, Biffi R, MacFie J, Pertkiewicz, M. ESPEN guidelines on parenteral nutrition: Central venous catheters (access, care, diagnosis, and therapy of complications). *Clin Nutr*. 2009;28:365–377.

Potter PA. Parenteral nutrition. In: Perry AG, Potter PA, eds. *Clinical Nursing Skills and Techniques*, 5th edn. St Louis, MO: Mosby;2002, pp. 683–699.

Prelack K, Sheridan RL. Micronutrient supplementation in the critically ill patient: Strategies for clinical practice. *J Trauma*. 2001;51:601–620.

Ruesch S, Walder B, Trammer M. Complications of central venous catheters: Internal jugular versus subclavian access—A systematic review. *Crit Care Med*. 2002;30:454–460.

Schleman KA, Tullis G, Blum R. Intracardiac mass complicating malassezia furfur fungemia. *Chest*. 2000;118:1828–1829.

Seidner DL, Mascioli EA, Istfan NW et al. Effects of long chain triglyceride emulsions on reticuloendothelial system function in humans. *J Parenter Enteral Nutr*. 1989;13:614–619.

Steiger E. Dysfunction and thrombotic complications of vascular access devices. *J Parenter Enteral Nutr* (*JPEN*). 2006;30:S70–S72.

Szeszycki EE, Benjamin S. Complications of parenteral feeding. In: Cresci G, ed. *Nutrition Therapy for the Critically Ill: A Guide to Practice*. Boca Raton, FL: CRC Press;2005, pp. 303–319.

Ulkeja A, Romano MM. Complications of parenteral nutrition. *Gastroenterol Clin N Am*. 2007;36:23–46.

Van den Berghe G, Wilmer A, Hermans G et al. Intensive insulin therapy in the medical ICU. *N Engl J Med*. 2006;354:449–461.

Van den Berghe G, Wouters P, Weekers F et al. Intensive inulin therapy in critically ill patients. *N Engl J Med*. 2001;354:1359–1367.

Whitmire SJ. Fluid, electrolytes, and acid-base balance. In: Matarese LE, Gottschlich MM, eds. *Contemporary Nutrition Support Practice: A Clinical Guide*, 2nd edn. Philadelphia, PA: Saunders Elsevier;2003, pp. 127–144.

Whitmire SJ. Nutrition-focused evaluation and management of dysnatremias. *Nutr Clin Pract*. 2008;23:108–121.

17 Enteral Feeding Challenges

Carol Rees Parrish, Joe Krenitsky, and Kendra Glassman Perkey

CONTENTS

INTRODUCTION

Nutrition support of the critically ill patient remains an area of controversy. Large, randomized, controlled trials have started to provide some data, but questions such as the timing of nutrition, nutrient needs, and specific nutrients that would best affect outcomes remain active research topics. The best available evidence is that enteral nutrition (EN) provides improved outcomes in the critically ill patient, compared to parenteral nutrition (PN) (Braunschweig et al. 2001).

TABLE 17.1
Barriers to EN Delivery in the Hospital Setting

- Diagnostic procedures
- High-dose Diprivan (propofol) use
- Enteral access problems (clogged/pulled tubes or obtaining postpyloric access)
- BRE < 30°
- Feedings held due to drug–nutrient interactions
- Hemodialysis
- Hypotensive episodes
- Inadvertent hypocaloric EN orders
- *NPO* at midnight for tests, surgery, or procedures
- Physical or occupational therapy
- Transportation of the unit
- *GI intolerance or dysfunction*

Source: Parrish, C.R. et al., *Nutrition Support Traineeship Syllabus*, Fully revised, University of Virginia Health System, Charlottesville, VA, July 2013. Used with permission.

There are many barriers encountered in the hospital setting that prevent adequate infusion of EN into patients. The literature reports that *gastrointestinal (GI) intolerance* is responsible for the majority of lost feeding time (De Beaux et al. 2001; De Jonghe et al. 2001; Sheean et al. 2012). See Table 17.1 for a list of barriers that alter effective infusion of EN in a typical intensive care unit (ICU).

The real barrier, however, may be the perceptions and misinformation regarding GI intolerance, due to the lack of evidence-based and uniform practice in assessing GI function during initiation and progression of EN. How do we effectively provide EN to a patient population with inherent *endogenous ICU barriers* that thwart our efforts to provide adequate feeding? This chapter will attempt to provide a review of GI function to better assess true *EN tolerance* in these patients. The most common GI intolerance issues facing clinicians will be addressed, specifically:

- Aspiration
- Bowel sounds (BSs)
- Residual volumes
- Nausea/vomiting
- Diarrhea
- Osmolality/dilution of EN
- Constipation
- Initiation and progression of EN
- Clogged feeding tubes

Suggestions to surmount EN intolerance will be provided.

ASPIRATION

Aspiration is defined as the passage of materials into the airway below the level of the true vocal cords (Teasell et al. 1994). The aspirated substance may be saliva, naso- or oropharyngeal secretions, bacteria, food, beverage, or gastric contents. Studies that investigate the risk or management of aspiration related to EN are unable to differentiate the source of the aspirated material unless the feeding is radioactively labeled (Heyland et al. 2001). However, few studies are so designed. The incidence of aspiration pneumonia in patients who receive EN is difficult to determine due to varying definitions of aspiration and pneumonia and varying ability to recognize aspiration events. Studies that have investigated methods to decrease aspiration pneumonia in tube-fed patients have described aspiration pneumonia rates between 5% and 36% (Drover et al. 2003; Kearns et al. 2000; Neumann and DeLegge 2002).

Detection of Aspiration

Several methods of monitoring patients for aspiration risk have been popularized through *conventional wisdom*. These include (1) the routine monitoring of gastric residual volumes (GRVs) (see the section "Residual Volume"), (2) checking tracheal secretions for the presence of glucose, and (3) the addition of blue food coloring (BFC) to feeding formulas.

The presence of glucose in tracheal secretions is not a specific or sensitive method of detecting aspiration of EN. Tracheal glucose can be positive in patients who are not receiving EN, and in one study, tracheal glucose correlated with serum glucose, but not aspiration (Kinsey et al. 1994; Metheny and Clouse 1997). Some enteral formulas will not trigger a positive result even when aspirated due to the low glucose content of the formula (Kinsey et al. 1994).

Several studies have provided data that the use of blue dye in enteral formulas had a very low sensitivity (Metheny and Clouse 1997; Montejo-Gonzalez et al. 1994; Potts et al. 1993). In addition, some food dyes are absorbed by critically ill patients and are mitochondrial toxins when absorbed (Czop and Herr 2002; FDA Public Health Advisory 2003). The use of food color or methylene blue to detect aspiration is not recommended due to low sensitivity and concern for toxicity in critically ill patients. On September 29, 2003, the Food and Drug Administration released a public health advisory regarding reports of toxicity associated with the use of FD&C Blue No. 1 (Blue 1) in EN solutions (FDA Public Health Advisory 2003).

Reducing Aspiration Risk

Body Position

There is evidence that the position of the patient is one of the primary factors that can influence aspiration risk. Several studies have demonstrated that aspiration and pneumonia are significantly more likely when patients are supine (Drakulovic et al. 1999; Li Bassi and Torres 2011). Semirecumbent position cannot guarantee absolute protection against all aspiration or pneumonia events, but it is a method that is not expensive or time consuming, and it is a variable that can be controlled. Strict use of semirecumbent position (backrest elevation [BRE] of 30°–45°) is the most consistent and potent means to reduce the likelihood of aspiration.

Tube Size and Placement Issues

The best available data suggest that the size of the nasal- or oral-placed feeding tube does not influence the incidence of aspiration or pneumonia (Dotson et al. 1994). It *is* critical that the placement of the feeding tube be properly confirmed via radiograph before feedings begin (Dotson et al. 1994; Krenitsky 2011).

Although a tube crossing the gastroesophageal junction might appear to increase the risk of aspiration, the evidence would suggest otherwise. Several studies have demonstrated that the incidence of aspiration does not differ between gastrostomy and nasogastric feedings (Gomes et al. 2012).

TABLE 17.2
Patients Who Should Be Considered for Jejunal Feeding Tubes

- Neuromuscular disease involving aerodigestive tract
- Structural abnormalities of aerodigestive tract
- Gastroparesis or severely delayed gastric emptying
- Persistently high gastric residuals
- Patients who require supine positioning

Source: Parrish, C.R. et al., *Nutrition Support Traineeship Syllabus*, Fully revised, University of Virginia Health System, Charlottesville, VA, July 2013. Used with permission.

It is not uncommon for clinicians to place the tip of feeding tubes beyond the pylorus, in the hope of decreasing aspiration events. However, placement of feeding tubes into the small bowel does not appear to reduce aspiration risk compared to gastric feeding (Davies et al. 2012; Krenitsky 2006; Marik and Zaloga 2003). There are a number of limitations in the available literature, not the least of which is the small size of most studies. In addition, not all of the studies positioned the tip of the feeding tube beyond the ligament of Treitz, and most did not regularly reconfirm feeding tube position during the study period (Marik and Zaloga 2003). If the feeding tube location is not monitored throughout the study, the question remains if a properly positioned tube would reduce aspiration events. Meta-analysis of these studies has been reported in an attempt to compensate for the small sample size of each individual study (Marik and Zaloga 2003). However, despite the increased numbers of patients available for analysis, it remains unclear if a properly positioned jejunal tube can reduce aspiration; therefore, from a purely evidence-based perspective, the question of jejunal placement of feeding tubes and aspiration risk remains unanswered.

One practical observation that can be gleaned from these studies is that taken together, a large number of critically ill patients appear to have received gastric tube feedings in a safe and effective manner. In studies where protocols for aspiration precautions were established, patients received full tube feedings with very low rates of aspiration pneumonia (Marik and Zaloga 2003). Considering the time and expense that can be associated with jejunal placement of feeding tubes, it would appear reasonable to routinely feed via the gastric route unless patients demonstrate intolerance to gastric feedings. Patients suspected to be at increased risk for aspiration of gastric contents due to altered anatomy or motility should be considered for jejunal placed tubes (see Table 17.2).

Feeding Delivery Methods

The delivery rate of the feeding formula may also influence aspiration and pneumonia. Bolus administration of 350 mL of EN into the stomach has been demonstrated to reduce lower esophageal sphincter pressure, which can trigger reflux of feeding (Coben et al. 1994). Continuous EN has been associated with improved EN tolerance and reduced aspiration events (Ciocon et al. 1992; Kocan and Hickisch 1986). One group reported reduced aspiration events in patients fed with cyclic drip feedings compared to a continuous feeding (Jacobs et al. 1990). The authors postulated that cyclic EN might allow for a reduction in gastric pH with reduced colonization of gastric contents. However, randomized trials have failed to find a difference in gastric pH or in gastric colonization or pneumonia incidence between patients fed with cyclic versus continuous feedings (Bonten et al. 1996; Spilker et al. 1996). The increased use

TABLE 17.3
Risk Reduction for Aspiration Pneumonia

- Maintain a semirecumbent position with the head (shoulders) elevated >30° to 45° or placing patient in reverse Trendelenburg at 30°–45° if no contraindication to that position. Patients with femoral lines can be at 30°
- Good oral care
- Minimize use of narcotics
- Verify appropriate placement of feeding tube
- Clinically assess
  - GI tolerance
  - Abdominal distention
  - Fullness/discomfort
  - Vomiting
  - Excessive residual volumes (see the section "Residual Volume")
- Remove nasoenteric or oroenteric feeding tubes as soon as possible

Source: Parrish, C.R. et al., *Nutrition Support Traineeship Syllabus*, Fully revised, University of Virginia Health System, Charlottesville, VA, July 2013. Used with permission.

of continuous insulin drips in many ICUs also raises the concern that cyclic feeding schedules may increase the chance of hypoglycemic episodes.

Pharmacological Interventions

Several prokinetic medications have been investigated for efficacy in improving EN tolerance. In critically ill patients, metoclopramide and erythromycin improve gastric emptying compared to placebo (Booth et al. 2001; Ridley and Davies 2011). Erythromycin and the combination of erythromycin and metoclopramide allow increased amounts of EN to be provided to the patient (Boivin and Levy 2001; Nguyen et al. 2007). There are limited data on the use of promotility agents in reducing the incidence of aspiration pneumonia. One prospective study in 305 ICU patients receiving nasogastric feedings investigated the use of metoclopramide on pneumonia incidence. No significant difference was noted in the incidence of pneumonia or mortality between the group receiving placebo and those receiving metoclopramide (Yavagal et al. 2000).

A recent study in mechanically ventilated patients receiving opioid analgesia reported that enteral use of the narcotic antagonist naloxone decreased gastric residual and the incidence of pneumonia (Meissner et al. 2003). The median volume of gastric residual (54 vs. 129 mL, $p = 0.03$) and frequency of pneumonia (34% vs. 56%, $p = 0.04$) were significantly lower in the naloxone group. The use of enteral naloxone did not change the requirement for opioid administration in this study (Meissner et al. 2003). See Table 17.3 for guidelines to help prevent aspiration pneumonia during EN.

BOWEL SOUNDS: TO HAVE OR HAVE NOT

Listening for BSs, a practice in use for many years, has been presumed a proxy for a patient's readiness to initiate oral or EN. This practice is based on the assumption that BSs are an indication of peristalsis and the lack of BS would indicate aperistalsis and without peristalsis, a functional ileus would exist. If gastric stasis should occur above the pylorus due to lack of peristalsis, then the 3–5 L of secretions produced daily would build up causing abdominal distension and ultimately emesis, unless nasogastric decompression is instituted.

TABLE 17.4
Suggested Guidelines in the Assessment of GI Function When BSs Are Absent

- Does patient require gastric decompression? If so, is it meaningful based on the clinical exam? (i.e., is the volume similar to normal secretions above the pylorus or is it a small volume every shift?) Distinguish severity by differentiating those patients requiring
  - Low constant suction
  - Gravity drainage
  - An occasional, random gastric residual check every 4–6 h (note: small bowel aspirates should not be checked)
- Abdominal exam—firm, distended, tympanic?
- Is the patient nauseated, bloated, feeling full, or vomiting?
- Is the patient passing gas or stool?
- What is the differential diagnosis? Are abdominal issues high on the list?
- If the aforementioned clinical parameters are benign, consider a trial of EN at low rate of 10–20 mL/h and observe for the symptoms listed earlier

Source: Parrish, C.R. et al., *Nutrition Support Traineeship Syllabus*, Fully revised, University of Virginia Health System, Charlottesville, VA, July 2013. Used with permission.

BSs are a function of the air/fluid interface within the bowel. Without air in the bowel, there will be no BSs. BSs are a nonspecific marker that reflects the presence of air in either the small bowel or the colon. In the presence of an ileus, BS can be nonexistent, hypoactive, louder, higher pitched, or hyperactive in the setting of an obstruction (Waxman 2003). Due to their nonspecific nature, BSs are not an accurate indicator of peristalsis nor a surrogate for GI tract function.

Peristalsis is propagated by two distinct waves of contractile patterns: fed and fasting (Livingston et al. 1990). Feeding activates several neural and humoral systems and elicits powerful propulsive contractions along the GI tract and provides a stimulus for secretion of GI hormones that have pro-motility effects. The second pattern, the migrating motor complex (or intestinal housekeeper), is responsible for moving luminal contents along the GI tract between meals. In the post-op setting, this is the only mechanism of importance if patients are not fed. In the post-op literature, there are reports of BSs being associated with the initiation of EN (Holte and Kehlet 2000; Luckey et al. 2003). EN may stimulate a reflex that results in coordinated propulsive activity and elicit GI hormone secretion enhancing bowel motility—"if you feed them, bowel sounds will follow," so to speak. One small study also demonstrated earlier time to flatus and stooling after EN initiation (Beier-Hogerson and Boesby 1996). There are several studies in the post-op setting that support early oral feeding despite the lack of BS (Madsen et al. 2005; Willcutts 2010). Despite the universal use of BS, there are no prospective, randomized, clinical trials comparing patients enterally fed with and without BS. Until further evidence is available, a common sense approach is suggested in Table 17.4.

RESIDUAL VOLUME

The Stomach as a Reservoir: A Brief Review of Gastric Function

GRV has been used as a surrogate marker for GI motility for decades, despite inadequate evidence to support the practice. In order to discuss GRV, one must appreciate the various factors that contribute to GRV. First, as a reminder, one of the main functions of the stomach is to act as a reservoir; the idea that the stomach should always be empty is physiologically unsound. Approximately 3–5 L enters the GI tract above the pylorus daily; this does not include *any* exogenous intake such as EN. Table 17.5 lists the contributions of endogenous GI secretions, and Table 17.6 demonstrates typical endogenous gastric volume produced and EN infused in the clinical setting. Clearly, if 200 mL (or even 500 mL) is obtained after 4 h, then significant emptying has occurred during that time period, especially if medications and water were also given.

TABLE 17.5
Absorption and Secretion of Fluid in the GI Tract

GI Fluid Movement	
Additions	**mL**
Diet	2000
Saliva	1500
Stomach	2500
Pancreas/bile	2000
Intestine	1000
Subtractions	
Colointestinal	8900
Net stool loss	**100**

Source: Harig, J.M., Pathophysiology of small bowel diarrhea, in: *American Gastroenterological Association Postgraduate Course Syllabus*, Kahrilas, P.J. and Vanagunas, A. (eds.), American Gastroenterological Association, Boston, MA, 1993, p. 199.

TABLE 17.6
Sample of Expected GRV with EN Infusing Checked Every 4 h

EN infusing at 100 mL/h × 4 h	400 mL
Endogenous secretions in next 4 h (8)	>500 mL
Approximate amount of fluid entering the stomach (does not include medication or water flushes)	>900 mL every 4 h
A GRV of 200 mL appears *insignificant*, as the majority of what has been delivered has emptied	

Source: Parrish, C.R. et al., *Nutrition Support Traineeship Syllabus*, Fully revised, University of Virginia Health System, Charlottesville, VA, July 2013. Used with permission.

OTHER FACTORS TO CONSIDER WHEN CHECKING RESIDUAL VOLUMES

Normal Gastric Emptying

Normal gastric emptying is estimated to be approximately 188 mL/h of endogenous secretions alone (gastric juice and saliva) (Lin and Van Citters 1997). Nutrient density will alter gastric emptying; for example, 500 mL of normal saline empties at a rate of 70%/h, 500 mL of 10% glucose at a rate of 35%/h, and enteral formulas range between 20%/h and 50%/h (Lin and Van Citters 1997). Theoretically then, if 120 mL/h of EN were to be infused in addition to the 188 mL/h of secretions per hour made, a total of ~290 mL/h would be crossing the pylorus per hour. If there were no gastric emptying after 4 h, then 1160 mL would remain.

Cascade Effect

In the supine position (predominant among hospitalized patients), the spine protrudes upward effectively breaking the stomach in half. A functional barrier is created by the spine, and gravity keeps secretions from leaving the fundus, or proximal section of the stomach, until it fills enough to *cascade over* the spine like a waterfall into the antrum, allowing secretions to then leave the

TABLE 17.7
Factors to Consider regarding Efficacy of GRV

1. Does checking GRV correlate with a decrease in aspiration events?
2. Furthermore, how does one check a GRV? Consider the following:
    - Type of tube (feeding tube vs. salem sump type)
    - Location of tube tip in stomach (fundus, antrum, or G-tube)
    - Position of patient (supine vs. right or left side vs. prone)
    - Method of aspirating (20–60 mL syringe vs. gravity drainage vs. low constant suction)

The volume withdrawn from the stomach may depend on any or all of the aforementioned considerations. Therefore, does the GRV mean something different depending on the setting, and if so, is validation and a different cutoff needed for each?

3. What volume is too much?
4. What effect does the use of histamine-2 receptor blockers and proton pump inhibitors (PPIs) play in the assessment of GRV?
5. What is done with the contents once they have been removed—reinfuse or discard?

Source: Parrish, C.R. et al., *Nutrition Support Traineeship Syllabus*, Fully revised, University of Virginia Health System, Charlottesville, VA, July 2013. Used with permission.

stomach. If the EN tube happens to sit in the fundus, then during EN infusion, an artificial residual can accumulate until it *cascades* over the spine into the pyloric region and on out of the stomach.

Just the words *gastric residual volume* conjure up the idea that having one is not acceptable, even though the stomach is essentially a reservoir. Assumptions are often made that any type of residual in the stomach is abnormal or that undesirable clinical consequences will follow such as fullness, nausea, vomiting, and aspiration followed by pneumonia. Table 17.7 lists other factors clouding the practice of checking GRV.

Throughout the literature, one of the primary reasons EN is held, decreased, or stopped altogether is due to a predetermined yet arbitrary GRV. This arbitrary GRV often results in inadequate delivery of nutrients (Martins et al. 2012; Rice et al. 2012). However, the GRV for which EN is often held is much lower than the combined volume of EN, medications, normal endogenous GI secretions, and the water given as flushes over the measured period. This suggests that *significant net emptying* has actually occurred (refer Table 17.6). Furthermore, there is no agreement among practitioners regarding the GRV at which EN needs to be held and is largely based upon practitioner experience and training. The maximum allowed GRV cited in the literature ranges from 60 to 500 mL (Parrish 2008). Due to decades of use, 100–150 mL is considered *standard practice* as it is one of the most common cutoff levels for GRV (Parrish 2008).

Clinical Relevance of Residual Volumes

Although the practice of checking GRV has existed for decades, the first study attempting to evaluate its utility as a reliable tool in the clinical setting was in 1992 (McClave et al. 1992). McClave compared GRV with physical exam and radiographic findings in enterally fed patients and healthy volunteers over an 8 h period. EN was infused continuously via 10 Fr nasogastric tubes (NGTs) to volunteers (N = 20), critically ill patients (N = 10), and floor patients with percutaneous endoscopic gastrostomies (PEG) (N = 8). The important findings of this study included the following:

1. GRV did not correlate with physical exam or radiographic evidence.
2. Physical exam and radiographic findings correlated significantly.
3. Forty percent of volunteers had a GRV of >100 mL during the study versus thirty-nine percent of subjects.
4. Because of the short duration of the study (8 h total), no conclusions can be made as to the safety or value of GRV > 100 to 200 mL, but it does raise the question of the validity of checking GRV.

Powell et al. hypothesized that checking GRV leads to the occlusion of small-bore feeding tubes (Powell et al. 1993). General medicine patients were continuously fed a polymeric formula through an 8 Fr NGT. Group A (N = 15) had GRV checked every 4 h; Group B's (N = 13) GRV was not checked. Occlusion rates were significantly higher in Group A than in Group B. Unfortunately, actual GRV was not reported, and the study was not designed nor powered to demonstrate sensitivity of GRV as a marker for aspiration.

Lukan et al. added yellow microspheres and BFC directly to tube feeding and obtained GRV and specimens from oropharynx and trachea from critically ill, ventilated patients fed via NGT (N = 13), PEG (N = 13), or NGT then PEG (N = 2) (Lukan et al. 2002). Aspiration and regurgitation events were defined by detection of yellow color on fluorometry. Although GRV reached greater than 400 mL in 0.7% of samples, they did not correlate with aspiration or regurgitation events. The authors concluded that a GRV less than 400 mL is an insensitive marker for risk of aspiration. Of note, *aspiration pneumonia* does not necessarily follow regurgitation and aspiration events.

In a prospective, randomized, multicenter study of 28 Spanish adult ICUs, Montejo evaluated 329 patients that required EN for at least 5 days (Montejo 2010). The GRV was set at 200 mL (control group) versus 500 mL (study group). The frequency of GI complications was higher in the control group, but the only difference was in the frequency of high GRV, yet ICU-acquired pneumonia was similar in both groups. The authors concluded that increasing limit for normal GRV to 500 mL is associated with an increase in EN volume delivered and is not associated with adverse effects in GI complications.

In a prospective study of 360 critically ill patients using the presence of pepsin in tracheal secretions as a surrogate marker for aspiration of gastric contents, Metheny described the frequency and outcomes associated with aspiration (Metheny et al. 2006). The most significant independent risk factors for pneumonia were frequency of pepsin (+) secretions, use of paralytic agents, and a high sedation level. The author noted that "increased GRV did not significantly correlate with aspiration or pneumonia." Of note in this oft-quoted study, the mean overall GRV reported was 41 mL in the *high aspiration* group and 31 mL in the *low aspiration* group. In addition, BRE was less than 30° in 54% of patients (hours between midnight and 08:00 were not monitored).

In another observational study, Metheny described the association between GRV and aspiration of gastric contents over 3 days (Metheny et al. 2008). High GRV and low level of consciousness were associated with aspiration events (not pneumonias). It is important to note that again the mean GRV for the total sample was 37 mL (range was 0.2–192 mL). Unfortunately, in this later study, an even greater percentage of patients (65%) had a BRE < 30°. The authors acknowledged that they "found no consistent relationship between GRV and aspiration."

Recently, Poulard compared checking GRV with threshold of 250 mL versus not checking in 205 adult mechanically ventilated medical–surgical ICU patients (Poulard et al. 2010). Patients without GRV monitoring received more EN without experiencing increased rates of vomiting or ventilator-associated pneumonia (VAP).

In a recent study, Rice et al. (2012) randomized 200 enterally fed, critically ill patients to either a full-energy group or an initial trophic EN. GRV was set at greater than 300 mL. Despite the higher threshold, very little vomiting, regurgitation, or aspiration was reported (one episode of aspiration occurred in the trophic group).

Mounting evidence is available to suggest that the standard practice of 150–200 mL GRV *cutoff* is overly conservative and results in unnecessary withholding of EN. What is becoming more apparent, however, is that GRV itself is not a validated tool to assess EN tolerance or aspiration risk, and in fact, nursing time may be better spent on those interventions that have supporting evidence to decrease aspiration risk such as BRE, good oral care, and minimizing the use of narcotics (Parrish 2008). A very large, prospective, controlled trial with adequate power will be necessary to put this controversy to rest. For now, the health-care team needs to be vigilant in good clinical judgment to ensure safe enteral feeding. For suggested strategies until further evidence is available, see Table 17.8.

TABLE 17.8
Suggested Guidelines to Evaluate Residual Volume

1. Wash your hands
2. Is it a GRV? (i.e., is it less than the flow rate?)
3. Confirm that the BRE is >30° to 40°. Maintain a semirecumbent position with the BRE (shoulders) elevated ≥30° to 45° or place the patient in reverse Trendelenburg at 30°–45° if no contraindication exists for that position. Patients with femoral lines can be elevated up to 30°
4. Do not consider automatic cessation of EN until a second high GRV is demonstrated at least 4 h after the first
5. Clinically assess patient for
   - Abdominal distension/discomfort
   - Bloating/fullness
   - N/V
6. Place the patient on their right side for 15–20 min before checking a GRV again (to take advantage of the effect of gravity and to avoid the cascade effect)
7. Consider diverting the level of infusion of EN lower in the GI tract (postpyloric)
8. Switch to a more calorically dense product to decrease the total volume infused
9. Avoid constipation
10. Review and minimize all fluids given enterally including medications and water flushes
11. Minimize use of narcotics or consider use of a narcotic antagonist to promote intestinal contractility
12. Verify appropriate placement of feeding tube
13. Switch from bolus feeding to continuous infusion
14. Initiate prokinetic therapy (or leave standing orders to allow the nurse to initiate a prescription if needed) typical doses for available prokinetics are as follows:
   - Metoclopramide—5–20 mg q.i.d (may need to give IV initially)
   - Erythromycin—125–250 mg q.i.d
   - Domperidone—10–30 mg q.i.d
15. Consider raising the threshold level or *cutoff* value for GRV for a particular patient
16. Consider stopping the GRV checks if the patient is *clinically stable*, has no apparent tolerance issues, and has shown relatively low GRV for 48 h. Should the clinical status change, GRV checks can be resumed
17. If consideration is given to increasing the time interval between GRV checks to >6 to 8 h, then the clinical situation may warrant cessation of GRV checks
18. Consider a PPI in order to decrease volume of endogenous gastric secretions (e.g., omeprazole, lansoprazole, esomeprazole, pantoprazole, rabeprazole)
19. Initiate aggressive regimen for oral hygiene

Source: Parrish, C.R. et al., *Nutrition Support Traineeship Syllabus*, Fully revised, University of Virginia Health System, Charlottesville, VA, July 2013. Used with permission.

NAUSEA/VOMITING

The idea of initiating EN in a patient experiencing nausea and vomiting (N/V) may appear somewhat counterintuitive. N/V is often the result of medication side effects, a procedure, surgery, or an underlying disease process; this is especially true in the critical care setting. Critically ill patients with persistent N/V are at a high risk for malnutrition (if not already present). After careful assessment, the underlying cause can often be identified and treated. While efforts at curtailing the N/V are initiated, EN can be started. Due to the subjective nature of nausea and intermittent bouts of vomiting, antiemetics are often ordered on a *PRN* basis. If N/V is significant enough to prevent EN, consider standing orders for medications aimed at providing symptomatic relief. See Table 17.9 for suggestions for the treatment of N/V. Additionally, an excellent review of the management of N/V is available (Garrett et al. 2003; Quigley et al. 2001).

TABLE 17.9
Suggestions to Overcome N/V in EN-Fed Patients

- Slow EN infusion (if practical—i.e., 24 h continuous infusion is rarely practical for patients going home on EN)
- Use a more calorically dense formula to decrease total volume required (*Note*: ensure adequate hydration)
- Glucose control (<150 mg/dL) to avoid gastroparesis from hyperglycemia
- Seek transpyloric tube placement
- Trial of a prokinetic agent or antiemetics; also consider
    - *PRN* vs. scheduled dosing
    - Tablet vs. elixir vs. IV
    - Route of medication delivery

Example: Gastric delivery of antiemetics with concurrent gastric decompression will most likely be a futile measure unless gastric port is clamped for some time after dose is given

Source: Parrish, C.R. et al., *Nutrition Support Traineeship Syllabus*, Fully revised, University of Virginia Health System, Charlottesville, VA, July 2013. Used with permission.

DIARRHEA

Management of diarrhea in critically ill, enterally fed patients can be challenging. Historically, the use of EN has been implicated as a primary cause of diarrhea in this population. Available evidence does not support these implications (Bittencourt et al. 2012; Bliss et al. 1992; Heimburger et al. 1994; Keohane et al. 1984; Levinson and Bryce 1993). Successful management of diarrhea in the critically ill patient depends on accurate identification and treatment of the source (Ferrie and East 2007; Garey et al. 2006). Manipulation of EN has often been a primary means of attempting to prevent or treat diarrhea. However, the vast majority of diarrhea in enterally fed patients has been associated with the use of medications or infectious agents (Bliss et al. 1192; Edes et al. 1990; Heimburger et al. 1994; Jones et al. 1983; Keohane et al. 1984). A newly identified contributor to diarrhea in EN fed patients may be fermentable oligo-, di-, and monosaccharides and polyols (FODMAP) (Gibson and Sheperd 2010; Halmos et al. 2010). Until further data are available, clinicians may want to consider the FODMAP content of EN formulas when evaluating patients with diarrhea, *after* the much more obvious sources of diarrhea such as laxatives, oral contrast, sorbitol, or other sugar alcohol–containing medications, and *Clostridium difficile* infection is ruled out. Therapies to treat diarrhea have included use of low fat or elemental feeds, slowing the feeding rate, using less concentrated solutions, or stopping EN altogether. These interventions are often implemented without investigation into the primary etiology of the diarrhea. Not only are these treatments often unnecessary, but they also may prevent the patient from receiving optimal EN and, even worse, an inappropriate switch to PN support.

Incidence of Diarrhea in EN

The reported incidence of diarrhea among tube-fed patients ranges from 2% to 68% (Bittencourt et al. 2012; Cataldi-Betcher et al. 1983; Kelly et al. 1983; Luft et al. 2006). Subjective measures such as stool frequency, consistency, and volume may not be clinically relevant. More objective, quantifiable measures are difficult to obtain and include stool weight (>300 g/day) or volume (>500 mL/day). In one EN-fed population, a 46% incidence of diarrhea was reported using subjective data, and a 0% incidence was reported using objective data (Benya et al. 1991). In the clinical setting, recording stool characteristics (volume, consistency, and frequency) while concomitantly looking for clinical signs and symptoms of diarrhea (dehydration, electrolyte imbalance, and sacral and perianal skin irritation) can assist with evaluation of need for treatment.

Flow Rate

EN has been customarily initiated at lower flow rates in an attempt to avoid abdominal *issues* including diarrhea. The need to use *starter*-type regimes (initiation of EN at a lower rate and/or osmolality) in order to give the GI tract a chance to *adapt* has been refuted (Keohane et al. 1984; Zarling et al. 1986). In normal volunteers, the GI tract has been shown to tolerate up to 150 mL/h gastrically and 267 mL/h transpylorically (Kandil et al. 1993; Zarling et al. 1986). Adjustment of flow rate has not been determined to be associated with increased incidence of abdominal discomfort, diarrhea, or malabsorption. Keep in mind that 60 mL/h = 1 drop/min infused.

Formula Composition

The use of elemental diets is not routinely indicated for use in patients with diarrhea (Silk and Grimble 1992). Patients with functional GI tracts tolerate polymeric formulas as well as elemental formulas (Jones et al. 1983). In a prospective, randomized, clinical trial, Heimburger et al. compared the use of peptide-containing formulas with intact protein formulas in 50 critically ill patients (Heimburger et al. 1994). Both formulas were well tolerated, and the incidence of diarrhea was attributed to medication (Edes et al. 1990).

While the GI tract may be affected in many ways by critical illness, its overall absorptive capacity is significant. For malabsorption to occur, 90% of organ function must be impaired (Silk and Grimble 1992). The use of elemental formulas should be limited to those patients with documented malabsorption of fat that cannot be treated or chyle leaks. In patients with short gut, highly osmotic, elemental formulas may aggravate stool output (McIntyre et al. 1986).

OSMOLALITY/DILUTION OF TUBE FEEDINGS

Osmolality is often blamed for GI intolerance of EN. Hypertonic formulas (>300 mOm) are sometimes diluted to make them *isotonic*. However, there are no data to support the practice of diluting EN in order to make it isotonic and more easily tolerated. Two studies have demonstrated that hypertonic formulas (ranging from 503–620 mOsm/kg), infused either gastrically or at the ligament of Treitz, achieve isotonicity or near isotonicity very rapidly within the jejunum (Hecketsweiler et al. 1979; Miller et al. 1978). In fact, the osmolality of EN formulas should not cause a clinical problem for several reasons. The osmolality of clear and full liquid diets routinely used by hospitalized patients is far greater than that of EN, but clinicians would not recommend a ½ or ¼ strength clear liquid diet. Consider also the osmolality of common medications delivered via the enteral route (see Table 17.10). The osmolality of medications is much higher than that of EN, yet most focus on the EN formula as the culprit. At times, patients have increased hydration needs that justify diluted tube feedings. Using diluted feedings (at increased rates) allows the delivery of both adequate nutrition and increased hydration without the need for the nurse or caregiver to frequently give water boluses.

Medications

The most common cause of diarrhea in EN-fed patients has consistently been found to be the use of liquid or hyperosmotic medications (Edes et al. 1990; Guenter et al. 1991). Once enteral access is achieved, it is common practice to switch medications from IV to enteral route due to cost. Liquid medications contain sugar alcohols that are highly osmotic, poorly absorbed, and very fermentable in the GI tract. Eads et al. reported a 26% incidence of diarrhea in a population of tube-fed patients; medications were determined to be responsible in 61% of the cases (Edes et al. 1990). Antibiotic use with its association with *C. difficile* has been cited as a primary cause of diarrhea (Bliss et al. 1998;

TABLE 17.10
Osmolality of Selected Liquids and Medications

Typical Liquids	(mOsm/kg)	Drug	(mOsm/kg)
EN formulas	250–710	Acetaminophen elixir	5400
Milk/eggnog	275/695	Diphenoxylate susp.	8800
Gelatin	535	KCl elixir (sugar-free)	3000
Broth	445	Multivitamin liquid	5700
Sodas	695	Furosemide (oral)	3938
Popsicles	720	Metoclopramide	8350
Juices	~990	Multivitamin liquid	5700
Ice cream	1150	Na phosphate	7250
Sherbet	1225	Nystatin susp.	3300

Source: Parrish, C.R. et al., *Nutrition Support Traineeship Syllabus*, Fully revised, University of Virginia Health System, Charlottesville, VA, July 2013. Used with permission.

Heimburger et al. 1994; Keohane et al. 1984). Examples of medications commonly associated with diarrhea and their osmolalities are listed in Table 17.10. Possible options for resolving medication-related diarrhea include changing to a different medication, or changing from the liquid form to a tab that can be crushed if available, or diluting the medication prior to administration, and/or changing the route of administration from enteral to IV.

Gastrointestinal

Diarrhea can be caused by malabsorption; however, diarrhea does not *cause* malabsorption. In a patient with persistent diarrhea, once the obvious culprits have been investigated, a review of anatomy, underlying disease states, concomitant problems, and secondary effects of treatments or medications is in order (Owens and Greenson 2007; Thomas et al. 2003). If malabsorption is suspected, it should be evaluated systematically, evaluated and treated. Manipulation of feeding regimes has not been proven to *treat* diarrhea, and commercial claims of such should be highly scrutinized. There are some patients whose diarrhea may be exacerbated by fiber and FODMAP (including fructooligosaccharides [FOS]), and hence, these formulations should be avoided (Gibson and Sheperd 2010; Halmos et al. 2010).

Treatment of Diarrhea

Once the most likely etiology of the diarrhea is determined, appropriate intervention can be initiated. See Table 17.11 for suggested strategies for treatment.

Diarrhea and Probiotics

The use of probiotic cultures to prevent or treat diarrhea remains an area of investigation. Lactobacillus probiotics have been shown to reduce the duration of diarrhea associated with rotavirus in children (Szajewska and Mrukowicz 2001) and to reduce the incidence of antibiotic-associated diarrhea (Hempel et al. 2012). Lactobacillus supplements have not been adequately tested in adults receiving tube feedings to assess if there are beneficial effects in terms of diarrhea or acquisition of *C. difficile*. A probiotic yeast, *Saccharomyces boulardii*, reduced the mean percentage of days with diarrhea multicenter in a double-blind trial in critically ill patients receiving EN (Bleichner et al. 1997).

TABLE 17.11
Systematic Approach When Addressing Diarrhea in EN-Fed Patients

1. Quantify stool volume—is it really diarrhea?
2. Review medication list (did medications switch from the IV to enteral route when enteral access achieved?) Common offenders include
   - Acetaminophen and guaifenesin elixir
   - Neutra Phos
   - Lactulose
   - Standing orders for stool softeners/laxatives
3. Check for *C. difficile* or other infectious cause (lactoferrin, leukocytes)
4. Try fiber
   - Few clinical studies
   - Supports the health of colonocytes
   - May aggravate diarrhea in some (see FODMAPs)
5. Once infectious causes are ruled out,
   - Try an antidiarrheal agent (may need standing order versus *PRN*)
6. No evidence that diluting EN is beneficial
7. Be mindful of those patients at risk for stooling around an impaction
   - Nursing home, patients with neuromuscular disease such as ALS pts, para- or quadriplegics
8. Finally, review anatomy and medical history—is it possible that there is an unappreciated pancreatic insufficiency or small bowel bacterial overgrowth present?
9. Continue to feed

Source: Parrish, C.R. et al., *Nutrition Support Traineeship Syllabus*, Fully revised, University of Virginia Health System, Charlottesville, VA, July 2013. Used with permission.

However, *S. boulardii* has been reported to be a potential pathological agent in the critically ill population (Lherm et al. 2002). Seven cases of fungemia with *S. boulardii* were reported over a 2-year period when mechanically ventilated patients were pretreated with the probiotic yeast. Investigators confirmed the genomic identity between isolates of blood culture and yeasts from the packets administered to the patients (Lherm et al. 2002).

A number of cases of sepsis from probiotic lactobacillus preparations in critically ill patients have been reported, and one randomized trial of lactobacillus supplements in critically ill patients demonstrated increased mortality in some subgroups of patients (Kochan et al. 2011; Land et al. 2005). A large, multicenter, randomized study of patients with severe pancreatitis that received a mixed-species probiotic revealed significantly increased mortality in the group receiving the probiotics (Besselink et al. 2008). A systematic review of probiotics in critical illness reported that probiotics were associated with reduced infectious complications only in lower-quality studies, with no difference in infections in high-quality studies, and concluded that further research is required (Petrof 2012). The routine use of probiotic supplements is not recommended in critically ill patients until additional data are available regarding efficacy and risks in populations with immune or gut barrier compromise.

CONSTIPATION

While bowel movement frequency is highly individual, less than or equal to two stools weekly have been included as one of the Rome consensus criteria for the symptom (Longstreth et al. 2006). When evaluating constipation in the critical care setting, several factors need to be considered, including patient's normal stool history, time since last bowel movement, and comprehensive assessment of the abdomen by an experienced practitioner. Factors contributing to the incidence of constipation in the critically ill patient include use of anticholinergics, narcotics, and sedatives and inadequate provision of fluid, immobilization, and neuromuscular or GI motility disorders.

Daily monitoring of GI function is important to help avoid more serious cases of constipation. Left untreated, stool can accumulate, filling the entire large bowel. Patients with signs and symptoms of constipation should be evaluated for impaction, bowel obstruction, and/or ileus. Treatment options include slow increase in fluid and fiber in the diet followed by inclusion of a saline agent such as milk of magnesia. If these interventions fail, inclusion of a stimulant agent should be considered (Longstreth et al. 2006).

INITIATION AND PROGRESSION OF TUBE FEEDINGS

The starting rate and advancement of EN has been dictated more by tradition than by objective evidence. Nutrition support texts generally recommend starting continuous EN at 10–40 mL/h and advancing by 10–20 mL every 8–12 h as tolerated (Bankhead et al. 2009). Intermittent feeding recommendations are generally to start with 60–120 mL of EN every 4 h and advance by 60–120 mL every 8–12 h. However, no references are given for these recommendations. Few investigators have attempted to study the question of the *ideal* start-up and advancement rate for EN. Healthy volunteers can tolerate infusion rates of 30–60 mL/min. Only at rates of 85 mL/min (5100 mL/h) did subjects show intolerance (Heitkemper et al. 1977).

Rees continuously infused 87 mL/h into 14 patients with impaired GI function and achieved 100% of prescribed volume in 9 patients (Rees et al. 1992). In a later study of patients with moderately impaired GI function, Rees did not use a starter regimen in his EN-fed patients (Rees et al. 1985). These patients were set to receive 2.25 L of either an intact or predigested EN product; patients *averaged* 1985 kcal/day, suggesting they tolerated EN well.

These studies were not designed to establish the limits of tolerance or the ideal tube feeding progression. Nevertheless, it is clear that many patients, even those with impaired GI function, will tolerate initiation and progression of feedings much faster than has traditionally been recommended. See Tables 17.12 and 17.13 for sample tube feeding protocols for initiation and advancement of EN. When discussing flow rates, it is important to keep the actual delivery volume in perspective. For example, 30 mL/h is only two tablespoons, and 60 mL/h is ¼ cup delivered over an *entire hour*.

OBSTRUCTED FEEDING TUBES

Feeding tube obstruction has been reported to occur in 16%–35% patients fed with a small-bore feeding tube (Bourgault et al. 2003; Marcuard et al. 1989). Factors that increase the incidence of clogging include pump malfunction, improper administration of medications, failure to adequately

TABLE 17.12
Typical Practices at UVAHS for Initiating EN after Feeding Tube Placement

- *Soft nasogastric feeding tubes*: x-ray confirmation of placement obtained prior to use
- *Transpyloric tubes, nasojejunal, orojejunal*: EN may begin after x-ray confirmation of correct placement
- *PEG*: EN may begin 3 h after PEG placement
- *PEJ or PEG with jejunal extension (PEG/J)*: EN may begin immediately via j port
- *Surgically placed tubes*: Initiation and advancement of EN dependent on surgeon and individual patient

Source: Parrish, C.R. et al., *Nutrition Support Traineeship Syllabus*, Fully revised, University of Virginia Health System, Charlottesville, VA, July 2013. Used with permission.

TABLE 17.13
UVAHS Protocol for Initiation and Advancement of EN

Continuous feeding	Begin at 50 mL/h × 4 h; advance by 20 mL q 4 h until goal rate is reached
	Also have the option to begin feeding at goal rate
	2 cal/mL products, start at half the aforementioned rate
Intermittent feeding	125 mL × 1 feeding; if tolerated, advance by 125 mL q feeding until goal is reached

Source: Parrish, C.R. et al., *Nutrition Support Traineeship Syllabus*, Fully revised, University of Virginia Health System, Charlottesville, VA, July 2013. Used with permission.

flush tube with water, and precipitation of tube feeding proteins. Precipitation of tube feeding occurs with gastric feedings more frequently than small bowel feedings due to its acidic environment (Marcuard et al. 1989). Small-bore feeding tubes require more care than larger-bore tubes as they are more likely to clog.

Carbonated beverages and various fruit juices have historically been misused in an attempt to unclog feeding tubes, but controlled studies demonstrate that cola is not better than water and cranberry juice was less effective than plain water for restoring tube patency (Dandeles and Lodolce 2011).

Prevention of clogging is important since placement of small-bore feeding tubes can be timely and costly. Giving lavage flushes of warm water may be enough to remove a clog and should be attempted first. If this method fails, the use of a pancreatic enzyme solution has been shown to be effective (Marcuard et al. 1989). A commercial product containing enzymes and surfactants has also demonstrated effectiveness for restoring tube patency from clots of feeding formula (Dandeles and Lodolce 2011). Different strategies for preventing tube clogging and declogging feeding tubes are listed in Table 17.14. In addition, commercially available decloggers can be found in Table 17.15.

TABLE 17.14
Preventing Feeding Tube Occlusion and Declogging Techniques Once Occluded

Prevention of clogging

- Use liquid medications whenever possible
- Adequately crush pills to powder form prior to administration
- Irrigate feeding tube with water before and after administration of medications
- Flush tube before and after aspirating for gastric residuals to eliminate acid precipitation of formula in the feeding tube
- Avoid mixing tube feedings with liquid medications having a pH value of 5.0 or less

Suggested technique for unclogging feeding tubes

- Attempt to unclog tube with lukewarm water
- If unsuccessful, mix Viokace and sodium bicarbonate mixture
  (1 crushed Viokace tablet, 1 non-enteric-coated 325 mg $NaHCO_3$ [or 1/8 teaspoon baking powder], dissolve in 5 mL lukewarm water)
- Gently aspirate the tube contents proximal to the clog to allow solution direct contact with clog
- Inject the pancreatic enzyme solution into the feeding tube, clamp it, and allow mixture to remain in tube for 30 min
- Unclamp feeding tube and gently flush tube with warm tap water to restore patency

Source: Parrish, C.R. et al., *Nutrition Support Traineeship Syllabus*, Fully revised, University of Virginia Health System, Charlottesville, VA, July 2013. Used with permission.

TABLE 17.15
Commercially Available Tube Decloggers

DeCloggers™ Bionix	Soft, flexible screw-threaded device to be inserted down the tube to clear buildup or clog Available in various lengths and sizes	Bionix Enteral Feeding Tube Declogger
Clog Zapper™ CORPAK Viasys MedSystems	Combines a *multienzyme cocktail*, acids, buffers, and antibacterial agents in its formulation. Will break up formula clogs but may not work with clogs from medications. Kit contains chemical powder, syringe, and applicator. Unopened kit has a shelf life of 12 months. Once reconstituted, should be used within 24 h	Corpak Medsystems Clog Zapper
PEG cleaning brush BARD	Flexible catheter with feather cut brush at distal end # 000396	Bard PEG Cleaning Brush

Source: Parrish, C.R. et al., *Nutrition Support Traineeship Syllabus*, Fully revised, University of Virginia Health System, Charlottesville, VA, July 2013. Used with permission.

CONCLUSION

The best available evidence indicates that EN is the preferred method for nourishing critically ill patients who are unable to eat on their own. Efforts to eliminate the barriers to EN delivery improve the delivery of EN to critically ill patients. This chapter has reviewed the evidence for many of the issues that impede effective EN delivery and attempted to make suggestions to overcome these barriers based on the evidence as well as the clinical experience of the authors.

CASE STUDY

A patient was admitted s/p myocardial infarction requiring mechanical ventilation.

Past history: chronic kidney disease, hypertension. Tube feedings of a 1.5 kcal/mL formula were started day 3 at 55 mL/h, well tolerated for 2 days. The patient was alert. Continuous renal replacement therapy needed for a 3-day period during which she experienced a residual volume of 150 mL. No c/o of abdominal distension, nausea, or discomfort. The primary team decided to send her down to fluoroscopy for transpyloric tube placement. Do you agree?

Answer:

A transpyloric tube is not indicated for a gastric residual volume of 150 mL in a patient who is tolerating tube feeds and does not complain of any abdominal distension, nausea, or discomfort. It is recommended to continue tube feeds at goal rate while monitoring for signs or symptoms of intolerance.

REFERENCES

Bankhead, R., Boullata, J., Brantley, S. et al. 2009. Enteral nutrition practice recommendations. *J Parenter Enteral Nutr* 33(2):122–167.

Bard PEG Cleaning Brush, http://www.bardaccess.com/feed-peg-brush.php (Accessed December 17, 2014.)

Beier-Holgersen, R., Boesby, S. 1996. Influence of postoperative enteral nutrition on postsurgical infections. *Gut* 39:833.

Benya, R., Layden, T.J., Mobarhan, S. 1991. Diarrhea associated with tube feedings: The importance of using objective criteria. *J Clin Gastroenterol* 13:167.

Besselink, M.G., Van Santvoort, H.C., Buskens, E. et al. 2008. Probiotic prophylaxis in predicted severe acute pancreatitis: A randomised, double-blind, placebo-controlled trial. *Lancet* Feb 23, 371(9613):651–659.

Bionix Enteral Feeding Tube Declogger, http://www.bionixmed.com/MED_Pages/DeClogger.html (Accessed December 17, 2014.)

Bittencourt, A.F., Martins, J.R., Logullo, L. et al. 2012. Constipation is more frequent than diarrhea in patients fed exclusively by enteral nutrition: Results of an observational study. *Nutr Clin Pract* 27(4):533–539.

Bleichner, G., Bléhaut, H., Mentec, H. et al. 1997. Saccharomyces boulardii prevents diarrhea in critically ill tube-fed patients. A multicenter, randomized, double-blind placebo-controlled trial. *Intensive Care Med* 23:517.

Bliss, D., Guenter, P.A., Settle, R.G. 1992. Defining and reporting diarrhea in tube-fed patients—What a mess! *Am J Clin Nutr* 55:753.

Bliss, D.Z., Johnson, S., Savik, K. et al. 1998. Acquisition of *Clostridium difficile* and *Clostridium difficile*-associated diarrhea in hospitalized patients receiving tube feeding. *Ann Intern Med* 129:1012.

Boivin, M.A., Levy, H. 2001. Gastric feeding with erythromycin is equivalent to transpyloric feeding in the critically ill. *Crit Care Med* 29:1916.

Bonten, M.J., Gaillard, C.A., Van der Hulst, R. et al. 1996. Intermittent enteral feeding: The influence on respiratory and digestive tract colonization in mechanically ventilated intensive-care-unit patients. *Am J Respir Crit Care Med* 15:394.

Booth, C.M., Heyland, D.K., Paterson, W.G. 2002. Gastrointestinal promotility drugs in the critical care setting: A systematic review of the evidence. *Crit Care Med* 30:1429.

Bourgault, A.M., Heyland, D.K., Drover, J.W. et al. 2003. Prophylactic pancreatic enzymes to reduce feeding tube occlusions. *Nutr Clin Pract* 18:398–401.

Braunschweig, C.L., Levy, P., Sheean, P.M. et al. 2001. Enteral compared with parenteral nutrition: A meta analysis. *Am J Clin Nutr* 74:534.

Cataldi-Betcher, E.L., Seltzer, M.H., Slocum, B.A. et al. 1983. Complications occurring during enteral nutrition support: A prospective study. *J Parenter Enteral Nutr* 7:546.

Ciocon, J.O., Galindo-Ciocon, D.J., Tiessen, C. et al. 1992. Continuous compared with intermittent tube feeding in the elderly. *J Parenter Enteral Nutr* 16:525.

Coben, R.M., Weintraub, A., Di Marino, A.J. Jr. et al. 1994. Gastroesophageal reflux during gastrostomy feeding. *Gastroenterology* 106:13.

Corpak Medsystems Clog Zapper, http://www.corpakmedsystems.com/Supplement_Material/SupplementPages/enteral/ClogZapper/ClogZap_Brochure.html (Accessed December 17, 2014.)

Czop, M., Herr, D.L. 2002. Green skin discoloration associated with multiple organ failure. *Crit Care Med* 30:598.

Dandeles, L.M., Lodolce, A.E. 2011. Efficacy of agents to prevent and treat enteral feeding tube clogs. *Ann Pharmacother* 45(5):676–680.

Davies, A.R., Morrison, S.S., Bailey, M.J. et al. 2012. A multicenter, randomized controlled trial comparing early nasojejunal with nasogastric nutrition in critical illness. *Crit Care Med* 40(8):2342–2348.

De Beaux, I., Chapman, M., Fraser, R. et al. 2001. Enteral nutrition in the critically ill: A prospective survey in an Australian intensive care unit. *Anaesth Intensive Care* 29:619.

De Jonghe, B., Appere-De-Vechi, C., Fournier, M. et al. 2001. A prospective survey of nutritional support practices in intensive care unit patients: What is prescribed? What is delivered? *Crit Care Med* 29:8.

Dotson, R.G., Robinson, R.G., Pingleton, S.K. 1994. Gastroesophageal reflux with nasogastric tubes. Effect of nasogastric tube size. *Am J Respir Crit Care Med* 149:1659.

Drakulovic, M.B., Torres, A., Bauer, T.T. et al. 1999. Supine body position as a risk factor for nosocomial pneumonia in mechanically ventilated patients: A randomized trial. *Lancet* 354:1851.

Drover, J.W., Dhaliwal, R., Heyland, D.K. 2003. Small bowel versus gastric feeding in the critically ill patient: Results of a meta-analysis. *Crit Care Med* 30:A44.

Edes, T.E., Walk, B.E., Austin, J.L. 1990. Diarrhea in tube-fed patients: Feeding formula not necessarily the cause. *Am J Med* 88:91.

FDA Public Health Advisory FDA/Center for Food Safety & Applied Nutrition. September 29, 2003. Reports of blue discoloration and death in patients receiving enteral feedings tinted with the dye, Acheson, D. (ed.), FD&C Blue No. 1.

Ferrie, S., East, V. 2007. Managing diarrhoea in intensive care. *Aust Crit Care* 20:7–13.

Garey, K.W., Graham, G., Gerard, L. et al. 2006. Prevalence of diarrhea at a university hospital and association with modifiable risk factors. *Ann Pharmacother* 40:1030–1034.

Garrett, K., Tsuruta, K., Walker, S. et al. 2003. Managing nausea and vomiting. *Crit Care Nurse* 23:31.

Gibson, P.R., Shepherd, S.J. 2010. Evidence-based dietary management of functional gastrointestinal symptoms: The FODMAP approach. *J Gastroenterol Hepatol* 25(2):252–258.

Gomes Jr., C.A., Lustosa, S.A., Matos, D. et al. 2012. Percutaneous endoscopic gastrostomy versus nasogastric tube feeding for adults with swallowing disturbances. *Cochrane Database Syst Rev* Mar, 14:3.

Guenter, P.A., Settle, R.G., Perlmutter, S. 1991. Tube feeding related diarrhea in acutely ill patients. *J Parenter Enteral Nutr* 15:277.

Halmos, E.P., Muir, J.G., Barrett, J.S. et al. 2010. Diarrhoea during enteral nutrition is predicted by the poorly absorbed short-chain carbohydrate (FODMAP) content of the formula. *Aliment Pharmacol Ther* 32(7):925–933.

Harig, J.M. 1993. Pathophysiology of small bowel diarrhea, in: *American Gastroenterological Association Postgraduate Course Syllabus*, Kahrilas, P.J., Vanagunas, A. (eds.). American Gastroenterological Association, Boston, MA, p. 199.

Hecketsweiler, P., Vidon, N., Emonts, P. et al. 1979. Absorption of elemental and complex nutritional solutions during a continuous jejunal perfusion in man. *Digestion* 19:213.

Heimburger, D., Sockwell, D.G., Geels, W.J. 1994. Diarrhea with enteral feeding: Prospective reappraisal of putative causes. *Nutrition* 10:392.

Heitkemper, M., Hanson, R., Hansen, B. 1977. Effects of rate and volume of tube feeding in normal subjects. *Commun Nurs Res* 10:71–89.

Hempel, S., Newberry, S.J., Maher, A.R. et al. 2012. Probiotics for the prevention and treatment of antibiotic-associated diarrhea: A systematic review and meta-analysis. *JAMA* May 9, 307(18):1959–1969.

Heyland, D.K., Drover, J.W., MacDonald, S. et al. 2001. Effect of postpyloric feeding on gastroesophageal regurgitation and pulmonary microaspiration: Results of a randomized controlled trial. *Crit Care Med* 29:1495.

Holte, K., Kehlet, H. 2000. Postoperative ileus: A preventable event. *Brit J Surg* 87:1480.

Jacobs, S., Chang, R.W., Lee, B. et al. 1990. Continuous enteral feeding: A major cause of pneumonia among ventilated intensive care unit patients. *J Parenter Enteral Nutr* 14:353.

Jones, B.J.M., Lees, R., Andrews, J. et al. 1983. Comparison of an elemental and polymeric enteral diet in patients with normal gastrointestinal function. *Gut* 24:78.

Kandil, H.E., Opper, F.H., Switzer, B.R. et al. 1993. Marked resistance of normal subjects to tube-feeding-induced diarrhea: The role of magnesium. *Am J Clin Nutr* 57:73.

Kearns, P.J., Chin, D., Mueller, L. et al. 2000. The incidence of ventilator-associated pneumonia and success in nutrient delivery with gastric versus small intestinal feeding: A randomized clinical trial. *Crit Care Med* 28:1742.

Kelly, T.W.J., Patrick, M.R., Hillman, K.M. 1983. Study of diarrhea in critically ill patients. *Crit Care Med* 11:7.

Keohane, P., Attrill, H., Love, M. et al. 1984. Relation between osmolality of diet and gastrointestinal side effects in enteral nutrition. *Br Med J* 288:678.

Kinsey, G.C., Murray, M.J., Swensen, S.J. et al. 1994. Glucose content of tracheal aspirates: Implications for the detection of tube feeding aspiration. *Crit Care Med* 10:1557.

Kocan, M.J., Hickisch, S.M. 1986. A comparison of continuous and intermittent enteral nutrition in NICU patients. *J. Neurosci Nurs* 18:333.

Kochan, P., Chmielarczyk, A., Szymaniak, L. et al. 2011. *Lactobacillus rhamnosus* administration causes sepsis in a cardiosurgical patient—Is the time right to revise probiotic safety guidelines? *Clin Microbiol Infect* 17(10):1589–1592.

Krenitsky, J. 2006. Gastric versus jejunal feeding: Evidence or emotion? *Pract Gastroenterol* XXX(9):46.

Krenitsky, J. 2011. Blind bedside placement of feeding tubes: Treatment or threat? *Pract Gastroenterol* XXXV(3):32–42.

Land, M.H., Rouster-Stevens, K., Woods, C.R., Cannon, M.L., Cnota, J., Shetty, A.K. 2005. Lactobacillus sepsis associated with probiotic therapy. *Pediatrics* 115(1):178–181.

Levinson, M., Bryce, A. 1993. Enteral feeding, gastric colonization and diarrhoea in the critically ill patient: Is there a relationship? *Anaesth Intens Care* 21:85.

Lherm, T., Monet, C., Nougière, B. et al. 2002. Seven cases of fungemia with *Saccharomyces boulardii* in critically ill patients. *Intensive Care Med* 28:797.

Li Bassi, G., Torres, A. 2011. Ventilator-associated pneumonia: Role of positioning. *Curr Opin Crit Care* Feb, 17(1):57–63.

Lin, H.C., Van Citters, G.W. 1997. Stopping enteral feeding for arbitrary gastric residual volume may not be physiologically sound: Results of a computer simulation model. *J Parenter Enteral Nutr* 21:286.

Livingston, E.H., Passaro Jr., E.P. 1990. Postoperative ileus. *Dig Dis Sci* 35:121.

Longstreth, G.F., Thompson, W.G., Chey, W.D. et al. 2006. Functional bowel disorders. *Gastroenterology* 130(5):1480–1491.

Luckey, A., Livingston, E., Taché, Y. 2003. Mechanisms and treatment of postoperative ileus. *Arch Surg* 138:206.

Luft, V.C., Beghetto, M.G., DeMello, E.D. et al. 2008. Role of enteral nutrition in the incidence of diarrhea among hospitalized adult patients. *Nutrition* 24(6):528–535.

Madsen, D., Sebolt, T., Cullen, L. et al. 2005. Listening to bowel sounds: An evidence-based practice project: Nurses find that a traditional practice isn't the best indicator of returning gastrointestinal motility in patients who've undergone abdominal surgery. *Am J Nurs* 105:40–49.

Marcuard, S.P., Stegall, K.L., Trogdon, S.1989. Clearing obstructed feeding tubes. *J. Parenter Enteral Nutr* 13:81.

Marik, P.E., Zaloga, G.P. 2003. Gastric versus post-pyloric feeding: A systematic review. *Crit Care* 7:R46.

Martins, J.R., Shiroma, G.M., Horie, L.M. et al. 2012. Factors leading to discrepancies between prescription and intake of enteral nutrition therapy in hospitalized patients. *Nutrition* 28(9):864–867.

McClave, S.A., Lukan, J.K., Stefater, J.A. et al. 2005. Poor validity of residual volumes as a marker for risk of aspiration in critically ill patients. *Crit Care Med* 33(2):324–330.

McClave, S.A., Snider, H.L., Lowen, C.C. et al. 1992. Use of residual volume as a marker for enteral feeding intolerance: Retrospective blinded comparison with physical examination and radiographic findings. *J Parenter Enteral Nutr* 16:99.

McIntyre, P.B., Fitchew, M., Lennard-Jones, J.E. 1986. Patients with a high jejunostomy do not need a special diet. *Gastroenterology* 91:25–33.

Meissner, W., Dohrn, B., Reinhart, K. 2003. Enteral naloxone reduces gastric tube reflux and frequency of pneumonia in critical care patients during opioid analgesia. *Crit Care Med* 31:776.

Metheny, N.A., Clouse, R.E. 1997. Bedside methods for detecting aspiration in tube fed patients. *Chest* 103:724.

Metheny, N.A., Clouse, R.E., Chang, Y.H. et al. 2006. Tracheobronchial aspiration of gastric contents in critically ill tube-fed patients: Frequency, outcomes, and risk factors. *Crit Care Med* 34:1007–1015.

Metheny, N.A., Schallom, L., Oliver, D.A. et al. 2008. Gastric residual volume and aspiration in critically ill patients receiving gastric feedings. *Am J Crit Care* 17:512–519.

Miller, L.J., Malagelada, J.R., Go, V.L.W. 1978. Postprandial duodenal function in man. *Gut* 19:699.

Montejo, J.C., Minambres, E., Bordeje, L. et al. 2010. Gastric residual volume during enteral nutrition in ICU patients. The REGANE study. *Intensive Care Med* 36(8):1386–1393.

Montejo-Gonzalez, J.C., Pérez-Cardenas, M.D., Fernández-Hernández, A.I. et al. 1994. Detecting pulmonary aspiration of enteral feeding in intubated patients. *Chest* 106:1632.

Neumann, D.A., DeLegge, M.H. 2002. Gastric versus small-bowel tube feeding in the intensive care unit: A prospective comparison of efficacy. *Crit Care Med* 30:1436.

Nguyen, N.Q., Chapman, M., Fraser, R.J. et al. 2007. Prokinetic therapy for feed intolerance in critical illness: One drug or two? *Crit Care Med* 35(11):2561–2567.

Owens, S.R., Greenson, J.K. 2007. The pathology of malabsorption: Current concepts. *Histopathology* 50:64–82.

Parrish, C.R., Krenitsky, J., McCray, S. July 2013. *Nutrition Support Traineeship Syllabus*, Fully revised. University of Virginia Health System, Charlottesville, VA.

Parrish, C.R., McClave, S. 2008. Checking gastric residual volumes: A practice in search of science? *Pract Gastroenterol* 32:33.

Petrof, E.O., Dhaliwal, R., Manzanares, W. et al. 2012. Probiotics in the critically ill: A systematic review of the randomized trial evidence. *Crit Care Med* Dec, 40(12):3290–3302.

Potts, R.G., Zaroukian, M.H., Guerrero, P.A. et al. 1993. Comparison of blue dye visualization and glucose oxidase test strip methods for detecting pulmonary aspiration of enteral feedings in intubated adults. *Chest* 103:117.

Poulard, F., Dimet, J., Martin-Lefevre, L. et al. 2010. Impact of not measuring residual gastric volume in mechanically ventilated patients receiving early enteral feeding: A prospective before-after study. *J Parenter Enteral Nutr* 34(2):125–130.

Powell, K.S., Marcuard, S.P., Farrior, E.S. et al. 1993. Aspirating gastric residuals causes occlusion of small-bore feeding tubes. *J Parenter Enteral Nutr* 17:243.

Quigley, E.M.M., Hasler, W.L., Parkman, H.P. 2001. AGA technical review on nausea and vomiting. *Gastroenterology* 120:263.

Rees, R.P.G., Hare, W.R., Grimble, G.K. et al. 1992. Do pts with moderately impaired gastrointestinal function requiring enteral nutrition need a predigested nitrogen source? A prospective crossover controlled trial. *Gut* 33:877.

Rees, R.P.G., Keohane, P.P., Grimble, G.K. et al. 1985. Tolerance of elemental diet administered without starter regimen. *Br Med J* 290:1869.

Rice, T., Wheeler, A.P., Thompson, B.T. et al. 2012. Initial trophic vs. full enteral feeding in patients with acute lung injury: The EDEN Randomized Trial. *JAMA* 307(8):795–803.

Ridley, E.J., Davies, A.R. 2011. Practicalities of nutrition support in the intensive care unit: The usefulness of gastric residual volume and prokinetic agents with enteral nutrition. *Nutrition* 27(5):509–512.

Sheean, P.M., Peterson, S.J., Zhao, W. et al. 2012. Intensive medical nutrition therapy: Methods to improve nutrition provision in the critical care setting. *J Acad Nutr Diet* 112(7):1073–1079.

Silk, D.A., Grimble, G.K. 1992. Relevance of physiology of nutrient absorption to formulation of enteral diets. *Nutrition* 8:1.

Spilker, C.A., Hinthorn, D.R., Pingleton, S.K. 1996. Intermittent enteral feeding in mechanically ventilated patients. The effect on gastric pH and gastric cultures. *Chest* 110:243.

Szajewska, H., Mrukowicz, J.Z. 2001. Probiotics in the treatment and prevention of acute infectious diarrhea in infants and children: A systematic review of published randomized, double-blind, placebo-controlled trials. *J Pediatr Gastroenterol Nutr* 33:S17.

Teasell, R.W., Bach, D., McRae, M. 1994. Prevalence and recovery of aspiration poststroke: A retrospective analysis. *Dysphagia* 9:35.

Thomas, P.D., Forbes, A., Green, J. et al. 2003. Guidelines for the investigation of chronic diarrhoea, 2nd edn. *Gut* 52(Suppl. V):v1–v15.

Waxman, K. 2000.The acute abdomen, in: *Textbook of Critical Care*, 4th edn., Grenvik, A. (ed.). W.B. Saunders, Philadelphia, PA, p. 1603.

Willcutts, K. 2010. Pre-op NPO and traditional post-op diet advancement: Time to move on. *Pract Gastroenterol* XXXIV(12):16.

Yavagal, D.R., Karnad, D.R., Oak, J.L. 2000. Metoclopramide for preventing pneumonia in critically ill patients receiving enteral tube feeding: A randomized controlled trial. *Crit Care Med* 28:1408.

Zarling, E.J., Parmar, J.R., Mobarhan, S. et al. 1986. Effect of enteral formula infusion rate, osmolality, and chemical composition upon clinical tolerance and carbohydrate absorption in normal subjects. *J Parenter Enteral Nutr* 10:588.

18 Drug–Nutrient Interactions

Rex O. Brown and Roland N. Dickerson

CONTENTS

INTRODUCTION

The interaction of drugs and nutrition is an extremely important component of clinical monitoring of patients (Santos and Boullata 2005). The number of drugs used in the critical care setting has increased recently, and early use of nutrition support is a reasonable standard for the critically ill patient. This creates an environment for many possible clinically significant drug–nutrient interactions. This chapter will address the clinically significant drug–nutrient interactions that may occur in the critical care setting. There are several clinically significant drug–nutrient interactions (e.g., grapefruit juice and many drugs metabolized by the CYP3A4 enzyme) that would likely not occur in the critical care setting, so they will not be addressed in this chapter.

Chan (2000) has suggested that drug–nutrient interactions be placed in four distinct categories: biopharmaceutical inactivations, absorption, systemic or physiologic dispositions, and alteration of elimination or clearance. While this categorization has not been universally accepted, it would allow for a systematic clinical evaluation of the different drug–nutrient interactions and possibly identify areas for concentrated clinical research. Drug-related problems in patients in an acute care setting receiving nutrition support were studied by Cerulli and Malone (1999). They reported 220 clinically important interventions in 440 patients. Another patient population that would be at high risk of drug–nutrient interactions because of the number of medications needed are solid-organ transplant patients (Chan 2001). This chapter will address clinically important drug–nutrient interactions using two major categories: drug affecting nutrition and nutrition affecting drugs.

DRUG EFFECTS ON NUTRITION THERAPY

Gastrointestinal Effects

Since enteral nutrition (EN) is advocated in critically ill patients, assessment of gastrointestinal tolerance is an important component of clinical monitoring. Drugs that cause gastrointestinal disorders need to be recognized, especially when one is trying to separate EN intolerance from a drug-induced gastrointestinal disorder (Table 18.1). Diarrhea that emanates in the intensive care unit (ICU) is often caused by EN and its accompanying pharmacotherapy. While *Clostridia difficile* has received most of the attention for infectious diarrhea, organisms like *Clostridium perfringens, Klebsiella oxytoca*, and *Bacteroides fragilis* should be considered as well (Polage et al. 2012). Drug vehicles have been under close scrutiny as etiologies of diarrhea because they are often hyperosmolar. Edes et al. (1990) reported that approximately 80% of diarrhea in acute care patients was caused by concomitant drug therapy. The major etiologies in this study were sorbitol used as a drug vehicle (48%) and diarrhea from *C. difficile* (17%). Liquid drug preparations would be logical choices for critical care patients who have small-bore feeding tubes or permanent enterostomies. Many of these liquid products have a substantial sorbitol content and osmolalities that exceed 1000 mOsm/L (Dickerson and Melnik 1988; Lutomski et al. 1993). Preparations like acetaminophen elixir can have an osmolality >5000 mOsm/L. See Table 18.2 for examples of osmolality for some liquid drug products. When hypertonic products are given by bolus administration via a tube, especially a jejunostomy tube, the osmotic load may cause diarrhea. In the case of acetaminophen, switching to crushed tablets followed by 15–30 mL water flushes will alleviate this problem. Other interventions include diluting the hyperosmotic liquid preparation with water to potentially improve gastrointestinal tolerance. Prokinetic drugs like metoclopramide and erythromycin are used for improving gastrointestinal emptying during EN in critically ill patients; however, they also act on the small bowel. These drugs can potentially cause gastrointestinal intolerance in some patients. When gastric emptying is improved with the administration of metoclopramide or erythromycin, the drug should then be discontinued, or the dose should be reduced as appropriate to prevent diarrhea in the patient receiving EN.

Fluid and Electrolytes

A major part of clinical monitoring of the critical care patient who is receiving EN or parenteral nutrition (PN) is treating fluid and electrolyte imbalances. These are problems that occur quite often in this patient care setting, and they may be even more common in patients receiving nutrition support (Driscoll 1989). There are many drugs that induce electrolyte imbalances, and an appreciation of these can markedly improve clinical monitoring. Some electrolyte imbalances may be inherited by the nutrition support service (NSS). Since most of the electrolyte components are in the PN or EN formulations, there is an expectation that the nutrient formulations will help treat these disorders.

Sodium imbalances are the most difficult to diagnose and treat. Dysnatremias are fairly prevalent in the critical care setting, especially when nutrition support is being administered (Whitmire 2008).

TABLE 18.1
Gastrointestinal Disorders Caused by Drug Therapy

Drug	Result
Hyperosmolar liquids	Diarrhea
Sorbitol-containing preparations	Diarrhea
Metoclopramide	Diarrhea
Erythromycin	Diarrhea

TABLE 18.2
Osmolality of Selected Liquid Drug Products Used in Critical Care

Drug	Osmolality (mOsm/kg)
Acetaminophen elixir (650 mg/10 mL)	5400
Acetaminophen with codeine elixir	4700
Amoxicillin suspension (250 mg/5 mL)	2250
Cimetidine elixir (300 mg/5 mL)	5550
Trimethoprim/sulfamethoxazole suspension	2200
Dexamethasone elixir (1 mg/10 mL)	3350
Dextromethorphan syrup (10 mg/5 mL)	5950
Docusate sodium syrup (100 mg/30 mL)	4700
Erythromycin ethylsuccinate suspension (200 mg/5 mL)	1750
Ferrous sulfate liquid (300 mg/5 mL)	4700
Furosemide solution (40 mg/4 mL)	2050
Lactulose syrup (20 g/30 mL)	3600
Metoclopramide syrup (10 mg/10 mL)	8350
Multivitamin liquid	5700
Phenytoin suspension (125 mg/5 mL)	1500
Potassium chloride liquid 10%	3550

Sources: Adapted from Dickerson, R.N. and Melnik G., *Am. J. Hosp. Pharm.*, 45, 832, 1988; Lutomski, D.M. et al., *Ann. Pharmacother.*, 27, 269, 1993.

Patients with hyponatremia need to be evaluated for extracellular volume status concurrently (Table 18.3). Hypovolemic hyponatremia requires replacement of salt and water, usually as normal saline or lactated ringers in the critical care setting. Euvolemic hyponatremia usually requires water restriction or administration of an antidiuretic hormone antagonist (e.g., conivaptan) in the critical care setting. Hypervolemic hyponatremia would require salt and especially water restriction. Some drugs like loop diuretics have an intended effect to increase the renal excretion of sodium, usually for an edematous state. Other drugs like trimethoprim–sulfamethoxazole (Kaufman et al. 1983) and cisplatin (Hutchison et al. 1988) cause renal wasting of sodium, but they are often overlooked as etiologies. In critical care patients, there are many causes of the syndrome of inappropriate secretion of antidiuretic hormone (SIADH) with drugs being a major contributor to this problem

TABLE 18.3
Hyponatremia and Nutrition Support

Type of Hyponatremia	Treatment
Hypotonic hypovolemic	• Continue PN or EN
	• Replace volume deficits with NS or LR
Hypotonic euvolemic	• Concentrate PN to decrease free water
	• Concentrate EN to decrease free water
	• Decrease other water intake (IVF)
	• Antidiuretic hormone antagonist
Hypotonic hypervolemic	• Eliminate sodium and concentrate PN
	• Concentrate EN by using 2 kcal/mL formulation
	• Discontinue IVF/water boluses

NS, normal saline; LR, lactated ringers; IVF, intravenous fluid.

(Belton and Thomas 1999). Carbamazepine (Lahr 1985), thiazide diuretics (Sonnenblick et al. 1993), and amiodarone (Patel and Kasiar 2002) have all been implicated to cause SIADH. Patients with hyponatremia from these drugs will need free water restricted by concentrating the nutrient formulation, especially if the drug cannot be changed. This would require higher concentrations of dextrose, amino acids, and lipid in the PN formulation, so the infusion rate could be decreased and still meet the patient's nutritional needs. With EN, administration of a 1.5 or 2 kcal/mL formulation would be used to minimize water and still meet nutritional needs. Antidiuretic hormone antagonists are approved for the treatment of euvolemic hyponatremia and can help correct this disorder by increasing the excretion of free water (Munger 2007).

Hypernatremia usually implies a deficit in water; however, extracellular volume status must be assessed so that proper treatment can be prescribed. Excessive administration of lactulose has resulted in hypovolemic hypernatremia, presumably from excessive stool losses of water (Nelson et al. 1983). Replacement with salt and water initially to perfuse vital organs should be followed by the administration of hypotonic fluid like water, D5 in ¼ normal saline, ½ normal saline, or D5W. Obviously, the dose of lactulose should be reduced to reduce stool losses to an acceptable volume (e.g., one to two soft stools per day).

Potassium balance in the critical care patient can be particularly challenging because multiple factors (e.g., urine output, pH) can change and influence the concentration of this cation. Potassium is particularly important in nutrition support patients because it is the major intracellular cation, so as new cells are synthesized, potassium will be incorporated into them. Many drugs affect potassium balance. Loop and thiazide diuretics, antipseudomonal penicillins, corticosteroids, and amphotericin B can all cause increased urinary excretion of potassium resulting in hypokalemia. Drugs like piperacillin have been shown to decrease not only potassium but also serum concentrations of magnesium and calcium (Polderman and Girbes 2002). Amphotericin B has been reported to increase urinary excretion of both potassium and magnesium. Other drugs like insulin and beta-2 agonists promote the movement of potassium into the intracellular space and can result in hypokalemia. Dickens et al. (1994) demonstrated a mean decrease of 0.8 mEq/L in serum potassium concentration following a single nebulized 2.5 mg dose of albuterol. Drugs that are used to induce a barbiturate coma in severe head trauma have been reported to cause hypokalemia during the administration of the drug. A rebound hyperkalemia has been reported when the drug has been discontinued (Ng et al. 2011). It is common to have patients in the critical care setting receiving nutrition support and several of the aforementioned drugs at one time. Standard amounts of potassium in PN or EN formulations will not maintain potassium balance in these patients when they are receiving these drugs. They will need frequent bolus doses of potassium as well as having the concentration increased in PN. See Table 18.4 for general guidelines for administering electrolytes for hypokalemia, hypophosphatemia, hypomagnesemia, and hypocalcemia. Oral liquid preparations of potassium are generally incompatible when admixed with enteral feeding formulations.

Several drugs are known to induce hyperkalemia. Hyperkalemia secondary to potassium-sparing diuretics, angiotensin-converting enzyme inhibitors, and angiotensin receptor blocking agents is well appreciated in all settings. Heparin can be a cause of hyperkalemia, especially with therapeutic doses in patients with diabetes or renal failure (Oster et al. 1995). Heparin is known to inhibit aldosterone, which normally causes sodium retention and potassium excretion. Antagonism of aldosterone results in sodium excretion and potassium retention. Trimethoprim, which is a component with sulfamethoxazole in an antibiotic product, is also a weak potassium-sparing diuretic (Velazquez et al. 1993). Two clinical studies have reported mean increases in the serum potassium concentration >1 mEq/L in patients receiving the sulfamethoxazole/trimethoprim combination (Alappan et al. 1996; Greenberg et al. 1993).

Calcium imbalances in the critical care setting are fairly common. One recent study of 100 critically ill patients reported a 21% and 6% incidence of hypocalcemia and hypercalcemia, respectively, using ionized calcium concentrations (Dickerson et al. 2004). It should be noted that it is very difficult to separate true hypocalcemia from hypocalcemia secondary to hypoalbuminemia using total

TABLE 18.4
Treatment of Common Electrolyte Disorders Requiring Replacement in Critically Ill Patients[a]

Hypokalemia

Lab Value	Intravenous Replacement Dose (mEq)
3.5–3.9	40
3–3.4	40 × 2
<3	40 × 3

Do not administer faster than 20 mEq/h.

Hypophosphatemia

	Intravenous Replacement Dose (mmol/kg)	
Lab Value	Medical–Surgical Patients	Trauma–Burn Patients
2.3–3	0.16	0.32
1.6–2.2	0.32	0.64
<1.5	0.64	1

Do not administer faster than 7.5 mmol/h.

Hypomagnesemia

Lab Value	Intravenous Replacement Dose (g/kg)
1.6–1.8	0.05
1–1.5	0.1
<1	0.15

Do not administer faster than 1 g/h.

Hypocalcemia

Lab Value (ionized Ca, mmol/L)	Intravenous Replacement Dose (g/kg)
1–1.12	2
<1	4

May give 1 g over 1 h.

These guidelines are only for patients with normal renal function.

[a] Intravenous replacement doses are usually required in critically ill patients secondary to the acuity of the patient and potential for serum concentrations to decrease further. Oral replacement may be appropriate for patients who are hemodynamically stable and have a functional/accessible gastrointestinal tract.

calcium concentrations because the common conversion equations are inaccurate in the ICU setting (Dickerson et al. 2004). In the critical care setting, ionized calcium concentrations should be used exclusively to assess calcium status if they are available. Foscarnet, a drug used for cytomegalovirus in patients with HIV infection, has a profound effect on ionized calcium concentrations resulting in hypocalcemia. Four of six patients receiving a 90 mg/kg dose developed hypocalcemia, while all 11 patients receiving a 120 mg/kg dose developed this electrolyte disorder (Jacobson et al. 1991). Patients receiving intravenous foscarnet should be monitored frequently and vigorously supplemented with calcium during and after administration of this drug. A nutrient (calcium carbonate) and a drug (levothyroxine) that are often given to geriatric patients may potentially interact (Singh et al. 2000). When administered concurrently, it has been shown in vitro that levothyroxine may adsorb to calcium carbonate. This could lead to increases in the dosing of the thyroid product. When patients are receiving both drugs, it would be prudent to space the administration times so that the levothyroxine is given 2–4 h apart from the calcium administration. Calcium gluconate and calcium chloride are products used commonly for parenteral treatment/replacement of hypocalcemia in the critically ill. It should be appreciated that 1 g of calcium chloride provides three times as much elemental calcium per gram as calcium gluconate (13.5 vs. 4.5 mEq/g). Most clinicians use calcium gluconate for parenteral replacement of calcium in the critical care setting. Recent parenteral drug shortages have included calcium gluconate. This results in clinicians using parenteral calcium chloride. It is imperative that institutions have a policy that clearly establishes replacement doses using calcium chloride. Oral calcium is used most frequently for bone health; however, these products could theoretically be used to treat hypocalcemia in patients who are hemodynamically stable with functional/accessible gastrointestinal tracts. The two products used most frequently are calcium carbonate (20 mEq of elemental calcium/g) and calcium acetate (12.7 mEq of elemental calcium/g).

Similar to potassium, the need for phosphorus will be markedly enhanced as new cells are synthesized during administration of nutrition support because phosphate is the major intracellular anion. It has been demonstrated that patients with hypophosphatemia also have a deficit of phosphorus in skeletal muscle (Fiaccadori et al. 1990). This issue would be particularly important in patients with underlying pulmonary disease (e.g., COPD) or in patients receiving mechanical ventilation in the critical care setting. Many clinicians begin the replacement of phosphorus when patients have serum concentrations of phosphorus in the low-normal range (Brown et al. 2006). This could theoretically prevent moderate to severe hypophosphatemia and the accompanying sequelae. With PN, the phosphorus concentration can be increased to 30 mmol/L safely in most formulations. With EN, phosphorus will need to be administered as an intravenous replacement dose in the critical care setting. Oral replacement of phosphorus is an option for patients with mild hypophosphatemia; however, the gastrointestinal tract is limited to what can be tolerated because phosphate is an osmotic laxative and can cause diarrhea. Hyperphosphatemia is rare outside of acute kidney injury or chronic kidney disease; however, a few cases of this disorder secondary to administration of oral phosphorus in patients with compromised renal function have been reported (Sutters et al. 1996). It should also be noted that colonic absorption of phosphorus can occur following administration of phosphate-containing enemas. Severe hyperphosphatemia (serum phosphorus concentration >6 mg/dL) invariably requires removal of all phosphorus from the PN formulation. Metastatic calcification of calcium phosphate in soft tissues can occur with severe hyperphosphatemia. This is particularly important in the patient that has any degree of renal compromise. With EN, formulations with lower concentrations of phosphorus can be used, or phosphate binders (e.g., calcium acetate or sevelamer) may be added to the pharmacotherapy regimen.

Hypomagnesemia is another electrolyte disorder that occurs fairly frequently in the critical care setting. While lower gastrointestinal losses and alcohol abuse are contributing causes of magnesium depletion, drugs are major factors in critical care patients. Several drugs have been identified to cause or contribute to hypomagnesemia through renal wasting of this electrolyte. Cisplatin (Schilsky and Anderson 1979), cyclosporine (Nozue et al. 1992), aminoglycosides (Zaloga et al. 1984), loop or thiazide diuretics (Sheehan and White 1982), proton pump inhibitors (Furlnatto and Faulhaber 2011; Gau et al. 2012), and amphotericin B have all been shown to increase urinary excretion of magnesium. It is clear that long-term use of proton pump inhibitors can result in hypomagnesemia, but less clear whether this disorder occurs acutely in the ICU (Hoorn et al. 2010). Elliott et al. (2000) demonstrated a significant increase in magnesium fractional excretion rate from 3.4% ± 0.8% to 11.8% ± 6.4% following the administration of gentamicin. In addition to effects on calcium status, foscarnet has been reported to cause hypomagnesemia (Gearhart and Sorg 1993). Considering that several of these drugs can be given to critical care patients concurrently, hypomagnesemia can become a major problem when serum electrolyte monitoring and appropriate supplementation are not implemented. Hypomagnesemia can also cause hypokalemia because it is important in maintaining proper functioning of the sodium/potassium ATPase pump. Also, magnesium is critically important in the function of parathyroid hormone, which maintains calcium balance. Therefore, moderate to severe hypomagnesemia can also cause hypocalcemia. With PN, the concentration of magnesium sulfate can be increased as high as 32 mEq/L in some formulations.

A standard concentration range used by many institutions is from 8 to 12 mEq/L. Intravenous replacement of magnesium sulfate is often needed in addition to increasing the concentration in the PN formulation. With EN, it is difficult to replace a large magnesium deficit via the gastrointestinal tract because of its cathartic properties. In the critical care setting, intravenous replacement is the most reliable method of treatment, especially for those patients with moderate to severe hypomagnesemia. Magnesium oxide and magnesium gluconate are oral forms of magnesium that can be administered orally or via tube in patients receiving EN with mild hypomagnesemia. Gastrointestinal tolerance needs to be monitored closely during administration of the aforementioned salts because they can be cathartic laxatives in some patients.

Glycemic Control

Critically ill patients often exhibit increased gluconeogenesis and insulin resistance resulting in hyperglycemia. Despite controversy regarding the optimal target blood glucose concentration range (Finfer et al. 2009; Van Den Berghe et al. 2001), unabated hyperglycemia and severe hypoglycemia are associated with detrimental clinical outcomes. Thus, medications that cause hyperglycemia or hypoglycemia need to be appreciated during nutrition therapy, and glycemic control may need to be altered. Table 18.5 lists the most common medications that may induce hyper- or hypoglycemia.

For patients with significant hyperglycemia, most clinicians will change the nutrition therapy to decrease the glucose or carbohydrate content and increase the lipid/fat content to keep the caloric intake constant. This is easily done with PN by altering the dextrose and lipid content and requires a formula change to a *diabetic-type formula* with EN. Any exogenous sources of glucose and carbohydrate are also eliminated. The implementation of more aggressive insulin therapy with either a continuous intravenous insulin infusion or *tightened sliding scale coverage* is also often required. It is important to ascertain if the drug therapy is a major etiology for the hyperglycemia as when the drug therapy changes, hypoglycemia may occur if the glycemic control therapy is not altered. For example, the most common drug-induced causes of hyperglycemia in our ICUs at our institution are corticosteroids and vasopressor adrenergic agents. As the pharmacotherapy is being weaned, insulin requirements are often reduced necessitating a change in glycemic management of the patient.

TABLE 18.5
Drugs That Can Potentially Alter Glucose Homeostasis in the Critical Care Setting

Hyperglycemia	Adrenergic	Epinephrine, norepinephrine, phenylephrine
	Atypical antipsychotics	Clozapine, olanzapine, quetiapine, risperidone
	Corticosteroids	Hydrocortisone, methylprednisolone, prednisone
	Calcineurin inhibitors	Cyclosporine, sirolimus, tacrolimus
	Diltiazem	
	Hydrochlorothiazide	
	Levofloxacin[a]	
	Protease inhibitors	Stavudine, didanosine, lamivudine, ritonavir, zidovudine
Hypoglycemia	Cotrimoxazole	Trimethoprim–sulfamethoxazole
	Disopyramide	
	Insulin	
	Levofloxacin[a]	
	Oral hypoglycemic agents	Glipizide, glyburide
	Pentamidine	

[a] Fluoroquinolones have been associated with dysglycemia and may cause either hyper- or hypoglycemia.

For patients receiving medications that cause hypoglycemia, it is important to use care when abruptly discontinuing continuous EN or PN. Additionally, caution is necessary when implementing glycemic control therapy as these patients may be at higher risk for the compounding effects of glucose-lowering pharmacotherapy.

VITAMINS

There are a number of clinically important drug–nutrient interactions involving vitamins; however, the majority of these will be encountered in chronic care and will not be covered in this chapter. Two independent studies have identified the risk of developing thiamine deficiency following the administration of the loop diuretic, furosemide (Brady et al. 1995; Seligman et al. 1991). It is thought that the loop diuretic enhances the urinary excretion of thiamine, leading to a deficient state. This is likely to occur when furosemide is prescribed in multiple doses for several days or as a continuous intravenous infusion. Since therapeutic doses of thiamine (100 mg BID) are relatively benign, supplementation of this vitamin when loop diuretics are used over several days appears to be prudent. It is appreciated that the absorption of vitamin B-12 (cyanocobalamin) is markedly decreased when patients are treated with proton pump inhibitors (Marcuard et al. 1994). While the development of a macrocytic anemia would take a few years to develop with chronic therapy, many patients are placed on proton pump inhibitors for acid suppression while in the ICUs, especially if they had been receiving the drug before admission. This is an excellent time to monitor the patient for anemia as part of routine clinical care. Some clinicians will monitor for macrocytic anemia using amino acid markers that are dependent on folic acid and cyanocobalamin. For instance, elevated serum concentrations of both homocysteine and methylmalonic acid or methylmalonic acid alone are consistent with cyanocobalamin deficiency in a patient with a macrocytic anemia. Intramuscular treatment of cyanocobalamin is the treatment of choice for these types of patients, especially if they must continue to receive proton pump inhibitors.

CALORIE INTAKE FROM DRUG VEHICLES

Drug vehicles can have important implications to the nutrition support clinician when a substantial dose of nutrition is delivered to the critically ill patient. Propofol, an intravenous anesthetic and sedative, is frequently used for a few days in selected patients in the critical care setting (Devlin et al. 2005; Kang 2002). This product is particularly useful in traumatic brain injury where frequent neurological evaluations are desired. The short half-life of propofol allows periodic stopping and evaluation of mental status. It is contained in a 10% lipid emulsion vehicle, so patients receive a continuous infusion of fat emulsion when this drug is given for sedation (Table 18.6). Several authors have identified the importance of including lipid calories from propofol when prescribing nutrition support (Lowrey et al. 1996; Roth et al. 1997). If the dose of lipid (e.g., 9–10 kcal/kg/day) from propofol approaches the desired lipid dose with PN, lipid can be omitted from the PN formulation until the propofol is weaned or discontinued. EN patients who are receiving a substantial number

TABLE 18.6
Lipid Calories Delivered from Different Doses of Propofol Infusion

Rate (mL/h)	Propofol Dose (mg/h)	Calories/24 h
10	100	264
15	150	396
20	200	528
25	250	660
30	300	792

of calories from propofol can be treated with a low-calorie, high-protein EN formulation, so the fat calories from the drug vehicle will be accounted for. Even though one group has suggested that propofol infusions do not increase serum triglyceride concentrations (McLeod et al. 1997), this has not been the experience of many clinicians (Lowrey et al. 1996; Roth et al. 1997). Therefore, serum triglyceride concentrations should be monitored frequently (e.g., two to three times per week) when patients are receiving higher doses of propofol (e.g., >5 mg/kg/h). If patients develop serum triglyceride concentrations >400 mg/dL during propofol infusions, an alternative sedative agent like lorazepam or midazolam should be considered. There are now several lipid preparations of amphotericin B marketed in the United States; however, their caloric contribution is negligible (Graybill 1996). It is notable that the calcium channel blocker, clevidipine butyrate, is manufactured in a 20% intravenous fat emulsion (Thompson 2008).

Metabolic Alterations

Numerous drugs, particularly those with sedative and paralytic properties, are known to reduce energy expenditure of critically ill patients. A concerted interdisciplinary effort by clinicians has resulted in a marked improvement in sedation and analgesia for the critically ill patient over the past decade. Continuous sedation with intravenous midazolam and fentanyl is common practice in many ICUs that care for surgical, trauma, and thermally injured patients. Effective analgesia and sedation can decrease measured resting energy expenditure by as much as 6%–27% during critical illness (Dickerson and Roth-Yousey 2005).

Propofol reduces oxygen consumption by 25%–40% when given for sedation after surgery. Its influence upon lowering energy expenditure for patients with traumatic brain injury has not been examined; however, a reduction is likely (Dickerson and Sachs 2011). Pentobarbital therapy, given in doses sufficient to render the patient comatose, is sometimes given to patients with traumatic brain injury who are refractory to conventional measures for lowering intracranial pressure. Pentobarbital therapy has been shown to reduce energy expenditure by 30% (590 kcal/day) (Fried et al. 1989). Skeletal muscle paralysis with a neuromuscular blocker, such as pancuronium, vecuronium, or atracurium, has been reported to reduce energy expenditure by 11%–17%. However, during heavy sedation, skeletal muscle paralysis may only have a modest and clinically irrelevant effect on energy expenditure for patients with traumatic brain injury (Fried et al. 1989). In the thermally injured patient, implementation of neuromuscular blockage has been reported to result in a 23% reduction (about 500 kcal/day) in measured energy expenditure despite the presence of sedation and analgesia pharmacotherapy (Dickerson and Roth-Yousey 2005). Propranolol and other beta-adrenergic receptor blockers, when given to acutely ill, thermally injured, or traumatic brain injured patients, may reduce energy expenditure by 6%–12%. The reader is referred to a systematic review of medication effects on metabolic rate for additional information (Dickerson and Roth-Yousey 2005).

Because the hypermetabolic response to critical illness coexists with hypercatabolism, it is possible that drug therapy that reduces hypermetabolism may conversely downregulate protein catabolism and nitrogen excretion. Unfortunately, clinical data investigating this phenomenon are limited. In a small study, Fried et al. (1989) demonstrated that nitrogen excretion was decreased from 19 to 11 g/day in patients with traumatic brain injury when given pentobarbital therapy. It also has been suggested that the lack of difference in protein requirements for trauma patients with or without traumatic brain injury (in contrast to older refuting data before the availability of propofol) may be partially explainable by implementation of propofol therapy for those with traumatic brain injury (Dickerson and Sachs 2011).

Corticosteroids such as hydrocortisone, prednisone, methylprednisolone, and dexamethasone increase proteolysis and muscle loss by upregulating the ubiquitin–proteasome proteolytic pathway as well as other autophagy genes and cathepsin. High-dose corticosteroids, now considered obsolete therapy for the management of traumatic brain injury, have been demonstrated to increase urinary nitrogen excretion 30%–50% (Dickerson and Sachs 2011).

These data are important for the clinician to recognize and incorporate into their plan when designing a nutrition regimen, particularly regarding calories and protein intakes, for a critically ill patient.

NUTRITIONAL EFFECTS ON DRUG THERAPY

There are substantial data involving the effect of nutrition on the metabolism of drugs (Walter-Sack and Klotz 1996); however, many of the clinically significant issues do not involve critical care patients like the grapefruit juice/drug interactions. Also, several of these interactions that are statistically significant are not really clinically important. It is known, however, that volume of distribution for many drugs is increased in severe starvation due to an expanded extracellular volume compartment. Also, conjugation of many drugs may be impaired in patients with malnutrition (Walter-Sack and Klotz 1996). It is very clear that the clearance of aminoglycoside antibiotics like gentamicin is enhanced with the administration of dietary protein (Dickson et al. 1986). Since these types of drugs have a narrow therapeutic index (i.e., small difference between drug failure, drug efficacy, and drug toxicity), appreciation of this drug–nutrient interaction is critical. Patients who are receiving aminoglycosides and have PN or EN started should have a marked increase in renal clearance of these drugs. This is especially true of critical care patients where high-protein formulations are the standard of practice provided patients have normal renal function. Clinicians managing these types of patients should expect to have to increase the dose of aminoglycosides to maintain or attain therapeutic drug concentrations.

DRUG ADMINISTRATION AND ENTERAL NUTRITION

The effects of EN on drug therapy have become an important issue in the critical care setting. EN is being promoted as the feeding method of choice, so many patients now have enteral access via small-bore feeding tubes that did not have this in the past. Therefore, drug therapy administration via tube becomes a reality in a lot of different scenarios (Dickerson and Sachs 2011; Williams 2008). There are several oral dosage forms that are prepared as sustained-release preparations. Generally, these should not be crushed and administered via a feeding tube. In some cases, the sustained-release capsule can be opened, and the intact pellets may be poured down the feeding tube followed by a water flush. This maintains the integrity of the sustained-release product but allows it to be administered via a tube if the patient cannot or will not swallow. The Institute for Safe Medication Practices has a list of medications that should not be crushed. This list is frequently updated and can be accessed at http://www.ismp.org/tools/donotcrush.pdf.

It used to be common practice when administering proton pump inhibitors (lansoprazole, pantoprazole) to coadminister it with an acidic juice when given into the stomach and a bicarbonate slurry with water when given via a jejunostomy feeding tube. However, studies have demonstrated the efficacy of using an alkalemic solution whether the drug was administered into the stomach or small bowel (Phillips et al. 2001) and commercially available preparations such as immediate-release omeprazole/sodium bicarbonate powder for oral suspension simplify this process.

When medications are given concurrently with enteral feeding, potential drug–enteral feeding interactions can occur resulting in medication bioavailability being decreased or the pharmacodynamic effect being decreased. Data demonstrating an adverse effect when the medication is coadministered with enteral feeding are summarized in the following.

It has been reported that approximately a threefold increase in amiodarone dosage was required to achieve therapeutic drug concentrations for 8 patients receiving the medication nasoduodenally compared to 85 patients given the medication by the oral route (Kotake et al. 2006). It is unclear whether this interaction was partially due to loss of the drug in the dosage process (tablet crushing, etc.), adherence to the enteral feeding formula, or due to the medication's delivery directly into the duodenum/jejunum.

Bioavailability of ciprofloxacin ranges from 33% to 75% when coadministered with continuous enteral feeding compared to intravenous medication delivery. Despite decreased gastrointestinal absorption of ciprofloxacin in critically ill, enterally fed patients, the use of a higher dose (750 mg every 12 h) given via a nasogastric tube resulted in plasma concentrations similar to 400 mg every 12 h given intravenously (Cohn et al. 1996). Ciprofloxacin may be given to patients receiving concurrent EN with the caveat of a dosage adjustment consideration. Additionally, the location of the feeding tube may be very important as it relates to the administration of fluoroquinolones. The major site of absorption is the duodenum, so administration of this drug via a jejunostomy feeding tube cannot be recommended at this time.

Despite holding the enteral tube feeding for a minimum interval of 2 h from the enteral feeding, plasma concentrations from itraconazole oral solution were about two-thirds of plasma concentrations when administered intravenously (Vandewoude et al. 1997). Doubling the enteral dosage achieved similar plasma concentrations to intravenous itraconazole; however, it resulted in an increased prevalence of diarrhea. Administration of itraconazole by the feeding tube should be avoided if possible.

The combination of levodopa and carbidopa is a drug used for the treatment of Parkinson's disease. It is well known that protein intake can interfere with the bioavailability of levodopa. Cooper et al. (2008) described a 77-year-old male patient who was hospitalized following an intracerebral hemorrhage. He required continuous EN providing 1.4 g protein/kg/day during his recovery and was restarted on his home dose of levodopa/carbidopa. The patient developed severe rigidity despite continuation of his home medications. His EN was changed to bolus feeding separating the enteral formulation and drug administration times. This resulted in improvement in his Parkinson's disease.

Levothyroxine is a common medication used for the treatment of hypothyroidism. It is well known that oral coadministration with antacids, iron, and calcium interferes with the absorption of this drug. The effect of continuous EN on levothyroxine bioavailability has been a reasonable question over several years. Dickerson et al. (2010) recently studied the coadministration of levothyroxine with continuous EN in 13 patients. Eleven of these patients were admitted to the hospital following trauma and required EN for support during recovery. Eight of the fourteen patients developed problems with levothyroxine during the coadministration with EN. Two developed subclinical hypothyroidism, and six developed overt hypothyroidism while receiving their home dose of the drug. Currently, it is unknown if holding the EN for an hour before and after the levothyroxine dose alleviates this problem. The authors suggested a modest dose escalation of 25 mcg/day when this problem is encountered (Dickerson et al. 2010).

One of the most appreciated drug–nutrient interactions is between phenytoin and EN formulations. Despite being recognized for over 30 years (Bauer 1982), there is still debate about the cause and the clinical significance of the interaction (Au Yeung and Ensom 2000; Gilbert 1996). Bauer (1982) demonstrated a significant decrease in phenytoin serum concentrations in neurosurgical patients who received both the drug and EN concurrently compared to patients receiving only the drug. Others have supported the recommendations of Bauer and suggest holding EN for 1–2 h prior to and after the phenytoin dose or doses (Gilbert 1996). In vitro data suggest that phenytoin suspension adheres to caseinate salts that are often used as the protein component of EN formulations (Smith et al. 1988). It is important from a nutritional standpoint to realize that the desired EN rate would need to be increased over a shorter time period if the EN is held before and after the administration. Close monitoring of serum phenytoin concentrations during enteral feeding is warranted.

Another potentially major drug–nutrient interaction occurs between warfarin and EN or PN formulations. There are some clinical data to suggest that this interaction occurs and that the drug may actually bind to the protein component of EN (Penrod 2001). In vitro data from Kuhn et al. (1989) would support this mechanism. Holding the EN 1 h before and after the daily dose is supported by clinical studies and case reports (Dickerson et al. 2008; Krajewski and Butterfoss 2011). Several reports of warfarin resistance during the administration of lipid-containing PN exist (Lutomski et al. 1987; MacLaren et al. 1997). It is interesting to note that 500 mL of 10% intravenous fat emulsion contains 154 mcg of vitamin K from the plant oils of the soybean used to make these products. Other formulations using a combination of soybean and safflower plant oils may provide less than

100 mcg of vitamin K. Some clinicians believe the vitamin K from these products will make anticoagulation very difficult. This becomes even more important as many institutions transition to new daily parenteral vitamin products that contain 150 mcg of vitamin K. Prothrombin time and INR monitoring during warfarin administration is imperative in the patient receiving concomitant PN, especially with intravenous fat emulsion and vitamins containing vitamin K.

Screening drug therapy for potential drug–nutrient interactions will always be an important part of clinical monitoring during delivery of PN or EN to critically ill patients. The clinically significant drug–nutrient interactions must be recognized so that clinicians can make rational decisions in caring for this patient population. The introduction of new drugs and nutritional products will undoubtedly increase the number of these interactions that will continually change the way clinicians practice during the provision of nutrition support.

CASE STUDY

LL is a 70-year-old male who is involved in a motor vehicle crash. He sustains a broken femur, traumatic brain injury, and pulmonary contusions. After undergoing a craniotomy and pinning of the femur, he requires mechanical ventilation and sedation with propofol. The patient is 6 ft tall and weighs 80 kg. He has a past medical history of heart failure and hypertension. Current medications in the critical care setting are the following:

Phenytoin 100 mg IV Q8H	Furosemide 40 mg IV BID
Esomeprazole 20 mg IV daily	Albuterol nebulized treatments Q6H
Enoxaparin 40 mg SQ daily	Propofol 20 mL/h

On hospital day 3, he has bowel sounds, so EN is started at 40 mL/h (1 kcal/mL, 63 g protein/L formula). On day 4, EN is advanced to 60 mL/h, and on day 5, it is advanced to 85 mL/h. The following laboratory values are available on day 5:

Sodium = 150 mEq/L	Potassium = 3.2 mEq/L
Chloride = 118 mEq/L	Bicarbonate = 22 mEq/L
Blood urea nitrogen = 10 mg/dL	Serum creatinine = 1 mg/dL
Ionized calcium = 1.05 mmol/L	Phosphorus = 1.5 mg/dL
Magnesium = 1.2 mg/dL	Triglycerides = 180 mg/dL

Arterial blood gas: pH = 7.5, pCO_2 = 30, pO_2 = 95, HCO_3 = 23.

Questions

1. What drugs/clinical conditions contributed to LL's hypokalemia?
2. What drug contributed to LL's hypocalcemia?
3. What drug contributed to LL's hypomagnesemia?
4. Design a regimen of electrolyte boluses for LL.
5. What drug likely contributed to LL's hypertriglyceridemia?
6. How many calories are being given via drug vehicles? How many calories/kg/day are being given via drug vehicles?
7. The patient had a seizure shortly after injury, so phenytoin will be continued beyond 1 week. It is changed to 300 mg daily as capsules. What intervention would allow absorption of the drug and deliver the desired nutrition support?

Answers

1. Furosemide by renal wasting of potassium, albuterol by promoting intracellular movement, and respiratory alkalosis.
2. Furosemide by renal wasting of calcium.
3. Furosemide by renal wasting of magnesium.
4. K phosphate 60 or 90 mmol IV over 8 or 12 h.
   Magnesium sulfate 8 g IV over 8 h.
   Ca gluconate 2 g IV over 2 h.
5. Propofol.
6. 528 cal or 6.6 kcal/kg/day.
7. Hold the EN 2 h before and after the daily phenytoin dose. Increase EN to run 100 mL/h × 20 h to deliver the desired nutrition support.

REFERENCES

Alappan, R., Perazella, M.A., Buller, G.K., 1996. Hyperkalemia in hospitalized patients treated with trimethoprim-sulfamethoxazole. *Ann Intern Med* 124: 316–320.

Au Yeung, S.C., Ensom, M.H., 2000. Phenytoin and enteral feedings: Does evidence support an interaction? *Ann Pharmacother* 34: 896–905.

Bauer, L.A., 1982. Interference of oral phenytoin absorption by continuous nasogastric feedings. *Neurology* 32: 570–572.

Belton, K., Thomas, S.H., 1999. Drug-induced syndrome of inappropriate antidiuretic hormone secretion. *Postgrad Med J* 75: 509–510.

Brady, J.A., Rock, C.L., Horneffer, M.R., 1995. Thiamin status, diuretic medications, and the management of congestive heart failure. *J Am Diet Assoc* 95: 541–544.

Brown, K.A., Dickerson, R.N., Morgan, L.M., Alexander, K.H, Minard, G., Brown, R.O., 2006. A new graduated dosing regimen for phosphorus replacement in patients receiving nutrition support. *J Parenter Enteral Nutr* 30: 209–214.

Cerulli, J., Malone, M., 1999. Assessment of drug-related problems in clinical nutrition patients. *J Parenter Enteral Nutr* 23: 218–221.

Chan, L.N., 2000. Redefining drug–nutrient interactions. *Nutr Clin Prac* 15: 249–252.

Chan, L.N., 2001. Drug–nutrient interactions in transplant recipients. *J Parenter Enter Nutr* 25: 132–141.

Cohn, S.M., Sawyer, M.D., Burns, G.A., Tolomeo, C., Milner, K.A., 1996. Enteric absorption of ciprofloxacin during tube feeding in the critically ill. *J Antimicrob Chemother* 38: 871–876.

Cooper, M.K., Brock, D.G., McDaniel, C.M., 2008. Interaction between levodopa and enteral nutrition. *Ann Pharmacother* 42: 439–442.

Devlin, J.W., Lau, A.K., Tanios, M.A., 2005. Propofol-associated hypertriglyceridemia and pancreatitis in the intensive care unit: An analysis of frequency and risk factors. *Pharmacotherapy* 25: 1348–1352.

Dickens, G.R., McCoy, R.A., West, R., Stapczynski, J.S., Clifton, G.D., 1994. Effect of nebulized albuterol on serum potassium and cardiac rhythm in patients with asthma or chronic obstructive pulmonary disease. *Pharmacotherapy* 14: 729–733.

Dickerson, R.N., Alexander, K.H., Minard, G., Croce, M.A., Brown, R.O., 2004. Accuracy of methods to estimate ionized and corrected serum calcium concentrations in critically ill multiple trauma patients receiving specialized nutrition support. *J Parenter Enteral Nutr* 28: 133–141.

Dickerson, R.N., Garmon, W.M., Kuhl, D.A., Minard, G., Brown, R.O., 2008. Vitamin K-independent warfarin resistance after concurrent administration of warfarin and continuous enteral nutrition. *Pharmacotherapy* 28: 308–313.

Dickerson, R.N., Maish, G.O., Minard, G., Brown, R.O., 2010. Clinical relevancy of the levothyroxine-continuous enteral nutrition interaction. *Nutr Clin Prac* 25: 646–652.

Dickerson, R.N., Melnik, G., 1988. Osmolality of oral drug solutions and suspensions. *Am J Hosp Pharm* 45: 832–834.

Dickerson, R.N., Roth-Yousey, L., 2005. Medication effects on metabolic rate: A systematic review (Part 1). *J Am Diet Assoc* 105: 835–843.

Dickerson, R.N., Sacks, G.S., Medication administration considerations with specialized nutrition support. In: DiPiro, J.T., Talbert, R.L., Yee, G.C., Matzke, G.R., Wells, B.T., Posey, L.M. (eds.), *Pharmacotherapy: A Pathophysiological Approach*, 8th edn. New York: McGraw Hill Companies, Inc. 2011, pp. 2493–2503.

Dickson, C.J., Schwartzman, M.S., Bertino, J.S., 1986. Factors affecting aminoglycoside disposition: Effects of circadian rhythm and dietary protein intake on gentamicin pharmacokinetics. *Clin Pharmacol Ther* 39: 325–328.

Driscoll, D.F., 1989. Drug-induced metabolic disorders and parenteral nutrition in the intensive care unit: A pharmaceutical and metabolic perspective. *DICP, Ann Pharmacother* 23: 363–371.

Edes, T.E., Walk B.E., Austin, J.L., 1990. Diarrhea in tube-fed patients: Feeding formula not necessarily the cause. *Am J Med* 88: 91–93.

Elliott, C., Newman, N., Madan, A., 2000. Gentamicin effects on urinary electrolyte excretion in healthy subjects. *Clin Pharmacol Ther* 67: 16–21.

Fiaccadori, E., Coffrini, E., Ronda, N. et al., 1990. Hypophosphatemia in course of chronic obstructive pulmonary disease. *Chest* 97: 857–868.

Finfer, S., Chittock, D.R., Su, S.Y. et al., 2009. Intensive versus conventional glucose control in critically ill patients. *N Engl J Med* 360: 1283–1297.

Fried, R.C., Dickerson, R.N., Guenter, P.A. et al., 1989. Barbiturate therapy reduces nitrogen excretion in acute head injury. *J Trauma* 29: 1558–1564.

Furlanetto, T.W., Faulhaber, G.A., 2011. Hypomagnesemia and proton pump inhibitors: Below the tip of the iceberg. *Arch Intern Med* 171: 1391–1392.

Gau, J.T., Yang, Y.X., Chen, R., Kao, T.C., 2012. Uses of proton pump inhibitors and hypomagnesemia. *Pharmacoepidemiol Drug Saf* 21: 553–559.

Gearhart, M.O., Sorg, T.B., 1993. Foscarnet-induced severe hypomagnesemia and other electrolyte disorders. *Ann Pharmacother* 27: 285–289.

Gilbert, S., 1996. How to minimize interaction between phenytoin and enteral feedings: Two approaches—A strategic approach. *Nutr Clin Prac* 11: 28.

Graybill, J.R., 1996. Lipid formulations for amphotericin B: Does the emperor need new clothes? *Ann Intern Med* 124: 921–923.

Greenberg, S., Reiser, I.W., Chou, S.Y., Porush, J.G., 1993. Trimethoprim-sulfamethoxazole induces reversible hyperkalemia. *Ann Intern Med* 119: 291–295.

Hoorn, E.J., van der Hoek, J., de Man, R.A., Kuipers, E.J., Bolwerk, C., Zietse, R., 2010. A case series of proton pump inhibitor-induced hypomagnesemia. *Am J Kidney Dis* 56: 112–116.

Hutchison, F.N., Perez, E.A., Gandara, M.D., Lawrence, H.J., Kaysen, G.A., 1988. Renal salt wasting in patients treated with cisplatin. *Ann Intern Med* 108: 21–25.

Jacobson, M.A., Gambertoglio, J.G., Aweeka, F.T., Causey, D.M., Portale, A.A., 1991. Foscarnet-induced hypocalcemia and effects of foscarnet on calcium metabolism. *J Clin Endocrinol Metab* 72: 1130–1135.

Kang, T.M. 2002. Propofol infusion syndrome in critically ill patients. *Ann Pharmacother* 36: 1453–1456.

Kaufman, A.M., Hellman, G., Abramson, R.G., 1983. Renal salt wasting and metabolic acidosis with trimethoprim-sulfamethoxazole therapy. *Mount Sinai J Med* 50: 238–239.

Kotake, T., Takada, M., Goto, T., Komamura, K., Kamakura, S., Morishita, H., 2006. Serum amiodarone and desethylamiodarone concentrations following nasogastric versus oral administration. *J Clin Pharm Ther* 31: 237–243.

Krajewski, K.C., Butterfoss, K., 2011. Achievement of therapeutic international normalized ratio following adjustment of tube feeds. *J Clin Pharmacol* 51: 440–443.

Kuhn, T.A., Garnet, W.R., Wells, B.K., Karnes, H.T., 1989. Recovery of warfarin from an enteral nutrient formula. *Am J Hosp Pharm* 46: 1395–1399.

Lahr, M.B., 1985. Hyponatremia during carbamazepine therapy. *Clin Pharmacol Ther* 37: 693–696.

Lowrey, T.S., Dunlap, A.W., Brown, R.O., Dickerson, R.N., Kudsk, K.A., 1996. Pharmacologic influence on nutrition support therapy: Use of propofol in a patient receiving combined enteral and parenteral nutrition support. *Nutr Clin Prac* 11: 147–149.

Lutomski, D.M., Gora, M.L., Wright, S.M., Martin, J.E., 1993. Sorbitol content of selected oral liquids. *Ann Pharmacother* 27: 269–273.

Lutomski, D.M., Palascak, J.E., Bower, R.H., 1987. Warfarin resistance associated with intravenous lipid administration. *J Parenter Enteal Nutr* 11: 316–318.

MacLaren, R., Wachsman, B.A., Swift, D.K., Kuhl, D.A., 1997. Warfarin resistance associated with intravenous lipid administration: Discussion of propofol and review of the literature. *Pharmacotherapy* 17: 1331–1337.

Marcuard, S.P., Albernaz, L., Khazanie, P.G., 1994. Omeprazole therapy causes malabsorption of cyanocobalamin (vitamin B12). *Ann Intern Med* 120: 211–215.

McLeod, G., Dick, J., Wallis, C., Patterson, A., Cox, C., Colvin, J., 1997. Propofol 2% in critically ill patients: Effects on lipids. *Crit Care Med* 25: 1976–1981.

Mitchell, J.F. Oral dosage forms that should not be crushed. http://www.ismp.org/tools/donotcrush.pdf (Accessed December 18, 2014).

Munger, M.A., 2007. New agents for managing hyponatremia in hospitalized patients. *Am J Health-Syst Pharm* 64: 253–265.

Nelson, D.C., McGrew, W.R., Hoyumpa, A.M., 1983. Hypernatremia and lactulose therapy. *JAMA* 249: 1295–1298.

Ng, S.Y., Chin, K.J., Kwek, T.K., 2011. Dyskalaemia associated with thiopentone barbiturate coma for refractory intracranial hypertension: A case series. *Intensive Care Med* 37: 1285–1289.

Nozue, T., Kobayashi, A., Uemasu, F. et al., 1992. Pathogenesis of cyclosporine-induced hypomagnesemia. *J Pediatr* 120: 638–640.

Oster, J.R., Singer, I., Fishman, L.M., 1995. Heparin-induced aldosterone suppression and hyperkalemia. *Am J Med* 98: 575–586.

Patel, G.P., Kasiar, J.B., 2002. Syndrome of inappropriate antidiuretic hormone-induced hyponatremia associated with amiodarone. *Pharmacotherapy* 22: 649–651.

Penrod, L.E., Allen, J.B., Cabacungan, L.R., 2001. Warfarin resistance and enteral feedings: 2 case reports and a supporting in vitro study. *Arch Phys Med Rehab* 82: 1270–1273.

Phillips, J.O., Olsen, K.M., Rebuck, J.A., Rangnekar, N.J., Miedema, B.W., Metzler, M.H., 2001. A randomized, pharmacokinetic and pharmacodynamic, cross-over study of duodenal or jejunal administration compared to nasogastric administration of omeprazole suspension in patients at risk for stress ulcers. *Am J Gastroenterol* 96: 367–372.

Polage, C.R., Solnick, J.V., Cohen, S.H., 2012. Nosocomial diarrhea: Evaluation and treatment of causes other than *Clostridium difficile*. *Clin Infec Dis* 55: 982–989.

Polderman, K.H., Girbes, A.R., 2002. Piperacillin-induced magnesium and potassium loss in intensive care unit patients. *Intensive Care Med* 28: 520–522.

Roth, M.S., Martin, A.B., Katz, J.A., 1997. Nutritional implications of prolonged propofol use. *Am J Health-Syst Pharm* 54: 694–695.

Santos, C.A., Boullata, J.I., 2005. An approach to evaluating drug–nutrient interactions. *Pharmacotherapy* 25: 1789–1800.

Schilsky, R.L., Anderson, T., 1979. Hypomagnesemia and renal magnesium wasting in patients receiving cisplatin. *Ann Intern Med* 90: 929–931.

Seligman, H., Halkin, H., Rauchfleisch, S. et al., 1991. Thiamine deficiency in patients with congestive heart failure receiving long-term furosemide therapy: A pilot study. *Am J Med* 91: 151–155.

Sheehan, J., White, A., 1982. Diuretic-associated hypomagnesemia. *Brit Med J* 285: 1157–1159.

Singh, N., Singh, P.N., Hershman, J.M., 2000. Effect of calcium carbonate on the absorption of levothyroxine. *JAMA* 283: 2822–2825.

Smith, O.B., Longe, R.L., Altman, R.E., Price, J.C., 1988. Recovery of phenytoin from solutions of caseinate salts and calcium chloride. *Am J Hosp Pharm* 45: 365–368.

Sonnenblick, M., Friedlander, Y., Rosin, A.J., 1993. Diuretic-induced severe hyponatremia: Review and analysis of 129 reported patients. *Chest* 103: 601–606.

Sutters, M., Gaboury, C.L., Bennett, W.M., 1996. Severe hyperphosphatemia and hypocalcemia: A dilemma in patient management. *J Am Soc Nephrol* 7: 2056–2061.

Thompson, C.A., 2008. FDA approves i.v. calcium-channel blocker. *Am J Health Syst Pharm* 65: 1686.

Van Den Berghe, G., Wouters, P., Weekers, F. et al., 2001. Intensive insulin therapy in critically ill patients. *N Engl J Med* 354: 1359–1367.

Vandewoude, K., Vogelaers, D., Decruyenaere, J. et al., 1997. Concentrations in plasma and safety of 7 days of intravenous itraconazole followed by 2 weeks of oral itraconazole solution in patients in intensive care units. *Antimicrob Agents Chemother* 41: 2714–2718.

Velazquez, H., Perazella, M.A., Wright, F.S., Ellison, D.H., 1993. Renal mechanism of trimethoprim-induced hyperkalemia. *Ann Intern Med* 119: 296–301.

Walter-Sack, I., Klotz, U., 1996. Influence of diet and nutritional status on drug metabolism. *Clin Pharmacokinet* 31: 47–64.

Whitmire, S.J., 2008. Nutrition-focused evaluation and management of dysnatremias. *Nutr Clin Prac* 23: 108–121.

Williams, N.T., 2008. Medication administration through enteral feeding tubes. *Am J Health-Syst Pharm* 65: 2347–2357.

Zaloga, G.P., Chernow, B., Pock, A., Wood, B., Zaritsky, A., Zucker, A., 1984. Hypomagnesemia is a common complication of aminoglycoside therapy. *Surg Gynecol Obstet* 158: 561–565.

Section IV

Nutrition Therapy throughout the Life Cycle

19 Nutrition Support during Pregnancy

Christina J. Valentine, Joy Lehman, and Carol L. Wagner

CONTENTS

INTRODUCTION

Nutrition support during pregnancy is complicated by the hypothalamic–pituitary–adrenal axis (HPA) changes of pregnancy [1] and the nutritional demands of the mother, placenta, and fetus. Women during the first two trimesters of pregnancy are in an anabolic state, which results in lipogenesis [2], whereas, later in pregnancy, a catabolic state predominates and subsequent insulin resistance results in a rise in lipolysis and free fatty acids [3]. The rise of progesterone, cortisol, and insulin in the first trimesters facilitates the anabolic systems [4]. In addition, the normal homeostatic mechanisms regulating appetite and food intake are modified to induce hyperphagia generated by a lack of hypothalamic response to leptin released from adipose tissue [5]. More specifically, free fatty acids can be used for beta-oxidation for acetyl CoA and glycerol used for glucose synthesis [6]. The placenta plays a key role in the release of placental lactogen, which may mediate the lack of hormonal response to leptin and therefore immediate supply of transfer of nutrients to the fetus [7,8]. In fact, glucose and amino acids are the most important substrates crossing the placenta [2]. Glucose is a major fuel for the growing fetus [9] and is transported by facilitated diffusion via glucose transporters (GLUTs) [10]. GLUT1 is the predominant rate-limiting transfer and is found in the microvillus and basal membrane of the syncytial barrier [10]. In a longitudinal examination of 6 women with normal glucose tolerance and 10 women with abnormal glucose tolerance, indirect calorimetry, endogenous glucose production examination (using [6-6$^2H_2$]-labeled glucose), and insulin sensitivity (using a hyperinsulinemic/euglycemic clamp) were performed [11]. Increased fat mass was significantly lower at 12–14 weeks of gestation in women with decreased pregravid insulin sensitivity ($r = -0.52$, $p = 0.04$). Diabetic pregnancies are associated with increased basal expression of GLUT1. Also positive expression is induced by ILGF1, placental GH, and hypoxia. Glucose and amino acid transfer adapts to maternal calorie intake, diet, and hormones [12]. Maternal plasma concentrations of amino acids fall during pregnancy, which is related to the metabolic flux via ketogenesis and gluconeogenesis in order to supply these critical nutrients to the fetus [13]. Maternal undernutrition however can impair this supply once the body stores are depleted resulting in not only intrauterine growth restriction of the fetus but also to adult risk of obesity, hypertension, and diabetes [7,14,15]. Conversely, maternal glucose intolerance results in fetal macrosomia and subsequent risks of delivery injuries and birth defects [16]. The complex nutritional process is summarized in the graphic demonstrated in Figure 19.1 and emphasizes the careful attention warranted in the dietary prescription in pregnancy. Energy expenditure and nitrogen assimilation is elevated for the growing fetal tissues; thus, macro and micronutrient needs are increased for the woman in pregnancy to meet the demands of the metabolic pathways involved.

Goal intake is based on the mother's body mass index (BMI) and additional factors to ensure adequate fetal growth velocity. Mothers that have GI illness such as hyperemesis gravidarum, biliary colic, pancreatitis, previous gastric bypass surgery, or inflammatory bowel disease are at risk for malnutrition and refeeding syndrome that can impact their health and also the growth of the fetus and thus require careful clinician evaluation and management of their nutrition support. This chapter will describe the background of current dietary recommendations for the mother while pregnant and highlight enteral and parenteral nutrition (PN) support consideration under special maternal conditions.

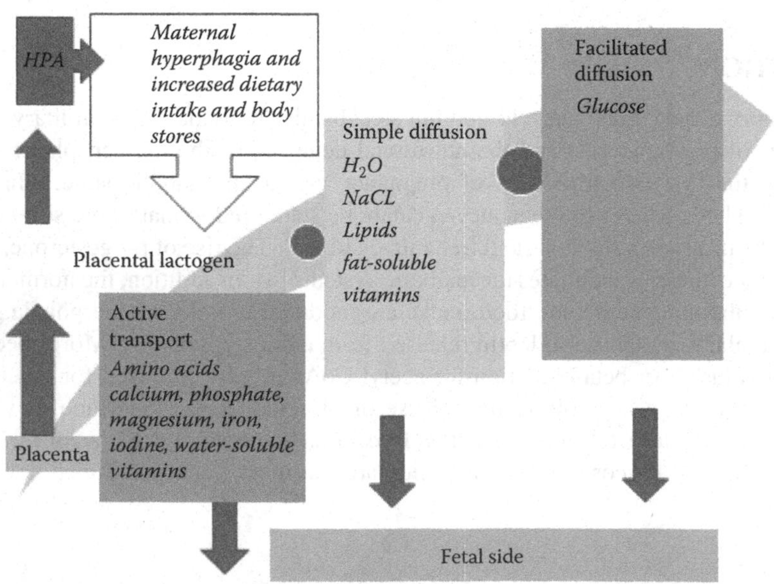

FIGURE 19.1 Nutrient delivery to the fetus.

BASIS FOR NUTRIENT RECOMMENDATIONS FOR THE PREGNANT MOTHER

A healthy weight gain is the most objective measure of adequate nutrition in the pregnant mother. The Institute of Medicine has provided weight if BMI < 18.5 (kg/m^2) then a women is suggested to gain 28–40 pounds. If BMI 18.5–24.9 then she should gain 25–35 pounds. If overweight with a BMI of 25–29.9 then a gain of 15–25 pounds is suggested. Finally, if the BMI is obese (>/=30 kg/m^2) then weight gain should total 11–20 pounds during pregnancy [17] gain guidelines based on the mother's pregravid BMI (BMI = weight in kilograms/[height in meters]^2) [17]. In addition, twin and triplet pregnancies should gain 15.9–20.5 kg [17] to avoid pregnancy complications.

RECOMMENDED DIETARY INTAKE

Nutrition support during pregnancy requires an individual prescription depending on maternal BMI and medical status. A systematic review of interventional studies based on physical activity and diet counseling combined with weight monitoring can reduce excessive weight gain and the morbidities associated [18]. Fundamentally, the incidence of intrauterine growth retardation is higher in women consuming too little nutrition [15], whereas large, macrosomic infants, cesarean sections, and preterm delivery are increased in women with a heightened velocity of weight gain [19]. Thus, education regarding nutrients in pregnancy becomes a public health priority. The following sections will provide a physiologic basis for nutrients and suggested target daily intakes to achieve the most optimal weight gain and health for the mother and fetus. A specific emphasis will be placed on human studies and the nutrients folate, DHA, and vitamin D because of the increased demands in pregnancy particularly in the last trimester. Furthermore, it is apparent that research remains lacking in many areas of pregnancy nutrition in the human model and emphasizes the importance of future dietary examinations with vital longitudinal follow-up.

MACRONUTRIENTS

CALORIES/PROTEIN

The energy needs of pregnancy are based on the assumptions of the weight gain required by a woman in adequate health and weight prepregnancy [20] to achieve a favorable outcome. Weight gain takes into account the fetus, placenta, amniotic fluid, uterus, and breasts and the increase in blood volume, extracellular fluid, and maternal fat storage [20]. Using a factorial approach to account for these changes, a cumulative increase of 12 kg is often used [21] and corresponds to a total energy cost of pregnancy based on the increment of basal metabolic rate to approximately 85 kcal/day in the first trimester, 285 kcal/day in the second trimester, and 475 kcal/day in the third trimester [22]. The 2002 Dietary Reference Intakes (DRI) for pregnancy estimates 340 kcal/day extra during the second trimester and 452 kcal/day during the third trimester [23]. It has been estimated that twin pregnancies magnify the depletion of glycogen and metabolism of fat [24] and thus require an additional 150 kcal/day more than that recommended for singletons [25]. Of interest, however, is that assessments of energy expenditure vary widely among geography and ethnic backgrounds [26–28]. Special attention should also be made for adolescent women that are pregnant to ensure their own growth and development. For more individualized prescription, the baseline estimated energy requirement (EER) should be determined by age (women >18 years of age: EER = 354 − [6.91 × age (years)] + PA × 9.36 × weight [kilograms] + 726 × height [meters]) and activity from sedentary to very active added using the physical activity coefficient (PA = 1 if sedentary, 1.12 if low active, 1.27 if active, 1.45 if very active) and then additional calories added for the median change of total energy expenditure of 8 kcal/week and an energy deposition of 180 kcal/day [23]. More recently, in a cohort of healthy Czech women (*n* = 152), a new equation was developed from the Harris–Benedict equation to predict energy expenditure (energy expenditure = 346.43943 + 13.962564 × weight [kilograms] + 2.700416 × height [centimeters] – 6.826376 × age [years]) [29] and then validated in a second group ($n = 121$) using REE indirect calorimetry [29] and corresponded closely with the measured values ($r = 0.84$, $p < 0.0001$).

Protein demands of the fetus increase as pregnancy progresses. The factorial method estimates the total protein gain in pregnancy is 925 g [30]. The protein concentration in maternal plasma therefore falls during pregnancy due to increased placental uptake, increased insulin levels, hepatic diversion of amino acids for gluconeogenesis, and transfer of amino acids to the fetus for glucose production [4]. In addition, there is a corresponding decrease in urea production, a lower rate of branched-chain amino acid transamination and an unchanged rate of weight-specific protein turnover [31]. The placenta and its structure and integrity play a major role in amino acid delivery to the fetus, and if impaired poor fetal growth is evident [32]. Paradoxically, protein supplementation to women in pregnancy at high concentrations (25% or calories) does not overcome this effect. A meta-analysis of 11 trials in protein supplementation during pregnancy indicated that a *balanced protein energy* diet significantly reduces the risk of a small for gestational age infant [33]. In fact when a mother experiences amino acid oxidation (grams of nitrogen per day) rather than synthesis, it accounted for 34% of the variation in infant birth weight [30]. The recommended dietary allowance (RDA) for protein in pregnancy based on these assumptions is 1.1 g/kg/day or 25 additional grams of protein per day to the normal diet [23] for a singleton pregnancy to total 71 g/day and an additional 50 g/day beginning in the second trimester for twins to total 96 g/day.

Lipids/Fatty Acids

Maternal hypertriglyceridemia increases during pregnancy through the enhanced activity of hepatic lipase and decreased adipose tissue lipoprotein lipase [34]. The lipoproteins VLDL cholesterol and LDL cholesterol increase, but these products cross the placenta with difficulty [2]. The free fatty acids liberalized are utilized primarily for ketogenesis by the mother, and the glycerol is used for glucose synthesis [6]. The transport of cholesterol remains to be defined, but HDL and LDL provide cholesterol for placental progesterone synthesis and are crucial for the growing fetal tissues [35]. In fact, cholesterol activates sonic hedgehog (Shh) proteins that propagate a series of events in transcription (Shh–Gli pathway) responsible for the development of organ systems including the heart [36]. In an examination of amniotic fluid of 126 healthy singleton pregnancies, total sterols characterized by mass spectrometry demonstrated that the fetus heavily relies on early maternal cholesterol [37]. During early gestation, the fetus receives free fatty acids from the mother but in fact relies primarily on de novo lipid synthesis from glucose in the latter parts of pregnancy to ensure approximately 16% fat as body weight by delivery [38]. The long-chain polyunsaturated fatty acids, DHA and arachidonic acid (ARA) are preferentially transported across the placenta in the last trimester compared to the other omega-3 and omega-6 fatty acids and contribute to the fetus approximately 50 and 400 mg/kg/day, respectively [6]. The LCPUFA are vital components of membrane phospholipids that are uniquely associated with 50% of brain deposition and vascular and prostaglandin formation [6]. The placenta itself contains lipoprotein receptors and lipase activity to capture the fatty acids from triglycerides in the maternal circulation [39]; whereas free fatty acids are facilitated by translocation involving a fatty acid–binding protein [40], DHA modulates ligands on extracellular membranes that produces the series 3 prostaglandins that are anti-inflammatory [41]. DHA and ARA can be synthesized from its precursor, omega-3 and omega-6 fatty acids—linolenic and linoleic acid—essential fatty acids, respectively, through a series of elongase and desaturase enzyme activities in the liver endoplasmic reticulum [42]; however, studies supplementing linolenic acid have not been found to result in increased DHA plasma, RBC, or whole blood concentrations [43] making dietary DHA sources important. Plasma and RBC phospholipids significantly increase as dietary DHA increases [44]. In addition, it is speculated from animal studies that if the essential fats are utilized as a caloric source or under conditions of glucocorticoid therapy, the delta 6 desaturase step may be limiting [45]. Of additional concern is that the fetal and cord blood concentrations of these important fatty acids vary according to maternal diet and body stores [46] thereby making specific dietary and supplementation recommendations important. Observational and secondary analysis of larger trials has demonstrated that the likelihood of infants born less than 34 weeks of gestation is reduced if dietary DHA is consumed through three or more fish sources per week [47]. In a large interventional, randomized controlled trial, significantly less infants were born less than 1500 g and significantly less infants less than 34 weeks of gestation when mothers received 600 mg per DHA compared to the placebo group [48], making this an important avenue to investigate for perinatal outcomes. When prescribing DHA in perinatal care, however, specific attention is to be made to the actual concentration of DHA in the product. Observational and experimental studies of DHA in adults employ variable doses and fish sources of DHA often making interpretation of the study outcomes difficult. The variability of DHA concentration in fish oil capsules is striking. In our own observations, prenatal vitamins can contain 0–200 mg of DHA, and fish oil sources contain 23 mg to 1 g depending on the product taken. We found that postnatal women in the Midwest taking variable supplements resulted in a mean intake of 23 mg/day [49] despite recommendations to ingest a minimum extra 200 mg to a 1 g/day in the diet while pregnant and lactating [50]. This is an important finding because dietary intake less than 200 mg/day results in low concentrations of both blood and breast milk DHA. We found that in a cross-sectional study, low dietary intake is prevalent across North America in postpartum women breast-feeding their infants with intakes less than 200 mg/day to produce milk concentrations of 0.1% DHA [51]. In a pilot, feasibility trial [52], we could safely and effectively increase breast milk concentrations by providing a single source of DHA at 1 g/day by an over-the-counter dietary supplement. Food sources from fatty fish such as mackerel* herring, salmon, anchovy, rainbow trout, halibut, cod, catfish, shrimp, or lobster three times per week can also suffice.

MICRONUTRIENTS

Folate and the B Vitamins

Folate is a B vitamin that is water soluble and functions in carbon metabolism for DNA synthesis [53] and is thus required at increased dietary concentrations in pregnancy [54]. Food sources predominate in green leafy vegetables, orange juice, and fortified grains. Food folate is however polyglutamated and requires cleavage for absorption, whereas folic acid the fully oxidized form found in fortification and supplements is more bioavailable [54]. Erythrocyte folate concentration is the primary indicator of adequacy [54], and concentrations greater than 906 nmol/L are associated with the lowest risk of neural tube defects (NTDs) in the fetus [54]. A meta-analysis of three randomized controlled trials of folate supplementation determined that NTD was reduced 70% in women with a prior NTD pregnancy and in one RCT 62% in primary prevention, respectively [55]. A population-based cohort study found that folate supplementation reduced cleft lip and palate [56]. In a systematic review that comprised 18 studies, it was apparent that folate deficiency was also associated with placental abruption, preeclampsia, and spontaneous abortion [57]. Women of childbearing age and during pregnancy are therefore recommended to take a minimum additional 400 mcg/day of folate via supplementation to their diet [58].

* EPA, USFDA, and AHA, however, recommend less than 12 oz/week of fish to limit potential mercury exposure.

Vitamin B6 (***pyridoxine***) is a component of pyridoxal 5′phosphate (PLP) that acts as a vital coenzyme for numerous reactions [59] involved in amino acid metabolism; heme, nucleic, hormonal, neurotransmission, carbohydrate, and lipid synthesis; transsulfuration of homocysteine to cysteine; and the release of stored glycogen to glucose. Food sources include cereals, potatoes, bananas, meat, fish, and poultry and are greater than 75% bioavailable [59]. ***B12*** (cobalamin) is essential for cell multiplication in pregnancy [59]. B12 relies on an intrinsic factor in the GI tract for absorption and during periods of malabsorption, gastric bypass, or just poor dietary intake, can develop signs of pernicious anemia [59]. Animal sources contain the highest natural source of B12 or fortification in grains and cereals. B12 concentrations fall in the maternal serum, whereas fetal concentrations rise [59]. Well-nourished women have adequate body stores to provide to the fetus, and only caution should be those with compromised GI tracts or in developing regions of the world on a poor intake of animal sources.

Antioxidants: Vitamin C/E

Vitamin C (***ascorbic acid***) is a naturally occurring antioxidant found in fruits and vegetables and is an important electron donor for enzymes involved with collagen synthesis, hormones, neurotransmitters, and carnitine biosynthesis [59]. In pregnancy, the placenta converts the oxidized form to the reduced form to provide to the fetus [59]. Maternal deficiency is noted when the serum or plasma ascorbic acid is less than 11 mmol and is more common in obesity, poor dietary intake, oral contraceptive use, and smokers [59]. A Cochrane review examining 5 trials that included 766 women did not find a positive effect on many outcomes, but in the combination of three trials, the effect was an increase in preterm delivery (RR 1.38, CI 1.04–1.82) [60].

Vitamin E, can be one of eight isomers of tocopherol or tocotrienols, is a fat-soluble vitamin (the most widely distributed form of vitamin E is alpha-tocopherol) found in plants and seed oils. Of interest is that the name tocopherol comes from the Greek origin tokos (childbirth) and phero (to bear) and was widely known historically as the antisterility vitamin that prevented fetal reabsorption in rats and testicular degeneration [61]. The main antioxidant role for vitamin E is preventing oxidant damage [62]. The placenta however appears to regulate fetal concentrations, and cord blood is lower than maternal concentration [63]; however, its metabolite, alpha-carboxyethyl-hydroxychroman, is increased suggesting maternal or fetal liver degradation of vitamin E [63]. Trials in humans investigating improved pregnancy outcomes related to preeclampsia have not been beneficial [64]. The RDA is therefore 15 mg/day of alpha-tocopherol, which is not different than that in the nonpregnant female [23].

Vitamin A

Vitamin A is a fat-soluble vitamin that functions to promote growth, produce red blood cells, and develop immunity [65]. The fetus receives vitamin A via facilitated diffusion [66]. It has been estimated that 19 million pregnant women in low-income areas are vitamin A deficient; however, examination of trials does not show supplementation to reduce preterm birth, stillbirths, miscarriage, or fetal loss [67].

The RDA for vitamin A is expressed in retinol activity equivalents (RAEs) because the amount of bioavailable vitamin A varies based on the source [23]. The conversion rates between mcg RAE and international units (IU) are as follows:

- 1 IU retinol = 0.3 mcg RAE
- 1 IU beta-carotene from dietary supplement = 0.15 mcg RAE
- 1 IU beta-carotene from food = 0.05 mcg RAE

Vitamin A recommendations are higher in pregnancy and lactation to support growth and cell differentiation [68]. The DRIs are dependent on age and range from 750 to 770 mcg/day RAEs for pregnant women 14–18 years and 19–50 years, respectively [23].

Vitamin D

Vitamin D is a precursor hormone, and unlike other nutrients that can only be obtained from diet, the vast majority of vitamin D is derived from its synthesis within the skin following ultraviolet B exposure and thermal conversion from 7-dehydrocholesterol to vitamin D_3 or cholecalciferol. About 10% of the daily requirement comes from the diet in one of two forms—vitamin D_3 (obtained mainly from fatty fish, organ meats such as liver, and eggs) and vitamin D_2 or ergocalciferol (derived from plants and fungi, e.g., mushrooms). In a recent National Institute of Child Health and Development (NICHD)-sponsored vitamin D supplementation trial during pregnancy by Hollis et al. [69], the average daily dietary vitamin D intake of women was approximately 200 IU/day compared to the 10,000–20,000 IU that are generated within 24 h of whole body sunlight exposure (without sunscreen) [70].

Vitamin D status during pregnancy varies by region throughout the world as a function of maternal sunlight exposure, degree of skin pigmentation, latitude, lifestyle, BMI, and the intake of oral vitamin D supplements [69,71–77]. What is well established is that if a woman is deficient during her pregnancy, then her fetus also will be deficient during gestation [69,78]. At the time of delivery, the newborn's total circulating 25(OH)D concentration, the indicator of vitamin D status, is approximately 0.7–0.8 that of the mother's [69,79], and maternal 25(OH)D is what crosses the placenta and becomes the substrate for fetal synthesis of $1,25(OH)_2D$, the active hormonal form of vitamin D. While evidence is mounting to support the premise of health effects of vitamin D as a function of status, whether such variation in vitamin D status can be associated with worse pregnancy outcomes still remains an open question. While vitamin D's effect on calcium homeostasis and its role in the prevention of rickets in children have been well established [80,81], advances made in the past decade using molecular techniques demonstrate the significant role that vitamin D plays in immune function, both innate and adaptive [82–84]. Yet, despite this expanded view of vitamin D, the role of vitamin D during pregnancy in immune modulation is just beginning to be understood [85,86]. As reviewed later, recent studies suggest that there is a link between maternal and fetal well-being and vitamin D status [79,86–89].

Studies conducted in the 1980s and 1990s found associations between maternal deficiency and abnormal fetal growth, dentition, and maternal health, yet the robustness of these findings was held in question as the studies were plagued by small sample sizes and the amount of vitamin D given was often low with few differences noted between women who had received placebo and those who had received treatment—typically 400 IU vitamin D/day [90–94]. Prior studies did not establish the optimal vitamin D requirements and blood levels during pregnancy. In addition, the effects of vitamin D during pregnancy were thought and continue to be thought by some to be limited to calcium and bone metabolism and that the daily requirements were met by casual outdoor sunlight exposure and a prenatal vitamin containing 400 IU [81]. In 2010, based on calcium and bone data, the Institute of Medicine listed the Estimated Average Requirement as 400 IU vitamin D/day and the RDA as 600 IU/day [81].

There is evidence, however, that a woman's vitamin D requirements are not 400 IU/day or even 600 IU/day, but rather 4000 IU/day. To begin to answer the question of what constitutes vitamin D sufficiency during pregnancy, two recent randomized clinical trials conducted by our group were presented and published [69,79]. The largest was an National Institute of Child Health and Development-sponsored randomized controlled trial of vitamin D supplementation beginning at 12–16 weeks of gestation where healthy women were randomized to one of three treatment groups—400, 2000, and 4000 IU vitamin D_3/day [69]. Of the 494 women enrolled, 350 women continued until delivery: mean 25(OH)D concentrations by group at delivery and 1 month before delivery were significantly different ($p < 0.0001$), and the percent who achieved sufficiency was significantly different by group, greatest in 4000 IU group ($p < 0.0001$). As mentioned earlier, circulating 25(OH)D had a direct influence on circulating 1,25$(OH)_2$D concentrations throughout pregnancy ($p < 0.0001$), with maximal production of 1,25$(OH)_2$D in all strata in the 4000 IU group. There were no differences between groups on any safety measure.

While it had been known for some time that the active hormone 1,25$(OH)_2$D rises twofold to threefold during pregnancy as early as 8–10 weeks of gestation, it was only recently shown that the optimal conversion of 25(OH)D to the active form the hormone—1,25$(OH)_2$D— is not attained until 25(OH)D concentration is at least 100 nmol/L (40 ng/mL) [69]. It remains unclear what the physiological significance of the more than two and a half times nonpregnant levels of 1,25$(OH)_2$D is during pregnancy with virtually no change in calcium levels. Various health effects of vitamin D deficiency during pregnancy continue to be reported, notably with increased risk of preeclampsia [87,88,95], infection [79,96–98], preterm labor and preterm birth [79,98], cesarean section [86,99], and gestational diabetes [100–102]. What do these seemingly diverse groups of disease states and events have to do with vitamin D? What is the plausible mechanism of action that links them to vitamin D? The link between these disease states and events appears to be vitamin D's effect on immune modulation of both the innate as well as adaptive immune systems [103–105].

In the second clinical trial sponsored by the Thrasher Research Fund, women were randomized at 12–16 weeks of gestation to either 2000 or 4000 IU vitamin D_3/day [79]. Vitamin D status and health characteristics were recorded for both studies. Maternal 25(OH)D in the 161 women who completed the study through delivery increased from 22.7 ng/mL (standard deviation (SD) 9.7) at baseline to 36.2 ng/mL (SD 15) and 37.9 ng/mL (SD 13.5) in the 2000 and 4000 IU groups, respectively. While maternal 25(OH)D change from baseline did not differ between groups, 25(OH)D monthly increase differed between groups ($P < 0.01$). No supplementation-related adverse events occurred. Mean cord blood 25(OH)D was 22.1 ± 10.3 ng/mL in 2000 IU and 27.0 ± 13.3 ng/mL in 4000 IU groups ($P = 0.024$). After controlling for race and study site, preterm birth, preterm labor, and infection were inversely associated with predelivery and mean 25(OH)D, but not baseline 25(OH)D. The overall conclusion of that study was that maternal supplementation with vitamin D 2000 and 4000 IU/day during pregnancy improved maternal/neonatal vitamin D status. While there was evidence of risk reduction in infection, preterm labor, and preterm birth, additional studies powered for these endpoints were recommended.

While there was sufficient power to detect health outcome differences in women during pregnancy as a function of treatment, the effect of nonadherence to vitamin D supplementation mitigated the potential effects of treatment in more than a third of the women in both the NICHD and the Thrasher Research Fund trials. As such, total circulating 25(OH)D then was more reflective of the true *group*—sufficient or insufficient—to which each mother belonged. Because both studies used a common data dictionary and the same lot number of vitamin D and placebo, datasets were combined for further analysis with results recently published [98]. When using 25(OH)D concentration as the outcome, rather than treatment group, which has the inherent bias of compliance or adherence, there was a strong association between combined comorbidities of pregnancy and final maternal 25(OH)D, an effect that persisted even after controlling for race and study. Using an a priori cut point of 20 and 32 ng/mL as the definitions of deficiency and sufficiency, respectively, there were statistically significant differences in the rates of comorbidities by both criteria for preeclampsia, infection, hypertensive disorders of pregnancy, and combined comorbidities. Maternal delivery 25(OH)D was inversely associated with any comorbidity of pregnancy, with fewer events as 25(OH)D increased.

The essence of these studies involving pregnant women and vitamin D is that deficiency is a global issue that cannot easily be fixed without increasing sunlight exposure or increasing vitamin D supplementation. A daily dose of 4000 IU vitamin D optimizes the conversion of 25(OH)D to 1,25$(OH)_2$D and safely improves the vitamin D status of women across diverse racial/ethnic groups. Additional studies will elucidate the specific effects of vitamin D on immune function during pregnancy. Until those studies are available, it is important for a woman to have her total circulating 25(OH)D concentration measured to ensure that she is vitamin D sufficient with a level of at least 40 ng/mL to achieve optimal conversion of 25(OH)D to $1,25(OH)_2D$.

Calcium

Calcium is best known as the nutrient responsible for the formation and metabolism of bone. It exists in the form of calcium hydroxyapatite ($Ca_{10}[PO_4]_6[OH]_2$) in bones and teeth, where it provides hard tissue with its strength [81]. The 1% of calcium that is dissolved in the blood as ionized calcium is essential to maintain homeostasis in the various compartments of the body—the circulatory system, extracellular fluid, muscle, and other tissues—where it is critical for mediating a multitude of functions within the body: vascular contraction and vasodilatation, muscle function, nerve transmission, intracellular signaling, and hormonal secretion, to name a few. The reservoir for calcium necessary for the various metabolic processes is bone tissue, where through the actions of parathyroid hormone (PTH) and $1,25(OH)_2D$, there is a rapid release of calcium in the form of ionized calcium from the bone into the circulation. Clearly, given the metabolism of calcium and its intimate link with vitamin D, women who are deficient in either calcium or vitamin D or both will have demineralization of their bone tissue in order to maintain calcium homeostasis. Over time, this leads to demineralization of bone, osteopenia, and eventually osteoporosis.

The neonate contains about 20–30 g calcium at birth, all accrued during fetal development and thus transferred from the mother. On average, about 200 mg Ca/day is secreted into breast milk at peak lactation and can be as much as 400 mg/day in some individuals [106,107]. The reference human fetus accretes about 30 g of calcium by term, 99% found within the skeleton [108]. During the third trimester, placental calcium transport averages 110–120 mg/kg/day [109]. With increasing fetal accretion of calcium as pregnancy progresses, maternal serum calcium falls; however, this fall in serum calcium does not appear to have significant consequences, as ionized calcium remains stable [110]. The fall is thought to be due to the concomitant fall in serum albumin caused by an expansion in plasma volume. Following pregnancy, during lactation, human breast milk generally will provide two to three times the amount of calcium to the infant during 6 months of lactation as the pregnant woman will have provided to the fetus during the preceding 9 months of pregnancy [106].

In the United States, most pregnant women receive adequate calcium intake from their diet [111]. This may not be true for the growing pregnant adolescent whose calcium requirements are significantly greater than her adult pregnant counterpart. The calcium requirements of the pregnant adolescent are ~300 mg higher than the adult woman, who is advised to take 1000 mg/day of dietary calcium [81]. Sources of calcium include dairy products such as milk, yogurt, and cheeses. According to the U.S. Department of Agriculture, dairy products provide the major share of dietary calcium, accounting for ~72% of the dietary calcium intake when including such foods to which dairy products have been added (e.g., pizza, lasagna, dairy desserts). The remaining calcium comes from vegetables (7%); grains (5%); legumes (4%); fruit (3%); meat, poultry, and fish (3%); eggs (2%); and miscellaneous foods that include those fortified with calcium, a common practice in the United States (3%) [111]. The most common forms of supplemental calcium are calcium carbonate and calcium citrate. Other forms of calcium dietary supplements include lactate, gluconate, glucoheptonate, and hydroxyapatite [81].

Human pregnancy and lactation are associated with changes in calcium and bone metabolism that support the transfer of calcium between mother and child [112,113]. The changes generally appear to be independent of maternal calcium intake in those areas of the world where maternal intake is close to dietary recommendations. Calcium intestinal absorption increases from

~50 mg/day at 20 weeks of gestation to ~330 mg/day at 35 weeks [108], which parallels the fetal requirements in the last trimester. Dieting reduces the fractional calcium absorption by 5% [114]. Those women who have undergone gastric bypass are at higher risk of calcium malabsorption and, therefore, have higher requirements for dietary calcium as well [115]. One word of caution concerning higher calcium consumption by pregnant women, however, is seen with those consuming moderate (800–1000 mg/day) [116,117] to high (1950 mg/day) [118] amounts of calcium: those women will have higher calcium excretion in their urine and may become hypercalciuric due to increased intestinal calcium absorption (i.e., absorptive hypercalciuria), and as such pregnancy itself may be a risk factor for kidney stones [81].

Iron and Zinc

Iron deficiency is associated with preterm birth, smaller babies, and subsequent infant developmental problems [119]. The fetal developing brain requires iron for myelination, monoamine neurotransmitter synthesis, and hippocampal energy metabolism in the late fetal/early neonatal period [120]. The heightened demand of iron in pregnancy and risk for deficiency is due to the expansion of maternal blood volume, the fetal needs, and postpartum blood loss [121] (see Table 19.1 for recommendations). Anemia of pregnancy is a global health problem [122]. The placenta transports iron across a concentration gradient utilizing predominately the transferrin receptor-1 (TfR) [121]. This tightly regulated iron transport is still under investigation but is speculated to be due to the demand of the fetus and yet also to avoid prooxidant damage [119].

Zinc is a vital component of many metalloenzymes and has been found in a review of 20 randomized trials to demonstrate a 14% relative reduction in preterm birth in zinc compared to placebo trials in low-income women [123]. The DRI is therefore increased in pregnancy to 12 mg/day in adolescents and 11 mg/day in older pregnant women [23].

TABLE 19.1
Dietary Reference Intake (DRI) for the Pregnant Mother*

Water-Soluble Nutrients (Per Day)	Maternal Age (14–18 Years)	Maternal Age (19–30 Years)	Maternal Age (30–50 Years)
Thiamin (B1) (mg)	1.4	1.4	1.4
Riboflavin (B2) (mg)	1.4	1.4	1.4
B6 (mg)	1.9	1.9	1.9
B12 (mcg)	2.6	2.6	2.6
Vitamin C (mg)	80	85	85
Folate (mcg)	600	600	600
Fat-Soluble Vitamins	***Age 15–18 Years***	***Age 19–30 Years***	***Age 30–50 Years***
A (mcg)	750	770	770
D (IU)	600	600	600
E (mg)	15	15	15
K (mcg)	75	90	90
Minerals			
Calcium** (mg)	1300	1000	1000
Phosphorus (mg)	1250	700	700
Iodine (mcg)	220	220	220
Zinc (mg)	12	11	11
Iron (mg)	27	27	27

Iodine

Iodine is a highly water-soluble trace element whose primary source is the sea and, thus, is found at highest concentrations in sea animals and plants. Iodine is an essential component of the thyroid hormones thyroxine and triiodothyronine, which modulate cellular metabolism—lipid, carbohydrate, and protein—as well as oxygen consumption and are important for temperature regulation. During fetal development, thyroid hormones are essential for normal development of the brain through its effect on myelination, on the heart, and on immune and reproductive systems [124].

Deficiency during pregnancy leads to a wide spectrum of disorders based on the degree and timing of deficiency during pregnancy. Complications during pregnancy include spontaneous abortion, intrauterine fetal demise, and endemic cretinism (characterized by mental deficiency, profound deafness, dwarfed stature, bone dystrophy, spastic diplegia and a low basal metabolism, and less commonly the myxedematous type of cretinism) [120,124–126]. An iodine-deficient diet in the pregnant woman has been strongly linked to mental retardation in her offspring. In their meta-analysis of 18 studies, Bleichrodt and Born estimated that maternal iodine deficiency lowered offspring IQ score by 13 points [127]. Thus, iodine deficiency is by far the most common preventable cause of mental deficits in the world.

The impact of iodine deficiency is mitigated if a mother is diagnosed preconception; clearly, the earlier the intervention, the more likely the serious sequelae will be lessened. While a 50–70 mg (µg) intake of iodine per day is sufficient to avoid hypothyroidism in women, an intake of 150 µg, the current RDA and what is the recommended concentration in a prenatal vitamin, will offset the adverse effects of dietary goitrogens, with an additional 25 µg/day recommended during pregnancy. Thus, for pregnant women, the RDA is 175 µg/day. The American Thyroid Association, however, recommends that pregnant women have an intake of at least 250 µg/day [126].

The iodine requirement during pregnancy is increased to provide for the needs of the growing fetus, who is completely dependent on maternal iodine stores, and to compensate for the increased loss of iodine in the urine resulting from an increased renal clearance of iodine during pregnancy [120,124,126]. After conception, maternal thyroid hormone production increases by about 50% due to increased utilization by the fetus (whose own thyroid does not begin to function until after ~20 weeks of gestation), increased renal clearance of iodide by about 30%–50%, and increased binding to thyroid-binding globulin (TBG) [120,124,125,128].

The main sources of iodine, as mentioned earlier, come from food from the sea, with the highest concentration in seaweed. Iodine also is added to salt labeled as *iodized*, but not to sea salt that is commonly used by gourmet cooks. According to the Office of Dietary Supplements of the NIH [129], recommended amounts of iodine can be obtained by eating a variety of foods, including the following:

- Fish (such as cod and tuna), seaweed, shrimp, and other seafood serve as the greatest sources of iodine, with the highest concentration in seaweed or kelp (varies from 16 to 2984 mcg per gram served).
- Dairy products (such as milk, yogurt, and cheese) and products made from grains (like breads and cereals), major sources of iodine in American diets.
- Certain fruits and vegetables, although the amount depends on the iodine in the soil where they grew and the fertilizer that was used.
- Iodized salt, which is readily available in the United States and many other countries. Interestingly, processed foods, however, such as canned soups, almost never contain iodized salt.

Women who live in endemic areas with low iodine and little access to seafood or sea plants are at greatest risk for iodine deficiency and, therefore, with the greatest need for supplementation. Surprisingly, as reported in the National Health and Nutrition Examination Survey (NHANES 2007–2008) report, based on urinary iodine concentration (the gold standard for assessing iodine status in the body), more than half of pregnant American women in the cohort were characterized as iodine insufficient [130]. About one in six pregnant women in this sample had moderate or severe deficiency. Such deficiency presents as hypothyroidism in the woman with elevated TSH levels and visualization of a goiter on physical examination. While repletion of iodine is essential in pregnant women, the sooner the problem is discovered, the better will be the fetal outcome; therefore, being aware of a woman's dietary pattern and her risk factors for iodine deficiency is the first step in diagnosis. The summary of dietary reference intakes (DRIs) can be seen in Table 19.1.

MATERNAL CONDITIONS THAT WARRANT SPECIAL DIETARY CONDITION CONSIDERATIONS

There has been an increase in the number of women who become pregnant after bariatric surgery. The Roux-en-Y (RNY) procedure remains one of the most common gastric bypass procedures in the United States [131]. The RNY creates a small gastric pouch, which is attached to the distal part of the small intestine, bypassing the duodenum and part of the jejunum. This procedure can result in several micronutrient deficiencies due to malabsorption [132], which include vitamin B12, folate, zinc, iron, copper, and, less commonly, calcium and vitamin D. Women who want to become pregnant following a gastric bypass or become pregnant should receive supplements totaling the minimum RDA for all of these micronutrients. Often, it is recommended that women take a prenatal vitamin in addition to a multivitamin [132]. Maternal dietary intake should be closely followed in patients who are post gastric bypass to make sure they are receiving appropriate nutrition. Fetal growth should also be measured on a regular basis as this can be an indicator of maternal deficiencies [131].

Hyperemesis gravidarum is a condition of protracted nausea and vomiting, typically diagnosed within the first 12 weeks of pregnancy. Hyperemesis gravidarum can lead to electrolyte disturbances and nutrient deficiency. The most effective treatment of hyperemesis is an enteral diet. Clinicians should maximize pharmacologic antiemetics and nonpharmacologic therapies to help achieve enteral diet [133]. Patients with electrolyte disturbance failing an oral challenge has been successfully managed with continuous iso-osmolar, jejunal feeding at low volumes (50 mL/h) [134–136].

Certain GI diseases, such as Crohn's disease, pancreatitis, and cholecystitis, may require bowel rest and PN [137–139]. The risks and benefits of PN should be carefully weighed prior to initiating PN in the pregnant patient. There is increased risk of line infection due to altered immune response in pregnancy [140]. However, a careful examination of fetal growth demonstrated reversal of growth abnormalities when a mother unable to eat orally was on a total parenteral regimen [141]. When calculating energy requirements for PN, no adjustment is needed for patients in their first trimester of pregnancy. During the second and third trimester, an additional 200–300 kcal/day and 10 g of protein per day may be required to support the pregnancy and appropriate fetal growth. Following initiation, the clinician should follow nitrogen balance and maternal and fetal weight gain to determine adjustments to the formula [142].

Nutritional Enteral Supplements

There are numerous vitamins, supplemental foods, and enteral products that should be investigated individually. Probiotics and the microbiome are in its infancy in trials in pregnancy and are beyond the scope of this chapter.

HERBS

While herbs hold a prominent place in the culinary arts and daily food consumption, herbs also are used as medicine [143]. Throughout the world and for the past several millennia, herbal preparations have been used to maintain health or to treat illness. In India, herbal medicine called Ayurvedic medicine dates back at least 6500 years, and in China, reports of herbal use date back at least 4000 years. For centuries in England and Australia, herbalists have practiced as primary health-care providers *tacitly protected under English common law* [144]. More than half of the medicines that are prescribed today have their link to plants, including herbs [144]. The time-honored use of herbs is widespread throughout the world, but in more Westernized countries, the knowledge base that accompanied herbal use was lost and the dangers of certain herbs during specific times during the life cycle unknown. During the past 30 years, there has been resurgence in herbal product use in the United States, for example, to the point where herbal products are a multibillion dollar industry. A total of 44% of all out-of-pocket costs for complementary and alternative medicine products, or about $14.8 billion, were spent on the purchase of nonvitamin, nonmineral, natural products, or herbal products [145]. Whenever possible, topical use of herbs for medicinal use is preferred instead of internal ingestion. It sometimes is confusing for a given herb or compound as some herbalists and naturopathic physicians recommend complete avoidance of certain medicinal herbs during pregnancy, while others recommend use on a limited basis [146]. There are precautions issued with certain herbs that are specific only during pregnancy because of potential deleterious effects on the fetus or the mother. For example, blue cohosh is an herb that has a long history of causing uterine contractions. Ceylon or true cinnamon at high doses can induce abortion. Herbs that are used for cooking are typically well tolerated with few side effects noted; however, certain herbs such as basil, sage, and fenugreek are listed as cautionary as they should not be ingested in large quantities. Spices added to cooking such as turmeric, cloves, coriander, ginger, and black peppercorns have been used for millennia and have positive health effects due to an abundance of phytonutrients, plant compounds that bestow health and promote healing in a variety of ways [143]. Many are powerful antioxidants and others have anti-inflammatory properties. Advice to pregnant women is that if she has been consuming a particular spice prior to pregnancy without difficulty, then it can be continued through pregnancy, taking care that if a particular ingredient imparts nausea, that it be avoided.

CONCLUSION

Pregnancy requires careful nutrition prescription by the dietitian to ensure adequate nutritional demands of the mother, placenta, and fetus are being met. Weight gain velocity goals during pregnancy should be targeted and special considerations made for maternal illness or obesity. Macro and micronutrient needs are specific and should be based on DRIs and evidence-based trials in humans. More work is needed to specifically understanding the nutrient demands in pregnancy related to fetal outcome. Vitamin supplements are imperative to include additional folate, iron, DHA, and vitamin D. Future trials will examine probiotic and herbal relationships to health outcome.

REFERENCES

1. Trainer, P.J., Corticosteroids and pregnancy. *Semin Reprod Med*, 2002. **20**(4): 375–380.
2. Herrera, E., Metabolic adaptations in pregnancy and their implications for the availability of substrates to the fetus. *Eur J Clin Nutr*, 2000. **54**(1): S47–S51.
3. Damjanovic, S.S. et al., Relationship between basal metabolic rate and cortisol secretion throughout pregnancy. *Endocrine*, 2009. **35**(2): 262–268.
4. Hadden, D.R. and C. McLaughlin, Normal and abnormal maternal metabolism during pregnancy. *Semin Fetal Neonatal Med*, 2009. **14**(2): 66–71.
5. Ladyman, S.R., R.A. Augustine, and D.R. Grattan, Hormone interactions regulating energy balance during pregnancy. *J Neuroendocrinol*, 2010. **22**(7): 805–817.
6. Herrera, E. and E. Amusquivar, Lipid metabolism in the fetus and the newborn. *Diabetes Metab Res Rev*, 2000. **16**(3): 202–210.
7. Burton, G.J. and A.L. Fowden, Review: The placenta and developmental programming: Balancing fetal nutrient demands with maternal resource allocation. *Placenta*, 2012. **33**: S23–S27.
8. Hay Jr., W.W., Placental transport of nutrients to the fetus. *Horm Res*, 1994. **42**(4–5): 215–222.

9. Novakovic, B. et al., Glucose as a fetal nutrient: Dynamic regulation of several glucose transporter genes by DNA methylation in the human placenta across gestation. *J Nutr Biochem*, 2013. **24**(1): 282–288.
10. Illsley, N.P., Placental glucose transport in diabetic pregnancy. *Clin Obstet Gynecol*, 2000. **43**(1): 116–126.
11. Catalano, P.M. et al., Longitudinal changes in body composition and energy balance in lean women with normal and abnormal glucose tolerance during pregnancy. *Am J Obstet Gynecol*, 1998. **179**(1): 156–165.
12. Vaughn, D.E. and D.B. Muchmore, Use of recombinant human hyaluronidase to accelerate rapid insulin analogue absorption: Experience with subcutaneous injection and continuous infusion. *Endocr Pract*, 2011. **17**(6): 914–921.
13. Assel, B., K. Rossi, and S. Kalhan, Glucose metabolism during fasting through human pregnancy: Comparison of tracer method with respiratory calorimetry. *Am J Physiol*, 1993. **265**(3 Pt. 1): E351–E356.
14. Barker, D.J. and C. Osmond, Infant mortality, childhood nutrition, and ischaemic heart disease in England and Wales. *Lancet*, 1986. **1**(8489): 1077–1081.
15. Belkacemi, L. et al., Early compensatory adaptations in maternal undernourished pregnancies in rats: Role of the aquaporins. *J Matern Fetal Neonatal Med*, 2011. **24**(5): 752–759.
16. Ford, C. and M.R. Genc, Optimized amniotic fluid analysis in patients suspected of intrauterine infection/inflammation. *J Perinat Med*, 2011. **40**(1): 33–37.
17. Institute of Medicine (IOM) and NRC (National Research Council). 2009. Weight gain during pregnancy: Reexamining the Guidelines. Washington DC: The National Academies Press.
18. Streuling, I., A. Beyerlein, and R. von Kries, Can gestational weight gain be modified by increasing physical activity and diet counseling? A meta-analysis of interventional trials. *Am J Clin Nutr*, 2010. **92**(4): 678–687.
19. Yee, L.M. et al., Effect of gestational weight gain on perinatal outcomes in women with type 2 diabetes mellitus using the 2009 Institute of Medicine guidelines. *Am J Obstet Gynecol*, 2011. **205**(3): 257.e1–257.e6.
20. FAO/WHO/UNU Expert Consultation, *Human Energy Requirements*, F.a.A.O.o.t.U. Nations, ed. 2001: Italy, Rome.
21. Hytten, F.E. and G. Chanberlain, *Clinical Physiology in Obstetrics*. 1980, Oxford, U.K.: Blackwell Scientific Publications.
22. Butte, N.F. and J.C. King, Energy requirements during pregnancy and lactation. *Public Health Nutr*, 2005. **8**(7A): 1010–1027.
23. Food and Nutrition Board, I.o.M.o.t.N.A., *Dietary Reference Intakes for Energy, Carbohydrate, Fiber, Fat, Fatty Acids, Cholesterol, Protein, and Amino Acids*, I.o. Medicine, ed. 2002, Washington, DC: The National Academies Press.
24. Luke, B., Nutrition and multiple gestation. *Semin Perinatol*, 2005. **29**(5): 349–354.
25. Rosello-Soberon, M.E., L. Fuentes-Chaparro, and E. Casanueva, Twin pregnancies: Eating for three? Maternal nutrition update. *Nutr Rev*, 2005. **63**(9): 295–302.
26. van Raaij, J.M. et al., Energy requirements of pregnancy in The Netherlands. *Lancet*, 1987. **2**(8565): 953–955.
27. Hronek, M. et al., Dietary intake of energy and nutrients in relation to resting energy expenditure and anthropometric parameters of Czech pregnant women. *Eur J Nutr*, 2013. **52**: 117–125.
28. Blumfield, M.L. et al., Systematic review and meta-analysis of energy and macronutrient intakes during pregnancy in developed countries. *Nutr Rev*, 2012. **70**(6): 322–336.
29. Hronek, M. et al., New equation for the prediction of resting energy expenditure during pregnancy. *Nutrition*, 2009. **25**(9): 947–953.
30. Duggleby, S.L. and A.A. Jackson, Protein, amino acid and nitrogen metabolism during pregnancy: How might the mother meet the needs of her fetus? *Curr Opin Clin Nutr Metab Care*, 2002. **5**(5): 503–509.
31. Kalhan, S.C., Protein metabolism in pregnancy. *Am J Clin Nutr*, 2000. **71**(5 Suppl.): 1249S–1255S.
32. Cleal, J.K. and R.M. Lewis, The mechanisms and regulation of placental amino acid transport to the human foetus. *J Neuroendocrinol*, 2008. **20**(4): 419–426.
33. Imdad, A., A. Jabeen, and Z.A. Bhutta, Role of calcium supplementation during pregnancy in reducing risk of developing gestational hypertensive disorders: A meta-analysis of studies from developing countries. *BMC Public Health*, 2011. **11**(3): S18.
34. Ghio, A. et al., Triglyceride metabolism in pregnancy. *Adv Clin Chem*, 2011. **55**: 133–153.
35. Knopp, R.H. et al., Lipoprotein metabolism in pregnancy, fat transport to the fetus, and the effects of diabetes. *Biol Neonate*, 1986. **50**(6): 297–317.
36. Wagner, M. and M.A. Siddiqui, Signal transduction in early heart development (I): Cardiogenic induction and heart tube formation. *Exp Biol Med (Maywood)*, 2007. **232**(7): 852–865.

37. Baardman, M.E. et al., The origin of fetal sterols in second-trimester amniotic fluid: Endogenous synthesis or maternal-fetal transport? *Am J Obstet Gynecol*, 2012. **207**(3): 202.e19–25.
38. Noble, N.A. et al., Hexose monophosphate shunt metabolism in sheep: Comparison of fetal, newborn and adult erythrocytes. *J Dev Physiol*, 1981. **3**(6): 333–341.
39. Coleman, R.A., The role of the placenta in lipid metabolism and transport. *Semin Perinatol*, 1989. **13**(3): 180–191.
40. Kuhn, D.C. and M. Crawford, Placental essential fatty acid transport and prostaglandin synthesis. *Prog Lipid Res*, 1986. **25**(1–4): 345–353.
41. Massaro, M. et al., The omega-3 fatty acid docosahexaenoate attenuates endothelial cyclooxygenase-2 induction through both NADP(H) oxidase and PKC epsilon inhibition. *Proc Natl Acad Sci USA*, 2006. **103**(41): 15184–15189.
42. Brenna, J.T. and A. Lapillonne, Background paper on fat and fatty acid requirements during pregnancy and lactation. *Ann Nutr Metab*, 2009. **55**(1–3): 97–122.
43. Herrera, J.A., M. Arevalo-Herrera, and S. Herrera, Prevention of preeclampsia by linoleic acid and calcium supplementation: A randomized controlled trial. *Obstet Gynecol*, 1998. **91**(4): 585–590.
44. Kuratko, C.N. and N. Salem Jr., Biomarkers of DHA status. *Prostaglandins Leukot Essent Fatty Acids*, 2009. **81**(2–3): 111–118.
45. Valentine, C.J., Maternal dietary DHA supplementation to improve inflammatory outcomes in the preterm infant. *Adv Nutr*, 2012. **3**(3): 370–376.
46. Innis, S.M., Essential fatty acid transfer and fetal development. *Placenta*, 2005. **26**(A): S70–S75.
47. Klebanoff, M.A. et al., Fish consumption, erythrocyte fatty acids, and preterm birth. *Obstet Gynecol*, 2011. **117**(5): 1071–1077.
48. Carlson, S.E. et al., DHA supplementation and pregnancy outcomes. *Am J Clin Nutr*, 2013. **97**(4): 808–815.
49. Valentine, C.J. et al., Docosahexaenoic acid and amino acid contents in pasteurized donor milk are low for preterm infants. *J Pediatr*, 2010. **157**(6): 906–910.
50. Koletzko, B., I. Cetin, and J.T. Brenna, Dietary fat intakes for pregnant and lactating women. *Br J Nutr*, 2007. **98**(5): 873–877.
51. Valentine, C.J., Morrow, G., Fernandez, S., Gulati, P., Bartholomew, D., Long, D., Welty, S.E., Morrow, A.L. and L.K. Rogers, Docosahexaenoic acid and amino acid contents in pasteurized donor milk are low for preterm infants. *J Pediatr*, 2010. Dec;**157**(6): 906–910.
52. Valentine, C.J. et al., Randomized controlled trial of docosahexaenoic acid supplementation in midwestern U.S. Human milk donors. *Breastfeed Med*, 2013. **8**(1): 86–91.
53. Hovdenak, N. and K. Haram, Influence of mineral and vitamin supplements on pregnancy outcome. *Eur J Obstet Gynecol Reprod Biol*, 2012. **164**(2): 127–132.
54. Lamers, Y., Folate recommendations for pregnancy, lactation, and infancy. *Ann Nutr Metab*, 2011. **59**(1): 32–37.
55. Blencowe, H. et al., Folic acid to reduce neonatal mortality from neural tube disorders. *Int J Epidemiol*, 2010. **39**(Suppl. 1): i110–i121.
56. Kelly, D., T. O'Dowd, and U. Reulbach, Use of folic acid supplements and risk of cleft lip and palate in infants: A population-based cohort study. *Br J Gen Pract*, 2012. **62**(600): e466–e472.
57. Ray, J.G. and C.A. Laskin, Folic acid and homocyst(e)ine metabolic defects and the risk of placental abruption, pre-eclampsia and spontaneous pregnancy loss: A systematic review. *Placenta*, 1999. **20**(7): 519–529.
58. Wilson, R.D. et al., Pre-conceptional vitamin/folic acid supplementation 2007: The use of folic acid in combination with a multivitamin supplement for the prevention of neural tube defects and other congenital anomalies. *J Obstet Gynaecol Can*, 2007. **29**(12): 1003–1026.
59. Dror, D.K. and L.H. Allen, Interventions with vitamins B6, B12 and C in pregnancy. *Paediatr Perinat Epidemiol*, 2012. **26**(Suppl. 1): 55–74.
60. Rumbold, A. and C.A. Crowther, Vitamin E supplementation in pregnancy. *Cochrane Database Syst Rev*, 2005(2): CD004069.
61. Evans, H.M., O.H. Emerson, and G.A. Emerson, The isolation from wheat germ oil of an alcohol, α-tocopherol, having the properties of vitamin E. *J Biol Chem*, 1936. **113**(1): 319–332.
62. Wong, R.S. and A.K. Radhakrishnan, Tocotrienol research: Past into present. *Nutr Rev*, 2012. **70**(9): 483–490.
63. Didenco, S. et al., Increased vitamin E intake is associated with higher alpha-tocopherol concentration in the maternal circulation but higher alpha-carboxyethyl hydroxychroman concentration in the fetal circulation. *Am J Clin Nutr*, 2011. **93**(2): 368–373.

64. Rumbold, A. and C.A. Crowther, Vitamin C supplementation in pregnancy. *Cochrane Database Syst Rev*, 2005 Apr 18;(2):CD004072. Review.
65. Azais-Braesco, V. and G. Pascal, Vitamin A in pregnancy: Requirements and safety limits. *Am J Clin Nutr*, 2000. **71**(5 Suppl.): 1325S–1333S.
66. Malone, J.I., Vitamin passage across the placenta. *Clin Perinatol*, 1975. **2**(2): 295–307.
67. Thorne-Lyman, A.L. and W.W. Fawzi, Vitamin A and carotenoids during pregnancy and maternal, neonatal and infant health outcomes: A systematic review and meta-analysis. *Paediatr Perinat Epidemiol*, 2012. **26**(Suppl. 1): 36–54.
68. Carlier, C. et al., A randomised controlled trial to test equivalence between retinyl palmitate and beta carotene for vitamin A deficiency. *BMJ*, 1993. **307**(6912): 1106–1110.
69. Hollis, B.W. et al., Vitamin D supplementation during pregnancy: Double-blind, randomized clinical trial of safety and effectiveness. *J Bone Miner Res*, 2011. **26**(10): 2341–2357.
70. Matsuoka, L.Y. et al., Clothing prevents ultraviolet-B radiation-dependent photosynthesis of vitamin D3. *J Clin Endocrinol Metab*, 1992. **75**(4): 1099–1103.
71. Hamilton, S.A. et al., Profound vitamin D deficiency in a diverse group of women during pregnancy living in a sun-rich environment at latitude 32 degrees N. *Int J Endocrinol*, 2010. **2010**: 917428.
72. Johnson, D.D. et al., Vitamin D deficiency and insufficiency is common during pregnancy. *Am J Perinatol*, 2011. **28**(1): 7–12.
73. Webb, A.R., L. Kline, and M.F. Holick, Influence of season and latitude on the cutaneous synthesis of vitamin D_3 synthesis in human skin. *J Clin Endocrinal Metab*, 1988. **67**: 373–378.
74. Moan, J. et al., Seasonal variation of 1,25-dihydroxyvitamin D and its association with body mass index and age. *J Steroid Biochem Mol Biol*, 2009. **113**(3–5): 217–221.
75. Dawodu, A. and C.L. Wagner, Mother–child vitamin D deficiency: An international perspective. *Arch Dis Child*, 2007. **92**(9): 737–740.
76. Dawodu, A. and C.L. Wagner, Prevention of vitamin D deficiency in mothers and infants worldwide—A paradigm shift. *Paediatr Int Child Health*, 2012. **32**(1): 3–13.
77. Dawodu, A., What's new in mother-infant vitamin D deficiency: A 21st century perspective. *Med Princ Pract*, 2012. **21**(1): 2–3.
78. Hollis, B. and C. Wagner, Assessment of dietary vitamin D requirements during pregnancy and Lactation. *Am J Clin Nutr*, 2004. **79**: 717–726.
79. Wagner, C.L. et al., A randomized trial of vitamin D supplementation in 2 community health center networks in South Carolina. *Am J Obstet Gynecol*, 2013. **208**(2): 137.e1–137.e13.
80. American Academy of Pediatrics. Committee on Nutrition. The prophylactic requirement and the toxicity of vitamin D. *Pediatrics*. 1963. 512–525.
81. Food and Nutrition Board. *Standing Committee on the Scientific Evaluation of Dietary Reference Intakes. Dietary Reference Intakes for Vitamin D and Calcium*. 2010, Washington, DC: National Academy Press.
82. Walker, V.P. et al., Cord blood vitamin D status impacts innate immune responses. *J Clin Endocrinol Metab*, 2011. **96**(6): 1835–1843.
83. Liu, P.T. et al., Toll-like receptor triggering of a vitamin D-mediated human antimicrobial response. *Science*, 2006. **311**(5768): 1770–1773.
84. Hewison, M., Vitamin D and the immune system: New perspectives on an old theme. *Endocrinol Metab Clin North Am*, 2010. **39**(2): 365–379.
85. Wagner, C.L. et al., Vitamin D and its role during pregnancy in attaining optimal health of mother and fetus. *Nutrients*, 2012. **4**(3): 208–230.
86. Hollis, B.W. and C.L. Wagner, Vitamin D and pregnancy: Skeletal effects, nonskeletal effects, and birth outcomes. *Calcif Tissue Int*, 2013. **92**(2): 128–139.
87. Bodnar, L.M. et al., Maternal vitamin D deficiency increases the risk of preeclampsia. *J Clin Endocrinol Metab*, 2007. **92**(9): 3517–3522.
88. Robinson, C.J. et al., Plasma 25-hydroxyvitamin D levels in early-onset severe preeclampsia. *Am J Obstet Gynecol*, 2010. **203**(4): 366 e1–e6.
89. Robinson, C.J. et al., Maternal vitamin D and fetal growth in early-onset severe preeclampsia. *Am J Obstet Gynecol*, 2011. **204**(6): 556.e1–556.e4.
90. Marya, R. et al., Effects of vitamin D supplementation in pregnancy. *Gynecol Obstet Invest*, 1981. **12**: 155–161.
91. Brooke, O.G. et al., Vitamin D supplements in pregnant Asian women: Effects on calcium status and fetal growth. *Br Med J*, 1980. **1**: 751–754.
92. Brooke, O.G., F. Butters, and C. Wood, Intrauterine vitamin D nutrition and postnatal growth in Asian infants. *Brit Med J*, 1981. **283**: 1024.

93. Brooke, O. et al., Observations on the vitamin D state of pregnant Asian women in London. *Br J Obstet Gynaecol*, 1981. **88**: 18–26.
94. Maxwell, J. et al., Vitamin D supplements enhance weight gain and nutritional status in pregnant Asians. *Br J Obstet Gynaecol*, 1981. **88**: 987–991.
95. Robinson, C.J. et al., Association of maternal vitamin D and placenta growth factor with the diagnosis of early onset severe preeclampsia. *Am J Perinatol*, 2013. **30**(3): 167–172.
96. Bodnar, L.M., M.A. Krohn, and H.N. Simhan, Maternal vitamin D deficiency is associated with bacterial vaginosis in the first trimester of pregnancy. *J Nutr*, 2009. **139**(6): 1157–1161.
97. Hensel, K.J. et al., Pregnancy-specific association of vitamin D deficiency and bacterial vaginosis. *Am J Obstet Gynecol*, 2011. **204**(1): 41.e1–41.e9.
98. Wagner, C. et al., Health characteristics and outcomes of two randomized vitamin D supplementation trials during pregnancy: A combined analysis. *J Steroid Biochem Mol Biol*, 2013 Jul;136:313–320.
99. Merewood, A. et al., Association between vitamin D deficiency and primary cesarean section. *J Clin Endocrinol Metab*, 2009. **94**(3): 940–945.
100. Lau, S.L. et al., Serum 25-hydroxyvitamin D and glycated haemoglobin levels in women with gestational diabetes mellitus. *Med J Aus*, 2011. **194**(7): 334–337.
101. Parlea, L. et al., Association between serum 25-hydroxyvitamin D in early pregnancy and risk of gestational diabetes mellitus. *Diabet Med*, 2012. **29**(7): e.25–e.32.
102. Burris, H.H. et al., Vitamin D deficiency in pregnancy and gestational diabetes mellitus. *Am J Obstet Gynecol*, 2012. **207**(3): 182.e1–182.e8.
103. Liu, N.Q. and M. Hewison, Vitamin D, the placenta and pregnancy. *Arch Biochem Biophy*, 2012. **523**(1): 37–47.
104. Bikle, D.D., Vitamin D regulation of immune function. *Vitam Horm*, 2011. **86**: 1–21.
105. Lagishetty, V., N.Q. Liu, and M. Hewison, Vitamin D metabolism and innate immunity. *Mol Cell Endocrinol*, 2011. **347**(1–2): 97–105.
106. Fairweather-Tait, S. et al., Effect of calcium supplements and stage of lactation on the calcium absorption efficiency of lactating women accustomed to low calcium intakes. *Am J Clin Nutr*, 1995. **62**: 1188–1192.
107. Prentice, A., Calcium in pregnancy and lactation. *Annu Rev Nutr*, 2000. **20**: 249–272.
108. Forbes, G.B., Letter: Calcium accumulation by the human fetus. *Pediatrics*, 1976. **57**(6): 976–977.
109. Kovacs, C.S., The role of vitamin D in pregnancy and lactation: Insights from animal models and clinical studies. *Annu Rev Nutr*, 2012. **32**(1): 97–123.
110. Pedersen, E.B. et al., Calcium, parathyroid hormone and calcitonin in normal pregnancy and preeclampsia. *Gynecol Obstet Invest*, 1984. **18**(3): 156–164.
111. U.S. Department of Agriculture/*Economic Research Service Nutrient Availability Data*. 2009.
112. Olausson, H. et al., Changes in bone mineral status and bone size during pregnancy and the influences of body weight and calcium intake. *Am J Clin Nutr*, 2008. **88**(4): 1032–1039.
113. Olausson, H. et al., Calcium economy in human pregnancy and lactation. *Nutr Res Rev*, 2012. **25**(1): 40–67.
114. Cifuentes, M. et al., Energy restriction reduces fractional calcium absorption in mature obese and lean rats. *J Nutr*, 2002. **132**(9): 2660–2666.
115. Riedt, C.S. et al., True fractional calcium absorption is decreased after Roux-en-Y gastric bypass surgery. *Obesity* (*Silver Spring*), 2006. **14**(11): 1940–1948.
116. Gertner, J.M. and M. Domenech, 25-hydroxyvitamin D levels in patients treated with high-dosage ergo- and cholecalciferol. *Clin Path*, 1977. **30**: 144–150.
117. Kent, G.N. et al., Acute effects of an oral calcium load in pregnancy and lactation: Findings on renal calcium conservation and biochemical indices of bone turnover. *Miner Electrolyte Metab*, 1991. **17**(1): 1–7.
118. Cross, N. et al., Calcium homeostasis and bone metabolism during pregnancy, lactation, and postweaning: A longitudinal study. *Am J Clin Nutr*, 1995. **61**: 514–523.
119. Gambling, L., C. Lang, and H.J. McArdle, Fetal regulation of iron transport during pregnancy. *Am J Clin Nutr*, 2011. **94**(6 Suppl.): 1903S–1907S.
120. Georgieff, M.K., Nutrition and the developing brain: Nutrient priorities and measurement. *Am J Clin Nutr*, 2007. **85**(2): 614S–620S.
121. Cetin, I. et al., Placental iron transport and maternal absorption. *Ann Nutr Metab*, 2011. **59**(1): 55–58.
122. Lee, A.I. and M.M. Okam, Anemia in pregnancy. *Hematol Oncol Clin North Am*, 2011. **25**(2): 241–259, vii.
123. Mori, R. et al., Zinc supplementation for improving pregnancy and infant outcome. *Cochrane Database Syst Rev*, 2012. **7**: CD000230.

124. Obican, S.G. et al., Teratology public affairs committee position paper: Iodine deficiency in pregnancy. *Birth Defects Res A Clin Mol Teratol*, 2012. **94**(9): 677–682.
125. Glinoer, D., The importance of iodine nutrition during pregnancy. *Public Health Nutr*, 2007. **10**(12A): 1542–1546.
126. Public Health Committee of the American Thyroid Association et al., Iodine supplementation for pregnancy and lactation—United States and Canada: Recommendations of the American Thyroid Association. *Thyroid*, 2006. **16**(10): 949–951.
127. Bleichrodt, N. and M. Born, eds. A metaanalysis of research on iodine and its relationship to cognitive development. In: *The Damaged Brain of Iodine Deficiency*, J. Stanbury, ed. 1994, Cognizant Communication Publication: New York. pp. 195–200.
128. Glinoer, D., Clinical and biological consequences of iodine deficiency during pregnancy. *Endocr Dev*, 2007. **10**: 62–85.
129. National Institutes of Health, Supplements, O.o.D., *Iodine. Quick Facts*. 2011, http://ods.od.nih.gov/factsheets/Iodine-HealthProfessional/.
130. Caldwell, K.L. et al., Iodine status of the U.S. population, National Health and Nutrition Examination Survey, 2005–2006 and 2007–2008. *Thyroid*, 2011. **21**(4): 419–427.
131. Dao, T. et al., Pregnancy outcomes after gastric-bypass surgery. *Am J Surg*, 2006. **192**(6): 762–766.
132. Kominiarek, M.A., ACOG practice bulletin No. 105: Bariatric surgery and pregnancy. *Obstet Gynecol*, 2009. **113**(6): 1405–1413. doi: 10.1097/AOG.0b013e3181ac0544.
133. Hastoy, A. et al., Hyperemesis gravidarum and pregnancy outcomes. *J Gynecol Obstet Biol Reprod* (*Paris*), 2014 Jan 16. pii: S0368-2315(13)00367-0. doi: 10.1016/j.jgyn.2013.12.003. [Epub ahead of print]
134. Pearce, C.B. et al., Enteral nutrition by nasojejunal tube in hyperemesis gravidarum. *Clin Nutr*, 2001. **20**(5): 461–464.
135. Saha, S. et al., Feeding jejunostomy for the treatment of severe hyperemesis gravidarum: A case series. *JPEN J Parenter Enteral Nutr*, 2009. **33**(5): 529–534.
136. Christodoulou, D.K. et al., Peripheral parenteral nutrition in protracted hyperemesis gravidarum—Report of two cases and a literature review. *Acta Gastroenterol Belg*, 2008. **71**(2): 259–262.
137. Jacobson, S. and L.O. Plantin, Concentration of selenium in plasma and erythrocytes during total parenteral nutrition in Crohn's disease. *Gut*, 1985. **26**(1): 50–54.
138. Weinberg, R.B. et al., Treatment of hyperlipidemic pancreatitis in pregnancy with total parenteral nutrition. *Gastroenterology*, 1982. **83**(6): 1300–1305.
139. Lockwood, C., R.J. Stiller, and R.J. Bolognese, Maternal total parenteral nutrition in chronic cholecystitis. A case report. *J Reprod Med*, 1987. **32**(10): 785–788.
140. Peled, Y. et al., The impact of total parenteral nutrition support on pregnancy outcome in women with hyperemesis gravidarum. *J Matern Fetal Neonatal Med*, 2014. **27**(11): 1146–1150.
141. Herbert, W.N. et al., Fetal growth response to total parenteral nutrition in pregnancy. A case report. *J Reprod Med*, 1986. **31**(4): 263–266.
142. Cimbalik, C. and J.D. Paauw, *The AS.P.E.N. Adult Nutrition Support Core Curriculum*, 2nd edn., C.M. Mueller et al., eds. 2012, Silver Spring, MD: A.S.P.E.N.
143. Aggarwal, B. and D. Yost, *Healing Spices*. 2011, New York: Sterling Publishing.
144. Foster, S. and R. Johnson, *National Geographic Desk Reference to Nature's Medicine*. 2006, Washington, DC: National Geographic Society.
145. Nahin, R. et al., Costs of complementary and alternative medicine (CAM) and frequency of visits to CAM practitioners: United States, 2007. In: *National Center for Health Statistics*. 2009: Hyattsville, MD.
146. Harrar, S. and S. O'Donnell, *The Woman's Book of Healing Herbs*. 1999, Emmaus, PA: Prevention Health Books for Women. Rodale Press, Inc.

20 Nutrition Support for the Critically Ill Neonate

Jatinder Bhatia and Cynthia Mundy

CONTENTS

INTRODUCTION

Preterm (PT) birth rates have slightly declined since 2009 and are currently at 11.55% in the United States [1]. Over the past several decades, advances in neonatal care have increased the survival of premature infants at lower gestational ages. This creates challenges for the clinician not only in terms of technological support but also in terms of nutritional support. In addition to the focus on somatic growth, the importance of aggressive nutritional support has recently been shown to have a significant and possibly independent effect, on improved neurodevelopmental outcomes in PT infants [2]. PT infants in this study who grew at the upper quartiles demonstrated lower incidences of cerebral palsy, neurodevelopmental impairment, and abnormal neurologic exams at long-term follow-up [2].

The traditional goal in nutrition for the term (T) infant is to assist in the transition from *in utero nutrition* to *ex utero nutrition*. Growth and biochemical responses in a healthy T breast-fed infant remains the gold standard. However, in the premature infant, the optimal nutritional requirements are not completely defined. Present recommendations are designed to approximate the rate of growth and composition of gain of a fetus of the same postmenstrual age [3]. The premature infant,

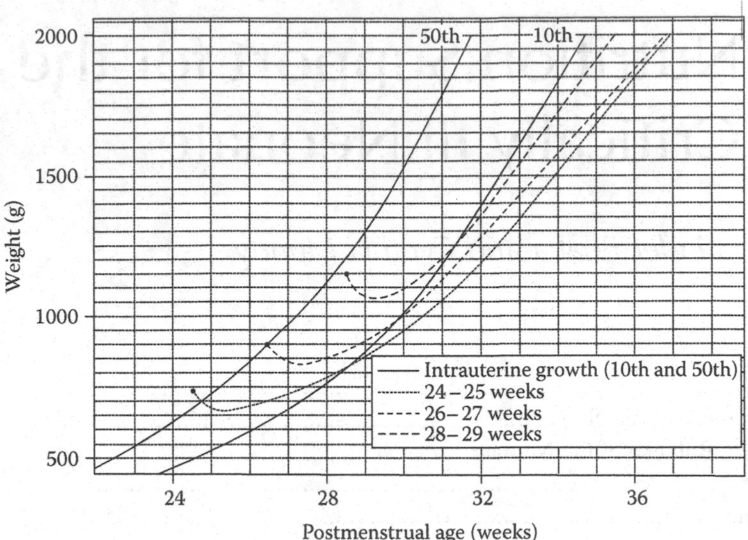

FIGURE 20.1 Postnatal growth in PT infants in relation to intrauterine growth curves. (From Ehrenkranz, R.A. et al., *Pediatrics*, 104(2 Pt. 1), 280, August 1999.)

depending on the extent of prematurity, will dictate different approaches to initiate, advance, and maintain appropriate nutrient delivery and growth. One needs to provide the appropriate mixture of nutrients to assist in reaching maturity, that is, T postconceptional age and beyond, but at the same time maintain appropriate growth. Determining the ideal growth pattern for the PT infants remains problematic. The *reference fetus* term created by Ziegler et al. [4] serves as a classic model for estimating nutrient requirements for extrauterine growth. Existing growth curves generated from measurements of infants born prematurely can help us to at least approximate their weight gain, linear growth, and head growth [5,6]. Based on these curves, a PT infant should gain 15–20 g/kg of body weight a day, 0.75–1.0 cm length/week, and 0.75–1.0 cm head circumference/week. Extrauterine growth has been described for a large cohort of premature infants from 24 to 29 weeks and compared to intrauterine growth curves using the data of Alexander et al. [7,8] (Figure 20.1). This may be a better representation of current neonatal growth data, since the previously published classical curves were mainly representing certain regions only [6].

ENERGY REQUIREMENT OF THE NEONATE

Energy provided by nutrition is distributed according to the classical energy balance equation:

$$E_{intake} = E_{expended} + E_{stored} + E_{excreted}$$

Energy expenditure includes the energy used for resting (or basal) metabolism, activity, thermoregulation, and energy utilized for new tissue synthesis. The basal metabolic rate (BMR) is the minimal energy needed to maintain life in the resting state. This is the largest portion of the total energy expenditure. Ideally, it should be measured in a thermoneutral environment and in a fasting state for 12–18 h. The latter would not be feasible to perform in PT infants; current estimates are based on measurements during sleep for 2–3 h. The estimated BMR for PT infants is 50 kcal/kg/day [9]. This BMR is somewhat lower initially when compared to T infants, but it gradually rises in both T and PT babies, and eventually PT infants demonstrate a higher BMR [10]. The energy expenditure during muscle activity is more important in the larger PT and T infant, since the smaller

TABLE 20.1
Estimated Caloric Requirement of the PT Infant

Energy Expenditure	kcal/kg/day
Resting metabolic rate	50
Activity	15
Thermoregulation	10
Synthesis	8
Energy stored	25
Energy excreted	12
Total	120

Source: American Academy of Pediatrics, Committee on Nutrition, *Nutritional Needs of the Preterm Infant: Pediatric Nutrition Handbook*, 5th edn., American Academy of Pediatrics, Elk Grove Village, IL, 2003, pp. 23–54.

and sick PT infant is usually less active. Cold stress and energy used for thermoregulation are major factors in PT infants; they show an increased energy need for thermoregulation compared to T infants because of a higher rate of heat loss from their relatively larger body surface area [11]. The advent of better technology to maintain thermoneutral environment with humidified incubators has minimized heat loss. The energy utilized during tissue synthesis is different from the stored energy, since this is not being retained in the tissue, but rather *burnt up* during growth. To achieve the 15 g/kg/day weight gain, about 20–30 kcal/kg energy will be stored in the tissue [12]. Energy excretion is mainly stool losses (and some minimal loss in urine), due to the fat and carbohydrate content that passes unabsorbed. As absorption improves, one can expect 85%–95% retention rate by 2–3 weeks of life, even in the low-birth-weight (LBW) infants [13] (Table 20.1).

Most infants show steady weight gain when provided this energy intake enterally. In certain condition such as chronic lung disease, for example, the energy intake needs to be increased to compensate for energy needed for the ongoing tissue remodeling and work of breathing [14]. Similarly, small for gestational age and very small premature infants may require higher energy intakes to maintain appropriate growth.

T infants show appropriate growth with an energy intake around 90–110 kcal/kg/day, with formula-fed babies requiring a slightly higher intake [15,16].

FLUID/ELECTROLYTE BALANCE OF THE NEONATE

After birth, there is a contraction of the extracellular fluid compartment that is followed by natriuresis, diuresis, and weight loss [17]. The typical weight loss is in the range of 7%–10% of body weight within the first 10–14 days of life. Most infants are oliguric initially, since it is not until the first 24–48 h of life before these fluid shifts occur. The initial renal sodium loss appears to be obligatory [18]; therefore, initial fluids should not contain any sodium, since this would put an extra burden on the kidneys. Restricting sodium intake in the first few days of life actually shows some other benefits, such as decreased oxygen requirement and lower incidence of bronchopulmonary dysplasia (BPD), without compromising growth [19,20].

After this initial fluid shift, infants will require sodium to maintain growth. The PT kidney shows a higher fractional excretion of sodium (FeNa) because of the immaturity of the tubular system. The FeNa appears to be correlated with the prematurity, where lower gestational age translates to higher FeNa. These infants are at risk for late hyponatremia [21] and may require higher sodium intake to maintain adequate growth. Extremely premature infants may need 4–8 mEq/kg/day of sodium intake during their growing phase [22], while older infants grow appropriately with 2–3 mEq/kg/day of sodium.

Potassium is the main intracellular cation. Its daily requirement is 2–3 mEq/kg/day, and does not show much variation between T and PT infants. PT infants are susceptible to hyperkalemia during the first few days of life even in the absence of overt renal failure [23].

Insensible water loss (IWL) takes up a major part in the fluid requirements for PT infants. LBW infants have a disproportionately larger loss because of their relatively larger body surface and the immaturity of their skin to prevent evaporation [24]. While most T infants can be started on 60–80 mL/kg/day of fluid maintenance, some of the extremely premature infants may require 100–120 mL/kg/day to prevent hypernatremia. The use of humidified incubators has significantly decreased the fluid requirements that were recommended prior to their use (over 200 mL/kg/day) in PT infants. Recent research has shown decreased fluid intake, improved electrolyte balance, and increased growth velocity when using humidification [25]. Factors that affect IWL are listed in Table 20.2.

For the infant less than 1000 g, a suggested fluid and nutrition regimen adapted from Parish and Bhatia [26] is provided in Tables 20.3 and 20.4.

TABLE 20.2
IWL

Factors that increase IWL
- Prematurity
- Radiant warmer heat
- Phototherapy
- Skin defects—omphalocele, gastroschisis
- Tachypnea
- Nonhumidified oxygen/environment

Factors that decrease IWL
- Mature skin
- Heat shields
- Topical skin agents—paraffin, Aquaphor
- Covering skin defects
- Humidified oxygen/environment

Source: Parish, A. and Bhatia, J., Nutritional considerations in the intensive care unit: Neonatal issues, in: *Nutritional Considerations in the Intensive Care Unit: Science, Rationale and Practice*, Shikora, S.A., Martindale, R.G., and Schwaitzberg, S.D. (eds.), ASPEN, Kendall/Hunt Publishing Company, Dubuque, IA, 2002, pp. 297–310.

TABLE 20.3
Maintenance Fluid Requirement by Birth Weight for the First Month of Life

		Water Requirement		
Birth Weight (g)	Insensible Losses (mL/kg/day)	Day 1–2 (mL/kg/day)	Day 3–7 (mL/kg/day)	Day 8–30 (mL/kg/day)
<750	100–200	100–200	150–200	120–180
75–1000	60–70	80–150	100–150	120–180
1001–1500	30–65	60–100	100–150	120–180
>1500	15–30	60–80	100–150	120–180

Source: Adapted from Fanaroff, A.A. (eds.), *Neonatal-Perinatal Medicine: Diseases of the Fetus and Infant*, 9th edn., Mosby, 2010.

TABLE 20.4
Suggested Nutrition Regimen for Infants <1000 g

	600–800 g	801–1000 g
Radiant warmer		
IVF, mL/kg/day	100–120	80–100
Dextrose%	5[a]	10[a]
AA, g/kg/day	1.0[b]	1.0[b]
Lipids,[c] g/kg/day	0.5	0.5
Incubator		
IVF, mL/kg/day	80–100	80
Dextrose%	7.5–10[a]	10[a]
AA, g/kg/day	1.5[b]	1.5[b]
Lipids,[c] g/kg/day	0.5	0.5

AA, amino acid—pediatric formulation.

[a] Infants less than 1000 g may be intolerant to higher concentrations of glucose and may need adjustment based on serum glucose. Advancing glucose delivery is also dictated by tolerance.

[b] Beginning on DOL1, increase by 0.5 g/kg/day to max of 2.5–3.0 g/kg/day.

[c] Starting on DOL 2, 0.5 g/kg/day, increase in 0.5 g/kg/day increments to a max of 2–3 g/kg/day; monitor triglycerides at every increase and max.

MACRONUTRIENTS

CARBOHYDRATE

For intensive care patients, the initial source of carbohydrate is glucose, since they are on intravenous fluids at least at the beginning of their course. The normal glucose requirement is about 6–8 mg/kg/min to maintain euglycemia. It should be increased in increments to maintain normal serum concentrations. The typical dextrose concentration used is D10W, with D5W being used in extremely LBW infants; the use of the latter is due to glucose intolerance exhibited by very small premature infants. Moreover, if higher fluid intakes are required, adjustments in glucose concentration to maintain appropriate glucose delivery should be made. It is not unusual for the extreme premature infant to only require 2–3 mg/kg/min of glucose to maintain serum glucose in the appropriate range. However, using <4 mg/kg/min may decrease glucose delivery to the brain and should be used with extreme caution. Hypoglycemia (blood glucose <40 mg/dL) and hyperglycemia (blood glucose >175 mg/dL) are not an infrequent finding in sick newborns. The use of insulin to treat extreme hyperglycemia (>250 mg/dL) while maintaining appropriate glucose delivery may be required.

The major source of carbohydrate in breast milk and in most T formulas is lactose. Lactase activity is deficient in PT infants compared to T babies. On the other hand, glycosidase enzymes are fully functional even in the very premature infants [27,28]. Therefore, commercial formulas prepared for PT infants contain 50%–60% of their carbohydrate in other forms, such as glucose polymers, which is easily digested by the premature gut.

PROTEIN

Mature human breast milk contains 0.9–1.0 g/dL of protein. The protein content of the colostrum (<5 days) is much higher (2.6 g/dL) and decreases to 1.6 g/dL in transitional milk (6–10 days). The whey-to-casein ratio is approximately 70:30, which helps digestion and absorption. Therefore, a typical T infant taking about 180 mL/kg of breast milk daily would receive around 2.2 g/kg/day of protein. Breast milk contains lactalbumin as the main nitrogen source. Commercially available preparations contain slightly more protein (1.4–1.6 g/dL), and the whey-to-casein ratio is 60:40. The predominant whey protein in cow milk is alpha-lactoglobulin. Compared to human milk-fed infants, infants fed whey-predominant formulas have higher serum concentrations of threonine, phenylalanine, valine, and methionine. There are differences in composition of human milk based on delivery of a T or PT infant (Table 20.5).

The optimal daily protein requirement for the PT infant is somewhat more problematic and probably best determined in relation to intrauterine growth rate and protein accretion rate. Another important factor in assessing dietary requirement for the PT infants is the protein/energy ratio. If energy intake is limited, the protein will go to the oxidative route to provide energy; on the other hand, providing too much protein might place a burden on the nitrogen-clearing capacity of the liver and kidneys without providing any benefit in terms of retention of more muscle body mass. Kashyap et al. [29] followed the growth of LBW infants divided into three groups. Group 1 and 2 received similar energy intakes (119 and 120 kcal/kg/day, respectively), while receiving different amounts of protein (2.8 and 3.8 g/kg, respectively). The third group was placed on high-calorie formula and received 142 kcal/kg and the higher amount of protein intake (3.8 g/kg). The growth rate and protein retention rate in group 1 were slightly higher than the intrauterine accretion rate, suggesting that this amount of intake is sufficient to maintain in utero growth rate. On the other hand, both groups 2 and 3 showed better growth compared to the lower protein group, showing the efficacy of higher protein intake to promote better growth. However, blood urea nitrogen and amino acid concentrations were also higher in both groups, reflecting lower protein utilization with the higher intake. Moreover, the higher energy intake in group 3 did not increase the weight gain significantly in comparison to group 2. Schulze et al. [30] monitored the growth of three groups of LBW infants with only a slightly different regimen. Group A had 2.24 g/kg/day protein with 113 kcal/kg/day, group B 3.6 g/kg/day and 115 kcal/kg/day, and group C 3.5 g/kg/day and 149 kcal/kg/day. While group A was still able to maintain in utero growth rate, both groups B and C showed better weight gain. While group C had significantly better weight gain compared to group B, the nitrogen retention rate was similar. This shows that the extra energy provided to this group was not associated with greater protein synthesis, but with storage of nonprotein energy such as lipids or glycogen.

TABLE 20.5
Nutritional Components of PT and T Breast Milk

	Days Postpartum									
	3		7		14		21		28	
Nutrient	PT	T	PT	T	PT	T	PT	T	PT	T
Energy (kcal/dL)	51.4	48.7	67.4	60.6	72.3	64.2	65.6	68.6	70.1	69.7
Protein (g/dL)[b]	3.24	2.29	2.44	1.87	2.17	1.57	1.82	1.52	1.81	1.42
Fat (g/dL)	1.63	1.71	3.81	3.06	4.40	3.48	3.68	3.89	4.00	4.01
Lactose (g/dL)[b]	5.96	6.16	6.05	6.52	6.21	6.78	6.49	7.12	6.95	7.26
Sodium (mEq/L)[b]	26.6	22.3	21.8	16.9	19.7	11.0	13.4	10.8	12.6	8.5
Potassium (mEq/L)	17.4	18.5	17.6	16.5	16.2	15.4	16.3	15.8	15.5	15.0
Chloride (mEq/L)[b]	31.6	26.9	25.3	21.3	22.8	14.5	17.0	15.2	16.8	13.1
Calcium (mg/dL)	208	214	247	254	219	258	204	266	216	249
Phosphorous (mg/dL)	95	110	142	151	144	168	149	153	143	158
Magnesium (mg/dL)	28	25	31	29	30	26	24	29	25	25

Source: Adapted from Gross, S.J. et al., *Pediatrics*, 68(4), 490, October 1981.

[a] Numbers are expressed as mean.

[b] Denotes significant difference ($P < 0.05$).

In summary, to provide the balance between adequate growth and optimal protein/energy ratio, the current recommendation for PT infants is in the range of 3.0–3.5 g/kg/day or 2.3–2.9 g/100 kcal of protein [10,13]. In short-term studies, Bhatia et al. [31] demonstrated similar growth but improved cognitive function in infants fed 3.2 g protein/100 kcal compared to 2.7 or 2.2 g/100 kcal. Infants on total parenteral nutrition (TPN) would need at least 2.5 g/kg/day of protein and 70 kcal/kg/day of nonprotein energy to maintain positive nitrogen balance. To achieve intrauterine growth rate (15 g/kg/of weight gain a day), they need 3.0 g/kg of protein and 80 kcal/kg nonprotein energy intakes daily [32].

Lipid

Lipids are the major energy source in both enteral and parenteral nutrition. Human milk lipid system provides approximately 50% of the energy, whereas fats in cow milk-based formulas make up 40%–50% of the energy content. Various fat blends are used to provide the essential, short-, medium-, and long-chain fatty acids (FAs), and more recently, docosahexaenoic (DHA) and arachidonic acids (AA) have been added to most formulas in the United States. The American Academy of Pediatrics (AAP) Committee on Nutrition recommends that at least 3% of total calories should be in the form of linoleic acid and linolenic acid to meet the essential FA requirement of the newborn.

Long-chain polyunsaturated fatty acids (LCPUFAs) have attracted considerable interest in recent years. The most important are AA and DHA. They are important components of membrane phospholipids and several biologically important mediators. Human milk contains both of them, but commercial formulas were supplemented only in the last decade. The current recommendations state that T infant formulas should include at least 0.2% of total FAs as DHA and 0.35% as AA. PT formulas should contain at least 0.35% DHA and 0.4% AA [33]. Several studies have demonstrated that T infants receiving LCPUFA-supplemented formula have more mature retinal function/cortical processing as measured by visual evoked potential [34,35], electroretinography [30], and visual acuity by behavioral methods [36]. A meta-analysis of 12 published trials supports the benefit of LCPUFAs on visual acuity [37]. Improved cognitive function with LCFUFA supplementation has been reported by some [38–40], but not others [41–44]. The differences in the results may be due to many factors including variations in FA supplementation and levels, testing age and procedures, and experimental design. None of the studies, however, have demonstrated adverse effects. PT infants delivered in the third trimester of pregnancy do not have the advantage of the placental transfer of these LCPUFAs and should benefit more from LCPUFA supplementation. O'Connor et al. [45] followed PT infants fed with supplemented formula and demonstrated improved visual acuity and better scores on the Fagan test of novelty preference at 6 months of age. Vocabulary comprehension was also greater at 14 months in supplemented infants after infants of Spanish-speaking families, and twins were excluded from the analyses. There were no demonstrable growth benefits or disadvantages. In contrast, Innis et al. [46] demonstrated significantly faster weight gain with supplemented PT formula feeding and weight: length ratios similar to those of T breast-fed infants at 48 and 57 weeks post-menstrual age (PMA). In a similar study, PT infants who were fed supplemented formulas for 92 weeks PMA were evaluated at 118 weeks; developmental scores using the BSID II were significantly better in the infants supplemented with a single-cell source of DHA and ARA [47]. In contrast, Fewtrell et al. [48] in a short-term study could not demonstrate differences in developmental scores in supplemented or control infants at 18 months of age; of concern is the shorter length of the supplemented infants at 18 months. The reasons for the latter are not clear.

In a systematic review, Simmer [49] found that supplementation of formula provides some increase in the early rate of visual development for PT infants, but not for T infants [50]. No long-term benefit has been shown so far in either group. Also, no adverse effects on weight or growth have been demonstrated.

MINERALS, VITAMINS, AND MINOR NUTRIENTS

The in utero accretion rate of calcium is about 120–140 and 60–75 mg/kg/day for the phosphorus [10]; this intake cannot be provided in parenteral solutions because of the limited solubility. Hypocalcemia is a frequent finding in premature infants; therefore, calcium supplementation is routinely started in infants <1800 g and adjusted based on serum levels. One of the biggest challenges in nutrition for the PT infant is to provide enough calcium and phosphorus for bone development. The recommended daily oral intake for PT infants is 200 mg/kg/day for Ca and 100 mg/kg/day for P, taking into consideration the limited gut absorption of these nutrients [10]. While prolonged parenteral nutrition and the use of unfortified human milk can lead to metabolic bone disease especially in the small PT infant, currently available PT formulas provide adequate amounts of calcium and phosphorus; human milk fortifiers also enhance the amounts of calcium and phosphorus when used appropriately. The risk of metabolic bone disease is inversely related to gestational age and birth weight and higher in the sicker infants [51].

Although a causal relationship has not been fully demonstrated, iron deficiency has been associated with lower psychomotor development, poorer cognitive and behavioral performance, and adverse effects on neurodevelopment [52]. The bulk of the iron stores in neonates are acquired transplacentally during the third trimester. T infants have sufficient reserve for 4–6 months [53], so it is recommended that exclusively breast-fed T infants begin 1 mg/kg/day iron supplementation at 4 months and continued until the infant has transitioned to complimentary foods. T formula-fed infants do not require supplementation since standard formulas contain 12 mg of iron/L [52]. No adverse effects, other than slightly increasing the risk of diarrhea, have been shown with iron supplementation [52]. SGA and PT infants have limited iron supplies and require supplementation in the first few weeks. Iron requirements for this population are higher, estimated to be between 2 and 4 mg/kg/day, and supplementation of at least 2 mg/kg/day should begin no later than 1 month in breast-fed infants [52]. PT formulas supply approximately 14.6 mg of iron/L, but iron-deficiency anemia has still been documented in PT infants receiving formula [54]. These infants may need supplementation although no formal recommendation exists at this time [52]. Supplementation for both T and PT infants should be continued through 12 months of age in the PT population [52].

Vitamin K is universally given to all newborns to prevent hemorrhagic disease. After that, the intestinal flora usually produces it, and deficiency is rare. Vitamin D deficiency can be seen in

TABLE 20.6
Trace Minerals and Vitamins in Parenteral Nutrition

Nutrient (amount/kg/day)	<14 day	>14 day
Manganese (μg)	0.0–0.75	1.0
Chromium (μg)	0.0–0.05	0.2
Selenium (μg)	0.0–1.3	2.0
Molybdenum (μg)	0	0.25
Iodine (μg)	0.0–1.0	1.0
Vitamin C (mg)	80	
Vitamin A (mg)	0.7	
Vitamin D (μg)	10 (400 IU)	
Vitamin B1 (mg)	1.2	
Vitamin B2 (mg)	1.4	
Vitamin B6 (mg)	1	
Niacin (mg)	17	

Provided as MVI (pediatric); each 5 mL provides amounts shown; not to exceed 2 mL/kg/day.

certain high-risk groups, such as totally breast-fed infants with limited sun exposure. The 2008 AAP guideline on vitamin D intake recommends a minimum of 400 IU/day intake beginning in the first few days of life [55]. Vitamin A deficiency has been associated with BPD [56], and vitamin E deficiency has been reported to cause hemolytic anemia [57]. However, with the change in vitamin E/PUFA ratio in infant formulas, the incidence of vitamin E deficiency anemia is extremely low. Typical nutritional management (both enteral and parenteral) provides enough supplements to maintain normal levels of these vitamins.

Recent data have raised concerns regarding zinc sufficiency in PT infants. The estimated fetal accretion of zinc is approximately 850 μg/day. Clinical zinc deficiency has been reported in human-milk-fed PT infants, and the concentration of zinc in human milk declines postpartum [58]. Current recommendation of 600 μg to 1 mg/kg/day can be met with the use of PT and T formulas and fortified human milk. Trace elements are usually sufficiently supplied by breast milk or formulas. For parenteral nutrition, suggested intakes are depicted in Table 20.6 [59].

TOTAL PARENTERAL NUTRITION

In the NICU, most of the admissions involve some kind of intravenous nutrition for a period of time. It is more prolonged in the very immature infants and most of the surgical patients because of the inability of enteral feeding. In certain cases, it can supplement enteral feeding until about 75%–80% of energy, and protein requirements are reached by the enteral route. TPN has been used in neonates for the past three decades. It evolved from experiences in adults with the appropriate adjustments considering the requirements of neonates.

Energy

In general, the energy requirement for a steady growth during TPN is 85–95 kcal/kg/day, because the energy loss related to absorption is bypassed, and there is no energy loss through stooling. About half of the calories are provided from glucose, 30%–40% from lipids and the rest from amino acids. Nonprotein energy intake should be at least 60–70 kcal/kg/day.

Glucose

The typical glucose concentration is 12.5%–15%. Peripheral administration cannot be more than 12.5% solution, because of the risk of sclerosis from extravasation. If higher delivery is needed, a central line should be placed. This provides a glucose delivery of 6–8 mg/kg/min, which is usually sufficient to maintain normoglycemia. Extremely LBW infants frequently show glucose intolerance in the first few days of life [60]. If glucose delivery is minimized by the lowest possible glucose concentration (4%–5%), insulin may be helpful and appears to be safe in these infants [61].

Protein

The initial goal immediately after birth, besides providing caloric intake to maintain basal metabolic processes, is to prevent nitrogen loss. Protein should be started early, preferably within the first few hours to prevent negative nitrogen balance. Providing at least 2–2.5 g/kg/day of protein from day 1 can maintain protein balance without any adverse effects. Paisley et al. reported a group of infants who were started at 3 g/kg/day and found it efficacious and safe. It can be increased in daily increments of 0.5–1.0 g/kg up to 3.5 g/kg/day, or not more than 10%–12% of total energy intake [62]. Numerous other studies have demonstrated the safety and efficacy of early amino acid intake as part of an aggressive nutrition regimen [63–66]. Protein is provided as a mixture of crystalline amino acids. Cysteine, an essential amino acid for the neonate, is added to the commercial preparation later (40 mg/g/AA), because it is unstable in solution. It has been shown to enhance nitrogen balance [67].

Lipids

The currently used lipid preparations are derived from safflower oil or soybean oil. They are available in 20% concentrations. LBW neonates tolerate the 20% concentration better since they show lower serum levels when given this preparation [68]. This may be explained by the lower phospholipid concentration in the 20% solution, since the phospholipid component competes for the lipoprotein lipase, therefore decreasing its clearance. It usually started at 0.5–1.0 g/kg/day and gradually increased up to 3.5–4.0 g/kg/day, or not more than 40% of total calories. To prevent essential FA deficiency, the minimal intake should be 0.5 g/kg/day. In small infants, daily measurements are necessary during advancement to ensure proper lipid clearance, and the dose needs to be held or decreased if triglyceride level is over 180–200 mg/dL. Intravenous lipids are better tolerated if infused over prolonged periods (at least 20 h).

Vitamins and Trace Elements

Vitamins and trace elements are added to the preparation from commercial formulas (see Table 20.6).

Complications

The complications of parenteral nutrition are related to the content of the solution (metabolic) and/or associated with the route of delivery. The most common metabolic complications are metabolic bone disease and liver dysfunction. Providing calcium intake that is comparable to intrauterine accretion rates is impossible through intravenous nutrition because of precipitation at higher concentrations. Therefore, infants maintained on TPN for prolonged time will develop metabolic bone disease to some extent. Currently, there are no good clinical markers of metabolic bone disease. Low phosphorus levels (<4 mg/dL) and increasing alkaline phosphatase levels, signifying extensive bone remodeling, are the best practical tools to monitor the evolving disease, since serum electrolyte levels are maintained by the expense of bone reabsorption.

The most prevalent sign of liver dysfunction is cholestasis. Signs usually develop after a few weeks of parenteral nutrition. Elevated direct bilirubin is a late sign, but probably the most cost-effective way to monitor periodically. The use of fish oils (omega-3 fatty acids [O3FA]), instead of safflower- and/or soybean-based intravenous lipid preparations, is currently under investigation as a preventative measure to reduce intestinal failure-associated liver disease [69]. O3FAs may offer hepatic protection by decreasing inflammation and thrombosis, stimulating biliary flow, and decreasing de novo lipogenesis [69]. Further research needs to be evaluated before formal recommendations can be made regarding fish oil use in PT infants. The prognosis for TPN-related liver dysfunction is good; the process is typically reversible once enteral feeding is started, even if it is only small volume enteral feedings. Every effort should be made to advance these infants to at least some partial feedings to limit the liver dysfunction. Periodic monitoring is needed to minimize and monitor complications while on parenteral nutrition (Table 20.7).

Catheter-related complications in infants requiring TPN include sepsis/bacteremia and tip misplacement with possible pericardial effusion, thrombosis, and extravasation. These can be minimized by proper sterile technique, avoidance of multiple manipulation of dressing and breaking up the continuity of the line, use of continuous fluids to prevent clot formation in the lumen or hub, and periodic radiographic monitoring of line position.

In infants maintained on parenteral nutrition, special attention should be paid for the possibility of metabolic acidosis, mainly because most of the salts are given in chloride form. Substituting chloride partially for acetate can prevent this problem [70].

TABLE 20.7
Suggested Monitoring during Parenteral Nutrition

Component	Initial	Later
Weight	Daily	Daily
Length	Weekly	Weekly
Head circumference	Weekly	Weekly
Na, K, Cl, CO_2	Daily until stable	Weekly
Glucose	Daily	PRN
Triglycerides	With every lipid change	Weekly or biweekly
Ca, PO_4	Daily until stable	Weekly or biweekly
Alkaline phosphatase	Initial	Weekly or biweekly
Bilirubin	Initial	Weekly or biweekly
Mg	Initial	Weekly or biweekly
Ammonia	PRN	PRN
Gamma GT	Initial	Weekly or biweekly
ALT/AST	Initial	Weekly or biweekly
Complete blood count	Initial	Weekly or PRN

FEEDING THE PRETERM INFANT

Although the suck reflex may be observed in many premature infants, the coordination of suck, swallow, and breathing is not present until 32–34 weeks of postconceptional age [71]. Other factors affecting the ability of feeding of the premature infant include delayed gastric emptying, low stomach volume, and weak esophageal sphincter leading to an almost universal gastroesophageal reflux [72–74]. If the infant is unable to feed per os, an oro- or nasogastric tube is placed to initiate feedings. Gastric feeding can be continuous or bolus. Continuous feeding, although it is not physiologic, is more energy efficient and allows reaching higher volumes when compared to bolus feedings [75,76]. A subgroup of infants cannot tolerate even continuous gastric feeding. For them, transpyloric feeding may be an option until gastric emptying improves. This should be as a last resort only, since it does not seem to provide much advantage in weight gain or caloric intake, but exposes the infant to a lot more radiation [77]. Table 20.8 shows characteristics of the commonly used feeding practices.

Studies have shown the benefit of providing minimal feeding for PT infant on parenteral nutrition to prevent atrophy of villi and to promote gut maturation [78,79]. The usual amount of feeding in these studies was ≤20 mL/kg/day. They demonstrated a shorter time to reach full volume of feeds, a decreased incidence of feeding intolerance without an increase in the incidence of necrotizing enterocolitis (NEC) [80–82].

Berseth et al. compared minimal feeding (where feeding was held at 20 mL/kg/day) and advancing feeding over a 10-day period. They showed an increased risk of NEC in the group where feedings were advanced [83].

Although we have more and more evidence to support early feeding, the controversy is not resolved. This is reflected in recent reviews in the Cochrane Database that concluded that there is still not enough clinical evidence to promote the universal use of early feeding in high-risk infants [84,85]. Therefore, the most common approach is to hold feeding in high-risk infants for a few days, start slowly with low volumes, and advance slowly (≤20 mL/kg/day) [86]. These infants require a high index of suspicion to withhold feeding, but it can be restarted if symptoms subside.

Human milk is superior to formula in several aspects. Although maternal milk is the most desirable, the AAP has recognized that donor breast milk is recommended when maternal milk is not available [87]. Studies have shown various benefits to the use of donor milk including prevention against NEC [88,89], less generalized feeding intolerance [88], and long-term health benefits

TABLE 20.8
Commonly Used Feeding Practices

Method	Advantages	Disadvantages
Nipple	Simple; physiologic; hormonal, digestive, and neurologic benefit	Consumes energy; possible aspiration; not feasible on CPAP or ventilator
Orogastric–nasogastric	Suck–swallow not required; can be used in intubated patients; decreased risk of aspiration; conserves energy	Inadvertent tracheal intubation; blocks nasal passage and increases airway resistance: vagal stimulation and gagging
Intermittent–bolus	Mimics nipple feeding with possible enteric hormone benefits	Gastric residuals, reflux, abdominal distention
Constant infusion	Better tolerated by infants with delayed gastric emptying; possible larger milk intake	Not physiologic; loss of cyclic hormonal effect
Transpyloric	Less residuals and reflux in infants with poor gastric emptying; possible larger milk intake	Multiple x-rays; catheter misplacement and complication; alters gut flora
Gastrostomy	Indicated for patients with severe neurologic damage	Morbidity/mortality with the procedure

Source: Adapted from Dweck, H.S., *Clin. Perinatol.*, 2, 183, 1975.

including lower blood pressure and lower cholesterol levels [90,91]. PT human milk has a higher content of nitrogen, sodium, vitamin, and lipids when compared to mature milk. Table 20.5 shows a comparison of PT and T human milk [92].

During the first few weeks, human milk can provide enough nutrient to meet the requirement for LBW infants, but later, especially for babies with <1800 g birth weight, supplementation is required. It can be fortified by adding commercially available human milk fortifiers that enhance human milk by adding more protein, fat, sodium, calcium, phosphorus, vitamins, and trace minerals [79]. Commercially available fortifiers add 0.8–1.1 g/dL of protein for a total of approximately 2.5 g/dL, which is higher than human milk alone (approximately 1.5 g/dL) but may still be inadequate for postnatal growth. Additional strategies are being investigated to target higher protein concentrations based on the protein content of the provided human milk. Human milk can be mixed to 22 kcal/oz (for infants less than 2500 g) or 26 kcal/oz (for infants less than 1800 g) preparations.

Soy-based formulas are not recommended for PT infants, because the phytic acid can bind calcium, lowering absorption. Infants fed soy-based formula also showed less nitrogen retention, lower levels of serum albumin, and total protein along with a diminished weight gain [93].

Feeding the Term Infant

T infants admitted to NICU are usually too unstable to be fed enterally/orally. The initial nutrition therefore has to be intravenous. When the infant becomes more stable and the gut function is appropriate (good bowel sounds, no distention, regular stooling pattern), enteral feeding can be started, even if the infant remains on the ventilator. If the infant condition allows, the feeding can be advanced faster than in PT infants (approximately 30 mL/kg/day). Once feasible, oral feeding is started. Most T infants are able to nipple after a short intensive care course. A subgroup of infants, who had more prolonged illness (such as CDH, post-ECMO), frequently show suck–swallow dysfunction and gastroesophageal reflux. These infants stay on tube feeding for a longer time, which may prolong their length of stay [94].

The AAP strongly recommends the use of breast milk [95]. Every effort should be made to provide support for mothers to pump while their baby is critically ill, and allow them to visit and nurse whenever possible. If breast milk is not available, most NICUs use T, cow milk–based formulas. If one encounters malabsorption as seen in short-gut syndrome, a more elemental formula could be used.

Regular diet sufficient in protein would provide enough glutamine, and supplementation is not needed. In conditions involving stress and catabolic processes, or intestinal disease, it has been shown to be *conditionally* essential [96]. It is not supplied during parenteral nutrition; therefore, PT infants maintained on prolonged TPN are high risk for gut atrophy and may benefit from its use. A randomized clinical trial in premature infants receiving parenteral nutrition is underway. Neu et al. conducted a randomized trial in 68 very-low-birth-weight (VLBW) infants (<1250 g), where they used a formula supplemented with 0.3 g/kg/day of glutamine. Decreased hospital-acquired infection, improved tolerance to enteral feeds, and a decrease in hospital costs were found in the glutamine-supplemented group without any safety concerns [97]. Vaughn et al. in a later study found no difference in nosocomial sepsis using the same dose of supplementation [98]. Tubman and Thompson reviewed the current literature for the Cochrane Database and concluded that there is not enough evidence in the randomized trials so far to support universal supplementation for PT infants [99].

Special Considerations

Corticosteroids became widely used in the 1990s to improve respiratory outcome in infants with severe respiratory failure. Later in the decade, reports appeared on follow-up studies showing abnormal neurodevelopment, especially in infants treated with early and prolonged corticosteroid regimens. Steroids have profound effect on many aspects of the metabolism as well. Administration of pharmacological doses promotes protein catabolism with subsequent protein wasting and induces lipid and glucose intolerance. This can put an extra burden on the metabolic needs of the PT infant, further compromising their growth. The benefit to use steroids should be strongly weighed against its risks and complications and restricted to very special circumstances as recently suggested by an AAP policy statement [100].

POST-DISCHARGE FEEDING OF THE PREMATURE INFANT

The challenge to provide appropriate nutritional support for PT infants continues beyond their hospital stay. Providing the currently recommended energy and protein intake might not be sufficient to replicate intrauterine growth rate. Ehrenkranz et al. [8] published data from a large cohort of PT infants (birth weight 500–1500 g) regarding their postnatal growth. These infants accrue a considerable amount of nutritional deficit during their first few weeks. They are frequently unstable initially; parenteral and enteral nutrition advances slowly because of concerns of complications. Therefore, full nutrition support might not be reached before the second or even third week of life. Despite some catch-up growth in the second month of their hospitalization, most infants born between 24 and 29 weeks did not reach the median weight of the reference fetus of the same gestational age. This *extrauterine growth restriction* seems to continue into the second year of life. The incidence of failure to thrive in infants less than 1000 g in the neonatal research cohort was more than 30% at 18 months of corrected age [101]. Lucas et al. [102] conducted a randomized, double-blind study of PT infant-fed fortified formula after discharge to see if post-discharge growth deficit can be improved with higher caloric intake in the first 9 months postterm. Significant increases in linear growth and weight gain were observed in the infants who received the enriched diet. There was no increase in diet-related complications in the group with the modified formula. Carver et al. [103] compared 22 kcal/fL enriched formula diet with regular T formula feeding up to 12 months of corrected age. They found improved growth in the nutrient-enriched formula-fed group, with the highest benefit for infants less than 1250 g birth weight. There have now been several studies published demonstrating the benefit of LCPUFAs in the post hospital discharge period as well. In a recent study, infants randomized to DHA (17 mg/100 kcal and ARA 34 mg/100 kcal) demonstrate greater weight gain than unsupplemented infants from 6 to 18 months of age; these infants also had greater lengths at 79 and 92 weeks postmenstrual age [104]. Innis et al. [46] demonstrated that PT infants fed DHA (0.14%) and AA (0.27%) gained weight significantly faster than unsupplemented infants and had weight/length ratios similar to those of T breast-fed infants at 48 and 57 weeks postmenstrual age. In addition, visual acuity and neurodevelopmental benefits have been demonstrated. Based on these data, it seems prudent to maintain LBW formula-fed infants on enriched formulas up to 6–9 months of corrected age.

SUMMARY

In summary, for the T infant, the growth and biochemical responses of a healthy infant breast-fed by a healthy mother remains the gold standard. Over the past few decades, continued improvement in formulas have been made with the addition of iron, altering whey-to-casein ratio and the fat blends, and addition of taurine, nucleotides, and, most recently, DHA and ARA. The AAP and the Canadian Pediatric Society have strongly recommended that breast-feeding be the preferred feeding for all infants and that donor milk is an appropriate substitute when maternal milk is unavailable. In the absence of human milk, currently available formulas are appropriate substitutes for feeding full-term infants during the first year of life. While we strive to increase breast-feeding rates in the United States, we need to continue to improve available formulas to be as close to human milk as possible. For the PT infant, a continuous strategy to nourish the infant from birth through the hospitalization period and beyond needs to be continually improved upon to enhance growth and development of this increasing cohort of infants. We need to continue to advocate for human milk feedings, appropriately fortify them as needed, and continue to make improvements in the commercially available formulas. The current generation of premature infant formulas was designed for the *larger* PT infant and may not be the ideal formulation for the very small premature infant. However, recently introduced *high-protein* formulas provide adequate amounts of protein and energy, so they should be used in the VLBW infants in the absence of human milk.

The strategies in feeding T and PT infants differ and need to be individualized. Although reliance on evidence should guide us in nourishing these infants, feeding infants is also an art and based on experience. Experience should then be molded by evidence to enhance our nutritional care of these fragile infants.

REFERENCES

1. Martin JA, Hamilton BE, Osterman MJK, Sally C. Curtin SC, Mathews TJ. Births: Final data for 2012. *Natl Vital Stat* 2013:62,9.
2. Eherankrantz RA, Dusick AM, Vorh BR, Wright LL, Wrage LA, Poole WK. Growth in the neonatal intensive care unit influences neurodevelopmental and growth outcomes of extremely low birth weight infants. *Pediatrics* 2006;117:1253–1261.
3. American Academy of Pediatrics, Committee on Nutrition. Nutritional needs of low-birth-weight infants. *Pediatrics* 1985;75:976.
4. Ziegler EE, O'Donnell AM, Nelson SE, Fomon SJ. Body composition of the reference fetus. *Growth* 1976;40:239.
5. Babson SG, Benda GI. Growth graphs for the clinical assessment of infants of varying gestational ages. *J Pediatr* 1976;89:814.
6. Lubchenco L, Hansman C, Boyd E. Intrauterine growth in length and head circumference as estimated from live births at gestational ages from 26 to 42 weeks. *Pediatrics* 1966;37:403.
7. Alexander GR, Himes JH, Kaufman RB, Mor J, Kogan M. A United States national reference for fetal growth. *Obstet Gynecol* 1996;87:163–168.
8. Ehrenkranz RA, Younes N, Lemons JA. Longitudinal growth of hospitalized very low birth weight infants. *Pediatrics* August 1999;104(2 Pt 1):280–289.
9. American Academy of Pediatrics, Committee on Nutrition. *Nutritional Needs of the Preterm Infant: Pediatric Nutrition Handbook*, 5th edn., American Academy of Pediatrics, Elk Grove Village, IL, 2003, pp. 23–54.
10. Hay WW Jr. (ed.) *Nutritional Requirement of the Extremely Low-Birth-Weight Infant*, Mosby Year Book, St. Louis, MO, 1991.

11. Sauer PJJ, Dane HF, Visser HKA. Longitudinal studies on metabolic rate, heat loss, and energy cost of growth in low birth weight infants. *Pediatr Res* 1984;18:254.
12. Ziegler EE, Thureen PJ, Carlson SJ. Aggressive nutrition of the very low birth weight infant. *Clin Perinatol* 2002;29:225–244.
13. Tsang RC, Lucas A, Uauy R, Zlotkin S. (eds.) *Nutritional Needs of the Preterm Infant: Scientific Basis and Practical Guideline*, William & Wilkins, Pawling, NY, 1993.
14. Brunton JA, Saigal S, Atkinson SA. Nutrient intake similar to recommended values does not result in catch-up growth by 12 mo of age in very low birth weight infants (VLBW) with bronchopulmonary dysplasia (BPD). *Am J Clin Nutr* 1997;66:221 (abs. 102).
15. Butte NF, Garza C, Smith EO, Nichols BL. Human milk intake and growth in exclusively breast-fed infants. *J Pediatr* February 1984;104(2):187–195.
16. Garza C, Butte NF. Energy intakes of human milk-fed infants during the first year. *J Pediatr* August 1990;117(2 Pt 2):S124–S131.
17. Lorenz JM, Kleinman LI, Ahmed G, Markarian K. Phases of fluid electrolyte homeostasis in the extremely low birth weight infant. *Pediatrics* 1995;96:484.
18. Schaffer SG, Meade V. Sodium balance and extracellular volume regulation in very low birth weight infants. *J Pediatr* 1989;115:285–290.
19. Hartnoll G, Betremieux P, Modi N. Randomized controlled trial of postnatal sodium supplementation on oxygen dependency and body weight in 25–30 week gestational age Infants. *Arch Dis Child Fetal Neonatal Ed* 2000;82:F19–F23.
20. Costarino AT, Gruskay JA, Corcoran L et al. Sodium restriction versus daily maintenance replacement in very low birth weight premature neonates: A randomized, blind therapeutic trial. *J Pediatr* 1992;120:99–106.
21. Sulyok E, Kovacs L, Lichardus B et al. Late hyponatremia in premature infants: Role of aldosterone and arginine vasopressin. *J Pediatr* 1985;106:990–994.
22. Baumgart S, Costarino AT. Water and electrolyte metabolism of the micropremie. *Clin Perinatol* 2000;27:131–146.
23. Gruskay J, Costarino AT, Polin RA et al. Non-oliguric hyperkalemia in the premature infant weighing less than 1000 grams. *J Pediatr* 1988;113:381–386.
24. Rutter N, Hull D. Water loss from the skin of term and preterm babies. *Arch Dis Child* 1979;54:858–868.
25. Kim SM, Lee EY, Chen J, Ringer SA. Improved care and growth outcomes by using hybrid humidified incubators in very preterm infants. *Pediatrics* 2010;125:e137–e145.
26. Parish A, Bhatia J. Nutritional considerations in the intensive care unit: Neonatal issues. In: *Nutritional Considerations in the Intensive Care Unit: Science, Rationale and Practice*, Shikora SA, Martindale RG, Schwaitzberg SD (eds.), ASPEN, Kendall/Hunt Publishing Company, Dubuque, IA, 2002, pp. 297–310.
27. MacLean WC Jr, Fink BB. Lactose malabsorption by premature infants: Magnitude and clinical significance. *J Pediatr* September 1980;97(3):383–388.
28. Mobassaleh M, Montgomery RK, Biller JA, Grand RJ. Development of carbohydrate absorption in the fetus and neonate. *Pediatrics* January 1985;75(1 Pt 2):160–166.
29. Kashyap S, Schulze KF, Forsyth M, Zucker C, Dell RB, Ramakrishnan R, Heird WC. Growth, nutrient retention, and metabolic response in low birth weight infants fed varying intakes of protein and energy. *J Pediatr* October 1988;113(4):713–721.
30. Schulze KF, Stefanski M, Masterson J, Spinnazola R, Ramakrishnan R, Dell RB, Heird WC. Energy expenditure, energy balance, and composition of weight gain in low birth infants fed diets of different protein and energy content. *Pediatrics* May 1987;110(5):753–759.
31. Bhatia J, Rassin DK, Cerreto MC et al. Effect of protein/energy ratio on growth and behavior of premature infants: Preliminary findings. *J Pediatr* 1991;119:103–110.
32. Zlotkin SH, Bryan MH, Anderson GH. Intravenous nitrogen and energy intakes required to duplicate in utero nitrogen accretion in prematurely born human infants. *J Pediatr* July 1981;99(1):115–120.
33. Koletzko B, Agostoni C, Carlson SE et al. Long chain polyunsaturated fatty acids (LC-PUFA) and perinatal development. *Acta Paediatricia* 2001;90:460–464.
34. Hoffman DR, Birch EE, Birch DG, Uauy R, Castaneda YS, Lapus MG, Wheaton DH. Impact of early dietary intake and blood lipid composition of long-chain polyunsaturated fatty acids on later visual development. *J Pediatr Gastroenterol Nutr* November 2000;31(5):540–553.
35. Makrides M, Neumann MA, Jeffrey B, Lien EL, Gibson RA. Randomized trial of different ratios of linoleic to alpha-linolenic acid in the diet of term infants: Effects on visual function and growth. *Am J Clin Nutr* January 2000;71(1):120–129.

36. Carlson SE, Ford AJ, Werkman SH et al. Visual acuity and fatty acid status of term infants fed human milk and formulas with and without docosahexaenoate and arachidonate from egg yolk lecithin. *Pediatr Res* 1996;39:882–888.
37. San Giovanni JP, Berkey CS, Dwyer JT, Colditz GA. Dietary essential fatty acids, long-chain polyunsaturated fatty acids, and visual acuity in healthy full term infants: A systematic review. *Early Hum Dev* 2000;57:165–188.
38. Birch EE, Garfield S, Hoffman DR, Uauy R, Birch DG. A randomized controlled trial of early dietary supply of long-chain polyunsaturated fatty acids and mental development in term infants. *Dev Med Child Neurol* March 2000;42(3):174–181.
39. Agostini C, Trojan S, Bellu R et al. Neurodevelopmental quotient of healthy term infants at 4 months and feeding practice: The role of long-chain polyunsaturated fatty acids. *Pediatr Res* 1995;38:262–266.
40. Wilatts P, Forsyth JS, DiMadugno MK et al. Effect of long-chain polyunsaturated fatty acids in infant formulas on problem solving at 10 months of age. *Lancet* 1998;352:688–691.
41. Makrides M, Neumann M, Simmer K et al. Are long-chain polyunsaturated fatty acids essential nutrients in infancy? *Lancet* 1995;345:1463–1468.
42. Markides M, Neumann M, Simmer K et al. A critical appraisal of the dietary long-chain polyunsaturated fatty acids on neural indices of term infants: A randomized controlled trial. *Pediatrics* 2000;105:32–38.
43. Auestad N, Halter R, Hall RT et al. Growth and development in term infants fed long-chain polyunsaturated fatty acids: A double-masked, randomized, parallel, prospective, multivariate study. *Pediatrics* 2001;108:372–381.
44. Lucas A, Stafford M, Morley R et al. Efficacy and safety of long-chain polyunsaturated fatty acid supplementation of infant-formula milk: A randomized trial. *Lancet* 1999;354:1948–1954.
45. O'Connor DL, Hall R, Adamkin D et al. Growth and development in preterm infants fed long-chain polyunsaturated fatty acids: A prospective, randomized controlled trial. *Pediatrics* August 2001;108(2):359–371.
46. Innis SM, Adamkin DH, Hall RT et al. Docosahexaenoic acid and arachidonic acid enhance growth with no adverse effects in preterm infants fed formula. *J Pediatr* 2002;140:547–554.
47. Clandinin M, VanArde J, Antonson D, Lim M, Stevens D, Merkel K, Harris J, Hansen J. Formulas with docosahexaenoic acid [DHA] and arachidonic acid [ARA] promote better growth and developmental scores in very-low-birth-infants [VLBW]. *Pediatr Res* 2002;51(4):1092.
48. Fewtrell MS, Morley R, Abbott RA, Singhal A, Isaacs EB, Stephenson T, MacFadyen U, Lucas A. Double-blind, randomized trial of long-chain polyunsaturated fatty acid supplementation in formula fed to preterm infants. *Pediatrics* July 2002;110(1 Pt 1):73–82.
49. Simmer K. Long chain polyunsaturated fatty acid supplementation in preterm infants. *Cochrane Database Syst Rev* 2000;2:CD000375. Review.
50. Simmer K. Longchain polyunsaturated fatty acid supplementation in infants born at term. *Cochrane Database Syst Rev* 2001;4:CD000376. Review.
51. Koo WWK, Gupta JM, Nayanar VV et al. Skeletal changes in preterm infants. *Arch Dis Child* 1982;57:447–452.
52. American Academy of Pediatrics, Committee on Nutrition. Iron supplementation. *Pediatrics* 2010;126:1040–1050.
53. American Academy of Pediatrics, Committee on Nutrition. Iron supplementation. *Pediatrics* 1976;58:765.
54. Griffin IJ, Cooke RJ, Reid MM, McCormick KP, Smith JS. Iron nutritional status in preterm infants fed formulas fortified with iron. *Arch Dis Child Fetal Neonatal Ed* 1991;81:F45–F49.
55. American Academy of Pediatrics. Prevention of rickets and vitamin D deficiency in infants, children and adolescents. *Pediatrics* 2008;122:1142–1152.
56. Shenai JP, Chytil F, Stahlman MT. Vitamin A status of neonates with bronchopulmonary dysplasia. *Pediatr Res* 1985;19:185.
57. Oski FA, Barnes LA. Vitamin E deficiency: A previously unrecognized cause of hemolytic anemia in the premature. *J Pediatr* 1967;70:211.
58. Zlotkin SH. Assessment of trace element requirements [zinc] in newborns and young infants, including the infant born prematurely. In: *Trace Elements in Nutrition of Children II*, Chandra RK (ed.), Raven Press, New York, 1991, pp. 49–64.
59. Bhatia J, Bucher C, Bunyapen C. Feeding the preterm infant. In: *Handbook of Nutrition and Food*, Berdanier CD (ed.), CRC Press, Boca Raton, FL, 2002, pp. 203–218.
60. Lilien DP, Rosenfeld RL, Baccaro MM et al. Hyperglycemia in stressed, small premature infants. *J Pediatr* 1979;94:454–459.

61. Collins JW Jr, Hoppe M, Browne K et al. A controlled trial of insulin infusion and parenteral nutrition in extremely low birth weight infants with glucose intolerance. *J Pediatr* 1991;118:921–927.
62. Paisley JE, Thureen PG, Baron KA, Hay WW. Safety and efficacy of low versus high parenteral amino acids in extremely low birth weight neonates immediately after birth. *Pediatr Res* 2000;47:293A.
63. Ibrahim HM, Jeroudi MA, Baier RJ et al. Aggressive early total parental nutrition in low-birth-weight infants. *J Perinatol* 2004;24:482–486.
64. Poindexter BB, Langer JC, Dusick AM et al. Early provision of parenteral amino acids in extremely low birth weight infants: Relation to growth and neurodevelopmental outcome. *J Perinatol* 2006;148:300–305.
65. te Braake FJ, Van Den Akker CP, Wattimena DL et al. Amino acid administration to premature infants directly after birth. *J Perinatol* 2005;147:457–461.
66. Thureen PJ, Hay WW. Early aggressive nutrition in preterm infants. *Semin Neonatol* 2001;6:403–415.
67. Rivera A, Jr., Bell EF, Stegink LD, Ziegler EE. Plasma amino acid profiles during the first three days of life in infants with respiratory distress syndrome: Effect of parenteral amino acid supplementation. *J Pediatr* 1989;115:465.
68. Haumont D, Deckelbaum RD, Richelle M et al. Plasma lipid and plasma lipoprotein concentration in low birth weight infants given parenteral nutrition with 20% compared to 10% intralipid. *J Pediatr* 1989;115:787.
69. Venick RS, Calkins K. The impact of intravenous fish oil emulsions on pediatric intestinal failure-associated liver disease. *Curr Opin Org Transplant* 2011;16:306–311.
70. Sugiura S, Inagaki K, Noda Y, Nagai T, Nabeshima T. Acid load during total parenteral nutrition: Comparison of hydrochloric acid and acetic acid on plasma acid-base balance. *Nutrition* April 2000;16(4):260–263.
71. Broussard DL. Gastrointestinal motility in the neonate. *Clin Perinatol* 1995;22:37.
72. Ittman PI, Amarnath I, Berseth CL. Maturation of antroduodenal activity in preterm and term infants. *Dig Dis Sci* 1992;37:14.
73. Siegel M, Lebenthal E, Krantz B. Effect of caloric density on gastric emptying in premature infants. *J Pediatr* 1984;104:118.
74. Cavell B. Gastric emptying in preterm infants. *Acta Paediatr Scand* 1979;68:725–730.
75. Grant J, Denne SC. Effect of intermittent versus continuous enteral feeding on energy expenditure in premature Infants. *J Pediatr* 1991;118:928.
76. Robertson AF, Bhatia J. Feeding premature infants. *Clin Pediatr* 1993;31:36.
77. Laing IA, Lang MA, Callaghan O et al. Nasogastric compared with nasoduodenal feeding in low birth-weight infants. *Arch Dis Child* 1986;61:138–141.
78. Berseth CL. Effect of early feeding on maturation of the preterm infant's small intestine. *J Pediatr* 1992;120:947–953.
79. Berseth CI, Nordyke C. Enteral nutrients promote postnatal maturation of intestinal motor activity in preterm infants. *Am J Phys* 1993;264:G1046–G1051.
80. Slagle TA, Gross SJ. Effect of early low-volume enteral substrate on subsequent feeding tolerance in very low birth weight Infants. *J Pediatr* 1988;113:526–531.
81. Troche B, Harvey-Wilkes K, Engle WD, Nielsen HC, Frantz ID 3rd, Mitchell ML, Hermos RJ. Early minimal feedings promote growth in critically ill premature infants. *Biol Neonate* 1995;67(3):172–181.
82. Ostertag SG, LaGamma EF, Reisen CE et al. Early enteral feeding does not affect the incidence of necrotizing enterocolitis. *Pediatrics* 1986;77:275–280.
83. Berseth CL, Bisquera JA, Paje VU. Prolonging small feeding volumes early in life decreases the incidence of necrotizing enterocolitis in very low birth weight infants. *Pediatrics* 2003;111:529–534.
84. Kennedy KA, Tyson JE, Chamnanvanikij S. Early versus delayed initiation of progressive enteral feedings for parenterally fed low birth weight or preterm infants. *Cochrane Database Syst Rev* 2000;2:CD001970.
85. Tyson JE, Kennedy KA. Minimal enteral nutrition for promoting feeding tolerance and preventing morbidity in parenterally fed infants. *Cochrane Database Syst Rev* 2000;2:CD000504.
86. La Gamma EF, Browne LE. Feeding practices for infants weighing less than 1500 gm at birth and the pathogenesis of necrotizing enterocolitis. *Clin Perinatol* 1994;21:271–306.
87. American Academy of Pediatrics. Policy statement. *Pediatrics* 115:496;2005.
88. Boyd CA, Quigley MA, Brocklehurst P. Donor breast milk versus infant formula for preterm infants: Systematic review and meta-analysis. *Arch Dis Child Fetal Neonatal Ed* 2007;92:F169.
89. Quigley MA, Henderson G, Anthony MY, McGuire W. Formula milk versus donor breast milk for feeding preterm or low birth weight infants. *Cochrane Database Syst Rev* 2007;4:CD002971.
90. Singhal A, Cole TJ, Lucas A. Early nutrition in preterm infants and later blood pressure: Two cohorts after randomized trials. *Lancet* 2001;357(9254):413–419.

91. Sisk PM, Lovelady CA, Dillard RG, Gruber KJ, O'Shea TM. Early human milk feeding is associated with a lower risk of necrotizing enterocolitis in very low birth weight infants. *J Perinatol* 2007;27(7):428–433.
92. Jensen RG (eds.). *Handbook of Milk Composition*, Academic Press, San Diego, CA, 1995.
93. Schanler RJ, Cheng SF. Infant formulas for enteral feeding. In: *Neonatal Nutrition and Metabolism*, Hay WW Jr (ed.), Mosby Year Book, St. Louis, MO, 1991, p. 303.
94. Van Meurs KP, Robbins ST, Reed VL, Karr SS, Wagner AE, Glass P, Anderson KD, Short BL. Congenital diaphragmatic hernia: Long-term outcome in neonates treated with extracorporeal membrane oxygenation. *J Pediatr* June 1993;122(6):893–899.
95. American Academy of Pediatrics, Committee on Nutrition. Encouraging breast-feeding. *Pediatrics* 1980;65:657.
96. Lacey JM, Wilomre DW. Is glutamine a conditionally essential amino acid? *Nutr Rev* 1990;48:397–409.
97. Neu J, DeMarco V, Weiss M. Glutamine supplementation in low-birth-weight-infants: Mechanism of action. *JPEN* 1999;23:s49–s51.
98. Vaughn P, Thomas P, Clark R, Neu J. Enteral glutamine supplementation and morbidity in low birth weight infants. *J Pediatr* June 2003;142(6):662–668.
99. Tubman TR, Thompson SW. Glutamine supplementation for prevention of morbidity in preterm infants. *Cochrane Database Syst Rev* 2001;4:CD001457.
100. American Academy of Pediatrics, Committee on Fetus and Newborn. Postnatal corticosteroids to treat or prevent chronic lung disease in preterm infants. *Pediatrics* Feb 2002;109(2):330–338.
101. Clark RH, Wagner CL, Merritt RJ, Bloom BT, Neu J, Young TE, Clark DA. Nutrition in the neonatal intensive care unit: How do we reduce the incidence of extrauterine growth restriction? *J Perinatol* June 2003;23(4):337–344.
102. Lucas A, Bishop NJ, King FJ et al. Randomized trial of nutrition for preterm infants after hospital discharge. *Arch Dis Child* 1992;67:324–327.
103. Carver JD, Wu PY, Hall RT et al. Growth of preterm infants fed nutrient-enriched or term formula after hospital discharge. *Pediatrics* April 2001;107(4):683–689.
104. Clandinin M, VanAerde J, Antonson D et al. Formulas with docosahexaenoic acid (DHA) and arachidonic acid (ARA) promote better growth and development scores in very-low-birth-weight infants (VLBW). *Pediatr Res.* 2002;51:187A–188A.
105. Fanaroff AA (eds.). *Neonatal-Perinatal Medicine: Diseases of the Fetus and Infant*, 9th edn., Mosby, St. Louis, MO, 2010.
106. Gross SJ, Geller J, Tomarelli RM. Composition of breast milk from mothers of preterm infants. *Pediatrics* October 1981;68(4):490–493.
107. Dweck HS. Feeding the premature born infant. *Clin Perinatol* 1975;2:183–202.

21 Nutrition Support for the Critically Ill Pediatric Patient

Jodi Wolff, Gerri Keller, and Deborah A. Carpenter

CONTENTS

INTRODUCTION

Pediatric patients are more susceptible than adults to the catabolism that occurs during the metabolic response to stress. Compared to adults, infants and children have less protein and lipid stores and higher baseline energy requirements per kilogram of body weight. Their limited reserves place them at high risk for malnutrition. Nutrition assessment with early nutrition intervention, followed by close monitoring, is important to help improve clinical outcome.

METABOLIC RESPONSE TO CRITICAL ILLNESS

During critical illness, a series of complex reactions takes place referred to as the metabolic stress response, which results in profound hormonal, metabolic, and immunological changes.

This *stress response* induces a hypercatabolic state proportional to the degree and severity of illness or injury and is characterized most notably by protein breakdown and turnover; however, increased usage of all macronutrients occurs. Until the precipitating factors of illness or injury are corrected, the catabolic phase of the metabolic response will continue (Mehta et al. 2009a).

As part of the inflammatory response, skeletal muscle is broken down and protein degradation predominates. The resulting free amino acids move through the circulation to the wound and other tissues to be used for the synthesis of inflammatory response proteins, for new protein synthesis and tissue repair (Mehta et al. 2009a). Glucose is the preferred fuel for the brain, renal medulla, and erythrocytes as well as the energy source for the tissues involved in the inflammatory response. Overall glucose oxidation is increased; however, aerobic oxidation of glucose may be impaired due to limited oxygen availability in injured tissue (Mehta et al. 2009a). Hyperglycemia is common due to insulin resistance (Faustino and Apkon 2005). The provision of exogenous glucose alone will not inhibit gluconeogenesis or muscle breakdown. Adequate protein intake along with glucose is necessary to prevent negative nitrogen balance and loss of lean tissue. If protein and energy are not supplied, then the progressive breakdown of muscle mass may lead to loss of diaphragmatic and intercostal muscle, altered respiratory function, and loss of cardiac muscle (Mehta et al. 2009b).

Lipolysis increases during stress with free fatty acids becoming the primary oxidative fuel. Due to the increased demand for lipid and the limited stores in a child, it is crucial to provide a fat source for energy, as well as for prevention of essential fatty acid deficiency (EFAD) (Mehta et al. 2009a). During the acute phase of illness, the goals of nutrition intervention are to support the catabolic state, control hyperglycemia, and preserve or limit loss of lean body mass (Szeszycki 2010).

NUTRITION ASSESSMENT

Nutrition screening and assessment should be completed for all critically ill infants and children. Unfortunately malnutrition is prevalent in children admitted to the pediatric intensive care unit (PICU) and for many this may worsen throughout hospitalization. A recent international prospective cohort study involving 500 patients from 8 countries revealed that 30% of the patients admitted to the PICU were severely malnourished (Mehta et al. 2012). Every infant, child, and adolescent should be screened for malnutrition upon admission to the ICU. Malnutrition during critical illness is associated with increased infection, poor wound healing, and increased morbidity and mortality (Mehta and Duggan 2009). Identification of malnutrition with timely nutrition intervention can improve outcome by decreasing medical complications, infection rate, length of stay, and hospital costs (Skillman and Mehta 2012a). Components of a complete nutrition assessment include medical history, anthropometric measurements, biochemical data, nutrition-focused physical exam, and food and nutrition–related history.

MEDICAL HISTORY

Pediatric medical conditions that exist prior to admission to the ICU should be considered during nutrition assessment as they may influence nutrient requirements. Premature infants with bronchopulmonary dysplasia or infants with heart disease may have increased energy requirements due to work of breathing. Patients with cystic fibrosis or short bowel syndrome with malabsorption may have increased nutrient needs. Renal disease may affect protein, fluid, and electrolyte requirements. Children with neurological impairment due to cerebral palsy, spina bifida, or other syndromes may have decreased energy needs due to lower muscle mass, lower activity, and decreased brain function. The risk of malnutrition is further increased when critical illness is superimposed on these conditions.

Anthropometric Measurements

Anthropometric measures are an essential component of pediatric nutrition assessment. Body weight, recumbent length or height, and head circumference (birth to 24 months) are the most common growth indices in pediatric patients. Individual measurements are compared to population data represented by percentile curves on a growth chart. The 2006 World Health Organization (WHO) growth charts should be used for all patients 0–24 months of age (Grummer-Strawn et al. 2010). The 2000 Center for Disease Control (CDC) growth charts should be used for ages 2–20 years. Poor weight gain may signify acute malnutrition, while inadequate linear growth may indicate chronic malnutrition or stunting. The Waterlow Criteria (Tables 21.1 and 21.2) are often used to help determine the degree of stunting or wasting in children aged 1–3 years (Waterlow et al. 1977). Atypical growth suggesting underweight or stunting may be suspected when the weight or height for age is below the second percentile when using the WHO charts or fifth percentile on the CDC charts. The CDC recommends using body mass index in children over the age of 2 to identify underweight (<5th percentile), overweight (85th–95th percentile), and obesity (equal to or >95th percentile).

Accurate heights and weights are often difficult to obtain in the ICU. Recumbent lengths or a reported stature measure from a caregiver are often used due to inability to measure standing height during critical illness. Trauma, burn, or surgical patients may require casting, traction, or dressings and obtaining a reliable weight is not possible. Initially, it may be necessary to use an estimated weight from a caregiver or the most recent weight from a medical visit. Obtaining previous growth charts to assess growth over time is optimal and may help identify preexisting malnutrition. Daily weights may be helpful to assess the adequacy of the nutrition regimen; however, in the presence of edema, ascites, fluid resuscitation, or diuresis weights may not reflect intake.

Head circumference is closely related to brain growth, and the American Academy of Pediatrics (AAP) recommends monitoring head circumference at each well child visit until 24 months of age. Decreases in head growth may occur in severely undernourished children who often have poor linear growth. A rapid increase in head circumference may indicate hydrocephalus (Allen 2012).

TABLE 21.1
Waterlow Criteria for Degree of Wasting

>120%	Obese
110%–120%	Overweight
90%–110%	Normal
80%–89%	Mild wasting
70%–79%	Moderate wasting
<70%	Severe wasting

Source: Waterlow, J.C. et al., *Bull. World Health Organ.*, 55(4), 1977, 489.

TABLE 21.2
Waterlow Criteria for Degree of Stunting

>95%	Normal
90%–95%	Mild
85%–89%	Moderate
<85%	Severe

Source: Waterlow, J.C. et al., *Bull. World Health Organ.*, 55(4), 1977, 489.

Biochemical Assessment

Laboratory parameters are part of a complete nutrition assessment that must be interpreted in the context of critical illness. Serum albumin, prealbumin, transferrin, and retinol binding protein may not reflect nutrition status during stress, inflammation, and infection (Mehta et al. 2009b). Production of these negative acute phase reactants are downregulated, while positive acute phase proteins, such as C-reactive protein and ferritin, are preferentially produced by the liver and necessary for recovery. Serum albumin also decreases with fluid resuscitation, liver disease, and increased capillary permeability and increases with albumin infusion and dehydration. Prealbumin has a half-life of 24–48 h and is decreased in liver disease and increased in renal failure. C-reactive protein measures the acute phase response and reflects the severity of injury. Decreasing levels may signify a return to the anabolic phase with a subsequent rise in prealbumin (Mehta et al. 2009b).

Food and Nutrition–Related History

A diet history is important in nutrition assessment as it may identify preexisting energy, protein, or micronutrient deficits or excess. Inquiry regarding formula preparation for infants is important because inaccurate mixing may contribute to altered growth, dehydration, or electrolyte abnormalities. Assessment of the typical volume tolerated may be helpful in developing enteral regimens for patients with gastroesophageal reflux. Infants and children may also have food allergies that should be identified upon admission. Allergens should be considered when selecting an infant formula or tube feeding as standard pediatric products are cow milk based and exposure to the allergen may result in respiratory distress or enterocolitis.

Nutrition-Focused Physical Exam

A nutrition-focused physical exam (NFPE) may help identify over- and undernutrition as well as clinical signs of nutrient deficiencies or excess. This is useful in critical illness when biochemical markers are affected by stress and inflammation and anthropometrics are difficult to obtain or inaccurate due to fluid status. NFPE may also identify dehydration, fluid overload, or edema. NFPE can be a thorough head to toe exam or may be focused on a particular system based on information obtained from the medical or diet history.

NUTRITIONAL REQUIREMENTS

Energy

Energy requirements during critical illness in pediatric patients are variable and are based on age, metabolic stress, comorbidities, preexisting nutritional status, and the need for resumed growth later in the course of illness. Accurate assessment of energy needs is important to prevent over- and underfeeding. Overfeeding is associated with fatty liver, increased carbon dioxide production, and difficulty weaning from mechanical ventilation (Mehta et al. 2009b). Hyperglycemia due to overfeeding has been shown to prolong mechanical ventilation and hospital length of stay (Alaedeen et al. 2006). Underfeeding may impair immune function, deplete muscle mass, and compromise respiratory status when the diaphragm and intercostal muscles are affected (Hulst et al. 2006).

It was previously thought that critically ill children become hypermetabolic due to an increased turnover of protein, carbohydrate, and fat. However, current pediatric research indicates the impact on metabolism is variable and the severity of illness does not always correspond with the effect on metabolism (Botran et al. 2011a). Children who suffer severe trauma or burns are hypermetabolic (Suman et al. 2006; Botran et al. 2011a), but most children are normometabolic or even hypometabolic during illness (Mehta et al. 2009a; Briassoulis et al. 2010). A study conducted by Framson measured resting energy expenditure via indirect calorimetry (IC) in critically ill children and found a

TABLE 21.3
Children at High Risk for Metabolic Alterations Who Are Suggested Candidates for Targeted Measurement of REE in the PICU

- Underweight (BMI < 5th percentile for age), at risk of overweight (BMI > 85th percentile for age), or overweight (BMI > 95th percentile for age).
- Children with >10% weight gain or loss during ICU stay.
- Failure to consistently meet prescribed caloric goals.
- Failure to wean or need to escalate respiratory support.
- Need for muscle relaxants for >7 days.
- Neurological trauma (traumatic, hypoxic, and/or ischemic) with evidence of dysautonomia.
- Oncological diagnoses (including children with stem cell or bone marrow transplant).
- Children with thermal injury.
- Children requiring mechanical ventilator support for >7 days.
- Children suspected to be severely hypermetabolic (status epilepticus, hyperthermia, systemic inflammatory response syndrome, dysautonomic storms, etc.) or hypometabolic (hypothermia, hypothyroidism, pentobarbital or midazolam coma, etc.).
- Any patient with ICU LOS (length of stay) >4 weeks may benefit from IC to assess adequacy of nutrient intake.

Source: Mehta, N.M. et al., *J. Parenter. Enteral Nutr.*, 33(3), 2009, 260. With permission.

hypometabolic pattern predominated during the early acute phase of the illness and hypermetabolism did not occur until convalescence. It was concluded that most forms of critical illness do not cause children to become hypermetabolic and EE may be close to or less than predicted basal metabolic rate (Framson et al. 2007). To explain the impact on metabolism and EE in children, it has been suggested that growth ceases during critical illness and the energy previously used for growth is redirected toward meeting the demands of the acute illness. Other factors that may decrease the REE include the use of mechanical ventilation, which will decrease the work of breathing; the use of sedatives which decrease brain function; and neuromuscular blockades, which paralyze the skeletal muscle.

Commonly used predictive equations are based on IC data in healthy children with added stress factors to account for illness. These equations have been shown to be inaccurate, resulting in both under- and overfeeding (Mehta et al. 2011). Indirect calorimetry is the gold standard to measure energy needs in this population; however, despite the known advantages, its use in clinical practice is often limited due to lack of resources, the expertise needed to administer and interpret the test, and the clinical condition of the patient. Inaccurate measurement may occur in patients with ventilatory leaks or high oxygen requirements ($FIO_2 > 50\%$). The American Society for Parenteral and Enteral Nutrition (ASPEN) recommends the use of indirect calorimetry to assess energy expenditure in pediatric patients at risk for metabolic alterations (Table 21.3) (Mehta et al. 2009b). If IC is not possible, then commonly used equations such as the World Health Organization (WHO) (Anonymous 1985) and the Schofield (1985), which estimate basal metabolic rate, may be used without the addition of stress or correction factors (Table 21.4). General guidelines for energy requirements based on kilogram of body weight are often used (Table 21.5). Regardless of the method used to estimate energy needs, reassessment throughout the course of the illness is necessary.

Protein Requirements

The provision of adequate protein may be the single most important nutrition intervention for critically ill children. The precise protein requirements of critically ill children have yet to be established but needs appear higher than healthy children in order to optimize protein synthesis, reduce catabolism, and facilitate wound healing and the inflammatory response (Mehta et al. 2009b). Protein loss can be significant if chest tubes and open wounds are present. Requirements vary depending upon age and diagnosis

TABLE 21.4
Common Equations to Predict Metabolic Rate

Age (Years)	Calories/Day World Health Organization	Schofield
Male		
0 to 3	60.9(*W*) − 54	0.167(*W*) + 15.174(*H*) − 617.6
>3 to 10	22.7(*W*) + 495	19.59(*W*) + 1.303(*H*) + 414.9
>10 to 18	17.5(*W*) + 651	16.25(*W*) + 1.372(*H*) + 515.5
Female		
0 to 3	61(*W*) − 51	16.252(*W*) + 10.232(*H*) − 413.5
>3 to 10	22.5(*W*) + 499	16.969(*W*) + 1.618(*H*) + 371.2
>10 to 18	12.2(*W*) + 746	8.365(*W*) + 4.65(*H*) + 200.0
W = weight in kg	*H* = height in cm	

Sources: Energy and protein requirements, Report of a joint FAO/WHO/UNU expert consultation, World Health Organization Technical Report Series, 724, 1985, 1–206; Schofield, W.N., *Hum. Nutr. Clin. Nutr.*, 39(Suppl. 1), 5–41, 1985.

TABLE 21.5
Daily Energy Requirements (Total kcal/kg) for Pediatric Patients

Preterm neonate	90–120
<6 months	85–105
6–12 months	80–100
1–7 years	75–90
7–12 years	50–75
>12–18 years	30–50

Source: Mirtallo, J. et al., *J. Parenter. Enteral Nutr.*, 28(6), S39, 2004.

(Premji et al. 2006). Based upon expert consensus, ASPEN recommends 0–2 years, 2–3 g/kg/day; 2–13 years, 1.5–2 g/kg/day; and 13–18 years, 1.5 g/kg/day (Mehta et al. 2009b). Several recent studies support protein requirements close to 3 g/kg/day in critically ill infants and children (van Waardenburg et al. 2009; Botrán et al. 2011b; de Betue et al. 2011). Care should be taken to avoid excessive intake, especially in the presence of altered hepatic or renal function. Intakes ≥4 g/kg/day have been associated with conditions such as azotemia and metabolic acidosis (Premji et al. 2006, CD003959).

Fluid and Electrolyte Requirements

Daily fluid needs vary with age, level of physical exertion, and disease state. Premature infants and patients with gastrointestinal (GI) losses, burns, or high fever have increased fluid needs. Patients with conditions such as oliguric renal failure, lung disease, or heart failure may have decreased fluid needs. Maintenance fluid needs are based on insensible losses from the respiratory tract and skin and sensible losses from urine and stool. One of the most commonly used methods to estimate fluid needs is the Holliday–Segar method (Table 21.6), which is based on weight or determination of body surface area multiplied by 1500–1700 mL (Holliday et al. 2007). Electrolyte management in critically ill children requires frequent monitoring and evaluation. Serum levels can be affected by intake and output, acid–base balance, hormone secretion, and disturbances in organ and gland function (Mehta and Duggan 2009). Electrolyte requirements vary according to age and are dosed according to body weight (Table 21.7).

TABLE 21.6
Holliday–Segar Fluid Calculation

Weight	Fluid Needs
1–10 kg	100 mL/kg
>10 to 20 kg	1000 mL for the first 10 kg, plus 50 mL/kg over 10 kg
>20 to 80 kg	1500 mL for the first 20 kg, plus 20 mL/kg over 20 kg up to 2400 mL/day

Source: Holliday, M.A. et al., *Arch. Dis. Child.*, 92(6) (Jun), 546, 2007.

TABLE 21.7
Electrolyte Dosing Guidelines[a]

	Preterm Neonates	Infants/Children	Adolescents and Children >50 kg
Sodium	2–5 mEq/kg	2–5 mEq/kg	1–2 mEq/kg
Potassium	2–4 mEq/kg	2–4 mEq/kg	1–2 mEq/kg
Calcium	2–4 mEq/kg	0.5–4 mEq/kg	10–20 mEq
Phosphorus	1–2 mmol/kg	0.5–2 mmol/kg	10–40 mmol
Magnesium	0.3–0.5 mEq/kg	0.3–0.5 mEq/kg	10–30 mEq
Acetate	As needed to maintain acid–base balance		
Chloride	As needed to maintain acid–base balance		

Source: Reprinted from Mirtallo, J. et al., *J. Parenter. Enteral Nutr.*, 28(6), S39, 2004. With permission.
[a] Assumes normal organ function and losses.

Micronutrient Requirements

The requirements of vitamins and minerals in the critically ill child have not been extensively studied. Generally, the dietary reference intakes (DRIs) are recommended as the goal for micronutrients unless there is a clinical condition that may increase losses and result in deficiencies (Mehta and Duggan 2009). It is important to determine the volume of formula required to meet the DRI for patients receiving enteral feeds and provide additional supplementation if needed.

Over the past few years, there has been a major focus on vitamin D due to the degree of deficiency being reported, as well as its potential role beyond bone health. Recent literature has investigated vitamin D status and critical illness. McNally et al. and Madden et al. found vitamin D deficiency was common among critically ill children and associated with an increased severity of critical illness (Madden et al. 2012; McNally et al. 2012). Both suggest further investigation regarding the role of vitamin D to improve clinical outcome. The best indicator of vitamin D status is the measurement of 25-hydroxy vitamin D. Goal serum levels are considered to be >30 ng/mL, insufficiency from 21 to 29 ng/mL and deficiency <20 ng/mL (Holick et al. 2011). Breastfed infants are at high risk for deficiency due to the low vitamin D content in human milk. AAP recommends breastfed infants and infants receiving less than 1000 mL infant formula per day supplement with 400 IU vitamin D daily (Wagner et al. 2008). Premature infants, children with dark skin, and children taking anticonvulsants are also at risk for deficiency. The recommendation for critically ill children receiving nutrition support is to screen and assess vitamin D status to determine the need for supplementation. Infants and children who are deficient should receive 1000–2000 IU per day of D2 or D3 or 50,000 IU of D2 per week for 6 weeks to achieve a blood level above 30 ng/mL (Holick et al. 2011). Current research suggests that at high doses vitamin D3 may be more effective than D2 (Institute of Medicine (US) 2011; Tripkovic et al. 2012).

Research investigating zinc status in critically ill children found that low serum zinc levels were associated with decreased survival in patients who developed septic shock (Cander et al. 2011). Cvijanovich et al. investigated zinc homeostasis and found a correlation between low serum zinc levels and organ failure (Cvijanovich et al. 2009). Both studies recommend the need for further investigation into the role and benefit of zinc supplementation in critically ill children. Currently, serum zinc is used to assess zinc status; however, it is not considered a sensitive indicator. Evidence-based guidelines are not yet available for zinc supplementation. Once zinc supplementation is started, levels should be reassessed every 10–14 days until the serum value is corrected. Excessive enteral zinc administration should be avoided as it may impair copper absorption resulting in anemia as copper is required for iron absorption.

NUTRITIONAL DELIVERY ROUTES

Enteral Nutrition

Enteral nutrition is the preferred mode of feeding in critically ill infants and children with a functioning gastrointestinal tract and respiratory and hemodynamic stability. Some advantages of enteral feeding over parenteral nutrition (PN) are lower cost, safety, preservation of gastric function, and fewer infectious complications (Skillman and Mehta 2012a). Early enteral feeding within 24–72 h of admission is considered safe and can be used in most pediatric patients.

Formula Selection

Enteral formula selection is dependent upon age, diagnosis, fluid allowance, and the nutrient needs of the infant or child. Currently, there are no enteral formulas that have been specifically designed for critically ill infants and children. For most infants, human milk is the feeding of choice due to a multitude of benefits including gastrointestinal health and motility as well as immunological properties (Schanler 2011). Standard cow milk–based infant formula is used as a supplement or substitute to human milk. If the infant is sensitive to lactose, then a cow milk–based, lactose-free infant formula or soy-based formula would be appropriate. Protein hydrolysates or an infant formula with free amino acids is intended for infants allergic to cow milk or soy protein or who have malabsorptive conditions such as short bowel syndrome. Disease-specific formulas are available for those infants with lipid disorders such as chylothorax, renal dysfunction, metabolic disorders, or those born prematurely. At standard dilution, infant formula provides 20 kcal/oz and variable protein. Human milk is generally considered 20 kcal/oz though exact caloric density as well as protein and fat content are not easily estimated as it has a dynamic nutrient composition.

Formulas are available for children 1–10 years of age. Standard polymeric formulas are well tolerated in most children. Cow milk–based, soy-based, meat-based, peptide-based, and free amino acid formulas are available. Peptide and amino acid–based formulas are appropriate for children with limited digestive and absorptive capacity or multiple food allergies. These formulas provide 20, 30, or 45 kcal/oz and variable protein. Some formulas have soy fiber added for those with constipation. Adult formulas can be used for children over the age of 10 years. The source of carbohydrate, protein, and fat is similar to those used in formulations intended for children less than 10 years of age, but the vitamin and mineral content is different and should be evaluated for adequacy. The routine use of immune enhancing formulas that contain a variety of nutrients such as arginine, glutamine, and omega 3 fatty acids is not recommended at this time. Reported benefits are mixed and primarily based on adult studies, and the safety and efficacy of their use in children is questionable (Mehta et al. 2009b).

The goal of enteral nutrition is to meet estimated caloric, protein, and vitamin and mineral requirements. If fluids are restricted in infants, then human milk or infant formula may not meet caloric or protein goals at standard dilution. Infant formula can be concentrated up to 27 cal/oz. Depending upon the needs of the infant, additional calories or nutrients can be added to infant formula or human milk in the form of infant formula concentrate, liquid carbohydrate, liquid fat, or human milk fortifier. Use of powdered components is not recommended for critically ill infants as these are not sterile. Since there is a range of caloric density available for those over the age of 1, it is easier to meet estimated caloric need. If, however, estimated energy requirements are low, then protein, sodium, and vitamin or mineral needs may not be met. Modular components are available to increase the caloric or protein content of pediatric formula and vitamin and mineral supplements can be added to specifically tailor a formula to meet individual need.

Enteral Administration

Nasogastric tube feeding is indicated if the infant or child is unable to orally feed due to altered neurological status and respiratory failure or if the airway cannot be protected due to depressed cough or gag (Mehta 2009). If the infant or child has increased gastric distention or is at high risk of aspiration due to delayed gastric emptying, then the tube may be placed transpylorically into the small bowel. There are insufficient data to support routine use of transpyloric feeding over nasogastric feeding (Mehta et al. 2009b).

Two methods are used for the delivery of enteral nutrition by tube. Intermittent bolus feedings deliver formula at timed intervals typically every 3, 4, or 6 h over a period of time similar to an oral feeding. Bolus feedings are initiated at small volume with slow increases until goal is met. A continuous infusion is necessary for transpyloric feeding or for those who do not tolerate bolus feeds. Continuous feedings can be started at 1–2 mL/kg/h in infants and small children and 25 mL/kg/h in older children with slow advancement to goal (Carney et al. 2010).

Monitoring

Barriers to achieving nutrition goals exist in the PICU. The most common reasons for feeding interruptions are medical procedures, feeding intolerance, and fluid restriction. At least 50% of these interruptions (Mehta 2009) have been found to be avoidable, which supports the need for the development of evidence-based guidelines and protocols (Mehta 2009). Brown et al. demonstrated that the use of a gastric feeding protocol improved feeding tolerance and decreased the length of time to achieve energy goals (Brown 2012). Protocols help maximize caloric intake, achieve goals, and improve feeding tolerance as they lead the practitioner through a decision-making process for enteral nutrition initiation and advancement (Skillman and Mehta 2012a). Protocols also provide guidelines for monitoring and managing the complications of enteral nutrition and feeding intolerance.

Feeding intolerance due to GI complications includes abdominal distention, diarrhea, constipation, gastroesophageal reflux disease (GERD), and emesis. Gastric residual volume (GRV) is often used as a measure for gastric emptying. An increased GRV is thought to correlate with an increased risk for aspiration. However, there is no evidence for an acceptable GRV in critically ill children, nor is the lower limit that will protect from aspiration known. The GRV measurement assumes that residual is only infused formula and does not take into consideration the contribution from gastric juice and salivary production. The decision to interrupt feeds should be based on a variety of factors such as abdominal distention, discomfort, vomiting, and diarrhea and not a GRV measurement (Mehta et al. 2010). If gastric feeds are not tolerated or if there is a high risk of aspiration, post-pyloric feeding may be warranted (Mehta et al. 2009b). The use of blue food dye for the diagnosis of aspiration is not recommended due to low sensitivity and association with increased mortality (Kattelmann et al. 2006). Constipation may become a significant problem especially in young children receiving opiates as they decrease transit time and increase water absorption resulting in dry, hard stools. The addition of fiber, adequate fluids, and the use of laxatives or stool softeners may be required. Diarrhea defined as >3 watery stools in 24 h may be related to the osmolarity of the formula, as well as microbial contamination. Preventative measures include proper hang time; use of sterile, liquid formula; and aseptic technique in handling formula and enteral feeding equipment (Lyman and Colombo 2010). Diarrhea may be due to nonformula factors, such as high sorbitol content of medications, withdrawal from opiates, or prolonged antibiotic use. The use of prebiotics or probiotics in pediatric critically ill patients is not yet supported by evidence (Mehta et al. 2009b). Other GI complications include nausea and vomiting, which may be related to medications or delayed gastric emptying (Bourgault et al. 2007).

Parenteral Nutrition

PN may be considered when the GI tract is nonfunctional or when nutritional needs cannot be met with enteral feeding. The length of time that an individual patient can tolerate inadequate nutrient intake is based on the patient's age, nutritional status, and underlying disease. In general, normally nourished children should be given PN after 5 days of suboptimal enteral nutrient intake (Skillman and Mehta 2012b). PN should be initiated sooner in malnourished patients or infants and neonates with anticipated suboptimal enteral nutrient intake greater than 3–5 days (Skillman and Mehta 2012a). PN should be used judiciously because of the increased risk of infection as well as liver damage associated with long-term use (Wylie et al. 2010).

Composition of PN

In pediatrics, a tailored PN solution is often used to meet the individualized needs of the infant or child versus a standard formula. The desired fluid volume is kept constant and macronutrients are increased to meet energy and protein goals. Dextrose (3.4 kcal/g) is initiated and advanced based on glucose infusion rate (GIR). Infants and children can tolerate a higher GIR than adolescents (Table 21.8). Dextrose should be initiated at 5–6 mg/kg/min for infants and 10% dextrose for children and adolescents (Carney et al. 2010). Gradual increases of 2.5%–5% dextrose per day to goal are usually well tolerated.

Crystalline amino acids (4 kcal/g) are the protein source in PN. Specialized pediatric AA products have been developed with high concentrations of histidine and tyrosine, which are essential amino acids for the young infant (Carney et al. 2010). They are formulated to promote growth in neonates and young infants and to achieve a plasma amino acid pattern similar to the amino acid pattern of postprandial breastfed infants. The pH is lower than standard products, which allows for the addition of more calcium and phosphorous that is necessary in infancy (Carney et al. 2010). These specialized AA products are often used in patients ≤1 year of age and long-term PN dependent children with cholestasis. Cysteine is a conditionally essential amino acid for premature infants

TABLE 21.8
Glucose Infusion Rate

Age Group	GIR Goal (mg/kg/min)	
Preterm infants	8–12	(Max 14–18)
Term infants	12	(Max 14–18)
Children (1–10 years)	8–10	
Adolescents	5–6	

Source: Carney, L. et al., Parenteral and enteral support: Determining the best way to feed, in: *The A.S.P.E.N. Pediatric Nutrition Support Core Curriculum*, Corkins, M. (ed.), American Society for Parenteral and Enteral Nutrition, Silver Spring, MD, 2010, pp. 433–447.

because unlike adults they are unable to synthesize it from methionine. The recommended amount of L-cysteine hydrochloride is typically 40 mg/g of AA and is typically given for the first year of life and must be added separately (Carney et al. 2010).

Fatty acids are an important energy source in critically ill children. The risk of EFAD in children receiving fat-free PN is greater because of the increased rate of fat oxidation and limited fat stores. Infants and children must receive at least 0.5–1.0 g/kg/day of lipid or 4.5% of linoleic and 0.5% of linolenic acid to prevent EFAD (Carney and Blair 2010). Intravenous fat emulsion (IVFE) is typically initiated at 0.5–1.0 g/kg/day and advanced by 0.5–1.0 g/kg/day to a maximum intake of 4 g/kg/day or 30%–40% of total calories with close monitoring of triglyceride levels. The maximum lipid infusion rate is 0.15 g/kg/h in term infants (Szeszycki 2010). The CDC recommends that intravenous lipid infusions not be infused longer than 12 h to avoid microbial growth (O'Grady et al. 2002). If a child has an egg allergy, a test dose of lipid should first be given as the long chain triglyceride contains egg phospholipid.

Vitamins and Trace Elements

Standard commercial vitamin and trace element preparations are generally used; however, certain medical conditions may require customization. For children with cholestasis, it is recommended to decrease copper intake by 50% and eliminate manganese (Carney et al. 2010). Additional zinc may be required for children with short bowel syndrome (SBS) or excessive GI loss (Carney et al. 2010). An ASPEN task force recently assessed scientific evidence in order to recommend changes in the manufacturing of parenteral and multitrace element solutions (Vanek et al. 2012). Limited pediatric research exists to support recommending changes to the pediatric multivitamin products at this time. The task force however did recommend adding 2 mcg/kg/day of selenium to all pediatric PN solutions and reducing manganese to 1 mcg/kg/day with a daily maximum dose of 55 mcg/day. Chromium is part of the pediatric TE solutions and is also found as a contaminant in PN solutions, which has resulted in elevated levels in pediatric patients (Buchman et al. 2001). These findings led the committee to recommend the creation of a pediatric product without chromium (Vanek et al. 2012). Carnitine is a compound responsible for transporting fatty acids into the mitochondria of the cell. Deficiency can result in impaired lipid metabolism with subsequent hypertriglyceridemia. Currently, the use of carnitine is limited to neonatal PN and in select pediatric cases. The committee recommended providing 2–5 mg/kg/day carnitine as part of a multivitamin or multiple trace element product or as individual product for neonates. Current practice is to monitor serum levels and adjust supplementation from 8 to 10 mg/kg/day and adjust to a maximum of 20 mg/kg/day (Carney et al. 2010).

Monitoring

PN monitoring is essential to prevent complications. Daily weights, evaluation of total fluid intake and output, physical exam, vital signs, and laboratory values can help determine if the patient is tolerating PN volume. Signs of dehydration may include a rapid decrease in weight, tachycardia, and increased BUN, sodium, albumin, hemoglobin, and urine-specific gravity. Physical examination in patients with dehydration may reveal dry skin, lips, and mucous membranes, whereas fluid overload may be accompanied by a rapid increase in weight, tachypnea, and decreased sodium, albumin, hemoglobin, and urine-specific gravity. Physical examination may reveal edema and increased abdominal girth (Szeszycki 2010).

Laboratory monitoring may help prevent metabolic complications. Baseline monitoring should include glucose, a basic chemistry panel, magnesium, phosphorous, triglycerides, prealbumin, and albumin. Laboratory values should be monitored daily until the patient is receiving their goal PN solution. As the patient stabilizes, the frequency may be decreased to twice weekly and then weekly. Liver function tests (alkaline phosphatase, ALT, AST, GGT) and total bilirubin should be ordered weekly and copper and manganese should be checked in patients with a total bilirubin >2 mg/dL (Szeszycki 2010). Glucose should be monitored as the dextrose concentration is increased to prevent hyperglycemia. If hyperglycemia is present, then a reduction in GIR should be considered. The use of insulin should be carefully evaluated. The adult literature recommends tight glucose control, but at this time evidence-based guidelines are not available for children and aggressive glycemic control is not recommended (Mehta et al. 2009b). Triglycerides should be monitored initially and with each increase until patients receive goal volume of lipid and then may be decreased to weekly. If hypertriglyceridemia occurs (>200 mg/dL), the lipids can be held until levels normalize and restarted at 0.5 g/kg/day (Szeszycki 2010).

CONCLUSION

Critically ill children are at high risk for malnutrition due to their limited nutrient reserves and associated catabolism that occurs as a result of the metabolic response to stress. Nutrition assessment with accurate evaluation of energy and protein needs is important to prevent over- and underfeeding. Close monitoring and frequent reassessment is required to adjust nutrition therapy throughout the phases of critical illness.

CASE STUDY

CE is a full-term infant admitted to the PICU on day 1 of life. Medical diagnosis includes transposition of the great arteries with need for a balloon atrial septostomy. When using the WHO growth chart, the birth weight of 3.1 kg fell at the 25th percentile, birth length of 50 cm fell at the 50th percentile, and head circumference of 34 cm at the 25th percentile. Growth parameters were appropriate for gestational age (AGA). Estimated parenteral caloric needs were 100 kcal/kg based on 90% of DRI as the patient was sedated on mechanical ventilation. Estimated protein needs were 2–3 g/kg based on ASPEN guidelines for critical illness. PN was initiated on day 1 of life. By day 4 of life, CE was meeting 70% of caloric goal, the lower end of estimated protein need, and meeting essential fatty acid need. CE developed hyperglycemia and the concentration of dextrose was lowered from 10 to 7 mg/kg/min with normalization of serum glucose. Serum triglyceride levels were within normal limits. By day 8 of life, PN met 100% of caloric and protein goals. A nasogastric tube was placed and continuous feeds of mother's milk were initiated. Nasogastric feeds were advanced per PICU protocol to full volume while PN was weaned. Fluids were restricted and caloric density of mother's milk was advanced to 27 cal/oz using a combination of human milk fortifier and term infant formula concentrate. CE was successfully weaned from mechanical ventilation on day 18 of life. Upon weaning from the ventilator, caloric goal was increased to 115 kcal/kg based on DRI for age. CE was transitioned from continuous nasogastric feeds to bolus feeds. He was then allowed to orally feed with supplemental tube feeding until he was able to consume 100% goal volume by mouth. Caloric density of feeds was decreased to 24 cal/oz in preparation for home. Parents were instructed on preparation of 24 cal/oz human milk using term formula powder. CE was discharged to home on day 25 of life.

REFERENCES

Alaedeen, D. I., M. C. Walsh, and W. J. Chwals. 2006. Total parenteral nutrition-associated hyperglycemia correlates with prolonged mechanical ventilation and hospital stay in septic infants. *Journal of Pediatric Surgery* 41 (1) (Jan): 239–244; discussion 239–244.

Allen, J. M. 2012. Vasoactive substances and their effects on nutrition in the critically ill patient. *Nutrition in Clinical Practice: Official Publication of the American Society for Parenteral and Enteral Nutrition* 27 (3) (Jun 13): 335–339.

Anonymous. Energy and protein requirements. Report of a joint FAO/WHO/UNU expert consultation. 1985. *World Health Organization Technical Report Series* 724: 1–206.

Botran, M., J. Lopez-Herce, S. Mencia, J. Urbano, M. J. Solana, A. Garcia, and A. Carrillo. 2011a. Relationship between energy expenditure, nutritional status and clinical severity before starting enteral nutrition in critically ill children. *The British Journal of Nutrition* 105 (5) (Mar): 731–737.

Botrán, M., J. López-Herce, S. Mencía, J. Urbano, M. J. Solana, and A. García. 2011b. Enteral nutrition in the critically ill child: Comparison of standard and protein-enriched diets. *The Journal of Pediatrics* 159 (1) (7): 27, 32.e1.

Bourgault, A. M., L. Ipe, J. Weaver, S. Swartz, and P. J. O'dea. 2007. Development of evidence-based guidelines and critical care nurses ' knowledge of enteral feeding. *Critical Care Nurse* 27 (4) (Aug): 17, 22, 25–29; quiz 30.

Briassoulis, G., S. Venkataraman, and A. Thompson. 2010. Cytokines and metabolic patterns in pediatric patients with critical illness. *Clinical and Developmental Immunology* 2010: 354047.

Brown, A. 2012. Effects of a gastric feeding protocol on efficiency of enteral nutrition in critically ill infants and children. *Infant and Child Adolescent Nutrition* 4: 175–180.

Buchman, A. L., M. Neely, V. B. Grossie Jr., L. Truong, E. Lykissa, and C. Ahn. 2001. Organ heavy-metal accumulation during parenteral nutrition is associated with pathologic abnormalities in rats. *Nutrition (Burbank, Los Angeles County, Calif.)* 17 (7–8) (Jul–Aug): 600–606.

Cander, B., Z. D. Dundar, M. Gul, and S. Girisgin. 2011. Prognostic value of serum zinc levels in critically ill patients. *Journal of Critical Care* 26 (1) (Feb): 42–46.

Carney, L., and J. Blair. 2010. Assessment of nutrition status by age and determining nutrient needs. In *The A.S.P.E.N. Pediatric Nutrition Support Core Curriculum*, ed. M. Corkins, p. 409. Silver Spring, MD: American Society for Parenteral and Enteral Nutrition.

Carney, L., A. Nepa, and S. Cohen. 2010. Parenteral and enteral support: Determining the best way to feed. In *The A.S.P.E.N. Pediatric Nutrition Support Core Curriculum*, ed. M. Corkins, pp. 433–447. Silver Spring, MD: American Society for Parenteral and Enteral Nutrition.

Cvijanovich, N. Z., J. C. King, H. R. Flori, G. Gildengorin, and H. R. Wong. 2009. Zinc homeostasis in pediatric critical illness. *Pediatric Critical Care Medicine: A Journal of the Society of Critical Care Medicine and the World Federation of Pediatric Intensive and Critical Care Societies* 10 (1) (Jan): 29–34.

de Betue, C. T., D. A. van Waardenburg, N. E. Deutz, H. M. van Eijk, J. B. van Goudoever, Y. C. Luiking, L. J. Zimmermann, and K. F. Joosten. 2011. Increased protein-energy intake promotes anabolism in critically ill infants with viral bronchiolitis: A double-blind randomised controlled trial. *Archives of Disease in Childhood* 96 (9) (Sep): 817–822.

Faustino, E. V. and M. Apkon. 2005. Persistent hyperglycemia in critically ill children. *The Journal of Pediatrics* 146 (1) (Jan): 30–34.

Framson, C. M., N. S. LeLeiko, G. E. Dallal, R. Roubenoff, L. K. Snelling, and J. T. Dwyer. 2007. Energy expenditure in critically ill children. *Pediatric Critical Care Medicine: A Journal of the Society of Critical Care Medicine and the World Federation of Pediatric Intensive and Critical Care Societies* 8 (3) (May): 264–267.

Grummer-Strawn, L. M., C. Reinold, N. F. Krebs, and Centers for Disease Control and Prevention (CDC). 2010. Use of World Health Organization and CDC growth charts for children aged 0–59 months in the United States. *MMWR. Recommendations and Reports: Morbidity and Mortality Weekly Report. Recommendations and Reports/Centers for Disease Control* 59 (RR-9) (Sep 10): 1–15.

Holick, M. F., N. C. Binkley, H. A. Bischoff-Ferrari, C. M. Gordon, D. A. Hanley, R. P. Heaney, M. H. Murad, C. M. Weaver, and Endocrine Society. 2011. Evaluation, treatment, and prevention of vitamin D deficiency: An Endocrine Society clinical practice guideline. *The Journal of Clinical Endocrinology and Metabolism* 96 (7) (Jul): 1911–1930.

Holliday, M. A., P. E. Ray, and A. L. Friedman. 2007. Fluid therapy for children: Facts, fashions and questions. *Archives of Disease in Childhood* 92 (6) (Jun): 546–550.

Hulst, J. M., K. F. Joosten, D. Tibboel, and J. B. van Goudoever. 2006. Causes and consequences of inadequate substrate supply to pediatric ICU patients. *Current Opinion in Clinical Nutrition and Metabolic Care* 9 (3) (May): 297–303.

IOM (Institute of Medicine). 2011. Dietary Reference Intakes for Calcium and Vitamin D. Washington, DC: The National Academies Press.

Kattelmann, K. K., M. Hise, M. Russell, P. Charney, M. Stokes, and C. Compher. 2006. Preliminary evidence for a medical nutrition therapy protocol: Enteral feedings for critically ill patients. *Journal of the American Dietetic Association* 106 (8) (Aug): 1226–1241.

Lyman B., J. Colombo, and J. Gamis. 2010. Implementation of the Plan. In *The A.S.P.E.N. Pediatric Nutrition Support Core Curriculum*, M. Corkins, (ed.) p. 455. SilverSpring, MD: American Society for Parenteral and Enteral Nutrition.

Madden, K., H. A. Feldman, E. M. Smith, C. M. Gordon, S. M. Keisling, R. M. Sullivan, B. W. Hollis, A. A. Agan, and A. G. Randolph. 2012. Vitamin D deficiency in critically ill children. *Pediatrics* 130 (3) (Sep): 421–428.

McNally, J. D., K. Menon, P. Chakraborty, L. Fisher, K. A. Williams, O. Y. Al-Dirbashi, D. R. Doherty, and on behalf of the Canadian Critical Care Trials Group. 2012. The association of vitamin D status with pediatric critical illness. *Pediatrics* 130 (3) (Sep): 429–436.

Mehta, N. M. 2009. Approach to enteral feeding in the PICU. *Nutrition in Clinical Practice: Official Publication of the American Society for Parenteral and Enteral Nutrition* 24 (3) (Jun–Jul): 377–387.

Mehta, N. M., L. J. Bechard, N. Cahill, M. Wang, A. Day, C. P. Duggan, and D. K. Heyland. 2012. Nutritional practices and their relationship to clinical outcomes in critically ill children-an international multicenter cohort study. *Critical Care Medicine* 40 (7) (Jul): 2204–2211.

Mehta, N. M., L. J. Bechard, M. Dolan, K. Ariagno, H. Jiang, and C. Duggan. 2011. Energy imbalance and the risk of overfeeding in critically ill children. *Pediatric Critical Care Medicine: A Journal of the Society of Critical Care Medicine and the World Federation of Pediatric Intensive and Critical Care Societies* 12 (4) (Jul): 398–405.

Mehta, N. M., L. J. Bechard, K. Leavitt, and C. Duggan. 2009a. Cumulative energy imbalance in the pediatric intensive care unit: Role of targeted indirect calorimetry. *JPEN: Journal of Parenteral and Enteral Nutrition* 33 (3) (May–Jun): 336–344.

Mehta, N. M., C. Compher, and A.S.P.E.N. Board of Directors. 2009b. A.S.P.E.N. clinical guidelines: Nutrition support of the critically ill child. *JPEN: Journal of Parenteral and Enteral Nutrition* 33 (3) (May–Jun): 260–276.

Mehta, N. M. and C. P. Duggan. 2009. Nutritional deficiencies during critical illness. *Pediatric Clinics of North America* 56 (5) (Oct): 1143–1160.

Mehta, N. M., D. McAleer, S. Hamilton, E. Naples, K. Leavitt, P. Mitchell, and C. Duggan. 2010. Challenges to optimal enteral nutrition in a multidisciplinary pediatric intensive care unit. *JPEN: Journal of Parenteral and Enteral Nutrition* 34 (1) (Jan–Feb): 38–45.

Mirtallo, J., T. Canada, D. Johnson, V. Kumpf, C. Petersen, G. Sacks, D. Seres, P. Guenter, and Task Force for the Revision of Safe Practices for Parenteral Nutrition. 2004. Safe practices for parenteral nutrition. *JPEN: Journal of Parenteral and Enteral Nutrition* 28 (6) (Nov–Dec): S39–S70.

O'Grady, N. P., M. Alexander, E. P. Dellinger, J. L. Gerberding, S. O. Heard, D. G. Maki, H. Masur et al. 2002. Guidelines for the prevention of intravascular catheter-related infections. Centers for disease control and prevention. *MMWR. Recommendations and Reports: Morbidity and Mortality Weekly Report. Recommendations and Reports/Centers for Disease Control* 51 (RR-10) (Aug 9): 1–29.

Premji, S. S., T. R. Fenton, and R. S. Sauve. 2006. Higher versus lower protein intake in formula-fed low birth weight infants. *Cochrane Database of Systematic Reviews (Online)* (1) (1) (Jan 25): CD003959.

Schanler, R. J. 2011. Outcomes of human milk-fed premature infants. *Seminars in Perinatology* 35 (1) (Feb): 29–33.

Schofield, W. N. 1985. Predicting basal metabolic rate, new standards and review of previous work. *Human Nutrition. Clinical Nutrition* 39 (Suppl 1): 5–41.

Skillman, H. E., and N. M. Mehta. 2012a. Nutrition therapy in the critically ill child. *Current Opinion in Critical Care* 18 (2) (Apr): 192–198.

Suman, O. E., R. P. Mlcak, D. L. Chinkes, and D. N. Herndon. 2006. Resting energy expenditure in severely burned children: Analysis of agreement between indirect calorimetry and prediction equations using the Bland-Altman method. *Burns: Journal of the International Society for Burn Injuries* 32 (3) (May): 335–342.

Szeszycki, E. 2010. Evaluation and monitoring of pediatric patients receiving nutrition support. In *The A.S.P.E.N. Pediatric Nutrition Support Core Curriculum*, ed. M. Corkins, pp. 460–476. Silver Spring, MD: American Society for Parenteral and Enteral Nutrition.

Tripkovic, L., H. Lambert, K. Hart, C. P. Smith, G. Bucca, S. Penson, G. Chope et al. 2012. Comparison of vitamin D2 and vitamin D3 supplementation in raising serum 25-hydroxyvitamin D status: A systematic review and meta-analysis. *The American Journal of Clinical Nutrition* 95 (6) (Jun): 1357–1364.

Vanek, V. W., P. Borum, A. Buchman, T. A. Fessler, L. Howard, K. Jeejeebhoy, M. Kochevar et al. 2012. A.S.P.E.N. position paper: Recommendations for changes in commercially available parenteral multivitamin and multi-trace element products. *Nutrition in Clinical Practice: Official Publication of the American Society for Parenteral and Enteral Nutrition* 27 (4) (Aug): 440–491.

van Waardenburg, D. A., C. T. de Betue, J. B. Goudoever, L. J. Zimmermann, and K. F. Joosten. 2009. Critically ill infants benefit from early administration of protein and energy-enriched formula: A randomized controlled trial. *Clinical Nutrition (Edinburgh, Scotland)* 28 (3) (Jun): 249–255.

Wagner, C. L., F. R. Greer, American Academy of Pediatrics Section on Breastfeeding, and American Academy of Pediatrics Committee on Nutrition. 2008. Prevention of rickets and vitamin D deficiency in infants, children, and adolescents. *Pediatrics* 122 (5) (Nov): 1142–1152.

Waterlow, J. C., R. Buzina, W. Keller, J. M. Lane, M. Z. Nichaman, and J. M. Tanner. 1977. The presentation and use of height and weight data for comparing the nutritional status of groups of children under the age of 10 years. *Bulletin of the World Health Organization* 55 (4): 489–498.

Wylie, M. C., D. A. Graham, G. Potter-Bynoe, M. E. Kleinman, A. G. Randolph, J. M. Costello, and T. J. Sandora. 2010. Risk factors for central line-associated bloodstream infection in pediatric intensive care units. *Infection Control and Hospital Epidemiology: The Official Journal of the Society of Hospital Epidemiologists of America* 31 (10) (Oct): 1049–1056.

22 Geriatrics

Ronni Chernoff

CONTENTS

INTRODUCTION

The American population is getting older rapidly due to the beginning of the 77 million *baby boomers* turning 65 starting in 2011.[1,2] The proportion of older persons admitted to an intensive care unit (ICU) is estimated to be between 25% and 50% and is likely to grow as a result of the increasing age of the U.S. population. This is particularly important because there seems to be a pattern of providing less life-sustaining treatment to patients aged 80 years and older. It has been suggested that long-term acute care hospitalization, as opposed to ICU placement, is more cost effective and survival rates are similar.[3–5]

Among hospitalized patients, the elderly constitute a majority of nutrition support recipients and it is therefore essential to address their specific needs. However, there is a paucity of quality research concerning optimal nutrition support of critically ill older persons. Much of the current standards of care have been extrapolated from younger and middle-aged adults.

Unlike younger or middle-aged adults, the elderly are more likely to manifest chronic health conditions such as diabetes, coronary heart disease, neurological disorders, renal disease cancer, and other comorbidities prior to their admission to the ICU.

As a result of these multiple comorbidities, body composition changes, physiology, and lifestyle changes that occur with aging, older patients are at greater risk for presenting with symptoms mimicking or actual nutritional deficiencies. Among many factors, social isolation, oral health problems, functional limitations, depression, and altered mental status can negatively impact the quantity and quality of dietary intakes. Polypharmacy, including prescription drugs, dietary supplements, and herbal remedies, may also exacerbate nutritional problems by interfering with nutrient intake, metabolism, and/or absorption.

Increasing age has been associated with a decline in muscle mass called sarcopenia.[6,7] This loss of muscle can adversely impact critical care outcomes secondary to decreased metabolic reserve for response to injury and inflammation. Old age is also associated with an increase in total body fat mass and deposition of intra-abdominal fat (visceral fat). Obesity is growing in prevalence among the U.S. older population. According to National Health and Nutrition Survey report, almost 75% of older men were overweight or obese and 67% of older women were overweight or obese.[8] At 80 years or greater, the prevalence of obesity fell off precipitously.[8,9] Excess weight and obesity are associated with medical comorbidities such as hypertension, diabetes mellitus, dyslipidemia, and coronary artery disease in old age.[10]

Undernutrition syndromes such as wasting, cachexia, failure to thrive, and protein energy undernutrition are routinely observed among hospitalized older patients. The proportion of hospitalized elderly people found to be undernourished may be over one-third or greater of all hospital admissions and may be even higher in a critical care setting.[11–13] Among these patients, undernutrition has been associated with an increased risk of adverse outcomes such as poor wound healing, increased pressure ulcers, higher rate of infections, and longer length of hospital stays and recovery periods.[14–17] Furthermore, nutritional status is likely to deteriorate as the catabolic response associated with critical illness takes place. It has been suggested that negative energy balance in critically ill patients puts them at particularly high risk for poor nutritional status and negative nitrogen balance.[18,19]

NUTRITION ASSESSMENT

It is important to undertake a comprehensive nutritional assessment of critically ill elderly patients to detect any suspected undernutrition syndrome or obesity. Based upon this assessment, appropriate interventions and monitoring must be initiated to maintain optimal nutrition status throughout the hospital stay. Nutrition status at time of discharge is a strong predictor of early nonelective hospital readmission.[20–22]

ANTHROPOMETRIC MEASURES

Anthropometric measurements are fundamental components of nutrition assessment. They include weight history, weight, height, body mass index (BMI), skinfolds, and circumferences.

Although difficult to obtain from critically ill patients, weight history provides useful information regarding a patient's nutritional status. Caregivers, family members, and medical records can be helpful resources although not necessarily factually accurate. Any weight loss of more than 5% of usual body weight in the last month or 10% in the past 6 months is prognostic of adverse clinical outcomes.[23,24] Weight should be closely monitored throughout the hospital stay using bed scales for bed bound patients if necessary. Note that fluid shifts and fluid retention can often mask lean body mass changes.

Height is useful for the calculation of anthropometric indices such as BMI. For bed-bound patients, segmental or recumbent measures may yield a height most closely matching an erect height if it were able to be measured. Loss of height occurs slowly over time due to kyphosis, spinal disc compression, and poor stature.[25]

In older persons, including the seriously ill elderly, BMI values under the 15th percentile (using cut-off points in the NHANES Follow-up Studies) have been associated with a higher risk of mortality.[24,25] According to the latest National Institute of Health (NIH) guidelines on body size, a BMI (defined as weight (kg)/height (m^2)) under 18.5 places the patient at high risk for being undernourished.[26] However, a lifetime history of weight is helpful to assess whether or not BMI is contributory as a measure of risk.

Reduced skinfold thickness and mid-arm circumference have been associated with risk of adverse outcomes in hospitalized elderly patients,[14] although there are no reference values for elderly individuals no matter the state of their health. Changes in body composition, skin elasticity, and muscle tone that occur with aging limit the reliability of these measurements and only trained clinicians should consider their use. One of the physiological changes associated with aging is a reduction of lean body mass, including muscle tissue, and a shift in fat deposition toward an increase in visceral fat. Monitoring changes over time, using each patient as his or her own control, is the optimal way of using these measurements. A detailed description of procedures for anthropometric measurements can be found in the NHANES III Anthropometric Procedures Video.[27] It is essential to note that there are no anthropometric reference values for elderly individuals.

Laboratory Data

Laboratory data are generally evaluated as part of routine nutritional assessment. In the critically ill elderly, laboratory tests and results can be affected by many factors unrelated to nutrition and should be interpreted with caution. They should also be used in combination with clinical judgment and with other indicators of nutritional status.

Serum albumin levels are generally well preserved among healthy older persons. Hypoalbuminemia is particularly useful as an indicator of risk of adverse outcomes among hospitalized patients, keeping in mind the potential impact of hydration status, prescription and over-the-counter medications, and comorbidities. Albumin levels have been linked with increased lengths of hospital stay, complications, readmissions, and mortality.[11,20,27] In the critical care setting, the prognostic value associated with hypoalbuminemia is related to cytokine-mediated response to injury, disease (cancer, renal, or hepatic disease), and inflammatory conditions.[14,28–31] Serum albumin levels less than 35 g/L are often seen in the critically ill elderly and are associated with adverse outcomes.[28,32] Transthyretin (prealbumin) may be a better indicator of short-term visceral protein status than albumin but otherwise suffers many of the same limitations as serum albumin as an indicator of nutritional status in critically ill elderly.[33] C-reactive protein was a better predictor of changes associated with an inflammatory state. It would, therefore, be a better indicator for recovery from an acute illness.[33]

Hypocholesterolemia (<160 mg/dL) is often observed among undernourished older persons presenting with serious underlying disease, although there has been speculation that it may be a secondary manifestation of the primary disease process.[34,35] It is a nonspecific indicator of poor health status that has been associated with increased complications and mortality. In many clinical settings, such as in the ICU, low cholesterol levels are independent from dietary intakes and nutritional deprivation. Most likely, they result from ongoing cytokine-mediated inflammatory response, particularly interleukin-6 (IL-6).[36]

Undernutrition is also associated with a decline in many cell-mediated immune functions including such indicators as total lymphocyte counts, helper/suppressor T-cell ratios, and skin test anergy. In the critically ill elderly patient, impaired immune response is a nonspecific marker for undernutrition and is more likely to reflect a variety of other conditions such as response to injury, underlying disease, and polypharmacy.[37–40]

Nutrition Screening Tools

There are no established gold standard measures to assess nutritional status of older individuals, much less those patients who are critically ill. Over the past decade, researchers have attempted to develop multi-item nutrition risk screening tools, particularly for application to geriatric populations.[41] For many of these tools, it is unknown whether they have appropriate specificity and sensitivity to correctly identify undernourished persons. This is particularly true in the critical care setting.[42] It also remains to be clarified whether people identified at high nutritional risk can be treated with interventions that result in more favorable outcomes.[43]

Table 22.1 summarizes nutrition screening tools and prediction equations that are commonly used in the hospital geriatric population.

TABLE 22.1
Nutrition Screening Tools

Tools	Purpose, Administration, and Description of Tool	Reference Measure and Validation Data
MNA-SF[a,70]	Assessment of nutritional status. *Trained clinician administered* 6 items, including appetite, weight loss, mobility, psychological and neuropsychological status, dementia, BMI.	Standard MNA score[71] Sensitivity: 97.9% Specificity: 100% PPV[i]: 98.7%
MNA[b,72,73]	Assessment of nutritional status. *Trained clinician administered* 18 items, including anthropometric and dietary assessment, weight loss, living environment, medication use, clinical global assessment, self-perception of health and nutritional status.	Clinical status, dietary intakes, laboratory data[74–76] Sensitivity: 96% Specificity: 98% Internal consistency ≥ 0.74 Intraclass correlation coefficient ≥ 0.89
NSI[c]—Level I Screen[77]	Assess for further evaluation and intervention. *Trained clinician administered* 31 items, including measures of height and weight as well as additional assessment items regarding weight change, dietary habits, functional status, and living environment.	No data
NSI[c]—Level II Screen[77]	Collect diagnostic information for evaluation and intervention. *Trained clinician administered* 46 items, including all items from level 1 plus additional biochemical and anthropometric measures, provision for more detailed evaluation of depression and mental status.	Hospital admissions[78] Eating problems and polypharmacy items Sensitivity: 58% Specificity: 56.3% PPV[i]: 17.9% Functional limitations[79] Items found to be significant predictors of functional limitations: age ≥ 75 years, use of ≥3 medications, albumin concentration <35.0 g/L, poor appetite, eating problems, income <$6000/year, eating alone, and depression
SGA[d,80]	Assess nutrition status. *Trained clinician administered* 11 items including weight loss, dietary intake, presence of gastrointestinal symptoms, functional capacity, physical assessment, subjective assessment of nutritional status.	Nutrition-related complications[81] Sensitivity: 82% Specificity: 72%
NRI[e,81]	Predict operative complications. *Predictive equation* 2 items: [1.59 (albumin) + 0.417 (current or usual weight)] × 100	Nutrition status using a combined index[82] Sensitivity: 100% Specificity: 46% PPV[i]: 87%
HPI[f,83]	Predict sepsis and mortality *Predictive equation* 4 items: 0.91 (albumin) – 1.00 (delayed hypersensitivity) – 1.44 (presence or absence of sepsis) + 0.98 (presence or absence of cancer cachexia) – 1.09	Sepsis and mortality[83] Sensitivity: 74% Specificity: 66% PPV[i]: 72%

(Continued)

TABLE 22.1 (*Continued*)
Nutrition Screening Tools

Tools	Purpose, Administration, and Description of Tool	Reference Measure and Validation Data
PNI[g,84]	Predict operative complications. *Predictive equation* 4 items: 158 – 16.6 (albumin in g/dL) – 0.78 (tricep skinfolds in mm) – 0.20 (transferring in mg/dL) – 5.8 (delayed hypersensitivity skin test).	Mortality[85] Sensitivity: 93% Specificity: 44%
PINI[h,86]	Predict mortality and risk of complication. *Predictive equation* 4 items: (a1-acid glycoprotein) × (C-reactive protein)/(albumin) × (prealbumin)	Hospital mortality RR = 4.34 with PINI score ≥ 25 Chronic institutionalization RR = 2.04 with PINI score ≥25

Source: Adapted from Reuben, D.B. et al., *J. Am. Geriatr. Soc.*, 43, 415, 1995.

a Mini nutritional assessment short-form.
b Mini nutritional assessment.
c Nutrition screening initiative.
d Subjective global assessment.
e Nutrition risk index.
f Hospital prognostic index.
g Prognostic nutritional index.
h Prognostic inflammatory and nutritional index.
i Positive predictive value.

NUTRITIONAL REQUIREMENTS

ENERGY

With aging, there is a decrease in energy needs as a consequence of a decline in lean body mass and physical activity.[44] Energy requirements should be estimated to ensure adequate nutritional support and avoid complications associated with over- or underfeeding. Overfeeding has been linked with severe adverse events such as difficulties in ventilator weaning, congestive heart failure, and refeeding syndrome.[3,45]

Several ways of estimating resting energy expenditure have been studied. Indirect calorimetry is considered the gold standard but is technically demanding, time consuming, and requires expensive equipment.[46,47] It is also not suitable for use with the high FIO_2 (>60 mmHg) requirements of many ventilated, critically ill patients.

The Harris–Benedict equation, which includes age as a variable in the estimation of energy requirements, is often used but has been shown to be less accurate than others.[48,49] Because Harris–Benedict may underestimate energy needs of highly stressed persons, it should be adjusted to account for additional requirements imposed by critical illness. There are other formulas, such as Mifflin-St Jeor, that yield a more accurate estimate of resting energy expenditure and can be used as a base for calculating energy needs in adults.[48,49] Using a correction factor between 1.00 and 1.55 is most likely to match true energy requirements of the critically ill elderly and avoid complications associated with overfeeding. Another common approach is to estimate needs at 25–35 kcal/kg/day. An adjusted body weight must be used for obese individuals.

Harris–Benedict equations:

In men: BEE (kcal/day) = 66.5 + (13.8 × weight (kg)) + (5 × height (cm)) – (6.8 × age (year))
In women: BEE (kcal/day) = 655.1 + (9.6 × weight (kg)) + (1.8 × height (cm)) – (4.7 × age (year))

Mifflin-St. Jeor[50]

In men: REE = 10 × weight (kg) + 6.25 × height (cm) – 5 × age (year) + 5
In women: REE = 10 × weight (kg) + 6.25 × height (cm) – 5 × age (year) – 161

Protein

According to recent research and studies conducted starting in the latter years of the twentieth century, the latest recommendations for protein needs in older adults (over age 65 years) are for at least 1.0 g/kg/day.[51] According to the most recent dietary reference intakes (DRIs)[52] recommendation of 0.8 g/kg/day for protein, the same as for middle-aged adults, there is evidence that healthy, free-living elderly require approximately 1 g/kg/day and this level is likely to be insufficient for patients with acute illness or chronic disease. The hypercatabolic response to serious stress increases requirements to 1.5–2 g/kg/day among critically ill older persons.[53,54] Evaluation of muscle catabolism and adequacy of protein replacement can be monitored with urinary nitrogen excretion and determination of nitrogen balance. Note that certain conditions such as renal or hepatic dysfunction may require protein restriction.

Nitrogen balance calculation

Nitrogen balance (g/24 h) = (protein intake (g/24 h)/6.25) – (urine urea nitrogen (g/24 h) + 4)

Micronutrient

The DRIs for micronutrients have been revised in the past few years.[55–57] The updated values now include life stages 51–70 years and 71 years and older. The DRIs include four subdivisions: recommended dietary allowance (RDA), adequate intake (AI), tolerable upper intake level (UL), and estimated average requirement (EAR). Table 22.2 describes the DRI for older persons.

These reference values have been developed for healthy individuals, and they have yet to be specifically addressed in the critically ill population. Decreased food intakes that occur with aging can result in vulnerable nutritional status before hospitalization. Reduced nutrient intake may be related to chronic disease, decreased financial resources, being housebound, increased medication needs, disability, and anorexia related to illness. Older persons are particularly at risk for developing nutrient deficiencies in calcium, vitamin D, B_{12}, B_6, folate, and iron. Severe nutritional deficiencies may be even more likely to develop as a result of increased needs associated with critical illness and its treatment.[58] Note that recent trends favoring pharmacological supplementation of vitamin A, vitamin C, vitamin E, and zinc, for patients with severe traumatic wounds or thermal injuries, should be approached with caution for older, critically ill patients. In particular, vitamin A intake should not exceed recommendations due to the potential toxic effects of excessive intake.

Fluid

Dehydration is a common fluid and electrolyte disorder among elderly hospital patients. Aging has been associated with a decline in thirst drive, impaired response to fluid deprivation, and lower urine concentration after water deprivation.[59] Although there is no consensus on fluid requirements

TABLE 22.2
Dietary Reference Intakes for Micronutrients for Older Persons

Nutrient	Male 51–70 years	Male >70 years	Female 51–70 years	Female >70 years
Calcium (mg)	1200*	1200*	1200*	1200*
Phosphorus (mg)	700	700	700	700
Magnesium (mg)	420	420	320	320
Vitamin D (μg)	10*	15*	10*	15*
Fluoride (mg)	4*	4*	3*	3*
Thiamin (mg)	1.2	1.2	1.1	1.1
Riboflavin (mg)	1.3	1.3	1.1	1.1
Niacin (mg)	16	16	14	14
Vitamin B_6 (mg)	1.7	1.7	1.5	1.5
Folate (μg)	400	400	400	400
Vitamin B_{12} (μg)	2.4	2.4	2.4	2.4
Pantothenic acid (mg)	5*	5*	5*	5*
Biotin (μg)	30*	30*	30*	30*
Choline (mg)	550*	550*	425*	425*
Vitamin C (mg)	90	90	75	75
α-Tocopherol (mg)	15	15	15	15
Selenium (μg)	55	55	55	55

Sources: Adapted from Institute of Medicine, *Dietary Reference Intakes for Calcium, Phosphorus, Magnesium, Vitamin D, and Fluoride*, National Academy Press, Washington, DC, 1997; Institute of Medicine, *Dietary Reference Intakes for Thiamin, Riboflavin, Niacin, Vitamin B6, Folate, Vitamin B12, Pantothenic Acid, Biotin, and Choline*, National Academy Press, Washington, DC, 1999; Institute of Medicine, *Dietary Reference Intakes for Vitamin C, Vitamin E, Selenium, and Carotenoids*, National Academy Press, Washington, DC, 2000.

Recommended dietary allowances (RDA) are presented in ordinary type and adequate intakes (AI) are followed by an asterisk (*).

in the elderly, dehydration can be prevented with an intake of 30 mL/kg actual body weight/day or 1 mL/kcal consumed.[60] It has been suggested that aiming for at least 1500 mL/day, even in small elderly women, will contribute to the maintenance of fluid balance.[60] Fluid needs may be higher when disease and infection are present or with the administration of medication such as diuretics and laxatives.

Fluid intakes should be closely monitored and patients showing any sign of dehydration such as rapid weight loss (greater than 3% of body weight), abnormal declines in orthostatic blood pressure, orthostatic pulse increases, decreased urine output, elevated body temperature, constipation, mucosal dryness, and/or mental confusion should be treated promptly. The American Medical Association guidelines in the management of dehydration in older adults may be useful in this case.[61] Laboratory parameters (electrolytes, osmolality, creatinine, serum urea nitrogen [SUN], SUN/creatinine ratio, hematocrit, and hemoglobin) can also be used to determine hydration status, although they can be altered by other medical conditions in the elderly.[61] Alternatively, volume overload is common among critically ill older persons with conditions like cardiac, hepatic, or renal failure. Overinfusion of intravenous fluids may be a contributing factor. In these states, fluid restriction may be indicated.

NUTRITIONAL INTERVENTION

Initiating Nutritional Support

Malnutrition in elderly persons admitted to subacute or ICUs should be considered at high risk for poor clinical outcomes. Many elderly patients are subclinically malnourished upon admission.[62] Table 22.3 describes patients admitted to the ICU who would most likely benefit from early nutrition support. Elderly patients may deteriorate more rapidly due to decreased lean body mass, sarcopenia, and decreased nutritional reserves.[42] Nutrition support should be considered within 2–3 days of onset of acute critical illness in elderly patients who are unable to eat adequately, less than 50% of their estimated needs, to avoid declines that contribute to increased morbidity, mortality, and prolonged hospital stays.[63] Nutritional support results in increased energy and nutrient intakes and may result in improvements in nutritional status as well as clinical and functional parameters in elderly patients.[63]

Nutrition Support Guidelines

There is remarkable agreement in nutrition support guidelines among various nutrition organizations, including the American Society for Parenteral and Enteral Nutrition, the European Society for Parenteral and Enteral Nutrition, and the Academy of Nutrition and Dietetics.[64–69]

A multitude of studies have explored using parenteral nutritional support in different populations with assorted diagnoses, but only a few of them have examined the tolerance for parenteral nutrition in elderly individuals.[70,71] Given the strength of the data supporting the benefits of enteral over parenteral nutrition, the situation in which the choice between the two is a consideration facing the patient should be the exception. Total parenteral nutrition (TPN) should only be initiated if the patient's gastrointestinal tract is not functional or cannot be used for an extended period, greater than 7–10 days.[72] In general, older patients without organ failure tolerate standard TPN formulations containing conventional amounts of macronutrients, electrolytes, and multivitamins with minerals. Adult onset diabetes mellitus is common among older persons; intensive insulin management and reduced dextrose loads should be considered among those with a history of diabetes or evident stress-related hyperglycemia.[70] Similarly, marked volume overload is common among critically ill older persons and should warrant consideration of concentrated TPN formulas.

Enteral nutrition is the preferred method of feeding for older critically ill persons and should be used whenever possible.[71,72] Standard enteral feeding formulations are generally well tolerated. Respiratory failure requiring ventilatory support is a common indication for enteral feeding in

TABLE 22.3
ICU Patient Who May Require Early Enteral Feeding

Respiratory failure requiring ventilatory support
Cerebrovascular accident, advanced dementia, head trauma
May have swallowing problems related to neurological injury, can be retrained to swallow, should be reevaluated often
Degenerative chronic diseases
Refusal or inability to sustain adequate intake of food
Acute hip fracture
Reduces rehabilitation time in undernourished patients hospitalized with acute hip fracture
Surgery, trauma, or acute disease states
Predicted intake to be inadequate for >5 days

Sources: Adapted from Sullivan, D.H. et al., *J. Am. Coll. Nutr.*, 17, 155, 1998; Karkeck, J.M., *Nutr. Clin. Pract.*, 8, 211, 1993.

the intensive care setting. Patients with cerebrovascular accidents or with degenerative chronic diseases such as Parkinson's disease or multiple sclerosis will often require enteral nutritional support. Patients with surgery, trauma, or acute disease states that leave them with anticipated inadequate intakes for more than 5 days should be evaluated for enteral nutritional support.[72] Elderly patients hospitalized with acute hip fracture may benefit from early nutritional support. Enteral feeding may reduce rehabilitation time in undernourished patients hospitalized with acute hip fracture.[63]

Nasoenteric feeding tubes are undesirable for use longer than 4–6 weeks, which is a requirement characteristic of many older critically ill patients.[63] Patients with advanced dementia or otherwise altered mental status are not good candidates for nasoenteric tubes due to the risk of aspiration from self-extubation.[63] Restraints can be used to reduce the risk of self-extubation, but are inappropriate for long-term use. Percutaneous endoscopic gastrostomy, percutaneous endoscopic jejunostomy, or surgical gastrostomy or jejunostomy tubes may be the best option for many elderly patients. Patients receiving nutritional support through these types of tubes versus nasoenteric tubes receive more of their prescribed feeds, suffer fewer treatment failures, and are often discharged earlier from the hospital.[73]

CONCLUSIONS

Advanced age is an independent risk factor for mortality in critically ill elderly patients.[74] If there is an opportunity to intervene early with appropriate nutrition support, it would seem reasonable to do so. Unfortunately there has been only limited investigation of nutrition support for older critically ill persons. Much of the current standards of care have been extrapolated from younger and middle-aged adults. Changes that occur with aging in body composition, physiology, and lifestyle factors place many older persons at nutritional risk. Because many elderly, critically ill patients are malnourished on admission,[75] an individualized approach to nutrition screening, assessment, and intervention is recommended. Nutrition support should be considered early in the critical care course with the level of care guided by advanced directive.

CASE STUDY*

A 87-year-old woman residing in a nursing home presented with fever, abdominal pain, and vomiting. Her past medical history was remarkable for coronary heart disease with class II angina pectoris, hypothyroidism, a paratracheal mass, organic brain syndrome, and fecal and urinary incontinence.

In the emergency department, she exhibited generalized marasmus. Her abdomen was distended. Laboratory results were within normal limits except for an albumin level of 2.8 g/dL (normal range, 4–5) and a white blood cell count of $13.2 \times 100/mm^2$ (normal range, 4.5–11). Obstruction series radiographs showed dilated loops of small bowel with air-fluid levels consistent with small bowel obstruction.

The patient was deemed a high-risk surgical candidate; therefore, conservative treatment measures were selected. Unfortunately, her condition did not improve. Peripheral intravenous nutrition was initiated on the fifth hospital day. A frank discussion was held with family members regarding risks and benefits, and the patient was taken to the operating room of the ninth hospital day. Exploratory laparotomy revealed a high-grade small bowel obstruction caused by adhesive bands of fibrous tissue. Lysis of adhesions was performed, and no other abnormalities

* Reproduced with permission from Talabiska, D.G. and Jensen, G.L., *News Lines*, 4, 1, 1995.

were identified. Peripheral parenteral nutrition was continued in anticipation of return of bowel function. By the fourth postoperative day, anasarca developed and bowel function had not resumed.

The Nutrition Support Service was consulted for further nutritional assessment and intervention. The patient had taken nothing by mouth for about 2 weeks. Her albumin level had decreased to 1.8 g/dL. The anasarca was attributed to the extravasation of fluids into the extracellular compartments due to hypoalbuminemia. TPN was recommended in view of deteriorating nutritional status, volume constraints imposed by fluid overload, and exhaustion of peripheral venous access. Actual body weight was 59 kg and height was 155 cm (corresponding ideal body weight was 58 kg). Preoperative weight was unrecorded, but was estimated to be 50 kg. Based on a protein intake of 1.5 g/kg/day and 25–30 kcal/kg/day, her nutritional needs were calculated at 87 g of protein and 1500 kcal daily.

A central venous catheter was placed and TPN was cautiously begun. Fluid intake and output, weight, and electrolyte levels were closely monitored. Her bowel function gradually returned to baseline. She remained on TPN for a total of 10 days and then resumed oral intake. Following the 24-day hospitalization, the patient returned to the nursing home in her usual state of health.[68]

ACKNOWLEDGMENTS

Alice E Buchanan, MS, RD; Marie-Andrée Roy, MSc; Gordon L Jensen, MD, PhD.

REFERENCES

1. U.S. Census Bureau, Current Population Reports, United States Department of Commerce, Washington, DC, 2010.
2. U.S. Census Bureau, 2008 Census Projections, August 2008.
3. Fuchs L, Chronaki CE, Park S et al. ICU admission characteristics and mortality rates among elderly and very eldery patients, *Intensive Care Medicine* 38:1654–1661, 2012.
4. Brandberg C, Blomqvist H, Jirwe M. What is the importance of age in treatment of the elderly in the intensive care unit? *Acta Anaesthesiologica Scandinavica.* 57(6):698–703, 2013.
5. Kahn JM, Werner RM, David G et al. Effectiveness of long-term acute hospitalization in elderly patients with chronic critical illness, *Medical Care* 51(1):4–10, 2013.
6. Arango-Lopera VE, Arroyo P, Gutiérrez-Robledo LM et al. Mortality as an adverse outcome of sarcopenia, *Journal of Nutrition Health and Aging* 17(3):259–262, 2013.
7. Boirie Y. Physiopathological mechanisms of sarcopenia, *Journal of Nutrition Health and Aging* 13(8):717–723, 2009.
8. Crescioni M, Gorina Y, Bilheimer L, Gillum RF. Trends in health status and health care use among older men, National Health Statistics Reports No 24, April 2010.
9. Flegal KM, Carroll MD, Ogden CL, Johnson, CL. Prevalence and trends in obesity among US adults, 1999–2000, *JAMA* 288:1723, 2002.
10. Li C, Balluz LS, Okoro CA et al. Surveillance of certain health behaviors and conditions among states and selected local areas—behavioral risk factor surveillance system, *MMWR Surveillance Summary* 60(9):1–250, August 19, 2011.
11. Constans T, Bacq Y, Brechot JF, Guilmot JL, Choutet P, Lamisse, F. Protein-energy malnutrition in elderly medical patients, *Journal of the American Geriatrics Society* 40:263, 1992.
12. Mowé M, Bøhmer T. The prevalence of undiagnosed protein-calorie undernutrition in a population of hospitalized elderly patients, *Journal of the American Geriatrics Society* 39:1089, 1991.
13. Sullivan DH, Moriarty MS, Chernoff R, Lipschitz DA. Patterns of care: An analysis of the quality of nutritional care routinely provided to elderly hospitalized veterans, *JPEN: Journal of Parenteral and Enteral Nutrition* 13(3):249–254, 1989.
14. Sullivan DH, Bopp MM, Roberson PK. Protein-energy undernutrition and life-threatening complications among the hospitalized elderly, *Journal of General Internal Medicine* 17:923, 2002.
15. Sullivan DH, Patch GA, Walls RC, Lipschitz DA. Impact of nutrition status on morbidity and mortality in a select population of geriatric rehabilitation patients, *American Journal of Clinical Nutrition* 51:749, 1990.

16. Potter J, Klipstein K, Reilly JJ, Roberts, M. The nutritional status and clinical course of acute admissions to a geriatric unit, *Age and Ageing* 24:131, 1995.
17. Naber TJ, Schermer T, de Bree A, Nusteling K, Eggink LJWK, Bakkeren J, van Heereveld H, Katan MB. Prevalence of malnutrition in nonsurgical hospitalized patients and its association with disease complications, *American Journal of Clinical Nutrition* 66:1063, 1997.
18. Monk DN, Planks LD, Franch-Arcas G et al. Sequential changes in the metabolic response in critically injured patients in the first 25 days after blunt trauma, *Annals of Surgery* 223:396–404, 1996.
19. Dickerson RN, Pitts SL, Maish GO III et al. A reappraisal of nitrogen requirements for patients with critical illness and trauma, *Journal of Trauma and Acute Care Surgery* 73(3):549–557, 2012.
20. Friedmann JM, Jensen GL, Smiciklas-Wright H, McCamish MA. Predicting early nonelective hospital readmissions in nutritionally compromised older adults, *American Journal of Clinical Nutrition* 65:1714, 1997.
21. Lim SL, Ong KCB, Chan YH et al. Malnutrition and its impact on cost of hospitalization, length of stay, readmission and 3-year mortality, *Clinical Nutrition* 32(5):737–742, 2013.
22. Agarwal E, Ferguson M, Banks M et al. Malnutrition and poor food intake are associated with prolonged hospital stay, frequent readmissions, and greater in-hospital mortality: Results from the Nutrition Care Day Survey 2010, *Clinical Nutrition* 31(1):41–47, 2012.
23. Miller S, Wolfe R. The danger of weight loss in the elderly, *Journal of Nutrition Health and Aging* 12:487–491, 2008.
24. Woods JL, Iuliano-Burns S, Walker KZ. Weight loss in elderly women in low level care and its association with transfer to high-level care and mortality, *Clinical Interventions Aging* 6:311–317, 2011.
25. Mitchell CO. In Chernoff R (ed.), Nutrition assessment of elderly adults, *Geriatric Nutrition*, 4th edn., Jones & Bartlett, Sudbury, MA, 2014, pp. 435–464.
26. National Institute of Health, Aim for a Healthy Weight, Bethesda, MD, 1998.
27. D'Erasmo E, Pisani D, Ragno A et al. Serum albumin level on admission: Mortality and clinical outcomes in the elderly, *American Journal of the Medical Sciences* 314:17, 1997.
28. Doweiko JP, Nompleggi DJ. Role of albumin in human physiology and pathophysiology, *JPEN: Journal of Parenteral and Enteral Nutrition* 15:476, 1991.
29. Rall C, Roubenoff R, Harris T. In Rosenberg IH (ed.), *Nutritional Assessment of Elderly Populations: Measure and Function*, Raven, New York, 1991.
30. Rothschild MA, Oratz M, Schreiber SS. Serum albumin, *Hepatology* 8:385, 1988.
31. Ňamendys-Silva SA, González-Herrera MO, Texcocano-Becerra RN et al. Hypoalbuminemia in critically ill patients with cancer: Incidence and mortality, *American Journal of Hospice and Palliative Medicine* 28(4):253–257, 2011.
32. Pan S-W, Kao H-K, Yu W-K et al. Synergistic impact of low serum albumin on intensive care unit admission and high blood urea nitrogen during intensive care unit stay on post intensive care unit mortality in critically ill elderly patients requiring mechanical ventilation, *Geriatrics and Gerontology International* 13:107–115, 2013.
33. Davis CJ, Sowa D, Keim KS et al. The use of prealbumin and C-reactive protein for monitoring nutrition support in adult patients receiving enteral nutrition in an urban medical center, *Journal of Parenteral and Enteral Nutrition* 36(2):197–204, 2012.
34. Vyroubal P, Chiarla C, Giovannini I et al. Hypocholesterolemia in clinically serious conditions—A review, *Biomedical Papers of the Medical Faculty of the University Palacky Olomouc Czech Republic* 152(2):181–189, 2008.
35. Peifung H, Seeman TE, Harris TB, Reuben DB. The effects of serum beta-carotene concentration and burden of inflammation on all-cause mortality risk in high-functioning older persons: MacArthur studies of successful aging, *Journal of the American Geriatrics Society* 51:80–84, 2003.
36. Ettinger WH, Jr., Harris TB, Verdery RB et al. Evidence of inflammation as a cause of hypocholesterolemia in older people, *Journal of the American Geriatrics Society* 43:264, 1995.
37. Seltzer MH, Fletcher HS, Slocum BA, Engler PE. Instant nutritional assessment in the intensive care unit, *JPEN: Journal of Parenteral and Enteral Nutrition* 5:70, 1981.
38. Mitchell CO, Lipschitz DA. Detection of protein-calorie malnutrition in the elderly, *American Journal of Clinical Nutrition* 36:340, 1982.
39. Kaiser FE, Morley JE. Idiopathic CD4+ lymphophenia in older persons, *Journal of the American Geriatrics Society* 42:1291, 1994.
40. Jayarajan S, Daly JM. The relationships of nutrients, routes of delivery, and immunocompetence, *Surgical Clinics of North America* 91(4):737–753, 2011.
41. Chernoff R. Nutrition screening tools. In Benardier C, Dwyer J, Heber D (eds.), Nutrition Screening Tools, *Handbook of Nutrition and Food*, 2nd edn., CRC Press, Boca Raton, FL, 2014, pp. 505–516.

42. Sheean PM, Peterson SJ, Chen Y et al. Utilizing multiple methods to classify malnutrition among elderly patients admitted to the medical and surgical intensive care units (ICU), *Clinical Nutrition* 32(5):752–757, 2013.
43. Sánchez Garcia E, Montero Errasquin B, Sánchez Castellano C, Cruz-Jentoft AJ. Importance of nutritional support in older people, *Nestle Nutrition Institute Workshop Series*, Karger AG, Basel, Switzerland, 2012.
44. Roubenoff R, Hughes VA, Dallal GE et al. The effect of gender and body composition method on the apparent decline in lean mass-adjusted resting metabolic rate with age, *Journal of Gerontology: Medical Science* 55A(12): M757–M760, 2000.
45. Schulman RC, Mechanick JI. Can nutrition support interfere with recovery from acute illness? *World Review of Nutrition and Dietetics* 105:69–81, 2013.
46. Weissman C, Kemper M, Askanazi J et al. Resting metabolic rate of the critically ill patients: Measured versus predicted, *Anesthesiology* 64:673, 1986.
47. Harris JA, Benedict FG. *A Biometric Study of Basal Metabolism in Man*, Carnegie Institution of Washington, Washington, DC, 1919.
48. Frankenfield D, Roth-Yousey L, Compher C. Comparison of predictive equations for resting metabolic rate in healthy nonobese and obese adults: A systematic review, *Journal of the American Dietetic Association* 105(5): 775–789, 2005.
49. Frankenfield D, Hise M, Malone A et al. Prediction of resting metabolic rate in critically ill adult patients: Results of a systematic review of the evidence, *Journal of the American Dietetic Association* 107:1552–1561, 2007.
50. Mifflin MD, St. Jeor ST, Hill LA et al. A new predictive equation for resting energy expenditure in healthy individuals, *American Journal of Clinical Nutrition* 51:241–247, 1990.
51. Wolfe RR, Miller SL, Miller KB. Optimal protein intake in the elderly, *Clinical Nutrition* 27:675–684, 2008.
52. Institute of Medicine. *Dietary Reference Intakes for Calcium, Phosphorus, Magnesium, Vitamin D, and Fluoride*, National Academy Press, Washington, DC, 2008.
53. Genton L, Pichard C. Protein catabolism and requirements in severe illness, *International Journal Vitamin Nutrition Research* 81(2–3), 143–152, 2011.
54. Biolo G. Protein metabolism and requirements, *World Review of Nutrition and Dietetics* 105:12–20, 2013.
55. Institute of Medicine. *Dietary Reference Intakes for Calcium and Vitamin D,* National Academy Press, Washington, DC, 2010.
56. Institute of Medicine. *Dietary Reference Intakes for Thiamin, Riboflavin, Niacin, Vitamin B6, Folate, Vitamin B12, Pantothenic Acid, Biotin, and Choline*, National Academy Press, Washington, DC, 2011.
57. Institute of Medicine. *Dietary Reference Intakes for Vitamin C, Vitamin E, Selenium, and Carotenoids*, National Academy Press, Washington, DC, 2011.
58. Cherry-Bukowiec JR. Optimizing nutrition therapy to enhance mobility in critically ill patients, *Critical Care Nursing Quarterly* 36(1):28–36, 2013.
59. Popkin BM, D'Anci KE, Rosenberg IH. Water, hydration and health, *Nutrition Reviews* 68(8):439–458, 2010.
60. Chidester JC, Spangler AA. Fluid intake in the institutionalized eldery, *Journal of the American Dietetic Association* 97(1):23–28, 1997.
61. Weinberg AD, Minaker KL. Evaluation and management in older adults, *Journal of the American Medical Association*, Council on Scientific Affairs of the American Medical Association, 274:1552, 1995.
62. Charlton K, Nichols C, Bowden N et al. Poor nutritional status of older subacute patients predicts clinical outcomes and mortality at 18-months of follow-up, *European Journal of Clinical Nutrition* 66:1224–1228, 2012.
63. Rubinsky MD, Clark AP. Early enteral nutrition in critically ill patients, *Dimensions in Critical Care Nursing* 31(5):267–274, 2012.
64. Clinical guidelines—Selection of appropriate enteral formulations. *Journal of Parenteral and Enteral Nutrition* 33(3):277–316, 2009.
65. 2009 Clinical guidelines—When indicated, maximize efficacy of parenteral nutrition. *Journal of Parenteral and Enteral Nutrition* 33(3):277–316, 2009.
66. 2009 Clinical guidelines—When to use parenteral nutrition. *Journal of Parenteral and Enteral Nutrition* 33(3):277–316, 2009.
67. Bozzetti F, Forbes A. The ESPEN clinical practice guidelines on parenteral nutrition: Present status and prespectives for future research, *Clinical Nutrition* 28:359–364, 2009.

68. Volkert D, Berner YN, Berry E et al. ESPEN guidelines on enteral nutrition: Geriatrics, *Clinical Nutrition* 25(2):330–360, 2006.
69. Ethical Framework for the Registered Dietitian in Decisions Regarding Withholding/Withdrawing Medically Assisted Nutrition and Hydration. *Journal of the American Dietetic Association* 106(2): 206–208, 2006.
70. Ferry M, Leverve X, Constans T. Comparison of subcutaneous and intravenous administration of a solution of amino acids in older patients, *Journal of the American Geriatrics Society* 45:857–860, 1997.
71. Lutz BH. Total parenteral nutrition in the older patient. *Home Healthcare Nurse* 14:123–125, 1996.
72. Chernoff R, Seres D. In Chernoff R (ed.), Nutritional support for the older adults, *Geriatric Nutrition: The Health Professional's Handbook,* Jones & Bartlett, Sudbury MS, 2014, pp. 465–485.
73. Norton B, Homer-Ward M, Donnelly MT et al. A randomized prospective comparison of percutaneous endoscopic gastrostomy and nasogastric tube feeding after acute dysphagic, *British Medical Journal* 312:13, 1996.
74. Fuchs L, Chronaki CE, Park S et al. *Intensive Care Medicine* 38:1654, 2012.
75. Talabiska DG, Jensen GL. *News Lines* 4:1, 1995.
76. Reuben DB, Greendale GA, Harrison GG. Nutrition screening in older persons. *Journal of the American Geriatrics Society* 43:415–425, 1995.
77. Institute of Medicine. *Dietary Reference Intakes for Calcium, Phosphorus, Magnesium, Vitamin D, and Fluoride*, National Academy Press, Washington, DC, 1997.
78. Institute of Medicine. *Dietary Reference Intakes for Thiamin, Riboflavin, Niacin, Vitamin B6, Folate, Vitamin B12, Pantothenic Acid, Biotin, and Choline*, National Academy Press, Washington, DC, 1999.
79. Institute of Medicine. *Dietary Reference Intakes for Vitamin C, Vitamin E, Selenium, and Carotenoids*, National Academy Press, Washington, DC, 2000.
80. Sullivan DH, Nelson CL, Bopp MM, Puskarich-May CL, Walls RC. *Journal of the American College of Nutrition* 17:155, 1998.
81. Karkeck J.M. *Nutrition in Clinical Practice* 8:211, 1993.

Section V

Nutrition Therapy for Special Interests Groups

23 Trauma and Acute Care Surgery

Michael D. Taylor and Kavitha Krishnan

CONTENTS

INTRODUCTION

INCIDENCE

Injury remains one of the largest public health problems worldwide. In 2014 in the United States, approximately 29 million people were treated in an emergency room for injuries. More than 2.8 million people were admitted to the hospital with an estimated 180,000 dying from their injuries. More than 2.8 million people will be admitted to the hospital, and nearly 180,000 will die from their injuries. The monetary cost in medical care and lost productivity exceeds $400 billion. Injury, whether intentional or unintentional, continues to be among the leading causes of death in all age groups. Table 23.1 outlines the leading causes of death in the United States [1].

ASSESSMENT OF SEVERITY OF INJURY

Injuries are typically categorized by mechanism and intent, and various scoring systems may be used to describe the severity of injury. Mechanism is broadly divided among several categories, including blunt, penetrating, blast, crush, exposure, ingestion, bites/stings, and burns. The International Classification of Disease (ICD) incorporates E-codes to provide detailed information regarding the circumstances associated with the injury [1]. A variety of different organ-specific injury scoring systems are used, as well as global assessments, including the revised trauma score (RTS), abbreviated injury score (AIS), injury severity score (ISS), and the trauma-injury severity score (TRISS).

TABLE 23.1
Leading Causes of Death in the United States

Ten Leading Causes of Death by Age Group, United States, 2010

Rank	Age										
	<1	1–4	5–9	10–14	15–24	25–34	35–44	45–54	55–64	65+	All
1	Congenital anomalies	Unintentional injury	Unintentional injury	Unintentional injury	Unintentional injury	Unintentional injury	Unintentional injury	Neoplasms	Neoplasms	Heart disease	Heart disease
2	Short gestation	Congenital anomalies	Neoplasms	Neoplasms	Homicide	Suicide	Neoplasms	Heart disease	Heart disease	Neoplasms	Neoplasms
3	SIDS	Homicide	Congenital anomalies	Suicide	Suicide	Homicide	Heart disease	Unintentional injury	Respiratory	Respiratory	Respiratory
4	Maternal pregnancy complications	Neoplasms	Homicide	Homicide	Neoplasms	Neoplasms	Suicide	Suicide	Unintentional injury	Cerebro-vascular	Cerebro-vascular
5	Unintentional injury	Heart disease	Heart disease	Congenital anomalies	Heart disease	Heart disease	Homicide	Liver disease	Diabetes	Alzheimer's	Unintentional injury
6	Placenta/cord	Influenza and pneumonia	Respiratory	Heart disease	Congenital anomalies	HIV	Liver	Cerebro-vascular	Cerebro-vascular	Diabetes	Alzheimer's
7	Sepsis	Sepsis	Cerebro-vascular	Respiratory	Cerebro-vascular	Diabetes	Cerebro-vascular	Diabetes	Liver	Influenza and pneumonia	Diabetes
8	Respiratory	Benign neoplasms	Benign neoplasms	Benign neoplasms	Influenza and pneumonia	Cerebro-vascular	HIV	Respiratory	Suicide	Nephritis	Nephritis
9	Circulatory system	Perinatal	Influenza and pneumonia	Cerebro-vascular	Diabetes	Liver	Diabetes	HIV	Nephritis	Unintentional injury	Influenza and pneumonia
10	Necrotizing enterocolitis	Respiratory	Sepsis	Sepsis	Complicated pregnancy	Congenital anomalies	Influenza and pneumonia	Hepatitis	Sepsis	Sepsis	Suicide

Source: Adapted from WISQARS™; Data Source: National Vital Statistics System, National Center for Health Statistics, CDC; Produced by: Office of Statistics and Programming, National Center for Injury Prevention and Control, CDC using WISQARS™. http://www.cdc.gov/injury/wisqars/leadingcauses.html, 2010.

TABLE 23.2
Abbreviated Injury Score

AIS Score	Injury
1	Minor
2	Moderate
3	Serious
4	Severe
5	Critical
6	Unsurvivable

TABLE 23.3
Example Calculation of Injury Severity Score

Region	Injury Description	AIS	AIS-Squared
Head and neck	Mild concussion, no loss of consciousness	1	1
Face	None		
Chest	Bilateral pulmonary contusions	4	16
Abdomen	Nonexpanding subcapsular liver hematoma	2	4
Extremity	None		
External	None		
Injury severity score			21

The AIS is an anatomical scoring system first described in 1969 by a joint committee of the American Medical Association, the Society of Automotive Engineers, and the Association for the Advancement of Automotive Medicine (Table 23.2). The AIS has undergone several revisions. Injuries are ranked from 1 to 6, in order of increasing severity. The ISS is an overall score across body regions (head and neck, face, chest, abdomen, extremity, and external). The AIS is assigned, and the three most severely injured body regions have their scores squared and then added together to produce the ISS (Table 23.3) [2].

PHYSIOLOGICAL RESPONSE TO INJURY

It has long been recognized that the physiological impact of major injury is a complex process involving a variety of local and systemic responses. Trauma and infection may alter metabolism and affect any organ system. The inflammatory response differs from the adaptive changes to starvation. A host of metabolic and circulatory changes occur to some degree in discrete phases, mediated by a number of cell types (including platelets, vascular endothelial cell, and leukocytes). In the 1930s, Cuthbertson described the ebb and flow phases. The benefit of nutrition support high in protein and calories was noted to be beneficial, although it was also observed that in the hypercatabolic phase protein losses inevitably occurred [3].

The ebb phase is characterized as a hypometabolic state. The core temperature may be lower, there is decreased energy expenditure, low cardiac output, and poor tissue perfusion. Elevated catecholamines and glucocorticoids lead to elevated blood glucose, decreased insulin, increased glucagon, and mild protein catabolism. The flow phase is one of hypermetabolism. Core temperature and overall energy expenditure are increased. The cardiac output may be elevated and tissue perfusion restored. There is often a persistent increase in catecholamines and glucocorticoids, elevated insulin and hyperglycemia. The protein catabolism is significantly accelerated [4]. The study of the molecular mechanisms of injury and recovery confirms this ebb and flow at a molecular level.

A systemic inflammatory response syndrome (SIRS) followed by a compensatory anti-inflammatory response syndrome (CARS) was initially described [5], but the sequence of molecular events does not appear to be adequately illustrated by this simple linear model. The metabolomic response is more like a number of subroutines being initiated simultaneously, and there is a complex array of pro- and anti-inflammatory processes. The persistent inflammation, immunosuppression, and catabolism syndrome (PICS) defines the pathobiology of prolonged critical care [6].

The altered metabolic function associated with tissue injury manifests in a wide variety of ways. Impaired macronutrient metabolism is typical and results from elevated catecholamines and cortisol, increased hepatic glycogenolysis and gluconeogenesis, altered insulin function, increased lipolysis, and increased muscle proteolysis. A increase in the respiratory quotient is often seen [7]. A number of micronutrients are lost in urine as well as wound effluent [8,9].

ENERGY REQUIREMENTS

A significant increase in energy expenditure (often 150% of resting energy expenditure or higher) is a hallmark of the metabolic response to injury (Table 23.4). This results from a number of factors, including hyperdynamic circulatory response, increased temperature, increased oxygen utilization, and carbon dioxide production. The injured patient is at risk for developing protein-calorie malnutrition, and that their energy requirements may exceed normal values by 50% or more [10].

When available, indirect calorimetry should be utilized to guide nutrition therapy. Otherwise, use of predictive equations is appropriately used. A detailed description is provided in Chapter 6. It is important to note that major trauma, particularly burns and other open wounds, can elicit a significant increase in protein and energy demands beyond what is typically seen in other ICU patients [11,12].

PROTEIN REQUIREMENTS

Trauma (including the controlled injury of elective surgery) leads to significant alterations of plasma and tissue protein content and metabolism. The metabolic distress of major tissue disruption is associated with protein losses in the first several days after injury. The systemic inflammatory response leads to variations in serum proteins that differ from the changes seen in simple starvation [13]. A rapid decrease in serum albumin, prealbumin, and total protein can be expected. This occurs due to multiple factors, including changes in hepatic function, increased capillary permeability, and altered insulin/glucose metabolism.

TABLE 23.4
Metabolic Response to Stress versus Simple Starvation

	Metabolic Stress	Starvation
Resting energy expenditure	↑↑	↓↓
Respiratory quotient	↑	↓
Proteolysis	↑↑↑	↑
Primary fuel	Mixed	Fat
Catecholamines	↑↑↑	—
Acute phase protein	↑↑↑	—
Gluconeogenesis	↑↑↑	↑
Urinary nitrogen losses	↑↑↑	↑
Weight loss	Rapid	Slow
Ketones	↑	↑↑↑

Source: Adapted from Kozar RA et al., *ACCP Crit. Care Board Rev.*, 2003.

Not only is the production and distribution of proteins affected, but protein loss also occurs. In addition to increased overall energy requirements, the injured patient can be expected to lose as much as 110 g protein/day [14]. Open wounds are a source of major ongoing protein, electrolyte, and fluid losses [15]. The protein loss across a burn wound can be estimated to be [1.2 × body surface area (m^2) × %burn] [16].

ROUTE OF NUTRITION SUPPORT

There remains little doubt that nutrition support should be provided via the enteral route. Total enteral nutrition is well tolerated in most patients and may favorably impact inflammatory cytokines and immune function, reduce septic complications, and promote wound healing [17–19]. All too often, enteral nutrition is not delivered at the prescribed amount. Interruption of tube feeds frequently occurs due to planned procedures [20]. In general, enteral nutrition should not be interrupted for procedures [21].

ROLE OF IMMUNE-MODULATING DIETS AND ADJUNCTIVE THERAPIES

A number of commercially available formulas contain combinations of two or more ingredients considered *immune modulating*. It is difficult to draw any firm conclusions as to the optimal composition of an immune-modulating diet, but current evidence supports the use of such formulas. The mechanisms and evidence regarding the use of various adjunctive nutrition support therapies in the critically ill patient (including glutamine, arginine, omega-3 fatty acids, antioxidants, trace minerals, probiotics, etc.) are discussed elsewhere. While glutamine and antioxidants in particular have been studied in the trauma population, their optimal utilization is unclear. While there are a number of studies supporting the use of these supplements, the REDOXs© study indicates that they should not be used in sicker patients [22–27].

SPECIAL POPULATIONS

Abdominal Compartment Syndrome and the Open Abdomen

Intra-abdominal hypertension (IAH) and abdominal compartment syndrome (ACS) are recognized complications of trauma and critical illness. They may occur primarily (as a direct result of abdominal or pelvic injuries) or secondarily (due to massive resuscitation). Abdominal wall and bowel edema lead to an increased pressure within the abdominal cavity. The abdominal perfusion pressure is the mean arterial pressure minus the intra-abdominal pressure. IAH is defined by a sustained intra-abdominal pressure ≥12 mmHg. Abdominal compartment syndrome is defined as a sustained IAP >20 mmHg that is associated with new organ dysfunction or failure [28].

The critically ill surgical patient may need to have the abdominal cavity left open for decompression or in anticipation of repeat laparotomies (e.g., damage-control) as an urgent, life-saving measure. A variety of methods are available to effect temporary coverage of the abdominal and pelvic contents, and definitive abdominal closure is delayed until the acute issues have sufficiently resolved. There continues to be reluctance among practitioners to initiate enteral nutrition in the patient with an open abdomen. In some cases, the bowel may be in discontinuity with stapled ends, and enteral nutrition is clearly not indicated. Impaired motility may be present, particularly if there is significant bowel edema. However, the mere presence of an open abdomen should not discourage attempts at enteral nutrition support. A number of published studies and reports illustrate the feasibility of early enteral support in the patient with an open abdomen [29–33]. Early enteral feeding in these patients does not appear to impair the rate for delayed fascial closure and may reduce the risk of nosocomial infection [34]. An association between enteral feeding and overall decreased complication rates, higher fascial closure rate, and decreased mortality in patients without bowel injury has been demonstrated [35].

Head Injury

Traumatic brain injury (TBI) has come to be recognized as a significant public health problem. An estimated 1.7 TBIs occur every year and are a contributing factor in almost a third of injury-related deaths [36]. The actual number of TBIs is almost certainly underreported as data are typically only collected on patients who are admitted to the hospital. The clinical consequences of TBI may persist long after the initial injury. Alterations on structure and function of the brain may continue for years.

Although there may be differences between focal and diffuse brain injury, the transfer of energy to brain tissue is a common feature. Depolarization of nerve cells leads to the release of the neurotransmitter glutamate and calcium. A number of cellular systems are affected. Mitochondrial function, membrane stability, blood flow, and cytoskeletal structure frequently exhibit dysfunction after TBI. A number of pharmacological agents intended to confer a neuroprotective effect (including selfotel, pegorgotein, magnesium, deltibant, and dexanabinol) have been studied, but none have been shown to improve outcomes [37,38].

Increases in cerebral and systemic energy requirements occur. Initiation of nutrition support in the first few days may have an important impact on mortality. A study of 797 patients with traumatic brain injury in New York state trauma centers showed an association between caloric debt and mortality; for each 10 kcal/kg reduction in caloric intake, there was an increase in mortality [39]. Patients with increased intracranial pressure appeared to benefit the most from early feeding. The results of a number of smaller studies also support early enteral nutrition support; a prospective, randomized, controlled study of 82 head-injured patients admitted to a British hospital showed that improved enteral nutrition support in the first week after injury reduced total complications and sped up the time to recovery [40]. A 2008 Cochrane Collaborative review indicated "that early feeding may be associated with fewer infections and a trend toward better outcomes in terms of survival and disability" [41].

The Institute of Medicine published a comprehensive review of the growing role of nutrition support to improve outcomes for patients with TBI. Although supplementation of specific micro- or macronutrients (such as n-3 fatty acids, creatine, choline, vitamin D, antioxidants, branched-chain amino acids) or other specialized nutrition support (e.g., ketogenic diet) show some promising possibilities, additional research is needed before any detailed recommendations can be endorsed. The recommendations include the following [42]:

Provision of nutrition support in the first 24 h after injury
Provide >50% of total energy expenditure for the first 2 weeks after injury
Provide 1–1.5 g/kg of protein in the first 2 weeks after injury

Spinal Cord Injury

According to the Centers for Disease Control and Prevention, ~200,000 people in the United States are living with a spinal cord injury (SCI), with an additional 12–20,000 new injuries each year. Alcohol use is a significant factor in ~25% of these cases [43]. Alcohol use was found to be more prevalent in patients with cervical SCI than those without [43,44]. Any body organ system may be affected, depending on the level and extent of SCI. Once injury occurs, treatment options are often limited. Therefore, prevention continues to be crucial. Blunt trauma is more common; motor vehicle crashes and falls account for about 2/3 of spinal cord injuries. Use of a seatbelt and airbag decreases the odds of injury by 80% [45]. Restraint devices also reduce the severity of injury and infectious morbidity [46]. The direct lifetime medical costs due to the SCI range from $500,000 to $3 million. Most cases occur in young people, ages 15–35.

The injury can cause metabolic changes similar to other causes of injury and inflammation; often, there are significant associated injuries. The presence of a SCI can present additional challenges due to a number of factors. Impaired sensation increases the risk of pressure ulcers, which can occur in mere hours. The alteration in autonomic tone can contribute to hypoperfusion and the inability to mount an appropriate physiological response to new stressors. Anemia, even in the absence of any obvious blood loss, is very common [47].

SCI is associated with increased visceral adipose tissue [48]. However, there does not appear to be an increased risk of metabolic syndrome [49]. There is increased risk of cardiovascular disease, diabetes, and hypertension [50]. Pressure ulcers are also more common, occurring in more than one-quarter of patients with SCI [51,52].

Nutrition support is increasingly recognized as an important element of recovery and rehabilitation from SCI. While focused nutrition support is typically a part of the postacute stay, it is not uncommon for the patient to proceed to acute rehabilitation very soon after the initial ICU stay. As with other ICU patients, enteral nutrition remains preferable to the parenteral route. However, when a cervical spine injury requires prolonged immobilization, alternate enteral access should be discussed early.

GUIDELINES

The following includes some of the pertinent guidelines for the trauma patient excerpted from the Guidelines for the Provision and Assessment of Nutrition Support Therapy in the Adult Critically Ill Patient [53].

Immune-modulating enteral formulations (supplemented with agents such as arginine, glutamine, nucleic acid, ω-3 fatty acids, and antioxidants) should be used for the appropriate patient population (major elective surgery, trauma, burns, head and neck cancer, and critically ill patients on mechanical ventilation), with caution in patients with severe sepsis (for surgical ICU patients, grade A).

Administration of probiotic agents has been shown to improve outcome (most consistently by decreasing infection) in specific critically ill patient populations involving transplantation, major abdominal surgery, and severe trauma (Grade: C).

The addition of enteral glutamine to an EN regimen (not already containing supplemental glutamine) should be considered in burn, trauma, and mixed ICU patients (Grade: B).

REFERENCES

1. Esposito TJ, Brasel KJ. Epidemiology, in *Trauma*, 7th edn., Mattox KL et al., eds. McGraw Hill Medical, New York, 2013, pp. 18–35.
2. Baker SP et al. The injury severity score: A method for describing patients with multiple injuries and evaluating emergency care. *J Trauma* 1974;14(3):187–196.
3. Cuthbertson DP. Further observations on the disturbance of metabolism caused by injury, with particular reference to the dietary requirement of fracture cases. *Br J Surg* 1936;23:505–520.
4. Hill AG, Hill GL. Metabolic response to severe injury. *Br J Surg* 1998;85:884–890.
5. Cavaillon JM et al. Immunodepression in sepsis and SIRS assessed by ex vivo cytokine production is not a generalized phenomenon: A review. *J Endotoxin Res* 2001;7:85–93.
6. Gentile LF et al. Persistent inflammation and immunosuppression: A common syndrome and new horizon for surgical critical care. *J Trauma Acute Care Surg* 2012;72:1491–1501.
7. Kudsk KA, Curtis C. Nutritional support and electrolyte management, in *Trauma*, 7th edn., Mattox KL et al., eds. McGraw Hill Companies, New York, 2013, pp. 1100–1127.
8. Askari A et al. Urinary zinc, copper, nitrogen, and potassium losses in response to trauma. *J Parenter Enteral Nutr* 1979;3:151–156.
9. Klein CJ et al. Trace element loss in urine and effluent following traumatic injury. *J Parenter Enteral Nutr* 2008;32:129–139.
10. Jones TN et al. Factors influencing nutritional assessment in abdominal trauma patients. *J Parenter Enteral Nutr* 1983;7:115–116.
11. Long CL et al. Metabolic response to injury and illness: Estimation of energy and protein needs from indirect calorimetry and nitrogen balance. *J Parenter Enteral Nutr* 1977;3:452–456.

12. Frankenfield D. Energy expenditure and protein requirements after traumatic injury. *J Parenter Enteral Nutr* 2006;21:430–437.
13. Holbrook IB et al. Response of plasma amino acids to elective surgical trauma. *J Parenter Enteral Nutr* 1979;3:424–426.
14. Hill GL. Rhoads Lecture. Body composition research: Implications for the practice of clinical nutrition. *J Parenter Enteral Nutr* 1992;16:197–218.
15. Hourigan LA et al. Loss of protein, immunoglobulins, and electrolytes in exudates from negative pressure wound therapy. *Nutr Clin Pract* 2010;25:510–516.
16. Waxman K et al. Protein loss across burn wounds. *J Trauma* 1987;27:136–140.
17. Moore EE, Jones TN. Benefits of immediate jejunal feeding after major abdominal trauma: A prospective randomized study. *J Trauma* 1986;26:874.
18. Moore FA et al. TEN versus TPN following major abdominal trauma—Reduced septic morbidity. *J Trauma* 1989;29:916–922.
19. Kudsk KA et al. Enteral versus parenteral feeding: Effects on septic morbidity after blunt and penetrating abdominal trauma. *Ann Surg* 1992;215:503–511.
20. Morgan LM et al. Factors causing interrupted delivery of enteral nutrition in trauma intensive care unit patients. *Nutr Clin Pract* 2004;19(5):511–517.
21. Pousman RM et al. Feasibility of implementing a reduced fasting protocol for critically ill trauma patients undergoing operative and nonoperative procedures. *J Parenter Enteral Nutr* 2009;33(2):176–180.
22. Burke DJ et al. Glutamine-supplemented total parenteral nutrition improves gut immune function. *Arch Surg* 1989;124:1396–1399.
23. Houdijk APJ et al. Randomised trial of glutamine-enriched enteral nutrition on infectious morbidity in patients with multiple trauma. *Lancet* 1998;352:772–776.
24. Blass SC et al. Time to wound closure in trauma patients with disorders in wound healing is shortened by supplements containing antioxidant micronutrients and glutamine: A PRCT. *Clin Nutr* 2012;31:469–475.
25. Collier BR et al. Impact of high-dose antioxidants on outcomes in acutely injured patients. *J Parenter Enteral Nutr* 2008:32:384–387.
26. Berger MM. Antioxidant micronutrients in major trauma and burns: Evidence and practice. *Nutr Clin Pract* 2006;21:438–449.
27. Heyland D et al. A randomized trial of glutamine and antioxidants in critically ill patients. *N Engl J Med* 2013;369:482.
28. Malbrain ML, Cheatham ML, Kirkpatrick A, Sugrue M, Parr M, De Waele J, et al. Results from the international conference of experts on intra-abdominal hypertension and abdominal compartment syndrome. I. Definitions. *Intensive Care Med.* 2006;32:1722–1732.
29. Tsuei BJ et al. Enteral nutrition in patients with an open peritoneal cavity. *Nutr Clin Pract* 2003;18(3):253–258.
30. Cothren CC et al. Postinjury abdominal compartment syndrome does not preclude early enteral feeding after definitive closure. *Am J Surg* 2004;188:653–658.
31. Byrnes MC et al. Early enteral nutrition can be successfully implemented in trauma patients with an "open abdomen." *Am J Surg* 2010;199:359–363.
32. McKibbin B et al. Nutrition support for the patient with an open abdomen after major abdominal trauma. *Nutrition* 2003;19:563–566.
33. Powell NJ, Collier B. Nutrition and the open abdomen. *Nutr Clin Pract* 2012;27(4):499–506.
34. Dissanaike S et al. Effect of immediate enteral feeding on trauma patients with an open abdomen: Protection from nosocomial infections. *J Am Coll Surg* 2008;207(5):690–697.
35. Burlew CC et al. Who should we feed? Western Trauma Association multi-institutional study of enteral nutrition in the open abdomen after injury. *J Trauma Acute Care Surg* 2012;73(6):1380–1387.
36. Faul M, Xu L, Wald MM, Coronado VG. Traumatic brain injury in the United States: Emergency department visits, hospitalizations, and deaths. Centers for Disease Control and Prevention, National Center for Injury Prevention and Control, Atlanta, GA, 2010.
37. McConeghy KW et al. A review of neuroprotection pharmacology and therapies in patients with acute traumatic brain injury. *CNS Drugs* 2012;26(7):613–636.
38. Bratton SL et al. Guidelines for the management of severe traumatic brain injury. XII. Nutrition. *J Neurotrauma* 2007;24(Suppl. 1):S77–S82.
39. Härtl R et al. Effect of early nutrition on deaths due to severe traumatic brain injury. *J Neurosurg* 2008;109(1):50–56.

40. Taylor SJ et al. Prospective, randomized, controlled trial to determine the effect of early enhanced enteral nutrition on clinical outcome in mechanically ventilated patients suffering head injury. *Crit Care Med* 1999;27(11):2525–2531.
41. Perel P, Yanagawa T, Bunn F, Roberts I, Wentz R, Pierro A. Nutritional support for head injured patients. The Cochrane Library 2008;Issue 4:CD001530.
42. IOM (Institute of Medicine). *Nutrition and Traumatic Brain Injury: Improving Acute and Subacute Health Outcomes in Military Personnel*. The National Academies Press, Washington, DC, 2011.
43. Beers MH, Kaplan JL, eds. *The Merck Manual of Diagnosis and Therapy*, 18th edn. Merck Sharp & Dohme Corp, Whitehouse Station, NJ, 2006.
44. Garrison A et al. Alcohol use associated with cervical spinal cord injury. *J Spinal Cord Med* 2004;27(2):111–115.
45. Clayton B et al. Cervical spine injury and restraint system use in motor vehicle collisions. *Spine* 2004;29(4):386–389.
46. Williams RF et al. Impact of airbags on a Level I trauma center: Injury patterns, infectious morbidity, and hospital costs. *J Am Coll Surg* 2008;206(5):962–968.
47. Huang CT et al. Anemia in acute phase of spinal cord injury. *Arch Phys Med Rehabil* 1990;71(1):3–7.
48. Edwards LA et al. Visceral adipose tissue and the ratio of visceral to subcutaneous adipose tissue are greater in adults with than in those without spinal cord injury, despite matching waist circumferences. *Am J Clin Nutr* 2008;87(3):600–607.
49. Liang H et al. Different risk factor patterns for metabolic syndrome in men with spinal cord injury compared with able-bodied men despite similar prevalence rates. *Arch Phys Med Rehabil* 2007;88(9):1198–1204.
50. Bauman WA et al. Risk factors for atherogenesis and cardiovascular autonomic function in persons with spinal cord injury. *Spinal Cord* 1999;37:601–616.
51. Salzberg CA et al. A new pressure ulcer risk assessment scale for individuals with spinal cord injury. *Am J Phys Med Rehabil* 1996;75(2):96–104.
52. Garber SL, Rintala DH. Pressure ulcers in veterans with spinal cord injury: A retrospective study. *J Rehabil Res Dev* 2003;40(5):433–441.
53. McClave SA, Martindale RG, Vanek VW, McCarthy M, Roberts P, Taylor B, Ochua JB, Napolitano L, Cresci G; the A.S.P.E.N. Board of Directors; the American College of Critical Care Medicine. Guidelines for the Provision and Assessment of Nutrition Support Therapy in the Adult Critically Ill Patient: Society of Critical Care Medicine (SCCM) and American Society for Parenteral and Enteral Nutrition (A.S.P.E.N.). *J Parenter Enteral Nutr* 2009;33:277.
54. Kozar RA et al. Nutritional support of the stressed ICU patient. *ACCP Crit Care Board Rev* 2003; pp. 440–458.

24 Nutrition Support for Burns and Wound Healing

Theresa Mayes and Michele M. Gottschlich

CONTENTS

BURNS AND WOUND HEALING

Wounds originate from a variety of sources. Burns, surgery, infectious disease, trauma, toxic epidermal necrolysis, radiation therapy, decubiti, diabetes, or vascular ulcers are only a few of the many causes of tissue destruction. Normal progression of tissue repair requires conditions that maximize vascular sufficiency, aseptic state, immunity, and nutritional balance. This chapter focuses on the metabolic alterations produced by burns and wounds, the nutritional components of tissue repair, methods for assessment of nutritional adequacy, and therapeutic modalities that enhance anabolism, and thus, the promotion of healing.

METABOLIC CONSEQUENCES

Wounds are classified according to the size and depth of skin layer injury (Figure 24.1). Alterations in metabolism positively correlate with the assessment of both of these parameters. Wound specification in this manner allows the clinician to determine the degree of heat, fluid, and nutrient losses as well as the comorbid risk of infection and mortality.

The classic injury response as described by Cuthbertson and Tilstone[1] is most obvious following a burn that covers a large surface area. Table 24.1 describes the dominant factors of the ebb and flow phases and how these responses are characterized clinically. The ebb phase is typically present for 24–48 h postburn but can last up to 5 days. The transition to the flow response is primarily driven by an increase in the catabolic hormones epinephrine, norepinephrine, and their metabolites, glucocorticoids and glucagon. The synergistic effects of these hormones accelerate proteolysis, gluconeogenesis, lipolytic activity, and most profoundly, energy expenditure.[2] The effects of these hormones on metabolic rate and catabolism are present until the wound achieves closure and the patient enters the convalescent state.

The etiology of hypermetabolism is driven not only by hormonal alterations, but also by a number of additional contributing factors. Increased evaporative water and heat loss from the burn wound appear to increase the metabolic response.[3] In addition, significant sleep pattern disruption in burn patients has been reported; suggesting that lack of deep sleep in the acute postburn period may contribute to hypermetabolism.[4] Furthermore, early enteral feeding has also been proposed as a means to reduce the postinjury surge in metabolism.[5–7] Finally, cytokines appear to indirectly affect metabolic rate by stimulating the endocrine system to release increased concentrations of the catecholamines, cortisol, and glucagon.[8,9]

Gradual wound closure provides the greatest effect on decreasing metabolic rate. Reduction in wound size serves to decrease catabolic hormone production, enhance sleep, and diminish evaporative heat loss. Interestingly, wound closure does not completely normalize metabolism as Hart and colleagues[10] denote an exaggerated metabolic and catabolic response up to 9 months following injury. Prevention of systemic infection, provision of adequate pain and anxiety relief, and promotion of restorative sleep are also important factors in lessening the metabolic response.

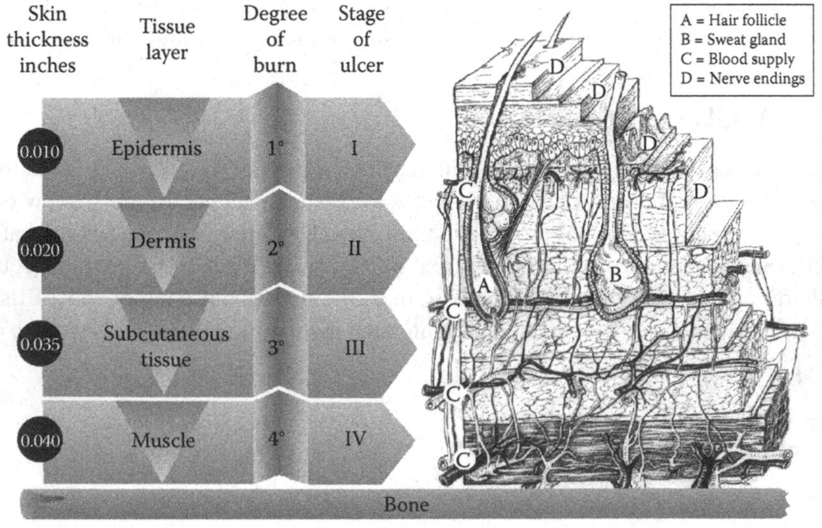

FIGURE 24.1 Classification of wounds.

TABLE 24.1
Metabolic Alterations Produced by Burns

Flow Response	Ebb Response	Acute Phase	Adaptive Phase
Dominant factors	Loss of plasma volume Poor tissue perfusion Shock Low plasma insulin levels	Increased total body blood flow Elevated catecholamines Elevated glucagon Elevated glucocorticoids Normal or elevated serum insulin High glucagon–insulin ratio	Stress hormone response subsiding Convalescence
Metabolic and clinical characteristics	Decreased oxygen consumption Depressed resting energy expenditure Decreased blood pressure Cardiac output below normal Decreased body temperature	Catabolism Hyperglycemia Increased respiratory rate Increased oxygen consumption and hypermetabolism Increased carbon dioxide production Increased body temperature Redistribution of polyvalent cations such as zinc and iron Increased urinary excretion of nitrogen, sulfur, magnesium, calcium, phosphorus, potassium, and creatinine Accelerated gluconeogenesis Fat mobilization Increased use of amino acids as oxidative fuels	Anabolism Normoglycemia Energy expenditure diminished Bone demineralization Nutrient requirements approaching preinjury needs

Source: Adapted from Gottschlich, M.M. et al., Enteral nutrition in patients with burns or trauma, in Rombeau, J.L. and Caldwell, M.D. (eds.), *Enteral and Tube Feeding*, Vol. 1, W.B. Saunders, Philadelphia, PA, 1990, p. 307. With permission.

MACRONUTRIENTS

Protein

The role of protein in tissue repair is irrefutable. Adequate protein ensures cell multiplication and collagen and connective tissue formation. Intact protein, particularly of whey source, has been proven to be superior to free amino acids in maintaining body weight and nitrogen retention.[11–13]

Protein requirements positively correlate with the total body surface area (TBSA) affected as well as the depth of injury. Patients with burn injuries greater than 25% TBSA benefit from approximately 23% of total calories as protein.[14] Given the hypermetabolic state of the burn patient, this may translate to 3–5 g/kg/day. Evidence-based guidelines are lacking for protein provision in patients with less than 25% open area. It is generally prudent, however, to begin protein replacement at slightly above the dietary reference intake[15] (DRI), at 1.2–1.5 g/kg for the adult patient that presents with less than 10% TBSA wound (as with small burns, decubitus,[16] etc.), and upward of 2 g/kg/day in patients whose wounds affect areas approaching the 20% TBSA marker (as with moderate burns). Increasing protein intake beyond 1.5 g/kg/day for smaller wounds may not increase protein synthesis, particularly in the elderly, and predispose to dehydration.[17] Despite etiology, size, and depth of the wound, the amount of protein should be modified based on routine evaluation of parameters noted in the section "Nutrition Assessment."

ARGININE

Arginine has a role in wound healing.[18–21] In addition to tissue repair, arginine augments the immune system through enhanced lymphocyte activity[22] and stimulates the release of anabolic hormones such as insulin, growth hormone, and insulin-like growth factor-1. Arginine levels are depleted in critical illness most likely from reduced intake, increased tissue uptake, and accelerated metabolism. Controversy exists regarding the production of nitric oxide from the delivery of arginine to hemodynamically unstable, critically ill patients. Nitric oxide can result in vasodilation and hypotension, enhancing instability. However, an argument exists that controlled vasodilation may be beneficial in sepsis and shock. For example, Yan et al.[23] noted that enteral provision of arginine during burn shock resuscitation promotes oxygen transport to injured tissue. In addition, studies have demonstrated that in combination with omega-3 fatty acid delivery, arginine supports wound healing and immune function.[24–26] The recommended dose of arginine replacement is at 2% of overall calories in burns.[24] The application of arginine replacement in lung injury,[27] medical and surgical patients, trauma, and sepsis is gaining acceptance as well.[28] Multiple studies also associate improved wound healing with supplementation of arginine in combination with vitamin C and zinc.[29–32]

GLUTAMINE

Glutamine enhances the proliferation of fibroblasts and macrophages, both of which are integral components of the wound healing process. Fibroblasts use glutamine as energy to produce collagen. Macrophages require glutamine for their role in growth factor production. In a preclinical study, glutamine was more effective than control in preventing apoptosis, improving total lymphocyte count and secretion of intestinal IgA, resulting in greater mucosal immunity.[33] Oral glutamine has been shown to improve healing of colonic anastomoses in rats.[34] Furthermore, evidence exists to support the supplementation of glutamine in patients with large burns as it has been shown to promote protein synthesis, reduce intestinal permeability, decrease length of stay, improve wound healing, and decrease infectious morbidity and overall mortality.[35–38]

Glutamine is also the major fuel source for immune cells and enterocytes, providing a protective effect on gut barrier function.[39–41] The optimal amount and form of glutamine required to achieve beneficial results is unknown. Gottschlich and colleagues[40] performed a prospective, randomized, double-blind study examining the clinical effect of adding 14.3 g of glutamine per liter of tube feeding versus control tube feeding lacking glutamine in pediatric patients with large burns. Four percent of patients in the control group experienced bowel necrosis and an additional 4% required laparotomy, whereas no patient in the treated group experienced such morbid outcome. In addition, the treated group had significantly less positive blood cultures for gram-negative bacteria. Trends toward reduced incidence of diarrhea, provision of exogenous albumin and insulin, and use of parenteral nutrition were associated with glutamine supplementation. The authors conclude that the decreased morbidity associated with glutamine enrichment may be the result of improved gut integrity, hemodynamic stability, or immune function. Glutamine supplementation is safe for patients (except those with hyperammonemia, hepatic or renal failure) and may be worth trialing as an adjunctive intervention especially in patients with large, nonhealing wounds. This study provides support for the work of Wischmeyer et al.[42] whereby reduced gram-negative bacteremia was noted following glutamine administration in the burn population.

Carbohydrate and Fat

Energy demands positively correlate to the size and depth of the wound as well. Energy in sufficient quantity to spare the increased protein requirement of wound healing is essential. The appropriate source of energy, either carbohydrate or fat, to be provided in the greatest quantity has been debated. Glucose is utilized efficiently as an energy source in tissue repair, and fat is a necessary component of cell membranes. A deficiency of essential fatty acids suppresses tissue repair. However, there is evidence that low-fat, high-carbohydrate provision enhances wound healing, suggesting that carbohydrate may be the preferred energy fuel.[24,43,44]

Lipid is an essential component of wound healing as it comprises cell membranes and acts as a carrier of the fat-soluble vitamins. Delayed wound healing has been shown in fatty acid deficiency.[45] Although the clinician may be attracted to fat as a concentrated means of supplying calories to the hypermetabolic patient, large amounts of fat have proven detrimental in wound recovery as a number of studies correlate high fat intake with a poor immune response.[24,43,44] In addition, fat does not stimulate insulin production nor does it assist with protein sparing. Mochizuki and colleagues recommend a diet containing 5%–15% of nonprotein calories as fat in order to optimally assist in the recovery from burn injury.[43]

In addition to the amount of fat, the type of fat provided to support wound healing is an essential component of the nutrition care plan.[46] Arachidonic acid is formed from linoleic acid and further metabolizes to the 1 and 2 series of prostaglandins, thromboxane, prostacyclin, and leukotrienes. These metabolites are associated with immunosuppression, inflammation, and proteolysis, thus impairment of the healing process. For these reasons, the diet of the patient with an open wound should be limited in linoleic acid, the precursor of arachidonic acid.

Eicosapentaenoic acid and docosahexaenoic acid are precursors of the triene prostaglandins and series 5 leukotrienes. These metabolites are known to have anti-inflammatory, immune-enhancing properties and prevent the linoleic to PGE1 and PGE2 cascade. The clinical contribution of Gottschlich and colleagues supports the laboratory work of Alexander and associates, deducing that an enteral diet that is low in fat and linoleic acid and supplemented with omega-3 fatty acids improves the immune response, significantly decreasing morbidity, wound infection, and length of stay.[24,46]

Choosing the appropriate enteral formula for the patient with large burns from the myriad of products available on the market takes a bit of scrutiny. For practical purposes, the formula should provide 20%–25% of calories as protein, be low in linoleic acid, contain omega-3 fatty acids (if not marketed as such, evaluate the alpha linolenic acid content), and have fairly low fat content (as low as 12%–15% of calories although most products are in the 20%–30% range). Administration of an enteral formula enriched with fish oil was associated with a significantly lower rate of new pressure ulcer development and lowered C-reactive protein levels when compared to subjects provided with a control tube feeding formula.[47] Generally, patients with wounds of any etiology covering less than 10% body surface area do not undergo a huge inflammatory response (unless other trauma invoked, e.g., smoke inhalation, fracture, blunt trauma); thus, the primary nutrition objective is provision of sufficient calories, protein, and micronutrients (Table 24.2).

MICRONUTRIENTS

Most micronutrients function as coenzymes and cofactors, which permit protein and calories to be utilized more efficiently. The role of various micronutrients in wound healing is outlined in Table 24.3. Inadequate intake, increased loss via wound exudate, malabsorption, and heightened metabolism impact micronutrient status postinjury. Experience suggests that for some nutrients, intake beyond that found in a standard multivitamin/mineral provision is beneficial to wound healing. For this reason, vitamins A and C and zinc are most commonly supplemented in burns according to the standards listed in Table 24.3.

TABLE 24.2
Micronutrient Summary Pertinent to Wound Healing

Micronutrient	Function in Wound Healing	Food Sources	Deficiency Symptoms	Test to Determine Deficiency State
Vitamin A	Enhances tissue regeneration by aiding in glycoprotein synthesis. Cofactor for collagen synthesis and cross-linkage.	Liver, fish liver oils, enriched dairy products, egg yolk, carrots, sweet potato, squash, apricots, peaches, and dark green leafy vegetables	Xerophthalmia (night blindness, conjunctival xerosis, Bitot's spots), respiratory ailments (pneumonia, bronchopulmonary dysplasia), affects epithelial tissues of the gut	Serum vitamin A
Thiamine (B_1)	Cofactor in collagen cross-linking.	Brewer's yeast, unrefined cereal grains, organ meats, pork, legumes, nuts, seeds	Beriberi, anorexia, fatigue, peripheral neuropathy, foot and wrist drop, cardiomegaly, hyperlactatemia	Serum or 24 h urinary thiamin
Riboflavin (B_2)	Cofactor in collagen cross-linking.	Broccoli, spinach, asparagus, turnip greens, meat, poultry, fish, yeast, egg whites, dairy products, milk, fortified grain products	Cheilosis, angular stomatitis, glossitis, scrotal dermatitis, cessation of growth, photophobia	Serum erythrocyte glutathione reductase
Pyridoxine (B_6)	Coenzyme that activates protein synthesis.	Chicken, fish, kidney, liver, pork, bananas, eggs, soy beans, oats, whole wheat products, peanuts, walnuts	Irritability, depression, stomatitis, glossitis, cheilosis, seborrhea of the nasal labial folds, normochromic, microcytic, or sideroblastic anemia	Serum erythrocytic glutamic-oxaloacetic transaminase (EGOT) and serum erythrocytic glutamic-pyruvic transaminase (EGPT)
Cobalamin (B_{12})	Coenzyme for protein and DNA synthesis.	Meat and meat products, fish, shellfish, poultry, eggs	Megaloblastic anemia, loss of appetite, weight loss, fatigue, glossitis, leukopenia, thrombocytopenia, achlorhydria	Serum cobalamin
Vitamin C	Necessary for hydroxylation of lysine and proline in collagen formation as well as cross-linking. Protects tissue from superoxide damage. Enhances tissue regeneration.	Citrus fruits, green vegetables, potatoes	Fatigue, anorexia, muscular pain, scurvy characterized by anemia; hemorrhagic disorders; weakening of collagenous structures in bone cartilage, teeth and connective tissue; degeneration of muscle; gingivitis; capillary weakness; and rheumatic leg pain	Serum vitamin C

(Continued)

TABLE 24.2 (*Continued*)
Micronutrient Summary Pertinent to Wound Healing

Micronutrient	Function in Wound Healing	Food Sources	Deficiency Symptoms	Test to Determine Deficiency State
Vitamin D	Regulates the synthesis of several structural proteins, including collagen type I.	Fortified dairy products, eggs, butter, fortified margarine	Bone demineralization	Serum 25 (OH) vitamin D
Vitamin E	Antioxidant properties promote cell membrane integrity.	Wheat germ, rice germ, vegetable oil, dark green leafy vegetables, nuts, legumes	Increased platelet aggregation, decreased red blood cell survival, hemolytic anemia, neurologic abnormalities, decreased serum creatinine levels, excessive creatinuria	Serum vitamin E
Vitamin K	Essential for coagulation that is a prerequisite for wound healing.	Green leafy vegetables, dairy products, meat, eggs, cereals, fruits	Hemorrhage	Plasma vitamin K, prothrombin time
Magnesium	Cofactor for enzymes involved in protein and collagen synthesis.	Nuts, legumes, unmilled grains, green vegetables, bananas	Nausea, muscle weakness, irritability, mental derangement	Serum magnesium
Calcium	Both the remodeling process and the degradation of collagen are accomplished through the action of various collagenases, all of which require calcium.	Dairy products, sardines, oysters, kale, greens, tofu	Osteoporosis	Serum calcium
Copper	Promotes the cross-linking reactions of collagen and elastin synthesis. Scavenges free radicals.	Whole grain breads and cereals, shellfish especially oysters, organ meats, poultry, dried peas and beans, dark green leafy vegetables	Skeletal demineralization, impaired glucose tolerance, anemia, neutropenia, leukopenia, changes in hair and skin pigmentation	Serum copper or ceruloplasmin
Iron	Necessary for hydroxylation of lysine and proline in collagen synthesis as well as transportation of oxygen to the wound bed.	Egg yolk, red meats, dark green leafy vegetables, enriched breads and cereals, legumes, dried fruits	Anemia, cheilosis, glossitis, atrophy of the tongue, hair loss, brittle fingernails, koilonychia, pallor, tissue hypoxia, exertional dyspnea, heart enlargement	Serum ferritin, hemoglobin, hematocrit

(*Continued*)

TABLE 24.2 (*Continued*)
Micronutrient Summary Pertinent to Wound Healing

Micronutrient	Function in Wound Healing	Food Sources	Deficiency Symptoms	Test to Determine Deficiency State
Selenium	Reduces intracellular hydroperoxides, thereby protecting membrane lipids from oxidant damage.	Seafood, kidney, liver, meats, grains	Growth retardation, muscle pain and weakness, myopathy, cardiomyopathy	Serum or plasma selenium
Zinc	A cofactor in over 100 different enzyme systems that promote protein synthesis, cellular replication, and collagen formation.	Oysters, dark meat turkey, liver, lima beans, pork	Hair loss, dermatitis, growth retardation, delayed sexual maturation, testicular atrophy, decreased appetite, depressed smell and taste acuity, depression, diarrhea, decreased dark adaptation	Serum or plasma zinc

Source: Adapted from Mayes, T. and Gottschlich, M.M., Burns and wound healing, in Gottschlich, M.M. (ed.), *American Society for Parenteral and Enteral Nutrition: The Science and Practice of Nutrition Support*, Kendall Hunt Publishing, Dubuque, IA, 2001, pp. 391–392. With permission.

TABLE 24.3
Micronutrient Guidelines after Thermal Injury

Adults and Children	Children
≥3 years of age	<3 years of age
>40 lb	≤40 lb
≥20% burn	≥10% burn
1 Multivitamin (qd)	1 Children's multivitamin (qd)
500 mg ascorbic acid (bid)	250 mg ascorbic acid (bid)
10,000 IU vitamin A (qd)	5000 IU vitamin A (qd)
220 mg zinc sulfate (qd)[a]	110 mg zinc sulfate (qd)[a]
1600 IU vitamin D_3 (qd)	800 IU vitamin D_3 (qd)

Source: Adapted from Mayes, T. et al., *J. Burn Care Rehabil.*, 18, 365, 1997. With permission.
qd, everyday; bid, twice a day; IU, international unit.
[a] Recommended delivery in suspension for tube feeding, because orally administered zinc in large doses may precipitate nausea or vomiting.

Clinical reports of prolonged hypocalcemia,[48–50] hypomagnesemia,[47,48,51] and hypophosphatemia[50,52,53] following burn injury are prevalent in the literature. Depressed vitamin D status has been confirmed in the postburn state as well.[54–57] Reduced stores of these nutrients may partially account for reports of decreased bone density,[55,57–60] increased fracture risk,[61] and pediatric growth delay[62] in burns. A recent randomized clinical trial comparing supplementation of vitamin D_2, D_3, and placebo in pediatric burns revealed that subjects receiving daily enteral vitamin D_3 in the acute postburn period had improved 25-hydroxyvitamin D levels at 1-year postburn time frame.[63]

Trends toward decreased length of stay, septic episodes, antibiotic days, surgical procedures, insulin requirement, wound healing time, and overall medical length of stay were evident in the group randomized to receive vitamin D_3. Interestingly, vitamin D_3 also appears to provide a protective bone effect as no patient in the D_3 supplemented group experienced long-bone fracture up to 2 years postinjury. This is in contrast to the 15% fracture occurrence that was reported in the combined vitamin D_2 and placebo groups.[64]

Micronutrients maintain an essential role in antioxidant defense and, therefore, enhanced immunity. Increasing evidence supports the role of micronutrients in the nutritional regimen postburn. Improved clinical outcomes such as fewer infection, improved wound healing, and reduction in skin graft requirement and mortality have been reported in burn patients receiving various trace element regimes.[65–68] In other less catabolic wound types, supplementation of micronutrients in patients without clinical symptoms of deficiency is contended.[77]

NUTRITIONAL ASSESSMENT

The process of nutritional assessment should include physical assessment of the condition of the skin. Changes in skin condition of the at-risk, long-term care resident, surgical patient, and burn victim provide essential information as to the adequacy of nutrition support. A thorough evaluation of skin condition is an essential component of nutritional adequacy and therefore should be completed minimally each week.

ENERGY

The provision of sufficient calories for wound repair is a major component of healing. Multiple equations exist to assist the clinician in the assessment of energy requirements for the burn patient (Table 24.4).[69–81] For other types of wounds, the use of a basal estimate calculation like the

TABLE 24.4
Formulas for Calculating Energy Requirements of Burn Patients

References	Age	% BSAB	Calories/Day
Curreri[69–71]	0–1 year	<50	Basal + (15 × % BSAB)
	1–3 years	<50	Basal + (25 × % BSAB)
	4–15 years	<50	Basal + (40 × % BSAB)
	16–59 years	Any	25W + (40 × % BSAB)
	>60 years	Any	Basal + (65 × % BSAB)
Long modification[72] of the Harris–Benedict[73] equation	Adult male	Any	(66.47 + 13.7W + 50H − 6.76A) × (activity factor) × (injury factor)
	Adult female	Any	(655.1 + 9.56W + 1.85H − 6.68 A) × (activity factor) × (injury factor)
Hildreth[74–76]	<15 years	>30	(1800/m² BSA) + (2200/m² burn)
Hildreth[77]	<12 years		(1800/m² BSA) + 1300/m² burn
Mayes[78]	0–3 years	10–50	108 + 68W + (3.9 × % BSAB)
	5–10 years		818 + 37.4W + (9.3 × % BSAB)
Parks[79]	Adult	Any	(1800/m² BSA) + (2200 kcal/m² BSAB)
Soroff[80]	Adult	Any	3500/m² BSA
Troell and Wretlind[81]	Adult	Any	40–60W

Source: Adapted from Kagan, R.J. et al., Nutritional support in the burn patient, in Robin, A.P. (ed.), *Problems in General Surgery*, Vol. 8, JB Lippincott, Philadelphia, PA, 1991, p. 65. With permission.

BSAB, body surface area burned; BSA, body surface area; W, weight in kg; A, age in years; H, height in cm.

TABLE 24.5
Potential Factors Affecting Metabolic Rate in Patients with Burns

Activity
Age
Anxiety
Application and removal of allograft
Body composition
Body temperature
Catecholamine production
Circadian rhythm
Dry heat loss (ambient temperature)
Energy cost of protein synthesis
Energy cost of respiratory stress
Extent of injury
Evaporative heat loss (wound coverage)
Gender
Graft loss
Immediate vs. delayed feeding
Infection
Medications
Pain
Sedation
Sleep vs. wakefulness
Specific dynamic action of food
Surgery
Wound healing

Source: Adapted from Gottschlich, M.M. et al., *J. Am. Diet. Assoc.*, 97, 132, 1997. With permission

Harris–Benedict[73] with added factors for activity, wound healing, and other variables (Table 24.5) is common practice. The reliability of equations is questioned because confounding factors that influence metabolic rate are not wholly inherent in any calculation. For example, formulas cannot accurately predict energy needs if weight is skewed by edema, amputation, or wound dressing or if additional stress factors such as fractures, smoke inhalation injury, head trauma, surgery, or infection are present.

For these reasons, indirect calorimetry remains the preferred method of determining energy needs for any stressed patient. Indirect calorimetry determines energy needs inherently accounting for changes in weight and wound size, the presence or absence of infection or inhalation injury, and other extraneous variables. For the burn patient, a factor of 20%–30% should be added to measured resting energy expenditure to account for increased demands from physical therapy, wound dressing changes, temperature spikes, anxiety, pain, and other conditions that serve to increase energy requirement but are not accounted for at the time of the resting measurement. For the mechanically ventilated, severely burned or hospitalized patient presenting with open wound, indirect calorimetry is recommended two times per week. Spontaneously breathing patients with wounds who require enteral nutrition support should have indirect calorimetry repeated a minimum of one time per week. The nutrition support regimen should be routinely adjusted in accordance with the metabolic cart measurement.

Respiratory quotient (RQ) is a parameter that accompanies standard indirect calorimetry measurements. RQ is helpful to the clinician as a means of determining overfeeding or underfeeding, both of which have deleterious stresses on the patient.

Acute and chronic wounds require nutrition support that is tailored to meet the individual requirement of the patient. Indirect calorimetry provides the optimal means of individualizing the nutrition care plan; however, it is recognized that not all institutions are privy to this technology. For this reason, estimates from equations are a practical alternative for projecting calorie needs. In either method of energy assessment, the nutrition support regimen should be reevaluated regularly and alterations made in concomitance with other assessment parameters.

Anthropometrics

Accurate height and weight assessment is important. These two variables are crucial in the initial assessment of calorie and protein requirement of any patient. Trends in weight are especially important as they provide insight into the adequacy of calorie provision. For this reason, weekly weights are recommended for any burn patient or long-term care resident with greater than second-stage pressure ulcer. As in any patient, caution is presumed in the assessment of weight fluctuation due to the impact of edema. Burn patients exhibit fluid retention well into their acute course, at times lasting for 4–6 weeks (or greater). Varying medical conditions inherently cause chronic edema as well. The effects of such must be considered in the weight assessment.

Guidelines for initiating intervention based on weight fluctuation have been established in the long-term care setting (Table 24.6). In addition, maintenance of 90%–110% of preburn weight is recommended for the burn patient. Furthermore, burned children have been reported to exhibit long-term growth delays—up to 2 years postburn.[62] This knowledge should be factored into the assessment of the pediatric burned patient in the outpatient setting.

Laboratory Indices

Different labs are important in the nutritional assessment of patients with wounds depending on severity and etiology. Patients with large burn wounds exhibit extremely low levels of albumin due to plasma leaks across the microvasculature. Exogenous albumin supplementation is routine in large burns, although guidelines have been established, which have lowered the albumin threshold, thus decreasing the supplement requirement.[82]

Due to the marked, immediate impact of the burn injury itself and other burn-mediated factors such as edema, surgery, excessive hydration, and blood loss on serum albumin and because the plummet is related to injury conditions, not the adequacy of nutrition support, albumin is not routinely used in the nutritional assessment of the acutely burned individual. Due to its long half-life (essentially 3 weeks) and insensitivity to acute changes in nutrition status, albumin is a more effective indicator of nutrition status during the rehabilitative phase of burn or in the long-term care resident. Albumin serves as a monitor of long-term trends in nutrition status or determining the impact of initiating or withdrawing nutrition intervention over time.

TABLE 24.6
Weight Status Conditions Prompting Nutrition Intervention in the Long-Term Care Setting

Unintended weight loss
≥5% in 30 days
≥7.5% in 90 days
≥10% in 180 days
Body mass index <21
(703 × weight in pounds/height in inches)

Prealbumin is an additional indicator of visceral protein synthesis. The half-life of prealbumin is 2 days, thus making it a more sensitive indicator of nutrition status than albumin. Surgery, wound exudate, fluid shifts, blood transfusions, and infection all negatively impact prealbumin level. Inclusion of prealbumin in the nutrition assessment is better suited for the convalescent stage of burn recovery or to monitor acute changes in the intake, weight, or skin condition of the long-term care resident.

Nitrogen balance is most often used in the acute setting following surgical stress or burn injury. Twenty-four hour nitrogen intake and urinary nitrogen losses must be calculated precisely to determine balance and thus the degree of anabolism or catabolism. The standard equation used to estimate nitrogen balance (24 h nitrogen intake [g] – 24 h urinary urea nitrogen [g] + factor for insensible losses) is modified to account for nitrogen losses in wound exudate following a burn injury.[83] As an option, completing nitrogen balance studies in patients with burns in excess of 25% TBSA using the aforementioned equation and targeting a goal (unadjusted for wound size) at +5 to +10 clinically supports wound healing (the larger the percent burn, the higher is the nitrogen balance goal in the noted range).

Special Conditions

The presence of diabetes is the most common condition that attenuates wound healing. Factors including wound hypoxia from poor circulation and increased infection risk are recognized in the diabetic patient. An elevated serum glucose is indicative of failure of glucose to enter the cell. This interferes with aerobic and anaerobic metabolism. Insulin deficiency suppresses collagen deposition in wounds. The work of Van Den Berghe et al.[84–86] indicates that tighter glucose control via increased insulin provision reduces infectious episodes and mortality in the critically ill population. As a result, most critical care and burn units have adopted intensive insulin therapy protocols. This topic is discussed in detail in next section of this chapter, "Pharmacologic Modulation of Metabolism."

Pressure ulcers are a common wound care issue in the immobilized elderly. Inadequate energy, protein and fluid intake, significant weight loss, and urinary and fecal incontinence contribute to development. The Braden scale is typically employed in the long-term care setting by the interdisciplinary team to predict a resident's risk of pressure ulcer development (Table 24.7).[87] A version for pediatric patients, the Braden Q scale,[88] is also available. These assessment tools include a nutrition component that identifies individuals requiring nutrition intervention. It is recommended that the interdisciplinary assessment of ulcer risk be completed monthly for long-term care residents, so that timely interventions to prevent ulcer development or minimize size and depth can be initiated.

PHARMACOLOGIC MODULATION WOUND HEALING

Pharmacologic agents such as anabolic steroids, recombinant growth hormone, insulin, and growth factors reportedly have positive effects on wound healing. The impact of other therapies including beta-blockers, sleep-enhancing agents, and probiotics on wound healing remains intriguing, but unknown.

Oxandrolone, a testosterone analog, when combined with a high protein diet, enhances weight gain and closure of previously nonhealing wounds.[89–91] Following acute burns, oxandrolone provision correlates with decreased length of stay,[92,93] enhanced lean body mass accretion,[92,94,95] accelerated wound healing,[89–91,93] greater bone mineral content,[95] and improved survival.[96] A study combining review of oxandrolone and exercise in the rehabilitative phase of burn injury noted significant improvements in lean body mass in comparison to independent exercise or oxandrolone use alone.[97] The known concern with oxandrolone use is increased liver enzymes[92,93]; therefore, routine monitoring is recommended.

While a positive relationship between recombinant human growth hormone provision and earlier donor site healing in patients with large burns has been previously established,[98] few institutions currently employ this intervention due to its extreme monetary cost as well as existing controversy over its safety.[99–101]

TABLE 24.7
Braden Scale for Predicting Pressure Sore Risk

Client's Name		Evaluator's Name		Date of Assessment	Score
Sensory perception: Ability to respond meaningfully to pressure-related discomfort.	1. *Completely limited*: Unresponsive (does not moan, flinch, or grasp) to painful stimuli, due to diminished level of consciousness or sedation. Or Limited ability to feel pain over most of body surface.	2. *Very limited*: Responds to only painful stimuli. Cannot communicate discomfort except by moaning or restlessness. Or Has a sensory impairment that limits the ability to feel pain or discomfort over 1/2 of body.	3. *Slightly limited*: Responds to verbal commands but cannot always communicate discomfort or need to be turned. Or Has some sensory impairment that limits ability to feel pain or discomfort in 1 or 2 extremities.	4. *No impairment*: Responds to verbal commands. Has no sensory deficit that would limit ability to feel or voice pain or discomfort.	
Moisture: Degree to which skin is exposed to moisture.	1. *Constantly moist*: Skin is kept moist almost constantly by perspiration, urine, etc. Dampness is detected every time patient is moved or turned.	2. *Moist*: Skin is often but not always moist. Linen must be changed at least once a shift.	3. *Occasionally moist*: Skin is occasionally moist, requiring an extra linen change approximately once a day.	4. *Rarely moist*: Skin is usually dry; linen requires changing only at routine intervals.	
Activity: Degree of physical activity.	1. *Bedfast*: Confined to bed.	2. *Chairfast*: Ability to walk severely limited or nonexistent. Cannot bear down weight and/or must be assisted into chair or wheelchair.	3. *Walks occasionally*: Walks occasionally during day but for very short distances, with or without assistance. Spends majority of each shift in bed or chair.	4. *Walks frequently*: Walks outside the room at least twice a day and inside room at least once every 2 h during waking hours.	
Mobility: Ability to change and control body position.	1. *Completely immobile*: Does not make even slight changes in body or extremity position without assistance.	2. *Very limited*: Makes occasional slight changes in body or extremity position but unable to make frequent or significant changes independently.	3. *Slightly limited*: Makes frequent though slight changes in body or extremity position independently.	4. *No limitations*: Makes major and frequent changes in position without assistance.	

(*Continued*)

TABLE 24.7 (*Continued*)
Braden Scale for Predicting Pressure Sore Risk

Client's Name		Evaluator's Name		Date of Assessment	Score
Nutrition: Usual food intake pattern.	1. *Very poor*: Never eats a complete meal. Rarely eats more than 1/3 of any food offered. Eats 2 servings or less of protein (meat or dairy products) per day. Takes fluids poorly. Does not take a liquid dietary supplement. Or Is NPO[a] and/or maintained on clear liquids or IV[b] for more than 5 days.	2. *Probably inadequate*: Rarely eats a complete meal and generally eats only 1/2 of any food offered. Protein intake includes only 3 servings of meat or dairy products per day. Occasionally will take a dietary supplement. Or Receives less than optimum amount of liquid diet or tube feeding.	3. *Adequate*: Eats over half of most meals. Eats a total of 4 servings of protein (meat or dairy products) each day. Occasionally refuses a meal, but will usually take a supplement if offered. Or Is on a tube feeding or TPN[c] regimen, which probably meets most of nutritional needs.	4. *Excellent*: Eats most of every meal. Never refuses a meal. Usually eats a total of 4 or more servings of meat and dairy products. Occasionally eats between meals. Does not require supplementation.	
Friction and shear	1. *Problem*: Requires moderate to maximum assistance in moving. Complete lifting without sliding against sheets is impossible. Frequently slides down in bed or chair, requiring frequent repositioning with maximum assistance. Spasticity, contractures, or agitation leads to almost constant friction.	2. *Potential problem*: Moves feebly or requires minimum assistance. During a move, skin probably slides to some extent against sheets, chair, restraints, or other devices. Maintains relatively good position in chair or bed most of the time but occasionally slides down.	3. *No apparent problem*: Moves in bed and in chair independently and has sufficient muscle strength to lift up completely during move. Maintains good position in bed or chair at all times.		
				Total score	

Source: Reprinted from Braden, B.J. and Maklesbust, J., *Am. J. Nurs.*, 105, 70, 2005. With permission.

Scoring: The maximum possible score is 23. A lower score reflects higher risk for pressure ulceration. The cutoff score to denote risk for pressure ulceration is ≤16.

[a] NPO, nothing by mouth.

[b] IV, Intravenously.

[c] TPN, total parenteral nutrition.

Recently, the therapeutic response to the stress-induced hyperglycemia of critical illness has been modified as studies report the adverse impact of hyperglycemia on wound healing, immunity, and mortality.[102–106] In addition, insulin provision has been shown to decrease the inflammatory response postburn.[107,108] As a result, successful intensive insulin therapy protocols are increasingly accepted in critical care and burn units.[109–114] The positive impact of postburn glycemic control on infectious, inflammatory, hepatic, renal, and survival outcomes has been noted with target blood glucose levels between 120 and 150 mg/dL. Caution must be conducted to prevent hypoglycemic episodes with the use of intense insulin therapy, particularly in patients whose enteral feeds are suspended for various clinical reasons.

The administration of beta-blockers as a means to attenuate metabolism and reduce muscle protein catabolism following severe burns has been introduced.[115,116] Beta-blocker therapy has the potential to reduce wound healing time; however, the full extent of the implications of this practice is unknown and is currently not mainstream.

Growth factors are a subgroup of cytokines that distinctively induce cellular proliferation.[117–120] Altered growth factor production has also been associated with poor wound healing. Numerous studies have demonstrated the ability of these cytokines to assist tissue repair.[121–125] The effect of growth factors on healing remains controversial as animal and clinical trials in the burn population have not produced consistent evidence to support application to routine care.[126–129] Risk factors to growth factor use include the possibility for increased scarring from enhanced granulation tissue accumulation and potentially malignant transformation. Growth factors have the potential for making significant enhancements to clinical care although application guidelines must be refined.

The impact of prolonged sleep deprivation and reduced restorative sleep reported in pediatric burns has far-reaching implications for wound healing, inflammation, and immune status.[4] Future research is required to determine the most appropriate therapeutic sleeping agent(s) for institutionalized patients with burns and other wound types. Finally, with the recent introduction of the concept of the intestinal microbiome,[130,131] the addition of prebiotics and/or probiotics to the nutritional regimen, whether stimulating a direct or indirect effect on wound healing, deserves investigative attention.

NUTRITION SUPPORT GUIDELINES

Oral nutrition can usually be enhanced to sufficiently increase calories and protein to a level that supports healing in previously well-nourished individuals who have acute wounds involving less than 20% open area. Combining provision of food preferences; supplementing high calorie, high protein commercial products; and concealing protein and carbohydrate modules in foods and beverages are useful in increasing calorie and protein intake. Before nutrition support is implemented in the long-term care resident with significant pressure ulcer, a review of patient goals by the health care team as well as the patient/family should be explored.

Enteral

Enteral nutrition is the preferred route of nutrient administration and is indicated in patients/residents exhibiting characteristics listed in Table 24.8, assuming ethical issues related to sustaining quality of life have been addressed (Chapter 38). Increased intestinal blood flow, preserved gastrointestinal function, decreased mucosal atrophy, and reduced bacterial translocation are associated with feeding the gut.[132–135] Acute wounds, such as burns, may be associated with gastric ileus and the tendency may be to withhold enteral support or initiate parenteral nutrition in response. Although the stomach may be affected by posttraumatic ileus, the small intestine maintains its functional and absorptive capabilities and therefore remains a viable alternative postburn. Gastric feedings are not supported in the patient with large burns because the ileus often prevents the initial advancement and optimal delivery of enteral feedings. In addition, heightened aspiration risk is recognized in the burn patient

TABLE 24.8
Indications for Consideration of Enteral Nutrition Support in Patients with Wounds

Acute or chronic weight loss
Chronic open wound
Greater than 20% TBSA burns
Inadequate oral intake for greater than 5 days
Oral/facial injury
Preexisting malnutrition
Prolonged ventilator dependence

due to multiple position changes during daily dressing changes, physical therapy sessions, and various postoperative position needs (e.g., prone, neck hyperextension, etc.). Furthermore, small bowel feedings permit minimal interruption of the nutrition regimen, thereby limiting chronic nutrient deficiencies, and preclude the need to withhold enteral feedings for respiratory treatments, intravenous line changes, or surgery, thus maximizing nutrient intake. Gastric feedings also interrupt the normal hunger response and therefore impact the intake of foodstuff orally. For the long-term care resident or stable surgical patient who is not subject to the multiple aspiration risks of a burn patient, routine gastric feedings via gastrostomy tube or nasogastric tube, respectively, are acceptable. Regardless of placement, alterations in the nutrition support regimen should occur (i.e., withhold feeds at meals or nocturnal feeds only) to maximize the oral intake of oriented individuals.

Feeding during Resuscitation

Feeding tube placement in the third segment of the duodenum, just beyond the ligament of Treitz, is recommended for the burn patient. This permits continuous drip feedings to be initiated within hours of admission and generally requires minimal to no interruption for care purposes.[136] For patients with uncomplicated resuscitation (i.e., usually ≤20% TBSA burns),[137] the initial hourly infusion should begin at one-half the goal and advance by 5–20 mL/h, dependent on age. As a precautionary means of preserving gastrointestinal integrity, patients with burns in excess of 20% TBSA should have an evaluation of fluid and hemodynamic stability prior to advancement of enteral nutrition. Patients who are underresuscitated, as evidenced by poor urine output or poor edematous response, or hemodynamically unstable during resuscitation or throughout the acute course are provided enteral trophic feeds sufficient to stimulate the gut but provide minimal nutrition support.[137] Tube feeds are advanced as fluid and hemodynamic stability is achieved.

Perioperative

Multiple studies support the role of nutrition and wound healing in the postoperative period.[138–142] However, it is common practice to allow patients nothing by mouth, with enteral feedings withheld, preceding and following surgical procedures. As a result, negligible nutrient intake is realized at a time when the body is most stressed, catabolic, and in need of nutrients that appropriately support healing.

Several authors have successfully accomplished continuous enteral feedings during operative procedures.[138,139] A significant reduction in caloric deficit accompanied by less need for exogenous albumin to maintain serum levels and decreased wound infection were noted in burn patients fed continuously through surgery. In addition, Andel and colleagues[139] promote continuous duodenal feedings through surgery to improve intraoperative splanchnic oxygen balance. Strict guidelines must be in place to ensure diligent monitoring of feeding tube position and gastric reflux throughout the operative procedure.

Parenteral

Instituting parenteral nutrition as a standard in patients with a functional gastrointestinal tract is unwarranted and not without complication. Parenteral nutrition is associated with a host of negative implications including increased prevalence of blood-borne pathogens, suppressed immunity, and increased mortality.[134,143] As a result, parenteral feeds are reserved for patients whose intestines are nonfunctioning or low functioning. Examples of such conditions include, but are not limited to, persistent intestinal ileus, abdominal trauma, intractable diarrhea, stress ulceration of the stomach or duodenum, pseudo-obstruction of the colon, and superior mesenteric artery syndrome.

Recent trials suggest beneficial effects of omega-3 fatty acid–supplemented parenteral nutrition. Studies indicate the magnitude of inflammatory response is decreased and host immune defense improved with intravenous omega-3 fatty acids.[144–146] Evaluation of the impact of parenteral nutrition augmented with omega-3 fatty acids on wound healing is emerging in the medical literature.[147,148] These studies suggest a promising role for this substrate in the nutrition regimen of patients with wound healing demands who require parenteral nutrition.

Parenteral nutrition should be viewed as a backup means of nutrition support with enteral nutrition always given primary consideration. When intravenous nutrition is necessitated, promotion of the following is recommended: gut stimulation via trophic feeds, conservative fat provision due to its hyperlipidemic and immunosuppressive effects, and routine attempts to progress enteral feeds, thereby limiting intravenous support.

SUMMARY

Wound healing is a multifactorial, complex process aided by appropriate nutrition support and the application of assessment methods that ensure wound healing progression is maximized. Studies undoubtedly support the role of high protein, high calorie intake in wound healing. Burn wounds require further diet alteration, with research suggesting a regimen consisting not only of increased calories and protein but of high-carbohydrate, low-fat, and omega-3 fatty acid supplementation. Micronutrient provision is to be carefully considered. Supplementation of vitamins A, C and zinc is fairly standard in large burns. Provision of vitamin D_3 and antioxidant therapies are gaining increased support following burn injury. It is beneficial to be prudent with supplementation in patients with other wound types. Given the positive effects on immunity, enteral feeding remains the preferred method of nutrient delivery in wound management. The role of nutrition support in wound healing has progressed significantly in the past 20 years. Appropriate nutrient provision is recognized as an intricate component to wound repair and as such should remain an irrefutable priority in the multidisciplinary plan of care.

CASE STUDY

History and Physical

TK is a 30-year-old male admitted to the burn unit 4 h postburn from a housefire. He had been intubated at the scene and is reliant upon mechanical ventilation. Upon exam, the patient appears neurologically intact and has suffered 60% TBSA burns to face, upper and lower extremities with 45% full thickness. Adequate urine output is established using the Parkland formula.[149]

The patient is hemodynamically stable, receiving adequate hydration, weighs 86 kg, and is 185 cm tall. Past medical history is unremarkable. A nasogastric tube is connected to low wall suction.

Nutrition Support Initiation

By postburn hour 6, the wounds have been cleansed and dressed and fluoroscopy is used to place the feeding tube into the third portion of the duodenum just beyond the ligament of Treitz. Once tube placement is confirmed, a 1 cal/mL; high, intact protein; moderately low fat; linolenic acid– and arginine-enriched enteral formula is initiated. The initial goal rate is established using the DRI[15] for energy for a normal, healthy adult as the patient will remain in the ebb response until approximately 48 h postburn. TK's DRI for calories is established at 3200 cal/day. It is estimated that dextrose in the maintenance fluid used following resuscitation will provide an additional 500 cal/day. As a result, the energy necessary from tube feeding is estimated at 2700 cal/day. The tube feeding rate will begin at one-half of this goal, or 65 mL/h, and advance by 20 mL/h to a goal rate of 135 mL/h. Indirect calorimetry is performed approximately 30 h postburn, and resting energy expenditure with a 30% activity/stress factor confirms the current goal of 3200 cal/day. The protein goal is established at 184 g/day (23% of total calories or 2 g/kg). Modular whey protein is added to the enteral formula to ensure protein provision at this level. A multivitamin/mineral supplement, vitamins C and D_3, zinc, and glutamine (if not inherent in the tube feeding) are provided according to guidelines listed in Table 24.3. Baseline transferrin and prealbumin labs are obtained. Twenty-four-hour urinary urea nitrogen lab tests are initiated the following morning and will continue daily until the urinary catheter is discontinued.

Surgery

TK is taken to the operating room postburn day 3 for excision of all clearly demarcated full-thickness areas. The following day, approximately 20% of the wounds are autografted and 25% of the wounds are covered in allograft. The allograft will remain on the wound until the donor site can be reharvested in approximately 10–14 days. TK requires two additional excision and grafting procedures before his wounds are covered by autograft. The enteral feeding regimen is not interrupted for any surgery and remains at goal rate postoperatively each time.

Sepsis

Approximately 5 days following his first surgical procedure, TK presents with a septic episode for which a 10-day course of antibiotics is initiated. Indirect calorimetry is routinely completed two times per week. The latest test indicates energy needs have soared to 4500 cal/day; RQ is low at 0.80 and the tube feeding rate is adjusted upward. Mean nitrogen balance over the past week has been steady around +3. The tube feeding rate increase provides additional protein at approximately 3 g/kg; therefore, nitrogen balance into postburn week 2 has improved appropriately to +7. Transferrin and prealbumin decline during this septic period, as is expected, due to their classification as acute phase reactants.

Diarrhea

Diarrhea develops on postantibiotic day 4. Stool is sent for *Clostridium difficile* culture and returns negative. Postpyloric feeding tube placement is checked and confirmed in the proper position. (Feeding tube placement should be a routine component of the care plan when diarrhea first develops. Often with postpyloric feeds, the feeding tube inadvertently advances significantly beyond the pylorus and simply retracting the tube by the appropriate amount of *x-ray indicated cm's* will resolve the issue.) Scheduled antidiarrheal medications are administered every 4–6 h. Diluted feeds are provided for 2 days and gradually advanced back to full strength. Loose stools are controlled by postantibiotic day 8. Antidiarrheal medications are weaned.

Progression toward Discharge

Over the next 7 weeks, TK progresses well and his wounds are now >95% healed. His tolerance of the enteral regimen (rate determined by biweekly indirect calorimetry) is good. TK is now free of edema, and his weight status is good at 95% of preburn weight. A gradual improvement in weekly transferrin and prealbumin levels is noted. TK is removed from the ventilator postburn week 5, and an oral diet is initiated 2 days later. As TK's oral intake has improved, tube feeding is tapered accordingly; held 2 h at meals when oral intake averages 25% of goal; held 7 a.m. to 7 p.m. when oral intake averages 50% of goal; and eventually discontinued postburn week 7 when oral intake consistently meets 75% of goal with the aid of a supplement. Indirect calorimetry was discontinued when the feeding tube was discontinued. TK is discharged postburn day 62 (1.03 days per percent burn) on a regular diet without the need for further protein or micronutrient enhancement as all wounds are covered. The standard length of stay per percent burn is generally accepted at 1.0. He is now 93% of preburn weight. He will be monitored in the outpatient department for the next month for weight fluctuations and on an as-needed basis thereafter.

REFERENCES

1. Cuthbertson, D., Tilstone, W.J. 1969. Metabolism during the post injury period. *Adv Clin Chem* 121:1.
2. Bessey, P.Q., Lowe, K.A. 1993. Early hormonal changes affect the catabolic response to trauma. *Ann Surg* 218:476.
3. Harrison, H.N., Moncrief, J.A., Duckett, J.W. Jr., Mason, A.D. Jr. 1964. The relationship between energy metabolism and water loss from vaporization in severely burned patients. *Surgery* 56:203.
4. Gottschlich, M.M., Khoury, J., Warden, G.D., Kagan, R.J. 1994. An evaluation of the neuroendocrine response to sleep in pediatric burn patients. *J Parenter Enteral Nutr* 33:317.
5. Mochizuki, H., Trocki, O., Dominioni, L., Brackett, K.A., Joffe, S.N. 1984. Mechanisms of prevention of postburn hypermetabolism and catabolism by early enteral feeding. *Ann Surg* 200:297.
6. Dominioni, L., Trocki, O., Mochizuki, H., Fang, C., Alexander, J.W. 1984. Prevention of severe postburn hypermetabolism and catabolism by immediate intragastric feeding. *J Burn Care Rehabil* 5:106.
7. Jenkins, M., Gottschlich, M.M., Mayes, T., Khoury, J., Kagan, R.J., Warden, G.D. 1994. An evaluation of the effect of immediate enteral feeding on the hypermetabolic response following severe burn injury. *J Burn Care Rehabil* 15:199.
8. Cerami, A. 1992. Inflammatory cytokines. *Clin Immunopathol* 62:S3.
9. Tredgett, E.E., Yu, Y.M., Zhong, S., Burini, S., Okusawa, S., Gelfand, J.A. et al. 1988. Role of interleukin-1 and tumor necrosis factor on energy metabolism in rabbits. *Am J Physiol* 255:E760.
10. Hart, D.W., Wolf, S.E., Micak, R., Chinkes, D.L., Ramzy, P.J., Obeng, M.K. et al. 2000. Persistence of muscle catabolism after severe burn. *Surgery* 128:312.
11. Prokop-Oliet, M., Trocki, O., Alexander, J.W., MacMillan, B.G. 1983. Whey protein supplementation of complete tube feeding in the nutritional support of thermally injured patients. *Proc Am Burn Assoc* 15:45.
12. Trocki, O., Mochizuki, H., Dominioni, L., Alexander, J.W. 1986. Intact protein versus free amino acids in the nutritional support of thermally injured animals. *J Parenter Enteral Nutr* 10:139.
13. Newport, M.J., Henschel, M.J. 1984. Evaluation of the neonatal pig as a model for infant nutrition. Effects of different proportion of casein and whey protein in milk on nitrogen metabolism and composition of digesta in the stomach. *Pediatr Res* 18:658.
14. Alexander, J.W., MacMillan, B.G., Stinnett, J.D., Ogle, C.K., Bozian, R.C., Fischer, J.E. et al. 1980. Beneficial effects of aggressive protein feeding in severely burned children. *Ann Surg* 192:505.
15. Trumbo, P., Schlicker, S., Yates, A.A., Poos, M.; Food and Nutrition Board of the Institute of Medicine, The National Academies. 2002. Dietary reference intakes for energy, carbohydrate, fiber, fat, fatty acids, cholesterol, protein and amino acids. *J Am Diet Assoc* 102(11):1621–1630.

16. Bergstrom, N., Allman, R.M., Carlson, C.E. 1994. Treatment of pressure ulcers (Clinical Practice Guide, No. 15), AHCPR, Publication No. 95-0652. Rockville, MD: US Department of Health and Human Services Public Health Service, Agency of Health Care Policy and Research.
17. Long, C.L., Nelson, K.M., Geiger, J.W., Merrick, H.W., Blakemore, W.S. 1990. Physiological basis for the provision of fuel mixtures in normal and stressed patients. *J Trauma* 30:1077.
18. Kirk, S.J., Hurson, M., Regan, M.C., Holt, D.R., Wasserkrug, H.L., Barbul, A. 1993. Arginine stimulates wound healing and immune function in elderly human beings. *Surgery* 114:155.
19. Barbul, A., Lazarou, S.A., Efron, D.T., Wasserkrug, H.L., Efron, G. 1990. Arginine enhances wound healing and lymphocyte immune responses in humans. *Surgery* 108:331.
20. Kirk, S.J., Barbul, A. 1990. Role of arginine in trauma, sepsis, immunity. *J Parenter Enteral Nutr* 14(5):226S–229S, 226S.
21. Cui, X., Iwasa, M., Iwasa, Y., Ohmori, Y., Yamamoto, A., Maeda, H. et al. 1999. Effects of dietary arginine supplementation on protein turnover and tissue protein synthesis in scald-burn rats. *Nutrition* 15(7/8):563.
22. Marin, V.B., Rodriguez-Osiac, L., Schlessinger, L., Villegas, J., Lopez, M., Castillo-Duran, C. 2006. Controlled study of enteral arginine supplementation in burned children: Impact on immunologic and metabolic status. *Nutrition* 22:705.
23. Yan, H., Peng, X., Huang, Y., Zhao, M., Li, F., Wang, P. 2007. Effects of early enteral arginine supplementation on resuscitation of severe burn patients. *Burns* 33:179.
24. Gottschlich, M.M., Jenkins, M., Warden, G.D., Baumer, T., Havens, P., Snook, J.T. et al. 1990. Differential effects of three enteral dietary regimens on selected outcome variables in burn patients. *J Parenter Enteral Nutr* 14:225.
25. Bansal, V., Syres, K.M., Makarenkova, V., Brannon, R., Matta, B., Harbrecht, B.G. et al. 2005. Interactions between fatty acids and arginine metabolism: Implications for the design of immune-enhancing diets. *J Parenter Enteral Nutr* 29:S75.
26. Alexander, J.W., Metze, T.J., McIntosh, M.J., Goodman, H.R., First, M.R., Munda, R. et al. 2005. The influence of immunomodulatory diets on transplant success and complications. *Transplantation* 79(4):460–465.
27. Murakami, K., Enkhbaatar, P., Yu, Y., Traber, L.D., Cox, R.A., Hawkins, H.K. et al. 2007. L-Arginine attenuates acute lung injury after smoke inhalation and burn injury in sheep. *Shock* 28:477.
28. Zhou, M., Martindale, R.G. 2007. Immune-modulating enteral formulations: Optimum components, appropriate patients, and controversial use of arginine in sepsis. *Curr Gastroenterol Rep* 9:329.
29. Cereda, E., Gini, A., Pedrolli, C., Vanotti, A. 2009. Disease-specific, versus standard, nutritional support for the treatment of pressure ulcers in institutionalized older adults: A randomized controlled trial. *J Am Geriatr Soc* 57:1395.
30. Frias, S.L., Lage Vazquez, M.A., Maristany, C.P., Xandri Graupera, J.M., Wouters-Wesseling, W., Wagenaar, L. 2004. The effectiveness of oral nutritional supplementation in the healing of pressure ulcers. *J Wound Care* 13:319.
31. Desneves, K.J., Todorovic, B.E., Cassar, A., Crowe, T.C. 2005. Treatment with supplementary arginine, vitamin C and zinc in patients with pressure ulcers: A randomized controlled trial. *Clin Nutr* 24:979.
32. Van Anholt, R.D., Sobotka, L., Meijer, E.P., Topinkova, E., Van Leen, M. 2010. Specific nutritional support accelerates pressure ulcer healing and reduces wound care intensity in non-malnourished patients. *Nutrition* 26:867.
33. Fan, J., Meng, Q., Guo, G., Xie, Y., Xiu, Y., Li, T. et al. 2009. Effects of enteral nutrition supplemented with glutamine on intestinal mucosal immunity in burned mice. *Nutrition* 25:233.
34. Raeder da Costa, M.A., Campos, A.C., Coelho, J.C., de Barros, A.M., Matsumoto, H.M. 2003. Oral glutamine and the healing of the colonic anastomoses in rats. *J Parenter Enteral Nutr* 27:186.
35. Zhou, Y.P., Jiang, Z.M., Sun, Y.H., Wang, X.R., Ma, E.L., Wilmore, D. 2003. The effect of supplemental enteral glutamine on plasma levels, gut function and outcome in severe burns: A randomized, double-blind, controlled clinical trial. *J Parenter Enteral Nutr* 27:241.
36. Peng, X., Yan, H., You, Z., Wang, P., Wang, S. 2005. Clinical and protein metabolic efficacy of glutamine granules-supplemented enteral nutrition in severely burned patients. *Burns* 31:342.
37. De-Souza, D.A., Greene, L.J. 2005. Intestinal permeability and systemic infections in critically ill patients: Effect of glutamine. *Crit Care Med* 33:1125.
38. Garrel, D., Patenaude, J., Nedelec, B., Samson, L., Dorais, J., Champoux, J. et al. 2003. Decreased mortality and infectious morbidity in adult burn patients given enteral glutamine supplements: A prospective, controlled, randomized clinical trial. *Crit Care Med* 31:2444.

39. O'Dwyer, S.T., Smith, R.J., Hwang, T.L., Wilmore, D.W. 1989. Maintenance of small bowel mucosa with glutamine-enriched parenteral nutrition. *J Parenter Enteral Nutr* 13:579.
40. Gottschlich, M.M., Mayes, T., Khoury, J., Kagan, R.J. 2004. Effect of enteral glutamine supplementation on selected outcome variables in burned children. *J Burn Care Rehabil* 25:572.
41. Tazuke, Y., Wasa, M., Shimizu Y., Wang, HS., Okada, A. 2003. Alanyl-glutamine supplemented parenteral nutrition prevents intestinal ischemia-reperfusion in rats. *J Parenter Enteral Nutr* 27:110.
42. Wischmeyer, P.E., Lynch, J., Liedel, J., Wolfson, R., Riehm, R., Gottlieb, L. et al. 2001. Glutamine administration reduces gram-negative bacteremia in severely burned patients: A prospective, randomized, double-blind trial versus isonitrogenous control. *Crit Care Med* 29:2075.
43. Mochizuki, H., Trocki, O., Dominioni L., Ray, M.B., Alexander J.W. 1984. Optimal lipid content for enteral diets following thermal injury. *J Parenter Enteral Nutr* 8:638.
44. Garrell, D.R., Razi, M., Lariviere, F., Jobin, N., Naman, N., Emptoz-Bonneton, A. et al. 1995. Improved clinical status and length of care with low-fat nutrition support in burn patients. *J Parenter Enteral Nutr* 19:482.
45. Hulsey, T.K., O'Neill, J.A., Neblett, W.R., Meng, M.C. 1980. Experimental wound healing in essential fatty acid deficiency. *J Pediatr Surg* 15:505.
46. Alexander, J.W., Saito, H., Trocki, O., Ogle, C.K. 1986. The importance of lipid type in the diet after burn injury. *Ann Surg* 204:1.
47. Theilla, M., Singer, P., Cohen, J., DeKeyser, F. 2007. A diet enriched in eicosapentaenoic acid, gamma-linolenic acid and antioxidants in the prevention of new pressure ulcer formation in critically ill patients with acute lung injury: A randomized, prospective, controlled study. *Clin Nutr* 26:752.
48. Klein, G.L., Nicolai, M., Langman, C.B., Cuneo, B.F., Sailer, D.E., Herndon, D.N. et al. 1997. Dysregulation of calcium homeostasis after severe burn injury in children: Possible role of magnesium depletion. *J Pediatr* 131:246.
49. Murphey, E.D., Chattopadhyay, N., Bai, M., Kifor, O., Harper, D., Traber, D.L. et al. 2000. Up-regulation of the parathyroid calcium-sensing receptor after burn injury in sheep: A potential contributory factor to postburn hypocalcemia. *Crit Care Med* 28:3885.
50. Loven, L., Nordstrom, H., Lennquist, S. 1984. Changes in calcium and phosphate and their regulating hormones in patients with severe burn injuries. *Scand J Plast Reconstr Surg* 18:49.
51. Klein, G.L., Herndon, D.H. 1998. Magnesium deficit in major burns: Role in hypoparathyroidism and end-organ parathyroid hormone resistance. *Magnes Res* 11:103.
52. Lennquist, S., Lindell, B., Nordstrom, H., Sjoberg, H.E. 1979. Hypophosphatemia in severe burns. *Acta Chir Scand* 145:1.
53. Loven, L., Larsson, L., Nordstrom, H., Lennquist, S. 1986. Serum phosphate and 2,3-diphosphoglycerate in severely burned patients after phosphate supplementation. *J Trauma* 26:348.
54. Gottschlich, M.M., Mayes, T., Khoury, J., Warden, G.D. 2004. Hypovitaminosis D in acutely injured pediatric burn patients. *J Am Diet Assoc* 104:931.
55. Klein, G.L., Langman, C.B., Herndon, D.N. 2002. Vitamin D depletion following burns in children: A possible factor in post-burn osteopenia. *J Trauma* 52:346.
56. Wray, C.J., Mayes, T., Khoury, J., Warden, G.D., Gottschlich, M. 2002. Metabolic effects of vitamin D on serum calcium, magnesium and phosphorus in pediatric burn patients. *J Burn Care Rehabil* 23:416.
57. Klein, G.L., Herndon, D.N., Langman, C.B., Rutan, T.C., Young, W.E., Pembleton, G. et al. 1995. Long-term reduction in bone mass after severe burn injury in children. *J Pediatr* 126:252.
58. Klein, G.L., Herndon, D.N., Langman, C.B., Rutan, T.C, Young, W.E., Pembleton, G. et al. 1995. Histomorphometric and biochemical characterization of bone following acute severe burns in children. *Bone* 17:455.
59. Edelman, L.S., McNaught, T., Chan, G.M., Morris, S.E. 2002. Bone mineral density changes following burn injury. *J Burn Care Rehabil* 23:S84.
60. Edelman, L.S., McNaught, T., Chan, G.M., Morris, S.E. 2003. Sustained bone mineral changes following burn injury. *J Surg Res* 114:172.
61. Mayes, T., Gottschlich, M., Scanlon, J., Warden, G.D. 2003. A four-year review of burns as an etiologic factor in the development of long bone fractures in pediatrics. *J Burn Care Rehabil* 24:279.
62. Rutan, R.L., Herndon, D.N. 1990. Growth delay in postburn pediatric patients. *Arch Surg* 125:392.
63. Gottschlich, M.M., Mayes, T., Khoury, J., Kagan, R.J. Clinical trial of vitamin D_2 versus D_3 supplementation in critically ill burn patients. *J Parenter Enteral Nutr,* submitted.
64. Mayes, T., Gottschlich, M.M., Brunner, C., Khoury, J., Kagan, R.J. An investigation of bone health following vitamin D supplementation following burn injury. *Nutr Clin Pract*, submitted.

65. Berger, M.M., Baines, M., Raffoul, W., Benathan, M., Chiolero, R.L., Reeves, C. et al. 2007. Trace element supplementation after major burns modulates antioxidant status and clinical course by way of increased tissue trace element concentrations. *Am J Clin Nutr* 85:1293.
66. Berger, M.M., Binnert, C., Chiolero, R.L., Taylor, W., Raffoul, W., Cayeux, M.C. et al. 2007. Trace element supplementation after major burns increases burned skin trace element concentrations and modulates local protein metabolism but not whole-body substrate metabolism. *Am J Clin Nutr* 85:1301.
67. Sahib, A.S., Al-Jawad, F.H., Alkaisy, A.A. 2010. Effect of antioxidants on the incidence of wound infection in burn patients. *Ann Burns Fire Disaster* 23:199.
68. Berger, M.M. 2006. Antioxidant micronutrients in major trauma and burns: Evidence and practice. *Nutr Clin Pract* 21:438.
69. Curreri, P.W., Richmond, D., Marvin, J., Baxter, C.R. 1974. Dietary requirements of patients with major burns. *J Am Diet Assoc* 65:415.
70. Day, T., Dean, P., Adams, M.C., Luterman, A., Ramenofsky, M.L., Curreri, P.W. 1986. Nutritional requirements of the burned child: The Curreri junior formula. *Proc Am Burn Assoc* (abstract) 18:86.
71. Adams, M.R., Kelley, C.H., Luterman, A., Curreri, P.W. 1987. Nutritional requirements of the burned senior citizen: The Curreri senior formula. *Proc Am Bur Assoc* (abstract) 19:83.
72. Long, C.L., Schaffel, N., Geiger, J.W., Schiller, W.R., Blakemore, W.S. 1979. Metabolic response to injury and illness: Estimation of energy and protein needs from indirect calorimetry and nitrogen balance. *J Parenter Enteral Nutr* 3(6):452.
73. Harris, J.A., Benedict, F.S. 1919. Biometric studies of basal metabolism in man, Pub. No. 279. Carnegie Institute of Washington, Washington, DC.
74. Hildreth, M., Carvajal, H.F. 1982. Caloric requirements in burned children: A simple formula to estimate daily caloric requirements. *J Burn Care Rehabil* 3:78.
75. Hildreth, M.A., Herndon, D.N., Desai, M.H., Duke, M.A. 1989. Calorie needs of adolescent patients with burns. *J Burn Care Rehabil* 10:523.
76. Hildreth, M.A., Herndon, D.N., Parks, D.H., Desai, M.H., Rutan, T. 1987. Evaluation of a caloric requirement formula in burned children treated with early excision. *J Trauma* 27:188.
77. Hildreth, M.A., Herndon, D.N., Desai, M.H., Broemeling, L.D. 1990. Current treatment reduces calories required to maintain weight in pediatric patients with burns. *J Burn Care Rehabil* 11:405.
78. Mayes, T.M., Gottschlich, M.M., Khoury, M.S., Warden, G. 1996. An evaluation of predicted and measured energy requirements in burned children. *J Am Diet Assoc* 96:24.
79. Parks, D.H., Carvajal, H.F., Larson, D.L. 1977. Management of burns. *Surg Clin North Am* 57:875.
80. Soroff, H.S., Pearson, E., Artz, C.P. 1961. An estimation of nitrogen requirements for equilibrium in burned patients. *Surg Gynecol Obstet* 112:159.
81. Troell, L., Wretlind, A. 1961. Protein and caloric requirements in burns. *Acta Chir Scand* 122:15.
82. Greenhalgh, D.G., Housinger, T.A., Kagan, R.J., Rieman, M., James, L., Novak, S. et al. 1995. Maintenance of serum albumin levels in pediatric burn patients: A prospective, randomized trial. *J Trauma* 39:67.
83. Kien, C.L., Young, V.R., Rohrbaugh, D.K., Burke, J.F. 1978. Increased rates of whole body protein synthesis and breakdown in children recovering from burns. *Ann Surg* 187:383.
84. Van Den Berghe, G., Wouters, P., Weekers, F., Verwaest, C., Bruyninckx, F., Schetz, M. et al. 2001. Intensive insulin therapy in critically ill patients. *N Engl J Med* 345:1359.
85. Van den Berghe, G., Wilmer, A., Milants, I., Wouters, P.I., Bouckaert, B., Bruyninckx, F. et al. 2006. Intensive insulin therapy in mixed medical/surgical intensive care units. *Diabetes* 55:3151.
86. Vlasselaers, D., Milants, I., Desmet, L., Wouters, P.J., Vanhorebeek, I., Heuvel, I.V. et al. 2009. Intensive insulin therapy for patients in pediatric intensive care: A prospective, randomized controlled study. *Lancet* 373:547.
87. Braden, B.J., Maklesbust, J. 2005. Preventing pressure ulcers with the Braden scale: An update on this easy-to-use tool that assesses a patient's risk. *Am J Nurs* 105:70.
88. Curley, M.A., Razmus, I.S., Roberts, K.E., Wypij, D. 2003. Predicting pressure ulcer risk in pediatric patients: The Braden Q scale. *Nurs Res* 52:22.
89. Demling, R.H., Desanti, L. 1997. Oxandrolone, an anabolic steroid, significantly increases the rate of weight gain in the recovery phase after major burns. *J Trauma* 43:47.
90. Demling, R.H., Desanti, L. 1999. Involuntary weight loss and the nonhealing wound: The role of anabolic agents. *Adv Wound Care* 12:1.
91. Demling, D.H. 1999. Comparison of the anabolic effects and complications of human growth hormone and the testosterone analog, oxandrolone, after severe burn injury. *Burns* 25:215.

92. Jeschke, M.G., Finnerty, C.C., Suman, O.E., Kulp, G., Micak, R.P., Herndon, D.N. 2007. The effect of oxandrolone on the endocrinologic, inflammatory, and hypermetabolic responses during the acute phase postburn. *Ann Surg* 246:351.
93. Wolf, S.E., Edelman, L.S., Kemalyan, N., Donison, L., Cross, J., Underwood, M. et al. 2006. Effects of oxandrolone on outcome measures in the severely burned: A multicenter prospective randomized double-blind trial. *J Burn Care Res* 27:131.
94. Porro, L.J., Herndon, D.N., Rodriguez, N.A., Jennings, K., Klein, G.L., Micak, R.P. et al. 2012. Five-year outcomes after oxandrolone administration in severely burned children: A randomized clinical trial of safety and efficacy. *J Am Coll Surg* 214:489.
95. Murphy, K.D., Thomas, S., Micak, R.P., Chinkes, D.L., Klein, G.L., Herndon, D.N. 2004. Effects of long-term oxandrolone administration in severely burned children. *Surgery* 136:219.
96. Pham, T.N., Klein, M.B., Gibran, N.S., Arnoldo, B.D., Gamelli, R.L., Silver, G.M. et al. 2008. Impact of oxandrolone treatment on acute outcomes after severe burn injury. *J Burn Care Res* 29:902.
97. Przkora, R., Herndon, D.N., Suman, O.E. 2006. The effects of oxandrolone and exercise on muscle mass and function in children with severe burns. *Pediatrics* 119:e109.
98. Gilpin, D.A., Barrow, R.E., Rutan, R.L., Bromelings, L., Herndon, D.N. 1994. Recombinant human growth hormone accelerates wound healing in children with large cutaneous burns. *Ann Surg* 220:19.
99. Takala, J., Ruokonen, E., Webster, N.R., Nielsen, M.S., Zandstra, D.F., Vundelinckx, G. et al. 1999. Increased mortality associated with growth hormone treatment in critically ill adults. *N Engl J Med* 341:785.
100. Svensson, J., Bengtsson, B. 2009. Safety aspects of GH replacement. *Eur J Endocrinol* 161:S65.
101. Ruokonen, E., Takala, J. 2002. Dangers of growth hormone therapy in critically ill patients. *Curr Opin Clin Nutr Metab Care* 5:199.
102. Gore, D.C., Chinkes, D., Heggers, J., Herndon, D.N., Wolf, S.E., Desai, M. 2001. Association of hyperglycemia with increased mortality after severe burn injury. *J Trauma Inj Infect Crit Care* 51:540.
103. Bochicchio, G.V., Sung, J., Joshi, M., Bochicchio, K., Johnson, S.B., Meyer, W. et al. 2005. Persistent hyperglycemia is predictive of outcome in critically ill trauma patients. *J Trauma Inj Infect Crit Care* 58:921.
104. Krinsley, J.S. 2003. Association between hyperglycemia and increased hospital mortality in a heterogeneous population of critically ill patients. *Mayo Clin Proc* 78:1471.
105. Umpierrez, G.E., Issacs, S.D., Bazargan, N., You, X., Thaler, L.M., Kitabchi, A.E. 2002. Hyperglycemia: An independent marker of in-hospital mortality in patients with undiagnosed diabetes. *J Clin Endocrinol Metab* 87:978.
106. Vogelzang, M., Nijboer, J.M., van der, H., Iwan, C.C., Zijlstra, F., ten Duis, H.J. et al. 2006. Hyperglycemia has a stronger relation with outcome in trauma patients then in other critically ill patients. *J Trauma Inj Infect Crit Care* 60:873.
107. Jeschke, M.G., Boehning, D.F., Finnerty, C.C., Herndon, D.N. 2007. Effect of insulin on the inflammatory and acute phase response after burn injury. *Crit Care Med* 35:S519.
108. Deng, H., Chai, J. 2009. The effects and mechanisms of insulin on systemic inflammatory response and immune cells in severe trauma, burn injury, and sepsis. *Int Immunopharmacol* 9:1251.
109. Vanhorebeek, I., Laungouche, L., Berghe, G.V. 2007. Tight blood glucose with insulin in the ICU. *Chest* 132:268.
110. Fram, R.Y., Cree, M.G., Wolfe, R.R., Micak, R.P., Qian, T., Chinkes, D.L. et al. 2010. Intensive insulin therapy improves insulin sensitivity and mitochondrial function in severely burned children. *Crit Care Med* 38:1475.
111. Jeschke, M.G., Kulp, G.A., Kraft, R., Finnerty, C.C., Micak, R., Lee, J.O. et al. 2010. Intensive insulin therapy in severely burned pediatric patients: A prospective randomized trial. *Thor Soc* 182(3):351–359.
112. Pham, T.N., Warren, A.J., Phan, H.H., Molitor, F., Greenhalgh, D.G., Palmieri, T.L. 2005. Impact of tight glycemic control in severely burned children. *J Trauma Inj Infec Crit Care* 59:1148.
113. Hemmila, M.R., Taddonio, M.A., Sama, A.E., Wahl, W.L. 2008. Safety and efficacy of an intensive insulin protocol in a burn-trauma intensive care unit. *J Burn Care Res* 29:187.
114. Gibson, B.R., Galiatsatos, P., Rabiee, A., Eaton, L., Abu-Hamdah, R., Christmas, C. et al. 2009. Intensive insulin therapy confers a similar survival benefit in the burn intensive care unit to the surgical intensive care unit. *Surgery* 146:922.
115. Arbabi, S., Campion, E.M., Hemmila, M.R., Barker, M., Dimo, M., Ahrns, K.S. et al. 2007. Beta-blocker use is associated with improved outcomes in adult trauma patients. *J Trauma Inj Infect Crit Care* 62:56.
116. Herndon, D.N., Hart, D.W., Wolf, S.E., Chinkes, D.L., Wolfe, R.R. 2001. Reversal of catabolism by beta-blockade after severe burns. *J Med* 345:1223.

117. Barrientos, S., Stojadinovic, O., Golinko, M.S., Brem, H., Tomic-Canic, M. 2008. Growth factors and cytokines in wound healing. *Wound Heal Soc* 16:585.
118. Schultz, G.S., Wysocki, A. 2009. Interactions between extracellular matrix and growth factors in wound healing. *Wound Repair Regen* 17:153.
119. Cross, K.J., Mustoe, T.A. 2003. Growth factors in wound healing. *Surg Clin* 83:531.
120. Serensen, O.E., Cowland, J.B., Theilgaard-Monch, K., Liu, L., Ganz, T., Borregaard, N. 2003. Wound healing and expression of antimicrobial peptides/polypeptides in human keratinocytes, a consequence of common growth factors. *J Immunol* 170:5583.
121. Robson, M.C., Phillips, L.G., Robson, L.E., Thomason, A., Pierce, G.F. 1992. Platelet-derived growth factor BB for the treatment of chronic pressure ulcers. *Lancet* 339:23.
122. Mustoe, T.A., Cutler, N.R., Allman, R.M., Goode, P.S., Deuel, T.F., Prause, J. et al. 1994. A phase II study to evaluate recombinant platelet-derived growth factor-BB in the treatment of stage 3 and 4 pressure ulcers. *Arch Surg* 129:213.
123. Robson, M.C., Phillip, L.G., Cooper, D.M., Lyle, W.G., Robson, L.E., Odom, L. et al. 1995. Safety and effect of transforming growth factor-beta 2 for treatment of venous stasis ulcers. *Wound Repair Regen* 3:157.
124. Steed, D.L. 1995. The Diabetic Ulcer Group: Clinical evaluation of recombinant human platelet-derived growth factor for the treatment of lower extremity diabetic ulcers. *J Vasc Surg* 21:71.
125. Robson, M.C., Phillip, L.G., Cooper, D.M., Lyle, W.G., Robson, L.E., Odom, L. et al. 1994. Safety and effect of topical recombinant human interleukin-1β in the management of pressure sores. *Wound Repair Regen* 2:177.
126. Galeano, M., Deodato, B., Altavilla, D., Squadrito, G., Seminara, P., Marini, H. et al. 2003. Effect of recombinant adeno-associated virus vector-mediated vascular endothelial growth factor gene transfer on wound healing after burn injury. *Crit Care Med* 31:1017.
127. Fang, C., Li, B., Wray, C., Hasselgren, P. 2002. Insulin-like growth factor-I inhibits lysosomal and proteasome-dependent proteolysis in skeletal muscle after burn injury. *J Burn Care Rehabil* 23:318.
128. Greenhalgh, D.G., Rieman, M. 1994. Effects of basic fibroblast growth factor on the healing of partial-thickness donor sites: A prospective, randomized double-blinded trial. *Wound Repair Regen* 2:113.
129. Cioffi, W.G., Gore, D.C., Rue, L.W., Carrougher, G., Guler, H.P., McManus, W.F. et al. 1994. Insulin-like growth factor-1 lowers protein oxidation in patients with thermal injury. *Ann Surg* 220:310.
130. Hattori, M., Taylor, T.D. 2009. The human intestinal microbiome: A new frontier of human biology. *DNA Res* 16:1.
131. Kinross, J.M., von Roon, A.C., Holmes, E., Darzi, A., Nicholson, J.K. 2008. The human gut microbiome: Implications for future health care. *Curr Gastroenterol Rep* 10:396.
132. Peng, Y.Z., Yuan, Z.Q., Xiao, G.X. 2001. Effects of early enteral feeding on the prevention of enterogenic infection in severely burned patients. *Burns* 27:145.
133. Chen, Z., Wang, S., Yu, B., Li, Y. 2006. A comparison study between early enteral nutrition and parenteral nutrition in severe burn patients. *Burns* 33:708.
134. Gramlich, L., Kichian, K., Pinilla, J., Rodych, N.J., Dhaliwal, R., Heyland, D.K. 2004. Does enteral nutrition compared to parenteral nutrition result in better outcomes in critically ill adult patients? A systematic review of the literature. *Nutrition* 20:843.
135. Saito, H., Trocki, O., Alexander, J.W. 1987. The effect of route of nutrient administration on the nutritional state, catabolic hormone secretion, and gut mucosal integrity after burn injury. *J Parenter Enteral Nutr* 11:1.
136. Gottschlich, M.M., Jenkins, M.E., Mayes, T., Khoury, J., Kagan, R.J., Warden, G.D. 2002. An evaluation of the safety of early vs delayed enteral support and effects on clinical, nutritional, and endocrine outcomes after severe burns. *J Burn Care Rehabil* 23:401.
137. Sonnier, D., Gottschlich, M.M., Kagan, R.J. Fluid resuscitation, inotropic agents and early enteral feeding after burn injury: Is there a risk for bowel necrosis? *J Burn Care Res*, submitted.
138. Jenkins, M.E., Gottschlich, M.M., Warden, G.D. 1994. Enteral feeding during operative procedures in thermal injuries. *J Burn Care Rehabil* 15:199.
139. Andel, D., Kamolz, L., Donner, A., Hoerauf, K., Schramm, W., Meissl, G. et al. 2005. Impact of intraoperative duodenal feeding on the oxygen balance of the splanchnic region in severely burned patients. *Burns* 31:302.
140. Schroeder, D., Gillanders, L., Mahr, K., Hill, G.L. 1991. Effects of immediate postoperative enteral nutrition on body composition, muscle function, and wound healing. *J Parenter Enteral Nutr* 15:376.

141. Farreras, N., Artigas, V., Cardona, D., Rius, X., Trias, M., Gonzalez, J. 2005. Effect of early postoperative enteral immunonutrition on wound healing in patients undergoing surgery for gastric cancer. *Clin Nutr* 24:55.
142. Braga, M., Gianotti, L., Gentilini, O., Parisi, V., Salis, C., DiCarlo, V. 2001. Early postoperative enteral nutrition improves gut oxygenation and reduces costs compared with total parenteral nutrition. *Crit Care Med* 29:242.
143. Simpson, F., Doig, S. 2005. Parenteral vs. enteral nutrition in the critically ill patient: A meta-analysis of trials using the intention to treat principle. *Intensive Care Med* 31:12.
144. Pscheidl, E., Schywalsky, M., Tschaikowsky, K., Bokeprols, T. 2000. Fish oil-supplemented parenteral diets normalize splanchnic blood flow and improve killing of translocated bacteria in a low-dose endotoxin rat model. *Crit Care Med* 28:1489.
145. Moriya, T., Fukatsu, K., Maeshima, Y., Ikezawa, F., Hashiguchi, Y., Saitoh, D. et al. 2012. The effect of adding fish oil to parenteral nutrition on hepatic mononuclear cell function and survival after intraportal bacterial challenge in mice. *Surgery* 151:745.
146. Sungurtekin, H., Degirmenci, S., Sungurterkin, U., Oguz, B.E., Sabir, N., Kaptanoglu, B. 2011. Comparison of the effects of different intravenous fat emulsions in patients with systemic inflammatory response syndrome and sepsis. *Nutr Clin Pract* 26:665.
147. Gercek, A., Yildirim, O., Konya, D., Bozkurt, S., Ozgen, S., Killic, T. et al. 2007. Effects of parenteral fish-oil emulsion (omegaven) on cutaneous wound healing in rats treated with dexamethasone. *J Parenter Enteral Nutr* 31:161.
148. McDaniel, J.C., Massey, K., Nicolaou, A. 2011. Wound repair and regeneration. *Wound Heal Soc* 19:189.
149. Warden, G.D. 1992. Burn shock resuscitation. *World J Surg* 16:16.

25 Solid Organ Transplantation

Jeanette Hasse and Srinath Chinnakotla

CONTENTS

TRANSPLANTATION BACKGROUND

The first successful kidney transplant was performed in 1954 by Dr. Joseph Murray in Boston. Since then, the field of organ transplantation has advanced rapidly. In 2013, more than 29,000 individuals received an organ transplant. In addition, based on Organ Procurement and Transplantation Network (OPTN) data as of March 6, 2015, more than 619,000 individuals have undergone transplantation in the United States in the last 26 years (OPTN 2015a). The first isolated pancreas transplant was performed by Dr. Lillihei in 1966 at the University of Minnesota. In 2013, 1018 adults received a pancreas transplant (Kandaswamy 2013). Since the first liver transplant was performed by Dr. Starzl in 1963 (Starzl 1968), liver transplantation has achieved incredible success, with over 5900 liver transplants being performed in the United States in 2013 (OPTN 2015a). Heart transplants are now actively performed in over 100 centers in the United States (OPTN 2015b). Lung transplants are increasingly being performed with 1923 lung transplants and 23 combined heart/lung transplants performed in 2013 (OPTN 2015a.). Since the first successful intestinal transplant in 1990 (Grant 1990), small intestinal transplant results have improved due to changes in immunosuppression, advances in surgical technique and postoperative care, and experience in the field (Garg 2011). Advances in surgical techniques have enabled transplant programs to broaden the indications for transplantation such that greater numbers of patients have benefited. Combined advances in critical care and immunosuppression are responsible for the vast improvements in allograft outcomes and, more importantly, prolonged patient survival.

Importance of Nutrition in Critically Ill Transplant Patients

Nutrition support is one of the integral parts in the management of critically ill transplant patients. Candidates with end-stage organ disease awaiting transplantation are often malnourished, and the operative stress of the transplant further decreases their metabolic stores. The efficacy of nutrition support after transplantation is well illustrated by prospective randomized clinical studies performed in liver transplant patients that are discussed later in this paper (Hasse 1995, Rayes 2002, 2005).

ROUTINE MEDICAL CARE OF UNCOMPLICATED TRANSPLANT PATIENTS

Kidney and Pancreas Transplantation

The most common indications for kidney transplantation are end-stage renal disease (ESRD) due to diabetes mellitus (DM), hypertension, glomerulonephritis, cystic kidney disease, and other miscellaneous diseases (Matas 2015.). The primary indication for a pancreas transplant is DM. If individuals with type 1 DM also have associated end-stage renal disease, a simultaneous pancreas and kidney (SPK) transplant may be performed.

In 60%–70% of renal transplant recipients with grafts from deceased donors and virtually 100% of renal transplant recipients with grafts from living donors, the transplanted kidney will function immediately. In recipients of a living kidney donor, as much as 6–10 L of urine output can be produced in the first 24 h posttransplant. In this situation, accurate fluid balance and supplementation of potassium and other electrolytes is necessary. About one-quarter of patients with deceased donor transplants and a few patients with living donor transplants develop delayed graft dysfunction due to acute tubular necrosis as a result of preservation injury. The rate of delayed graft function is increased in those patients who receive a kidney from an extended criteria donor (ECD) or donation after cardiac death (DCD). These patients will have oliguria or anuria and may require renal replacement therapy (RRT) until the graft function improves.

All kidney transplant grafts are placed in an extraperitoneal location, so bowel function returns upon recovery from anesthesia. Therefore, an oral diet is initiated as early as the first day posttransplant. The SPK transplant operation is significantly larger in scope than the kidney transplant. It is usually performed in an intraperitoneal fashion. There is more dissection and bowel manipulation during the operation. The return of bowel function often is delayed for several days. Also, many of these patients may have associated diabetic gastroparesis and a prolonged ileus. A majority of the time, the exocrine secretions are drained into the bowel. However, if the exocrine secretions of the pancreas graft are drained via the bladder, the transplant recipients also may lose significant amount of fluids due to loss of exocrine secretions rich in bicarbonate. Uncomplicated pancreas transplant patients typically do not require nutrition support; however, if they have a prolonged ileus, nutrition support may be indicated.

Liver Transplantation

Common indications for liver transplantation in the United States are cirrhosis of the liver due to viral hepatitis (B and C) and Laennec's (alcoholic) cirrhosis as well as cholestatic diseases such as primary biliary cirrhosis and primary sclerosing cholangitis. In addition, metabolic diseases, hepatic cancer, and cirrhosis from nonalcoholic fatty liver disease (NAFLD) are prevalent causes of liver disease. As treatment for hepatitis C improves (Bacon 2011, Jacobson 2011, Poordad 2011, Zeuzem 2011, Ghany 2013), it is expected that fewer individuals with this disease will require transplantation. However, since NAFLD has become the leading cause of liver disease in the United States (Younossi 2011), there will be a surge in NAFLD as a leading indicator for transplantation. After a successful liver transplant, liver function usually steadily improves and most patients achieve *good* liver function quickly. Once the new liver graft's physiologic makeup is sufficiently intact to handle basic synthesis and clearance of metabolic wastes, the intensive care unit (ICU) management mainly consists of replacing ongoing fluid losses and avoiding injury to the graft liver during the period of recovery. Advances in liver transplant surgical techniques have resulted in shortened ICU stay (median ICU stay for a liver transplant recipient at our center is 1 day) with early resumption of oral diet. The liver transplant operation usually does not involve a bowel anastomosis except in patients with primary sclerosing cholangitis or other patients who have indications for a Roux-en-Y bile duct anastomosis. Thus, the return of bowel function occurs within 1 or 2 days. Based on a global assessment of patient nutritional status, many liver transplant recipients demonstrate malnutrition and sarcopenia. A practice in some transplant programs is to place a nasojejunal feeding tube at the time of the liver transplant operation so that enteral feeding can be initiated within 12 h after transplantation (Hasse 1995, Ikegami 2012). Oral diet is initiated after return of bowel function. Once a patient has adequate oral calorie intake, the feeding tube is removed.

Small Bowel Transplantation

Common indications for small bowel transplantation are short gut syndrome, necrotizing enterocolitis, and pseudoobstruction (OPTN/SRTR 2011 Annual Data Report). In all small bowel transplant recipients, the distal transplant bowel is always brought out as an ostomy. After the operation, the small bowel starts functioning within the first few postoperative days. Ostomy losses of up to 100 mL/kg are acceptable and can be compensated for with supplemental intravenous fluids (IVFs). Parenteral nutrition (PN) is usually required in the early postoperative period. However, enteral nutrition is provided as soon as there is a return of intestinal function. In the absence of other clinical complications, enteral feedings are started on the third to seventh postoperative day (Colomb 2009, Matarese 2011). Potential surgical complications such as ischemia–reperfusion injury, denervation, and absence of lymphatic drainage of the transplanted intestine can compromise tube feeding (TF) tolerance (Colomb 2009). As patients recover, nutrition support is transitioned to oral diet (Garg 2011).

Heart Transplantation

The sine qua non consideration for heart transplantation is refractory congestive heart failure and severe functional limitation despite maximal medical therapy. Ischemic heart disease has become the number one indication after cardiomyopathy (OPTN/SRTR 2011 Annual Data Report). Most patients require inotropic support for the first 12–24 h after heart transplantation. Oral diets may begin as early as 1–2 days postoperatively.

Lung Transplantation

UNOS has developed four categories of lung disease for transplantation (OPTN/SRTR 2011 Annual Data Report):

Group A = Obstructive lung disease (e.g., emphysema)
Group B = Pulmonary vascular disease (e.g., primary pulmonary hypertension)
Group C = Cystic fibrosis or immunodeficiency disorder
Group D = Restrictive lung disease (e.g., idiopathic pulmonary fibrosis)

Double lung transplants are performed 70% of the time with the remainder being single lung transplants (OPTN/SRTR 2011 Annual Data Report). Patients undergoing lung transplantation can be at risk of malnutrition due to increased calorie needs from increased work of breathing and malabsorption as in cystic fibrosis. On the other hand, obesity can be prevalent in those patients who were treated with corticosteroids for their lung disease prior to transplantation. An oral diet is usually initiated following extubation; however, prolonged ventilation necessitates the initiation of TFs.

NUTRITION THERAPY

Effects of Malnutrition

Malnutrition is a risk factor for surgery and transplantation (Schwebel 2000, Merli 2002). It is known to prolong posttransplantation ventilatory support (Pikul 1994, Schwebel 2000, Hade 2003) and increase posttransplant hospital length of stay (Pikul 1994, Hade 2003), infection rates (Hade 2003), and mortality before (Snell 1998) and after (Plochl 1996, Schwebel 2000, Madill 2001, Aggrwal 2013) transplantation. Malnutrition has been measured in transplant patients in a variety of ways.

Molnar et al. utilized a 10-component *malnutrition-inflammation score* (MIS) in nearly 1000 kidney transplant recipients to analyze the relationship between the score and the mortality (Molnar 2011). The MIS was a significant predictor of mortality.

Some studies have found a relationship between subjective global assessment (SGA) and clinical variables of liver disease such as Child–Pugh score, ascites, edema, and encephalopathy (Ferreira 2010). One study (Merli 2009) found that malnutrition defined by SGA criteria in 38 liver transplant recipients was the only independent risk factor for increased ICU and hospital length of stay, whereas malnutrition, hemoglobin levels, and disease severity were associated with the number of infectious episodes in the hospital (Merli 2009).

Sarcopenia measured as psoas area determined by computed tomography (CT) scan has more recently been identified as a risk factor for mortality in liver transplant recipients

(Englesbe 2010). One-year survival in a group with psoas area at the lowest quartile was 49.7% versus 87% survival in those patients whose psoas muscle area was in the top quartile. This finding was corroborated by a study in patients with cirrhosis (Montano-Loza 2012). Forty-five of 112 patients with cirrhosis evaluated for liver transplantation were sarcopenic based on CT scan to determine L3 skeletal muscle index. In a multivariate analysis, only sarcopenia, Child–Pugh score, and model for end-stage liver disease (MELD) score were associated with increased mortality risk. The increase in mortality in sarcopenic patients was related to sepsis, not liver-related death. Sarcopenia was not correlated with MELD and Child–Pugh scores. A third study by Tandon et al. evaluated sarcopenia in patients awaiting liver transplantation (Tandon 2012). Sarcopenia (based on MRI/CT scan images of L3 skeletal muscle area) was identified in 41% of 142 patients listed for liver transplantation. Increased sarcopenia was associated with Child–Pugh class, but not MELD score, BMI, or SGA rating. Sarcopenia, as in other studies, was a predictor of mortality after age and MELD adjustments.

Nutrition Support Indications

While nutrition support is not necessary for transplant recipients who recover from surgery quickly and begin eating, it is almost always necessary for the critically ill, ICU-bound transplant patient. Transplant recipients who require ICU care are likely to be suffering from organ (possibly multiorgan) failure, sepsis, and/or neurologic compromise. A few of these patients may be allowed to eat or drink if they are not intubated, but even in this situation, oral intake usually is not adequate.

If a patient is well nourished and is expected to eat in less than 3 days, it is probably acceptable to wait to start nutrition support. However, many transplant recipients are malnourished and nutrition support should not be delayed in those patients. Figure 25.1 outlines a decision tree to determine the need for nutrition support in critically ill transplant recipients.

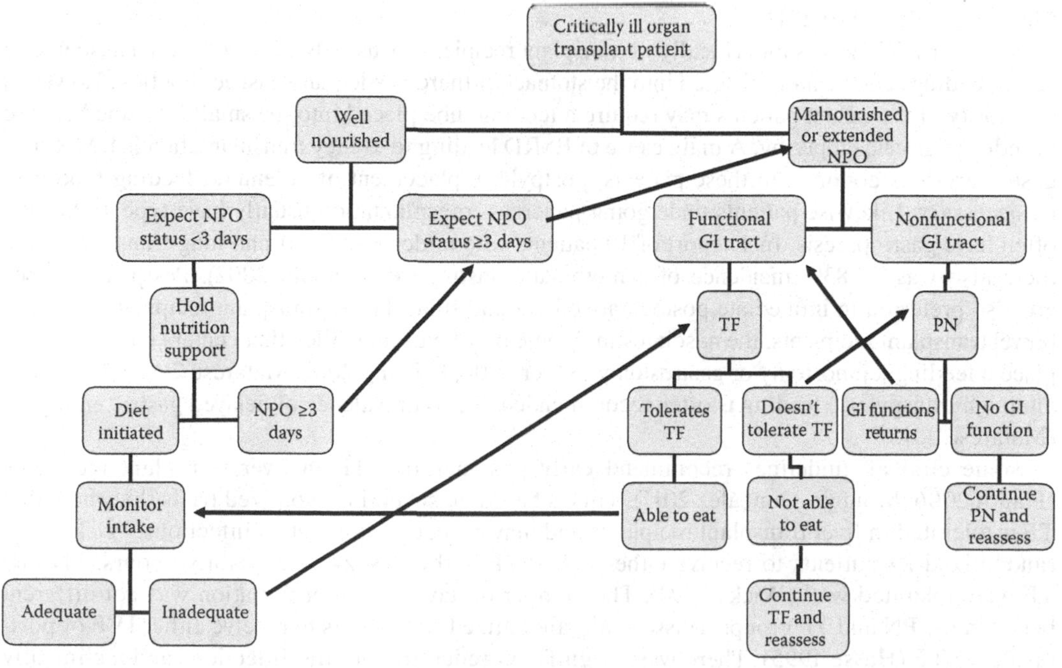

FIGURE 25.1 Algorithm for providing nutrition support to a critically ill organ transplant recipient. *Note:* GI, gastrointestinal; PN, parenteral nutrition; TF, tube feeding.

The mode of nutrition support depends on gastrointestinal (GI) function. Parenteral nutrition is reserved for patients without normal GI function (e.g., ileus, bowel obstruction, high-output fistula, GI bleeding). Small bowel transplant recipients require PN until the transplanted graft recovers (Colomb 2009, Matarese 2010, Garg 2011). While the goal is to establish enteral and oral nutrition in small bowel transplant recipients, PN may need to be reinstituted for severe intestinal graft rejection, major lymphatic leak, cytomegalovirus (CMV) enteritis, and graft dysmotility. Increased stomal output and severe diarrhea may improve with administration of antidiarrheal agents such as kaolin–pectin, loperamide, and opiates. At the other end of the spectrum, prokinetics may help gastroparesis when it occurs (Matarese 2010).

Postoperative Tube Feeding

TF is indicated for early postoperative feedings or supplementation when oral intake is not adequate (Figure 25.1). Most transplant recipients tolerate a standard isotonic formula. A high-nitrogen formula may be needed to meet protein needs, a concentrated formula may be helpful if a patient is hyponatremic or needs fluid restriction, and a fiber-containing formula may be helpful if a patient has constipation or diarrhea.

For small bowel transplant patients, TF can be initiated and PN tapered as TF and oral diet advance. The ideal TF formula for small bowel transplant recipients is yet to be determined. Some centers use an elemental or semielemental formula, while others use isotonic, intact-protein formulas. Some transplant centers support the idea of giving insoluble fiber to small bowel transplant recipients (to help reduce bacterial translocation) as well as soluble fiber (to promote the restoration of villous functional capacity) (Silver 2000). Although glutamine is considered a prime fuel for enterocytes, there have been no clinical studies to support giving glutamine to small bowel transplant recipients. Because the lymphatics are disrupted during organ procurement, there is a risk for intestinal transplant recipients to develop chylous ascites. Some programs preemptively use low-fat formulas and others choose standard formulas and switch to a low-fat formula only if chylous ascites develops (Weseman 2007, Colomb 2009, Matarese 2010, Garg 2011).

Short-term TF access for critically ill transplant recipients is usually achieved with a nasoenteral tube. Feedings can be administered into the stomach if there is adequate gastric function. However, a majority of transplant patients may require a feeding tube placed into the small intestine because of reduced gastric emptying. A main cause of ESRD leading to kidney transplantation is DM. Since gastroparesis is common in these patients, postpyloric placement of an enteral feeding tube may be necessary. Likewise patients undergoing pancreas transplantation usually have type 1 DM and often have gastroparesis. In 1 report of 10 patients who underwent heart and lung transplantation, there also was an 83% incidence of symptomatic gastroparesis (Sodhi 2002). Postpyloric tubes are also preferred in immediate postoperative liver and small bowel transplant recipients. In small bowel transplant recipients, the nasointestinal route may be used, while other centers will surgically place a feeding jejunostomy or gastrostomy (Silver 2000, Colomg 2009, Matarese 2010, Garg 2011) although transpyloric feeding is often recommended due to prevalence of delayed gastric emptying (Matarese 2010).

Some clinical guidelines recommend early postoperative TF in liver transplant recipients (Plauth 2006, Montejo-González 2011). This is based on several randomized trials that show that TF is tolerated in liver transplant recipients and may reduce postoperative infections. Wicks et al. randomized 24 patients to receive either PN or TF within 18–24 postoperative hours; PN and TF were tolerated well (Wicks 1994). The number of days until diet initiation was not different between the PN and TF groups. Hasse et al. randomized 50 patients to receive either IVF or postoperative TF (Hasse 1995). There was a significant reduction in viral infections and a clinically relevant reduction in bacterial infections in the tube-fed versus control group. Another transplant group evaluated the effect of probiotics and TF in liver transplant recipients (Rayes 2002).

Thirty-two patients (group 1) were enterally fed with a 1.0 kcal/mL formula along with small bowel decontamination. Thirty-one patients (group 2) received a fiber-containing formula and *Lactobacillus plantarum 299*. Thirty-two patients (group 3) received the same fiber-containing formula with a placebo probiotic. Infection rates were 48% in group 1, 34% in group 3, and 13% in group 2. These same researchers (Rayes 2005) did a follow-up study with 33 patients receiving high-nitrogen TF via a nasointestinal tube with a synbiotic containing four probiotics and four fibers. The control group of 33 patients received the same TF and fiber without the probiotic. The major finding was a reduction of infection from 48% in the control group to 3% in the study group.

Three studies have evaluated TF specifically in recipients of living donor liver transplants (Ikegami 2012, Kaido 2012, Yoshida 2012). Early postoperative TF was also found to reduce bacterial sepsis in liver transplant recipients in a retrospective study. Ikegami et al. retrospectively analyzed 345 adult living donor transplant recipients to identify risk factors for bacterial sepsis, since the 2-year graft survival rate was only 45.7% in the 46 patients who had bacterial sepsis (Ikegami 2012). The incidence of bacterial sepsis was 5.9% in patients who received TF within 48 h of transplantation and 21% in those who did not ($p = 0.002$). In addition, early graft loss was eightfold higher in patients who did not receive early postoperative TF and had a massive interoperative bleed compared with the other patients in the study.

The study by Yoshida and colleagues evaluated effectiveness of providing branched-chain amino-acid supplements during the perioperative period on outcomes in living donor liver transplant recipients (Yoshida 2012). Twelve patients received an oral branched-chain amino acid supplement before transplantation and again from postoperative day 3 to 28. Oral diet was started 1 week posttransplant. The control patients ($n = 12$) received diet only. There were no differences between the groups with regard to surgical outcomes or infection rates.

Kaido et al. reported benefits of providing a special immunomodulating TF formula to living donor liver transplant recipients (Kaido 2012). Seventy-six patients undergoing living donor liver transplantation also underwent jejunostomy tube placement at the time of transplantation. TF was started within 24 h of surgery; 40 patients received a hydrolyzed whey protein formula and 36 patients received an elemental formula. All patients received a synbiotic three times daily consisting of glutamine, fiber, and oligosaccharide as well as a once-daily beverage containing *Lactobacillus casei* Shirota strain. Those who received the whey formula had a 15% rate of bacteremia versus a 47% rate in controls ($p = 0.002$).

Postoperative Parenteral Nutrition

Parenteral nutrition is used less frequently than enteral nutrition in transplant recipients. As discussed earlier, PN is a bridge to TF or oral diet in intestinal transplant recipients. Other general indications for PN in transplant recipients include ileus, high-output fistula, small bowel obstruction, GI bleeding, and small bowel transplant failure.

Few studies in literature evaluated PN in transplant recipients (Reilly 1990, Wicks 1994, Zhu 2013). The study by Wicks et al. was discussed earlier. In the investigation by Reilly et al., 28 liver transplant patients were divided into three groups: one group received no specific nutrition therapy, the second received standard PN with 35 kcal/kg/day, and the third received PN with a branched-chain-enriched amino acid solution (Reilly 1990). At the end of 7 days, the PN groups had superior nitrogen balance, required a shorter period of posttransplant mechanical ventilation, and had shorter ICU stays. Also, the total hospital charges were the greatest in the group that received no nutrition support. It is unfortunate that this well-designed study did not include a treatment arm that used TF, which could be delivered at a fractional cost of PN; nevertheless, this study demonstrated the benefits of nutrition support in the ICU.

Zhu and colleagues compared effects of diet alone versus oral diet plus PN containing a standard 20% intravenous fat emulsion (IVFE) containing long-chain and medium-chain triglyceride or oral diet plus PN containing an *n*-3 fish oil lipid emulsion. The amino acid content of the PN was composed of a branched-chain amino acid solution. Oral diet was started around day 3 or 4 postoperatively, and PN was given for 7 days postoperatively. The researchers concluded that the *n*-3 IVFE reduced hepatic cell injury (as determined by liver biopsy on day 9). In addition, there was a reduction in hospital stay by an average of 2–4 days compared with the other groups. Infectious complications were also reduced in the *n*-3 PN group (9% of patients had infection versus 18% of patients with standard PN or 25% of patients receiving oral diet alone). There are some significant limitations to this study. The mean hospital length of stay (18–24 days) was about double that of many U.S. centers. The PN products used in this study are not readily available in the United States. Finally, early postoperative TF was not evaluated in this study and the patients did not meet generally accepted criteria for PN use.

NUTRIENT NEEDS

Nutrient needs of transplant recipients have been outlined for the immediate posttransplant phase. However, nutrient requirements have not been delineated in transplant patients who develop medical or surgical complications and require ICU care. One could conjecture that the nutrient needs in a transplant patient during critical illness would mimic those of other types of patients with a critical illness (Table 25.1).

Calories

Measuring caloric needs via indirect calorimetry is preferred over estimating caloric needs. Underfeeding can lead to weight loss, muscle wasting (including respiratory muscles), and reduced immune defense. Overfeeding may lead to hyperglycemia and potentiate increased infection rates in an immunosuppressed host. Providing excess energy may also cause steatosis or difficulty in weaning from the ventilator.

Protein

Critically ill transplant patients have heightened protein requirements (up to 1.5–2.0 g/kg). Protein catabolic rate increases with surgical stress and administration of corticosteroids. Protein needs are also increased owing to losses from open wounds, negative pressure wound therapy, surgical drains or chest tubes, dialysis, ostomy output, and para- or thoracentesis. Nitrogen balance studies may be helpful if renal function is adequate and it is possible to collect all losses.

Carbohydrate

Patients undergoing transplantation may have preexisting DM. As discussed earlier, DM is the primary indication for pancreas transplantation and is one of the leading causes of renal failure resulting in transplantation. In addition, patients with cystic fibrosis awaiting lung transplantation may have DM. DM is considered a comorbid condition that may complicate transplantation, but by itself is not a contraindication for transplantation. Risk factors for new-onset diabetes after transplantation (NODAT) include ethnicity, family history, increased age, BMI $\geq$ 25 kg/m^2, hepatitis C, alcoholic cirrhosis, and use of calcineurin inhibitors and corticosteroids (Bodziak 2009, Sarno 2013, Therasse 2013).

Even in patients without previous DM history, posttransplant hyperglycemia frequently occurs in part due to a metabolic stress response. However, immunosuppressive medications also cause hyperglycemia. Calcineurin inhibitors (tacrolimus and cyclosporine) decrease insulin secretion via a direct toxic effect on the β-cell or inhibition of DNA synthesis and increase in insulin (Bodziak 2009, Sarno 2013, Therasse 2013). Corticosteroids precipitate hyperglycemia by

TABLE 25.1
Nutrient Considerations in Critically Ill Organ Transplant Recipient

Nutrition Recommendation	Comments
1.5–2.0 g protein/kg/day	• Protein is needed for postoperative recovery and wound healing. • Surgical stress and corticosteroids increase protein catabolic rate. • Consider protein losses from surgical drains, fistulas, wounds, and dialysis.
130%–150% of calculated basal energy expenditure	• If estimating calories, provide the upper limit of calories for underweight patients; provide the lower limit for overweight patients. • Measure energy needs by indirect calorimetry in critically ill patients.
50% of calories as carbohydrate	• Metabolic stress, infection, and medications (e.g., corticosteroids, cyclosporine, and tacrolimus) can elevate serum glucose levels. • Attain glucose control with insulin if needed; consider insulin drip for blood glucose levels consistently >150–200 mg/dL. • Long-term, a combination of long- and short-acting insulin may be required for glucose control. • Oral hypoglycemic agents can be considered if the patient can absorb, metabolize, and excrete the drug. • Control glucose levels before advancing nutrition support.
30% of calories as lipid	• Increased lipid concentrations may be helpful temporarily when hyperglycemia is severe and not yet under control with insulin. However, there may be an inflammatory effect of *n*-6 fatty acids. • Patients with cystic fibrosis and patients' immediate post–small bowel transplant may malabsorb fat. • There is no research on supplementation of fish oil (*n*-3 fatty acids) in critically ill transplant patients.
1 mL fluid per calorie; adjust based on output	• Monitor losses from urine, drains, wounds, diarrhea, nasogastric tube suction, fistulas, para/thoracentesis. • Urine output from a newly transplanted kidney may initially be as high as 6–10 L/day. • Exocrine secretions from a pancreas drained via the bladder can be as high as 2–3 L/day. • Ostomy output from a small bowel transplant can be as high as 4 L/day. • Restrict fluid if hyponatremia/excess water exists.
2 g sodium per day	• Restrict if ascites or edema is severe. • Correct hyponatremia slowly with fluid restriction and/or hypertonic sodium solution. There is a strong association with rapid resolution of hyponatremia and central pontine myelinolysis.
Individualize potassium prescription	• Serum levels may increase with administration of tacrolimus, cyclosporine, or potassium-sparing diuretics; renal insufficiency; or metabolic acidosis. Infusion of red blood cells and fresh frozen plasma can contribute to hyperkalemia as can hemolysis. • Metabolic acidosis may also contribute to hyperkalemia. • Serum levels may decrease with administration of potassium-wasting diuretics or amphotericin, refeeding syndrome, diarrhea, or fistulas. • University of Wisconsin (UW) solution is an organ preservation solution high in potassium. The solution is usually washed out of the liver before reperfusion, but can still contribute to hyperkalemia.
1000–1500 mg calcium per day	• Renal and hepatic diseases lead to abnormal pretransplant calcium metabolism. If large amounts of citrated blood products are given to patients, there may be a low serum ionized calcium level.

(Continued)

TABLE 25.1 (*Continued*)
Nutrient Considerations in Critically Ill Organ Transplant Recipient

Nutrition Recommendation	Comments
Individualize phosphorus prescription	• Serum levels may increase with renal insufficiency. • Serum levels may decrease with refeeding syndrome or administration of corticosteroids.
Individualize magnesium prescription	• Hypomagnesemia can occur due to • Increased gastrointestinal losses from diarrhea, nasogastric tube suction, and fistula Increased urinary losses during diuretic phase of acute tubular necrosis and from calcineurin inhibitors Refeeding syndrome Losses from continuous renal replacement therapy Redistribution as in sepsis, massive blood transfusions Hypermagnesemia occurs less often and is usually iatrogenic (e.g., administration of magnesium-containing antacids or renal insufficiency).
Evaluate acid–base status	• Serum levels of bicarbonate often decrease due to exocrine losses of transplanted pancreas (bladder drainage) or losses from transplanted small intestine.

causing insulin resistance perhaps through decreasing insulin receptor affinity and defects at the postreceptor level, impairing peripheral glucose uptake in muscle, or increasing hepatic gluconeogenesis (Bodziak 2009, Sarno 2013, Therasse 2013). Sirolimus is also thought to contribute to NODAT through impairment of insulin-mediated suppression of hepatic glucose production, toxic effect on β-cells, and triglyceride deposition with insulin resistance (Johnston 2008, Bodziak 2009, Yates 2012).

Optimal glucose control has been shown to improve outcomes and survival in critically ill patients. One could theorize that tight glucose control would be important in transplant recipients who are prone to hyperglycemia and are at increased risk of infection (and increased mortality from infection) because of their immunosuppressed status. Postoperative hyperglycemia has been found to be a risk factor for transplant rejection. In a retrospective study of 230 nondiabetic kidney transplant recipients, those with hyperglycemia (>8 mmol/L or 144 mg/dL) had a 71% rate of rejection versus 42% in patients without hyperglycemia (Thomas 2000). Postoperative kidney transplant patients with DM with a mean blood glucose level >11.2 mmol/L (202 mg/dL) in the first 100 postoperative hours had an increased rate of rejection and infection compared with patients with lower glucose levels (Thomas 2001). A retrospective study of liver transplant patients found that elevated rates of postoperative infection and mortality occurred in patients with intraoperative hyperglycemia (Ammor 2007). Elevated glucose levels (>200 mg/dL) has also been found to be associated with increased rates of rejection in liver transplant patients (Wallia 2010).

LIPID

There are no studies in critically ill transplant patients that have evaluated effects of different levels or types of enterally or parenterally administered fats. One potential benefit of an increased fat diet would be better glucose control (due to the lower carbohydrate content). A theoretical downside would be further immune impairment and inflammatory state cause by *n*-6 fatty acids. A few studies evaluated *n*-3 fatty acids in stable transplant recipients and suggest that *n*-3 fatty acids may reduce posttransplant hyperlipidemia (Tatsioni 2005, Celik 2008, Filler 2012).

Another consideration of lipids relates to fat absorption. In the initial stages after small bowel transplantation, fat malabsorption will occur due to disruption of the lymphatic system. Regeneration of the lymphatic vessels occurs over time. Some, but not all, centers recommend a low-fat diet for

TABLE 25.2
Vitamin and Mineral Considerations for Critically Ill Transplant Recipients

Nutrient	Considerations
Fat-soluble vitamins	• Possible deficiency due to fat malabsorption and bile diversion. • Vitamin A necessary for wound healing. • Active form of vitamin D may be deficient especially with prior liver or renal failure. • Vitamin K is necessary for normal blood clotting; short-term supplementation (e.g., 3 days) may be necessary after liver transplantation.
B vitamins and folate	• Hyperhomocysteinemia in kidney transplant recipients is correlated with renal function and folate, vitamin B_6, and vitamin B_{12} status. • Alcoholism can cause deficiency of B vitamins. • B_6 deficiency has been reported in intestinal transplant recipients and can be associated with neuropathy.
Vitamin C	• Necessary for wound healing.

the first 4–6 weeks after intestinal transplantation (Weseman 2007, Colomb 2009, Matarese 2010, Garg 2011). If a liver transplant patient's bile is being diverted away from the intestine (such as via an external biliary drain), fat absorption may be impaired. Lung transplant recipients with cystic fibrosis may have malabsorption of long-chain fatty acids.

Fluid

General fluid needs are approximately 30 mL/kg, but determination of fluid rates must be individualized. Fluid restriction is indicated for cases of volume overload, reduced urine output, and hyponatremia. Fluid resuscitation is necessary if a patient has increased losses (from ostomy, drains, chest tubes, high urine output, gastric tube output, emesis, diarrhea) or hypernatremia.

Vitamins and Minerals

There are no studies delineating vitamin requirements for stable transplant recipients let alone critically ill patients. Nutrient levels are affected by original diagnosis, prehospitalization condition, medication therapy, and comorbid conditions. General considerations are outlined in Table 25.2.

DRUG–NUTRIENT INTERACTIONS IN ORGAN TRANSPLANTATION

One cannot discuss nutrition therapy for transplant recipients without reviewing the nutritional implications of immunosuppressive drugs. While immunosuppressive drugs are mandatory, the type and combination of drugs are individualized according to transplant type, patient characteristics, and transplant center protocols. Table 25.3 outlines the major immunosuppressive drugs and the nutritional ramifications.

COMPLICATIONS AND NUTRITION CONSIDERATIONS IN CRITICALLY ILL TRANSPLANT RECIPIENTS

While the medical course of each transplant patient cannot be fully predicted, there are several potential complications that can occur. Transplant patients are at risk for graft dysfunction and rejection, infection, renal failure, respiratory failure, GI complications, hyperglycemia, and other complications.

TABLE 25.3
Major Side Effects of Commonly Used Immunosuppressive Medications

	Alemtuzumab	Antilymphocyte serum	Azathioprine	Corticosteroids	Cyclosporine	Mycophenolate mofetil	Sirolimus	Tacrolimus
Bone marrow suppression	√		√			√	√	
Diarrhea		√	√			√		
Dysgeusia			√					
Fever and chills	√	√						
Gastrointestinal distress						√	√	√
Hyperglycemia				√	√			√
Hyperkalemia					√		√	√
Hyperlipidemia				√	√			
Hyperphagia				√				
Hypertension				√	√			√
Hypomagnesemia					√			√
Impaired wound healing				√			√	
Macrocytic anemia			√					
Nausea and vomiting	√	√	√					√
Neurotoxicity					√			√
Osteoporosis				√				
Pancreatitis			√	√				
Sodium retention				√				
Ulcers				√				

Source: Adapted from Hasse, J. and Robien, K., Nutrition support guidelines for therapeutically immunosuppressed patients, in Pichard, C. and Kudsk, K.A., eds., *From Nutritional Support to Pharmacologic Nutrition in the ICU*, Springer-Verlag, Berlin, Germany, 2000, pp. 361–383.

Graft Dysfunction

Medical Considerations

The causes of graft dysfunction can be classified into early and late causes. The common early causes include (1) primary nonfunction, (2) preservation injury, (3) vascular thrombosis, and (4) acute rejection. The late causes include (1) chronic rejection, (2) recurrence of primary disease, and (3) posttransplant lymphoproliferative disorder.

Primary nonfunction is defined as a transplant that has not functioned. These patients will have severe organ failure. For example, a patient with primary nonfunction after liver transplantation will manifest failure to regain consciousness and a sustained elevation in transaminases (increasing coagulopathy, acidosis, and poor bile production). Primary nonfunction is rarely seen since improved organ preservation solutions such as University of Wisconsin (UW) solution have been introduced. The treatment of primary nonfunction is retransplantation with a new organ.

Preservation injury is associated with preservation of an organ to transport it from donor to recipient. The organs after procurement from deceased donors are transported in cold preservation solution. The time from the organ procurement to the implantation into a recipient is called the cold ischemia time. The optimal cold ischemia time for a kidney is <24 h, <17 h for pancreas, <12 h for liver, <4 h for hearts, <6–8 h for lungs, and <12 h for a small intestine (Committee on OPTN 2013). Longer cold ischemia times can result in organ dysfunction, due to preservation injury.

Vascular thrombosis often presents acutely, and immediate surgical operative intervention is required. Acute rejections are common in all organs. The first line of treatment for acute rejection often is an increased dose of calcineurin inhibitor or the administration of high-dose corticosteroids. If this fails, antibody preparations such as antithymocyte globulin may be used.

Chronic rejection is less common, but is difficult to treat; retransplantation is the solution in most patients. Recurrent disease can be addressed with standard medical therapy but may require retransplantation. Due to prolonged immunosuppression, transplant patients are prone to lymphomas. The B-cell lymphomas are driven by the Epstein–Barr virus. The treatment of posttransplant lymphomas may be successfully treated with reduction or withdrawal of immunosuppression with specific chemotherapy (Murukesan 2012).

There are several immunosuppressive drug protocols in use in solid organ transplantation. They usually are developed by an individual center taking into account the local experience and preferences. Most protocols will include a calcineurin inhibitor (tacrolimus or cyclosporin) with or without corticosteroids. Mycophenolate and sirolimus are often used as third agents. The side effects of the various drugs are listed in Table 25.3.

Mycophenolate can cause significant GI side effects such as diarrhea and nausea. The GI side effects are typically dose dependent. When these side effects are significant and other etiology is ruled out, the first step would be to adjust the drug dose by giving the same daily dose by dividing it into three or four doses per day. This step alone frequently reduces the GI side effects. If the change in dosing frequency does not result in improvement of side effects, reducing the dosage by 50% is advised. Most patients would tolerate a dose reduction; discontinuation of the drug is rarely necessitated for control of side effects.

Nutrition Considerations

If a patient experiences primary nonfunction or complete graft failure, end-stage organ failure is present and nutrition therapy guidelines should correspond to those for the specific organ dysfunction. For example, if a kidney transplant graft fails, dialysis will be required and potassium and phosphorus restriction may be needed. If a small bowel transplant fails, PN needs to be resumed. If pancreas transplantation fails, then insulin therapy must be resumed.

Preservation injury may cause delayed graft function. For example, if urine output is low following renal transplantation due to delayed graft function, fluid intake may need to be limited as well. Since preservation injury will resolve given enough time, there is no permanent nutrition therapy adjustment needed in these instances.

As mentioned earlier, when a transplant graft rejects, the traditional rejection therapy is to heighten corticosteroid doses over a few days, starting with a high dose and tapering down to a maintenance dose. As mentioned earlier, this results in protein catabolism and increased protein needs. In addition, an increase in dose of corticosteroids or calcineurin inhibitors can also cause blood glucose elevation. If immunosuppressive drugs are added or changed, it may create GI symptoms or cause other drug or nutrient interactions (see Table 25.3).

If chronic rejection ensues, the patient may exhibit symptoms of organ dysfunction. If organ dysfunction is great enough, nutrition therapy may need to be adjusted. For example, chronic rejection of a kidney will lead to dialysis and nutrition therapy adjustments for hyperkalemia, hyperphosphatemia, and reduced urine output.

Infection/Sepsis

Medical Considerations

Infections continue to be the leading cause of mortality in solid organ transplantation. Immunosuppression is the main risk factor. A well-defined temporal sequence of infections is present in the posttransplant period (Fishman 2007, Pagalilauan 2013). The typical time table is divided into three parts: first month, 1–6 months, and the late period. In the first month after transplant, the major infectious complications include nosocomial infections such as postsurgical bacterial and *Candida* wound infections, postoperative pneumonia, and central line infections. The early infections can be donor or recipient derived. These infectious complications are later followed by opportunistic infections unique to the transplant patients. These include viral infections, mainly cytomegaolovirus (CMV), Epstein–Barr virus, herpes simplex virus, and recurrent hepatitis virus. It is also during this time that *Clostridia difficile*, *Pneumocystis carinii*, and *Cryptococcus neoformans* infection can occur. The late period (>6 months posttransplant) is the opportune time for community-acquired infections including community-acquired pneumonia, urinary tract infections, *Aspergillus* or *Nocardia*, and late viral infections. CMV infection is one of the more common viral infections in transplant patients. It usually presents with fever, malaise, leukopenia, and pneumonitis. Invasive CMV of the GI tract may present with diarrhea. Confirmation is obtained by checking a blood polymerase chain reaction (PCR) level of CMV. For invasive GI disease, a biopsy of the stomach or colon will reveal diagnostic CMV inclusion bodies.

A very aggressive approach is used for the treatment of infections in transplant recipients. Intravenous antibiotics with broad spectrum covering both gram-positive and gram-negative bacterial organisms are initiated immediately, and upon receipt of culture reports and sensitivities, specific antibiotics are used. Fungal prophylaxis is also used in high-risk patients. CMV infections are treated with intravenous antiviral medication for 2–4 weeks. Drugs such as sulfamethoxazole/trimethoprim are commonly used for prophylaxis of *P. carinii*. Fluconazole, micafungin, and amphotericin B are the commonly used antifungal agents.

Nutritional Considerations

Malnourished patients have an increased risk of developing infection. In addition, many antimicrobial agents cause GI symptoms including diarrhea, nausea, and vomiting. Antidiarrheal agents, fiber, or pectin-containing substances (such as banana flakes) may help minimize diarrhea and potential skin breakdown.

Acute Renal Failure

Medical Considerations

Acute renal failure is usually defined as an abrupt decrease in glomerular filtration rate caused by intrinsic renal disease or alteration in intrarenal hemodynamics resulting in the accumulation of waste products (urea, creatinine, and potassium) in the blood. Renal failure complicates the medical management of the transplant patient leading to increased morbidity and mortality (Clajus 2012).

The causes of renal failure may be prerenal (dehydration, fluid losses, or surgical hemorrhage), renal (preexisting chronic kidney disease, drug toxicity from medications including tacrolimus and cyclosporine, acute tubular necrosis from sepsis or another insult), or usually a combination of both.

Infection may also indirectly contribute to renal failure. The treatment will depend on the etiology—fluid resuscitation and correction of hypovolemia in dehydration, and in case of drug toxicity, stopping the offending drug. Temporary dialysis is often necessary especially when hypervolemia, hyperkalemia, metabolic acidosis, or uremic symptoms occur.

Nutritional Considerations

When a critically ill transplant recipient develops renal insufficiency, adjustments in nutrition therapy may be required. Acid–base and electrolyte requirements may be altered. If RRT is employed, restrictions of fluid, potassium, and phosphorus may be needed. If continuous RRT (CRRT) is used, patients may actually need additional potassium, magnesium, or phosphorus to replace that removed with CRRT. Fluid restriction may not be necessary if the RRT can remove adequate fluid amounts. Occasionally, renal failure may not require RRT, but potassium, phosphorus, magnesium, or fluid restrictions may be necessary. Generally, transplant patients who develop acute renal failure are catabolic and protein is not restricted.

Respiratory Failure

Medical Considerations

Patients after liver, small bowel, heart, and lung transplantation are usually received from the operating room to the ICU intubated. Often, after an uncomplicated posttransplant recovery, patients are extubated within 24 h. However, if patients develop graft dysfunction or sepsis and hemodynamic instability, they may require prolonged respiratory support. The other indications for respiratory support include primary lung infections like severe bacterial pneumonia, CMV pneumonia, and acute respiratory distress syndrome as part of sepsis.

Nutritional Considerations

When patients require mechanical ventilation, TF will be required. If mechanical ventilation is prolonged, it may be prudent to have a swallow evaluation prior to allowing a patient to eat. If aspiration occurs, pneumonia will develop and further compromise the patient's respiratory status.

Gastrointestinal Complications

If an ileus develops in a critically ill patient who requires nutrition support, PN should be initiated. An active GI bleed, high output fistula, small bowel obstruction, or nonfunctioning transplanted intestinal graft would also warrant PN. Diarrhea can occur as a result of mycophenolate, antibiotics, or other drugs. Diarrhea is common following small bowel transplantation due to rapid transit from loss of the ileocecal valve and/or extrinsic neuronal control as well as malabsorption and bacterial overgrowth (Dionigi 2001). Treatment of diarrhea in a transplant patient may include changing medications; adding antidiarrheal medications, fiber, or pectin; and replacing fluid and electrolyte losses.

Acid–Base Balance Disorders

Acid–base disorders are caused by clinical circumstances that lead to biochemical dysfunction and accumulation of acid or loss of base. The most common acid–base balance disorder in transplant patients is metabolic acidemia of septic shock where there is failure to supply tissue with sufficient blood flow and oxygen to meet the mitochondrial aerobic metabolism. The treatment is to correct the etiology of septic shock, and if the pH is less than 7.2, give a slow intravenous infusion of bicarbonate. Acidosis can also occur from loss of sodium salt in a fluid with high bicarbonate, such as with the loss of exocrine secretions in pancreas transplant or with severe diarrhea or losses from ostomy in a small bowel transplant. The treatment is replacement of bicarbonate. Metabolic alkalosis can occur in patients with prolonged vomiting or nasogastric drainage. When gastric juices rich in hydrochloric acid are lost and extracellular water and sodium become depleted, hormonal responses increase aldosterone. With more of the mineralocorticoid influence, more bicarbonate is transported to the already alkalemic plasma. This alkalosis problem is easily corrected by infusion of saline solution to restore intravascular volume and the administration of supplemental potassium chloride if potassium levels are low.

Hyperglycemia

Medical Considerations

As mentioned several times, immunosuppressed patients are at increased risk for infection. When infection occurs, it is a serious complication. Poorly controlled glucose levels are a risk factor for infection.

Causes of hyperglycemia include drugs (discussed earlier) and metabolic distress. Type 2 DM is common in transplant patients, especially renal transplant patients who may have required a kidney transplant for end-stage renal disease due to diabetic nephropathy.

Nutritional Considerations

Adequate glucose control is imperative. If a patient has a persistently high glucose level, an insulin drip may be necessary. Otherwise, a combination of long-acting insulin and short-acting insulin should be used to treat hyperglycemia. Oral agents can be considered if patients have the ability to absorb, metabolize, and excrete them normally.

CASE STUDY

History and Background

The case study patient is a 27-year-old man with cirrhosis due to primary sclerosing cholangitis and autoimmune hepatitis and a history of ulcerative colitis. The patient presented to the hospital with ascites, jaundice, cholangitis with biliary stones, portal hypertension with esophageal varices, iron-deficiency anemia, vitamin A and D deficiencies, and coagulopathy. The patient underwent evaluation for liver transplantation.

At his initial evaluation, the patient weighed 140 lb (height, 68 in.). His usual weight was 140 lb, with a lowest recent weight of 135 lb. At the time of evaluation, the patient had a good appetite and only complained of occasional nausea. He was counseled on a 2 g sodium, high-calorie diet and was prescribed vitamin supplements. After removal of bile duct stones, the patient was discharged from the hospital.

Over the next several days, the patient's condition declined necessitating rehospitalization. His nutrition status had also declined owing to a headache, poor appetite, and nausea. A nasojejunal feeding tube was placed to provide adequate nutrition. The patient's condition worsened requiring a transfer to ICU; he developed hepatic encephalopathy and acute respiratory failure requiring mechanical ventilation, acute kidney injury requiring CRRT, and anemia requiring transfusions. The patient was listed for liver transplantation with a MELD score of 27; it increased rapidly over the next 4 days to a maximum score of 40.

Postoperative Days 1–7: Immediate Postsurgical Period

The patient underwent a liver transplant with a Roux-en-Y hepaticojejunostomy 14 days after being listed for transplantation. After surgery, the patient returned to the ICU intubated, sedated,

TABLE 25.4
Nutrition Support Regimen in a Critically Ill Transplant Case Study Patient

Posttransplant Day	Tube Feeding Formula and Rate	Tube Feeding Intake Goal Intake = 2100–2300 Cal, 90–120 g protein (Cal/g protein)	Oral Intake (Cal/g protein)	Comments
–6	2 Cal/mL formula at 45 mL/h	2160/90	Minimal	
–1	2 Cal/mL formula at 45 mL/h	2160/90	NPO	Patient was intubated, undergoing CRRT. TF goal was 45 mL/h but patient was bleeding from mouth and nose.
1	1.2 Cal/mL high-nitrogen formula restarted postoperative at 20 mL/h	576/27	NPO	Patient still intubated being weaned from one of two vasopressors.
4	2 Cal/mL formula at 50 mL/h	2400/100	NPO	Patient was extubated, off pressors and sedation. Still undergoing CRRT.
7	1.2 Cal/mL high-nitrogen formula at 75 mL/h	2160/100	NPO—to undergo swallow evaluation	Patient transferred out of ICU on postoperative day (POD) 4, but returned to ICU on POD 7 for fever. TF formula changed to add free water.
12	1.2 Cal/mL high-nitrogen formula at 65 mL/h	1872/87	Passed swallow evaluation; ate small amounts of soft diet	
15	1.2 Cal/mL high-nitrogen formula at 80 mL/h × 16 h	1536/72	Eating 900 kcal/40 g pro	Undergoing corticosteroid recycle for rejection; transferred to rehabilitation hospital.

and requiring two pressor agents. Sedation and pressors were weaned, and the patient was extubated on postoperative day 4. CRRT was discontinued on postoperative day 5, and the patient did not require further dialysis. To prevent rejection, the immunosuppressive drugs mycophenolate and corticosteroids were initiated as well as thymoglobulin for 4 days after which tacrolimus was started. To prevent infection, antimicrobial agents including meropenem, vancomycin, amphotericin, ganciclovir, and bactrim were added to the patient's medication regimen. Over a period of a few days, the pressors were weaned. An elevation in liver function tests (LFTs) reflected preservation injury from the organ preservation.

Nutrient needs were calculated to be 2100–2300 cal (130%–140% basal energy expenditure calculated by Mifflin-St Jeor equation) and 90–120 g pro/day (1.5–2 g pro/kg). On postoperative day 1, TFs were restarted via the nasoduodenal tube that was placed prior to surgery (Table 25.4).

Postoperative Days 8–14: Recovery

The patient was transferred to the floor on postoperative day 8. Despite a declining serum total bilirubin level, other LFTs were slightly increased (Table 25.5). A liver biopsy confirmed acute

TABLE 25.5
Serum Laboratory Values in a Critically Ill Liver Transplant Case Study Patient: Preoperatively to 3 Months Postoperatively

Relation to Transplant Date	Total Bilirubin[b] (0.2–1.0 mg/dL)	Alkaline Phosphatase[b] (50–136 U/L)	Aspartate Aminotransferase[b] (15–37 U/L)	Alanine Aminotransferase (12–78 U/L)	γ-Glutamyl Transpeptidase[b] (15–85 U/L)	Sodium[b] (136–145 mEq/L)	Potassium[b] (3.5–5.1 mEq/L)	Blood Urea Nitrogen[b] (7–18 mg/dL)	Creatinine[b] (0.6–132 mg/dL)	Glucose[b] (75–110 mg/dL)
−1 week	70.0	316	251	54		138	3.3	69	5.8	101
Transplant day (preoperatively)[a]	73.6	745	501	80		143	3.6	40	2.5	87
Transplant day (postoperatively)[a]	43.6	407	1856	1013	141	147	3.9	38	2.1	105
+2 days[a]	46.5	218	387	454	108	143	4.1	44	1.7	153
+4 days[a]	38.4	373	148	265	355	144	3.8	38	1.6	105
+1 week	17.9	194	124	155	183	149	3.6	93	4.5	132
+2 weeks	4.4	181	61	141	156	140	3.7	143	3.8	112
+3 weeks	3.1	158	33	61	92	143	4.2	61	2.6	83
+1 month	2.1	272	22	45	156	140	3.0	49	2.2	83
+2 months	0.9	110	10	30	27	144	4.2	20	1.8	85
+3 months	0.5	83	34	76	27	146	4.3	1.6	1.6	84

[a] Undergoing renal replacement therapy.
[b] Normal values listed in parentheses.

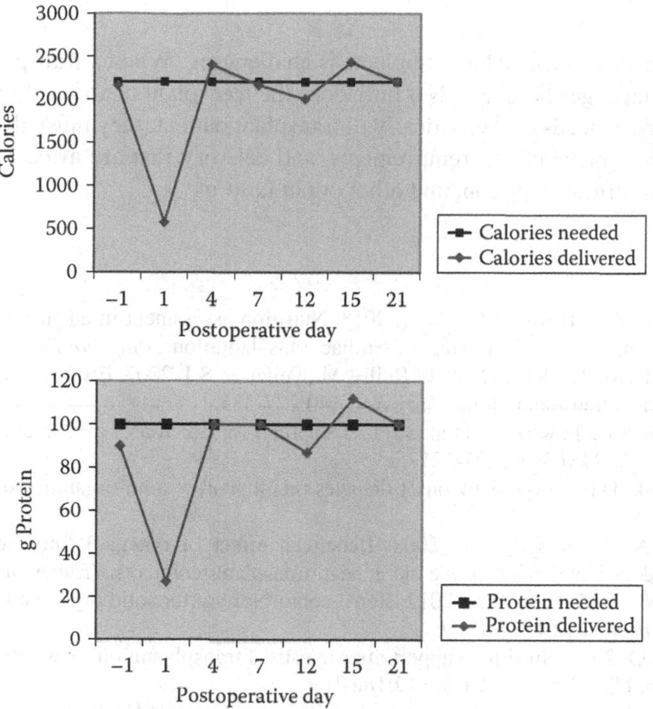

FIGURE 25.2 Calories required and delivered in a man with severe liver disease undergoing liver transplantation.

cellular rejection. The patient received IV corticosteroids tapering from 1 g on the first day to 40 mg 7 days later. A follow-up biopsy showed mild residual rejection requiring three additional every-other-day boluses of corticosteroids. During that time, the serum glucose level increased from normal to a range of 160–280 mg/dL (non-fasting). A single daily injection of glargine insulin was prescribed in addition to the regular insulin given via sliding scale four times per day.

The patient had continued to receive TF with a concentrated formula (to reduce volume) as the patient was not deemed to have adequate and safe swallow by the speech therapist until 11 days after transplantation. Once a diet was started, the TF was cycled over 16 h decreasing to 12 h/day 2 days later as the patient began to eat increased amounts. Figure 25.2 summarizes the patient's calorie and protein intake from the day before transplantation to 21 days after transplantation.

Postoperative Days 15–60: Rehabilitation

The patient was transferred to a rehabilitation facility for intensive physical therapy. His feeding tube was eventually removed when he was able to eat adequate amounts via an oral diet with supplements. The patient's blood glucose level normalized when the corticosteroid dose was reduced. The patient discharged from the rehabilitation hospital 1 week from arrival. The patient continued to be seen by the transplant team in the liver transplant clinic one to two times weekly. His appetite remained adequate. An anabolic steroid, oxandrolone, was added to help support weight and muscle repletion during this recovery phase. He and his mother attended a series of required outpatient transplant nutrition classes to learn about long-term nutrition needs. Three months after his transplant, the patient was discharged home to be under the medical care of his primary care physician. After reaching a low weight of 125 lb after transplant, the patient weighed 145 lb at the time of clinic discharge.

SUMMARY

Providing nutrition care to transplant recipients is challenging. When a transplant patient becomes critically ill, the challenges heighten. Not only does the transplant team need to consider the nutrition status and nutrient needs of the critically ill transplant patient, they must also consider all of the alterations in nutrient metabolism, requirements, and delivery that are affected by graft function, immunosuppressive drugs, infection, and other organ failures.

REFERENCES

Aggarwal, A., Kumar, A., Gregory, M.P., et al. 2013. Nutrition assessment in advanced heart failure patients evaluated for ventricular assist devices or cardiac transplantation. *Nutr Clin Pract.* 28:112-119.

Ammori, J.B., Sigakis, M., Englesbe, M.J., O'Reilly, M., Pelletier, S.J. 2007. Effect of intraoperative hyperglycemia during liver transplantation. *J Surg Res.* 140:227-233.

Bacon, B.R., Gordon, S.C., Lawitz, E., et al. 2011. Boceprevir for previously treated chronic HCV genotype 1 infection. *N Engl J Med* 364:1207-1217.

Bodziak, K.A., Hricik, D.E.. 2009. New-onset diabetes mellitus after solid organ transplantation. *Transpl Int* 22:519-530.

Celik, S., Doesch, A., Erbel, C., et al. 2008. Beneficial effect of omega-3 fatty acids on sirolimus- or everolimus-induced hypertriglyceridemia in heart transplant recipients. *Transplantation* 86:245-250.

Clajus, C., Hanke, N., Gottlieb, J., et al. 2012. Renal comorbidity after solid organ and stem cell transplantation. *Am J Transplant* 12:1691-1699.

Colomb, V., Goulet. O. 2009. Nutrition support after intestinal transplantation: how important is enteral feeding? *Curr Opin Clin Nutr Metab Care* 12:186-189.

Committee on Organ Procurement and Transplantation Policy, Division of Health Sciences Policy, INSTITUTE OF MEDICINE. Organ failure and patient survival. IN: Organ Procurement and Transplantation. Assessing Current Policies and the Potential Impact of the DHHS Final Rule. Washington DC: National Academy Press. 2013. 91-122. Available at: http://www.gao.gov/special.pubs/organ/chapter6.pdf.

Dionigi, P., Alessiani, M., Ferrazi, A. 2001. Irreversible intestinal failure, nutrition support, and small bowel transplantation. *Nutrition* 17:747-750.

Englesbe, M.J., Patel, S.P., He, K., et al. 2010. Sarcopenia and mortality after liver transplantation. J Am Coll Surg 211:271-278.

Ferreira, L.G., Anastacio, L.R., Lima, A.S., Correia, M.I.T.D. 2011. Assessment of nutritional status of patients waiting for liver transplantation. *Clin Transplant* 25:248-254.

Filler, G., Weiglein, G., Gharib, M.T., Casier, S. 2012. Ω3 fatty acids may reduce hyperlipidemia in pediatric renal transplant recipients. *Pediatr Transplant.* 2012 16:835-839.

Fishman, J.A. 2007. Infection in solid-organ transplant recipients. *N Engl J Med* 357:2601-2614.

Garg, M., Jones R.M., Vaughan R.B., Testro, A.G. 2011. Intestinal transplantation: current status and future directions. *J Gastroenterol Hepatol.* 26:1221-1228.

Grant, D., Wall, W., Zhong, R., et al. 1990. Experimental clinical intestinal transplantation: initial experience of a Canadian centre. Transplant Proc. 22:2497-2498.

Hade, A.M., Shine, A.M., Kennedy, N.P., McCormick, P.A. 2003. Both under-nutrition and obesity increase morbidity following liver transplantation. *Ir Med J.* 96:140-142.

Hasse, J.M., Blue, L.S., Liepa, G.U., et al. 1995. Early enteral nutrition support in patients undergoing liver transplantation, *J. Parenter. Enteral. Nutr* 19:437-443.

Ikegami, T., Shirabe, K., Yoshiya, S., et al. 2012. Bacterial sepsis after living donor liver transplantation: the impact of early enteral nutrition. *J Am Coll Surg.* 214:288-295.

Jacobson, I.M., McHutchison, J.G., Dusheiko, G., et al. 2011. Telaprevir for previously untreated chronic hepatitis C virus infection. *N Engl J Med* 364:2405-2416.

Johnston, O., Rose, C.L., Webster, A.C., Gill, J.S. 2008. Sirolimus is associated with new-onset diabetes in kidney transplant recipients. *J Am Soc Nephrol* 19:1411-1418.

Kaido, T., Ogura, Y., Ogawa, K., et al. 2012. Effects of post-transplant enteral nutrition with an immunomodulating diet containing hydrolyzed whey peptide after liver transplantation. *World J Surg* 36:1666-1671.

Kandaswamy, R., Skeans, M.A., Gustafson, S.K., Carrico, R.J., Tyler, K.H., Israni, A.K., Snyder, J.J., Kasiske, B.L. OPTN/SRTR 2013. Annual data report: Pancreas. 2015. *Am J Transplant* 15(Suppl 2):1–20.

Liang, T.J., Ghany, M.G. 2013. Current and future therapies for hepatitis C virus infection. *N Engl J Med* 368:1907-1917.

Madill, J., Gutierrez, C., Grossman, J., et al. 2001. Nutritional assessment of the lung transplant patient: body mass index as a predictor of 90-day mortality following transplantation. *J Heart Lung Transplant* 20:288-296.

Matarese, L E. 2010. Nutrition interventions before and fter adult intestinal transplantation: the pittsburgh experience. *Nutrition Issues in Gastroenterology*. 89:11-26.

Matas, A.J., Smith, J.M., Skeans, M.A., Thompson, B., Gustafson, S.K., Stewart, D.E., Cherikh, W.S., Wainright, J.L., Boyle, G., Snyder, J.J., Israni, A.K., Kasiske, B.L. OPTN/SRTR 2013. Annual data report: Kidney. 2015. *Am J Transplant* 15(Suppl 2):1–34.

Merli, M., Giusto, M., Gentili, F., et al. 2010. Nutritional status: its influence on the outcome of patients undergoing liver transplantation. *Liver Int* 30:208-214.

Merli, M., Nicolini, G., Angeloni, S., Riggio, O. 2002. Malnutrition is a risk factor in cirrhotic patients undergoing surgery. *Nutrition* 18:978-986.

Molnar, M.Z., Czira, M.E., Rudas, A., et al. 2011. Association of the malnutrition-inflammation score with clinical outcomes in kidney transplant recipients. Am J Kidney Dis 58:101-108. Montano-Loza, A.J., Meza-Junco, J., Prado, C.M.M., et al. 2012. Muscle wasting is associated with mortality in patients with cirrhosis. Clin Gastroenterol Hepatol. 10:166-173.

Montejo González, J.C., Mesejo, A., Bonet Saris, A. 2011. Guidelines for specialized nutritional and metabolic support in the critically-ill paients. Update. Consensus SEMICYUC-SENPE: Liver failure and liver transplantation. *Nutr Hosp* 26(Supl.2):27-31.

Murekesan, V., Mukherjee, S. 2012. Managing post-transplant lympoproliferative disorders in solid-organ transplant recipients. A review of immunosuppressant regimens. *Drugs* 72:1631-1643.

OPTN. 2015a. Transplants by donor type. U.S. transplants performed: January 1, 1988–November 30, 2014. Based on OPTN data as of February 27, 2015. http://optn.transplant.hrsa.gov (accessed March 6, 2015).

OPTN. 2015b. Adult recipient transplants by donor type, Center U.S. transplants performed: January 1, 1988–November 30, 2014. Based on OPTN data as of February 27, 2015. http://optn.transplant.hrsa.gov (accessed March 6, 2015).

OPTN Organ Procurement and Transplantation Network. 2013. http://optn.transplant.hrsa.gov.

Organ Procurement and Transplantation Network (OPTN) and Scientific Registry of Transplant Recipients (SRTR). OPTN / SRTR 2011 Annual Data Report. Department of Health and Human Services, Health Resources and Services Administration, Healthcare Systems Bureau, Division of Transplantation; 2012. Available at http://www.srtr.org/annual_Reports/2011/. Accessed June 28, 2013.

Pagalilauan, G.L., Limaye, A.P. 2013. Infections in transplant patients. *Med Clin N Am* 97:581-600.

Pikul, J., Sharpe, M.D., Lowndes, R., Ghent, C.N. 1994. Degree of preoperative malnutrition is predictive of postoperative morbidity and mortality in liver transplant recipients. *Transplantation* 57:469-472.

Plauth, M., Cabré, E., Riggio, O., et al. 2006. ESPEN Guidelines on Enteral Nutrition: Liver disease. *Clin Nutr* 25:285-294.

Plöchl,W., Pezawas, L., Artemiou, O., Grimm, M., Klepetko, W., Hiesmayr, M. 1996. Nutritional status, ICU duration and ICU mortality in lung transplant recipients. *Intensive Care Med* 22:1179-1185.

Poordad, F., McCone, J. Jr, Bacon, B.R., et al. 2011. Boceprevir for untreated chronic HCV genotype 1 infection. *N Engl J Med* 364:1195-1206.

Rayes, N., Seehofer, D., Hansen, S., et al. 2002. Early enteral supply of lactobacillus and fiber versus selective bowel decontamination: a controlled trial in liver transplant recipients.*Transplantation* 74:123-127.

Rayes, N., Seehofer, D., Theruvath, T., et al. 2005. Supply of pre- and probiotics reduces bacterial infection rates after liver transplantation--a randomized, double-blind trial. Am J Transplant 5:125-130.

Reilly J, Mehta R, Teperman L, Cemaj S, Tzakis A, Yanaga K, Ritter P, Rezak A,Makowka L. Nutritional support after liver transplantation: a randomized prospective study. JPEN J Parenter Enteral Nutr. 1990 14:386-391.

Sarno, G., Mehta, R.J., Guardado-Mendoza, R., Jimenez-Ceja, L.M., De Rosa. P., Muscogiuri, G. 2013. New-onset diabetes mellitus: predictive factors and impact on the outcome of patients undergoing liver transplantation et al. *Curr Diab Rev*. 9:78-85.

Sarno, G., Muscogiuri, G., De Rosa, P. 2012. New-onset diabetes after kidney transplantation: prevalence, risk factors, and management. *Transplantation* 93:1189-1195.

Schwebel, C., Pin, I., Barnoud, D., et al. 2000. Prevalence and consequences of nutritional depletion in lung transplant candidates. *Eur RespirJ*. 16:1050-1055.

Silver, H.J., Castellanos, V.H. 2000. Nutritional complications and management of intestinal transplant. *J Am Diet Assoc* 100:680-684, 687-689.

Snell, G.I., Bennetts, K., Bartolo, J., et al. 1998. Body mass index as a predictor of survival in adults with cystic fibrosis referred for lung transplantation. *J Heart Lung Transplant*. 17:1097-1103.

Sodhi, S.S., Guo, J.P., Maurer, A.H., O'Brien, G., Srinivasan, R., Parkman, H.P. Gastroparesis after combined heart and lung transplantation. 2002. *J Clin Gastroenterol.*34:34-39.

Starzl, T.E., Groth, C.G., Brettschneider, L., et al. 1968. Orthotopic homotransplantations of the human liver. *Ann. Surg.* 168: 392-415.

Tandon, P., Ney, M., Irwin, I., et al. 2012. Severe muscle depletion in patients on the liver transplant wait list: its prevalence and independent prognostic value. Liver Transpl 18:1209-1216.

Tatsioni, A., Chung, M., Sun, Y., et al. 2005. Effects of fish oil supplementation on kidney transplantation: a systematic review and meta-analysis of randomized, controlled trials. *J Am Soc Nephrol* 16:2462-2470.

Therasse, A., Wallia, A., Molitch, M.E. 2013. Management of post-transplant diabetes. *Curr Diab Rep* 13:121-129.

Thomas, M.C., Mathew, T.H., Russ, G.R., Rao, M.M., Moran, J.2001. Early peri-operative glycaemic control and allograft rejection in patients with diabetes mellitus: a pilot study. *Transplantation*72:1321-1324.

Thomas, M.C., Moran, J., Mathew, T.H., Russ, G.R., Rao, M.M. 2000. Early peri-operative hyperglycaemia and renal allograft rejection in patients without diabetes. *BMC Nephrol* 4;1:1.

Wallia, A., Parikh, N.D., Molitch, M.E., et al. 2010. Posttransplant hyperglycemia is associated with increased risk of liver allograft rejection. *Transplantation* 89:222-226.

Weseman, R.A. 2007. Review of incidence and management of chylous ascites after small bowel transplantation. *Nutr Clin Pract* 22:482-484.

Wicks, C., Somasundaram, S., Bjarnason, I., et al.1994. Comparison of enteral feeding and total parenteral nutrition after liver transplantation. *Lancet* 344:837-840.

Yates, C.J., Fourlanos, S., Hjelmesaeth, J. Colman, P.G., Cohney, S.J. 2012. New-onset diabetes after kidney transplantation – changes and challenges. *Am J Transplant* 12:820-828.

Yoshida, R., Yagi, T., Sadamori, H., et al. 2012. Branched-chain amino acid-enriched nutrients improve nutritional and metabolic abnormalities in the early post-transplant period after living donor liver transplantation. *J Hepatobiliary Pancreat Sci* 19:438-448.

Younossi, Z.M., Stepanova, M., Afendy, M., et al. 2011. Changes in the prevalence of the most common causes of chronic liver diseases in the United States from 1988 to 2008. *Clin Gastroenterol Hepatol* 9:524-530.

Zeuzem, S., Andreone, P., Pol, S., et al. 2011. Telaprevir for retreatment of HCV infection. *N Engl J Med* 364:2417-2428.

Zhu, X., Wu, Y., Qiu, Y., Jiang, C., Ding, Y. 2013. Effects of ω-3 fish oil lipid emulsion combined with parenteral nutrition on patients undergoing liver transplantation. JPEN J Parenter Enteral Nutr. 37:68-74.

Section VI

Specific Organ System Failure

26 Nutrition in the Critically Ill Patient with Intestinal Failure

Cassandra Pogatschnik, Neha Parekh, and Ezra Steiger

CONTENTS

INTRODUCTION

The intestine, an organ divided into the small and large bowel, is a long hollow cylinder lined with epithelial cells and smooth muscle layers. Enteric neurons, endocrine and paracrine agonists, regulate epithelia motor activity during digestive and postprandial phases, triggering fluid movement through the lumen, thus providing nutrient, electrolyte, and fluid absorptive and secretion functions. Uniquely, the small intestine lining is composed of villus-crypt organizations, which heighten the organ's responsibly of nutrient absorption alone. The large intestine or colon lacks villi and therefore primarily provides fluid and electrolyte absorptive and secretion function (Binder 2005). Intestinal failure (IF) is defined as a lack of functional gut mass, which limits digestion and absorption, leading to the inability to maintain protein-energy, fluid, electrolyte, or micronutrient balance (Carlson and Dark 2010). The term IF, often used interchangeably with short bowel syndrome (SBS), encompasses several malabsorptive states or phases, temporary or permanent (Carlson and Dark 2010). Associated with poor prognosis and increased mortality in the intensive care unit (ICU), IF is difficult to evaluate due to the intestine's depth inside the body habitus, immune and vascular complexity, and the critically ill patient's inability to communicate gastrointestinal (GI) symptoms (Piton et al. 2011). A prominent symptom of IF, diarrhea, which has been defined as stool weight exceeding 250 g/mL, may be used as a predictor of intestinal ischemia, particularly in patients experiencing GI symptoms post cardiac arrest (Harrell and Chang 2008, Piton et al. 2011, Wierdsma et al. 2011).

ACUTE INTESTINAL FAILURE

Piton et al. defines acute phase malabsorption or acute IF as an acute reduction of enterocyte mass or acute enterocyte dysfunction, which may be associated with loss of gut barrier function. Acute intestinal failure (AIF) is exceedingly common and is endured in the immediate postoperative period following abdominal surgery. AIF often presents within 3 days after surgery and is suspected with symptoms of diarrhea, GI bleeding, abdominal distention, and/or feeding tolerance (Piton et al. 2011). Its duration is short-lived and its treatment course ranges from weeks to months with latter duration due to complications such as fistulization (Carlson and Dark 2010). AIF is expected to resolve upon removal of offending factors or with standard intervention.

Interestingly, a standardized IF diagnostic tool is nonexistent, and multiorgan failure assessment tools fail to consider GI dysfunction in the critically ill (Reintam et al. 2006, 2008). Recent studies have investigated GI/IF assessment tools and have measured their accuracy and efficacy in determining the relationship between IF and mortality. Reintam's group developed a GI failure score (GFS) in an attempt to grade the severity of intestinal dysfunction (see Table 26.1). Scores combined food intolerance, defined as high gastric residual (defined as gastric residual greater than enteral product administered) upon enteral nutrition (EN), vomiting, bowel distention, and/or severe diarrhea (which lacked numeric definition), with intra-abdominal pressure (IAP). Interval IAP was measured indirectly via indwelling urinary catheter and bedside manometer. Serial measurements detected intra-abdominal hypertension (>12 mmHg) and abdominal compartment syndrome (>20 mmHg). Abdominal compartment syndrome is the accumulation of tissue fluid (edema, blood, or free fluid) within the peritoneal or retroperitoneal space in which the abdominal wall can no longer expand which results in organ failure. Though IAP alone has not been proven to adequately measure GI function and GI issues do not always coexist with intra-abdominal hypertension, measurement of IAP has been obtained and has strong correlation with mortality (Reintam et al. 2006, 2008). The group tested the accuracy of the GFS system and found it to be highly prognostic of mortality during the first 3 days of ICU stay and appeared more predictive of ICU mortality when combined with the sequential organ failure assessment (SOFA) score. Weaknesses include subjectivity of defining food intolerance (difference in residual volumes, adjustment of EN with diarrhea, definition of diarrhea, etc.) and its single center model (Reintam et al. 2008). Other centers have based IF solely on acute intestinal distress syndrome (intra-abdominal hypertension or abdominal compartment syndrome). Critics mention that IAP is influenced by other organs; therefore, it is nonspecific to small bowel function (Reintam et al. 2006, 2008, Berger et al. 2008).

CLINICAL PRESENTATION

Postoperative presentation of AIF is characterized by symptoms of abdominal distention, vomiting, and constipation. AIF usually resolves quickly unless further surgical complications develop. Ten percent of postabdominal surgical patients develop mechanical obstruction. Mechanical obstructions are most common after open infracolic compartment surgery, resultant of postsurgical adhesions,

TABLE 26.1
GIF Score

Points	Symptom
0	Normal GI function
1	Enteral feeding <50% of calculated needs or no feeding 3 days after abdominal surgery
2	Food intolerance or intra-abdominal hypertension
3	Food intolerance and intra-abdominal hypertension
4	Abdominal compartment syndrome

and tend to resolve spontaneously within 14 days (Sajja and Schein 2004, Carlson and Dark 2010). Postsurgical obstructions are likely to be treated conservatively with nasogastric decompression and bowel rest. Paralytic ileus, the impairment of coordinated intestinal motility, is a common complication among both nonabdominal and abdominal surgeries. Its pathogenesis is affected by a series of relations that inhibit GI motility including: the activation of sympathetic nervous system, the suppression of the parasympathetic nervous system, and the release of inflammatory mediators and neurotransmitters during surgical manipulation and trauma of tissue (Carlson and Dark 2010). The small bowel usually recovers first, followed by the stomach and colon. Colonic motility remains critical in postoperative ileus (POI) resolution. Attempts to reduce prolonged POI include: minimizing abdominal trauma during surgery, use of epidural anesthesia, and reduction of opioid use (Herbert and Holzer 2008, Zeinali 2009).

Seventy percent of the critically ill who undergo abdominal surgery develop abdominal sepsis and/or fistulization, with 10% of this population further developing SBS as a direct result of their surgical complication (Carlson and Dark 2010). Abdominal sepsis is more often found in postsurgical patients with underlying Crohn's or mesenteric vascular disease states. Computed tomography with contrast is used to diagnose and localize sepsis and can be utilized to determine if percutaneous drainage of fluid collection or abscess is warranted. A second look exploration may be indicated if the infectious source is unreachable. In cases of anastomotic dehiscence, a creation of proximal stoma and a defunctionalized intestinal loop may reduce septic contamination. In the worst cases, an open abdomen may be left to control an extensively contaminated abdomen (Carlson and Dark 2010).

Patients postintestinal resection present with symptoms of acute phase malabsorption and high enteric effluent (Sundaram et al. 2002). Gastric hypersecretion occurs due to increased gastrin production and occurs to a greater extent post jejunal resection versus ileal resection. Hypersecretion increases the acidity in the duodenum, which may damage intestinal mucosa, inactivate digestive enzymes, and stimulate hyperperistalsis (Sundaram et al. 2002). Immediately and up to 3 months postsurgery, secretory losses are high and patients are at an increased risk for the development of dehydration, electrolyte derangement, and caloric deficit.

Through intestinal resection rodent models, postsurgical commencement of intestinal adaptation has shown to be immediate (Levin and Rubin 2008). Early phase adaptation has been observed as an increase in paneth and goblet cells within 12 h following resection. Rapid cell proliferation with villi lengthening has begun within 14–16 h postsurgery, and the transport of nutrients has escalated by 48 h (Levin and Rubin 2008).

CHRONIC INTESTINAL FAILURE

Defining a patient's GI anatomy may distinguish SBS and determine the likeliness for chronic intestinal failure versus AIF. SBS has various definitions, but anatomically is traditionally defined as less than 200 cm of small intestine remaining (Parekh and Steiger 2007, Ramsey and Buchman 2008, Efsen and Jeppesen 2011, Thompson et al. 2011). Beyond the ligament of Treitz, average small intestinal length is 600 cm, divided into 150–300 cm of jejunum and 300–450 cm of ileum (Sundaram et al. 2002). Normal colon length is an estimated 150 cm depending on the body habitus. Upon jejunal resection (<75% of total jejunum remaining), the ileum has the capacity to adapt, absorbing macro- and micronutrients that the jejunum would typically absorb. However, the lack of jejunal inhibitory enterohormones leads to increased gastric hypersecretion, which causes inactivation of digestive enzymes, diminished pH, mucosal damage, and hastened peristalsis. In most cases, transit time should remain normal and bile salt absorption, along with vitamin B12, would be preserved with intact terminal ileum (Parekh and Steiger 2007). Although the ileum has limited contribution to macronutrient absorption if the jejunum is intact, ileal resection contributes largely to oral–cecal transit times. Particularly, preservation of the terminal ileum, the last 50–100 cm, is appreciated given its ability to preserve bile salts and vitamin B12. Loss of the terminal ileum leads to failure to release hormones to stimulate the ileal break mechanism. The ileal break is defined as inhibitory measures limiting proximal GI secretion, motility, mucosal growth, and intestinal blood flow, thereby maximizing absorption in the proximal bowel. Lack of hormone release (glucagon-like peptide 1, glucagon-like peptide 2, peptide YY, and neurotensin) leads to rapid transit of food and fluids through the intestine (Scolapio 1997, Efsen and Jeppesen 2011). The ileocecal valve, a sphincter which controls the delivery of chyme into the colon, prevents the reflux of colonic bacteria into the small intestine. The loss of the valve greatly increases the risk for small bowel bacterial overgrowth and worsens malabsorption. Though rare, duodenal resection impairs concentrated sugars and lactose absorption. Malabsorption of calcium, iron, and folic acid is also common. The preservation of colon is vital in maintaining hydration and absorbing additional calories. The colon has the ability to increase its surface area by threefold to fivefold, maximizing absorption (Sundaram et al. 2002). Short chain fatty acids, the fermented byproducts of undigested carbohydrate by gut microbiota, are absorbed in the distal intestine to account for upward of an additional 1000 cal/day. However, short small intestinal length with intact colon increases the risk for D-lactic acidosis, which may cause neurological syndrome.

Intestinal resection, often leading to SBS, is precipitated by multiple underlying diagnoses. Resection is often a result of active inflammatory bowel disease (IBD). Crohn's disease patients who have undergone abscess or fistula repair have demonstrated frequent disease recurrence and require more resections than those who develop obstruction, stricture, or perforation (Ramsey and Buchman 2008). Other conditions requiring surgical intestinal resection include complications of post malabsorptive surgeries (gastric bypass, duodenal switch, and gastric sleeve, etc.), radiation enteritis, Gardner's syndrome (desmoids), Ogilvie's syndrome, and chronic intestinal pseudoobstruction. Inadequate perfusion to overcome capillary pressure in the bowel wall or inadequate blood flow due to mechanical obstruction increases intestinal wall tension and can lead to intestinal ischemia. The celiac trunk supplies blood flow to the stomach, duodenum, and proximal jejunum. The superior mesenteric artery delivers blood flow to the small and large bowel up to the splenic flexure, while the inferior mesenteric artery supplies the transverse, descending, and sigmoid colon. The surgical aim in impeded venous outflow is to decrease IAP, increasing blood flow with embolectomy and resecting nonviable intestine (Sax 2008).

INTESTINAL MALABSORPTION

Malabsorption in the ICU is loosely defined as ≤85% of normal intestinal absorptive capacity and is the most prominent clinical symptom of IF (Keur et al. 2010). Though difficult to identify, adequate nutrient absorption is vital in improving patient outcomes and morbidity (Wierdsma et al. 2011). Several tests have been used to measure the intestine's functionality. Saccharide absorption testing (SAT) provides an assessment of the bowel's permeability and determines the ratio of large to small saccharide absorption (Keur et al. 2010). However, this test is unreliable in ICU patients with multisystem organ failure and in patients with oliguria or anuria. Fat excretion studies (FES) quantify fecal fat or steatorrhea. Steatorrhea is defined as ≥7 g fecal fat per 24 h stool collection. Enteral delivery of 75–100 g fat, followed by stool collection for 48–72 h, makes this test labor intensive. FES is not ideal, failing to detect all macronutrient malabsorptive states. The gold standard of intestinal function, bomb calorimetry, is a 72 h measurement of enteral calories consumed versus calories excreted in stool (Keur et al. 2010). A study was conducted in 48 critically ill patients in a mixed medical/surgical ICU without clinically evident GI dysfunction, to validate fecal weight as a marker for malabsorption and to calculate the intestinal absorption capacity of the critically ill (Wierdsma et al. 2011). Patients with fecal weight of >350 g/day had statistically significant energy malabsorption, validating an inverse relationship between fecal weight and energy absorption. Fecal fat, carbohydrate, and protein losses were significantly higher in those with diarrhea or fecal weight >350 g. Caloric loss on an average for the malabsorptive group was 627 cal in comparison to neutral balance with stool <350 g/day group. It was concluded that fecal weight was applicable to ICU patients and that caloric deficiency should be considered in nutritional support planning (Wierdsma et al. 2011).

The amino acid glutamine is metabolized to citrulline by the intestinal mucosal enterocytes. Chronic and acute reduction of enterocyte mass has correlated with low plasma citrulline; therefore, fasting plasma citrulline testing is used to predict remaining enterocyte mass and SBS. Unfortunately in septic or systemic inflammatory immune responses syndrome (SIR) conditions, the enterocyte may suffer acute dysfunction and may not synthesize citrulline, and hence, the lab result may result in inaccurate lower value and not reflect actual enterocyte mass (Piton et al. 2011). Kidneys convert citrulline into arginine; therefore, impaired renal function may increase citrulline levels, giving a false impression of increased enterocyte mass. The recently developed citrulline generation testing (CGT) measures the conversion time of glutamine to citrulline. The test challenges the conversion of glutamine to citrulline by slow administration of Dipeptiven, a glutamine–alanine dipeptide (100 mL intravenously or 20 g enterally). With decreased enterocyte mass, the metabolic pathway is overwhelmed and plasma levels of citrulline and other amino acids concentrations are determined using reverse phase liquid chromatography. Incremental serum citrulline levels assist in predictability of enterocyte function, mass, and severity of disease (Keur et al. 2010).

Medical Management of Intestinal Malabsorption

Malabsorption is quantified by fecal weight greater than 350 g/day; however, more practically, malabsorption may be identified as enteral loss greater than enteral intake. Early management of acute intestinal malabsorption includes controlling sepsis, maintaining hemodynamic stability, and maintaining electrolyte and fluid balance (Sundaram et al. 2002, Thompson et al. 2011). Cautious clinical, laboratory, and radiological tests for intestinal ischemia are essential to optimize positive outcomes. The critically ill patient requires careful measurement of enteric intake and enteric output, vital signs, central venous pressures, and frequent laboratory draws due to rapid metabolic changes. Extensive sodium losses subsequent to malabsorption may cause prerenal azotemia and hypotension. Aggressive fluid and electrolyte replacement are warranted, particularly the first days following resection when enteric losses are large to avoid life-threatening dehydration and dysrhythmias (Thompson et al. 2011).

Assessment of medications which may exacerbate malabsorption is essential to reduce the incidence of iatrogenic diarrhea. Antibiotic-associated diarrhea occurs in 3%–29% of all hospitalized patients (Harrell and Chang 2008), while residence in the ICU is a risk factor for developing *Clostridium difficile* infection alone. *C. difficile* should be screened for in patients with unexplained or massive diarrhea (Harrell and Chang 2008). Antibiotics should be utilized sparingly and specifically to target infection. Hyperosmolar medications, such as magnesium-containing antacids, lactulose, and liquid elixirs containing sugar alcohols, should be discontinued. Consider administering medications in intravenous (IV) form or crushing tablets if enteral access is obtained. Other medications that may produce malabsorption include nonsteroidal anti-inflammatory drugs and diuretics. Immune suppressants used in transplant, such as tacrolimus, may also worsen enteric loss (Harrell and Chang 2008).

Proton pump inhibitors and histamine 2 receptor antagonists (H2 blockers) (often compatible with parenteral nutrition infusions) regulate gastric hypersecretion, prevent peptic ulcer disease, and decrease secretory output (Thompson et al. 2011). Proton pump inhibitors also lead to increased intestinal pH that favors the development of small intestinal bacterial overgrowth (SIBO) with resultant diarrhea (Martin et al. 2000). Octreotide, a somatostatin analog, may increase the absorption of water, sodium, and nutrients and reduce gastric and biliary hypersecretion, reducing enteric losses, and decrease GI motility (Efsen and Jeppesen 2011). However, octreotide may also promote symptoms of obstruction, impair hepatic and pancreatic functions, cause gall bladder sludge backup, and may inhibit bowel adaptation. In some cases, octreotide has caused hypermotility (Efsen and Jeppesen 2011). Antidiarrheals may be commenced cautiously in the ICU to slow intestinal motility as patients are often at high risk for development of ileus or small bowel obstruction due to inflammation after surgery.

NUTRITION THERAPY IN INTESTINAL FAILURE

Parenteral Nutrition

Intestinal adaptation begins immediately postoperatively and most often occurs within the first year. In some cases, the intestine may take 2 years or more for full adaptation (Parekh and Steiger 2007). Upon first arrival to the ICU, control of respiration and hemodynamic stability are top priorities. Assessment of loss origin (stomach, pancreas/biliary tract, small intestine, large intestine, etc.) and volume determines the composition of fluid administered and protects the function of multiple organ systems. Aggressive hydration should be provided, replacing measured enteral and obligatory losses. Depending on bowel length and function, enteric losses, and anticipated length of therapy, PN will often be used for the IF patient. A short-term goal for parenteral nutrition (PN) provision is to prevent deterioration of nutritional status until the bowel improves with rehabilitation or if the patient later undergoes intestinal transplantation (Borges et al. 2011). Severely malnourished patients benefit from PN for 7–10 days after extensive bowel resection regardless of residual intestine length. This critically ill population suffers from small bowel atrophy, and absorption can be very challenging (Parekh and Steiger 2007). Severely malnourished patients who commence PN in the ICU are at high risk for refeeding syndrome and may require slow caloric increase and high doses of intravenous electrolyte repletion. GI losses tend to be the highest for the first few days after intestinal resection and poor absorption warrants PN. Jejunum, ileocecal valve, and functional colon determine the indefinite need for PN. The absorptive capacity of the residual length of intestine can be doubled with the presence of ileocecal valve (Sundaram et al. 2002). Patients who have <100–150 cm of small bowel to their ileostomies or jejunostomies and those with <50 cm of small bowel (jejunum or ileum) to colon in continuity will most likely necessitate prolonged PN (Sundaram et al. 2002, Parekh and Steiger 2007, Efsen and Jeppesen 2011).

Enteral Nutrition

Although PN is predominately used in early postintestinal resection, EN may be used to complement therapy, as enteral and parenteral therapies are nonexclusive. Trophic EN may be started to stimulate mucosal adaptation, though it may not be realistic in patients with short intestinal anatomies as described previously (Thompson et al. 2011). Benefits of providing luminal nutrients with EN include maintaining integrity of the intestinal barrier, stimulating blood blow, releasing normal GI hormones, maintaining intestinal pH, preventing bacterial translocation, and allowing normal hepatic digestive function (Lloyd and Powell-Tuck 2004).

Motor complexes are disturbed after intestinal resection, mechanical ventilation, and analgesic administration; which limit gastric emptying and intestinal motility. Small bowel function recovers quickly than gastric function; therefore, intra-duodenal or intra-jejunal delivery may be preferred. Unlike gastric and duodenal feedings, jejunal feeding fails to stimulate pancreatic secretion; therefore, cholecystokinin (CCK) and gastrin levels are reduced and do not contribute to high enteric losses (Lloyd and Powell-Tuck 2004). Duodenal delivery increases peptide YY that facilitates the ileal break properties, reduces pancreatic secretion, and maximizes oral cecal transit time (Lloyd and Powell-Tuck 2004).

EN should be administered at a low, continuous rate, with slow advancement pending tolerance and malabsorption. Standard, isotonic polymeric and primarily long chain fatty acids should be well tolerated and should stimulate villi and crypt cell proliferation. This formulation mimics normal oral intake and may lead to quicker adaptation. Soluble fiber containing products benefit patients with an intact colon, prolonging transit times and providing an additional energy source from short chain fatty acids. Isotonic, semielemental formulas may be trialed if polymeric formula is not tolerated (Parekh and Steiger 2007). High lactose or high fat products may contribute to copious enteral losses.

Bacterial contaminations due to formula hang-times >24 h or expired formulations should be avoided. This may contribute to the development of bacterial overgrowth in which the IF patient is predisposed to Lloyd and Powell-Tuck (2004). Bacterial overgrowth symptoms include abdominal distention, excessive flatus, nausea, malodorous stool, and increased malabsorption.

Fistuloclysis

Patients who develop peritonitis, necessitate open abdomen, and/or require repeated laparotomies often develop intestinal dehiscence, leak, and enteric fistula. Intestinal fistula or spontaneous communication between the bowel and the skin may be used as a modality for EN infusion, by utilizing defunctionalized bowel loops (Ham et al. 2007). Fistuloclysis, the refeeding of intestinal chyme and enteral product via the distal limb of the intestinal fistula, is thought to be a safe option for nutrition support (Peer et al. 2008). Though less popular, EN may be considered in this population after 2 or more weeks of stabilizing patients on PN and for patients who develop abnormal hepatic function, have poor intravenous access, and who have high infection risk (septicemia) (Ham et al. 2007). In most complex postsurgical cases, fistulae are not expected to close spontaneously and insertion of an enteral feeding tube is not contraindicated (Ham et al. 2007, Peer et al. 2008). A fistulogram is warranted to establish length of bowel and to exclude distal obstruction. Bowel length of 100 cm or greater is desired for effective nutrition support, regardless of the presence of the colon (Peer et al. 2008). Complications of fistuloclysis include abdominal pain, diarrhea, increased proximal fistula output, and migration of enteric tube to the distal small bowel. Addition of chyme is not necessary for nutrition adequacy and may be omitted due to hygienic and esthetic issues (Ham et al. 2007). The reduction of PN in this population reduced sepsis and hepatic dysfunction.

Glutamine Supplementation

Glutamine, a nonessential amino acid, becomes a conditionally essential amino acid during critical illness. The body is unable to maintain adequate amounts of glutamine during stressful states, resulting in adverse clinical outcomes (Vanek et al. 2011). Studies have suggested that PN glutamine supplementation would be best utilized in the postsurgical patients (Vanek et al. 2011). In an analysis of studies, further divided into surgical subgroup, there was no significant impact on mortality, although a significant decrease in infectious complications was noted in patients receiving glutamine (Vanek et al. 2011). In most analyses, length of stay was reduced in the glutamine-supplemented group. Weaknesses of the analyses include administration of PN to patient who did not have indication for the therapy as well as authors bias by conducting smaller studies to achieve stronger results. American Society of Parenteral and Enteral Nutrition (ASPEN) has no graded evidence at this time and European Society of Parenteral and Enteral Nutrition (ESPEN) simply states that PN containing glutamine and arginine may benefit the surgical patient (Vanek et al. 2011). Stronger evidence is needed to recommend glutamine provision to the critically ill, postsurgical patient.

Probiotics

Probiotic strains shown to facilitate motility and prevent intestinal bacterial overgrowth may be promising in surgical patients. Surgical infection contributes widely to postoperative mortality. Certain probiotic strains may limit pathogen adherence to the mucosal lining by competitive site binding. Intestinal bacterial translocation to lymph nodes and other organs can trigger tissue inflammation and damage. Potentially providing probiotics prophylactically to manipulate the gut microbiota to prevent a postoperative infection is intriguing (Correia et al. 2012). However, this requires further investigation.

SURGICAL THERAPY IN SHORT BOWEL SYNDROME

Intestinal Transplantation

Thought to be the most difficult organ to transplant, the intestine is rich in immune-competent cells which result in higher graft rejection. Presently no survival advantage exists with transplantation over living with PN dependence in those patients having no major home parenteral nutrition (HPN) complications. The inability to biopsy the outside of the bowel limits rejection diagnosis (Moon and Kishore 2012).

The Centers for Medicare and Medicaid Services (CMS) recognized isolated intestine and multivisceral transplant as an ideal therapy for irreversible IF and PN failure. As success and popularity of intestinal transplant grows, it is hopeful that CMS will recognize intestinal transplant as an option prior to PN failure. PN failure is defined as significant liver damage, limited central vascular access, multiple catheter-related blood stream infections, and/or frequent episodes of dehydration (Matarese et al. 2007, Moon and Kishore 2012). Irreversible IF is most common in SBS; however, it may occur among motility disorders, cancers (familial adenomatous polyposis), and enterocyte deficiencies (Matarese et al. 2007). Of note patients with SBS and radiation enteritis have a higher probability of developing recurrent sepsis and hepatic failure before and after receiving an intestinal graft, which may lead to repeated intestinal transplant candidacy. Unresectable or active cancers and active infection will contraindicate transplantation.

Careful monitoring of liver disease is essential to determine if liver damage may be reversed once PN is discontinued after receiving sole intestinal graft. If damage is thought to be too significant, the candidate will likely need liver-intestine transplant. Other visceral organ function must be measured to determine what organs may be indicated for a full or modified multivisceral transplant (stomach, pancreas, spleen, liver, kidneys).

Care Post Transplant

Generous fluid resuscitation to promote adequate blood flow to graft is essential. Magnesium and calcium are poorly absorbed by the new graft, with low magnesium potentiating tacrolimus neurotoxicity. High amounts of bicarbonate, sodium, and fluid are lost with high volume stomal losses. Aggressive IV correction of electrolytes is recommended. Serum pH and lactate should be assessed for acute injury and intestinal ischemia. Hemoglobin and hematocrit should be monitored for acute GI bleed. After transplant, patients may require higher protein and calories. Most transplant patients are malnourished prior to surgery due to their underlying diagnosis and SBS; and during their immediate postoperative phase, patients are at large risk for increased protein loss and negative nitrogen balance. Posttransplant patients also have large wound healing requirements. Nutrient expenditure is estimated to be 1.2–1.5 g protein/kg/day, and 25–30 kcal/kg/day (Matarese et al. 2007); with recommended needs estimated at 1.7–2 g protein/kg/day and 30–35 kcal/kg/day. Serial citrulline levels may also be useful to assess graft viability and detect onset of rejection or functionality (Pappas et al. 2002).

Postoperatively, the transplanted ICU patient may have edematous bowel due to preservation injury or positive lymphocytic cross match, producing reduced villus height and crypt death, causing decreased mucosal surface area and malabsorption. Inflammation also increases intestinal barrier permeability and disrupts the epithelial tight junctions. The disruption of the migrating motor complex also leads to impaired motility in both the small bowel and the stomach, leaving the patient at risk for aspiration if receiving EN via the stomach. The use of promotility agents in such cases may be helpful (Matarese et al. 2007).

Nutrition Therapy Post Transplant

PN should be started in the immediate postoperative phase once hemodynamic stability has been established. At some centers, PN independence is achieved by 4 weeks postoperatively; however, it often depends on the functionality of the graft and its acceptance of EN. Continuous isotonic trophic feeds can be started within 3–7 days and with evidence of bowel function, to stimulate the grafts' enterocytes (Moon and Kishore 2012). Stoma output and bowel function often guide the medical team when to start trophic feeding. Surgical jejunostomy tubes are often placed during transplantation to decrease aspiration risk and enhance patient acceptance and comfort. Polymeric enteral products are preferred as intestinal grafts have not been predisposed to malnutrition and do not need predigested formulas (Matarese et al. 2007). Products with soluble fiber or soluble fiber modular may help thicken high volume of watery stoma output or diarrhea. If chylous ascites occurs following transplantation, low fat formulations should be considered. Goal enteral feedings should not be attempted until several weeks posttransplantation. Gut lymphatics need time to adjust to absorption of lipid, and bowel patency should be assessed with computed tomography 1 week post-transplant to rule out anastomotic dehiscence or bowel leak.

REFERENCES

Berger, M.M., Oddo, M., Lavnchy, J., Longchamp, C., Delodder, F., and Schaller, M.D. 2008. Gastrointestinal failure score in critically ill patients. *Crit Care* 12: 436.

Binder, H.J. 2005. Intestinal fluid and electrolyte movement. In *Medical Physiology*, Updated Edition, eds. W.F. Boron and E.L. Boulpaep. Philadelphia, PA: Elsevier Saunders.

Borges, V.C., Teixeira da Silva, M.L., Goncalves Dias, M.C., Gonzalez, M.C., and Waitzberg, D.L. 2011. Long-term nutritional assessment of patients with severe short bowel syndrome managed with home enteral nutrition and oral intake. *Nutr Hosp* 26(4): 834–842.

Carlson, G.L. and Dark, P. 2010. Acute intestinal failure. *Curr Opt Crit Care* 16: 347.

Correia, M.I.T.D., Liboredo, J.C., and Consoli, L.D. 2012. The role of probiotics in gastrointestinal surgery. *Nutrition* 28: 230–234.

Efsen, E. and Jeppesen, P.B. 2011. Modern treatment of adult short bowel syndrome patients. *Minerva Gastroenterol Dietol* 54: 405–417.

Ham, M., Horton, K., and Kaunitz, J. 2007. Fistuloclysis: Case report and literature review. *Nutr Clin Pract* 22: 553–557.

Harrell, L.E. and Chang, E.B. 2008. Diarrhea. In *Intensive Care Medicine*, 6th edn., eds. R.S. Irwin and J.M. Rippe. Philadelphia, PA: Williams & Wilkins.

Herbert, M.K. and Holzer, P. 2008. Standardized concept for the treatment of gastrointestinal dysmotility in critically ill patients—Current status and future options. *Clin Nutr* 27: 25–41.

Keur, M.B., Beishuizen, A., and van Bodegraven, A. 2010. Diagnosing malabsorption in the intensive care unit. *F1000 Med Rep* 2: 7.

Levin, M.S. and Rubin, D.C. 2008. Intestinal adaptation: The biology of the intestinal response to resection and disease. In *Intestinal Failure: Diagnosis, Management and Transplantation*, eds. A.N. Langnas, O. Goulet, E.M. Quigley, and K.A. Tappenden. Malden, MA: Blackwell Publishing.

Lloyd, D.A. and Powell-Tuck, J. 2004. Artificial nutrition: Principles and practice of enteral feeding. *Clin Colon Rectal Surg* 17(2): 107–118.

Martin, R.M., Dunn, N.R., Freemantle, S., and Shakir, S. 2000. The rates of common adverse events reported during treatment with proton pump inhibitors used in general practice in England: Cohort studies. *Br J Clin Pharmacol* 50(4): 366–372.

Matarese, L.E., Guilherme, C., Bond, G. et al. 2007. Therapeutic efficacy of intestinal and multivisceral transplantation: Survival and nutrition outcome. *Nutr Clin Pract* 22: 474.

Moon, J. and Kishore, I. 2012. Intestinal rehabilitation and transplantation for intestinal failure. *Mt Sinai J Med* 79: 256–266.

Pappas, P.A., Saudubray, J.M., and Tzakis, A.G. 2002. Serum citrulline as a marker of acute cellular rejection for intestinal transplantation. *Transplant Proc* 14(3): 915–917.

Parekh, N.R. and Steiger, E. 2007. Short bowel syndrome. *Curr Treat Opt Gastroenterol* 10: 10–23.

Peer, S., Moodley, M.S., Cassimjee, H.M., and Singh, B. 2008. Fistuloclysis-A valuable option for a difficult problem. *S Afr J Surg* 46(2): 56–57.

Piton, G., Manzon, C., Cypriani, B., Carbonnel, F., and Gilles, C. 2011. Acute intestinal failure in critically ill patients: Is plasma citrulline the right marker? *Intens Care Med* 37: 911.

Ramsey, U.K. and Buchman, A.L. 2008. Inflammatory bowel disease and the short bowel syndrome. In *Intestinal Failure Diagnosis, Management, and Transplantation*, eds. A.N. Langnas, O. Goulet, E.M. Quigley, and K.A. Tappenden. Malden, MA: Blackwell Publishing.

Reintam, A., Parm, P., Redlich, U. et al. 2006. Gastrointestinal failure in intensive care: A retrospective clinical study in three different intensive care units in Germany and Estonia. *BMC Gastroenterol* 6: 19.

Reintam, A., Parm, P., Kitus, R., Starkopf, J., and Kern, H. 2008. Gastrointestinal failure score in critically ill patients: A prospective observational study. *Crit Care* 12: 90.

Sajja, S.B.S. and Schein, M. 2004. Early postoperative small bowel obstruction. *Br J Surg* 91: 683–691.

Sax, H.C. 2008. Causes of intestinal failure in the adult. In *Intestinal Failure Diagnosis, Management, and Transplantation*, eds. Langnas, A.N., Goulet, O., Quigley, E.M., and Tappenden, K.A. Malden, MA: Blackwell Publishing.

Scolapio, J.S. 1997. Gastrointestinal motility considerations in patients with short bowel syndrome. *Digest Dis* 15: 253–263.

Sundaram, A., Koutkia, P., and Apovian, C.M. 2002. Nutritional management of short bowel syndrome in adults. *J Clin Gastroenterol* 34(3): 207–220.

Thompson, J.S., Weseman, R., Rochling, F.A., and Mercer, D.F. 2011. Current management of short bowel syndrome. *Surg Clin N Am* 91: 493–510.

Vanek, W.V., Matarese, L.E., Robinson, M., Sacks, G.S., Young, L.S., and Kochevar, M. 2011. A.S.P.E.N. Position paper: Parenteral nutrition glutamine supplementation. *Nutr Clin Pract* 26: 479–494.

Wierdsma, N.J., Peters, J.H.C., Weijs, P.J.M. et al. 2011. Malabsorption and nutritional balance in the ICU: Fecal weight as a biomarker: A prospective observational pilot study. *Crit Care* 15: R2364.

Zeinali, F. 2009. Pharmacological management of post-operative ileus. *Can J Surg* 52: 2.

27 Nutrition Support for Pulmonary Failure

Alfredo A. Matos, William Manzanares, and Víctor Sánchez Nava

CONTENTS

INTRODUCTION

Ventilatory impairment is often associated with malnutrition. This seems to follow a logical progression of diminished intake and increased energy demands. However, the pathophysiology of this phenomenon is more complex. An interplay exists wherein malnutrition may induce ventilatory failure, and conversely, ventilatory may lead to malnutrition. Nutritional support is an important adjunct to the care of the pulmonary patient in the intensive care unit (ICU). Malnutrition and respiratory failure are integrally linked.

The overlap of these entities produces a group of patients whose illness is the combination of pulmonary disease and malnutrition. It is important to identify such individuals, because they require both respiratory and nutritional therapies. These patients can be expected to benefit greatly by the addition of nutritional support to their pulmonary regimen.

Whether respiratory failure is chronic and a consequence of primary pulmonary disease (e.g., chronic obstructive pulmonary disease [COPD]) or occurs as part of the spectrum of acute lung injury (ALI) ranging from mild pulmonary edema to adult respiratory distress syndrome (ARDS) that results from inflammation, sepsis, or injury, malnutrition is frequently a problem. In addition, the critically ill patient with respiratory failure is especially vulnerable to complications of underfeeding or overfeeding.

Furthermore, the effects of nutritional status on metabolism and pulmonary physiologic are evident in all patients with ventilatory impairment. Adequate management of chronic lung disease and mechanical ventilation requires attention in addition to the patient's nutritional requirements.

Numerous studies have shown that the adherence to good practice in the use of artificial nutrition in ventilated patients can improve the quality of this intervention and possibly clinical outcomes such as hyperglycemia, duration of mechanical ventilation, and even mortality.[1–4]

RESPIRATORY FAILURE: CAUSES

Respiratory failure is not a disease *per se* but a consequence of the problems that interfere with the ability to breathe. The term refers to the inability to perform adequately the fundamental functions of respiration: to deliver oxygen to the blood and to eliminate carbon dioxide from it. Respiratory failure involves the inability of the respiratory muscle to generate the negative inflation pressure necessary to overcome the high impedance to ventilation associated with certain parenchymal disorders.

Respiratory failure has many causes and can develop abruptly (acute respiratory failure [ARF]) or slowly (chronic respiratory failure) when it is associated over months or even years with a progressive underlying process. Typically, respiratory failure initially affects the ability either to take up oxygen (referred to as *oxygenation failure*) or to eliminate carbon dioxide (referred to as *ventilatory failure*). Eventually, both functions cease when the respiratory failure becomes severe enough.

Because so many underlying causes contribute to it, respiratory failure is a common and major cause of illness and death. It is the main cause of death from pneumonia and COPD, which together comprise the third leading cause of death in the United States today. It is also the main cause of death in many neuromuscular diseases, such as Lou Gehrig disease (amyotrophic lateral sclerosis [ALS]), because these diseases weaken the respiratory muscles, rendering them incapable of sustaining breathing. Epidemiologic studies suggest that respiratory failure will become more common as the population ages, increasing by as much as 80% in the next 20 years.[5,6]

Because respiratory failure is such a common cause of illness and death, the cost to society in terms of lost productivity and shortened lives is enormous. However, it is hard to quantify because the cause of death is more likely to be listed as pneumonia, COPD, or another underlying condition, rather than respiratory failure.

- *Muscle weakness*: It is a frequent cause of respiratory failure due to metabolic causes: hypophosphatemia, hypomagnesemia, hypokalemia, or hypothyroidism. Hypophosphatemia occurs with excessive use of aluminum-containing antacids, also from peritoneal dialysis with hypertonic dextrose solutions and insulin provided in the dialysate. It is also common with inadequate replacement in total parenteral nutrition solutions.

  Passive breathing on the ventilator will contribute to muscle weakness and subsequent respiratory failure with muscle atrophy secondary.
- *Increased work of breathing*: Airway obstructions from airway edema, foreign bodies, bronchospasm, thick secretions will contribute to excessive work of breathing. Small or obstructed endotracheal tubes will have a negative impact on the work of the breathing.
- *Inadequate respiratory drive*: Large doses of narcotic analgesic or sedatives will suppress the ventilatory drive; cerebrovascular accident will inevitably lead to ARF due to a lack of hypoxic or hypercapnic sensitivity. Figure 27.1 shows different causes and mechanisms leading to respiratory failure. Table 27.1 summarizes the causes of acute and chronic respiratory failure.
- *ALI/ARDS*: ALI and acute respiratory distress syndrome (ARDS) represent the most serious form of acute hypoxic respiratory failure. ALI/ARDS represents the expression of an acute, diffuse, inflammatory process in the lungs consequent to a variety of infections and noninfectious conditions. It is characterized pathologically by damage to pulmonary epithelial and endothelial cells, with subsequent alveolar-capillary leak and exudative pulmonary edema.

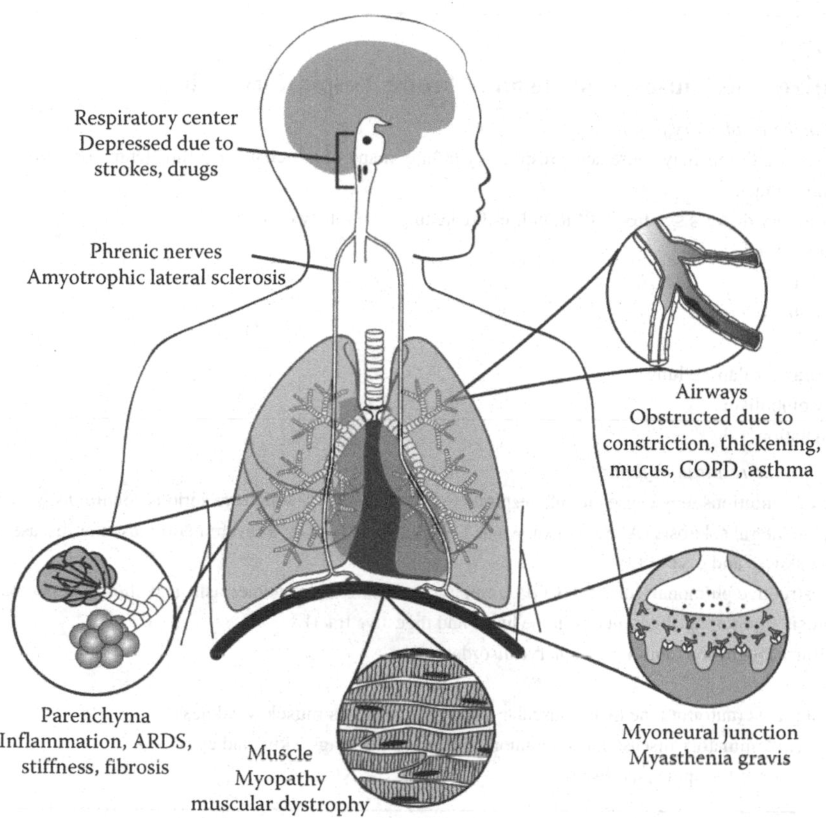

FIGURE 27.1 Several possible defects contribute to respiratory failure. The signal to breathe originates in the respiratory center and is sent by nerves via the myoneural junction to the respiratory muscles (such as the diaphragm). Respiratory function also depends on the integrity of the airways, lung structure, and blood vessels within the lungs. A few examples of diseases arising from the different defects are listed.

The main clinical features of ALI/ARDS include rapid onset of dyspnea, severe defects in gas exchange with imaging studies demonstrating diffuse pulmonary infiltrates. The role of nutrition in the management of ALI/ARDS has demonstrated the potential of certain dietary oils (e.g., fish oil, borage oil) to modulate pulmonary inflammation, thereby improving lung compliance and oxygenation, and reducing time on mechanical ventilation.[7]

SCIENTIFIC BACKGROUND

The concept that malnutrition can promote respiratory dysfunction was introduced in classic studies performed before 1950[8] where Benedict demonstrated that prolonged fasting produced a decrease in respiratory rate, tidal volume, and metabolic rate. The Jewish physicians of the Warsaw ghetto revealed that starvation was associated with premature emphysema and decreased total lung expansion. This, in turn, may produce atelectasis and segmental collapse. In malnutrition, the combination of atelectasis and an impaired immune response increases the incidence and severity of pulmonary infections. This results in increased destruction of lung tissue and eventually leads to the development of chronic lung disease.[9]

The process of respiration includes exchange of air between the atmosphere and the lung alveoli, diffusion of oxygen and carbon dioxide between the alveoli and blood,[10] and transport of oxygen and carbon dioxide in blood and body fluids to the cells. The respiratory muscles (diaphragm, intercostals, and accessory muscles of respiration) are subject to the same catabolic starvation. Ventilator

TABLE 27.1
Summarizes the Causes of Acute and Chronic Respiratory Failure

Causes of acute respiratory failure
A number of conditions may cause acute respiratory failure, many of which are life-threatening or serious conditions
Acute asthma attack
Acute respiratory distress syndrome (ARDS life-threatening respiratory condition)
Carbon dioxide poisoning
Chest trauma
Drug or alcohol overdose
Pneumonia
Pneumothorax (collapsed lung)
Pulmonary embolism
Smoke inhalation
Causes of chronic respiratory failure
A number of conditions may cause chronic respiratory failure, many of which are serious conditions.
Amyotrophic lateral sclerosis (ALS, also known as Lou Gehrig's disease; a severe neuromuscular disease that causes muscle weakness and disability)
Chronic obstructive pulmonary disease (COPD, emphysema, asthma, bronchiectasis, and chronic bronchitis)
Cystic fibrosis (buildup of thick mucus in the lungs and digestive tract)
Guillain–Barré syndrome (autoimmune nerve disorder)
Morbid obesity
Myasthenia gravis (autoimmune neuromuscular disorder that causes muscle weakness)
Sarcoidosis (inflammatory disease most commonly affecting the lungs, skin, and eyes)
Severe curvature of the spine (scoliosis)

dependence occurs when the patient cannot satisfactorily maintain oxygenation, carbon dioxide removal, or acid–base balance spontaneously. Respiratory insufficiency is a common feature of critical illness, especially sepsis, and persists in up to 20% of patients after the precipitating disease is resolved.

EFFECTS OF MALNUTRITION ON THE PULMONARY SYSTEM

A substantial proportion of patients with COPD are malnourished with incidence depending largely upon disease severity. As many as 25% of outpatients with COPD may be malnourished, while almost 50% of patients admitted to hospital have evidence of malnutrition.[11] Critically ill COPD patients with ARF have a 60% incidence of malnutrition. Disease severity can be assessed by the degree of pulmonary function and gas exchange abnormalities. Malnutrition occurs in 50% of patients with chronic hypoxemia and normoxemic patients with severe airflow obstruction (forced expiratory volume in one second [FEV1] <35% of predicted); however, it is also present in 25% of patients with moderate airflow obstruction.

Poor nutritional status can adversely affect thoracopulmonary function in spontaneously breathing as well as mechanically ventilated patients with respiratory disease by impairment of respiratory muscle function, ventilatory drive, and pulmonary defense mechanisms. The adverse effects of malnutrition occur independently of the presence or absence of primary lung disease; however, they can be additive in some patients with acute renal failure. In COPD, primary abnormalities of decreased inspiratory pressure and increased work of breathing are found. Inspiratory muscle weakness, as assessed by maximal inspiratory pressure, results both from mechanical disadvantage to inspiratory muscles consequent to hyperinflation and generalized muscle weakness. In COPD, inspiratory muscle weakness must be severe for hypercapnia to occur. In patients with myopathy, hypercapnia occurs when inspiratory pressures are less than one-third. However, hypercapnia is found in the majority of COPD patients when inspiratory pressures are only less than half normal.

Effects on Respiratory Musculature

The physiologic stress of starvation or critical illness induces the deterioration of lean body mass. The liberated amino acids are used for protein homeostasis and to provide energy via gluconeogénesis.[12] Since this results in loss of muscle mass, it was first thought that the body had a mechanism by which it could spare certain critical muscles such as the diaphragm and myocardium during starvation. It is now clear that this is not the case and that the respiratory muscle (diaphragm, intercostals, and accessory muscles of respiration)[13,14] is subject to the same catabolic conditions as other skeletal muscles during starvation or stress. Studies show that the myosin content of the diaphragm in patient with mild to moderate COPD is reduced, compromising diaphragm contractile performance. The mechanism for reduced contractile protein content is unknown. Ottenheljm et al.[15] hypothesized that the loss of contractile protein content is associated with activation of the ubiquitin-proteosomal pathway in the diaphragm of patients with mild to moderate COPD.

Effects on Respiratory Drive

Starvation is associated with a decreased metabolic rate and minute ventilation. Doekel administered hypocaloric feeding (500 kcal/day) to normal volunteers for 10 days and noted a 42% reduction in ventilatory response to hypoxia. In contrast, amino acid infusion following hypocaloric feedings increased neuromuscular drive. Since CO_2 productions remained relatively unchanged during amino acid infusion, increased CO_2 production could not have accounted for the increase in minute ventilation. Rather, there appeared to be a resetting of the chemoreceptors to respond to a lower $PaCO_2$. Askanazi[16] showed that increased nitrogen intake caused a leftward shift in the minute ventilation–$PaCO_2$ curve, suggesting that there is a change in the ratio of tryptophan to its amino acid competitors (valine, leucine, isoleucine, tyrosine, phenylalanine) that alters transport across the blood–brain barrier. This decreased central serotonin production, which, in turn, increased ventilatory sensitivity.

Effects on Pulmonary Defense Mechanisms

Death from starvation is often due to pneumonia. Malnutrition associated with critical illness impairs the immune response. Anergy is commonly observed as an impaired T-lymphocyte response to mitogens. These effects may be reversed with refeeding. These effects have an impact on alveolar defenses. The respiratory epithelium of malnourished patients has increased bacterial adherence and decreased IgA secretion. Lung aspirates taken shortly after death demonstrated a high recovery rate of bacteria, especially gram-negative organism in malnourished patients. The lung matrix is a dynamic structure that is continually undergoing a process of fiber repair and replacement. These fibers are composed of elastins, fibronectins, and collagens that provide structure and allow for elasticity. Damaged fibers are removed by enzymes such as proteinases and collagenases, which are activated in the immune response process. These destructive enzymes are normally kept in check by enzyme inactivators such as alpha-1-antitrypsin. The balance of activation and inactivation ensures a graded response to lung inflammation. However, malnutrition or critical illness may deplete circulating antiproteinases, resulting in unopposed proteinase activity. Each pulmonary infection is then met with an exaggerated amount and structurally abnormal lung matrix.

Effects on Pulmonary Metabolism

Substrate metabolism plays an important role in governing physiologic responses within the lung. The ratio of carbon dioxide production to oxygen consumption is expressed as the respiratory quotient (RQ). RQ is lower (0.7) when fat is oxidized and higher (1.0) during carbohydrate metabolism compared with fat metabolism. Since the lung must increase ventilation to eliminate this CO_2, a higher RQ is associated with greater minute ventilation.[17,18]

While these changes may be insignificant in healthy people, they may be detrimental to patients with ventilatory insufficiency. Such individuals cannot increase alveolar ventilation without a marked increase in the work of breathing. This eventually results in exhaustion and respiratory failure.

Septic and injured patients who may be hypermetabolic are also at risk of respiratory failure induced by a change in RQ. These patients are already overproducing CO_2. These conditions are associated with a preference for the utilization of lipid calories and the development of carbohydrate intolerance. Excess carbohydrates increase CO_2 production and work of breathing in these patients and may cause respiratory failure. This may also be the reason for worsening hypermetabolism during overfeeding in these patients.

CONSIDERATIONS FOR NUTRITION INTERVENTION

Nutrition is an important aspect of patient care in any patient with respiratory disease. Malnutrition adversely effects lung function by diminishing respiratory muscle strength, altering ventilatory capacity, and impairing immune function. Repletion of altered nutritional status or refeeding results in improvement of altered function and may be important in improving outcome. When spontaneous oral intake is inadequate, enteral feeding is preferred over parenteral feeding in all but those with nonfunctional gastrointestinal tracts. Unfortunately, as with any therapy, complications of nutritional support exist. Those complications presenting special problems to the patient with respiratory disease are nutritionally related hypercapnia and aspiration of enteral feedings.

CARBOHYDRATES

The protein-sparing effect of exogenous carbohydrates is well known. However, these nutrients must be used with caution in patients with respiratory failure. The idea is to provide sufficient calories to maximize protein sparing while minimizing the complications of overfeeding. The brain requires approximately 120 g/day of glucose and the blood cells 30–40 g/day of glucose. Carbohydrate administration to meet these requirements is imperative in order to minimize conversion of muscle protein into glucose via gluconeogenesis. Energy supplied in the form of fat also has nitrogen-sparing ability. Once the carbohydrate requirement is met (600–800 kcal/day in a normal adult), glucose and fat are equally effective in sparing nitrogen.

The requirement for glucose may be greater in injured or septic patients because wound tissue is also dependent on glucose (20–60 g/day). In a study of postoperative patients, increasing the glucose infusion rate from 4 to 7 mg/kg/min was associated with an increased rate of glucose oxidation.[19]

Patients with respiratory failure should receive glucose in amount sufficient to meet obligatory glucose needs (2–4 g/kg/day) without exceeding them. In an average patient, this amounts to approximately 200 g/day of glucose.

LIPIDS

Once glucose requirements are met, supplying additional calories as fat or glucose has an equal nitrogen-sparing effect. During uncomplicated starvation, the infusion of glucose will suppress lipolysis. However, glucose administration in the stressed patient has less effect on lipolysis. In the stressed patient, fat utilization continues despite the availability of adequate amounts of glucose. Lipids should be administered in a dosage range of 1–2 g/kg/day. The infusion of intravenous fat emulsion (IVFE) should be infused over a minimum of 10–12 h and preferably over 24 h. This permits optimal uptake and utilization. Such a protocol can be nicely achieved by means of the *triple mix* system, in which IVFE, dextrose, and amino acids are mixed together.

Infusion of lipids is often mistakenly thought to increase the complication rate of TPN therapy. In fact, the opposite is true, in that IVFE reduces the incidence of osmolar and vascular complications.

Proteins

The ventilatory response to CO_2 is increased by the infusion of amino acids. This may elevate minute ventilation in patients with respiratory failure who are already breathing at a high percentage of their maximal voluntary ventilation. Particular caution should be exercised when combining high glucose with a high protein mixture. The combination of increase CO_2 production with an increased ventilatory response to CO_2 may be overwhelming. Branched chain enriched amino acid preparations may cause an even greater increase in respiratory drive.

Micronutrients

Vitamins, trace elements, and minerals are very important in the prevention and management of critical patient's respiratory failure. However, of particular interest in patients with respiratory failure is hypophosphatemia, which can influence respiration in patients receiving nutritional support. Phosphate is transported intracellularly, predominantly into liver and muscle during heightened glucose utilization. Hypophosphatemia may be associated with altered red blood cell O_2 transport (increased hemoglobin–oxygen affinity with impaired release of O_2 to tissues) secondary to low levels of 2,3-diphosphoglycerate. Hypophosphatemia has been described in ARF.

CHRONIC OBSTRUCTIVE PULMONARY DISEASE (COPD)

COPD is the term that is known to emphysema, chronic bronchitis, chronic asthma, and bronchiectasis. The lower airways begin at the terminal bronchiole and extend through the respiratory bronchioles and alveolar ducts to the alveoli.[20] Lungs are perfused with blood via the pulmonary and bronchial arteries, through the pulmonary capillaries in the alveolar walls, leaving the lungs via the pulmonary veins. In COPD, inflammation causes direct destruction of lung tissues and also impairs defense mechanisms used to repair damaged tissues. This results in not only destruction of the lung parenchyma (i.e., emphysema) but also mucus hypersecretion and airway narrowing and fibrosis.[21]

COPD is a systemic disease in which manifestations are beyond the airflow obstruction, is associated with malnutrition, and also includes *pulmonary cachexia*.[22,23]

A wide range of inflammatory cells and mediators are involved in the pathogenesis of COPD, namely, neutrophils, macrophages, and CD8+ T cells in different areas of the lungs. Molecules that play a role in pulmonary cachexia are TNF-alpha, IL-1B, IL-6, C-reactive protein (CRP), reactive oxygen species, and reactive nitrogen species.[24,25]

Precipitating factors include smoking, air pollution, occupational exposure, repeated respiratory infections, heredity, aging, and allergies.

COPD and asthmatic patients use a substantial proportion of mechanical ventilation in the ICU, and their overall mortality with ventilatory support can be significant. From the pathophysiological standpoint, they have increased airway resistance, pulmonary hyperinflation, and high pulmonary dead space, leading to increased work of breathing.[26] If ventilatory demand exceeds work output of the respiratory muscles, ARF follows. The main goal of mechanical ventilation in this kind of patient is to improve pulmonary gas exchange and to allow for sufficient rest of compromised respiratory muscles to recover from the fatigued state.

Disease severity can be assessed by the degree of pulmonary function and gas exchange abnormalities. Malnutrition occurs in 50% of patients with chronic hypoxemia and normoxemia patients with severe airflow obstruction (forced expiratory volume in 1 s [FEV1] <35% of predicted); however, it is also present in 25% of patients with moderate airflow obstruction. Inadequate protein and caloric intake may further contribute to primary lung parenchymal disease, immunocompromise, and respiratory muscle wasting and dysfunction that result in the need for intubation and mechanical ventilation. Weight loss and body mass is a common complication of advanced COPD patients, mainly emphysematous type. The median survival of patients with cachexia and an FEV1 < 50% is approximately 2–4 years, considerably less than in noncachexic patients.[27] In addition, the low weight (corporal mass index or body mass index [BMI] < 20 kg/m^2) or recent weight loss and muscle atrophy value, measured by the index of fat-free mass, are independent predictors of mortality.[28] Patients with COPD who have respiratory failure and require mechanical ventilation should be given early enteral nutrition, gastrically or postpylorically, within 24–48 h of admission to ICU[29] if there are no contraindications to the use of the digestive tract.

Up to 60% of patients with COPD have increased basal energy expenditure, especially when they lose weight. Empirically, it seems reasonable to use the recommendation of 25–30 kcal/kg/day.

In patients requiring mechanical ventilation, it is recommended that the carbohydrate intake be 50%–70% and lipid intake be 30%–50% of energy requirements. Glucose infusion should not exceed 4 g/kg/day because higher contributions clearly increase the VCO_2, with 5 mg/kg/min hindering ventilator disconnection. Some randomized controlled studies have compared the effect of diets rich in carbohydrates (50%–100% of total energy) with lower percentage (30% of total energy), and adverse effects occurred only in cases where the amount of power calculated needed exceeded those administered.[30] Therefore, it is not necessary to use specific enteral formulas with low carbohydrate content and high content of lipids. The most important thing is to remember that the responsibility of increased caloric overload CO_2 is not the proportion of macronutrients in the diet, because when the total calories are administered in moderate amounts, manipulating macronutrients has little effect on the production CO_2.[31]

With respect to protein intake in critically ill patient on ventilator, a high protein intake is recommended. The proteins increase the minute volume, VO_2, and the ventilatory response to hypoxia and hypercapnia, irrespective of the pH and VCO_2. It's recommended contributions 1.0–1.5 g/kg/day in patients not hypercatabolic and 1.5–2.0 g/kg/day in hypercatabolic.

With regard to micronutrients, for the proper functioning of the respiratory muscles, it is important to maintain adequate levels of phosphorus, magnesium, calcium, iron, zinc, and potassium; their values should be normal during weaning from mechanical ventilation. It also requires provision of antioxidants selenium, vitamins A, C, and E.[32]

A review of the different societies of clinical nutrition and its proposals on nutritional therapy of patients with COPD with respect to high-fat intake in enteral formula suggests the following (European Society for Parenteral and Enteral Nutrition [ESPEN] 2006): "In stable COPD, there is no additional advantages of disease-specific low-carbohydrate, high fat oral nutrition supplements compared with standard high-protein or high-energy oral nutrition supplements."[33,34] American Dietetic Association Evidence Analysis Library (ADA) 2008: "Registered dietitians should advise that the selection of medical food supplements for individual with COPD be influenced more by patient preference than by the percentage of fat or carbohydrate."[35] Canadian Clinical Practice Guidelines 2009: "There are insufficient data to recommend high-fat/low-carbohydrates diets for critically ill patients."[36] Society of Critical Care Medicine and American Society for Parenteral and Enteral Nutrition (SCCM/ASPEN) 2009: "Speciality high-lipid, low-carbohydrate formulations designed to manipulate the respiratory quotient and reduce carbon dioxide production are not recommended for routine use in ICU patient with acute respiratory failure."[37] The Guidelines SCCM/ASPEN 2009 recommend immune-modulating enteral formulations (supplemented with agents such as arginine, glutamine nucleic acid, ω-3 fatty acids, and antioxidants in critically ill patient on mechanical ventilation).

ACUTE LUNG INJURY AND ACUTE RESPIRATORY DISTRESS SYNDROME (ALI/ARDS)

ARDS and its milder form ALI are a spectrum of lung diseases characterized by a severe inflammatory process causing diffuse alveolar damage and resulting in a variable degree of ventilation perfusion mismatch, severe hypoxemia, and poor lung compliance.[38,39] Patients with ARDS are often mechanically ventilated during the course of their illness. Morbidity and mortality remain high and early recognition of patients is a vital step in providing appropriate care. Due to the broad range of precipitating conditions, patients can present to any medical or surgical specialty with acute respiratory deterioration. Prompt appropriate management with ICU provision is essential to improve outcome.

ARDS was first reported by Ashbaugh et al. in 1967.[40] They described a rapid onset of tachypnea and hypoxemia, with loss of lung compliance and bilateral infiltrates on chest radiograph, in otherwise healthy young individuals. Although the ARDS precipitating illnesses differed between patients, they had similar clinical and pathological features. Differentiating pulmonary edema secondary to heart failure from ARDS is difficult, and in the subsequent decades, the pulmonary artery catheter was widely used to measure pulmonary artery wedge pressure to facilitate diagnosis and management. Furthermore, the advent of the specialty of intensive care medicine resulted in improved survival and enabled greater understanding of ARDS. However, much of this early work is difficult to interpret due to the lack of a consistent definition of ARDS.

In 1994, *The American-European Consensus Conference (AECC)* proposed a definition, which is now widely accepted as a simple diagnostic tool for patient characterization and research trial conduct. There are four diagnostic criteria for ARDS[41]:

1. Acute onset
2. Presence of acute severe hypoxemia (defined as a ratio of arterial oxygen tension over fractional inspired oxygen [PaO_2/FiO_2] < 200 mmHg [26.7 kPa])
3. Bilateral infiltrates on chest radiography (CXR) (Figure 27.2)
4. Absence of raised pulmonary artery wedge pressure

If the PaO_2/FiO_2 is >200 mmHg (26.7 kPa) and <300 mmHg (40 kPa), the correct name is ALI.

Clinical conditions associated with etiology of ARDS are direct lung injury and indirect lung injury, sepsis being the most frequent cause (Table 27.2). Most often it is shown that the genetic background can determine a patient's progress.[42]

A study of critical care units in the United States in 2005 estimated the incidence of ARDS to be 58/100,000 person years with 141,500 new cases per year and an annual death rate of 59,000/year.[43] European estimates are more conservative, ranging between 4.2 and 13.5/100,000 persons/year.

The patient with ARDS is undoubtedly a critical patient at high risk of malnutrition. This is due to many factors resulting in acute malnutrition rather than calorie protein including decreased

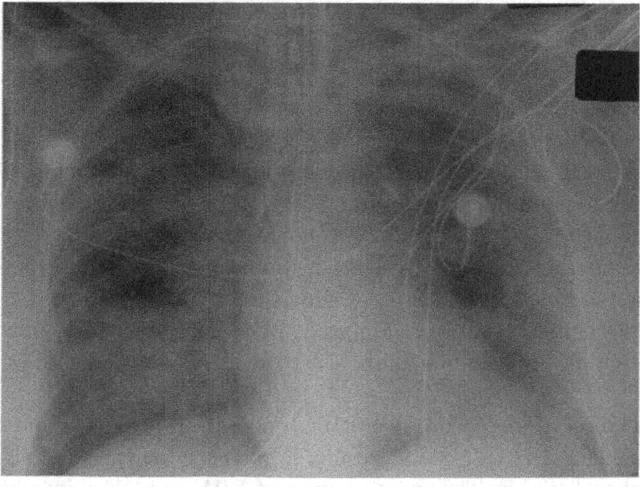

FIGURE 27.2 Chest radiography showing infiltrators *patchy* in the four quadrants of ARDS typical.

TABLE 27.2
Most Common Causes of ARDS

Direct Lung Injury	Indirect Lung Injury
Common causes	
Pneumonia	SEPSIS
Aspiration of gastric content	Severe trauma
	Multiple transfusions
Less common causes	
Pulmonary contusion	Cardiopulmonary bypass
Fat emboli	Drug overdose
Near-drowning	Acute pancreatitis
Inhalational injury	Transfusions of blood products

intake of macro- and micronutrients by anorexia; fasting and degradation; increased nutrient turnover, mainly proteins, by hypermetabolism and self-cannibalism; and decreased metabolism of carbohydrates and lipids as primary energy source. This type of malnutrition has adverse effects on respiratory function by decreasing respiratory muscle mass and contractility, decreasing the connective tissue lung surfactant production and compromised immune function.

With regard to altered immunity in this syndrome, it is due to a response of excessive local inflammation culminating in systemic immunosuppression.[44] Pulmonary inflammation is mediated by the activation of alveolar macrophage cells, and when activated, these immune cells are capable of altering the intermediate metabolism and the physiological lung function by releasing a variety of proinflammatory mediators including eicosanoid derivatives of arachidonic acid (thromboxanes and leukotrienes) and cytokines such as tumor necrosis factor and interleukin 1.

This syndrome is associated with a number of metabolic abnormalities, which should be monitored during the treatment of these patients. After pulmonary physiology stabilizes and hemodynamic stability is achieved, nutritional therapy should be initiated as calorie and protein requirements are high in these patients. Nutritional management is generally established with a protein 1.5–2.0 g/kg/day with a ratio of nonprotein calories nitrogen ranging from 80:1 to not more than 100:1. This is to give a total calorie intake of 25–30 kcal/kg/day. It is important to consider the quality of proteins such as conditionally essential amino acids glutamine and arginine.[45]

Glutamine, a semiessential amino acid, which becomes essential in critically ill patients on mechanical ventilation, has been very useful because in these patients, endothelial cells require large amounts of glutamine, increasing its consumption, a response mediated by TNFα and IL-1. It is useful to use the single amino acid arginine as a precursor of nitric oxide, which can play an important role as a substrate in the synthesis of nitric oxide by pulmonary endothelial cells, achieving also interest in pulmonary vasodilation in ARDS.

The carbohydrate intake must not exceed the rate of glucose oxidation (no more than 7 g/kg/day or 5 mg/kg/min trying to maintain an appropriate RQ); this is generally achieved by giving a contribution of 50% carbohydrates and 50% lipids as nonprotein calories.

One of the most important advances in the nutritional management of these patients has been the input modification of lipid type since it has been shown that if only used ω-6 these deleterious effects in the pathophysiology syndrome (Figure 27.3). Numerous studies in animals and humans have demonstrated significant benefits with the use of ω-3 fatty acids as well as the use of the combination of MCT/LCT.[46–48]

Increased consumption of long-chain n-3 PUFA, such as eicosapentaenoic acid (EPA;20:5 n-3) and docosahexaenoic acid (DHA;22:6 n-3), results in increased proportions of those fatty acids in inflammatory cell phospholipids. The incorporation of EPA and DHA into human inflammatory cells occurs in a dose-response fashion and is partly at the expense of arachidonic acid. Because less

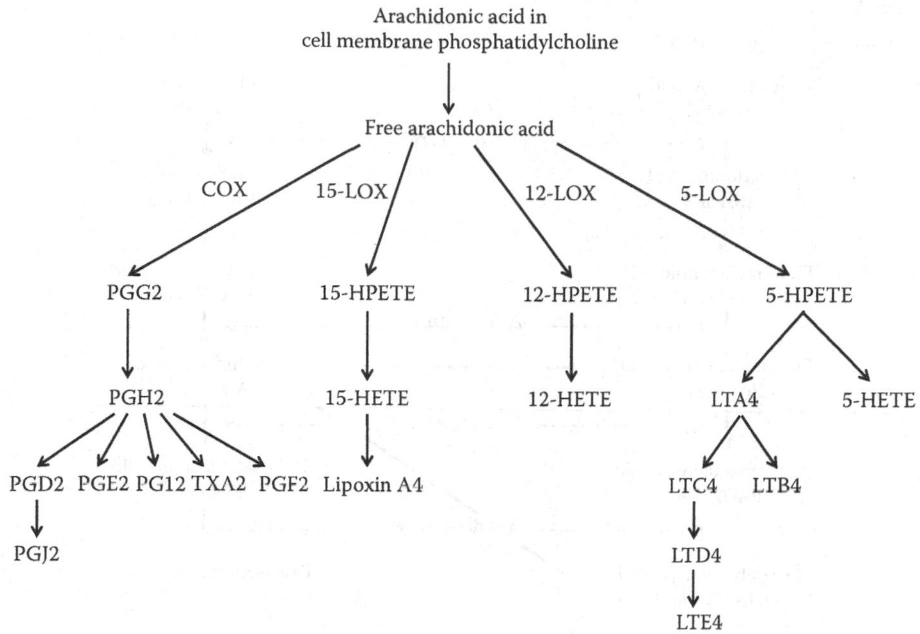

FIGURE 27.3 Metabolism of arachidonic acid and conversion to eicosanoids. COX, cyclooxygenase; HETE, hydroxyeicosatetraenoic acid; HPETE, hydroperoxyeicosatetraenoic acid; LOX, lipoxygenase; LT, leukotriene; PG, prostaglandin; TX, thromboxane.

substrate is available for synthesis of eicosanoids from arachidonic acid, fish oil supplementation of the human diet has been shown to result in decreased production of PGE2, thromboxane B2, LTB4, 5-hydroxyeicosatetraenoic acid, and LTE4, by inflammatory cells (Figure 27.4). n-3 fatty acid shows a potent anti-inflammatory effect, plus decreased leukocyte chemotaxis, decreased production of reactive oxygen species chemotaxis, decreased proinflammatory cytokines, and decreased adhesion molecule expression. EPA has protective actions against the damaging effect of TNF-α on C2C12 myogenesis.[49]

In ARDS, different studies using EPA (eicosapentaenoic acid) and GLA (gamma linolenic acid) associated with antioxidant agents have shown a decrease in pulmonary inflammation, which facilitates vasodilation in the pulmonary circuit, and improves PaO_2/FiO_2 ratio with improved oxygen supply, achieving a reduction in mechanical ventilation time, ICU length of stay, decreased appearance of new faults[7,50–52] in addition to improved strength in endotoxemia diaphragm.[53]

Gadek et al.[54] published the first report of beneficial effects in using a formula specialized in patients with ALI. Ninety-eight patients, as having ALI, were randomized to receive either a modified lipid formula for ARDS or control within 24 h after enrolling into the study. Patients receiving the specialized formula showed a significant improvement in oxygenation ($p < 0.05$), required significantly fewer days of mechanical ventilator support ($p = 0.01$), and demonstrated a decreased ICU length of stay ($p = 0.016$) compared with the control group. There was no difference in mortality between both groups. The main difference between the two enteral formulas was the type of lipid and the higher amount of antioxidants in the specialized formula. Patch et al.[55] designed a prospective, double-blind, controlled clinical trial, including 67 patients with ALI/ARDS. A total of 43 of 67 evaluable patients randomly received either EPA + GLA or an isonitrogenous, isocaloric standard diet, showing a decreased in bronchoalveolar lavage fluid (BALF) levels of IL-8, leukotrienes B4, and neutrophils in the study group.

Singer et al.[56] studied one hundred ventilated patients meeting the criteria for ALI who were randomized to receive either a formula containing EPA, GLA, and antioxidant or a control

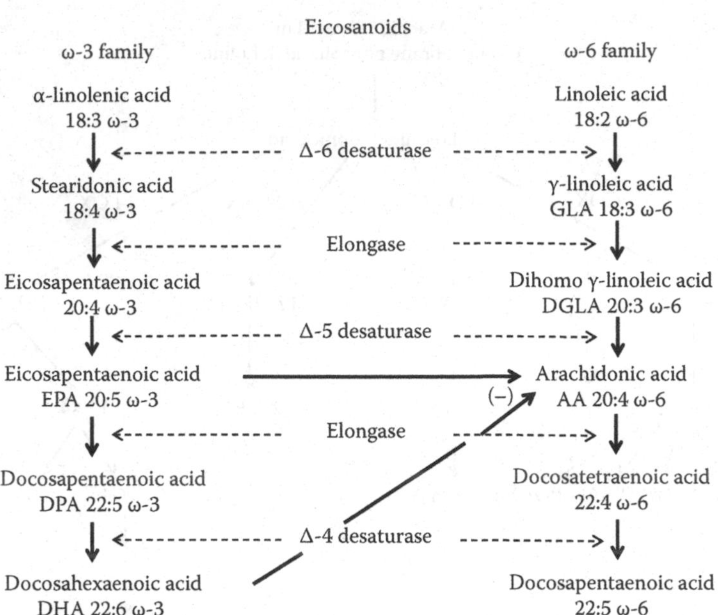

FIGURE 27.4 Metabolic conversion of ω-6 and ω-3 polyunsaturated fatty acids. Eicosapentaenoic acid (EPA) and docosahexaenoic acid (DHA) decreased the amounts of arachidonic acid available as a substrate for eicosanoid synthesis and also inhibit the metabolism of arachidonic acid.

pulmonary formula within 24 h of ICU admission. Patients who received the EPA/GLA formula had a significantly shorter length of ventilator time ($p < 0.05$) as well as a reduced ICU length of stay ($p < 0.05$) compared with the control patients. There was no difference in either hospital length of stay or mortality between the two groups. Pontes-Arruda et al.[57] reported their results in 165 patients with sepsis. Study patients were enrolled if they required mechanical ventilation and demonstrated an oxygenation measurement of $PaO_2/FIO_2 < 200$. Patients were randomized to receive a control standard pulmonary formula or a formula with EPA, GLA, and antioxidants, which was initiated within 6 h of study entry. Out of 103 patients, those who received the EPA/GLA formula experienced improved oxygenation on study days 4 and 7 compared with the control group. In addition, a greater number of ventilator-free days, a greater number of ICU-free days, and a significant reduction in new organ failure were demonstrated in those who received the lipid-modulated formula. The use of the EPA/GLA formula was associated with an increased survival rate, unlike in the previously cited trials.

Pontes-Arruda et al.[58] conducted a meta-analysis on the cumulative evidence comparing EPA/GLA formula versus control. Three randomized controlled trials met inclusion and quality criteria, providing a total simple size of 411 patients, of whom 296 were evaluable. The use of an EPA/GLA formula was associated with a 60% reduction in the risk of 28 day mortality ($OR = 0.40$, $p = 0.001$) with significant reductions in the risk of developing new organ failures ($OR = 0.17$, $p < 0.0001$), time on mechanical ventilation ($p < 0.0001$), improved oxygenation ($p < 0.0001$), and ICU stay ($p < 0.0001$). The authors concluded that patients with ALI/ARDS who were given an EPA/GLA formula had a significant reduction in mortality risk as well as improvements in oxygenation and clinical outcomes compared with those who received a standard formula. Sabater et al.[59] conducted a small study in 16 patients, of which 8 were supplemented with an ω-3 fatty acid–enriched lipid emulsion. In this study, the authors concluded that the ω-3-containing emulsion was safe and well tolerated in short-term (12 h) infusion to patients with ARDS. Furthermore, this type of parenteral formula was not able to produce any significant change in hemodynamic and gas exchange parameters. However, these studies[54,56,57] supplemented control diets containing high amounts of fat (up to 50% of energy requirements in two of them), with a high percentage of linoleic acid (an ω-6 fatty acid derived from soybean oil and safflower oil).

Immunonutrition using different mixtures of pharmaconutrients is a nutritional strategy, which has been largely used in the critical care setting. However, this type of strategy although clearly beneficial in the ICU does not allow to define the real benefit of each pharmaconutrient as a single strategy.

Three recent studies have intended to address this important issue. Rice et al.[60] compared the effect of supplements of ω-3 fatty acid plus antioxidants, given as a bolus every 12 h with standard enteral diet, compared to placebo formula and was stopped for it gave no result with 272 patients. Besides the study group received a formula with protein 3.8/240 mL and control groups 20/240 mL. The second study by Stapleton et al.[61] analyzed the inflammatory response in BALF of patients with ALI; the study group received 9.75 g EPA + DHA 6.75 g/day or saline placebo for 14 days in the control group. Fish oil did not reduce biomarkers of pulmonary or systemic inflammation in patient with ALI. The third study by Grau-Carmona et al.[62] studied a commercial diet with ω-3 fatty acids, EPA, GLA, and antioxidants in the treatment of patients with sepsis and ARDS. They showed in the study group a trend toward a decreased SOFA score, but it was not significant. No differences were observed in the PaO_2/FIO_2 ratio or the days on mechanical ventilation between the groups. Incidence of infections was similar in the groups. The control group stayed longer in the ICU than the EPA-GLA diet group (16 vs 18, p = 0.02).

According to current evidence, fish oil supplementation in critically ill patients with ARDS is still a subject of debate, which has been evaluated in a few numbers of randomized trials. Unpublished data from Heyland and coworkers demonstrated that fish oil containing emulsions may be associated with a tendency to reduce mortality and ventilation days, without any effect on infectious complications in the critically ill. Barbosa et al.[63] evaluated the effect of parenteral ω-3 containing lipid emulsion in 23 septic patients (fish oil group, 13 vs MCT/LCT, 10). In the fish oil group, the authors found a tendency to decrease hospital length of stay (22 vs 55, p = 0.079), which became significant (28 vs 82 days, p = 0.044) after including the patients who survived. Furthermore, the authors demonstrated an increase in plasma EPA levels and an improvement in gas exchange. Nonetheless, ventilation days, ICU length of stay, and mortality were not different between the two groups. Pontes-Arruda et al.[64] in the INTERSEPT study enrolled 115 patients with early sepsis (systemic inflammatory response syndrome with confirmed or presumed infection and without any organ dysfunction) and demonstrated that those fed with EPA/GLA diet developed less severe sepsis and/or septic shock than other patients (26.4% vs 50%, respectively, p = 0.02). The ITT analysis demonstrated that patients in the study group developed less cardiovascular failure (36.2% vs 21%, p = 0.03) and respiratory failure (39% vs 24%, p = 0.03) when compared with the control group. Finally, the authors concluded that EPA/GLA may play a beneficial role in the treatment of enterally fed patients in the early stages of sepsis, decreasing the progression of sepsis-related organ dysfunction, especially decreasing the incidence of hemodynamic and pulmonary dysfunctions.

To summarize, the current literature demonstrates an important role of fish oils (EPA and DHA) in the control of the inflammatory process, which is a major characteristic in patients with sepsis, severe sepsis, and ARDS. Enteral nutrition, including specialized diets rich in EPA, DHA, and GLA, may be able to improve clinical outcomes in ICU patients with ALI/ARDS. Large, rigorously designed, randomized controlled trials are required to elucidate the efficacy of enteral and parenteral fish oil in ALI/ARDS patient population.

The truth is that the ASPEN-SCCM guidelines[65] recommend that patients with ALI/ARDS be given a formula characterized by an anti-inflammatory lipid profile (i.e., ω-3 fish oils, borage oil) and antioxidants (grade A).

CONCLUSIONS

There is a close relationship between malnutrition and respiratory failure and often leads to another one. There are different causes of respiratory failure, some more difficult to correct, such as COPD, having greater negative impact on the patient's ventilation. This leads to progressive muscle weakness. Increased work of breathing and respiratory inadequacy impair the immune response. COPD patients, because of the high risk of malnutrition, have respiratory failure, requiring nutritional support that guarantees at least 1.5 g/kg/day protein, no carbohydrates 4 g/kg/day over. Ensuring an adequate supply of micronutrients, phosphorus cannot be given in optimal levels. Patients with ALI/ARDS have an active inflammatory process, which may be modulated through the provision of fatty acids derived from fish oil, but in the context of immunonutrition.

Immunonutrition is important to use early in the syndrome because the anti-inflammatory effects of ω-3 can take several days to act; we should not wait for this syndrome, once diagnosis is established and whether the patient is able to tolerate either enteral or parenteral. The potential benefits of immunonutrition include among other phagocytic function improvement, improvement in cell physiology, lower incidence of infections, improved healing, reduced antibiotic use, fewer days of mechanical ventilation, and shorter stay in the ICU and hospital.[66]

REFERENCES

1. Esteban A, Anzueto A, Frutos F et al. Mechanical ventilation international study group. Characteristics and outcome in adult patients receiving mechanical ventilation: A 28-day international study. *JAMA* 2002;287:345–355.
2. Doig GS, Simpson F, Finfer S. Nutrition guidelines investigators of the ANZICS clinical trial group. Effect of evidence-based feeding guidelines on mortality of critically ill adults: A cluster randomized controlled trial. *JAMA* 2008;300:2731–2741.
3. Barr J, Hecht M, Flavin KE et al. Outcomes in critically ill patients before and after the implementation of an evidence-based nutritional management protocol. *Chest* 2004;125:1446–1457.
4. Heyland DK, Dhaliwal R, Day A et al. Validation of the Canadian clinical practice guideline for nutrition support in mechanically ventilated, critically ill adult patients: Results of a prospective observational study. *Crit Care Med* 2004;32:2260–2266.
5. Carson SS, Cox CE, Holmes GM, Howard A, Carey TS. The changing epidemiology of mechanical ventilation: A population-based study. *J Intensive Care Med* 2006;21:173–182.
6. Nava S, Hill N. Non-invasive ventilation for acute respiratory failure. *Lancet* 2009;374:250–259.
7. Mizock BA, DeMichele SJ. The acute respiratory distress syndrome: Role of nutritional modulation of inflammation through dietary lipids. *Nutr Clin Pract* 2004;19:563–574.
8. Rothkopf MM, Stanislaus G, Haverstick L, Kvetan V, Askanazi J. Invited review: Nutritional support in respiratory failure. *Nutr Clin Pract* 1989;4:166–172.
9. Brug J, Schols A, Mesters I. Dietary change, nutrition education and chronic obstructive pulmonary disease. *Patient Educ Couns* 2004;52:249–257.
10. Ireton-Jones C, Borman KR, Turner WW, Jr. Nutrition considerations in the management of ventilator-dependent patients. *Nutr Clin Pract* 1993;8:60–64.
11. Sahebjami H, Stahianpitayakul E. Influence of body weight on the severity of dyspnea in chronic obstructive pulmonary disease. *Am J Respir Crit Care Med* 2000;161:886–890.
12. Schols AMW. Nutrition and respiratory disease. *Clin Nutr* 2001;20(Suppl.):173–179.
13. Orozco-Levi M, Lloreta J, Minguella J et al. Injury of the human diaphragm associated with exertion and chronic obstructive pulmonary disease. *Am J Respir Crit Care Med* 2001;164:1734–1739.
14. Tobin MJ, Laghi F. Disorders of the respiratory muscles. *Am J Respir Crit Care Med* 2003;168:10–48.
15. Ottenheljm CAC, Heunks LMA, Li YP et al. Activation of the ubiquitin-proteosome pathway in the diaphragm in chronic obstructive pulmonary disease. *Am J Respir Crit Care Med* 2006;174:997–1002.
16. Askanazi J, Weissman C, LaSala P et al. Effects of increasing protein intake on ventilatory drive. *Anesthesiology* 1984;60:106.
17. Pingleton SK. Enteral nutrition in patients with respiratory disease. *Eur Respir J*, 1996;9:364–370.
18. Collins PF, Stratton RJ, Elia M. Nutritional support in chronic obstructive pulmonary disease: A systematic review and meta-analysis. *Am J Clin Nutr* 2012;95:1385–1395.
19. Buyken AE, Flood V, Empson E et al. Carbohydrate nutrition and inflammatory disease mortality in older adults. *Am J Clin Nutr* 2010;92:634–643.
20. Barnes PJ. Chronic obstructive pulmonary disease. *N Engl J Med* 2000;343:269–280.
21. Chung KF, Adcok IM. Multifaceted mechanism in COPD: Inflammation, immunity, and tissue repair and destruction. *Eur Respir J* 2008;31:1334–1356.

22. Schols AM. Pulmonary cachexia. *Int J Cardiol* 2002;85:101–110.
23. Fabbri LM, Luppi F, Berghe B et al. Complex chronic comorbidities of COPD. *Eur Respir J* 2008;31:204–212.
24. Agusti A, Morla A, Sauleda J et al. NF-kappaB activation and iNOS upregulation in skeletal muscle of patient with COPD and low body weight. *Thorax* 2004;59:483–487.
25. Barnes PJ. The cytokine network in asthma and chronic obstructive pulmonary disease. *J Clin Invest* 2008;118:3546–3556.
26. Fabbri LM, Rabe KF. From COPD to chronic systemic inflammatory syndrome? *Lancet* 2007;370: 797–799.
27. Rabe FK, Hurd S, Anzueto A et al. Global initiative for chronic obstructive lung disease. Global strategy for the diagnosis, management, and prevention of chronic obstruction pulmonary disease: GOLD executive summary. *Am J Respir Crit Care Med* 2007;176:532–555.
28. Vestbo J, Prescott E, Almdal T, Dahl M et al. Body mass, fat-free body mass, and prognosis in patient with chronic obstructive pulmonary disease from a random population simple finding from the Copenhagen City Heart Study. *Am J Rspir Crit Care Med* 2006;173:79–83.
29. Doig GS, Heighes PT, Simpson F et al. Early enteral nutrition, provide within 24 h of injury or intensive care unit admission, significantly reduces mortality in critically ill patients: A meta-analysis of randomised controlled trials. *Int Care Med* 2009;35:2018–2027.
30. Creutzberg EC, Shols AM, Weling-Scheepers CA et al. Characterization of nonresponse to high caloric oral nutritional therapy in depleted patients with chronic obstructive pulmonary disease. *Am J Respir Crit Care Med* 2000;161:745–752.
31. King DA, Cordova F, Scharf SM. Nutritional aspects of chronic obstructive pulmonary disease. *Proc Am Thorac Soc* 2008;5:519–523.
32. Planas M, Alvarez J, Garcia-Peris PA et al. Nutritional support and quality of life in stable chronic obstructive pulmonary disease (COPD) patients. *Clin Nutr* 2005;24:433–441.
33. Malone AM. Specialized enteral formulas in acute and chronic pulmonary disease. *Nutr Clin Pract* 2009;24:666–674.
34. Kreyman KG, Berger MM, Deutz NE et al. ESPEN guidelines on enteral nutrition: Intensive care. *Clin Nutr* 2006;25:210–223.
35. The American Dietetic Association. Critical illness recommendations. http://www.adaevidencelibrary.com/template, accessed on October 26, 2012.
36. Critical Care Nutrition. Canadian clinical practice guidelines for nutrition support in adult critically patients. http://www.criticalcarenutricion.com/docs/cpg, accessed on October 26, 2012.
37. Martindale RG, McClave SA, Vanek VW et al. Guidelines for the provision and assessment of nutrition support therapy in the adult critically ill patient: Society of Critical Care Medicine and American Society for Parenteral and Enteral Nutrition: Executive Summary. *Crit Care Med* 2009;37:1757–1761.
38. Ware LB, Matthay MA. The acute respiratory distress syndrome. *N Engl J Med* 2000;342:1334–1349.
39. Dushianthan A, Grocott MPW, Postle AD et al. Acute respiratory distress syndrome and acute lung injury. *Postgrad Med J* 2011;87:612–622.
40. Ashbaugh DG, Bigelow DB, Petty TL et al. Acute respiratory distress in adults. *Lancet* 1967;2:319–323.
41. Bernard GR, Artigas A, Brigham KL et al. The American-European Consensus Conference on ARDS. Definitions, mechanisms, relevant outcomes, and clinical trial coordination. *Am J Respir Crit Care Med* 1994;149:818–824.
42. Vadász I, Sznajder JI. Update in acute lung injury and critical care 2010. *Am J Respir Crit Care Med* 2011;183:1147–1152.
43. Rubenfeld GD, Caldwell E, Peabody E et al. Incidence and outcomes of acute lung injury. *N Engl J Med* 2005;353:1685–1693.
44. Munford RS. Normal responses to injury prevent systemic inflammation and can be immunosuppressive. *Am J Respir Crit Care Med* 2001;163:316–321.
45. Mizock BA. Pharmaconutrients in the management of acute respiratory distress syndrome and acute lung injury. *US Respir Dis* 2008;36:24–26.
46. Calder PC. n-3 Polyunsaturated fatty acids, inflammation, and inflammatory disease. *Am J Clin Nutr* 2006;83(Suppl.):1505S–1519S.
47. Kalish BT, Fallon EM, Puder M. A tutorial on fatty acid biology. *JPEN* 2012;36:380–388.
48. Calder PC. Use of fish oil in parenteral nutrition: Rationale and reality. *Proc Nutr Soc* 2006;65:264–277.
49. Magee P, Pearson S, Allen J. The omega-3 fatty acid, eicosapentaenoic acid (EPA), prevents the damaging effects of tumour necrosis factor (TNF)-alpha during murine skeletal muscle cell differentiation. *Lipids Health Dis* 2008;7:24–35.

50. Mizock BA. Nutritional support in acute lung injury and acute respiratory distress syndrome. *Nutr Clin Pract* 2001;16:319–328.
51. Saito M, Kubo K. Relationship between tissue lipid peroxidation and peroxidizability index after alpha-linolenic, eicosapentaenoic, or docosahexaenoic acid intake in rats. *Br J Nutr* 2003;89:19–28.
52. Hasselmann M, Hasselmann C. Benefits of parenteral lipids emulsions in acute respiratory failure. *Crit Care Shock* 2003;6:151–155.
53. Calder P. A novel effect of eicosapentaenoic acid: Improved diaphragm strength in endotoxemia. *Crit Care* 2010;14:143–144.
54. Gadek JE, DeMichele SJ, Karistad MD et al. Effect of feeding with eicosapentaenoic acid, gamma-linoleic acid, and antioxidant in patients with acute respiratory distress syndrome. Enteral Nutrition in ARDS Study Group. *Crit Care Med* 1999;27:1409–1420.
55. Patch ER, DeMichele SJ, Nelson JL et al. Enteral nutrition with eicosapentaenoic acid, γ-linolenic acid, and antioxidants reduces alveolar inflammatory mediators and protein influx in patients with acute respiratory distress syndrome. *Crit Care Med* 2003;31:491–500.
56. Singer P, Theilla M, Fisher H et al. Benefit of an enteral diet enriched with eicosapentaenoic acid and gamma-linolenic acid in ventilated patients with acute lung injury. *Crit Care Med* 2006;34:1033–1038.
57. Pontes-Arruda A, Albuquerque AM, Albuquerque JD et al. The effects of enteral feeding with eicosapentaenoic acid, γ-linolenic acid and antioxidants in mechanically ventilated patients with severe sepsis and septic shock. *Crit Care Med* 2006;34:2325–2333.
58. Pontes-Arruda A, DeMichele S, Seth A et al. The use of an inflammation-modulating diet in patients with acute lung injury or acute respiratory distress syndrome: A meta-analysis of outcome data. *JPEN* 2008;32:596–605.
59. Sabater J, Masclans JR, Sacanell J et al. Effects on hemodynamics and gas Exchange of omega-3 fatty acid-enriched lipid emulsion in acute respiratory distress syndrome (ARDS): A prospective, randomized, double-blind, parallel group study. *Lipids Health Dis* 2008;7:39–48.
60. Rice TW, Wheeler AP, Thompson BT et al. Enteral omega-3 fatty acid, γ-linolenic acid, and antioxidant supplementation in acute lung injury. *JAMA* 2011;306:1574–1581.
61. Stapleton RD, Martin TR, Weiss NS et al. A phase II randomized placebo-controlled trial of omega-3 fatty acids for the treatment of acute lung injury. *Crit Care Med* 2011;39:1655–1662.
62. Grau-Carmona T, Moran-Garcia V, García de Lorenzo A et al. Effect of an enteral diet enriched with eicosapentaenoic acid, gamma-linolenic acid and anti-oxidants on the outcome of mechanically ventilated, critically ill, septic patients. *Clin Nutr* 2011;30:578–584.
63. Barbosa VM, Miles EA, Calhau C et al. Effect of fish oil containing lipid emulsion on plasma phospholipid acids, inflammatory markers, and clinical outcomes in septic patients: A randomized, controlled clinical trial. *Crit Care* 2010;14:R5–R16.
64. Pontes-Arruda A, Ferreira LM, de Lima SM et al. Enteral nutrition with eicosapentaenoic acid, γ-linoleic acid and antioxidants in the early treatment of sepsis: Results from a multicenter, prospective, randomized, double-blinded, controlled study: The INTERSEPT study. *Crit Care* 2011;15:R144–R150.
65. McClave SA, Martindale RG, Vanek VW et al. Guidelines for the provision and assessment of nutrition support therapy in the adult critically ill patient: Society of Critical Care Medicine (SCCM) and American Society for Parenteral and Enteral Nutrition (ASPEN). *JPEN* 2009;33:277–316.
66. Sanchez Nava VM. Nutricion en insuficiencia respiratoria aguda. In: Anaya RP, Arenas H, Arenas D (eds.), *Nutrición enteral y parenteral*, 2nd edición. Mexico: McGraw-Hill, 2012, pp. 347–349.

28 Renal Failure

Tom Stone McNees

CONTENTS

INTRODUCTION

The kidney regulates fluid, electrolyte, acid–base, and metabolite balance and disorders of renal function will usually manifest with disruptions of homeostasis in these systems. Renal failure is often accompanied by severe malnutrition and inflammatory processes. In the critical care setting, as many as one in three admissions will develop some form of acute kidney injury (AKI).[1] Those cases severe enough to require renal replacement therapy (RRT) suffer high mortality, a situation which has persisted despite advances in medical technology and treatments.[2] This discussion of renal failure in critical care will address AKI in particular with consideration given to maintenance of dialysis patients seen in critical care.

ACUTE KIDNEY INJURY

A lack of widespread agreement regarding the definition of acute renal failure (ARF) and the hope for improving collaboration between international agencies led to the use of the term *acute kidney injury* (AKI) and formation of the Acute Kidney Injury Network (AKIN) in 2004.[3] Although the term *acute renal failure* (or ARF) is still in use, AKI will be preferred here. AKI may be better understood as a syndrome rather than a disease in itself, which may be marked by uremia, electrolyte abnormalities, acid–base disturbances, or fluid overload.[3,4] Few patients may be admitted to the ICU solely on the basis of renal failure, yet sources estimate 3%–30% of these admissions will develop AKI.[5] In Hoste et al., 16.2% of 185 septic patients developed AKI and 70% of these required RRT.[6] This is concerning for high morbidity and mortality in this group. Researchers report 60%–70% mortality in critically ill patients developing AKI severe enough to require RRT.[7–11] There is also good news in these data, however. In a very large, multicenter study, Metnitz et al. showed by multivariate analysis that most interventions (including mechanical ventilation, vasoactive medications, cardiopulmonary resuscitation, treatment for complicated metabolic alkalosis or acidosis, and parenteral nutrition) were independently predictive of increased mortality. Only one of the interventions studied—enteral nutrition support—was associated with improved survival. The possibility that this could be due to a lower severity of illness in patients receiving enteral nutrition was ruled out by statistical analysis. In the authors' words, "Instead, our results demonstrate an additional effect of enteral nutrition on survival."[10]

Categories and Etiology of Acute Kidney Injury

AKI may be described as *prerenal*, from causes related to hypovolemia or hypotension that lead to decreased renal perfusion, *postrenal*, resulting from urinary obstruction, or *intrinsic*, due to disorders of renal physiology.[12] Historically, AKI has been attributed to three predominate causes, all associated with acute tubular necrosis (ATN): intraoperative ischemia/hypotension, nephrotoxin exposure, and sepsis.[9] Investigations suggest more complex etiologies arising out of interactions between the initial insult(s) to the kidney and subsequent inflammatory and coagulopathic processes that may result.[3]

Decreased Renal Perfusion

Loss of blood or other intravascular fluid losses, including volume lost to extravascular space due to hypoproteinemia and low oncotic pressure, lead to decreased arterial blood volume and pressure. Hypotension and inflammation associated with sepsis, cardiac failure, or other causes impair delivery of blood and oxygen to the body's organs, including the kidneys. Regardless of cause, the effect is the same: decreased perfusion of the kidney and reduced glomerular filtration rate (GFR) with resulting impairment of renal function.[13]

Nephrotoxic Medication

Toxic causes of AKI have increased, but prognosis for survival in these cases is good—by one review, near 80%.[4] According to their mechanism of action, different drugs may impair renal function in different ways. It is possible for a medication to defeat intrinsic homeostatic mechanisms. With mild hypovolemia or hypotension, compensatory mechanisms may defend GFR, but medications including nonsteroidal anti-inflammatory drugs (NSAIDs), acetylcholine esterase (ACE) inhibitors, and angiotensin receptor blockers (ARBs) may limit the ability to restore hemodynamics.[13]

Some drugs may impair intrarenal circulation and GFR by vasoconstriction in the kidney without affecting overall hemodynamics; these include the immunosuppressives tacrolimus and cyclosporine.[14] While not drugs, conditions of sepsis and hypercalcemia may reduce GFR and lead to AKI in the same manner.[13]

TABLE 28.1
Medications May Alter Glomerular Hemodynamics

Agent	Action	Predisposing Factors
NSAIDs	Inhibit prostaglandin-mediated renal vasodilation	CHF, cirrhosis, ASVD, CRF, hypovolemia
ACE inhibitors	Inhibit renal vasoconstriction	As with NSAIDs
Calcineurin inhibitors (tacrolimus, cyclosporine)	May induce preglomerular vasoconstriction Possible irreversible effects	Hypovolemia, possible interaction with antihypertensives/anti-infectives
Amphotericin B	Disrupts tubular function, limiting urine concentration	Some diuretics, ↓GFR
Radiographic contrast	Acute vasoconstriction	GFR < 35mL/min, severe heart failure, diabetic nephropathy, large amounts of contrast
Cocaine	Vasoconstriction; rhabdomyolysis, acid–base, or electrolyte imbalance	Cocaine use

Sources: Information from Albright, R.C., *Mayo Clin. Proc.*, 76, 67, 2001; Tedesco, D. and Haragsim, L., *J. Transplant.*, 230386, 2012.

NSAID, nonsteroidal anti-inflammatory drugs; CHF, congestive heart failure; ASVD, atherosclerotic vascular disease; CRF, chronic renal failure; GFR, glomerular filtration rate.

Acyclovir nephrotoxicity was once relatively common but has become less so since high-dose bolus administration of the drug has been replaced by continuous infusions.[13] The nephrotoxic effects of cisplatin, amphotericin, and aminoglycoside antibiotics are related to cumulative dose history and the same is true for radiocontrast agents.[13] See Table 28.1 for a presentation of potentially nephrotoxic medications.

Sepsis and AKI

Hoste et al. studied the incidence of AKI in septic patients to identify characteristics of those patients who would later develop renal failure.[6] Patients who did develop AKI tended to have lower mean arterial blood pressure despite normal or higher central venous pressure or pulmonary artery occlusion (wedge) pressure. These patients were more likely to have received aggressive fluid loading and more likely to have received vasoactive medications.[6]

Looking at the patients who would go on to develop AKI, on the first day of sepsis, they were six times more likely to have pH less than 7.35 and 7.5 times more likely to have serum creatinine greater than 1.0 mg/dL.[6]

Nutritional Effects of Acute Kidney Injury

From a nutrition standpoint, consider that some treatments a patient may receive in the early stages of renal insufficiency can lead to difficulty in subsequent AKI. Fluids and vasoactive medications intended to be therapeutic in early stages of renal insufficiency could become problematic. Fluid given with hope of increasing GFR and urine output may later be in excess.[5] Diuretics given to remove fluid can fail if the fluid has already escaped to the extravascular or *third space* due to decreased oncotic pressure. This may leave the patient intravascularly *dry* yet still fluid overloaded.

Hyponatremia is often seen with AKI.[5] This may be dilutional, relating to fluid overload, but in cases of excessive fluid loss due to *third spacing* or gastrointestinal losses, a patient may exhibit hypovolemic hyponatremia.[5] Hyperkalemia is frequently present in AKI.[5] Accumulation of potassium may be due to impaired renal excretion secondary to nephrotoxic drugs or tissue damage, release

TABLE 28.2
Enteral Phosphate Binders

Drug Name	Sevelamer Carbonate (Renvela®)[a]	Sevelamer Hydrochloride (Renagel®)[a]	Lanthanum Carbonate (Fosrenol®)[b]	Calcium Acetate (Eliphos™, [c]PhosLo®, Phoslyra™ Liquid[d])	Calcium Carbonate Antacids
Route of administration	Oral; swallow whole	Oral; swallow whole	Oral; crush or chew	Oral; swallow whole	Oral; crush or chew
Initial dose	800 or 1600 mg three times daily	800 mg three times daily	1500 mg in divided doses	1334 mg three times daily	N/A
Dosage form and strengths	800 mg tablet; 800 and 2400 mg packets	400 and 800 mg tablet; 403 mg capsule	500, 750, and 1000 mg tablet	667 mg gelcap; 667 mg/5 mL oral solution	Chewable tablet
Elemental calcium per dosage form	N/A	N/A	N/A	168 mg	200 mg (500 mg tablet)

Data from manufacturers' published package insert information. (a) Sanofi-Aventis, Cambridge, MA. (b) Shire US, Wayne, PA. (c) Hawthorn Pharmaceuticals, Madison, MS. (d) Fresenius Medical Care, Waltham, MA. Table preparation assistance Joyce Marshall, PharmD.

of potassium from cells lost to catabolism or lysis, or it may simply result from exogenous potassium delivery through nutrition support or medical overcorrection.[5] AKI interferes with homeostasis of phosphorous, calcium, and magnesium.[15] Phosphorous and magnesium can accumulate to high levels, which may be managed by limiting exogenous sources.[15] Hyperphosphatemia may be improved by RRT, although difficult or severe cases may prove refractory to dialysis. Absorption of phosphorous from the GI tract may be inhibited by the use of phosphate binders concurrent with enteral feeding, see Table 28.2 for information on selected phosphate-binding products. Note that one calcium acetate product is available as an oral solution, a form better suited for administration per feeding tube. Aluminum-based phosphate binders were omitted from the table due to concerns regarding the possibility of adverse effects that could be related to aluminum administration. Hypocalcemia is typical with AKI, and in many cases, this will be mild to moderate.[16] Calcium supplementation will usually be indicated only if hypocalcemia is severe or symptomatic, as may be the case with rhabdomyolysis or pancreatitis, or after the patient has received large amounts of bicarbonate.[15]

Impaired carbohydrate metabolism is characteristic of AKI.[17,18] Hyperglycemia in AKI is often associated with insulin resistance and hyperinsulinemia; insulin-mediated glucose uptake into skeletal muscle can be decreased by as much as 50%.[5,17] High serum glucose is exacerbated by accelerated gluconeogenesis, which is supported by catabolism and, unfortunately, cannot be suppressed by provision of exogenous glucose.[5,17,18] Effective insulin therapy is the key to maintaining euglycemia during administration of appropriate carbohydrate loads. Disturbances in lipid metabolism may lead to hypertriglyceridemia with AKI, due in large part to impaired lipolysis.[18] Serum levels of low-density and very-low-density lipoproteins are increased and high-density lipoproteins commonly decreased.[17] Limits on lipid clearance have been shown to affect both long- and medium-chain triglycerides given as parenteral emulsions.[17,18]

Of all the nutrition-related factors associated with AKI, a dominant feature is increased protein catabolism. In ARF, hepatic gluconeogenesis is stimulated and amino acids that are released from skeletal muscle catabolism are the substrates for this pathway. At the same time, protein synthesis is impaired and amino acid transport into skeletal muscle is inhibited as well.[19] An important catabolic stimulus in AKI is metabolic acidosis, and correction of acidosis is likely to improve protein and amino acid metabolism present in AKI.[19] Other causes also stimulate protein breakdown in AKI. Catabolic hormones, including catecholamines, glucagon, and glucocorticoids, are released along with proinflammatory cytokines, creating a hypercatabolic effect.[19,20]

The catabolic insult from AKI is exacerbated with RRT. Not only are nutritional substrates (serum proteins, amino acids) lost to dialysis, but production of inflammatory mediators in response to bioincompatibility with dialyzer membranes—as well as those arising out of the primary disease process—can stimulate further breakdown of somatic proteins.[19]

Unfortunately, limits to catabolism that defend lean mass in fasting healthy individuals do not protect those with critical illness, trauma, or sepsis whose loss of serum, somatic, and visceral proteins may be very great.[21] If it is understood that net protein loss is obligatory and irreversible by the administration of exogenous substrate proteins, then a primary goal of nutrition therapy should be to provide optimal support so that adverse effects of losses may be minimized.[19]

RENAL REPLACEMENT THERAPY (RRT)

RRT may be indicated in AKI with severe uremia, hyperkalemia, fluid overload, or metabolic acidosis.[13] RRT will not shorten the duration of renal failure; rather, it is utilized to ease metabolic consequences until renal recovery can take place.[13,15] Recovery will usually begin from 7 to 21 days following renal injury, but it may take as long as 6 months.[13] Different modes of RRT have been developed to accomplish the same goals in significantly different ways.

Modes of RRT

Intermittent hemodialysis (IHD) was the first mechanical form of RRT developed as an alternative to PD (see the following text) and a cornerstone of treatment in AKI for over 30 years.[15] IHD is usually applied 3–4 h daily or on alternate days, depending on the needs of the patient.[13,15] The need to remove water and solutes in a relatively short time requires removal and processing of large volumes of blood, which can result in interdialytic hypotension.[13,15] This may be especially problematic in critically ill patients with concurrent hypoalbuminemia, intravascular fluid loss, and septic vasodilatation, leading to hypotension even without RRT. In these cases, a continuous treatment modality may be employed.

A number of continuous renal replacement therapies (CRRTs) have been developed that vary in specific technical details of operation but share common features.[13] By removing and treating blood slowly over an extended period of time, these processes control uremia and fluid, electrolyte, and acid–base imbalances with minimal disruption of hemodynamic stability or plasma osmolality.[13]

PD is accomplished by the infusion of fluid into the peritoneum that is relatively isotonic but contains a lower concentration of electrolytes that are to be removed so that uremic wastes and high concentration electrolytes will diffuse across the peritoneal membrane into it, which is subsequently drained and eliminated.[22] Like continuous RRT, PD takes place slowly and therefore is less likely to cause hypotension.[13,22] Although the use of PD has declined in contemporary acute care settings, it can be accomplished with the use of simpler technologies, which makes it practicable in remote or disadvantaged areas where IHD or CRRT may be less available.[13,15]

Nutritional Effects of RRT

Hemodialysis and hemofiltration remove amino acids at rates from 3 to 5 g/h, and these losses have been considered in published nutrient recommendations for patients receiving RRT.[5,17,23–25] Bellomo reports there is little information available regarding nutrient losses in critically ill patients receiving IHD but has found support for recommendations in patients treated by CRRTs.[23] There is no significant loss of serum lipids in CRRT or in other forms of extracorporeal RRT.[18,23] If the replacement fluid used in RRT is rich in glucose (significantly higher in glucose concentration than blood levels), then the patient may be expected to gain approximately 500 kcal/day from glucose absorption at a dialysate flow rate of 1 L/h and proportionately more with higher flow rates or dialysate concentration.[23] Dialysate containing very low levels of glucose with patients receiving parenteral dextrose has resulted in a mean loss of infused glucose from the patient to the replacement fluid of 4%.[24]

The use of lactate as a buffer in CRRT replacement fluid can contribute to caloric gain by the patient, estimated to be from 300 to 400 additional kcal per day, with this variable influenced by not only the rate of dialysate flow but also the site of administration.[23]

NUTRITION MANAGEMENT IN ACUTE KIDNEY INJURY

Doctor Wilfred Druml wrote: "…there can be no doubt that nutritional therapy presents a cornerstone in the in the treatment of patients with ARF. Preexisting and/or hospital-acquired malnutrition have been identified as important factors contributing to the persisting high mortality in acutely ill patients with ARF."[17] Guidelines for nutrition management traditionally applied in cases of chronic renal failure (CRF) have been replaced by an approach that is intended to address more specifically the needs of the patient with AKI.[17] Recommendations for nutrition support with patients in AKI generally parallel those for other critically ill patients without AKI.[18] Table 28.3 compares guidelines for nutrition support in AKI published since 2000, and reflects a significant departure from the traditional norm whereby protein restriction was commonly applied. The kidney in a healthy state provides many homeostatic influences on metabolism that may be impaired or disabled in acute injury. For this reason, careful monitoring and accurate therapy targets are particularly important in this patient population.

ENERGY

Recommendations for energy intake for patients with AKI published by Druml in 1998 are the most restrictive shown in Table 28.3.[19] The author pointed out that hypermetabolic conditions rarely exceed 130% of *calculated basic energy expenditure* and any complications there may be from slightly underfeeding would be less significant than those resulting from overfeeding. For this reason, it was advised that patients with AKI should receive 25–30 kcal/kg of body weight per day.[17] Kapadia et al.[5] conclude that higher energy intakes are required in severe AKI than in

TABLE 28.3
Digest of Recommendations for Nutrition Support in Acute Kidney Injury with RRT

Author	Publication Date	Protein/AA (g/kg)	Energy (kcal/kg)	Micronutrient Supplement	Notes
Druml[17]	2001	1.0–1.5	25–35	Water-soluble vitamins	Ascorbate < 200 mg
Bellomo[23]	2002	1.5–2.0	30–35	Ascorbate, B6, folate, Zn, Se	IED "yes," early feeding "yes," renal-specific formulas "no"
Kapadia[5]	2003	1.5	35 (NPC)	Water-soluble vitamins IED "yes," early as feasible	NPC: 60% CHO, 40% lipid
Scheinkestel[24]	2003	2.5	100% as measured or predicted		
Cano[28]	2006	1.0–1.5, up to 1.7	25–30 (NPC)	Ascorbate not to exceed 30–50 mg/day	EN preferred; std. high-protein formula vs. IED unclear
Brown[49]	2010	Based on individualized assessment considering PCR, GFR, and markers of inflammation			std. parenteral AA formulations recommended
Fiaccadori[20]	2011	1.5–2.0	25–30	Water-soluble vitamins	Close attention to changing needs essential

RRT, renal replacement therapy; IED, immune-enhancing diet; NPC, nonprotein calories; SNS, specialized nutrition support; PCR, protein catabolic rate; GFR, glomerular filtration rate; AA, amino acids.

isolated or uncomplicated disease and recommend 35 *nonprotein* kcal per kg in addition to whatever energy may be contributed by protein. Bellomo recommends early (and enteral) administration of 30–35 kcal/kg and does not specifically exclude the contribution of protein from calculations of energy provided.[23] Scheinkestel et al. determined energy requirements of AKI patients in their study by direct measurement with a metabolic cart whenever possible, which they were able to do in 68% of subjects.[24] In the remaining 32%, energy needs were calculated by the use of predictive equation. The group attempted to provide each patient with 100% of measured or calculated energy needs as early in their treatment as they could. They highlight the relationship between energy intake and nitrogen balance and the likelihood that energy insufficiency will make achievement of positive or even neutral nitrogen balance very difficult. In the authors' words: "The difference between a surplus and a deficit in supplied energy may be critical in achieving a positive nitrogen balance."

Amino Acids and Protein

Given the hypercatabolic nature of severe AKI and the risk presented by loss of muscle and solid organ mass, protein requirements for these patients receive a great deal of attention. In 1998, Druml reviewed the literature of the time and found no support for delivery of protein in excess of 1.3–1.5 g/kg except in cases of continuous hemofiltration or peritoneal dialysis (PD) where an additional 0.2 g/kg was allowed, or up to a total of 1.7 g/kg.[19] He emphasized that protein in excess of these recommendations would only increase uremia and need for dialysis, a position which is reinforced in a 2001 publication by the same author.[17] Nevertheless, study results show that protein losses in severe AKI can exceed 150 g/day, and increasing protein delivery from less than 1 to as much as 2.5 g/kg improves nitrogen balance in a nearly linear manner.[23] Macias et al.[26] found that positive nitrogen balance could be achieved in patients with AKI receiving CRRT with a protein delivery of 1.5–1.8 g/kg/day. Kierdorf[18] reports similar findings of positive nitrogen balance in groups receiving 1.5 and 1.74 g of amino acids per kg per day and azotemia in these patients was well controlled by CRRT. (Kierdorf's subjects in all groups received 30 non-protein kcal per kg per day.)

In their study reported in 2003, Scheinkestel et al. tested nutrition support providing 1.5, 2.0, and 2.5 g of protein or amino acids per kg.[24] Recall that these subjects, as described earlier, were provided energy as close as possible to their measured (when available) or calculated needs. Nitrogen balance was assessed as protein delivery was increased for each experimental subject. Investigators found that nitrogen balance was very significantly more likely to be achieved when protein intake was greater than 2 g/kg/day. Nitrogen balance in these subjects was not just a technical success but associated directly with positive hospital and ICU outcomes. In fact, statistical analysis in this study revealed that for every gram increase in daily nitrogen balance, the probability of patient survival increased by 21%.

Micronutrient Supplementation

Reports to date have found no controlled trials to provide firm support for micronutrient supplementation in AKI.[18,24,27] Given such lack of evidence, it may seem reasonable to provide at least the recommended daily allowance (RDA) for vitamins and minerals.[23,27] Water-soluble vitamins are lost with RRT, and some sources recommend additional supplements.[5,17,18,23] Ascorbic acid, however, is a precursor of oxalic acid and excessive vitamin C may lead to oxalosis, aggravating AKI.[17,18] Supplemental vitamin C doses should be limited, but specific recommendations for ascorbate in AKI do range widely. Specifications vary from *not more than 30 to 50 mg*[28] to *at least 100 mg*[23] to *not more than 250 mg*.[18] It is noteworthy that the lowest dose recommendation for ascorbate, less than 50 mg daily, is a consensus guideline published by the European Society for Clinical Nutrition and Metabolism (ESPEN) in 2006.[28] Significant losses of folic acid and vitamin B6 have been documented with CRRT, and additional supplementation of these nutrients has been recommended.[23]

Levels of fat-soluble vitamins A, D, and E are found to be decreased in AKI (for A and E, this is unlike CRF), while vitamin K may be normal or even higher with AKI.[17]

Enteral Nutrition in AKI

In a study of critically ill patients with AKI, enteral feeding was singled out as the one factor independent of any other intervention that was clearly associated with improved outcomes.[24] Benefits of enteral feeding in the critically ill are well recognized and include preservation of intestinal barrier function and gut-mediated immunity; risk for infectious complications is lower in patients who are enterally fed. Enteral feeding has been shown to improve renal function when AKI is induced in experimental animals and is generally accepted as the preferred modality for nutrition support in critically ill patients with AKI.[29,30]

Commercially available enteral feeding formulas designed for renal failure patients on dialysis are included in Table 28.4, which provides a view of two products designed for use in AKI and two intended for use with CRF patients. In view of the preceding discussion regarding optimal protein and energy dosing for patients with AKI, a review of the nutrient composition of available renal formulas shows that products on the market show improvements over their predecessors. The two formulas designed for AKI are similar in caloric density, providing 1.8–2 kcal/mL. The protein content in both of these products is 18% of calories provided. Feeding one of these formulas at a rate sufficient to provide 30 kcal/kg will deliver approximately 1.2–1.4 g of protein per kg, and increasing the feeding rate to provide 35 kcal/kg will yield approximately 1.6–1.7 g of protein per kg. Reformulation of these *condition-specific* formulas in recent years enables practitioners to adhere more closely to contemporary guidelines for treatment using unmodified products, potentially improving the accuracy, efficiency, and safety of delivery.

An option for enteral support of the patient with AKI is the use of an *immune-enhancing diet* (IED) formula with 80–90 or more grams of protein per liter and 1.3–1.5 kcal energy per milliliter. With an IED delivering 30–35 kcal/kg, the regimen can meet a goal of 2 or more grams of protein per kilogram. Supplemental arginine as these products may contain is a metabolic precursor to nitric oxide, which has been associated with increased renal perfusion and oxygenation.[31,32] The emerging view of AKI as an immune or toxic state rather than a hemodynamic one suggests another possible benefit may be derived from the anti-inflammatory and immune-modulating properties of the IED.[33] In this respect, marine-sourced lipids or *fish oils* in these products may provide inflammation-reducing benefit. However, higher levels of antioxidant vitamins, ascorbate in particular, could exceed recommendations. Authors have advocated the use of IED in AKI, and as with any product, consideration of appropriateness for a particular patient should be of primary concern.

TABLE 28.4
Selected Characteristics of Renal-Specific Enteral Formulas

Product	kcal/mL	Protein (per L)	Potassium (per L)	Phosphorous (per L)	Water (per L)	n-6:n-3 Lipids
[a]Nepro®	1.8	81 g	27.2 mEq	720 mg	727 g	5.2:1
[b]Novasource® Renal	2.0	90.7 g	24 mEq	819 mg	717 g	2.2:1
[b]Renalcal®	2.0	34.4 g	2 mEq	100 mg	700 g	3.4:1
[a]Suplena®	1.8	45 g	29.1 mEq	717 mg	738 g	5.2:1

Manufacturers' published data. (a) Abbott Nutrition, Columbus, OH. (b) Nestle Clinical Nutrition, Deerfield, IL.

In the event that metabolic needs cannot be met with enteral feeding alone, parenteral nutrition support may be indicated.[5,23] See Chapter 15 for further discussion on renal enteral formulations.

Parenteral Nutrition (PN) in AKI

In the previously discussed study reported by Scheinkestel et al., 54% of the AKI patients were supported enterally, 30% with a combination of EN and PN, and in 16% of their subjects, the authors conclude, "…the enteral route failed completely."[24] In a survey of Canadian ICU practices, 12% of patients on nutrition support received parenteral only.[34] Some patients inevitably will exhibit a degree of intolerance to enteral feeding, and for them, it will be necessary to provide at least part of their metabolic needs parenterally.

Parenteral nutrition has the advantage of being readily adjustable to meet specific macro- or micronutrient needs of an individual patient and can be formulated to provide the balance of metabolic requirements when provision of adequate enteral support is not possible. In a 2007 report, a small group of subjects receiving 150 g parenteral amino acids daily versus 75 g in isocaloric PN (2000 kcal for both groups) had improved nitrogen balance and improved fluid balance with less diuretic requirement.[35]

Preparation of a parenteral nutrition formula for the patient with AKI should take into account the volume status of the patient and the frequency and intensity of RRT the patient may be receiving. If volume status is at risk for overload and facility capabilities permit, nutrients can be delivered in minimal volume, maximally concentrated form. Recall that patients with AKI typically exhibit some degree of carbohydrate intolerance.[17,18] To decrease the rate of parenteral dextrose infusion, a greater part of the nonprotein energy in the formula may be provided by lipid emulsion; however, exogenous insulin may still be necessary to control glycemia.

Automatic compounding simplifies parenteral nutrition ordering, as specifications may be easily accommodated, but it is not available in every hospital. Premixed PN solutions gaining acceptance in many facilities may be suitable for use with AKI patients if macronutrient and fluid dosing compromise yields a formula consistent with guidelines. Some cases of AKI presenting with particularly challenging electrolyte balance will require use of electrolyte-free versions of premixed PN so that micronutrient needs can be met with no excess. When available capabilities are limited, a model for renal PN has been suggested that is simply ordered: 500 mL each of glucose, lipids, and amino acids, concentration of each determined by patient requirements. Water- and fat-soluble vitamins are recommended daily, limiting total ascorbate to 200 mg or less. Trace minerals twice weekly are recommended, and electrolytes and insulin should be added as needed.[17]

Glutamine and Arginine in AKI

The possibility that supplemental arginine or enteral formulas containing added arginine may be beneficial in various disease states has been the subject of study and debate for several years. Arginine and nitric oxide (NO) for which it serves as substrate have been shown to improve renal function when impairment is related to vasoconstriction and reduced perfusion, and to reduce the nephrotoxic effects of cyclosporine.[32] On the other hand, inflammatory conditions may result in production of large amounts of NO sufficient to cause tissue damage. This is a key feature of the host response to infection, but has raised questions about the appropriateness of arginine supplementation in AKI associated with inflammation as in glomerulonephritis.[32,36] Schramm et al.[37] looked at this question and found the pathological actions of NO were not related to supplemental arginine administration. Arginine retains potential as an adjunct to therapy for AKI based primarily on animal studies; therefore, clinical utility of the supplement remains undetermined.[38]

With regard to glutamine, Druml reports that a post hoc (after the study was published) analysis of data from a study in critically ill patients suggested patients with AKI showed benefit from glutamine supplementation more than other patients.[17,39] Of the survivors in this study, patients with AKI numbered 4 out of 24 in the group that did not receive glutamine, but 14 of 23 survivors in the glutamine group had AKI.[17] These data are suggestive of benefit, while firm recommendations await the publication of conclusive clinical trials.[23]

CHRONIC AND END-STAGE RENAL FAILURE PATIENT IN THE ICU

Critically ill patients with renal failure should not be restricted from adequate nutrition intervention.[23] Recommendations from a 2002 report to the *6th International Conference on CRRT* specify that full nutrition support should be provided to all critically ill patients with renal failure including acute, chronic, and end-stage renal failure.[23] In order to follow these recommendations, appropriate dialysis therapy must be available.

Maintenance Dialysis and Albumin

The patient with severe CRF or end-stage renal disease (ESRD), typically receiving maintenance dialysis treatments on a routine schedule prior to admission to the ICU, commonly exhibits both protein-energy malnutrition and multiple micronutrient deficiencies.[40,41] This state of being has been attributed to poor dietary intake, loss of substrate to RRT, hypermetabolism, and inflammatory response; it is often marked by hypoalbuminemia.[40] Albumin depletion in maintenance dialysis patients has been related less to protein intake or protein catabolic rate (PCR) than to inflammation as marked by C-reactive protein (CRP) or other measures.[40] In Pifer et al. decreased serum albumin was independently associated with mortality but protein intake or PCR was not.[42] This supports the use of serum albumin as a prognostic indicator in renal failure patients but not as a marker of nutrition status or adequacy of nutrition support.

Nutrient Deficiencies and Recommendations in Maintenance Dialysis Patients

Low serum albumin may be seen concurrently with decreased nutrient intake and hepatic reprioritization of synthesis due to inflammation, however, and the National Cooperative Dialysis Study reveals average protein and energy intake of chronic dialysis patients is far less than recommended to maintain nitrogen and energy balance.[40,43,44]

Maintenance dialysis patients commonly suffer from micronutrient deficiencies, with the most prominent among vitamin deficiencies being ascorbate, folate, B-6, and calcitriol.[41] Trace element deficiencies of iron, zinc, and possibly selenium are noted in this population, and toxicity from aluminum and copper is seen.[41] If studies with dialysis patients suggest inadequate intake or greater needs are frequently seen in this population, then this should be taken into account when the maintenance dialysis patient is seen in critical care. See Table 28.5 for micronutrient recommendations for the maintenance dialysis patient.

The provision of full nutrition support to chronic and end-stage renal failure patients in critical care, as recommended, requires prioritizing each patient's concurrent medical problems and designing the optimal nutrition care plan accordingly.[23] Traditionally, limiting fluid intake to prevent overload and restricting protein to reduce accumulation of nitrogenous wastes created significant obstacles to nutrition support. Contemporary renal replacement therapies enable control of fluid balance and azotemia so that metabolic needs of critically ill patients with renal failure can be more fully met.

MONITORING NUTRITION INTERVENTION IN AKI

If it is given that the exact cause of hypercatabolism in AKI cannot be clearly stated, and that net nitrogen loss is unavoidable, then achieving the goal of minimizing protein loss requires some practicable method of measuring nitrogen balance in order to provide optimal support.[16,19]

TABLE 28.5
Micronutrient Daily Recommendations for Maintenance Dialysis (MD) Patients

Micronutrient	Daily Recommendation	Note
Vitamin B-1	1.1–1.2 mg	Same as for non-MD patients
Vitamin B-2	1.1–1.3 mg	Same as for non-MD patients
Pantothenic acid	5 mg	Same as for non-MD patients
Biotin	30 μg	Same as for non-MD patients
Niacin	14–16 mg	Same as for non-MD patients
Vitamin B-6	10 mg	Removed by hemodialysis
Vitamin B-12	2.4 μg	Same as for non-MD patients
Ascorbate	75–90 mg	Risk for oxalosis with excessive intake
Folic acid	1 mg	Removed by hemodialysis
Vitamin A	800–1000 μg	Vulnerable to toxicity, do not exceed RDA
Vitamin D	0.25–1.0 μg	MD patients often deficient unless supplemented
Vitamin E	400–800 IU (optional)	Effectiveness uncertain, apparently safe
Vitamin K	Not specified	Supplement IF not eating AND receiving antibiotic therapy
Iron	Not specified	Deficiency common in MD patients, parenteral supplementation preferred
Zinc	RDA (15 mg enteral)	More definitive studies needed
Selenium	Not specified	Losses to dialysate, low serum levels typical in MD patients
Copper	Not specified	Essential but excess can cause hemolytic anemia

Source: Information from Kalantar-Zadeh, K. and Kopple, J.D., *Adv. Ren. Replace. Ther.*, 10(3), 170, 2003.

In some cases, it may be possible to monitor and track blood urea nitrogen (BUN) levels as they respond to changes in protein delivery and removal by RRT although antibiotics such as tigecycline work by inhibiting protein synthesis and may elevate measured BUN levels beyond nutritional influences and without inhibiting renal function.[45,46]

A number of factors confound interpretation of serum protein levels in AKI. Fluid gains reduce measured serum levels and fluid losses increase them; in both cases, these changes are unrelated to protein nutriture and nitrogen balance. Diversion of protein synthesis into acute-phase products may be reflected by lower levels of albumin and prealbumin despite provision of adequate protein; at the same time, decreased renal clearance of proteins may lead to exaggerated serum levels and a false confidence with inadequate support.

In order to measure the effectiveness of nutrition support, nitrogen balance is calculated and can provide a useful guide to therapy. It should be noted, however, that nitrogen balance studies are limited in AKI by loss of urinary nitrogen excretion.[22] They must be interpreted with careful awareness of potentially significant confounding factors.

Nitrogen Balance

A method for assessing nitrogen balance is suggested in Suleiman and Zaloga, where nitrogen output is estimated from urea nitrogen appearance (UNA).[47]

To calculate UNA, sum

- Urinary urea nitrogen (g/day) +
- Dialysate urea nitrogen (g/day) +
- Change in body urea nitrogen (CBUN), where CBUN(g/day) = SUN2(g/L) − SUN1(g/L) × BW2 × (0.6 L/kg) + (BW2 − BW1) × SUN2 × (1.0 L/kg)

In this equation, 1 (as in SUN1, BW1) identifies the initial value for the study period and 2 is the final value. Serum urea nitrogen (SUN) is functionally equivalent to BUN, and BW is weight in kilograms.

Once UNA has been calculated in this manner, then *total nitrogen output* is estimated to be the sum of UNA + 2. The patient's net *nitrogen balance* = total nitrogen output – total nitrogen intake (where nitrogen intake is calculated from protein intake in grams by multiplying by 0.16).

CASE REPORT

The measure of a patient's response to care is their outcome. In the following example, extreme obesity complicated estimation of the patient's metabolic needs under RRT. Forty-year-old patient *Mrs. D.* had a history of reasonably good health except for her weight, which had been a problem for her since childhood. With a BMI of 66, the patient elected to undergo a sleeve gastrectomy, where the capacity of the stomach is limited by removing a section along the greater curvature, which is then stapled or sutured back together. This procedure has gained popularity because it is associated with infrequent complications and favorable outcomes.[48] Unfortunately in this case, the patient developed a gastric leak postoperatively and required transfer to the surgical intensive care unit (SICU) for intubation and mechanical ventilation.

Assessment

Mrs. D. was reassessed in the SICU with a weight just over 200 kg and height of 69 in. In discussion with the surgeon, concerns were expressed that delivery of calculated energy needs could result in weight maintenance for the patient who was, after all, hoping to lose weight. With the possibility of RRT on the horizon and the reality of nonhealing surgical wounds becoming apparent, the importance of adequate nutrition support was emphasized. It was agreed that the team would attempt to provide 25 kcal and 1.5 g protein per kg of *ideal body weight* in this case to start.

Intervention

The surgeon had wisely provided jejunostomy access during the original gastrectomy procedure so the patient was able to receive enteral nutrition soon after arrival in the ICU. A peptide-based critical care formula with fish oil met the macronutrient targets at a rate of 65 mL/h with sterile water flushes provided at 25 mL/h, for an approximate total of 1750 kcal, 105 g protein, and 1750 mL water daily.

Response

Net fluid balance was negative for the first few days, and hypophosphatemia (2.0 mg/dL) as well as ionized hypocalcemia (0.94 mg/dL) were addressed. Blood glucose over 180 mg/dL demanded treatment and a trial of subcutaneous insulin proved ineffective as expected, with glycemia climbing to over 275 mg/dL. An intravenous insulin infusion was begun and euglycemia established soon after. By the fourth day in the SICU, the patient's serum creatinine was over 6 mg/dL and the need for RRT was becoming apparent. Initiation of RRT was delayed by difficulties obtaining vascular access, and a new hyperphosphatemia developed with levels now over 7 and 8 mg/dL. The enteral formula was changed to a renal-specific product containing minimal phosphorous. While awaiting dialysis, ionized hypocalcemia developed again (0.97 mg/dL), which was treated with 2 g calcium gluconate by a very slow intravenous drip over 12 h. Enteral feeding was held almost 24 h pending placement of the dialysis access catheter, but this was eventually accomplished and feeding with the original critical-care formula resumed immediately after. Enteral feeding continued with IHD as needed until a suspicious abdominal fluid collection caused a hold and the patient was transitioned to total parenteral nutrition (TPN) for 7 days until it could be surgically confirmed that the leak was gastric in origin. The jejunostomy feeding resumed to replace TPN and continues. IHD continued while complications including intra-abdominal sepsis and the persistent gastric leak were treated.

A stent was placed around the remnant stomach in order to reapproximate the surgical borders and remained until recovery was complete. At the time of this writing, antibiotic therapy continues but the need for RRT is steadily decreasing and abdominal wounds are healing well. Phosphorous levels were stable within normal limits for a time then rose again, to be treated enterally this time with calcium acetate, two 667 mg tablets per jejunostomy tube *qid* (see Table 28.2). The patient remains NPO with continuous drainage per nasogastric tube and ventilated per tracheostomy but shows clear signs of improvement. The entire care team expects Mrs. D.'s transfer to a rehabilitation facility with continuing treatment and her full recovery in due time.

SUMMARY

The critically ill patient who has developed severe AKI may be among the more difficult and complicated to support by enteral nutrition, but evidence is clear that no other aspect of their care is equally and independently associated with improving their chances for survival. Not only enteral but also adequate medical support is essential. To know that every gram increase in nitrogen balance for these patients improves probability of survival, 21% should give clinicians a sense of empowerment and responsibility to advocate for timely and appropriate therapy. In few clinical scenarios, interdisciplinary communication and cooperation is so necessary and overcoming traditional barriers is as important as it is when caring for the patient with severe AKI.

REFERENCES

1. Lipsey, M. and Bellomo, R., Septic acute kidney injury: Hemodynamic syndrome, inflammatory disorder, or both? *Crit. Care*, 15(6), 1008, 2011.
2. Singbartl, K. and Kellum, J.A., AKI in the ICU: Definition, epidemiology, risk stratification, and outcomes, *Kidney Int.*, 81(9), 819–825, 2012.
3. Mehta, R.L. et al., Acute kidney injury network, report of an initiative to improve outcomes in acute kidney injury, *Crit. Care*, 11(2), R31, 2007.
4. Chew, S.L. et al., Outcome in acute kidney injury, *Nephrol. Dial. Transplant.*, 8, 101, 1993.
5. Kapadia, F.N., Bhojani, K., and Shah, B., Special issues in the patient with renal failure, *Crit. Care Clin.*, 19, 233, 2003.
6. Hoste, A.J. et al., Acute kidney injury in patients with sepsis in a surgical ICU: Predictive factors, incidence, comorbidity, and outcome, *J. Am. Soc. Nephrol.*, 14, 1022, 2003.
7. Strejc, J.M., Considerations in the nutritional management of patients with acute kidney injury, *Hemodial. Int.*, 9, 135–142, 2005.
8. Uchino, S. et al., Beginning and ending supportive therapy for the kidney (BEST Kidney) investigators: Acute renal failure in critically ill patients: A multinational, multicenter study, *JAMA*, 294(7), 813–818, 2005.
9. Chertow, G.M. et al., Prognostic stratification in critically ill patients with acute kidney injury requiring dialysis, *Arch. Intern. Med.*, 155, 1505, 1995.
10. Metnitz, G.H. et al., Effect of acute kidney injury requiring renal replacement therapy on outcome in critically ill patients, *Crit. Care Med.*, 30, 2051, 2002.
11. Clermont, G. et al., Renal failure in the ICU: Comparison of the impact of acute kidney injury and end-stage renal disease on ICU outcomes, *Kidney Int.*, 62, 986, 2002.
12. Albright, R.C., Acute kidney injury: A practical update, *Mayo Clin. Proc.*, 76, 67, 2001.
13. Lennon, A.-M., Coleman, P.L., and Brady, H.R., Management and outcome of acute kidney injury, in *Comprehensive Clinical Nephrology*, Johnson, R.J. and Feehally, J., Eds. Harcourt Publishers Limited, Edinburgh, U.K., Chap. 19, 2000.
14. Tedesco, D. and Haragsim, L., Cyclosporine: A review, *J. Transplant.*, 2012, Article ID 230386, 2012.
15. Brady, H.R. et al., Acute kidney injury, in *Brenner and Rector's the Kidney*, Brenner, B.M., Ed. W.B. Saunders, Philadelphia, PA, p. 1241, 2000.
16. Anderson, R.J. and Schrier, R.W., Acute kidney injury, in *Diseases of the Kidney and Urinary Tract*, 7th edn., Schrier, R.W., Ed. Lippincott Williams & Wilkins, Philadelphia, PA, p. 1119, 2001.
17. Druml, W., Nutritional management of acute kidney injury, *Am. J. Kidney Dis.*, 37, S89, 2001.

18. Kierdorf, H.P., The nutritional management of acute kidney injury in the intensive care unit, *New Horiz.*, 3, 699, 1995.
19. Druml, W., Protein metabolism in acute kidney injury, *Miner. Electrolyte Metab.*, 24, 47, 1998.
20. Fiaccadori, E., Cremaschi, E., and Regolisti, G., Nutritional assessment and delivery in renal replacement therapy patients, *Semin. Dial.*, 24, 169–175, 2011.
21. Hoogerwerf, M., Nutritional aspects of acute kidney injury, *EDTNA/ERCA J.*, (Suppl. 2), 54, 2002.
22. Gennari, F.J. and Rimmer, J.M., The dialysis patient, in *Massry and Glassock's Textbook of Nephrology*, 4th edn., Massry, S.G. and Glassock, R.J., Eds. Lippincott Williams & Wilkins, Philadelphia, PA, p. 1387, 2001.
23. Bellomo, R., How to feed patients with renal dysfunction, *Blood Purif.*, 20, 296, 2002.
24. Scheinkestel, C.D. et al., Prospective randomized trial to assess caloric and protein needs of critically ill, anuric, ventilated patients requiring continuous renal replacement therapy, *Nutrition*, 19, 909, 2003.
25. Cerra, F.B. et al., Applied nutrition in ICU patients: A consensus statement of the American College of Chest Physicians, *Chest*, 111, 769, 1997.
26. Macias, W.L. et al., Impact of the nutritional regimen on protein catabolism and nitrogen balance in patients with acute kidney injury, *JPEN*, 20, 56, 1996.
27. Wolk, R., Nutrition in renal failure, in *The Science and Practice of Nutrition Support: A Case-Based Core Curriculum*, M. Gottschlich, (Ed.), A.S.P.E.N./Kendall Hunt, Dubuque, IA, Chap. 28, 2001.
28. Cano, N. et al., ESPEN guidelines on enteral nutrition: Adult renal failure, *Clin. Nutr.*, 25, 295–310, 2006.
29. Druml, W. and Mitch, W.E., Enteral nutrition in renal disease, in *Enteral and Tube Feeding*, Rombeau, J.L. and Rolandelli, R.H., Eds. Saunders, Philadelphia, PA, Chap. 26, 1997.
30. Roberts, P.R., Black, K.W., and Zaloga, G.P., Enteral feeding improves outcomes and protects against glycerol-induced acute kidney injury in the rat, *Am. J. Respir. Crit. Care Med.*, 156, 1265, 1997.
31. Herselman, M., Protein and energy requirements in patients with acute kidney injury on continuous renal replacement therapy, *Nutrition*, 19, 813, 2003.
32. Efron, D.T. and Barbul, A., Arginine and nutrition in renal disease, *J. Ren. Nutr.*, 9, 142, 1999.
33. Wan, L. et al., The pathogenesis of septic acute kidney injury, *Curr. Opin. Crit. Care*, 9, 496, 2003.
34. Heyland, D.K. et al., Nutrition support in the critical care setting: Current practice in Canadian ICUs—Opportunities for improvement? *JPEN*, 27, 74, 2003.
35. Singer, P., High-dose amino acid infusion preserves diuresis and improves nitrogen balance in non-oliguric acute renal failure, *Wien Klin. Wochenschr.*, 119(7–8), 218–22, 2007.
36. Marletta, M.A. and Spierling, M.M., Trace elements and nitric oxide function, *J. Nutr.*, 133, 1431S, 2003.
37. Schramm, L. et al., L-Arginine deficiency and supplementation in experimental acute kidney injury and in human kidney transplantation, *Kidney Int.*, 61, 1423, 2002.
38. Chan, L.-N., Nutritional support in acute renal failure, *Curr. Opin. Clin. Nutr. Metab. Care*, 7, 207–212, 2004.
39. Griffiths, R.D., Outcome of critically ill patients after supplementation with glutamine, *Nutrition*, 13, 752, 1997.
40. Burl, R.D. and Kaysen, G.A., Assessment of inflammation and nutrition in patients with end-stage renal disease, *J. Nephrol.*, 13, 249, 2000.
41. Kalantar-Zadeh, K. and Kopple, J.D., Trace elements and vitamins in maintenance dialysis patients, *Adv. Ren. Replace. Ther.*, 10(3), 170, 2003.
42. Pifer, T.B. et al., Mortality risk in hemodialysis and changes in nutritional indicators: DOPPS, *Kidney Int.*, 62, 2238, 2002.
43. Kaysen, G.A. et al., Relationships among inflammation nutrition and physiologic mechanisms establishing albumin levels in hemodialysis patients, *Kidney Int.*, 61, 2240, 2002.
44. Schoenfeld, P.Y. et al., Assessment of nutritional status of the National Cooperative Dialysis Study population, *Kidney Int. Suppl.*, (13), S80–S88, 1983.
45. Doan, T.L. et al., Tigecycline: A glycycline antimicrobial agent, *Clin. Ther.*, 28(8), 1079–1106, 2006.
46. Shin, J.A. et al., Clinical outcomes of tigecycline in the treatment of multidrug-resistant *Acinetobacter baumannii* infection, *Yonsei Med. J.*, 53(5), 974–984, 2012.
47. Suleiman, M.Y. and Zaloga, G.P., Renal failure, in *Nutrition in Critical Care*, Zaloga, G.P., Ed. Mosby-Year Book, St. Louis, MO, Chap. 36, 1994.
48. Saber, A.A., Feasibility of single-access laparoscopic sleeve gastrectomy in super-super obese patients, *Surg. Innov.*, 17(1), 36–40, 2010.
49. Brown, R.O., Compher, C., and the ASPEN Board of Directors, A.S.P.E.N., Clinical guidelines: Nutrition support in adult acute and chronic renal failure, *J. Parenter. Enteral. Nutr.*, 34, 366–377, 2010.

29 Nutrition for the Critically Ill Patient with Hepatic Failure

Mazen Albeldawi, Peggy Hipskind, and Dian J. Chiang

CONTENTS

INTRODUCTION

The liver is the largest metabolic organ in the human body, and this organ integrates a wide variety of complex biochemical processes including carbohydrate, fat, and protein metabolism, vitamin storage and activation, and detoxification and excretion of endogenous and exogenous waste products. Severe liver injury leads to a wide variety of metabolic derangements that proceed to the development of protein calorie malnutrition (PCM). Consequently, it is not surprising that PCM is a common complication of advanced liver disease (DiCecco et al. 1989, Lautz et al. 1992). The demonstration that PCM is an independent risk factor for predicting clinical outcomes in hepatic failure, and the fact that nutritional intervention may improve survival, surgical outcome, liver function, and hepatic encephalopathy (HE), has made the recognition of PCM an important factor in the management of liver disease (Caregaro et al. 1996, Alberino et al. 2001).

ACUTE LIVER FAILURE

Acute liver failure (ALF) refers to the rapid deterioration of hepatic function characterized by the onset of HE and coagulopathy in a patient without any prior liver disease (Trey and Davidson 1970). Hepatic failure occurs as a result of severe liver injury from either hepatocellular necrosis and/or apoptosis depending on the etiology. In the United States, acetaminophen (APAP) is the most common etiology of ALF (46%), followed by non-APAP etiologies: indeterminate cause (14%), drug-induced injury (11%), acute hepatitis B (7%), and autoimmune hepatitis (5%) (Lee et al. 2008). With an estimated 2000 cases per year in the United States, patients with ALF have a high mortality rate and can develop cerebral edema, infections, and multiorgan failure (Hoofnagle et al. 1995). Before orthotopic liver transplantation (OLT), survival from ALF was only 20%. Currently, with the advent of OLT, overall survival rates approach 67%, and spontaneous survival without receiving OLT rates has risen to 45% (Ostapowicz et al. 2002).

CLINICAL FEATURES

The hallmark of ALF is the development of HE in the setting of acute and severe liver injury (Ware et al. 1971). Unlike HE of decompensated cirrhosis, HE of ALF responds poorly to therapy and often masks the development of cerebral edema, a catastrophic complication of ALF. Cerebral edema is characterized by systemic hypertension, hyperventilation, increased muscle tone, decorticate or decerebrate posturing, abnormal papillary reflexes, and eventually altered brainstem reflexes in the event of uncal or cerebellar herniation. Furthermore, ALF usually affects all organ functions, resulting in cardiovascular instability, respiratory failure, renal insufficiency, coagulopathy, severe malnutrition, and life-threatening infections (Table 29.1).

TABLE 29.1
Clinical Features of Acute Liver Failure

Clinical Features of Acute Liver Failure
Hepatic encephalopathy
Cerebral edema
Hepatocellular dysfunction
Coagulopathy
Hypoglycemia
Metabolic acidosis
Cardiovascular abnormalities
Hypoxia
Hypotension
Renal dysfunction
Acute tubular necrosis
Hepatorenal syndrome
Multiple organ dysfunction syndrome

TABLE 29.2
Staging of Encephalopathy

Stage	Clinical Manifestations
Stage 0	No change in consciousness, no degree of encephalopathy present
Stage 1	Impaired attention, mild confusion, insomnia/sleep disturbance, agitation, euphoria, or depression
Stage 2	Lethargy, disorientation, bizarre behavior, anxiety, slurred speech, personality change
Stage 3	Marked confusion, somnolence but arousable, asterixis
Stage 4	Stupor and coma, no response to painful stimuli

Hepatic Encephalopathy

HE is a defining criterion for ALF. The severity of HE, which manifests as neuropsychiatric dysfunction, has been stratified into four stages (Table 29.2) (Polson and Lee 2005). Cerebral edema occurs mostly in stages 3–4 of HE and is one of the principal causes of death in ALF. The pathogenesis of the cerebral edema in ALF is poorly understood. It has been proposed to result, in part, from increased cerebral interstitial fluid, increased permeability of the blood–brain barrier, and cellular edema. Cellular edema from astrocyte swelling appears to be the primary etiology of cerebral edema in the ALF patient (Blei 2008). If nutritional intake is insufficient to maintain requirements, then artificial nutrition should be commenced with enteral feeding preferred over parenteral feeding. Importantly, the risk of aspiration pneumonia in patients with advanced HE during enteral feeding must be weighed against the potential complications of parenteral nutrition (PN).

Coagulopathy and Bleeding

The liver is the major site of synthesis of coagulation factor (other than factor VIII) and related inhibitory proteins of fibrinolysis. In ALF, the abnormal prothrombin time found in all patients confirms the loss of liver synthetic function and is used as an indicator for the severity of hepatic injury. Patients with ALF frequently have a multifactorial coagulopathy and a resultant increased risk of bleeding and clotting. Critically ill patients with ALF have an increased risk of major hemorrhage (gastrointestinal and intrapulmonary) secondary to acute portal hypertension and coagulopathy (Boks et al. 1986).

Infection

Bacterial infections may develop in up to 80% of patients with ALF, because of compromised immune function, which is related to complement and opsonin deficiency and impaired neutrophil function. Furthermore, use of invasive intensive care unit (ICU) instrumentation increases the patient's exposure to potential pathogens. Not surprisingly, the most common isolated bacteria are *Staphylococci*, *Streptococci*, and gram-negative bacilli. One-third of the patients develop fungal infections, specifically *Candida* species (Vaquero et al. 2003).

Multiple Organ Failure Syndrome

The inflammatory response to massive liver injury can lead to widespread and progressive inflammatory injury. Frequently, sepsis contributes to this insult with endotoxemia leading to circulatory collapse, tissue hypoxia, and increased bacterial translocation across leaky intestinal mucosa. Subsequently, multiple organ failure can develop which manifests clinically as hypotension, pulmonary edema, renal failure, and disseminated intravascular coagulopathy (DIC).

Metabolic Abnormalities

The liver is the site of many biochemical processes (gluconeogenesis, glycogenolysis, and lactate metabolism). In the presence of severe hepatic necrosis, the liver is rendered ineffective as a source of glucose. Early recognition of hypoglycemia is paramount. Rapid correction of hypoglycemia can be achieved with continuous intravenous 10% dextrose infusion. Other metabolic abnormalities may include hypokalemia, hypophosphatemia, and hypomagnesemia. Moreover, severe lactic acidosis may complicate the metabolic acidosis associated with renal failure (Bihari et al. 1985).

MEDICAL MANAGEMENT OF ACUTE LIVER FAILURE

The management of patients with ALF should include rapid identification of the cause of ALF, with emphasis on treatable conditions (i.e., acetaminophen toxicity), supportive care, and early evaluation for OLT. Due to the possible rapid neurological deterioration, medical care should be provided in an ICU for any patient presenting with encephalopathy. Management of patients with ALF consists of aggressive supportive as well as surveillance for and treatment of complications while awaiting liver transplantation or until spontaneous liver function recovery occurs.

CHRONIC LIVER FAILURE

PCM is common in patients with chronic liver disease, with a prevalence of at least 20% in compensated liver disease to more than 80% in those patients with decompensated cirrhosis (Nompleggi and Bonkovsky 1994). PCM is associated with a number of complications including development of variceal bleeding and ascites, reduced survival, and increased surgical morbidity and mortality (Lautz et al. 1992, Siriboonkoom and Gramlich 1998). Frequently, patients with end-stage hepatic failure will present with muscle wasting, decreased fat stores, and overt cachexia. There are a number of factors that contribute to PCM in patients with chronic liver disease (Cheung et al. 2012): (1) anorexia secondary to central appetite suppression in the setting of proinflammatory cytokine production, (2) diagnostic and therapeutic procedures that interrupt eating and contribute to low intake, (3) early satiety caused by gastric compression from ascites and splenomegaly, (4) dysgeusia likely related to zinc deficiency and unpalatable diets, (5) fat malabsorption mainly due to reduced intestinal bile acids, and (6) increased intestinal protein losses.

Nutrition Assessment

Physical assessment of patients with liver failure is the primary means of assessing for malnutrition. Biochemical markers such as albumin, prealbumin, and transferrin are of limited use in the assessment of nutrition status. This is largely due to influences of edema, ascites, renal insufficiency, altered metabolic function, and presence of acute or chronic inflammation (Chadalavada et al. 2010, Mueller et al. 2011, Jensen and Wheeler 2012). Patients in the ICU frequently have an inflammatory process that contributes to exacerbation of malnutrition and inhibits the potential positive effects of nutrition interventions (Jensen and Wheller 2012). Examination of body composition based on weight changes, loss of subcutaneous fat, and loss of muscle mass are the key components of nutrition-focused physical assessment. A head-to-toe inspection of the patient's hair, skin, and nails can provide evidence of potential vitamin and mineral deficiencies. Changes in functional status, increased fatigue, and complaints of muscle and/or joint pain are supportive data that can substantiate macro- and micronutrient deficiencies. Frequent weight fluctuations are common in patients with liver disease due to edema and ascites and should be taken into account during the physical exam. An estimation of dry weight may be necessary if the medical record, patient, and family are unable to provide this information. The medical record may be used to confirm physical findings or provide information that may not otherwise be obtained from the patient or family.

TABLE 29.3
Physical Signs of Malnutrition in Patients with Liver Disease

	Area of Exam	Normal Attributes	Abnormal Attributes
Face	Orbital area	Slight fat pad bulge under the eye	Dark circles, sunken.
	Temporalis	Flat	Hollowed.
Chest	Pectoralis/deltoids	Clavicles nonprominent or not visible	Clavicles prominent/visible.
Back	Trapezius/deltoids	No scapula bone protrusion	Scapula bone protrusion.
	Latissimus dorsi	No rib bone protrusion	Rib bone protrusion.
Arms	Deltoids	Rounded, no bone protrusion	Bone protrusion.
	Triceps	Large amount of fatty tissue with pinch	Small amount of fatty tissue with pinch. **For patients with upper extremity edema, this cannot be assessed.
Abdomen	Midaxillary line superior to the iliac crest	Large amount of fatty tissue with pinch	Small amount of fatty tissue with pinch. **For patients who have ascites, this cannot be assessed.
Legs	Quadriceps	Well rounded	Thin with poor muscle tone.
	Gastrocnemius	Well developed	Thin with poor muscle tone. **For patients with lower extremity edema, this cannot be assessed.

Sources: Detsky, A.S. et al., *JPEN*, 11, 8, 1987; Secker, D.J. and Jeejeebhoy, K.N., *J. Acad. Nutr. Diet.*, 112, 424, 2012.

Determination of energy intake prior to ICU admission is useful to assess for malnutrition. Poor oral intakes compared to estimated energy requirements over a prolonged period of time will help determine the severity of malnutrition (Jensen and Wheeler 2012, White et al. 2012). Hydration status, presence of edema, ascites, hydrothorax, and renal insufficiency all affect interpretation of the patient's current weight related to weight history. In the presence of edema, assessment for signs of subcutaneous fat loss and muscle mass loss can be used to determine the existence and severity of malnutrition (Jensen and Wheeler 2012, White et al. 2012). Patients with chronic liver failure are often deficient in fat-soluble vitamins and zinc due to poor oral intakes, malabsorption, and decreased synthesis by the liver (Abbott-Johnson et al. 2011).

Moderate-to-severe malnutrition often results in physical changes. The physical assessment has been validated as a useful, accurate tool in the form of subjective global assessment (Detsky et al. 1987, Secker and Jeejeebhoy 2012). Taking this one step further, a more comprehensive evaluation of body fat and muscle can be evaluated (Table 29.3). Loss of subcutaneous fat can be assessed from the orbital fat pads below the eye and at the triceps. If ascites is not present, subcutaneous fat can be assessed at the midaxillary line superior to the iliac crest (Secker and Jeejeebhoy 2012). Evidence of muscle wasting can be determined by observation of hollowing of the temples, protrusion of the clavicles and/or scapula, squaring of the shoulder bones, and thinning of the thigh or calves. Fat mass and muscle mass can be measured by means of tools such as skin fold calipers to measure subcutaneous fat and hand dynamometers to measure muscle strength. A decrease in measured muscle strength has been linked to a decline in muscle mass (Norman et al. 2010).

Nutrition Requirements

Energy

In advanced liver disease, patients are often hypermetabolic and have high nutritional requirements (Plauth et al. 2009, Chadalavada et al. 2010). Literature suggests a late evening snack is beneficial to slow the onset of hypermetabolism. In patients with liver failure, an overnight fast accelerates

TABLE 29.4
Predictive Equations and Recommendations

Source	Calories	Protein	Carbohydrate	Fat
ASPEN	25–35 kcal/kg/day (compensated stable) 30–40 kcal/kg/day (stable/ malnourished)	1.0–1.2 g/kg body weight w/o HE 0.6–0.8 g/kg cirrhosis w/HE-temporary until cause of HE can be eliminated 0.6–0.8 g/kg/day cirrhosis w/chronic HE		
ESPEN	1.3 × REE (liver cirrhosis/ acute liver failure)	1.2–1.5 g/kg body weight for liver cirrhosis 0.8–1.2 g/kg for acute liver failure	50%–55% of calories ≤10% simple carbohydrates	30%–35% of calories
AHA				<7% of total fat as saturated fat
FDA				<2 g/day trans fatty acids

Sources: Frazier, T.H. et al., Liver disease, in: Mueller, C.M. (ed.), *ASPEN Adult Nutrition Support Core Curriculum*, 2nd edn., ASPEN, Silver Spring, MD, 2012, pp. 454–471; Plauth, M. et al., *Clin. Nutr.*, 28, 436, 2009.

starvation with an early shift toward lipid utilization (Owen et al. 1981, Bianchi et al. 2005, Tsien et al. 2012). Estimates of energy requirements for patients with hepatic failure vary widely (25–40 kcal/kg/day) in the literature. The predictive equations (Table 29.4) are commonly used to estimate energy requirements. Dry weight and ideal body weight have both been used to determine estimated energy needs. Measured resting energy expenditure (REE) is ideal for patients with liver failure due to altered body composition, changes in functional status, and metabolic disturbances associated with liver failure. In the absence of indirect calorimetry, predictive equations (Table 29.4) have been used as a quick and easy way to estimate REE (MacDonald and Hildebrandt 2003).

Protein

Contrary to earlier beliefs, a diet low in protein is not beneficial for patients who have HE (Cordoba et al. 2004, Chadalavada et al. 2010, Cabral and Burns 2011, Kachaamy and Bajaj 2011, Antar et al. 2012). Malnourished patients actually benefit from additional protein supplementation. In the absence of dietary protein sources, skeletal muscle is utilized to meet the increase in demand for amino acids. The increased release of amino acids may worsen HE secondary to the production of ammonia that is derived from their release (Cordoba et al. 2004). Nutrition support should provide adequate nutrients and substrates for protein and energy syntheses. High protein supplements have been shown to improve nitrogen balance (Cabral and Burns 2011).

Branched-chain amino acids (BCAAs) include valine, leucine, and isoleucine. BCAAs function as a substrate for protein synthesis and thus conserve muscle mass (Bianchi et al. 1993). During liver failure, the liver is unable to utilize aromatic amino acids, but skeletal muscle can still utilize BCAA. Therefore, a BCAA deficiency could result due to increased uptake and insufficient delivery (Hayaishi et al. 2011). Studies reveal patients with advanced cirrhosis have decreased levels of BCAA (Les et al. 2010). While providing high BCAA and low aromatic amino acid diets to treat HE makes logical sense, randomized trials fail to support that a diet with supplemental BCAAs effectively treats HE (Holecek 2010, Cabral and Burns 2011) or decreases HE reoccurrence (Chadalavada et al. 2010, Les et al. 2010). However, supplementation of BCAAs has been shown to have some benefits in improving cognition (Les et al. 2010), slowing progression of liver disease, prolonging survival (Bianchi et al. 1993, Muto et al. 2005), increasing muscle mass and nitrogen balance (Chadalavada et al. 2010, Les et al. 2010), reducing prevalence of ascites and edema, improving quality of life, reducing number of hospital readmissions, and increasing hand grip strength and improving anthropometric measurements (Bianchi et al. 1993, Marchesini et al. 2003, Poon et al. 2004). Leucine in particular has been shown to stimulate protein synthesis, insulin secretion, and liver regeneration (Holecek 2010). Feasibility of providing BCAA orally is limited as they are bitter-tasting, resulting in poor patient compliance, and they are costly (Chadalavada et al. 2010, Holecek et al. 2010).

Vegetable and dairy protein may be beneficial due to the higher fiber and bacterial content which can facilitate increased frequency of bowel movements (Cabral and Burns 2011). Additionally, foods containing vegetable and dairy protein are generally well tolerated (Chadalavada et al. 2010) and contain low levels of aromatic amino acids. Patients consuming a vegetable protein diet exhibit improved nitrogen balance (Bianchi et al. 1993) which gives the same benefit as BCAA supplements.

Carbohydrate

Glucose intolerance is found in up to 96% of cirrhotics (Holstein et al. 2002). Insulin is a hormone that is released by the pancreas when serum glucose levels are high. After ingestion and digestion of carbohydrates, glucose is absorbed from the intestine into the bloodstream. Insulin is secreted and signals the uptake of glucose into cells. With insulin resistance, there is cellular peripheral insulin receptor dysfunction which results in an increase in release of insulin from the pancreas due to increased levels of glucose in the blood. This results in hyperglycemia as a result of hyperinsulinemia. Hypoglycemia also should be avoided, in particular for patients in the ICU due to increased risk for life-threatening events and prolonged hospitalization (Brunkhorst et al. 2008). Therefore, provision of nutrition with moderate calories from complex carbohydrates will meet nutrition needs (Table 29.4).

Fat

Saturated and trans fatty acids have been linked to increased risk for cardiovascular disease, obesity, and diabetes (Aranceta 2012). Those with non-alcoholic fatty liver disease (NAFLD) are at high risk for cardiovascular disease due to a fatty liver, which is one of the components of metabolic syndrome along with obesity, hypertension, and elevated lipids. A diet high in saturated fatty acids may contribute to insulin resistance, and therefore, it is recommended to provide nutrition with low saturated fat content. A recent study was conducted in rats to determine if the fat source in enteral nutrition would affect the progression of NAFLD (Ronis et al. 2012). The authors concluded that the type of fat strongly influenced the progression of NAFLD with olive oil, a monounsaturated fatty acid, potentially reducing the risk of NAFLD progression to nonalcoholic steatohepatitis. A dietary intake limited in saturated fat and trans fatty acids is recommended. Refer to Table 29.4 for predictive equation for fat intake and recommendation for saturated and trans fat limitations.

Micronutrients

Fat-soluble vitamin deficiencies are common in patients with end-stage liver disease and can be associated with increased mortality rates (Institute of Medicine 2002, Abbott-Johnson et al. 2011). These deficiencies are common in this patient population due to decreased oral intakes, malabsorption (due to medications such as lactulose, gastrointestinal disturbances, bacterial overgrowth, pancreatic insufficiency, decreased bile formation in cholestatic forms of liver failure), alcohol consumption, reduced synthesis of carrier proteins, zinc deficiency, and liver process of vitamin conversion (Institute of Medicine 2002, Chadalavada et al. 2010). The high incidence of malnutrition in patients with liver disease is a contributing factor in micronutrient deficiencies.

Vitamin A

Vitamin A plays an important role in the vision cycle and maintenance of skin and skeletal muscles. Malabsorption of vitamin A can occur with diarrhea, which is common with patients who have gastroenteritis or who are on a hyperosmotic agent for the treatment of HE. It is important to avoid inappropriate vitamin A supplementation by carefully interpreting low vitamin A levels. Serum levels of vitamin A may be depleted as a result of zinc deficiency in the malnourished population (Christian and West 1998) since zinc is required for the mobilization of vitamin A from the liver to circulation as it is required in the synthesis of the carrier proteins for vitamin A. Inadequate protein and energy intakes also may lead to low levels (Institute of Medicine 2002) and therefore may affect the interpretation of vitamin A deficiency and result in inappropriate supplementations. In patients with liver disease, vitamin A deficiency may result in xerophthalmia, follicular hyperkeratosis, impaired immunity, increased infections, and eventual increased morbidity and mortality (Institute of Medicine 2002). Low serum retinol levels are prevalent in patients with liver disease (de Paula et al. 2010). Serum retinol depletion has been correlated to increased total bilirubin, increased prothrombin time, HE, and ascites (Peres et al. 2011). Approximately 90% of vitamin A is stored in the liver in a healthy population, but only 50% or less is stored in those with a deficiency (Institute of Medicine 2002, Dancygier et al. 2010). Prealbumin and retinol-binding proteins are both synthesized by the liver. Diminished synthesis of these carrier proteins by the liver can result in a vitamin A deficiency. Patients with liver disease are often unaware of changes to night vision (Institute of Medicine 2002, Abbott-Johnson et al. 2011).

Vitamin D

Vitamin D is a hormone that is obtained from the diet and exposure to sunlight. It increases intestinal calcium and phosphate absorption for the maintenance of bone formation (Institute of Medicine 2002, Holick 2011), and plays a role in immune health and insulin secretion (Lim and Chalasani 2012). Vitamin D deficiency is highly prevalent in patients with liver disease (Miroliaee et al. 2010, Cholongitas et al. 2012, Lim and Chalasani 2012). In addition to decreased oral intake or lack of sun exposure, patients with liver failure may be deficient due to decreased hydroxylation of cholecalciferol to hydroxycholecalciferol (Holick 2011), increased extrahepatic uptake by adipose tissue, malabsorption (Lim and Chalasani 2012), or decreased synthesis of carrier proteins. These patients may complain of bone pain, muscle pain, and muscle weakness. However, it is often identified by biochemical values (depleted hydroxycholecalciferol) prior to the patient's awareness of the symptoms.

Vitamin E

As an antioxidant, vitamin E prevents lipid oxidation of polyunsaturated fatty acids (PUFAs) (Institute of Medicine 2002). Vitamin E deficiency is rare; however, in liver disease and cholestatic disease, a deficiency may be related to decrease oral intakes, depletion of antioxidants due to increased oxidative stress, or prolonged fat malabsorption and steatorrhea (Erhardt et al. 2011, Singal et al. 2011). A deficiency can be characterized by neuromuscular disorders, hemolytic anemia, and ataxia (Institute of Medicine 2002). Supplementation of vitamin E may be of benefit due to its antioxidant properties.

Vitamin K

The gut microbiota synthesizes vitamin K, but not in high enough quantities to match the physiologic need of the body (Institute of Medicine 2002). Vitamin K controls the formation of coagulation factors in the liver (Institute of Medicine 2002). For patients with liver disease, a deficiency is related to decreases in bile salt synthesis that leads to impaired absorption of vitamin K or fat malabsorption. Vitamin K deficiency should be considered in patients with liver disease when prothrombin time is increased. Patients may bruise easily or have increased incidence of bleeding as a result of a decrease in clotting factor (Institute of Medicine 2002).

Zinc

Zinc is a trace element that has an important role in catalytic reactions as an electron acceptor (i.e., alcohol dehydrogenase and carbonic anhydrase), structural integrity of proteins, regulation of gene expression (Institute of Medicine 2002), and hepatic synthesis of retinol-binding protein

(Christian and West 1998). Although a deficiency is rare in the general population, in liver disease, it is more prevalent due to increased frequency of malabsorption syndromes, use of diuretics, diabetes mellitus, renal failure, sepsis, and age-related physiologic or socioeconomic issues (Smith et al. 1973, Christian and West 1998, Institute of Medicine 2002, Tuerk and Fazel 2009). Zinc deficiency is characterized by impaired immune function, alopecia, diarrhea, skin rashes, anorexia, hypogeusia, anemia, mental lethargy, and hyperammonemia (Institute of Medicine 2002, Tuerk et al. 2009). Liver disease may result in hypoalbuminemia, increased infection, and acute stress that may skew biochemical markers for zinc. Biochemical markers do not necessarily reflect a deficiency since it is estimated that only 0.1% of whole body zinc is in circulation (Tuerk et al. 2009). Impaired zinc absorption is common in alcoholics (Institute of Medicine 2002). Since the liver is key in maintaining zinc homeostasis, hepatic diseases can impair zinc availability and affect liver function and regeneration (Tuerk et al. 2009).

B-Vitamins

Deficiencies of thiamin and riboflavin are commonly found in alcoholic and nonalcoholic liver diseases. A deficiency of thiamin may be related to the use of diuretics, malabsorption, altered metabolism, and increased utilization (Sica 2007, Clark 2012). Riboflavin deficiency may be seen in patients with poor intake of animal protein (milk, eggs, and meat) or malabsorption (Clark 2012). Other B-vitamins that may be deficient are folate and pyridoxine. These are more commonly seen in alcoholic liver disease. Patients with alcoholism are often deficient in folate due to decreased oral intake and decreased absorption of this nutrient (Clark 2012). Due to the risk of encephalopathy or neuromuscular weakness, folate and thiamin should be supplemented in patients with alcoholic liver disease (ALD) (Chadalavada et al. 2010).

Oral Nutrition Therapy

Nutrition therapy in hepatic failure should attempt to optimize oral intake and prevent or treat malnutrition. Frequent small meals and snacks help reduce the muscle catabolism between meals, and improve nitrogen balance. A bedtime carbohydrate- and protein-rich snack is recommended to reduce breakdown of lean muscle mass during the overnight fast (Chang et al. 1997, Kondrup and Muller 1997). For a summary of recommended guidelines for enhancing oral intake, see Table 29.5. A 2 g (88 mmol/L) sodium-restricted diet is recommended to minimize the diuretic dose to control ascites and peripheral edema.

Enteral Nutrition

If nutritional supplementation is insufficient to maintain desired nutrient intake, then nutrition support therapy should be commenced with enteral feeding given first consideration. A nasoenteric (nasoduodenal or nasojejunal) feeding tube is considered a better option, due to a reduced risk of regurgitation and aspiration (McClave et al. 2002). However, feeding may be delayed trying to gain optimal tube positioning and fluoroscopic and endoscopic guidance methods may be necessary; thus, nasogastric tubes are commonly used initially. Randomized trials have provided evidence that enteral feeding provides increased dietary intake over conventional oral diet, is well tolerated, and leads to improvements in liver function (Cabre et al. 1990, Kearns et al. 1992, de Ledinghen et al. 1997).

TABLE 29.5
Guidelines for Improving Oral Intake

Guidelines for Improving Oral Intake
Avoid prolonged periods of nothing by mouth.
Frequent small meals (4–7/day).
Encourage an evening snack to reduce duration of overnight fast.
Encourage oral nutritional supplements.
Avoid unnecessary diet restrictions.

In hospitalized patients with inadequate dietary intake, enteral nutrition should be commenced as soon as possible, ideally within 24–48 h of admission. In a prospective study, Campillo et al. showed that a decrease in dietary intake was an independent predictor of hospital mortality and corresponded with a deterioration of liver function (Campillo et al. 2003). Traditionally, a restricted protein diet has been recommended; however, patients with cirrhosis exhibit increased protein requirements to achieve balanced nitrogen metabolism (Chang et al. 1997), and normal protein diets have been given safely in HE (Cordoba et al. 2004). Insertion of nasogastric tubes in patients with esophageal varices has been addressed in only one study in which 22 patients with esophageal varices after bleeding and endoscopic therapy were randomized to either nasogastric feeding or no oral diet for 3 days (de Ledinghen et al. 1997). This study showed that nasogastric tubes did not appear to cause a greater incidence of rebleeding from varices compared to no feeding tube.

Parenteral Nutrition

PN, containing lipids, amino acids, dextrose, electrolytes, vitamins, and minerals, is associated with increased risk of mechanical (e.g., pneumothorax) and infectious complications compared to enteral feeding. It is essential that PN is administered via a dedicated line to reduce incidence of sepsis. Also, parenteral solutions require high fluid volumes to provide significant calories and protein which may not be tolerated in liver failure patients. Thus, enteral feeding is preferred in liver disease reserving PN for those patients intolerant to enteral feeding (e.g., prolonged ileus). However, a randomized clinical trial comparing enteral versus parenteral feeding liver disease is lacking. However, overly aggressive nutritional therapy can have adverse clinical consequences, known as refeeding syndrome, in malnourished ALF patients. Daily monitoring of body weight, fluid intake, urine output, and plasma glucose and electrolytes (including magnesium and phosphate) is critical during early refeeding (first 3–5 days) so that appropriate adjustments can be made (Cordoba et al. 2004) (see Chapter 16).

Novel Intervention

A range of extracorporeal supportive devices have been promoted to replace liver function in patients with ALF; however, conclusive evidence of benefits to patients has not been reported (Demetriou et al. 2004). Hepatocyte transplantation has also been proposed for the treatment of ALF. In this technique, human hepatocytes are infused into the splenic or hepatic portal vascular beds or peritoneal cavity to provide adjunctive hepatic function for the failing liver. Although experience has suggested the technique is practical to undertake, a review of reported cases shows survival without conventional emergency transplantation to be 35% (Fisher and Strom 2006). Emerging data suggest that omega-3 PUFA may play a beneficial role in liver regeneration. Omega-3 PUFA is thought to decrease the expression of proinflammatory cytokines and increase the expression of anti-inflammatory cytokines. In one study, Qiu et al. showed that intravenous injection of omega-3 PUFA slowed the progress of ALF through and significantly promoted liver regeneration after 90% hepatectomy (Qiu et al. 2012).

CASE VIGNETTE

A 23-year-old female has a 2-week history of jaundice and a 24 h history of somnolence. She became sexually active with her boyfriend 6 months ago. Physical exam shows jaundice, disorientation, and asterixis. Laboratory results revealed AST 1510, ALT 1807, INR 3.2, total bilirubin 4.5 mg/dL, and serum creatinine 2.0 mg/dL.

In ALF,

A. Liver failure caused by drug toxicity has the worst prognosis
B. The most common viral etiology is hepatitis B virus
C. The slower the progression, the better is the outcome
D. Patients always need liver transplant because of the associated high mortality

The answer is B. Among viral infections, HBV is the most common cause of ALF.

What would be a suitable nutritional care plan?

A. Enteral nutrition with low protein feed
B. Enteral nutrition with BCAAs
C. Total parental nutrition
D. Enteral nutrition with high protein feed

The answer is D. Nutrition is important and enteral feedings should be initiated early. Severe restrictions of protein should be avoided; 60 g/day of protein is reasonable in most cases. BCAAs have not been shown to be superior to other enteral preparations. If enteral feedings are contraindicated, then PN is an option, although the risks of infection, particularly with fungal pathogens, should be considered.

REFERENCES

Abbott-Johnson WJ, Kerlin P, Abiad G, Clague AE, Cuneo RC. Dark adaptation in vitamin A-deficient adults awaiting liver transplantation: Improvement with intramuscular vitamin A treatment. *Br J Opthamol* 2011;4:544–548.

Alberino F, Gatta A, Amodio P et al. Nutrition and survival in patients with liver cirrhosis. *Nutrition* 2001;17(6):445–450.

Antar R, Wong P, Ghali P. A meta-analysis of nutritional supplementation for management of hospitalized alcoholic hepatitis. *Can J Gastroenterol* 2012;26:463–467.

Aranceta J. Recommended dietary reference intakes, nutritional goals and dietary guidelines for fat and fatty acids: A systematic review. *Br J Nutr* 2012;107(Suppl. 2):S8–S22.

Bianchi GP, Marchesini G, Fabbri A et al. Vegetable protein versus animal protein diet in cirrhotic patients with chronic encephalopathy: A randomized cross-over comparison. *J Intern Med* 1993;233:385–392.

Bianchi GP, Marzocchi R, Agostini F, Marchesini G. Update on nutritional supplementation with branched-chain amino acids. *Curr Opin Clin Nutr Metab Care* 2005;8:83–87.

Bihari D, Gimson AE, Lindridge J et al. Lactic acidosis in fulminant hepatic failure. Some aspects of pathogenesis and prognosis. *J Hepatol* 1985;1(4):405–416.

Blei AT. Brain edema in acute liver failure. *Crit Care Clin* 2008;24(1):99–114.

Boks AL, Brommer EJ, Schalm SW et al. Hemostasis and fibrinolysis in severe liver failure and their relation to hemorrhage. *Hepatology* 1986;6(1):79–86.

Brunkhorst FM, Engel C, Bloos F et al. Intensive insulin therapy and pentastarch resuscitation in severe sepsis. *N Engl J Med* 2008;358:125–139.

Cabral CM, Burns DL. Low-protein diets for hepatic encephalopathy debunked: Let them eat steak. *Nutr Clin Pract* 2011;26:155–159.

Cabre E, Gonzalez-Huix F, Abad-Lacruz A et al. Effect of total enteral nutrition on the short-term outcome of severely malnourished cirrhotics. A randomized controlled trial. *Gastroenterology* 1990;98(3): 715–720.

Campillo B, Richardet JP, Scherman E et al. Evaluation of nutritional practice in hospitalized cirrhotic patients: Results of a prospective study. *Nutrition* 2003;19(6):515–521.

Caregaro L, Alberino F, Amodio P et al. Malnutrition in alcoholic and virus-related cirrhosis. *Am J Clin Nutr* 1996;63(4):602–609.

Chadalavada R, Sappati Biyyani RS, Maxwell J, Mullen K. Nutrition in hepatic Encephalopathy. *Nutr Clin Pract* 2010;25:257–264.

Chang WK, Chao YC, Tang HS et al. Effects of extra-carbohydrate supplementation in the late evening on energy expenditure and substrate oxidation in patients with liver cirrhosis. *JPEN J Parenter Enteral Nutr* 1997;21(2):96–99.

Cheung K, Lee SS, Raman M. Prevalence and mechanisms of malnutrition in patients with advanced liver disease, and nutrition management strategies. *Clin Gastroenterol Hepatol* 2012;10(2):117–125.

Cholongitas E, Theocharidou E, Goulis, J, Tsochatzis E, Akriviadis E, Burroughs AK. Review article: The extra-skeletal effects of vitamin D in chronic hepatitis C infection. *Aliment Pharmacol Ther* 2012;35:634–646.

Christian P, West KP. Interactions between zinc and vitamin A: An update. *Am J Clin Nutr* 1998;68:435S–441S.

Clark SF. Vitamins and trace elements. In: Mueller CM (ed.), *ASPEN Adult Nutrition Support Core Curriculum*, 2nd edn. Silver Spring, MD: ASPEN, 2012, pp. 121–151.

Cordoba J, Lopez-Hellin J, Planas M et al. Normal protein diet for episodic hepatic encephalopathy: Results of a randomized study. *J Hepatol* 2004;41:38–43.

Dancygier H, Merle U, Stremmel W, Niederau C. Hepatic metabolism. In: *Clinical Hepatology: Principles and Practice of Hepatobiliary Diseases*. Dandygier, H. (ed.) Berlin, Germany: Springer Verlag, 2010, pp. 75–102.

de Ledinghen V, Beau P, Mannant PR et al. Early feeding or enteral nutrition in patients with cirrhosis after bleeding from esophageal varices? A randomized controlled study. *Dig Dis Sci* 1997;42(3):536–541.

Demetriou AA, Brown RS Jr, Busuttil RW et al. Prospective, randomized, multicenter, controlled trial of a bioartificial liver in treating acute liver failure. *Ann Surg* 2004;239(5):660–667; discussion 667–670.

de Paula TP, Ramalho A, Braulio VB. The effectiveness of relative dose response to retinol intake as an evaluation of vitamin A status of cirrhotic patients. *J Hum Nutr Diet* 2010;23:583–589.

Detsky AS, McLaughlin JR, Baker et al. What is subjective global assessment of nutritional status? *JPEN* 1987;11:8–13.

DiCecco SR, Wieners EJ, Wiesner RH et al. Assessment of nutritional status of patients with end-stage liver disease undergoing liver transplantation. *Mayo Clin Proc* 1989;64(1):95–102.

Erhardt A, Stahl W, Sies H, Lirussi F, Donner A, Haussinger D. Plasma levels of vitamin E and carotenoids are decreased in patients with nonalcoholic steatohepatitis (NASH). *Eur J Med Res* 2011;16:76–78.

Fisher RA, Strom SC. Human hepatocyte transplantation: Worldwide results. *Transplantation* 2006;82(4):441–449.

Frazier TH, Wheeler BE, McClain CJ, Cave M. Liver disease. In: Mueller CM (ed.), *ASPEN Adult Nutrition Support Core Curriculum*, 2nd edn. Silver Spring, MD: ASPEN, 2012, pp. 454–471.

Hayaishi S, Chung H, Kudo M et al. Oral branched-chain amino acid granules reduce the incidence of hepatocellular carcinoma and improve event-free survival in patients with liver cirrhosis. *Dig Dis* 2011;29:326–332.

Holecek, M. Three targets of branched-chain amino acid supplementation in the treatment of liver disease. *Nutrition* 2010;26:482–490.

Holick, MF. Vitamin D: A d-lightful solution for health. *J Investig Med* 2011;59:872–880.

Holstein A, Hinze S, Thiessen E, Plaschke A, Egberts EH. Clinical implications of hepatogenous diabetes in liver cirrhosis. *J Gastroenterol Hepatol* 2002;17:677–681.

Hoofnagle JH, Carithers RL, Shapiro C et al. Fulminant hepatic failure: Summary of a workshop. *Hepatology* 1995;21(1):240–252.

Institute of Medicine. Food and Nutrition Board. Vitamin A. In: *Dietary Reference Intakes for Vitamin A, Vitamin K, Arsenic, Boron, Chromium, Copper, Iodine, Iron, Manganese, Molybdenum, Nickel, Silicon, Vanadium, and Zinc*, Washington, DC, National Academy Press, 2002, pp. 82–161.

Jensen, GL, Wheeler D. A new approach to defining and diagnosing malnutrition in adult critical illness. *Curr Opin Crit Care* 2012;18:206–211.

Kachaamy T, Bajaj JS. Diet and cognition in chronic liver disease. *Curr Opin Gastroenterol* 2011;27:174–179.

Kearns PJ, Young H, Garcia G et al. Accelerated improvement of alcoholic liver disease with enteral nutrition. *Gastroenterology* 1992;102(1):200–205.

Kondrup J, Muller MJ. Read energy and protein requirements of patients with chronic liver disease. *J Hepatol* 1997;27:239–247.

Lautz HU, Selberg O, Korber J et al. Protein-calorie malnutrition in liver cirrhosis. *Clin Investig* 1992;70(6):478–486.

Lee WM, Squires RH, Nyberg SL et al. Acute liver failure: Summary of a workshop. *Hepatology* 2008;47(4):1401–1415.

Les I, Doval E, Garcia-Martinez R et al. Effects of branched-chain amino acids supplementation in patients with cirrhosis and a previous episode of hepatic encephalopathy: A randomized study. *Am J Gastroenterol* 2010;106:1081–1088.

Lim LY, Chalasani N. Vitamin D deficiency in patients with chronic liver disease and cirrhosis. *Curr Gastroenterol Rep* 2012;14:67–73.

MacDonald A, Hildebrandt L. Comparison of formulaic equations to determine energy expenditure in the critically ill patient. *Nutrition* 2003;19:233–239.

Marchesini G, Bianchi G, Merli M et al. Nutritional supplementation with branched-chain amino acids in advanced cirrhosis: A double-blind, randomized trial. *Gastroenterology* 2003;124:1792–1801.

McClave SA, DeMeo MT, DeLegge MH et al. North American summit on aspiration in the critically ill patient: Consensus statement. *JPEN J Parenter Enteral Nutr* 2002;26(6 Suppl.):S80–S85.

Miroliaee A, Nasiri-Toosi M, Khalilzadh O, Esteghamati A, Abdollhi A, Mazloumi M. Disturbances of parathyroid hormone-vitamin D axis in non-cholestatic chronic liver disease: A cross-sectional study. *Hepatol Int* 2010;4:634–640.

Mueller C, Compher C, Druyan ME. A.S.P.E.N. Clinical guidelines. *JPEN* 2011;35:16–24.

Muto Y, Sato S, Watanabe A et al. Effects of oral branched-chain amino acid granules on event-free survival in patients with liver cirrhosis. *Clin Gastronterol Hepatol* 2005;3:705–713.

Nompleggi DJ, Bonkovsky HL. Nutritional supplementation in chronic liver disease: An analytical review. *Hepatology* 1994;19(2):518–533.

Norman K, Stobaus N, Gonzalez MC, Schulzke JD, Pirlich M. Hand grip strength: Outcome predictor and marker of nutrition status. *Clin Nutr* 2010;30:135–142.

Ostapowicz G, Fontana RJ, Schiodt FV et al. Results of a prospective study of acute liver failure at 17 tertiary care centers in the united states. *Ann Intern Med* 2002;137(12):947–954.

Owen OE, Reichle FA, Reichard GA Jr et al. Hepatic, gut, and renal substrate flux rates in patients with hepatic cirrhosis. *J Clin Invest* 1981;68:240–252.

Peres WA, Chaves GV, Goncalves JC, Ramalho A, Coelho HSM. Vitamin A deficiency in patients with hepatitis C virus-related chronic liver disease. *Br J Nutr* 2011;11:1724–1731.

Plauth M, Cabre E, Campillo B et al. ESPEN guidelines on parenteral nutrition: Hepatology. *Clin Nutr* 2009;28:436–444.

Polson J, Lee WM; American Association for the Study of Liver Disease. AASLD position paper: The management of acute liver failure. *Hepatology* 2005;41(5):1179–1197.

Poon RT, Yu WC, Fan ST, Wong J. Long-term oral branched chain amino acids in patients undergoing chemoembolization for hepatocellular carcinoma: A randomized trial. *Aliment Pharmacol Ther* 2004;19:779–788.

Qiu YD, Wang S, Yang Y et al. Omega-3 polyunsaturated fatty acids promote liver regeneration after 90% hepatectomy in rats. *World J Gastroenterol* 2012;18(25):3288–3295.

Ronis MJ, Baumgardner JN, Marecki JC et al. Dietary fat source alters hepatic gene expression profile and determines the type of liver pathology in rats overfed via total enteral nutrition. *Physiol Genomics* 2012;44:1073–1089.

Secker DJ, Jeejeebhoy KN. How to perform subjective global nutritional assessment in children. *J Acad Nutr Diet* 2012;112:424–431.

Sica DA. Loop diuretic therapy, thiamin balance, and heart failure. *Congest Heart Fail* 2007;13:244–247.

Singal AK, Jampana C, Weinman SA. Antioxidants as therapeutic agents for liver disease. *Liver Int* 2011;31:1432–1448.

Siriboonkoom W, Gramlich L. Nutrition and chronic liver disease. *Can J Gastroenterol* 1998;12(3):201–207.

Smith JC, McDaniel EG, Fan FF, Halsted JA. Zinc: A trace element essential in vitamin A metabolism. *Science* 1973;181:954–955.

Trey C, Davidson CS. The management of fulminant hepatic failure. *Prog Liver Dis* 1970;3:282–298.

Tsien C, McCullough AJ, Dasarathy S. Late evening snack: Exploiting a period of anabolic opportunity in cirrhosis. *J Gastroenterol Hepatol* 2012;27:430–441.

Tuerk MJ, Fazel N. Zinc deficiency. *Curr Opin Gastroenterol* 2009;25:136–143.

Vaquero J, Polson J, Chung C et al. Infection and the progression of hepatic encephalopathy in acute liver failure. *Gastroenterology* 2003;125(3):755–764.

Ware AJ, D'Agostino AN, Combes B. Cerebral edema: A major complication of massive hepatic necrosis. *Gastroenterology* 1971;61(6):877–884.

White JV, Guenter P, Jensen G, Malone A, Schofield M. Consensus statement: Academy of Nutrition and Dietetics and American Society for Parenteral and Enteral Nutrition: Characteristics recommended for the identification and documentation of adult malnutrition (undernutrition). *JPEN* 2012;36:275–283.

30 Nutrition for the Critically Ill Cardiac Patient

A. Christine Hummell

CONTENTS

INTRODUCTION

Heart disease continues to remain the leading cause of mortality in the United States.[1] It is anticipated that the number of persons with heart failure will increase due to longer life expectancy and better treatment of heart failure.[2] Average length of stay in a hospital is 4.6 days,[1] but the length of stay and therefore hospital costs rise dramatically if critical illness develops.

The purpose of nutrition therapy for critically ill cardiac patients is to provide adequate and appropriate nutrition to maintain lean body mass, to replenish nutrient losses, to promote wound healing, and to regain strength for participation in rehabilitation.[3] In providing medical nutrition therapy to this critically ill patient population at risk for multisystem organ failure, it must do no harm.

ACUTE HEART FAILURE

Heart failure is the inability of the heart to work as a pump.[4] When the heart fails, water is retained throughout the body and blood perfusion is diminished.[5] Congestion occurs, resulting in pulmonary edema, hepatomegaly, bowel edema, and cardiorenal syndrome.[4] Consequently, the critically ill cardiac patient is at risk for developing multiple organ system failure.

Acute heart failure occurs during acute coronary syndromes, life-threatening arrhythmias, decompensating chronic heart failure, abrupt valvular dysfunction, and as a complication following cardiac surgery.[6] Myocardial infarctions and sometimes endocarditis will cause acute heart failure. Acute heart failure can also be the result of noncardiac etiologies.[6] Severity of acute heart failure and response to treatment will determine medical treatment. Anticoagulants, diuretics, and vasodilators will be utilized and if these are insufficient, then inotropes and vasopressors will be needed.[6] As a last resource for survival, mechanical circulatory support may be implanted.[6]

CARDIOGENIC OR CIRCULATORY SHOCK AND VASOPRESSORS

Patients in cardiogenic or circulatory shock often will have multiple organ failure. During shock, blood flow is diverted away from the heptatosplanchnic bed to the vital organs to promote survival.[6] Vasopressors increase blood pressure by their vasoconstricting action that exacerbates the reduction in blood flow to the peripheral organs and the splanchnic bed.[7] Organs that are impacted by the reduced blood flow include the gastrointestinal tract, kidneys, and skin.[6] Under normal circumstances, about 25% of the cardiac output is dedicated to the hepatosplanchnic circulation and it is doubled postprandially.[6] Consequently, during shock, this area can be significantly deprived of oxygen, resulting in the potential for bowel ischemia and bacterial translocation.[6]

MECHANICAL CIRCULATORY SUPPORT

Several mechanical devices are available to support the heart during failure. The most common device is the cardiopulmonary bypass pump. The cardiopulmonary bypass pump (CBP) is frequently used during open heart surgery when the beating heart is stopped; it provides oxygenated blood while bypassing the heart and lungs.[6] CBP is associated with undesirable outcomes, likely due to its ability to trigger systemic inflammation.[6] These adverse events range from mildly altered mental status to multiple organ dysfunction syndrome.[6] Ischemic-reperfusion injury of the bowel can occur, resulting in bacterial translocation.[6]

The intra-aortic balloon pump (IABP) may be used to improve blood circulation as a short-term therapy, usually not lasting more than 1 week.[3] Patients must be immobile in bed in a prone position.[3] Use of this device is associated with higher risks of leg and bowel ischemia and renal injury.[6]

Extracorporeal membrane oxygenation (ECMO) is the last resource for severe life-threatening cardiac or pulmonary failure when all other treatments have been unsuccessful.[6] It is similar to CBP in function but can be used for weeks, if needed, rather than the few hours CBP is utilized.[6] Like IABP, patients must remain immobile in bed in a prone position. Complications arising from use of ECMO are coagulopathy, leg ischemia, altered mental status, deep vein thrombosis, and air embolism.[6] Gastrointestinal complications include bleeding, ulcers, and perforations in addition to hepatic injury.[6]

Ventricular assist devices (VAD) are used for chronic heart failure, either as a *bridge* to heart transplantation or as a permanent device. VADs replace the pumping function of the heart.[2] They require a power source that is administered through *drive lines*.[3] Strokes, infections, and gastrointestinal bleeding, and device malfunctions are common complications.[2]

NUTRITIONAL STATUS

The nutritional status of cardiac patients ranges from overnutrition to malnutrition upon admission to the ICU.[3] Having a patient with morbid obesity or cardiac cachexia is not unusual in the coronary ICU.[3] Patients with acute cardiac disorders such as acute myocardial infarction are more likely to be well nourished than the person with chronic heart failure or chronic valvular disease.[3,6] Cardiac cachexia develops in about 10% of the patients with chronic heart or valvular disease, resulting in 50% survival rate in 18 months.[6] For persons undergoing cardiothoracic surgery, malnutrition increases mortality and morbidity rates, and patients with very low body fat stores will have higher mortality rates than those without fat depletion.[6] Excess fat stores associated with morbid obesity may impede cardiac surgery and delay recovery. Persons with endocarditis frequently have significant weight loss due to inflammation, impaired oral intake, and appetite-suppressing antibiotics.[3]

NUTRITIONAL ASSESSMENT

The nursing staff screens patients' nutritional status upon admission. Several simple screening tools have been developed in Europe, one of which is designed specifically for cardiac surgery patients. Components of Short Nutritional Assessment Questionnaire (SNAQ) are unintentional weight loss, loss of appetite, and use of nutritional supplements or enteral nutrition. Malnutrition Universal Screening Tool (MUST) incorporates body mass index, unintentional weight loss, acute disease effect, and lack of nutrition for at least 5 days. Investigators compared SNAQ and MUST to Subjective Global Assessment in identifying malnutrition in cardiac surgery patients and then to determine influence of malnutrition on outcomes.[7] SNAQ and MUST successfully identified malnutrition in 894 patients.[7] Malnutrition seemed to have an inconsistent impact on predicted postoperative infections, hospital and intensive care unit (ICU) length of stay, or mortality.[7–9] Later, a Cardiac-Surgery Specific Screening Tool was developed, which is MUST with the addition of age greater than 65 years, female gender, diminished food intake, and physical activity.[10] The authors of this tool identified malnutrition in a group of 325 cardiac surgery patients, and malnutrition was not associated with postoperative infection or mortality.

Nutritional assessment in the critically ill cardiac patient can be difficult due to edema, the use of resuscitating fluids, and the inflammatory nature of myocardial infarctions and cardiogenic shock.[3] An admitting weight should be obtained and then compared to subsequent weights while monitoring fluid intakes and outputs.[3] Diuresis is frequently one goal of treatment.[3] Patients who do not have congestive heart failure may know their usual weights.[3] However, due to frequent fluid imbalances, the person with congestive heart failure most likely will not know his usual weight.[3] A 10% unintentional preoperative weight loss has been associated with complications following cardiac surgery.[6] Fluid overload and the stress of myocardial infarctions and cardiogenic shock will render serum albumin useless as a nutritional parameter.[3]

In one study of 5168 cardiac surgery patients, the authors evaluated preoperative serum albumin and body mass index as predictors of postoperative complications.[11] Preoperative hypoalbuminemia was correlated with undesirable outcomes, and the lower the serum albumin, the worse the outcome. Serum albumin less than 3.5 g/dL was associated with increased risk of renal injury, atrial fibrillation, and length of stay. Increased mortality, low cardiac output, and greater likelihood of postoperative bleeding occurred in those with a serum albumin less than 2.5 g/dL. Body mass indexes outside of relatively normal range correlated with adverse outcomes. In patients whose body mass index was less than 20 kg/m^2, mortality, strokes, renal failure, pneumonia, and postoperative bleeding were increased. Obese patients with a body mass index greater than 30 kg/m^2 had more sternal wound and saphenous vein harvest site infections.

If possible, a brief diet history should be obtained from the patient or the family members. Usually, the person with an acute cardiac event was eating well prior to admission, whereas the person with chronic disease may have impaired oral intake due to illness and adverse effects of some cardiac medications.[3] Incidentally, some patients may have poor oral intake preoperatively due to anxiety about the upcoming surgery.[3]

A nutrition-focused physical examination should be performed but edema and critical care medicine may limit its value.[3] Edema masks the loss of muscle mass and fat stores; temporal muscle wasting, if present, will be visible. Due to poor blood circulation in persons with chronic cardiac disease, persons who have been bedfast are at high risk for developing decubiti.[3]

Most persons undergoing cardiac surgery do well, but there will be a few who have complications, usually related to preoperative problems, surgery, and CBP.[12] Postoperative cardiac problems can be arrhythmias, poor cardiac output, and hypotension.[12] Edema and pulmonary edema occur due to fluid retention during surgery.[12] Cardiac surgery is associated with more bleeding, neurological disturbances, and gastrointestinal issues than any other major surgical procedure.[12] Acute kidney injury is not uncommon and it correlates with increasing mortality due to its association with increased infection rates.[12] Water and sodium are retained and potassium is excreted due to the fluid and electrolyte shifts caused by CPB.[13] Hyperglycemia and insulin resistance occur due to elevated levels of epinephrine as a consequence of CBP.[13] Consequently, the risk of developing multiple organ system dysfunction is a real possibility following cardiac surgery.[3]

ORAL THERAPY

Many patients are able to eat, and the patient who had cardiac surgery will likely be allowed oral intake by postoperative day 1 or 2.[3] The diet will frequently be a heart-healthy diet that is restricted in cholesterol, saturated fats, and total fat.[3] A 2–4 g sodium restriction will be prescribed.[3] Other therapeutic diets may be necessary, depending on comorbidities, such as a consistent carbohydrate diet for those with diabetes.[3] Because heart failure can cause multiple organ failure, short-term modifications may be needed such as restrictions during acute renal failure.[3] Fluid restrictions are often prescribed in varying amounts, depending on the severity of fluid retention and the response to diuretics.[3]

Adequacy of oral intake can vary.[3] Some persons will eat well whereas other patients will have nearly no appetite.[3] Nausea, vomiting, diarrhea, anorexia, ascites, and early satiety can occur due to poor blood perfusion to the gastrointestinal tract during heart failure so adjusting the cardiac medications may help improve gastrointestinal function.[3] Cardiac medications may alter taste.[3] Loss of appetite may occur following cardiac surgery. Depression may occur postoperatively and it may suppress appetite. For those who are not eating well, providing only the diet restrictions needed to promote recovery may assist in enhancing food palatability, increasing provision of nutrients, and promoting patient satisfaction.[3] For example, if the patient is eating very little food, there is no need for diet restrictions until oral intake significantly improves. Patients with poor appetites may benefit from frequent, small, meals, a daily multivitamin, and liquid oral supplements. Lastly, critically ill cardiac patients may complain about the food, partly because of its blandness without salt and fat, but also due to their frustration and anger about being in the ICU.[3]

ENTERAL NUTRITION

Patients who remain on ventilators or have impaired swallowing will need alternate routes of nutrition. If the gastrointestinal tract is functional, enteral nutrition should be administered; otherwise, parenteral nutrition will be necessary. The type of enteral product and concentration of the parenteral nutrition will depend on cardiac status, severity of impairment of other organs, and treatment of organ failure. These critically ill patients are also at risk for developing refeeding syndrome, particularly those with cardiac cachexia.

Ideally, enteral nutrition should be started within 24–48 h of admission to the ICU; however, that may not be feasible for the critically ill unstable patient. When to initiate enteral nutrition has been a topic of considerable discussion because of the low flow state to the gastrointestinal tract during hemodynamic instability. Hypoperfusion limits oxygen supply to the splanchnic bed and vasopressors can worsen hypoperfusion, resulting in potential risk for bowel ischemia, increased gut permeability, bacterial translocation, worsening organ failure, and ultimately, elevated mortality.[6] Also, bowel ischemia can occur if there is insufficient oxygen to digest and absorb nutrients.[6] On the other hand, nutrients in small quantities may be beneficial during low flow states because they improve blood flow in the splanchnic bed.[6] Several studies examined tolerance of enteral nutrition in critically ill unstable patients, including those who had cardiac surgery, and found that it could be administered while on low-dose vasopressors but not tolerated as well if the vasopressors were increased.[6]

Critical care nutrition guidelines recommend initiating enteral nutrition after the patient has been resuscitated and stabilized,[14,15] but that is sometimes difficult to determine. Risk factors for developing bowel ischemia are a history of vascular insufficiency, use of mechanical circulatory devices, vasopressor administration, reduced cardiac output, and mechanical ventilation.[6]

Patients with mean arterial pressures of at least 60–70 mmHg should be stable enough to tolerate enteral nutrition.[4] Another potential marker of bowel ischemia is intra-abdominal pressure; a pressure of at least 15 mmHg could indicate risk of bowel ischemia, and bowel ischemia is probably occurring if the pressure is 20 mmHg or greater.[6] Enteral feedings should be initiated at a low rate (10–20 mL/h) and tolerance should be monitored, assessing abdominal distension, increase in nasogastric tube output or gastric residual volumes, decreased stool or flatus, diminished bowel sounds, worsening metabolic acidosis or base deficit.[6] Enteral nutrition should be stopped if there is an abrupt change for the worse in hemodynamic status or gastrointestinal function.[6]

Early enteral nutrition was shown to be beneficial in a small group of patients who needed cardiopulmonary resuscitation following cardiopulmonary arrest.[16] Of the 57 patients who survived 24 h after the arrest, 22 patients were started on enteral nutrition within 48 h of the arrest. In this retrospective study, the authors found that early enteral nutrition was a favorable predictor for 3 month survival. Patients receiving early enteral nutrition may not have been as sick as those fed later, having a lower APACHE II score. The study did not indicate if the patients receiving enteral feeding were receiving vasopressors or were on mechanical circulatory devices; also, the feeding tube placement, type of enteral formula, feeding rates, and feeding volumes were not identified.

Critically ill patients on ECMO or ventricular assist devices can be hemodynamically unstable. There is a paucity of research about enteral nutrition for this group of patients, partly because it is a very small and unique population. One study demonstrated successful enteral feeding in seven patients on ECMO requiring several vasopressors.[17] Mean duration of ECMO was 7 days. Enteral nutrition was initiated within 24–48 h, starting with 21 mL/h after the patient's demonstrated tolerance to enteral fluids. The feeding rate was advanced every 24 h so the goal rate was achieved by day 4. The head of the bed was maintained at a 30° angle at all times. Nasogastric feeding tubes terminating in the stomach were used for feeding and prokinetic medications were not needed. Patients received at least 70% of the recommended feeding by the end of the first week; the only complication was constipation in 4 patients.

Critical care nutrition guidelines state that feeding tube placement can be either gastric or post-pyloric.[14,15] Patients with impaired cardiac function and those with cardiac surgery may tolerate enteral nutrition better if the feeding tube is in a post-pyloric location rather than in the gastric location[6]; this should increase the likelihood of receiving adequate nutrition. Anesthesia, sedatives, opioids, and mechanical ventilation used during and after cardiac surgery promote gastric dysmotility.[6] Placing feeding tubes in patients with VADS could be challenging because some types of VADs are located in the abdominal area and thus hide the stomach.[3]

The choice of enteral product is dependent on the patient's medical condition, including cardiac function. It can be challenging to select the appropriate enteral product if the patient has multiple organ dysfunction syndrome. Cardiac surgery patients should benefit from immune-enhancing formulas.

PARENTERAL NUTRITION

Parenteral nutrition is reserved only for those patients with dysfunctional gastrointestinal tracts. Patients with mesenteric ischemia, abdominal aortic aneurysms that disrupt blood flow to the gastrointestinal tract, or abdominal compartment syndrome may need parenteral nutrition.[6] Also, patients who are not tolerating adequate enteral nutrition after all therapies have been attempted may be candidates for parenteral nutrition.[6] Like enteral nutrition, the patient needs to be resuscitated and hemodynamically stabilized before initiating parenteral nutrition.[6]

Cardiac patients tend to have abnormal lipid profiles that may limit the use of parenteral lipids. Lipids should be restricted if serum triglyceride levels exceed 400 mg/dL; otherwise, parenteral lipids will worsen hypertriglyceridemia.[6]

Cardiac patients tend not to tolerate large amounts of fluids well so parenteral nutrition volume may need to be concentrated.[6] However, it should not be so restrictive as to impair provision of adequate nutrition. Symptoms of volume overload should be monitored while receiving parenteral nutrition, assessing for edema, pulmonary congestion, worsening heart failure, urinary output, and ascites.[6]

NUTRITIONAL REQUIREMENTS

Nutritional requirements for critically ill cardiac patients are similar to other critically ill patients. Ideally, indirect calorimetry is used to determine energy requirements. If it is not available or feasible, then predictive equations such as the Penn State equations can be used for patients on mechanical ventilation.[6] Congestive heart failure is an inflammatory, hypermetabolic state in which levels of tumor necrosis factor and proinflammatory cytokines are elevated.[18] Consequently, patients will have high caloric and protein requirements.[3] Recommended protein requirements are 1.5–2.0 g protein/kilogram body weight (or ideal body weight if body mass index is 30 kg/m^2 or greater).[6] Protein requirements may need to be adjusted, depending on renal and hepatic functions.[6]

Due to losses and possibly poor oral intake, a multivitamin supplement is recommended. Patients receiving thiazide diuretics may need potassium and magnesium supplementation.[19]

GLYCEMIC CONTROL FOR CARDIAC SURGERY PATIENTS

Stress hyperglycemia occurs in cardiac surgery patients due to the inflammatory process associated with surgery.[6] Several large studies examined the effects of hyperglycemia with tight glucose control on the outcomes of cardiac surgery, and, because of conflicting results, it is difficult to make a recommendation at this time. In a study by van den Berghe et al. (n = 1548 ICU patients, mostly cardiac surgery patients), patients who received intensive insulin therapy to normalize blood glucose levels had lower mortality and morbidity rates than those whose blood glucose levels were maintained at 180–200 mg/dL.[20] Patients in this study were fed 200–300 g intravenous dextrose on the first postoperative day and then were advanced to either enteral nutrition, parenteral nutrition, or both on the second day, receiving 20–30 nonprotein calories/kilogram body weight. This practice may have resulted in overfeeding patients and it may not be usual procedure following cardiac surgery. In a second study (n = 6104), the Normoglycemia in Intensive Care Evaluation-Survival Using Glucose Algorithm Regulation, patients with intensive insulin therapy to maintain normal blood glucose levels had a higher mortality rate than those whose blood glucose levels were 180 mg/dL or less.[21] Patients in this study may have been underfed, receiving about 900 nonprotein calories for the first 14 days. Other studies noted reduced mortality when blood glucose levels were below 158 mg/dL.[22,23] Concerns in these trials have been the frequency of hypoglycemia with the attempts to normalize blood glucose levels. Considering the results of these studies, perhaps the goal of normal blood glucose levels is the ideal, but if it is not possible, then aiming for levels of 140–180 mg/dL should be acceptable.[6]

ANTIOXIDANTS

Systemic inflammation is characteristic of cardiac surgery patients and those with atrial fibrillation. Atrial fibrillation is triggered in part by inflammation and oxidative stress.[6] Studies examining the effects of supplemental vitamins C and E, selenium, and zinc in cardiac patients have shown mixed results in preventing atrial fibrillation, reducing number of ventilator days and length of stay, and improvement in inflammatory markers; there is either benefit or no benefit in these supplements.[6,24,25] Only omega-3 fatty acids have shown promise in preventing atrial fibrillation.[26] At this time, physicians seem not to be routinely prescribing these supplemental antioxidants.

REFERENCES

1. Centers for Disease Control. Heart disease faststats. http://www.cdc.gov/nchs/faststats/heart.disease.htm. Accessed August 2014.
2. Dunlay, S. M. et al., Contemporary strategies in the diagnosis and management of heart failure, *Mayo Clin Proc*, 89, 662, 2014.
3. Hummell, A. C., Nutrition for the critically ill cardiac patient, in *Nutrition Support for the Critically Ill Patient: A Guide to Practice*, Cresci, G. Ed., CRC Press, Boca Raton, FL, 2005, p. 519.
4. Porth, C., Heart failure, in *Pathophysiology*, Lippincott Company, Philadelphia, PA, 1982, p. 216.
5. Zile, M. R. and Brutsaert, D. L., New concepts in diastolic dysfunction and diastolic heart failure: Part I, *Circulation*, 105, 1387, 2002.
6. Cresci, G. et al., Nutrition intervention in the critically ill cardiothoracic patient, *Nutr Clin Pract*, 27, 323, 2012.
7. Lomivorotov, V. V. et al., Evaluation of nutritional screening tools for patients scheduled for cardiac surgery, *Nutrition*, 29, 436, 2013.
8. Van Venrooij, L. M. W. et al., Accuracy of quick and easy undernutrition screening tools—Short Nutritional Assessment Questionnaire, Malnutrition Universal Screening Tool, and Modified Malnutrition Universal Screening Tool—In patients undergoing cardiac surgery, *J Am Diet Assoc*, 11, 1924, 2011.
9. Chermesh, I. et al., Malnutrition in cardiac surgery: Food for thought, *Eur J Prev Cardiol*, 21, 475, 2014.
10. Van Venrooij, L. M. W. et al., Cardiac surgery-specific screening tool identifies preoperative undernutrition in cardiac surgery, *Ann Thorac Surg*, 95, 642, 2013.
11. Engelman, D. et al., Impact of body mass index and albumin on morbidity and mortality after cardiac surgery, *J Thorac Cardiovasc Surg*, 118, 866, 1999.
12. Mehta, S. and Pae, W. D., Complications of cardiac surgery, in *Cardiac Surgery in the Adult*, Edmunds, L. H. Ed., McGraw-Hill, New York, 1997, p. 369.
13. Bojar, R. J., Fluid management, renal and metabolic problems, in *Perioperative Care in Cardiac Surgery*, 3rd edn., Blackwell Science, Malden, MA, 1999, p. 337.
14. McClave, S. et al., Guidelines for the provision and assessment of nutrition support therapy in the adult critically ill patient: Society of Critical Care Medicine (SCCM) and American Society for Parenteral and Enteral Nutrition (A.S.P.E.N.), *J Parenter Enteral Nutr*, 33, 277, 2009.
15. Evidence Analysis Library, Academy of Nutrition and Dietetics, Initiation of enteral nutrition. http://www.andeal.com. Accessed August 2014.
16. Lee, H.-K. et al., Factors influencing outcome in patients with cardiac arrest in the ICU, *Acta Anaesthesiol Scand*, 57, 784, 2013.
17. Makikado, L. D. U. et al., Early enteral nutrition in adults receiving venoarterial extracorporeal membrane oxygenation: An observational case series, *J Parenter Enteral Nutr*, 37, 281, 2013.
18. Kirklin, J. K. et al., Pathophysiology and clinical features of heart failure, in *Heart Transplantation*, Churchill-Livingstone, Philadelphia, PA, 2002, p. 107.
19. Kirklin, J. K. et al., Nutritional management of the heart transplant recipient, in *Heart Transplantation*, Churchill-Livingstone, Philadelphia, PA, 2002, p. 139.
20. van den Berghe, G. et al., Intensive insulin therapy in the critically ill patients, *N Engl J Med*, 345, 1359, 2001.
21. Anonymous, Intensive versus conventional glucose control in critically ill patients, *N Engl J Med*, 19, 1283, 2009.
22. Frioud, A. et al., Blood glucose level on postoperative day 1 is predictive of adverse outcomes after cardiovascular surgery, *Diabetes Metab*, 36, 36, 2010.
23. Giakoumidakis, K. et al., Effects of intensive glycemia control on outcomes of cardiac surgery, *Heart Lung*, 42, 146, 2013.
24. Bjordahl, P. M. et al., Perioperative supplementation with ascorbic acid does not prevent atrial fibrillation in coronary artery bypass graft patients, *Am J Surg*, 204, 862, 2012.
25. Colby, J. A. et al., Effect of ascorbic acid on inflammatory markers after cardiothoracic surgery, *Am J Health Syst Pharm*, 68, 1632, 2011.
26. Costanzo, S. et al., Prevention of postoperative atrial fibrillation in open heart surgery patients by preoperative supplementation of n-3 polyunsaturated fatty acids: An updated meta-analysis, *J Thorac Cardiovasc Surg*, 146, 906, 2013.

31 Nutrition Support in Neurocritical Care

Arlene Escuro and Mary Rath

CONTENTS

INTRODUCTION

The brain is one of the largest and most complex organs in the human body. It consists of the cerebral cortex, brain stem, and cerebellum that control emotions, thoughts, memories, as well as basic vital life functions such as breathing, heartbeat, and blood pressure. A brain injury can affect one or many parts of the brain that may result in lifelong neurological deficits that can have a significant impact on a person's quality of life. The metabolic responses to the injury may be severe and prolonged especially when complicated by multiple organ failures. Therefore, along with prompt medical care, nutrition intervention is critical to optimize the best outcome following brain injury. This chapter will review two common types of brain injuries, traumatic brain injuries (TBIs) and stroke, and discuss appropriate nutritional intervention to prevent and/or treat malnutrition during critical illness.

TRAUMATIC BRAIN INJURY

According to the Department of Defense, the definition of TBI is "a traumatically induced structural injury or physiological disruption of brain function resulting from an external force that is indicated by new onset or worsening of symptoms involving level of consciousness, memory, mental state or neurological deficits (such as weakness, loss of balance, sensory loss, aphasia) or intracranial lesion" (Department of Defense 2009). Severity of a brain injury is determined by Glasgow Coma Score (GCS). The GCS comprises three tests, including eye, verbal, and motor responses (Table 31.1). A patient is assessed against the criteria of the scale and the resulting points give a patient score between 3 and 15, in which a score less than 8 is considered coma and defines a severe brain injury, with significant risk of mortality (Coronado et al. 2009).

The Center for Disease Control estimates that 1.7 million sustain a TBI annually (Faul et al. 2010). Falls continue to be the leading cause of TBI (35.2%) in the United States. Among all age groups, motor vehicle crashes and traffic-related incidents are the second leading cause of TBI (17.3%), resulting in the largest percentage of TBI-related deaths (31.8%) (Faul et al. 2010).

MEDICAL TREATMENT

TBI initially can include skull fractures, brain tissue disruption, and torn cerebral vessels that are managed by specific medical and surgical strategies. Within minutes, hours, or days of the primary injury, a secondary brain injury can occur. This secondary injury involves multiple metabolic mechanisms that result from interruption of blood flow and oxygen to undamaged cells, producing anaerobic metabolism, inadequate synthesis of adenosine triphosphate or cellular acidosis. Ideal medical management of severe TBI patients begins with early intervention and rapid stabilization of the patient's respiratory function. This requires attention to maintaining normal intracranial pressure (ICP), optimizing cerebral perfusion pressure, improving brain issue oxygenation, and preventing other organ system injuries (Tang and Lobel 2009). Patients with severe TBI will often require intubation for airway protection and mechanical ventilation to ensure adequate oxygenation and optimal carbon dioxide levels. Fluid resuscitation and vasopressor agents, such as norepinephrine, may be needed to maintain the cerebral perfusion pressure above 60 mmHg (Cook et al. 2007).

TABLE 31.1
Glasgow Coma Scale

Eye response	4. Opens eyes spontaneously
	3. Opens eyes in response to speech
	2. Opens eyes in response to pain
	1. Does not open eyes in response to pain
Motor response	6. Follow commands
	5. Localizes pain
	4. Moves to pain but not purposefully
	3. Flexes upper extremities to pain
	2. Extends all extremities to pain
	1. No motor response to pain
Verbal response	5. Oriented to person, place, and time
	4. Confused speech
	3. Replies with inappropriate words
	2. Incomprehensible sounds
	1. No verbal sounds

Metabolic Response

The brain's function as the regulator for metabolic activity leads to a complexity of metabolic alterations in TBI such as hormonal changes, irregular cellular metabolism, and cerebral and systemic inflammatory response. The end results of these alterations are systemic catabolism, protein wasting, and increased energy demand, which lead to hyperglycemia (Cook et al. 2008). The degree of the hypermetabolic state is directly related to the severity of injury and motor dysfunction (Fruin et al. 1986). After brain injury, secretion of many hormones that affect metabolic function such as adrenocorticotropic hormone (ACTH), growth hormone, prolactin, vasopressin, and cortisol are stimulated as a response to stress (Cresci et al. 2007). Glucagon and catecholamines are also released (Cherian et al. 2004). While catecholamines help to regulate cardiac output and support blood pressure, they also increase basal metabolism, oxygen consumption, glycogenolysis, hyperglycemia, proteolysis, and muscle wasting (Cook et al. 2007). Effective nutrition support can attenuate the catabolic response and avoid the potentially harmful effects of prolonged hypermetabolism (Cook et al. 2008).

Nutrition Assessment in TBI Patients

The goal of providing adequate nutrition support in TBI patients is to meet the needs of the hypermetabolic demands and minimize the loss of lean body mass. As with all critically ill patients, indirect calorimetry is the preferred method for determining energy requirements for TBI patients (Brunner 2007). However, the daily caloric requirements of brain-injured patients that have intermittent muscle contractions, sympathetic alterations, or fever may not be accurately represented using indirect calorimetry (Cook et al. 2008). The high cost of the metabolic cart is also a limiting factor hindering its availability in many critical care facilities. Therefore, various calculations have been used to predict the estimated expenditure, such as Harris–Benedict (HBE), Ireton–Jones, Penn State, weight-based calculations, and current ADA-endorsed Mifflin St. Jeor equations (Frankenfield et al. 2007 and Academy of Nutrition and Dietetics 2012). TBI patients exhibit 120%–250% of their BEE, using the Harris–Benedict Equation (HBE) (Kolpek et al. 1989; Koukiasa et al. 2014). However, medications, such as sedatives, paralytics, and barbiturates, often alter metabolism by 76%–120% of BEE. The Brain Trauma Foundation recommends providing 120%–140% calculated BEE using HBE, which will meet the needs of most TBI patients (Brain Trauma Foundation 2000). The American Society of Parental and Enteral Nutrition (ASPEN) recommend the use of Mifflin-St Jeor equation for basal energy expenditure (ASPEN 2002). However, the equation has not been validated for use in TBI population (McClave et al. 2009). Regardless of which method is used, no single method of estimating energy expenditure is flawless; therefore, close monitoring of each patient is needed to prevent over- or underfeeding.

Excessive proteolysis and skeletal muscle wasting is hallmark of TBI, which is stimulated by inflammatory mediators and catecholamines. Catabolism appears to peak 8–14 days after injury with retention by the third week (Young et al. 1992). Dickerson and Associates studied patients with acute head injury and found that protein oxidation accounted for ~30% of REE (Dickerson et al. 1990). However, supplementation of excessive calories or protein to abate protein loss does not appear to be effective (Bivins et al. 1986). Currently, the Brain Trauma Foundation recommends providing 1.5–2 g/kg/day protein for acute TBI patients to account for the excess catabolism (Hatton 2001). However, high protein doses may cause azotemia in patients with renal insufficiency; therefore, monitoring of blood urea nitrogen concentrations should be performed until the protein dose and renal function are stabilized (Rajpal and Johnston 2009).

Shortly after injury, TBI patients often require intravascular fluid resuscitation to maintain adequate mean arterial and cerebral perfusion pressures. Patients with elevated ICP may also receive osmotic diuretics, which also potentiate the need for intravenous fluid supplementation. However, excess fluid volumes may decrease cerebral compliance and increase brain edema (Hariri et al. 1993). The optimal fluid for use in TBI patients in not well defined. The Brain Trauma Foundation guidelines do not make a definitive statement on fluid choice from intravenous resuscitation for TBI (Brain Trauma Foundation 2000). Therefore, when providing fluid replacement for TBI patients, several factors, such as crystalloid versus colloid use, glucose content, free water content, and serum sodium imbalances, should be considered. Fluid and sodium balance disorders are further discussed in the section "Fluid and Electrolyte Balance in CNS Injuries."

STROKES

There are two types of strokes: ischemic and hemorrhagic. Ischemic stroke, which occurs when a clot or particle clogs a blood vessel, cutting off the blood flow to a part of the brain, can be either thrombotic or embolic. Hemorrhagic strokes include intracerebral hemorrhage (ICH) or subarachnoid hemorrhage (SAH). ICH occurs when blood vessels bleed into the tissue deep within the brain. SAH occurs when a blood vessel on the surface of the brain ruptures and bleeds into the space between the brain and the skull. Risk factors are listed in Table 31.2. Severity of stroke is also determined by the GCS as discussed with TBI injuries.

Stroke was the fourth leading cause of death in 2008 after more than five decades at number 3 in the ranking (Miniño et al. 2011). Ischemic strokes are the most common type of stroke, representing about 87% of all strokes, and about a quarter of all strokes occur under the age of 65 (Roger et al. 2011). Demographically, men experience a higher incidence of strokes than women, and African-Americans are significantly more likely to have a stroke than Caucasians (Roger et al. 2011). See Table 31.2 for common risk factors for stroke.

Medical Treatment

On admission, stroke location, stroke size, and stroke type are usually confirmed by either MRI or CT imaging. Stroke severity is assessed using GCS as well as National Institute of Health (NIH) stroke scale (NIHSS). NIHSS is a standardized method used by physicians and other health-care professionals to measure the level of impairment caused by stroke. Its main use in clinical medicine is to determine whether or not the degree of disability caused by a given stroke merits treatment with or tissue plasminogen activator (tPA), a potent blood thinner. Treatment with hemorrhagic strokes is similar to the treatment in TBI patients including the control of bleeding and reducing pressure within the brain. ICP can be monitored with a bolt or ventriculostomy placement. Medications are usually given that help to reduce blood pressure and prevent seizures (referred to later in this chapter). Surgery may include clipping of the aneurysm, coiling of the aneurysm, and/or surgical removal. However, despite the medical interventions, complications may include paralysis, dysphagia, aphasia, memory loss, pain, and loss of independence.

Metabolic Response

After neurological insult, metabolic demands are altered with elevation of peripheral plasma catecholamines, cortisol, glucagon, interleukin-6, interleukin-IRA, and acute phase proteins (Finestone et al. 2003). Hypermetabolism is well documented in TBI but not well defined in the stroke patient population. Infection, age, severity of stroke and comorbidities, medication, ventilator status, mobility, activity levels, and weight status can alter metabolic requirements. Early medical

TABLE 31.2
Risk Factors for Stroke

Family history	HTN
DM	BMI >25 kg/m^2
Physical inactivity	Cigarette smoking
Alcohol or drug abuse	

treatments in the acute care setting to decrease ICP such as the use of barbiturates or induced hypothermia also decrease caloric requirements.

Nutrition Assessment in the Stroke Patient

Patients admitted to the ICU following a CVA may require specialized nutritional support, depending on the severity of the event and the patient's baseline nutritional status (Dennis et al. 2005). Brain injury resulting from stroke has metabolic consequences, and the presence of preexisting malnutrition and malnutrition after stroke contributes to clinical outcomes. The prevalence of malnutrition-associated post-stroke, using validated tools such as Subjective Global Assessment and the Mini Nutritional Assessment, ranged from 16% to 26% in the first week after the event (Davis et al. 2004; Crary et al. 2006).

In the absence of indirect calorimetry, predicted equations are used to estimate energy requirements. Resting energy expenditure (REE) in stroke patients has been shown to have a 10%–15% elevation in energy needs regardless of type of stroke, gender, or age (Weekes and Elia 1992). Finestone and colleagues used indirect calorimetry on poststroke days 7, 11, 14, 21, and 90 to study energy demands over time after stroke. REE was shown to be approximately 10% higher than predicted by the HBE, but did not differ by type of stroke, and changes in REE were not statistically significant over time (Finestone et al. 2003). It was presumed that energy requirements were not elevated due to physical inactivity and changes in muscle tone related to the neurological injury (Finestone et al. 2003). A more recent prospective, observation study on ICU patients with spontaneous ICH found that compared with BMR (predicted by HBE), measured REE values (using IC) showed a statistically significant increase in energy needs from day 0 to day 10 with mean REE 117.5% of BMR. There was also a trend toward an increase in REE over time up to 126% of BMR by days 7 and 10. The patients in the study were sedated on mechanical ventilation and free of infectious or other complications that could interfere with metabolic requirements (Koukiasa et al. 2014). In summary, no single formula to calculate nutritional requirements has been validated with a large sample size in the stroke population. Factors such as infection, age, severity of stroke, comorbidities, medication, ventilator status, mobility, activity levels, and weight status can alter caloric requirements, necessitating frequent reassessment by nutrition clinicians (Academy of Nutrition and Dietetics 2012). See Chapter 6 for evaluation of predictive equations.

Protein provision is important in stroke recovery because cerebral ischemia initiates repression of protein synthesis, which can lead to cell death. Restoration of protein can allow cells to repair ischemic damage and recover function (Raschen 2003). Recommended protein needs are 1.0–1.5 g/kg preinjury weight or 1.5–2.0 g/kg per ideal weight in obese populations with BMI >30 kg/m^2 (Brunner 2007).

NUTRITION SUPPORT MANAGEMENT IN CENTRAL NERVOUS SYSTEM INJURIES

Timing of Feeding

The intense catabolic response immediately after a critical neurological injury is well documented. Effective nutrition support can play a major role in attenuating the catabolic response and avoiding the potentially harmful effects of prolonged hypermetabolism (Cook et al. 2008). Once it is determined that a patient with acute brain injury cannot be fed orally, initiation of enteral nutrition (EN) clearly becomes an important goal for nutrition support. Provision of early EN, particularly within 48 h, forestalls the breakdown of protein and fat stores, blunts the innate inflammatory response, promotes immune competence, decreases intensive care unit (ICU) infections, limits the risk of bacterial translocation, and improves neurological outcome at 3 months (Taylor et al. 1999; Perel et al. 2006). The Brain Trauma Foundation recommends achieving full caloric replacement by day 7 following a brain injury (Bratton et al. 2007). The Society for Critical Care Medicine (SCCM) and the American Society for Parenteral and Enteral Nutrition (A.S.P.E.N.) suggest providing >50%–65%

of goal calories in enteral nutrition over the first week of hospitalization to support quicker return of cognitive function in patients with head injury (ASPEN 2002 and McClave et al. 2009). Taylor and associates examined the effect of early enhanced EN on clinical outcome of head-injured patients requiring mechanical ventilation in a randomized, controlled trial of 82 patients (Taylor et al. 1999). Significant reductions in infectious complications as well as overall complications were noted in the early EN group, and the metabolic response, measured by a blunted rise in levels of the acute phase protein, C-reactive protein, seemed to indicate a beneficial outcome. Overall, they noted a slight improvement ($p = 0.08$) in neurological outcome at 3 months in the patients fed early EN, but no difference in ultimate outcome at 6 months. They concluded that the improvement in infectious complications and the reduction in the inflammatory response noted with early EN justified its administration (Taylor et al. 1999). More recent work demonstrated that patients who were not fed within 5 and 7 days after TBI had a two- and fourfold increase likelihood of death (Hartl et al. 2008). Every 10 kcal/kg decrease in caloric intake was associated with a 30%–40% increase in mortality rates (Hartl et al. 2008). Chiang et al. found EN initiated within 48 h postinjury in patients with severe TBI is associated with greater survival rate, GCS recovery, and a better clinical outcome at 1-month postinjury (Chiang et al. 2012).

Route of Feeding

Many early studies of nutrition support in acute brain injury patients favored parenteral nutrition due to issues of intolerance and delayed initiation of feeding with EN (Vizzini and Aranda-Michel 2011). These studies often utilized nasogastric tubes for EN shortly after brain injury (Cook et al. 2008). Advances in obtaining early enteral access have shown improved tolerance to enteral feeds, making it the preferred route of feeding for TBI patients. The impact of gastric feeding compared with small bowel feeding on nutrition and clinical outcomes was evaluated in a multicenter observational study of 1495 critically ill neurologically injured patients (Saran et al. 2014). The study showed that gastric feeding was associated with better adequacy of EN delivery despite increased likelihood of EN interruptions due to gastrointestinal (GI) complications, but neither feeding route showed clinically significant benefits to clinical outcomes (duration of mechanical ventilation and ICU and hospital length of stay; Saran et al. 2014). Nasoenteric tubes are intended for short-term use (less than 4 weeks). Long-term enteral access devices, such as gastrostomy or jejunostomy tubes, should be considered for patients requiring enteral nutrition greater than 4 weeks (Bankhead et al. 2009). Refer to Chart 31.1 for feeding algorithm to help determine the most appropriate route of feeding for neurocritical patients.

Enteral Formula Selection

Most studies evaluating enteral nutrition in brain-injured patients utilized isotonic, isocaloric formulas; a few studies involved the use of a disease-specific formula. Patients with brain injury experience accelerated muscle wasting from immobility, decreased protein synthesis, and development of undernutrition while hospitalized. Weight gain is often in fat-free mass and not muscle (Scherbakov and Doehner 2011). Whey protein is a source of branch-chain amino acids, including leucine; therefore, whey-based formulas have been evaluated in elderly stroke patients to potentially delay the development of sarcopenia that affects mortality and ICU length of stay (Aguilar-Nascimento et al. 2011). However, the double-blind randomized trial results were not statistically significant and mortality and ICU length of stay did not vary between the casein formula and whey formula groups.

Mineral and amino acid supplementation has been studied in central nervous system (CNS)–injured patient; however, limited current evidence supports the benefits of supplementation (Nishizawa 2001). Zinc, a cofactor for substrate metabolism, immune function, and *N*-methyl-D-aspartate (NMDA)

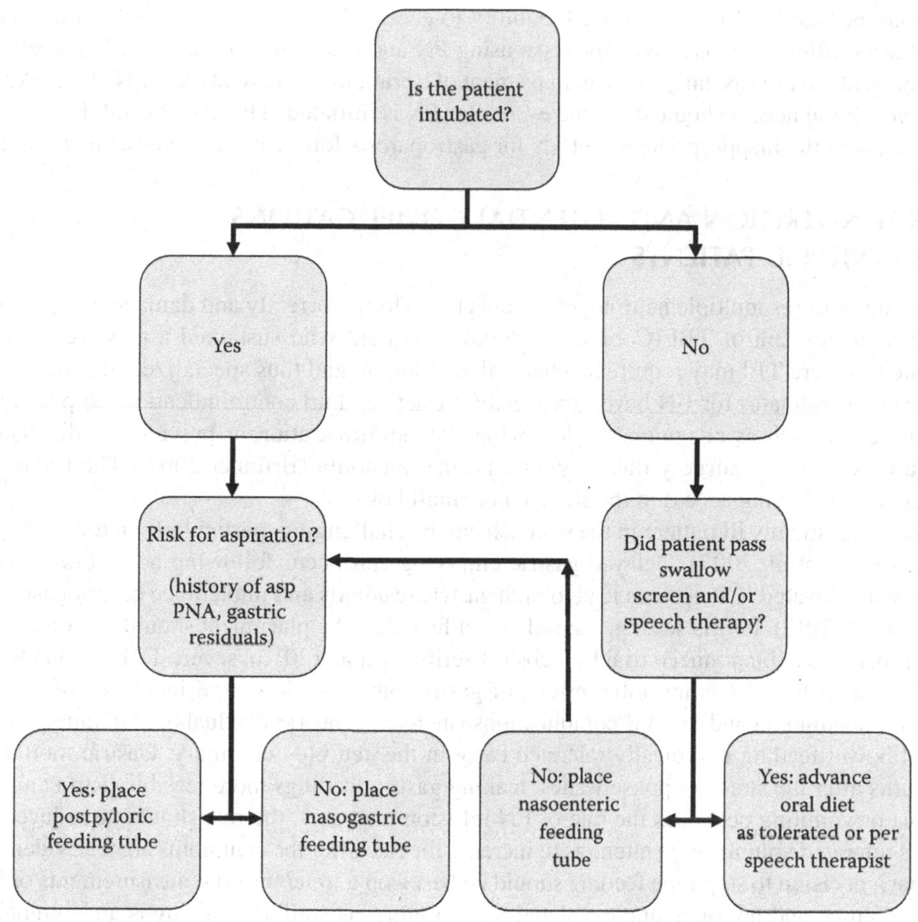

CHART 31.1 Feeding algorithm in neurocritical care.

receptor function, is diminished in brain injury due to liver sequestration and increased renal clearance (Young et al. 1996). Supplementation of zinc improved protein metabolism and neurological outcome at 1 month after TBI (Young et al. 1996). In a retrospective study, low serum zinc concentrations in patients following a stroke was associated with more severe strokes (NIHSS > 8) on admission and poor functional status at discharge (Bhatt et al. 2010). Magnesium was shown in animal studies to be neuroprotective due to activity at the NMDA receptor and modulation of cellular energy production and calcium influx (McKee et al. 2005). Despite these findings, human studies have yet to yield definitive benefits of zinc and magnesium supplementation in brain-injured patients.

With the information available to date, there are insufficient data to suggest that the use of a specialty formula can change CNS outcomes or disease-related sarcopenia. Every patient needs to be assessed on an individual basis and enteral formulas should be selected to optimally meet nutritional needs with goal to preserve lean body mass and prevent malnutrition during hospitalization.

Parenteral Nutrition Support

While enteral nutrition is preferred over parenteral nutrition, a critically ill patient who presents with a nonfunctioning GI tract or unable to ingest or absorb adequate nutrients from enteral nutrition may require PN (Mirtallo and Patel 2012 and Skipper 2003). In the acute brain injury patient, the use of PN may be indicated with prolonged inability to access the GI tract depending on the patient's premorbid nutritional status. Given the risks using PN and the relative efficacy of EN, every effort should be made to use EN early in the management of a brain injury patient (ASPEN 2002). Attempts to achieve enteral access should continue even after PN is initiated. The use of small bowel feeding tubes can avoid the inappropriate use of PN for gastroparesis following stroke or acute brain injury.

ENTERAL NUTRITION AND POTENTIAL COMPLICATIONS IN CNS-INJURED PATIENTS

Swallowing requires multiple neurological inputs to perform correctly and damage to these circuits may occur as a result of TBI (Cook et al. 2008). A patient who sustained a massive stroke or a moderate to severe TBI may require mechanical ventilation, and thus specialized nutrition support. Appropriate candidates for EN have functional GI tracts and no contraindications to placement of a feeding tube, such as coagulopathy following tPA administration or previous medical/surgical procedures such as GI surgery that may alter normal anatomy (Brunner 2007). The use of EN is contingent upon having access to the stomach or small bowel.

Feeding a critically ill patient in the stomach can be challenging, particularly in the acute phases of illness (Koc et al. 2007). Delayed gastric emptying can occur following acute brain injury in patients with elevated ICP and can lead to high gastric residuals and intolerance of nasogastric feeding (Ruf et al. 2012). In this setting, a small bowel feeding tube placement should be considered.

In a prospective, randomized trial by Acosta-Escribano et al. (2010), severe TBI patients fed early through a small bowel feeding tube instead of gastric tube had decreased incidence of ventilator-associated pneumonia and less GI complications (increased gastric residuals). Continuous infusion of small bowel feeding is typically tolerated early in the neurological injury. Gastric motility usually returns after the stress response wanes, making gastric feedings more feasible (Ruf et al. 2012). If nausea or vomiting occurs as the rate of EN infusion increases, the rate should be reduced to the previous tolerated volume, with attempts to increase the rate after the symptoms abate. Evidence suggests that a decision to stop tube feeding should be based on a trend in serial measurements of gastric residual volume and not on a single isolated high volume, as well as other signs and symptoms of intolerance (Malone et al. 2012). Concomitant use of promotility agents (metoclopramide and erythromycin) and enteral feeds may be beneficial in providing nutrition to acute brain injury patients with gastroparesis. Promotility agents are not without adverse effects, so these agents should be used for a short duration until the desired effect is obtained and maintained (Cook et al. 2008). Patients who may exhibit EN intolerance in the first few days after injury are still likely to benefit from some EN even at a low rate of 10–20 mL/h with improved mucosal blood flow (Cook et al. 2008).

Patients with acute brain injury may require high doses of vasopressors. EN should not be initiated until a patient is adequately resuscitated and hemodynamically stable. Signs to delay EN are abdominal distention, increasing gastric residual volumes, rising lactate, and escalating dose of vasopressors (McClave et al. 2009). Bowel necrosis is a rare complication that has been most often described in patients receiving EN via the jejunum (Wells 2012). For the majority of ICU patients, administration of EN into the stomach during the provision of low and stable doses of pressors with close monitoring of feeding intolerance or worsening hemodynamic stability poses very little risk for bowel necrosis (Wells 2012). For a critically ill patient on stable or declining doses of vasopressors, low-dose EN at 10–20 mL/h with a standard, polymeric, fiber-free formula can be initiated. It is important to closely monitor the patient for EN tolerance and adjust the EN feeding rate accordingly. If the patient is tolerating the slow EN rate and the clinical condition is improving, continue to increase the feeding infusion rate toward that goal.

Diarrhea can be challenging and is the most commonly reported GI complication of EN. Brain-injured patients often receive enterally delivered elixirs, electrolyte supplements, and other medications that are extremely hypertonic. Many liquid medications are mixed or suspended in sorbitol diluents (Cook et al. 2008). As little as 8–10 g/day of sorbitol may result in cramping and abdominal bloating with higher doses of >10 g/day frequently contributing to diarrhea (Cook et al. 2008). ICU patients with diarrhea should be evaluated and treated in a stepwise approach before using PN. Medications should be reviewed and those that contribute to increased diarrhea or bowel motility should be changed or eliminated if possible. Once infection and drug-related factors have been ruled out as causes of diarrhea, alterations in the EN formula may be a means to lessen diarrhea. If these initial interventions fail, the tube feeding rate can be decreased and antidiarrheal agents can be trialed once *Clostridium difficile* infection has been ruled out.

Critically ill stroke and acute brain injury patients frequently require narcotics, paralytic agents, and other anticholinergic agents that may contribute to constipation and poor motility. A standing bowel regimen (docusate and senna) can be instituted in the absence of diarrhea. Abdominal distention and ileus can often inhibit the patient from reaching and tolerating the EN goal and PN may be necessary.

FLUID AND ELECTROLYTE BALANCE IN CNS INJURIES

Fluid balance is a well-known concern in neurological critical care due to the extent of brain injury and subsequent swelling and medications that affect hydration status. Enteral formula selection process may need to take into account patient's fluid restriction or volume requirements.

Patients with neurological disease and patients treated with drugs that affect the CNS are more likely to develop disorders of sodium and water homeostasis (Bhardwaj 2006). Sodium and volume are regulated by neural, humoral, and renal mechanisms. These systems integrate information regarding extracellular fluid (ECF) osmolality, intravascular volume, circulatory hemodynamics, as well as sodium and water intake. If not treated properly, electrolyte disturbance can vastly increase morbidity and can even lead to death (Murphy-Human 2010). Appropriate diagnosis and treatment requires an understanding of the pathophysiological and physiological mechanisms involved in sodium and water homeostasis. Refer to Table 31.3 for a summary of the three main sodium and fluid disorders discussed in this section.

Hypernatremia is defined as serum sodium greater than 145 mEq/L, which results when there is a shift in the ratio of sodium to water, which the blood favors less water and/or more sodium (Murphy-Human 2010). This may be caused by increase in free water loss without adequate replacement such as diarrhea or osmotic diarrhea, or neurogenic diabetes insipidus (DI). Other causes of hypernatremia include excessive sodium retention as seen with primary hyperaldosteronism, Cushing's syndrome, or with administration of hypertonic solutions. Neurogenic DI is a failure of adequate release of arginine vasopressin (AVP), also known as antidiuretic hormone (ADH). The incidence of DI in a neurotensive care unit has been reported to be approximately 3.7% (Wong et al. 1998). DI is common following head trauma and is often seen in patients who progress to brain death (Agha et al. 2004; Smith 2004). Clinical symptoms include low urine osmolality (<300 mOsm/kg and specific gravity <1.005), high serum osmolality, and subsequent elevations in serum sodium

TABLE 31.3
Sodium and Fluid Disorders

Sodium/Fluid Disorder	Diagnostic Criteria	Therapy
Hypernatremia due to DI	Elevated sodium, sodium retention; low urine osmolality; may be caused by hypertonic fluids	Replace fluids after calculation of water deficit
Euvolemic hyponatremia (SIADH)	Dilutional hyponatremia; absence of adrenal, thyroid, or pituitary insufficiency	Water restriction; loop diuretics; vasopressin receptor antagonists
Hypovolemic hyponatremia (CSW)	Reductions in both total body water and sodium through renal or extrarenal sodium losses	Fluids and sodium administration

levels (Robertson 1988). Treatment with hormone and fluid replacement is generally successful to normalize serum sodium levels.

Hyponatremia is defined as a serum sodium less than 135 mEq/L and is the most common electrolyte abnormality in hospitalized patients (Anderson 1982). It is important to determine the possible etiology in order to treat appropriately with brain-injured patients. Syndrome of inappropriate secretion of diuretic hormone (SIADH) is generally considered the etiology of euvolemic hyponatremia and is the major cause of hyponatremia in patients with CNS disease (Bartter and Schwartz 1967; Baylis 2003). In SIADH, excessive plasma levels of AVP are not adequately suppressed in response to low plasma osmolality. This leads to excessive water retention by the kidney, which produces ECF volume expansion and ultimately dilutional hyponatremia. Clinically, the increase in ECF volume is not sufficient to cause peripheral or pulmonary edema. Treatment typically involves water restriction and/or loop diuretics.

Patients who demonstrate excretion of large volumes of urine with high-sodium content, volume contraction, and worsening hyponatremia despite usual therapies may be considered to have cerebral salt wasting (CSW). CSW is a manifested as hypovolemic hyponatremia. CSW has been predominately associated with SAH and other neurological disorders including TBI and brain tumors (Wijdicks 1985; Betjes 2002). These cases of hyponatremia are characterized by excessive renal sodium loss, which is suspected to be caused by disruption of sympathetic input to the kidneys and increased production of circulating natriuretic factors (Berendes et al. 1997; Betjes 2002; Rabinstein and Wijdicks 2003). This can be corrected by administration of large amounts of fluid and sodium. While it is beneficial to restrict fluids in SIADH, this is not recommended in patients with CSW hyponatremia. Treatment in CSW involves volume resuscitation.

MONITORING NUTRITION SUPPORT

To date, visceral protein labs are no longer considered reliable indicators of nutritional status in critically ill patients. In the critical care setting, the traditional protein markers (albumin, prealbumin, transferrin, retinol binding protein) are a reflection of the acute phase response (increases in vascular permeability and reprioritization of hepatic protein synthesis) and do not accurately represent nutrition status in the ICU setting. According to the ASPEN 2009 guidelines, anthropometrics are not reliable in assessment of nutrition status or adequacy of nutrition therapy in the critical care (Raguso et al. 2003; Martindale and Maerz 2006). It has been suggested that nitrogen balance studies may be useful in assessing the effectiveness of nutrition support regimens (Chalela et al. 2004).

MEDICATIONS AFFECTING DELIVERY OF NUTRIENTS

Propofol is a short-acting anesthetic and sedative commonly used in neurocritical patients because it is easily titrated to desirable clinical effects, and its actions are rapidly terminated with drug discontinuation (de-Leon Knapp 2009). It may also be used to decrease cerebral metabolic activity (Cook et al. 2008). The oil source of propofol is soybean, composed of long-chain triglycerides (LCTs) and omega-6 fatty acid. This 10% lipid vehicle provides 1.1 kcal/mL (0.1 mg/mL) calories in the form of fat, primarily linoleic acid. The extra calories provided are taken into consideration during assessment of nutrition support regimens. It should also be used with caution in patients who have known allergy to soy or eggs. ICUs with sedation protocol in place should include a nutrition component, such as routine measurement of serum triglycerides and routine adjustment of nutrition support recommendations, to avoid overfeeding and ensure protein adequacy.

Pentobarbital-induced coma is a treatment strategy reserved for the traumatic brain-injured patient with refractory intracranial hypertension. This treatment modality decreases the tone and amplitude of contractions of the GI tract and is mediated centrally and peripherally (Bochicchio et al. 2006). Patients on pentobarbital-induced coma can develop a significant ileus that is refractory to promotility agents (Bochicchio et al. 2006). Feeding tolerance may improve with small bowel feedings, and routine use of bowel regimens with stool softeners and stimulants can delay or eliminate the development of a drug-induced ileus. In addition, patients receiving pentobarbital may have diminished energy requirement due to decreased cerebral and peripheral energy demands (Cook et al. 2008). Patients tend to require 76%–86% of the predicted energy expenditure with less protein requirements as reflected by a 40% decrease in urinary nitrogen excretion (Dempsey et al. 1985; Fried et al. 1989).

Phenytoin represents a classic drug–nutrient interaction within the TBI population. Phenytoin is an anticonvulsant used for the prevention and treatment of posttraumatic epilepsy. Formulations commonly used include a phenytoin sodium salt injection and a phenytoin acid suspension (Cook et al. 2008). Concomitant administration of the acid suspension with EN solutions may inhibit absorption (Yeung and Ensom 2000). Practitioners have recommended that EN be held 1–2 h before and after each phenytoin dose to avoid concomitant administration, whereas others adjust the phenytoin suspension dose or use the injection solution enterally while administering simultaneously with EN (Gilbert et al. 1996). In our institution, EN is held for 1 h before and after each dose of the phenytoin acid suspension. The EN infusion rate is adjusted to reflect this interruption in feedings. To avoid routine EN interruptions, the intravenous route for phenytoin administration may be a better option.

SUMMARY

Nutrition support in acute brain injury can be effective in achieving best possible outcomes in this patient population. Proper assessment of each patient's needs, timing of interventions, and frequent monitoring of tolerance and adequacy of nutrition must be performed due to the demands of metabolic needs in brain injury and to prevent further complications resulting from injury.

CASE STUDY

History of present illness: This is a 54-year-old female h/o depression, obsessive-compulsive disorder who presents as transfer from outside hospital with unresponsiveness. CT head was performed, which demonstrates R hemispheric acute SAH. The patient was transferred to this facility for further management. History obtained from OSH records 2/2 patient's status and family unavailable. Prior to transfer, the patient was noted to have R fixed/dilated pupil, GCS of three requiring emergent intubation.

Anthropometrics:

Ht: 5′2″
Admit weight: 49.5 kg (109 lb)
Usual weight: unknown
BMI: 20 kg/m^2

Diet history (per family report): normal eating habits prior to motor vehicle accident.
Physical assessment: appears thin, no muscle wasting, adequate fat stores. Abdomen soft, +BS, last BM today. Skin intact. No edema.
Medications: vasopressin, colace, mannitol
Vitals: Tmax 37.5, HR 65, BP 112/86, Ve: 8.6

1. Based on patient's physical assessment, what route of feeding due to recommend?
   a. Patient should be able to tolerate gastric enteral feeding due to functioning GI tract. kidneys, ureters and bladder x ray should be done to confirm placement of OG or NG tube in distal stomach. Maintaining head of bed >30° will help to prevent the risk of ventilated associated aspiration.

2. What are the patient's estimated needs? What TF formula do you recommend?
   a. Since patient is intubated, the Penn State equation has been a validated tool to be used in the absence of indirect calorimetry.
   Penn State 2003b: Mifflin (0.96) + Ve (31) + Tm (167) – 6212.
   Estimated protein needs 1.0–1.5 g/kg
   TF formula should be high protein, isocaloric TF such as Promote or Replete.
3. Day #5: Patient started on a paralytic to help control seizures. New weight: 47.6 kg. What do you recommend?
   a. Reestimated needs to be done to account for decreased metabolic needs due to paralysis. Patients tend to require 76%–86% of the predicted energy expenditure with less protein requirements as reflected by a 40% decrease in urinary nitrogen excretion.
4. Day #10: Patient has improved, off paralytics/sedation. Remains intubated; however, started on phenytoin (oral) ordered BID. What do you recommend?
   a. Reestimate nutritional needs and adjust TF regimen for medication dosage. Holding TF 1 h before and after phenytoin dose. Make sure nursing staff is aware and documents appropriate medical record.
5. Day #14: Patient extubated, still has NG tube in place due to failed swallow evaluation. However, having high gastric residuals >500 mL. What do you recommend in regard to feeding?
   a. Each facility has its own policy when it comes to holding TF for gastric residual volume. This protocol should be updated based on current evidence. Based on our protocol, a GRV >500 mL should result in holding enteral nutrition and reassessing tolerance by the use of an established algorithm including physical assessment, GI assessment, evaluation of glycemic control, minimization of sedation, and consideration of promotility agent use, if not already prescribed. Consideration of a feeding tube placed below the ligament of Treitz when GRVs are consistently measured at >500 mL.
6. Day #21: Small bowel feeding tube placement and patient has improved neurologically, alert/oriented. Average TF intake meeting estimated needs. Failed swallow evaluation. What do you recommend at this point in time?
   a. A PEG tube placement should be discussed with the patient and family for long-term nutrition support.

REFERENCES

Academy of Nutrition and Dietetics. 2012. Critical Illness Determination of Resting Metabolic Rate (RMR): Recommendation Summary. Evidence Analysis Library.

Acosta-Escribano J, Fernandez-Vivas M, Grau Carmona T et al. 2010. Gastric versus transpyloric feeding in severe traumatic brain injury: A prospective, randomized trial. *Intensive Care Medicine* 36:1532–1539.

Agha A, Thornton E, O'Kelly P et al. 2004. Posterior pituitary dysfunction after traumatic brain injury. *Journal of Clinical Endocrinology Metabolism* 89(12):5987–5992.

Aguilar-Nascimento JE, Silveira BR, Dock-Nascimento DB. 2011. Early enteral nutrition with whey protein or casein in elderly patients with acute stroke: A double blind randomized trial. *Nutrition* 27:440–444.

Anderson RJ. 1982. Hyponatremia disorders due to vasopressin excess. *Schweizerische Medizinische Wochenschrift* 112(49):1755–1758.

A.S.P.E.N. Board of Directors and Clinical Guidelines Task Force. 2002. Guidelines for the use of parenteral and enteral nutrition in adult and pediatric patients. *Journal of Parenteral and Enteral Nutrition* 26:1SA–136SA.

Bankhead R, Boullata J, Brantley S et al. 2009. Enteral nutrition practice recommendations. *Journal of Parenteral and Enteral Nutrition* 33:122–167.

Bartter FC, Schwartz WB. 1967. The syndrome of inappropriate secretion of antidiuretic hormone. *American Journal of Medicine* 42(5):790–806.

Baylis PH. 2003. The syndrome of inappropriate antidiuretic hormone secretion. *International Journal of Biochemistry and Cell Biology* 35(11):1495–1499.

Berendes E, Walter M, Cullen P et al. 1997. Secretion of brain natriuretic peptide in patients with aneurysmal subarachnoid hemorrhage. *Lancet* 349(9047):245–249.

Betjes MG. 2002. Hyponatremia in acute brain disease: The cerebral salt wasting syndrome. *European Journal of the Internal Medicine* 13(1):9–14.

Bhardwaj A. 2006. Neurological impact of vasopressin dysregulation and hyponatremia. *Annals of Neurology* 59(2):229–236.

Bhatt A, Farooq SE, Pillainayagam BM et al. 2010. Clinical significance of serum zinc levels in cerebral ischemia. *SAGE: Stroke Research and Treatment.* Department of Neurology and Opthalmology, Michigan State University, East Lansing, MI.

Bivins BA, Twyman DL, Young AB. 1986. Failure of nonprotein calories to mediate protein conservation in brain-injured patient. *Neurosurgery* 14:784–791.

Bochicchio GV, Bochicchio K, Nehman S, Casey C, Andrews P, Scalea TM. 2006. Tolerance and efficacy of enteral nutrition in traumatic brain-injured patients induced into barbiturate coma. *Journal of Parenteral and Enteral Nutrition* 30(6):503–506.

Brain Trauma Foundation. 2000. Management and prognosis of severe traumatic brain injury. *Journal of Neurotrauma* 147:457–627.

Bratton SL, Chestnut RM, Ghajar J et al. 2007. Brain Trauma Foundation guidelines: Nutrition. *Journal of Neurotrauma* 24:S77–S82.

Brunner CS. 2007. Neurologic impairment. In: *The A.S.P.E.N. Nutrition Support Core Curriculum: A Case Based Approach—The Adult Patient*, Gottschlich MM, DeLegge MH, Mattox T, Mueller C, Worthington P, eds. Silver Springs, MD: American Society for Parenteral and Enteral Nutrition, pp. 424–439.

Chalela JA, Haymore J, Schellinger D et al. 2004. Acute stroke patients are underfed a nitrogen balance study. *Neurocritical Care* 3:331–334.

Cherian L, Hlatky R, Roberstson CS. 2004. Nitric oxide in traumatic brain injury. *Brain Pathology* 14:195–201.

Chiang YH, Chao DP, Chu SF et al. 2012. Early enteral nutrition and clinical outcomes of severe traumatic brain injury patients in acute stage: A multi-center cohort study. *Journal of Neurotrauma* 29:75–80.

Cook AM, Hatton J. 2007. Neurological impairment. In: *The A.S.P.E.N Nutrition Support Core Curriculum: A Case-Based Approach—The Adult Patient*, Gottschlich MM, Delegge MH, Mattox T, Mueller C, Worthington P, eds. Silver Spring, MD: American Society for Parental and Enteral Nutrition, pp. 425–435.

Cook AM, Peppard A, Magnuson B. 2008. Nutrition considerations in traumatic brain injury. *Nutrition in Clinical Practice* 23:608–620.

Coronado VG, Thurman DJ, Greenspan AI et al. 2009. Epidemiology. In: *Neurotrauma and Critical Care of the Brain*, Jallo J, Loftus C, eds. New York: Thieme.

Crary MA, Carnaby R, Mann GD et al. 2006. Dysphagia and nutritional status at the time of hospital admission for ischemic stroke. *Journal of Stroke and Cerebrovascular Disease* 15:164–171.

Cresci GA, Gottschlick MM, Mayes T et al. 2007. Trauma, surgery, and burns. In: *The A.S.P.E.N Nutrition Support Core Curriculum: A Case-based Approach—The Adult Patient*, Gottschlisch MM, DeLegge MH, Mattox T et al., eds. Silver Spring, MD: American Society for Parenteral and Enteral Nutrition, pp. 455–466.

Davis JP, Wong AA, Schluter PJ et al. 2004. Impact of premorbid undernutrition on outcome in stroke patients. *Stroke* 35:1930–1934.

De-Leon Knapp I. 2009. The effect of propofol on nutrition support. *Support Line* 31(6):12–19.

Dempsey DT, Guenter PA, Mullen JL et al. 1985. Energy expenditure in acute trauma to the head with and without barbiturate therapy. *Surgery, Gynecology and Obstetrics* 160:128–134.

Dennis MS, Lewis SC, Warlow C. 2005. Effect of timing and method of enteral tube feeding for dysphasic stroke patients: A multicentre randomized controlled trial. *Lancet* 365:764–722.

Department of Defense (DOD). 2009. *Traumatic Brain Injury Care in the Department of Defense*. Washington, DC: Department of Defense.

Dickerson RN, Guenter PA, Gennarlli TA et al. 1990. Increased contribution of protein oxidation to energy expenditure in head injured patients. *Journal of American College of Nutrition* 9:86–88.

Faul M, Xu L, Wald MM, Coronado VG. 2010. *Traumatic Brain Injury in the United States: Emergency Department Visits, Hospitalizations, and Deaths*. Atlanta, GA: Centers for Disease Control and Prevention, National Center for Injury Prevention and Control.

Finestone HM, Greene-Finestone LA, Foley N et al. 2003. Measuring longitudinally the metabolic demands of stroke patients. *Stroke* 34:502–507.

Frankenfield D, Hise M, Malone A et al. 2007. Prediction of resting metabolic rate in critically ill adult patients: Results of a systemic review of the evidence. *Journal of American Dietetic Association* 107:1552–1561.

Fried RC, Dickerson RN, Guenter PA et al. 1989. Barbiturate therapy reduces nitrogen excretion in acute head injury. *Journal of Trauma* 29:2449–2454.

Fruin AH, Taylor C, Pettis MS. 1986. Caloric requirements in patients with severe head injury. *Surgical Neurology* 25:25–28.

Gilbert S, Hatton J, Magnuson B. 1996. How to minimize interaction between phenytoin and enteral feedings: Two approaches. *Nutrition in Clinical Practices* 11:28–31.

Gottschlich MM, DeLegge MH, Mattox T, Mueller C, Worthington P, eds. Silver Spring, MD: American Society for Parenteral and Enteral Nutrition, pp. 425–435.

Hariri RJ, Firlick AD, Shepard SR et al. 1993. Traumatic brain injury, hemorrhagic shock, and fluid resuscitation: Effects on intracranial pressure and brain compliance. *Journal of Neurosurgery* 78:421–427.

Hartl R, Gerber LM, Quanhong NI, Ghajar J. 2008. Effect of early nutrition on deaths due to severe traumatic brain injury. *Journal of Neurosurgery* 109:50–56.

Hatton J. 2001. Pharmacological treatment of traumatic brain injury. *CNS Drugs* 15:553–581.

Koc D, Gercek A, Gencosmanoglu R, Tozun N. 2007. Percutaneous endoscopic gastrostomy in the neurosurgical intensive care unit: Complications and outcome. *Journal of Parenteral and Enteral Nutrition* 31:517–520.

Kolpek JH, Ott LG, Record KE et al. 1989. Comparison of urinary urea nitrogen excretion and measured energy expenditure in spinal cord injury and nonsteroid-treated severe head trauma patients. *Journal of Parenteral and Enteral Nutrition* 13:277–280.

Koukiasa P, Bitzani V, Papaioannou V, Pnevmatikos, I. 2014. Resting energy expenditure in critically ill patients with spontaneous intracranial hemorrhage (SICH). *Journal of Parental and Enteral Nutrition* published online June 13, 2014. DOI: 10:1177/0148607114539352.

Malone A, Seres D, Lord L. 2012. Complications of enteral nutrition. In: *The A.S.P.E.N. Adult Nutrition Support Core Curriculum*, 2nd edn., Mueller CM, Kovacevich DS, McClave SA, Miller SJ, Schwartz DB, eds. Silver Springs, MD: American Society for Parenteral and Enteral Nutrition, pp. 218–233.

Martindale RG, Maerz LL. 2006. Management of perioperative nutrition support. *Current Opinion in Critical Care* 12:290–294.

McClave SA, Martindale RG, Vanek VW et al. 2009. Guidelines for the provision and assessment of nutrition support therapy in the adult patient: Society for Critical Care Medicine (SCCM) and American Society for Parenteral and Enteral Nutrition (A.S.P.E.N.). *Journal of Parenteral and Enteral Nutrition* 33:277–316.

McKee JA, Brewer RP, Macy GE et al. 2005. Analysis of the brain. *Critical Care Medicine* 33:661–666.

Miniño AM, Sherry LM, Jiaquan Xu MD, Kenneth D, Kochanek MA. 2011. Deaths: Final data for. *National Vital Statistics Report 2008* 59:1–127.

Mirtallo JM, Patel M. 2012. Overview of parenteral nutrition. In: *The A.S.P.E.N. Adult Nutrition Support Core Curriculum*, 2nd edn., Mueller CM, Kovacevich DS, McClave SA et al., eds. Silver Springs, MD: American Society for Parenteral and Enteral Nutrition, pp. 235–244.

Murphy-Human T and Diringer M. 2010. Sodium disturbances commonly encounters in the neurologic intensive care unit. *Journal of Pharmacy Practice* 23:470.

Nishizawa Y. 2001. Glutamate release and neuronal damage in ischemia. *Life Science* 69:369–381.

Perel P, Yanagawa T, Bunn F, Roberts I, Wentz R, Pierro A. 2006. Nutritional support for head-injured patients. *Cochrane Database System Review* 4:CD001530.

Rabinstein AA, Wijdicks EF. 2003. Hyponatremia in critically ill neurological patients. *Neurologist* 9(6):290–300.

Raguso CA, Dupertuis YM, Pichard C. 2003. The role of visceral proteins in the nutritional assessment of intensive care unit patients. *Current Opinion in Clinical Nutrition and Metabolic Care* 6:211–216.

Rajpal V, Johnston J. 2009. Nutrition management of traumatic brain injury patients. *Dietitians in Nutrition Support: Support Line* 31:10–18.

Raschen W. 2003. Shutdown of translation: Lethal or protective? Unfolded protein response versus apoptosis. *Journal of Cerebral Blood Flow Metabolism* 23:773–779.

Robertson GL. 1988. Differential diagnosis of polyuria. *Annual Review of Medicine* 39:425–442.

Roger VL, Go AS, Lloyd-Jones DM et al. 2011. Heart disease and stroke statistics—2011 update: A report from the American Heart Association. *Circulation* 123(4):e18–e209.

Ruf K, Magnuson B, Hatton J, Cook AM. 2012. Nutrition in neurologic impairment. In: *The A.S.P.E.N. Adult Nutrition Support Core Curriculum*, 2nd edn., Mueller CM, Kovacevich DS, McClave SA et al., eds. Silver Springs, MD: American Society for Parenteral and Enteral Nutrition, pp. 363–376.

Saran D, Brody RA, Stankorb SM, Parrott SJ, Heyland DK. 2014. Gastric vs small bowel feeding in critically ill neurologically injured patients: Results of a multicenter observational study. *Journal of Parenteral and Enteral Nutrition* published online June 19, 2014. DOI: 10.1177/01486071145003.

Scherbakov N, Doehner W. 2011. Sarcopenia in stroke-facts and numbers on muscle loss accounting for disability after stroke. *Journal of Cachexia Sarcopenia Muscle* 2:5–8.

Skipper A. 2003. Parenteral nutrition. In: *Contemporary Nutrition Support Practice: A Clinical Guide*, 2nd edn., Matarese LE, Gottschlich MM, eds. St Louis, MO: Saunders, pp. 227–262.

Smith M. 2004. Physiologic changes during brain stem death—Lessons for management of the organ donor. *Journal of Heart and Lung Transplantation* 23(9):S217–S222.

Tang M, Darlene L. 2009. Severe traumatic brain injury: Maximizing outcomes. *Mount Sinai Journal of Medicine* 76:119–128.

Taylor SJ, Fettes SB, Jewkes C et al. 1999. Prospective, randomized, controlled trial to determine the effect of early enhanced enteral nutrition on clinical outcome in mechanically ventilated patients suffering from head injury. *Critical Care Medicine* 27:2525–2531.

Vizzini A, Aranda-Michel J. 2011. Nutritional support in head injury. *Nutrition* 27:129–132.

Weekes E, Elia M. 1992. Resting energy expenditure and body composition following cerebrovascular accident. *Clinical Nutrition* 11:18–22.

Wells DL. 2012. Provision of enteral nutrition during vasopressor therapy for hemodynamic instability: An evidence-based review. *Nutrition in Clinical Practice* 27:527–532.

Wijdicks EF, Vermeulen M, tenHaaf JA et al. 1985. Volume depletion and natriuresis in patients with a ruptured intracranial aneurysm. *Ann Neurology* 18(2):211–216.

Wong MF, Chin NM, Lew TW. 1998. Diabetes insipidus in neurosurgical patients. *Annals Academy of Medicine Singapore* 27(3):340–343.

Yeung CS, Ensom MH. 2000. Phenytoin and enteral feedings: Does the evidence support an interaction? *Annals of Pharmacotherapy* 34:896–905.

Young B, Ott L, Kasarkis, E et al. 1996. Zinc supplementation is associated with improved neurological recovery rate and visceral protein levels of patients with severe closed head injury. *Journal of Neurotrauma* 13:25–34.

Young B, Ott L, Yingling B et al. 1992. Nutrition and brain injury. *Journal of Neurotrauma* 9:S375–S383.

32 Nutritional Support in Acute Pancreatitis

R.F. Meier

CONTENTS

INTRODUCTION

Acute pancreatitis is an inflammatory disease of the pancreas with different degrees of severity. Often the nutritional status declines due to the acute systemic inflammatory response, catabolism, and the lake of appropriate nutritional support. Under normal condition, the pancreas plays an important role for digestion and absorption of nutrients. An impaired pancreatic function has negative consequences for the host. Nutritional deficiencies can occur rapidly.

Adequate fluid and food administration can be a major medical problem in patients with severe acute pancreatitis. Despite the increasing knowledge from research in the fields of metabolism, clinical nutrition and intervention is still controversial with respect to the optimal nutritional treatment regimens for acute pancreatitis. For many years, textbooks have advocated the concept that oral or enteral feeding is harmful in acute pancreatitis because it was thought that feeding stimulates exocrine pancreatic secretory responses and consequently autodigestive processes. This concept has been shown to be wrong. It is known that specific nutritional deficiencies can occur in patients with a prolonged and complicated course of acute necrotizing pancreatitis. The development of nutrient deficiencies is clearly associated with a negative outcome. Numerous studies have demonstrated that the nutritional support is different in acute mild and severe pancreatitis. Although there is much more evidence available on which to base rational management in acute pancreatitis, there are still areas of controversy that may depend on variations in experience and on the type of patients being treated.

ACUTE PANCREATITIS

Acute pancreatitis occurs in different clinical patterns ranging from a mild to severe necrotizing disease with local and systemic complications. Acute pancreatitis involves a systemic immuno-inflammatory response to a localized process of autodigestion of the pancreatic gland with variable involvement of the peri-pancreatic tissue and remote organ systems.

Alcohol abuse in men and gallstone disease in women are the most important underlying conditions for acute pancreatitis. The mechanisms by which these factors cause acute pancreatitis are still not exactly known.

The major pathological processes in acute pancreatitis are inflammation, edema, and necrosis of the pancreatic tissue and as well inflammation and injury of extrapancreatic organs [1].

In total, 75%–80% has mild, edematous, and about 20%–25% severe necrotizing pancreatitis.

The mortality rate for mild to moderate pancreatitis is low (1%). The mortality rate for severe pancreatitis increases to 19%–30% [2]. Mortality approaches 50% if necrosis of the gland is greater 50% and can further increase up to 80% if sepsis occurs [3]. Approximately half of the deaths in acute pancreatitis occur within the first 2 weeks of illness and are mainly attributed to organ failure. The other 50% of deaths occur weeks to months after this period, and are related to organ failure associated with infected necrosis.

Nutritional support in severe necrotizing pancreatitis is essential because these patients develop rapidly nutritional deficiencies. This is even more fatal if patients are already malnourished at the time of the initial attack.

OUTCOME PREDICTORS

Two factors, the severity of pancreatitis and the nutritional status, can be used to predict the outcome in acute pancreatitis.

Assessment of the Severity of the Acute Pancreatitis

Several prognostic scoring systems, which include clinical (Ranson Score, Glasgow Score, APACHE II-Score, Atlanta Classification), laboratory, and radiological criteria, are available [4–8]. The Atlanta Classification of severity defines severe acute pancreatitis on the basis of standard clinical manifestations: a score of 3 or more in the Ranson Criteria (Table 32.1) [4] or a score of 8 or more in the APACHE II-Score [6] and evidence of organ failure and intrapancreatic pathological findings (necrosis or interstitial pancreatitis) [7]. This classification is helpful because it also allows comparison of different trials and methodologies. The severity of acute pancreatitis based on imaging procedures is based on the Balthazarscore, which predicts severity on computed tomography (CT) appearance, including presence or absence of necrosis (Table 32.2) [8]. Failure of pancreatic parenchyma to enhance during the arterial phase of intravenous contrast-enhanced CT indicates necrosis, which predicts a severe attack if more than 50% of the gland is affected. The measurement of concentrations of serum C-reactive protein (CRP) is useful in clinical practice. CRP concentration has an independent prognostic value. A peak of more than 210 mg/L on day 2–4, or more than 120 mg/L at the end of the first week, is as predictive as multiple-factor scoring systems [9]. In some

TABLE 32.1
Ranson's Criteria of Severity for Acute Pancreatitis

Criteria
Admission criteria
Age >55 years
WBC >16.0 × 10^9/L
Glucose >10 mmol/L
Lactate dehydrogenase (LDH) >350 IU/L
Aspartamine transaminase (AST) >250U/L
Following initial 48 h criteria
Hematocrit decrease of >10%
BUN increase of >1.8 mmol/L
Calcium <2 mmol/L
PaO_2 <60 mmHg
Base deficit >4 mEq/L
Fluid sequestration >6 L

Source: Ranson, J.H. et al., *Surg. Gynecol. Obstet.*, 139, 69, 1974.

TABLE 32.2
Computed Tomography (CT) Grading System of Balthazar

CT Grade		Quantity of Necrotic Pancreas
Grade A = 0	Normal appearing pancreas	
Grade B = 1	Focal or diffuse enlargement of the pancreas	
Grade C = 2	Pancreatic gland abnormalities accompanied by mild parapancreatic inflammatory changes	<33% = 2 33%–50% = 4
Grade D = 3	Fluid collection in a single location, usually within the anterior pararenal space	>50% = 6
Grade E = 4	Two or more fluid collections near the pancreas or gas either within the pancreas or within parapancreatic inflammation	

Source: Balthazar, E.J. et al., *Radiology*, 174, 331, 1990.
Note: Total score = CT grade (0–4) + necrosis (0–6).

institutions, serum levels of creatinine and blood urea nitrogen are included in the assessment. At the moment, it seems that the existing scoring systems have reached their maximal efficacy in predicting persistent organ failure in acute pancreatitis until more sophisticated tools are developed [10].

Nutritional Status

Undernutrition and overweight is often seen in patients with acute pancreatitis. Both are well-known risk factors for more complications and higher mortality. Undernutrition is present in 50%–80% of chronic alcoholics and alcohol is a major etiological factor in male patients with acute pancreatitis (30%–40%) [11].

In one small study, the relationship of underweight and complication risk in acute pancreatitis found that underweight had no increased risk for developing more complications in comparison with those with a normal weight [12]. If this is true, it has to be studied in a larger prospective trial.

For nutritional support, it is necessary to assess the severity of acute pancreatitis and the nutritional status at the time of admission and during the course of the disease. Both factors are necessary to plan nutrition interventions in patients with acute pancreatitis.

Physiology and Pathophysiology with respect to Nutrition and Fluid Resuscitation

Specific and nonspecific metabolic changes occur during acute pancreatitis. A variety of proinflammatory cytokines increase the basal metabolic rate. This can result in increased energy consumption. The resting energy expenditure varies according to the severity and the length of disease. If patients develop sepsis, 80% of them show an elevation in protein catabolism and an increased nutrient requirement. A prolonged negative nitrogen balance determines negative clinical outcome [13]. Whether negative nitrogen balance is the principal factor for outcome is not clear. The relationship between nitrogen balance and outcome may only reflect the relationship between nitrogen balance and severity of disease. There is no study available in which patients were stratified according to the disease severity.

Metabolism of Carbohydrates

Glucose metabolism in acute pancreatitis is determined by an increase in energy demand. Endogenous gluconeogenesis is increased as a consequence of the metabolic response to the severe inflammatory process. Glucose is an important source of energy and can partially counteract the intrinsic gluconeogenesis from protein degradation. This can counteract, to a certain degree, the deleterious and unwanted effect of protein catabolism [14]. The maximum rate of glucose oxidation is approximately 4 mg/kg/min. The administration of glucose in excess can be harmful, and even wasteful, because of lipogenesis and glucose recycling. Furthermore, hyperglycemia and hypercapnia can occur. Hyperglycemia is a major risk factor for infections and metabolic complications. Monitoring and blood glucose control is therefore essential.

Protein Metabolism

A negative nitrogen balance is often seen in severe acute pancreatitis. The protein losses must be minimized and the increased protein turnover must be compensated. If acute pancreatitis is complicated by sepsis, up to 80% of patients are in a hypermetabolic state with an increase of the resting energy expenditure. A negative nitrogen balance is associated with adverse clinical outcome. Nitrogen losses are as much as 20–40 g/day in some patients with acute pancreatitis.

Lipid Metabolism

Hyperlipidemia is a common finding in acute pancreatitis. The mechanism of altered lipid metabolism is not entirely clear. After an acute attack, serum lipid concentration returns to normal ranges. It is also known that in some patients with severe hyperlipidemia an acute pancreatitis can develop [15].

Fluid Derangements

During the early acute state, there is only a narrow limit between mild disease and a transition to severe impairment. Especially at this stage, depletion of intravascular volume due to fluid sequestration, without obvious changes in arterial blood pressure and with additional disturbance of pancreatic and splanchnic microcirculation has been demonstrated. Moreover, according to some studies, pancreatic blood flow decreases by 73% immediately after the onset of acute pancreatitis. The resulting ischemia is probably responsible for further derangement in acinar cells with subsequent intracellular activation of digestive enzymes by lysosomal hydrolases and for progression of mild pancreatitis to parenchymal necrosis. Another consequence of splanchnic hypoperfusion is intestinal injury with damage to barrier function with subsequent infective complications and development of multiorgan failure. It has been shown repeatedly that early fluid resuscitation can prevent these disturbances. For example, lactated Ringer solution administered intravenously at infusion rates of 6.5 mL/kg/h, for 4 h prevented a decrease in pancreatic blood flow in dogs with experimental pancreatitis [16].

In patients with acute pancreatitis, early fluid resuscitation was associated with a reduced incidence of systemic inflammatory response syndrome (SIRS) and organ failure at 72 h. These effects were most pronounced in patients admitted with interstitial rather than severe pancreatitis [17]. In addition, patients treated with lactated Ringer's solution had a reduced systemic inflammation compared with those who were resuscitated with normal saline [18]. Unfortunately, all these studies are small and so the optimal fluid resuscitation is still unclear. Larger randomized controlled trials to assess different fluid solutions and infusion rates are needed.

TREATMENT OF ACUTE PANCREATITIS

Early Fluid Resuscitation

Hypovolemia with subsequent splanchnic ischemia is a very important factor in the pathogenesis and progression of acute pancreatitis. All patients presenting with abdominal pain, high CRP levels, and a high amylase should be considered as potentially progressing to severe pancreatitis. The patient should be admitted to a high dependency area and intensive fluid resuscitation should be started without delay according to the following scheme:

- Lactated Ringer's solution should be given at an initial rate of 1–2 L/h to maintain urinary output between 100 and 200 mL/h.
- If urinary output is low after 2–4 L of fluid, a urinary catheter should be inserted.
- If urinary production does not increase, a central venous catheter should be inserted for fluid replacement and central venous pressure (CVP) measurements.
- Lactated Ringer's solution should be given at a rate of 6–10 L/day (or even more) according to urinary output and CVP.

During the first 3 days, patients can accumulate 6–12 L of fluid and 600–1200 mmol of sodium. Throughout the succeeding period, remarkable fluid and sodium mobilization is frequently observed together with clinical improvement (bowel motility, decrease in CRP and amylases). Fluid mobilization is delayed in the complicated form of severe acute pancreatitis and the patient therefore remains edematous unless measures are taken.

Energy Requirements

Patients with severe acute pancreatitis are hypermetabolic. The more severe acute pancreatitis is, the more excessive is hypermetabolism. Resting energy expenditure can be variable in these patients. A range between 77% and 158% of the predicted energy expenditure was reported [19]. If the disease is complicated by sepsis or multiorgan failure, the resting energy expenditure is significantly increased.

It was shown that in severe acute pancreatitis, the Harris–Benedict equation is not sensitive enough to estimate the caloric expenditure. In these cases, indirect calorimetry is recommended to avoid over- or underfeeding.

For enteral or parenteral nutrition, 25–35 kcal/kg BW/day is recommended. Overfeeding and hyperglycemia should be avoided. Blood glucose concentration should not exceed 10 mmol/L. Insulin treatment is recommended, but the doses should not be higher than 4–6 units/h. The impaired glucose oxidation rate cannot be normalized by insulin administration. Normally, 3–6 g/kg BW/day of carbohydrates can be recommended.

The optimal goal of protein supply is between 1.2 and 1.5 g/kg BW/day. Lower protein intake should only be given to patients with renal or severe hepatic failure.

Fat can be given up to 2 g/kg BW/day, but blood triglyceride levels must be monitored carefully. Triglycerides are tolerated up to 12 mmol/L (Table 32.3).

TABLE 32.3
Recommended Dosages of Nutrients in Severe Acute Pancreatitis

Substrate	Quantity
Energy	25–35 kcal/kg BW/day[a]
Protein	1.2–1.5 g/kg BW/day
Carbohydrates	3–6 g/kg BW/day corresponding to blood glucose concentration (aim: <10 mmol/L)[a]
Lipids	Up to 2 g/kg BW/day corresponding to blood triglyceride concentration (aim: <12 mmol/L)[a]

[a] Overfeeding should be avoided, especially in obese patients possibly according to measured REE (indirect calorimetry).

Nutritional Support

Nutritional support in acute pancreatitis shifted from total parenteral nutrition (TPN) to enteral nutrition. TPN was used in the past to avoid stimulation of exocrine pancreatic secretion. For TPN alone, a clear beneficial effect was never shown. TPN did not change the course of the disease, but TPN was more expensive or accompanied with an increase in catheter-related infections and a longer hospital stay. In the last years, it became clear that some of these complications were often the consequence of overfeeding. Van den Berghe et al. showed, irrespective of the route of nutritional support, that the control of hyperglycemia with insulin reduced mortality in critical care patients [20]. This has changed after the patients with severe acute pancreatitis were fed by the enteral route.

Enteral feeding in acute pancreatitis may reduce catabolism and loss of lean body mass and may modulate the acute phase response and preserve visceral protein metabolism with the potential to downregulate splanchnic cytokine response [21] (Table 32.4).

Several prospective, randomized clinical trials have been performed comparing enteral with parenteral nutrition in patients with acute pancreatitis [22–35]. In only two trials, there was no difference on outcome [25,33]. In all other trials, enteral nutrition was found to be superior compared to TPN. In addition, in four trials, mortality was improved by the enteral route [30,31,34–36].

In mild to moderate acute pancreatitis, neither enteral nor parenteral nutrition showed a positive effect on outcome in these patients [22].

In the trials comparing enteral with parenteral nutrition in severe acute pancreatitis, the results were different from them in mild to moderate pancreatitis. In the first prospective study by Kalferanzos et al., comparing either a nasojejunal tube feeding with a semi-elemental diet with TPN started 48 h after admission showed that enteral feeding was well tolerated without adverse effects. In addition, the patients on enteral nutrition experienced fewer septic complication and fewer total complications compared to those receiving parenteral nutrition. Furthermore, the costs of nutritional support were three times higher in patients receiving TPN [23]. These findings are supported by several

TABLE 32.4
Benefits of Early Enteral Feeding

Maintain gut integrity (reduce bacterial challenge)
Set tone for systemic immunity (downregulate immune response)
Attenuate oxidative stress
Lessen disease severity
Promote faster resolution of disease process
Reduce complications (less infection and need for surgical intervention, shorter hospital length of stay, and possibly less multiorgan failure)

other trials [24,26–32,34,35]. The trial of Windsor et al. [24] showed that enteral nutrition attenuates the acute phase response in acute pancreatitis and improves disease severity and clinical outcome, despite the fact that pancreatic injuries were virtually unchanged in CT scan. In the enteral feeding group, SIRS and sepsis were reduced, resulting in a beneficial clinical outcome (APACHE II-score and CRP). Abou-Assi et al. treated 156 patients with acute pancreatitis initially with intravenous fluid and analgesics. Those who improved rapidly were fed orally afterward. The nonresponders were randomized to receive either enteral nutrition by a nasojejunal tube or TPN. Seventy percent of the initially enrolled patients improved with the oral regimen and were discharged within 4 days. The randomized patients in the enteral group were fed for a significantly shorter period (6.7 vs. 10.8 days), had significantly fewer metabolic and septic complications. In addition, hyperglycemia requiring insulin therapy was significantly higher in the parenteral-fed patients [27]. Petrov et al. randomized 70 patients out of 466 patients with acute pancreatitis to enteral or parenteral nutrition. They showed again that enteral nutrition was superior to parenteral nutrition by decreasing complications, single and multiorgan failure and mortality [30]. Two further trials recently published confirm the superiority of enteral nutrition again. Wu et al. randomized 107 patients to enteral or parenteral nutrition. In the enteral group as well, morbidity and mortality was significantly lower than in the TPN group [34]. Hegazi et al. found that early initiation of distal jejunal feeding was associated with reduced mortality in patients with severe acute pancreatitis. Early achievement of jejunal feeding goal was associated with a shorter ICU length of stay, irrespective of the severity of acute pancreatitis [35].

Today, there is no doubt that enteral nutrition should be the first attempt to feed patients with severe acute pancreatitis. The first meta-analysis from McClave et al. [37] already showed that the use of enteral nutrition was associated with a significant reduction in infectious morbidity, a reduction in hospital length of stay, and a trend toward reduced organ failure when compared with the use of parenteral nutrition. There was no effect on mortality. These results have changed including more trials in several meta-analyses [38–42]. In severe acute pancreatitis, enteral nutrition reduces significantly the risk for infectious complication, pancreatic infections, and mortality [38], and enteral nutrition is more effective than parenteral nutrition in reducing the risk of multiorgan failure, pancreatic infectious complication, and mortality [39]. Al-Omran et al. found that enteral nutrition significantly reduced not only mortality and systemic infections but also multiorgan failure and the need for operative intervention compared to parenteral nutrition [40]. It seems that the timing to start enteral nutrition is important. In the meta-analysis of Petrov et al., the positive effect of enteral nutrition was only found if nutrition was started within the first 48 h. There was no difference when nutrition was started after this time [41]. Compared with TPN, enteral nutrition was associated with a significantly lower incidence of pancreatic infection complication, surgical intervention, and mortality. There was no statistic difference in nonpancreatic-related complication. In enteral nutrition, a significantly higher incidence of noninfection-related complications was found [42].

Nutritional Support in Mild to Moderate Pancreatitis

There is no evidence that a nutritional support (enteral or parenteral) has a beneficial effect on clinical outcome in patients with mild acute pancreatitis [43,44]. Enteral nutrition is unnecessary if the patients can consume normal food after 5–7 days (ESPEN Guidelines: Grade B).

Enteral or parenteral nutrition within 5–7 days has no positive effect on the course of the disease and is therefore not recommended (ESPEN* Guidelines: Grade A). Early enteral nutrition support can be of importance in patients with pre-existing severe malnutrition or in patients when early refeeding in 5–7 days is not possible. A frequently used approach for these patients is shown in Figure 32.1.

The same recommendations are also given by the international consensus guidelines for nutrition therapy in pancreatitis [45].

* ESPEN guidelines. http://www.espen.org/education/guidelines.htm/pancreas.

1. Step (2–5 days)	- Fasting - Treat the cause of pancreatitis - i.v. fluid and electrolyte replacement - Analgesics
↓	
2. Step (3–7 days) No pain Enzymes regredient	- Refeeding - Diet: - Rich in carbohydrates - Moderate in protein - Moderate in fat
↓	
3. Step	- Normal diet

FIGURE 32.1 Nutritional treatment of mild to moderate pancreatitis.

Nutritional Support in Severe Acute Pancreatitis

In patients with severe pancreatitis, who have complications or need surgery, early nutritional support is necessary to prevent the adverse effect of nutrient deprivation. In severe necrotizing pancreatitis, enteral nutrition is indicated first if possible (ESPEN Guidelines: Grade A) [43,44]. In the last decade, the nutritional strategy in acute pancreatitis has changed. The nutritional management has shifted from parenteral to enteral nutrition. Enteral feeding in acute pancreatitis have shown to reduce catabolism and loss of lean body mass, modulation of the acute phase response, and preserve visceral protein metabolism, with the potential to downregulate the splanchnic cytokine response [24]. Furthermore, enteral nutrition has been shown in many studies to be safe and well tolerated. In general for patients with severe acute pancreatitis, enteral nutrition is recommended to start first if it is possible. In patients with severe necrotizing pancreatitis, the full amount of nutrient delivery by the enteral route is not always possible. If complete enteral nutrition is not possible, the nutritional support should be combined with parenteral nutrition. Usually, the combined nutritional support allows that the patient reach the nutritional goals. The administration of fat in parenteral nutrition can be regarded as safe if hypertriglyceridemia (<12 μmol/L) is avoided [43,44]. A practical approach for nutrition in severe acute pancreatitis is outlined in Figure 32.2.

The same recommendations are also given by the international consensus guidelines for nutrition therapy in pancreatitis [45].

Route of Feeding

The route of nutrient delivery (parenteral/enteral) should be determined by patients' tolerance. Tube feeding is possible in the majority of patients, but some patients need a combination with parenteral nutrition (ESPEN Guidelines: Grade A). Several prospective studies have shown that jejunal tube

- Patients with severe disease, complications, or the need for surgery require early nutrition support to prevent the adverse effects of nutrient deprivation.

  ↓

  - Start with aggressive fluid resuscitation
  - Try to start with a continuous early enteral jejunal feeding over 24 h with a polymeric or an elemental- or maybe immunenhancing diet
  - When side effects occur or the caloric goal cannot be achieved, TPN should be combined with enteral nutrition
  - When enteral nutrition is not possible (e.g., prolonged paralytic ileus) TPN should be given with a small amount of an elemental diet infused continuously into the jejunum according to tolerance (up to 10–30 mL/h).
- The use of intravenous lipids is safe when hypertriglyceridemia is avoided.

FIGURE 32.2 Nutritional treatment of severe pancreatitis.

feeding is possible in most patients with acute pancreatitis [43]. Placing a jejunal feeding tube distally to the ligament of Treitz can easily be performed. The tubes are placed either with fluoroscopic help or more and more with the endoscope. Normally, jejunal tubes are well tolerated [22,46–48]. Rarely, proximal migration of the feeding tube and subsequent pancreatic stimulation can aggravate acute pancreatitis [49]. Partial ileus is not a contraindication for enteral feeding because these patients frequently tolerate continuous low-volume jejunal nutrients. Several single or multilumen tubes are available. Multilumen tubes are very popular because you can switch the feeding site (gastral or jejunal) according to the patient tolerance. In case of pancreatic surgery, an intraoperative jejunostomy for postoperative tube feeding is feasible if a jejunal tube is not already in place [50].

Gastral versus Jejunal Feeding

Whether the jejunal feeding is absolutely necessary is not completely clear. Minimizing stimulation of the exocrine pancreatic secretion would support the jejunal feeding route. It is, however, controversial whether stimulation of pancreatic secretion is important for the outcome in this disease. Four randomized studies comparing nasogastric versus nasojejunal feeding or nasogastric versus TPN in severe acute pancreatitis were published [51–54]. It was found that nasogastric feeding was as safe as nasojejunal feeding. There was little difference between the two methods with respect to pain, analgesic requirements, nutritional intolerances, serum CRP concentration, or mortality. Compared to parenteral nutrition, there were significantly more complications in the first 3 days in the nasogastric group, but there was a better control of blood glucose levels. A systematic review including all studies found that in the majority (79%) the gastric feeding was safe and well tolerated without a statistically difference on clinical outcome [55]. A clear recommendation cannot be given yet. An often used approach today is to use a multilumen tube with one port in the stomach and one port in the jejunum. First feeding through the gastral port is started. If this is not tolerated, the switch to the jejunal port can be done. More clinical trials using such concepts are warranted.

Which Formula Should Be Used in Acute Pancreatitis?

Most studies have been done using peptide-based formulae. The use of peptide-based formulae showed beneficial effects (ESPEN Guidelines: Grade A) [43]. Nowadays in most institutions polymeric formula are used. A direct comparison of a peptide-based formula with the polymeric formula showed that there was no difference on outcome [56]. Today, it is common to start with a standard polymeric formula and if this is not tolerated, a peptide-based formula is tried. Petrov et al. performed a meta-analysis on the different formulas used and found no difference between polymeric- and (semi) elemental formulas. There was no difference on feeding intolerance, infectious complication, or death in patients with acute pancreatitis [57].

Several published trials used also formulas containing immune modulating substrates (glutamine, arginine, n-3 polyunsaturated fatty acids) or pre- and probiotics [37]. Until now, these formulas cannot be generally recommended because these studies need confirmation with studies including larger number of patients [57]. The concept of using pre- and probiotics to prevent intestinal bacterial translocation is very attractive. Two studies by Olah et al. examined the efficacy of enteral administration of probiotics in patients with severe acute pancreatitis [58,59]. In the first study, 22 patients received life *Lactobacillus plantarum* and oat fiber and 23 patients the same formulation with heat-killed bacteria. In the group with life bacteria, they found less positive cultures, less need of antibiotics, less pancreatic infections, and requiring surgical interventions ($p = 0.046$). Furthermore, the length of hospital stay was shorter (13.7 vs. 21.4 days) [58]. In the second study, they randomized 62 patients with acute pancreatitis that were fed with a nasojejunal tube. Twenty-seven patients received only enteral nutrition with fiber. Thirty-four patients were treated with enteral nutrition with fiber and a combination of four different lactobacilli. The treatment group again had significant lower complication rates ($p = 0.049$). The control group had higher multiorgan failure, pancreatic septic complications, surgical intervention, and mortality [59]. These observations were exciting until the large multicenter controlled trial by Besselink et al. was published [60].

They randomized 298 patients with severe acute pancreatitis with either a combination six probiotics (four strains lactobacilli and two strains bifidobacteria) or placebo.

A multifiber enteral solution was given in both groups through a nasojejunal tube. There were no differences in infectious complications between the probiotic and placebo groups (30% vs. 28%). Unfortunately, mortality was significantly higher in the probiotic group (16% vs. 6%). Nine patients in the probiotic group developed bowel ischemia. At the moment, it is not clear whether these complications are due to the combination of probiotics administered to the gut or whether other underlying factors have played a role. The two groups have not been fully comparable. Organ failure during admission was more common in the probiotic group than in the placebo group (27.0% vs. 16.0%; $p = 0.02$). Intestinal ischemia can also be found more often during vasopressor treatment. In the probiotic group, more patients received vasopressor drugs than in the placebo group. This could be another explanation for the developing of bowel ischemia. In addition in a hemodynamically compromised gut, a high-fiber diet in the jejunum together with high dose of probiotics could have led to a high fermentation rate. Increasing gas production can lead to more distension and may be so to more ischemia. In the Besselink study, no adverse events were shown in the group receiving only prebiotics. This is in line with a new study published by Karakan et al. [61]. They found that nasojejunal enteral nutrition with prebiotic fiber supplementation in patients with severe acute pancreatitis improved hospital stay, duration of nutrition therapy, acute phase response, and overall complications compared to standard enteral nutrition. For the moment, probiotics in severe acute pancreatitis cannot be recommended until more trials have shown that probiotics are effective and save.

Several studies were done by supplementation TPN with n-3 polyunsaturated fatty acids or glutamine. Wang et al. found that patients treated with n-3 polyunsaturated fatty acids had significantly higher EPA concentrations, lower CRP levels, and better oxygenation index after 5 days of TPN than the control group. In addition, the number of days of continuous renal replacement therapy was significantly decreased [62]. All of the glutamine studies demonstrated beneficial effects [37]. This was also confirmed by the study of Fuentes-Orozco et al. [63]. The group with glutamine supplementation had a significant increase in serum IL-10 levels, total lymphocyte and lymphocyte subpopulations counts, and albumin serum levels. Nitrogen balance improved to positive levels in the study group and remained negative in the control group. Infectious morbidity was more frequent in the control group. The duration of hospital stay and the mortality were similar between the two groups. It can make sense in the future to add n-3 polyunsaturated fatty acids and/or glutamine if patients with severe acute pancreatitis need TPN treatment.

Oral Refeeding

There are only few data available on oral refeeding. In mild pancreatitis, a soft diet is gradually advanced to normal food once gastric outlet obstruction has resolved, provided it does not result in pain, and if complications are under control. The start with a soft diet was more beneficial than a start with a liquid diet [64]. If this is tolerated well, a normal diet with a moderate fat content can be given.

Tube feeding can be gradually withdrawn as intake improves. Currently, there are only two studies investigating oral refeeding [65,66]. In the study of Levy et al., 21% of patients experienced a pain relapse on the first and second day of refeeding. Serum lipase concentration greater than three times the upper limit of the normal range and higher Balthazar's CT-scores at the onset of refeeding were identified as risk factors for pain relapse [65]. In general, if enteral feeding can be stopped, the same regimens as in mild pancreatitis with a soft diet gradually advanced to normal food with a moderate fat content can be recommended.

NUTRITIONAL SUPPORT IN PATIENTS WITH PANCREATIC SURGERY

Postoperative feeding can be done with a nasojejunal tube or a needle catheter jejunostomy.

Postoperative feeding with a needle catheter jejunostomy was successful in several small studies [47,50,67]. Hernandez-Aranda et al. found no difference between groups of patients who received postoperative parenteral nutrition or enteral nutrition via jejunostomy [41]. Furthermore, in patients undergoing surgery for severe acute pancreatitis, needle catheter jejunostomy for long-term enteral nutrition was safely applied with no nutritional risk [50]. In general, in these patients, nutritional support has to be planned before the operation according to the clinical situation and the course of the disease.

Currently, no randomized large trial has specifically addressed early enteral nutrition after pancreatic surgery because of acute pancreatitis. In principle, the same approach as in abdominal surgery can be used.

SUMMARY

In total, 75%–80% of patients with acute pancreatitis have mild to moderate disease and do not need specific nutritional support. Early oral refeeding can be started within a few days if the patients have no pain and gastrointestinal disturbances. There is no evidence that a specific enteral or parenteral nutrition is of benefit in these patients. There are only few data available to give a nutritional recommendation in patients with severe pre-existing malnutrition or obesity. These patients are at the same risks for complication as in other diseases. Therefore, the nutritional status has to be considered.

Patients with severe disease, complications, or the need for surgery require early nutritional support. In patients with severe pancreatitis, an enteral jejunal approach should be established, but parenteral nutrition is an alternative method, when enteral nutrition is insufficient. If jejunal feeding is always necessary is under discussion. Several studies have shown that also gastric feeding is possible. For the future, several factors have to be clarified: the optimal timing of nutritional therapy, the optimal feeding site (oral, gastric, jejunal, or TPN), and the optimal nutrient formulation (semi-elemental diet, polymeric diet, immune-enhancing diet, pre- and probiotics). Furthermore, in future studies, a clear stratification of the patients according to their nutritional status on admission should be performed.

REFERENCES

1. Pandol SJ, Saluja AK, Imrie CW, Banks PA. Review in basic and clinical gastroenterology. *Gastroenterology*, 2007;132:1127–1151.
2. Baron TH, Morgan DE. Acute necrotizing pancreatitis. *N Engl J Med* 1999;340:1412–1417.
3. Renner IG, Savage WT, Pantoja JL, Renner VJ. Death due to acute pancreatitis: A retrospective analysis of 405 autopsy cases. *Dig Dis Sci* 1985;30:1005–1018.
4. Ranson JH, Rifkind KM, Roses DF, Fink SD, Eng K, Spencer FC. Prognostic signs and the role of operative management in acute pancreatitis. *Surg Gynecol Obstet* 1974;139:69–81.
5. Blamey SL, Imrie CW, O'Neill J, Gilmour WH, Carter DC. Prognostic factors in acute pancreatitis. *Gut* 1984;25:1340–1346.
6. Knaus WA, Draper EA, Wagner DP, Zimmermann JE. APACHE II: A severity of disease classification system. *Crit Care Med* 1985;13:819–829.
7. Bradley EL. A clinically based classification system for acute pancreatitis. *Arch Surg* 1993;128:586–590.
8. Balthazar EJ, Robinson DL, Megibow AJ, Ranson JH. Acute pancreatitis: Value of CT in establishing prognosis. *Radiology* 1990;174:331–336.
9. Wilson C, Heads A, Shenkin A, Imrie CW. C-reactive protein, antiproteases and complement factors as objective markers of severity in acute pancreatitis. *Br J Surg* 1989;76:177–181.
10. Mounzer R, Langmead C, Wu BU et al. Comparison of existing clinical scoring systems to predict persistent organ failure in patients with acute pancreatitis. *Gastroenterology* 2012;142:1476–1482.
11. Robin AP, Campbell R, Palani CK et al. Total parenteral nutrition during acute pancreatitis: Clinical experience within 156 patients. *World J Surg* 1990;14:572–579.
12. Vanmierlo B, De Waele E, De Waele B, Delvaux G. The relationship of body underweight to complication risks in acute pancreatitis. *J Pancreas* 2009;10:67–68.
13. Sitzmann JV, Steinborn PA, Zinner MJ, Cameron JL. Total parenteral nutrition and alternate energy substrates in treatment of severe acute pancreatitis. *Surg Gynecol Obstet* 1989;168:311–317.
14. Alpers DH. Digestion and absorption of carbohydrates and protein. In: Johnson LR et al. (eds.), *Physiology of the Gastrointestinal Tract*, 2nd edn., Raven Press, New York, 1987, pp. 1469–1487.

15. Greenberger NJ. Pancreatitis and hyperlipidemia. *N Engl J Med* 1973;289:586–587.
16. Knol JA, Inman MG, Strodel WE, Eckhauser FE. Pancreatic response to crystalloid resuscitation in experimental pancreatitis. *J Surg Res* 1987;43:387–392.
17. Warndorf MG, Kurtzman JT, Bartel MJ et al. Early fluid resuscitation reduces morbidity among patients with acute pancreatitis. *Clin Gastroenterol Hepatol* 2011;9:705–709.
18. Wu BU, Hwang JQ, Gardner TH et al. Lactated Ringer's solution reduces systemic inflammation compared with saline in patients with acute pancreatitis. *Clin Gastroenterol Hepatol* 2011;9:710–717.
19. Dickerson RN, Vehe KL, Mullen JL, Feurer ID. Resting energy expenditure in patients with pancreatitis. *Crit Care Med* 1991;19:484–490.
20. Van Den Berghe G, Wouters P, Weekers F et al. Intensive insulin therapy in critically ill patients. *N Engl J Med* 2001;345:1359–1367.
21. Jabbar A, Chang WK, Dryden GW, McClave SA. Gut immunology and the differential response to feeding and starvation. *Nutr Clin Pract* 2003;18:461–482.
22. McClave SA, Greene LM, Snider HL et al. Comparison of the safety of early enteral vs. parenteral nutrition in mild acute pancreatitis. *J Parenter Enteral Nutr* 1997;21:14–20.
23. Kalfarentzos F, Kehagias J, Mead N, Kokkinis K, Gogos CA. Enteral nutrition is superior to parenteral nutrition in severe acute pancreatitis: Results of a randomized prospective trial. *Br J Surg* 1997;84:1665–1669.
24. Windsor AC, Kanwar S, Li AG et al. Compared with parenteral nutrition, enteral feeding attenuates the acute phase response and improves disease severity in acute pancreatitis. *Gut* 1998;42:431–135.
25. Powell JJ, Murchison JT, Fearson KC et al. Randomized controlled trial of the effect of early enteral nutrition on markers of the inflammatory response in predicted severe acute pancreatitis. *Br J Surg* 2000;87:1375–1381.
26. Olah A, Pardavi G, Belagyi T et al. Early nasojejunal feeding in acute pancreatitis is associated with a lower complication rate. *Nutrition* 2002;18:259–262.
27. Abou-Assi S, Craig K, O'Keefe SJD. Hypocaloric jejunal feeding is better than total parenteral nutrition in acute pancreatitis: Results of a randomized comparative study. *Am J Gastroenterol* 2002;97:2255–2262.
28. Gupta R, Patel K, Calder PC, Yaqoob P, Primrose JN, Johnson CD. A randomised clinical trial to assess the effect of total enteral and total parenteral nutritional support on metabolic, inflammatory and oxidative markers in patients with predicted severe acute pancreatitis (APACHE II >or = 6). *Pancreatology* 2003;3(5):406–413.
29. Louie BE, Noseworthy T, Hailey D et al. Enteral or parenteral nutrition for severe pancreatitis: A randomized controlled trial and healthy assessment. *Can J Surg* 2005;48:298–306.
30. Petrov MS, Kukosh MV, Emelyanov NV. A randomized controlled trial of enteral versus parenteral feeding in patients with predicted severe acute pancreatitis shows a significant reduction in mortality and in infected pancreatic complications with total enteral nutrition. *Dig Surg* 2006;23:336–345.
31. Targarona Modena J, Barreda Cevasco L, Arroyo Basto C et al. Total enteral nutrition as a prophylactic therapy for pancreatic necrosis infection in severe acute pancreatitis. *Pancreatology* 2006;6:58–64.
32. Casas M, Mora J, Fort E et al. Total enteral nutrition vs total parenteral nutrition in patients with severe acute pancreatitis. *Rev Esp Enferm Dig* 2007;99:264–269.
33. Doley RP, Yadav TD, Wig JD et al. Enteral nutrition in severe acute pancreatitis. *J Pancreas* 2009;10:157–162.
34. Wu XM, Ji KQ, Wang HY et al. Total enteral nutrition in prevention of pancreatic necrotic infection in severe acute pancreatitis. *J Pancreas* 2010;39:248–251.
35. Hegazi R, Raina A, Graham T et al. Early jejunal feeding initiation and clinical outcomes in patients with severe acute pancreatitis. *J Parenter Enteral Nutr* 2011;35:91–96.
36. Olah A, Romics L. Evidence-based use of enteral nutrition in acute pancreatitis. *Langenbecks Arch Surg* 2010;395:309–316.
37. McClave SA, Chang WK, Dhaliwal R, Heyland DK. Nutrition support in acute pancreatitis: A systemic review of the literature. *J Parent Enteral Nutr* 2006;30:143–156.
38. Petrov MS, Santvoort HC, Besselink MG et al. Enteral nutrition and the risk of mortality and infectious complications in patients with severe acute pancreatitis: A meta-analysis of randomized trials. *Arch Surg* 2008;143:1111–1117.
39. Petrov MS, Pylypchuck RD, Uchugina AF. A systematic review on the timing of artificial nutrition in acute pancreatitis. *Br J Nutr* 2009;101:787–793.
40. Al-Omran M, Albalwi ZH, Tashkandi MF et al. Enteral versus parenteral nutrition in acute pancreatitis. *Cochrane Database Syst Rev* 2010;20:CD002837.

41. Petrov MS, Whelan K. Comparison of complications attributable to enteral and parenteral nutrition in predicted severe acute pancreatitis: A systematic review and meta-analysis. *Br J Nutr* 2010;103:1287–1295.
42. Quan H, Wang X, Guo C. A meta-analysis of enteral and total parenteral nutrition in patients with acute pancreatitis. *Gastroenterol Res Pract* 2011;2011:698248.
43. Meier R, Ockenga J, Pertkiewicz M et al. ESPEN guidelines on enteral nutrition: Pancreas. *Clin Nutr* 2006;25:275–284.
44. Gianotti L, Meier R, Lobo DN et al. ESPEN guidelines on parenteral nutrition: Pancreas. *Clin Nutr* 2009;28:428–435.
45. Mirtallo JM, Forbes A, McClave SA et al. International consensus guidelines for nutrition therapy in pancreatitis. *J Parenter Enteral Nutr* 2012;36:284–291.
46. Cravo M, Camilo ME, Marques A, Pinto Correia J. Early tube feeding in acute pancreatitis: A prospective study. *Clin Nutr* 1989;7(Suppl.1):A8–14.
47. Kudsk KA, Campbell SM, O'Brian T, Fuller R. Postoperative jejunal feedings following complicated pancreatitis. *Nutr Clin Pract* 1990;5:14–17.
48. Nakad A, Piessevaux H, Marot JC et al. Is early enteral nutrition in acute pancreatitis dangerous? About 20 patients fed by an endoscopically placed nasogastrojejunal tube. *Pancreas* 1998;17:187–193.
49. Scolapio JS, Malhi-Chowla N, Ukleja A. Nutrition supplementation in patients with acute and chronic pancreatitis. *Gastroenterol Clin North Am* 1999;28:695–707.
50. Weimann A, Braunert M, Muller T, Bley T, Wiedemann B. Feasibility and safety of needle catheter jejunostomy for enteral nutrition in surgically treated severe acute pancreatitis. *J Parenter Enteral Nutr* 2004;28:324–327.
51. Eatcock FC, Brombacher GD, Steven A, Imrie CW, McKay CJ, Carter R. Nasogastric feeding in severe acute pancreatitis may be practical and safe. *Int J Pancreatol* 2000;28:23–29.
52. Eatock FC, Chong P, Menezes N et al. A randomized study of early nasogastric versus nasojejunal feeding severe acute pancreatitis. *Am J Gastroenterol* 2005;100:432–439.
53. Kumar A, Singh N, Prakash S et al. Early enteral nutrition in severe acute pancreatitis: A prospective randomized controlled trial comparing nasojejunal and nasogastric routes. *J Clin Gastroenterol* 2006;40:431–434.
54. Eckerwall GE, Axelsson JB, Andersson RG. Early nasogastric feeding in predicted severe acute pancreatitis. A clinical randomized study. *Ann Surg* 2006;244:959–965.
55. Petrov MS, Correia MI, Windsor JA. Nasogastric tube feeding in predicted severe acute pancreatitis. A systematic review of the literature to determine safety and tolerance. *J Pancreas* 2008;9:440–448.
56. Tiengou LE, Gloro R, Pouzoulet J, Bouhier K, Read MH, Arnaud-Battandier F, Plaze JM, Blaizot X, Dao T, Piquet MA. Semi-elemental formula or polymeric formula: Is there a better choice for enteral nutrition in acute pancreatitis? Randomized comparative study. *J Parenter Enteral Nutr* 2006;30:1–5.
57. Petrov MS, Loveday BP, Pylypchuck RD et al. Systematic review and meta-analysis of enteral nutrition formulations in acute pancreatitis. *Br J Surg* 2009;96:1243–1252.
58. Olah A, Belagyi T, Issekutz A, Gamal ME, Bengmark S. Randomized clinical trial of specific lactobacillus and fibre supplement to early enteral nutrition in patients with acute pancreatitis. *Br J Surg* 2002;89:1103–1107.
59. Oláh A, Belágyi T, Pótó L, Romics L Jr, Bengmark S. Symbiotic control of inflammation and infection in severe acute pancreatitis: A prospective, randomized, double blind study. *Hepatogastroenterology* 2007;54:590–594.
60. Besselink MG, van Santvoort JC, Buskens E et al. Probiotic prophylaxis in predicted severe acute pancreatitis: A randomised, double-blind, placebo-controlled trial. *Lancet* 2008;371:651–659.
61. Karakan T, Ergun M, Dogan I, Cindoruk M, Unal S. Comparison of early enteral nutrition in severe acute pancreatitis with prebiotic fiber supplementation versus standard enteral solution. A prospective randomized double-blind study. *World Gastroenterol* 2007;13:2733–2737.
62. Wang X, Li W, Li N, Li J. ω-3 fatty acids-supplemented parenteral nutrition decreases hyperinflammatory response and attenuates systemic disease sequelae in severe acute pancreatitis: A randomized and controlled study. *J Parenter Enteral Nutr* 2008;32:236–241.
63. Fuentes-Orozco C, Cervantes-Guevara G, Muciño-Hernández I et al. L-alanyl-L-glutamine-supplemented parenteral nutrition decreases infectious morbidity rate in patients with severe acute pancreatitis. *J Parenter Enteral Nutr* 2008;32:403–411.
64. Rajkumar N, Karthikeyan VS, Ali SM et al. Clear liquid diet vs soft diet as the initial meal in patients with mild acute pancreatitis: A randomized interventional trial. *Nutr Clin Pract* 2013;28:365–370.

65. Lévy P, Heresbach D, Pariente EA et al. Frequency and risk factors of recurrent pain during refeeding in patients with acute pancreatitis: A multivariate multicentre prospective study of 116 patients. *Gut* 1997;40:262–266.
66. Pandey SK, Ahuja V, Joshi YK, Sharma MP. A randomized trial of oral refeeding compared with jejunal tube refeeding in acute pancreatitis. *Indian J Gastroent* 2004;23:53–61.
67. Hernandez-Aranda JC, Gallo-Chico B, Ramirez-Barba EJ. Nutritional support in severe acute pancreatitis. Controlled clinical trial. *Nutr Hosp* 1996;11:160–166.

Section VII

General Systemic Failures

33 Nutrition Support in the General Surgery ICU Patient

Amy Berry and Kenneth A. Kudsk

CONTENTS

INTRODUCTION

Multiple complications can send the surgical patient into the intensive care unit (ICU). Factors contributing include an inability to maintain hemodynamic stability postoperatively, an inability to maintain oxygen saturation, or even intra-operative complications that require additional monitoring. If the patient does not require immediate ICU care postoperatively, a sudden change in mental status, tachycardia, hypotension, fevers, and/or leukocytosis can alert the team to impending systemic inflammatory response syndrome (SIRS) and/or sepsis. Finding the source and effective treatment of the underlying problem is imperative for recovery, whether it is a surgical bleed, anastomotic leak, abscess, or other source of infection. Further, it may make a difference for the need of ICU care if the patient undergoes emergent versus elective surgery. Emergent surgery patients often meet criteria for SIRS preoperatively and often have a longer hospital stay with increased complications [1,2].

In addition to the risks of surgery, a high prevalence of preexisting malnutrition further complicates the scenario. Studies have reported 40%–50% prevalence of malnutrition prior to surgery in this patient population [3,4]. Malnourished surgical patients are shown to have a significantly higher complication rate, including morbidity and mortality, compared to those well-nourished preoperatively [3,5,6]. Many variables predicting a higher morbidity and mortality in the general surgery patient cannot be controlled (i.e., interoperative blood loss), while there is a defined preoperative window where it is possible to alter outcome by early nutritional intervention. In addition to identifying and intervening preoperatively, there may be a significant benefit to feeding in the early postoperative period. Feeding early postoperatively has been associated with a decreased risk of surgical complications [7,8]. Early enteral feeding appears to provide significant benefit to those who are severely injured and/or malnourished and at a higher risk of infectious complications [9]. Regardless, those at risk of malnutrition have a diminished lean body mass, decreased ability to heal, and decreased ability to resist infections all which would worsen outcomes for the surgical patient. This chapter will address how to provide and optimize the impact of nutrition support on the general surgery ICU patient.

IMPORTANCE OF PREEXISTING NUTRITIONAL STATE

The importance of a well-nourished state preoperatively and its significant effect to a successful surgery is not new. In 1936, patients undergoing peptic ulcer disease (PUD) surgery with a 20% preoperative weight loss had a 33% higher mortality compared to 4% mortality in the well-nourished patients [10]. In major gastrointestinal (GI) surgery, endotoxemia occurs, initiating a proinflammatory cascade leading to increased TNF-α levels [11]. Increased proinflammatory cytokines (e.g., TNF-α, IL-6) are related to accelerated acute-phase response leading to increased inflammation and catabolism [11]. In the malnourished patient, multiple immunologic pathways are severely impaired, thus creating a cumulative immunosuppressive effect in the malnourished, surgical patient [12]. Even if a patient is considered well-nourished on admission, they can become malnourished throughout their hospital course despite the clinician's best efforts [13].

The risk of postoperative morbidity and mortality increases when lean body mass decreases [12]. Depletion of lean body mass contributes to diaphragmatic muscle and respiratory muscle weakness, predisposing the patient to prolonged mechanical ventilation and a higher risk of developing aspiration pneumonia [12]. Malnutrition is considered to be a risk factor in the development of postoperative surgical complications, and preserving and/or increasing nutritional status have been shown to improve healing from complications such as wound dehiscence and anastomotic leaks [5,12].

A depressed albumin, although affected by a multitude of factors other than nutrition (such as inflammation and fluid status), can be evaluated preoperatively as a prognostic indicator. There is a linear increase in complications in patients undergoing elective GI surgery as preoperative albumin decreases from normal levels to below 2.0 g/dL [9]. Complications increase in esophagectomy patients with an albumin <3.75 g/dL, and in gastric and pancreatic surgery, complications increase with an albumin <3.25 g/dL. Unfortunately, albumin is also an indicator of how ill the patient is, and often until their inflammatory cascade diminishes by the illness resolving, albumin levels are not likely to significantly improve. Studies have shown that giving nutrition support for at least 5–7 days preoperatively in severely malnourished patients can significantly decrease complications [14,15]. Providing immune nutrition (either by mouth or as a tube feeding) preoperatively could have an additional advantage [11,15,16]. However, providing nutrition support much less than a week preoperatively, and in any population that is less than severely malnourished, may not produce any obvious clinical benefit [14,17].

As severe malnutrition is associated with poor surgical outcomes, what indicates that a patient is indeed severely malnourished? This also has become a greater area of interest as reimbursement is now tied into the diagnosis of severe malnutrition. Unfortunately, many studies promoting the benefits of nutrition intervention in the malnourished patient include serum albumin levels as an indicator for malnutrition, which, as mentioned before, may simply be an indicator of severity of illness and not a direct correlation with nutritional status. Prealbumin is often utilized to evaluate nutrition, as it has a shorter half-life and is less variable than albumin. However, prealbumin is an acute phase reactant, so it too becomes void in determining nutritional status or nutritional adequacy during critical illness. A recent study showed that the amount of serum prealbumin level change in the critically ill significantly correlated with changes in C-reactive protein (an acute phase reactant), not with nutrition provision [18]. A commonly used technique

TABLE 33.1
Methods of Identifying Nutrition Risk

	Subjective Global Assessment SGA	Nutritional Risk Screening 2002 NRS-2002	Consensus from ADA and ASPEN
Variables	Recent weight loss Recent enteral intake GI dysfunction Functional status Metabolic demand of disease state	1. Undernutrition: a. Weight loss b. BMI c. Recent enteral intake 2. Severity of underlying disease. With score adjustment for age.	Recent enteral intake. Weight lost over a recent time period. Body fat loss. Lean muscle loss. Fluid accumulation. Reduced grip strength.
Criteria for diagnosis	Score of A, B, or C C indicates severe malnutrition	Rate each category 0–3 Total score of 3 or more indicates presence of severe malnutrition, with a score of 2 indicating moderate malnutrition.	Categories include acute, chronic, or environmental malnutrition, and each is differentiated as moderate or severe. Must have two components of the designated area for diagnosis.

Sources: White, J.V. et al., *J. Parenter. Enter. Nutr.*, 36(3), 275, April 24, 2012; Jeejeebhoy, K.N. et al., *JPEN J. Parenter. Enteral. Nutr.*, 14(5 Suppl), 193S, October 1990; Kondrup, J. et al., *Clin. Nutr.*, 22(3), 321, June 2003.

to evaluate nutrition status is subjective global assessment (SGA). This tool includes multiple variables that can affect nutritional status [19]. SGA has been validated and is easy to use in the clinical setting. The Nutritional Risk Screening 2002 (NRS-2002) often is used as an assessment tool and has been advocated by the European Society of Enteral and Parenteral Nutrition [20]. Recently, the Academy of Nutrition and Dietetics along with the American Society of Enteral and Parenteral Nutrition developed a consensus statement creating criteria to differentiate acute and chronic illness, and severe and moderate malnutrition, using a combination of indicators [13]. See Table 33.1 for details on various methods of identifying malnutrition in the hospitalized patient.

METABOLIC EFFECT IN THE SURGICAL ICU PATIENT

Complicating a common existence of preoperative malnutrition, the critically ill general surgical patient undergoes hypermetabolism and hypercatabolism, which exacerbate lean tissue degradation [21].

Nutrition support, preferably in the enteral form, provides substrates and micronutrients, which may help blunt excessive hypermetabolism before irreparable damage is done. In deciding on energy provision in the critically ill patient, it appears that increased energy intake is not able to completely prevent catabolism and thus loss of lean body mass [22]. Preserving lean body mass and minimizing nitrogen loss are a primary goal of nutrition support in the critically ill surgical population. However, determining and providing optimal energy can be a balancing act, as both overfeeding and underfeeding are detrimental to the critically ill patient. Overfeeding is linked to prolonged time on the ventilator, increased infectious risk, electrolyte abnormalities, and hyperglycemia. Overall, increased caloric provision potentially gives the patient a metabolic load they are unable to handle in a stressed state. Alternatively, an energy deficit often occurs in the critically ill patient, especially early in the hospital admission [23]. Due to surgical procedures, GI intolerance, diagnostic testing, or multiple other reasons, feedings are commonly held, and patients do not come close to meeting their estimated goals.

In addition to receiving inadequate energy, patients also receive inadequate protein. Protein helps with nitrogen retention, provides substrate for metabolic pathways and acute phase proteins, and additionally provides fuel for the gut and immune factors. Protein also maintains a positive nitrogen balance even in the absence of adequate calories [24,25]. There is a peak in protein hypercatabolism at 2–3 days postoperatively, which diminishes by 7–10 days if no complications develop. The restorative or anabolic phase can last 6 months up to a year [26,27]. Creating a positive nitrogen balance is the goal for surgical patients, but this may not be completely attainable during these early periods of postoperative hypercatabolism. In conditions such as sepsis and infection, the systemic inflammatory response and thus hypercatabolism may persist (see Chapter 1). Adequate protein provision in this state does help reduce nitrogen deficits, with one study showing a protein provision of ~2 g/kg/day having a greater propensity of creating a nitrogen equilibrium in the critically ill during the first 5–14 days of hospitalization [28]. Careful monitoring of renal function and implementation of medical intervention (e.g., kidney dialysis) are necessary when providing higher doses of protein to the critically ill patient.

DETERMINING APPROPRIATE CALORIC PROVISION IN THE SURGICAL ICU PATIENT

Multiple studies have attempted to find the ultimate goal for feeding the critically ill patient. Most clinicians agree that indirect calorimetry (IC) is the gold standard for assessing energy expenditure in the critically ill. However, taking these results and appropriately applying them to the patient can be difficult. Singer et al. found that resting energy expenditure (REE) varies significantly in the first few days of critical illness [29]. When REE was measured every 48 h during the first 10 days of ICU admission, values were significantly different. However, while this is important to consider when developing a nutritional plan for the critically ill surgical patient, it is impractical to measure REE that frequently (see Chapter 6). One study compared IC versus Harris–Benedict equation plus an activity factor versus calorie per kilogram (cal/kg/day) method using adjusted body weight and found no significant differences between the three methods [30]. Another study showed that even the best predictive equation was equal to IC only 60%–70% of the time [31]. To confound the issue further, it is important to note that the majority of critically ill patients actually *receive* only approximately 58%–70% of calculated and prescribed requirements [32,33].

The most important aspect in determining energy needs in the critically ill surgical patient is whether a benefit would be obtained if energy requirements were actually *supplied*. There has been no study showing that providing nutrition equal to the amount the critically ill patient is expending provides improved outcomes. The TICACOS study compared a *tight caloric control group*, which included IC performed every 48 h, daily follow-up, and nutrition adjustments for inadequate caloric provision, with the *standard group* of 25 kcal/kg/day, who did not receive daily nutrition adjustment [29]. The tight calorie-controlled group obtained a positive caloric balance, but was associated with prolonged duration on the ventilator and ICU stay. The authors did report a trend toward lower mortality in the tight calorie control group [29]. The results may have been confounded as the tight calorie control group did receive more total parenteral nutrition (TPN) than the control group. Rice et al. compared those who received full feeds (>80% goal) in the first week to trophic feeding and found no difference in vent-free days, ICU length of stay, infection, or between the groups [34]. Most notably, Caesar et al. concluded that TPN started by day 3 of the ICU admission to achieve caloric balance actually led to an increase in mortality [35]. This study had several criticisms including concerns that the patients were not severely ill and the majority of the subjects were cardiac surgery, not surgery or trauma, patients [36].

Determining goal feedings is problematic, but specifically underfeeding and exacerbating malnutrition in the critically ill patient continues to be of concern. Villet et al. showed that a significant caloric deficit occurs in the first week following critical illness with the second week's delivery still significantly less than target provision [23]. Cumulative energy deficit (>10,000 total calories) was associated with an increased ICU stay, ventilator requirement, infections, and antibiotic use [23]. This group felt this was a further reason for the need of early feeding in ICU patients. Heidegger et al. performed a randomized study of 123 ICU patients, using supplemental TPN to meet caloric needs of patients who were going to stay in the ICU at least 5 days *and* were able to tolerate only ≤60% of enteral feeds. This group found a reduced incidence of nosocomial infections by days 9–28 of hospitalization [37]. Alberda et al. examined the effect of early caloric provision in the critically ill intensive care patient, specifically comparing the outcomes between various BMI groups. They found that increasing nutrition provision in the first 12 days, by 1000 cal/day, was associated with a significant decrease in 60-day mortality rate and vent-free days in the patient groups with a BMI <25 and ≥35 [38]. This study noted that the highest BMI category received only 8–9 kcal/kg and 0.4 g protein/kg. They also brought up two important points in feeding the ICU patient: (1) overall patients received only 59.2% prescribed calories and 56% prescribed protein and (2) patients that did not receive caloric provision also did not receive protein provision [38]. All the studies reporting caloric deficit due to insufficient caloric provision comment on concurrent deficient protein provision; therefore, the benefit of increasing caloric provision may be related to increased protein intake in the ICU patient [38].

PROTEIN REQUIREMENTS FOR THE SURGICAL ICU PATIENT

A protein provision of at least 1.2 g protein/kg of preadmission weight has been suggested for the critically ill patient. However, as mentioned previously, a target rate does not assure that the patient actually receives this amount. The importance of protein is exemplified by a recent study associating adequate energy *plus* adequate protein provision with a decreased risk of 28-day and hospital mortality [39]. The group that reached energy targets but not the protein target did not have this positive outcome. Therefore, careful attention should be paid when assessing studies determining the effectiveness of nutrition support in the critically ill, assuring protein, not just calories, was provided in adequate amounts.

In addition to the hypercatabolism of critical illness, surgical patients have potential sources for ongoing nitrogen loss. Nitrogen balance studies attempt to quantify these losses, but accurately obtaining these studies are difficult; they require nutrition support being appropriately administered during the same 24 h as the urine collection for measurement. This test essentially is a reflection of the balance between exogenous nitrogen administration and renal removal of nitrogenous-containing compounds [40]. Therefore, if renal function is compromised in any way, this result will not be accurate. The concept of achieving a positive nitrogen balance is nitrogen *in* should exceed nitrogen *out*. However, this is still based on an estimate, as part of the equation includes an *insensible loss* factor of 2–4 g to account for additional losses in stool, sweat, etc. (see Figure 33.1). Surgical patients may also have abdominal and thoracic fluid losses through chest tubes, surgical drains, open wounds, open abdomens, and diarrhea. Recently, a study determined protein losses from an open abdomen and suggested adding 2 g of nitrogen per liter of open abdomen fluid loss [41]. As the use of negative pressure wound therapy has become common practice, another study examined nitrogen loss from both open abdomens and soft tissue wounds using this treatment method [42]. They found no differences in total protein, albumin, or urea nitrogen between the two

$$(\text{Protein in}^{*} \div 6.25) - (\text{nitrogen out}^{**} + 4^{***})$$

FIGURE 33.1 Nitrogen balance formula. *Note:* * How many grams of protein patient actually received during the same 24 h as the urine collection. ** Total grams of nitrogen from 24-h urine collection. *** Insensible loss.

sites and found a nitrogen loss of 4.6 g/L/day, which should be taken into account when estimating the patient's protein needs [42]. The open abdominal wall nitrogen loss was greater, simply due to the higher daily volume lost.

Often surgical ICU patients develop acute kidney injury (AKI) requiring the clinician to reanalyze the amount of protein that can be provided. In some circumstances, the medical goal may be to delay or avoid dialysis; therefore, the amount of protein the patient is able to tolerate without worsening kidney function will be questioned. However, this practice is not desirable for great lengths of time as the importance of adequate protein in this population has been demonstrated, and additionally, AKI without dialysis can worsen metabolic alterations (e.g., acidosis). In the critically ill patient, net protein synthesis is stimulated by protein provision *without* increasing whole-body protein catabolism [43]. A very small study in non-oliguric AKI patients' predialysis compared administration of 75 g protein versus 150 g protein, with both groups receiving 2000 kcal/day, and found no significant differences in blood urea nitrogen between the two [44]. A recent review of the literature reported providing protein at 1.3–1.5 g/kg predialysis did not increase urea generation compared with protein restriction when receiving adequate calories, while providing 2–2.5 g protein/kg improved nitrogen balance but came with the price of increasing urea [45]. Further protein loss comes from hemodialysis, which studies have reported a 6–12 g protein and 2–3 g peptide loss at each session, while CRRT (depending on the method) has been reported to cause losses of 1.2–7.5 g protein in 24 h [43,45]. Therefore, during dialysis, providing higher levels of protein is usually well tolerated.

In summary, in the critically ill postsurgical patient, it seems prudent to supply at least 1.5 g protein/kg/day, and with additional protein losses, needs may increase to 2–2.5 g protein/kg/day.

GLUCOSE AND FAT REQUIREMENTS IN THE SURGICAL ICU PATIENT

A maximum of 4–5 mg/kg/min of glucose can be oxidized by the liver [46]. With current caloric recommendations in the critically ill patient, this is not often exceeded unless a nutrition regimen is cycled over a shorter time period. In addition to the avoidance of overfeeding, current practice has shifted to emphasizing strict control of blood glucoses in the ICU. A large study of surgical ICU patients found that using intensive insulin therapy with tight target glucose control (keeping glucoses between 80 and 110 mg/dL) resulted in decreased ICU length of stay, decreased ventilator support, renal replacement therapy, septicemia, antibiotic use, and bacteremia and also found a significant decrease in mortality [47]. However, caloric levels seemed to be high in this study (giving up to 30 cal/kg of nonprotein calories); there was a higher-than-normal reliance on intravenous (IV) glucose and parenteral nutrition, and the majority of patients who benefited were recovering from cardiac surgery. This patient selection makes it impossible to extrapolate to general patient populations. Subsequently, a larger multi-institutional, multinational study of both surgical and medical ICU patients [48] was conducted on those patients expected to be in the ICU > 3 days and prioritized enteral nutrition, with a lower median nonprotein caloric level (~872–891 ± 490–500 kcal). Using the same glucose/insulin protocols, this study found no difference in mortality, number of days on the ventilator, renal replacement therapy use, or positive blood cultures, but *did* find increased mortality in the treatment/tight glucose control group [48]. Further, the treatment group suffered significantly more episodes of hypoglycemia (glucoses ≤ 40 mg/dL). Therefore, majority of ICUs currently endorse protocols to keep glucoses ≤ 150 mg/dL and to keep adequate glucose control, but not quite as tight as originally suggested in the first trial to help reduce the risk of hypoglycemic events.

Currently, only soybean oil–based lipid formulations are available in the United States. Soybean-based lipid emulsions contain 50% omega-6, which not only prevent fatty acid deficiency but also have the potential to increase inflammation in the critically ill patient [49]. The use of IV lipid avoids excessive dextrose administration, which has been linked to hyperlipidemia, cholestasis, prolonged ventilator weaning, and hyperglycemia in an already insulin-resistant patient population. The negative effects of IV lipids are minimized if administered at a rate ≤1 g/kg/day. Patients receiving IV lipids should have their serum triglyceride levels monitored, and if the levels are >400 mg/dL, the IV lipids should be discontinued and reevaluated in 1–2 weeks. In most enteral formulas, the calorie-to-nitrogen ratio and fat composition are predetermined and are well below these levels.

OPTIMAL FEEDING TUBE PLACEMENT

Beyond supplying calories and protein, the provision of enteral feeding to the critically ill ICU patient has its own benefit. The GI tract has important immune, barrier, and endocrine functions in addition to the ability to digest and absorb nutrients [50]. In the early stages of critical illness, the unfed gut undergoes mucosal atrophy, increased intestinal permeability, and a reduction in gut-associated lymphoid tissue [51]. In this condition, the gut becomes limited in its ability to prevent attachment and invasion of pathogenic bacteria, which further stimulates the release of inflammatory cytokines. Although the importance of gut stimulation through enteral feeding is known, clinical concerns of feeding a postsurgical patient with postoperative ileus or a critically ill patient with GI dysfunction lead to inadequate nutritional delivery [50,52]. These factors may predispose the patient to prolonged ICU and hospital stays, development of organ failure, and increased risk of mortality.

Gastroparesis is common in critically ill patients and after GI surgery. Delays in feeding are often attributed to fear of aspiration or causing an anastomotic leak. However, these are not absolute contraindications to gastric feeds. The Enhanced Recovery after Surgery (ERAS) group advocates feeding within 24 h after colorectal surgery and starting a diet within a few days following pancreaticoduodenectomy [53,54]. Studies examining early feeding in the ICU using a gastric versus post-pyloric route found no difference in aspiration pneumonia, length of stay, or complications. A post-pyloric tube can delay initiation of enteral feeding if completely dependent on its use for initiation of feeding [55,56]. A large multicenter randomized study investigated nasojejunal versus nasogastric feedings in critical illness, specifically in patients with mildly elevated residuals. They found that nasojejunal nutrition did not increase caloric delivery or decrease rates of pneumonia [57].

A more recent study looked at specific factors in assessing post-pyloric versus gastric feeding and risk of aspiration, including severity of illness, level of sedation, degree of head of bed (HOB) elevation, and use of gastric suction [58]. Pepsin-positive tracheal secretions were used to monitor for aspiration of gastric contents, and Clinical Pulmonary Infection Score was used to assess for pneumonia. The study groups were equal in APACHE II scores and sedation. They reported no significant difference in HOB elevation between the two groups, but the gastric feeding group had a mean HOB elevation of 26.2% ± SD 13 versus 38.6% ± SD 11. They found that each 10° increase in HOB elevation resulted in a 3.8% reduction in the percentage of pepsin-positive secretions. They found a lower incidence of pepsin-positive tracheal secretions the more distal the feeding tube tip was located in the GI tract (13.6% decrease with tube tip just post-pyloric and 26.8% decrease with the tip at the fourth portion of the duodenum/jejunum compared to the stomach). In addition, small bowel feeding with gastric suction resulted in 7.1% lower pepsin-positive tracheal secretions compared to patients with no gastric suction. They reported a significantly lower incidence of pneumonia once the feeding tube was in the second portion of the duodenum or beyond, compared to gastric feeding.

In most institutions, blind placement of small bore feeding tubes is a common and routine procedure. Unfortunately, this procedure carries a 1.5%–2% complication rate, many of which can be fatal. In a recent study, blind placement of feeding tubes placed resulted in advancement into the respiratory tree in 3.2% of patients, many of whom had multiple tubes placed during their hospitalization increasing their risk of injury. Nine patients sustained a pneumothorax as a result of this misadventure, and four of these patients died [59]. The rate of respiratory tract malposition was 1.5% for each attempt at feeding tube placement. Mandatory radiography of the tube after advancing the tube 30–35 cm does not eliminate this complication [60]. The creation of a *feeding tube team* and use of electromagnetic technology have been shown to eliminate these complications [61]. Initially, blind tube placement was allowed in non-ICU patients who were alert and oriented (and presumably capable of providing feedback to the individual placing the tube). Any neurologically compromised or intubated/patients in an intensive care setting mandated placement by the team. Airway placements were completely eliminated as well as the associated complications and deaths. The number of radiographs obtained for this procedure dropped by almost 50%, and fluoroscopic placement dropped from 11% of all patients to 2.1% with electromagnetic tracking. Surprisingly, airway placement and pneumothoraxes occurred in 2% of low-risk alert patients but without any deaths. The researchers recommend that blind placement of feeding tubes with stylets should be avoided even in awake patients, and tubes are best placed by a trained team using electromagnetic tracking to eliminate unnecessary morbidity, which reduces radiology costs. Contraindications to small bore placement include anatomic upper intestinal anomalies or proximal GI blockage or need to pass the tube through a recent anastomosis.

Several methods are available to gain access for small bowel feeding at the time of laparotomy. First, a small bore tube can be advanced through the nose or mouth and guided by the surgeon beyond the ligament of Treitz. These tubes require commitment of the nursing staff to avoid dislodgement during patient movement. If it is imperative that the tube stays jejunal or the patient has a history of agitation, it may be best to bridle the tube. Nasoenteric tubes also have the potential of flipping back into the stomach. Direct small bowel tube access with a 14–18 French catheter jejunostomy may be more reliable. If a complication occurs with this tube, it can be exchanged after the tract is formed, approximately 6–8 days. Once nasojejunal tubes are lost, a trip to fluoroscopy is often required, which may not be an option if dislodged early on postoperatively. A transgastric jejunal or percutaneous endoscopic gastrostomy–jejunal tube is another option that can be placed at the time of surgery. This tube allows for the decompression of the stomach, while feeding the small bowel. Considering the patient's anatomy is important when planning placement of feeding tubes. An insertion site in the small bowel should have a long mesentery and adequate length beyond the ligament of Treitz to preclude tethering and dislodgement if the patient develops distention. Second, a Witzel tunnel should be created for approximately 3–5 cm to preclude dislodgement into the peritoneal cavity. This segment should be sutured to the anterior abdominal wall with three to four sutures just lateral to the rectus sheath to eliminate the chance of torsion or volvulus at the attachment site and minimize the opportunity for small bowel to lineate over the site. The external portion of the catheter should be short to reduce dislodgement of the catheter by patients. No communication should exist between any part of the tube and peritoneal cavity.

Once the decision has been made for what part of the GI tract is safe to feed, starting at a lower rate of 20 mL/h in a postoperative patient may be prudent. Slow advancement and careful monitoring of tolerance should be ongoing. The HOB should be elevated to 30° no matter where the tip of the tube is located. If tube feeding is tolerated via a Salem-sump-type NGT, this should be replaced with a small bore tube to prevent sinusitis, minimize reflux, and increase patient comfort.

TIMING OF FEEDING

In the general surgery patient, small bowel motility returns in 0–24 h, gastric motility in 24–48 h, and colonic motility in 48–72 h [62]. There is no reason to wait for signs of *return of bowel function* such as stool passage, flatus, or bowel sounds, as none of these have been validated as proof that bowel function has returned. The ERAS protocol focuses on what methods can be employed in the surgical patient to decrease functional loss and facilitate functional recovery postoperatively [53,54]. Many factors are analyzed, and recommendations include avoidance of preoperative fasting, oral feeding as early as possible postoperatively, decreasing factors that impair GI function (e.g., anesthesia and opioids), and early mobilization. In the colorectal group, early feeding decreased the risk of infections and shortened the length of hospital stay with no increase in anastomotic dehiscence [53]. In colorectal surgery, they suggest that clear liquids be started within hours of surgery.

Enhanced recovery after surgery (ERAS) guidelines for pancreaticoduodenectomy reports early diets being safe and the archaic sips/chips progressed to clears progressed eventually to regular is not any safer and provide no additional benefit than allowing foods at will, as long as the patient is educated on the signs of GI intolerance [54,63]. The concern for anastomotic integrity after upper GI surgery often results in delayed feeding or early feeding distal to the anastomosis. However, this practice has not been supported by the literature. Oral intake creates a propulsive, reflex response, and several studies have shown that patients fed earlier tolerated a regular diet faster [62–65].

Feeding a postoperative patient early may be more readily achievable in the less complicated patient. Multiple studies have documented starting enteral nutrition within 24 h of surgery after upper and lower GI surgery [66]. A meta-analysis reported decreased risk of infectious complications, length of hospital stay, and possibly mortality when enteral feeds are started within 24 h of surgery [66]. Another meta-analysis examined early enteral nutrition specifically in the critically ill patient population, including studies initiating enteral feeding within 24 h of injury or admission to the ICU [51]. They found a statistically significant reduction in mortality and pneumonia in those started on early enteral nutrition [51]. Therefore, obtaining appropriate access and initiation of early enteral nutrition may include reduced postoperative infectious complications, anastomotic healing, decrease in weight loss, protein catabolism, and shortened hospital stay [64,65].

The more malnourished a patient is preoperatively, the more an impact early feeding may have. Kondrup et al. examined both these variables and found that with increasing severity of injury or greater degree of malnutrition, these patients had increasingly positive results with nutrition support [20]. Other literature has concluded that enteral nutrition instituted within 24–48 h of major abdominal surgery provides benefits, such as shorter hospital stays, fewer complications, and reduced infectious complications, which are not gained when enteral nutrition is delayed. Both ESPEN and ASPEN guidelines promote the use of early enteral nutrition within 24–48 h after surgery if oral nutrition is not feasible [67,68].

OPTIMAL FORMULA CHOICE

Complex formulas with intact protein, carbohydrates, and fat can be used without significant absorptive problems in the surgical ICU patient. Standard, high-protein formulas are available to meet the needs of surgical patients. Additionally, different modular components are available to provide additional protein. Specialized, partially hydrolyzed, or low-fat formulas for ease of digestion are needed only in those with significant absorptive problems, such as those with existing mucosal disease, a small surface area of functional gut, or a significant pancreatic resection. Fiber-containing formulas are usually well tolerated and have been associated with supporting gut mucosal cells as well as serving as a substrate for bacteria in the colon, which can convert fiber to short-chain fatty acids, which then can be used as a fuel for colonocytes and increase water absorption [69,70]. However, there also seems to be an increased use of FODMAPS (fermentable, oligo–di–monosaccharides and polyols) in these formulas, which have been reported to increase GI distress [71,72]. The safety of using a fiber-containing formula in an ICU patient with more tenuous hemodynamic stability has also been questioned [73].

Immune-modulating components added to the enteral formulation support the metabolic and immunologic functions of the surgical ICU patient. Immune-modulating formulas (IMFs) contain various combinations of omega-3 fatty acids, glutamine, branched-chain amino acids, nucleotides, and arginine. In trauma, the formulas have been shown to be effective in the most severely injured patients with severe chest, intra-abdominal, and musculoskeletal injuries requiring intubation and resuscitation but are not necessary in the less severely injured patients [9,74]. There is evidence in surgical patients that preoperative feeding (at least 5 days) and continuation of these diets postoperatively reduce infectious complications [11,15,75,76]. A meta-analysis suggested that both perioperative and postoperative immune nutrition reduces secondary infections, wound complications, and hospital length of stay and should be initiated preoperatively if possible [77]. A more recent meta-analysis reviewed arginine-dominant IMF use in general surgery and found no benefit to these diets over standard enteral supplementation preoperatively. However, when given peri- and postoperatively, these formulas had a potential benefit to length of stay and reduction in infectious complications [78]. There is a possible increase in mortality when diets enriched in arginine are used during sepsis, but there is no consensus on this topic. Until further data are available to clarify this issue, caution should be taken in using these formulas in a septic patient.

MONITORING FOR TOLERANCE

The literature reports that approximately 60% of ICU patients have GI symptoms, and GI dysfunction is related to worsening outcomes in critically ill patients [50]. Aspiration, abdominal distention, intestinal intolerance, and diarrhea are the most common complications of enteral feeding. If residuals remain high, GI agents can be administered [79,80]. If gastroparesis persists, post-pyloric or even jejunal small bore tube placement may be a good option. Caution should be made in relying on gastric residuals as a sole source of enteral feeding intolerance. Most of the literature agrees that gastric residual volumes are a poor measure of gastric function and correlate poorly with aspiration pneumonia [81]. Based on this, many facilities have raised their gastric residual cutoff for holding feedings to 300–500 mL [82]. Attention should be paid to the patient's physical exam, keeping the HOB elevation to >30° and appropriate oral care of the patient to prevent aspiration pneumonia. It is also important to note that often in the ICU, patients are being fed in the intestine with suction or gravity of the stomach. If the patient is having high gastric residuals in this case, checking the placement of the post-pyloric feeding tube would be prudent to ensure that the tip had not slipped back into the stomach.

See Chapter 7 for further discussion.

NECESSITY AND POTENTIAL DETRIMENT WITH PARENTERAL FEEDING

There is substantial evidence that enteral delivery of nutrients improves immunologic defenses and clinical outcome, compared to parenteral feeding (TPN) [9,65,83,84]. However, contraindications to enteral feeding exist especially in the critically ill surgical patient population. Relative contraindications include increasing abdominal distention particularly when other symptoms such as severe discomfort, cramping, pain, and tachycardia are present. Absolute contraindications include intestinal obstruction, bowel ischemia, short gut, high-output fistulas with inadequate distal functional gut, GI bleeding with potential need for reoperation, and anastomotic leak or suspected one. Therefore, if a patient is truly unable to tolerate enteral feeding, how is it best to feed them? Clinicians are increasingly aware of infectious risk related to TPN use, and the pendulum has swung in the complete opposite direction from the 1980s when giving high doses of TPN were felt to be in the patient's best interest. Clinicians may risk exacerbation of malnutrition in order to avoid its use and its risk of infectious complications. ASPEN guidelines published in 2009 state that if a critically ill patient cannot be fed enterally, the clinician should wait 7 days prior to initiating TPN [68]. However, this recommendation had the weakest rating of evidence-based literature supporting it. There is more support for providing TPN earlier in severely malnourished patients. This recommendation is based on the VA study published in 1991, where marginally and mildly malnourished patients that were provided TPN before and after surgery developed increased infectious complications [14]. However, severely malnourished patients receiving TPN sustained a decrease in noninfectious complications, a decrease in overall major complications, and no increase in infectious complications compared to the control group [14].

In addition to the malnourished patient, is it advisable to delay feeding in critically ill surgical patients for 7 days creating a severe caloric deficit? A study of 4640 patients compared early TPN supplementation versus withholding TPN until day 8 [35]. The early TPN group was provided 20% dextrose (D20) infusion for the first 2 days, with full nutrition provided by day 3 (TPN plus enteral feeding). TPN was continued until enteral nutrition met 80% of estimated caloric needs. Delaying TPN resulted in fewer ICU infections, a risk reduction in mechanical ventilation, a reduced need for renal replacement therapy, and an increased likelihood of being discharged alive earlier from the ICU and the hospital [35]. The subgroup of postsurgery patients with contraindications for enteral feeding had fewer infections by delaying TPN until day 8. There were several criticisms to this study [36,85]. Perhaps the D20 given the first 2 days of hospitalization with no protein provision had a negative impact. In addition, the protein provision was low overall compared to current recommendations for the critically ill patient. Many took issue with the short ICU stay of the patients, since the majority had length of stays of only 3–4 days. Many clinicians would not consider a group with such low mortality risk to be candidates for such extreme nutritional intervention. Patients at nutritional risk were included, but severely malnourished patients were excluded from the study. Subsequent to the Caesar et al. study's publication, Heidegger et al. published a smaller, randomized study examining the same question: should we utilize TPN in the first week of ICU stay to provide goal caloric and protein needs? This study required patients to have an expected ICU stay of at least 5 days and was used only if enteral nutrition was providing ≤60% of goal needs [37]. This group reported an improvement in nosocomial infections by day 9. Other studies are underway to help answer the question of increasing caloric provision in the ICU by utilizing supplemental TPN.

SUMMARY

Nutrition support is an integral part of ICU care and essential to the recovery of the general surgery patient. It is important to identify patients at nutritional risk early to help decrease the risk of surgery and institute therapy prior to surgery. Since this is not always achievable, initiating enteral feeding <48 h from the time of surgery may improve the outcome of the surgical patient. Caloric goals should minimize an extensive caloric deficit early while avoiding overfeeding. Adequate protein provision is essential for healing and recovery, and the clinician should consider losses from wounds and drains. Gastric feeding can be safe and effective in this patient population with appropriate HOB elevation. A small bore feeding tube with a stylet should be placed by a team of trained and competent clinicians; use of a device for guidance may be helpful with obtaining safe and accurate placements. General surgery patients tolerate a standard, high-protein formula well, and certain situations may warrant the use of an immune-enhancing formula. Enteral feeding is recommended over parenteral nutrition, but continued underfeeding may warrant use of parenteral nutrition to avoid the severe detriments to continued nutritional deficit.

CASE STUDY

GW was a 76-year-old male with a past history of PUD, in which he had previously undergone an antrectomy and gastrojejunostomy. Since this time, he has developed gastric outlet obstruction and/or gastroparesis. Due to these issues, he further has developed esophagitis with a distal esophageal stricture, providing difficulty to even pass a scope through for preoperative evaluation. This patient has been on jejunal tube feedings at home, which has been his primary source of nutrition.

GW went to the OR for a planned subtotal gastrectomy, but due to an esophageal leak identified intraoperatively (from dilation for insertion of a scope), he ended up undergoing a total gastrectomy with esophageal–jejunal anastomosis, with a roux-en-Y reconstruction. A drain was placed in the area of the anastomosis. During the OR case, there was bleeding from the spleen requiring splenectomy. Approximately 25–30 cm distal to the anastomosis, a jejunal feeding tube was placed and brought through the previous J-tube site. Blood loss was approximately 1 L and, although the patient remained hemodynamically stable throughout the case, was transported to SICU post-op for observation.

Post-op day (POD) 1, the patient was successfully extubated. A semi-concentrated (1.5 cal/mL) standard formula was initiated for the patient at a trophic rate of 20 mL/h.

ANTHROPOMETRICS

Ht, 5′11; Wt, 66 kg; IBW, 78.2 kg; UBW, 84.1 kg (1-year ago); BMI, 20.36.

GW was assumed to be at least moderately malnourished, as he was receiving enteral feeding at home and had reports of weight maintenance, but no weight regain.

GW was stable, and the ICU team was planning to transfer to the floor in the next couple of days. Our nutrition goal was for weight gain and adequate protein for healing; we assessed him as needing approximately 25–30 kcal/kg and 1.5 g protein/kg.

By POD 3, GW was receiving goal enteral feeding. He was transferred to the floor. He was newly confused and felt this was due to ICU delirium. GW had not started stooling yet, but his abdomen was soft and non-distended, and he was tolerating enteral feedings.

On POD 5, GW decompensated on the floor experiencing tachycardia, tachypnea, and confusion. GW had an episode of bilious emesis, and his abdomen was noted to be markedly distended. GW underwent a bronchoscopy, which suctioned out bile. He was also noted to have bile in his intra-abdominal drain.

The patient emergently returned to the OR. Once the fascia was reopened, large amounts of green fluid poured out of his abdomen (after suction complete, about 2 quarts in total). Two areas of leaking were noted: one at the jejunostomy tube site and the other at the esophageal anastomosis. The bowel proximal to the jejunostomy tube was markedly dilated, and it was felt the transition point was where the small bowel passed through the transverse colon mesentery; sutures here were cut to help relieve any obstruction. The jejunostomy tube was then removed, and this area sutured closed. About 2 cm lower, a new jejunostomy tube was placed. The second site was a leak at the esophagojejunal anastomosis, which was repaired by sutures.

Postoperatively, he returned to the SICU intubated.

On POD 7, custom TPN was initiated proving approximately 25 kcal/kg and 1.8 g protein/kg. GW was requiring multiple vasopressors for hemodynamic support at this time. GW continued to remain intubated in the SICU for several more days; his vasopressors were eventually weaned off.

On POD 12, trophic feedings were initiated. Over the next day, GW's enteral feedings were advancing to goal, stools were passed, and TPN was discontinued. Stools noted to be melanotic, but hemoglobin/hematocrit had remained stable. Pleural effusion noted on a chest radiograph, and a chest tube was placed, which immediately drained 1 L. His enteral feeds were providing 26 kcal/kg and 1.5 g protein/kg.

Later on this day, leakage was noted around the feeding tube. Tube feedings were held, and a tube study in fluoroscopy was done showing no leak so tube feedings were resumed.

Two days later, GW was extubated and doing well. The patient was changed to a standard high-protein formula as he was tolerating feeds well and had no needed volume restriction and the goal rate provided 27 kcal/kg and 1.8 g protein/kg.

At this time, the patient was transferred to the floor. However, 3 days later, the patient again became tachycardic, had an increased white blood cell count and was febrile, and confused. There was concern of bile coming from his midline wound. The wound care team placed a wound manager on his abdominal wound to collect and quantify the drainage. Enteral feeds had been started and stopped for a few days, and were now held due to concern for anastomotic leak versus fistula. TPN was restarted on POD 20. The patient then underwent a J-tube study in fluoroscopy and a small bowel follow-through. The follow-through was somewhat inconclusive due to contrast in the colon. No leak was appreciated. Over the next week, enteral feedings were still held, and TPN continued. Wound output decreased to almost nothing. Enteral feeds were restarted, and methylene blue was given via the J-tube on POD 29 and 30, which showed no leak. However, on POD 32, green drainage was noted around the J-tube site. Again TF were held, and TPN restarted. Trophic feeds were restarted on POD 35 and very slowly advanced to goal over the next few days, at which time TPN was discontinued. GW tolerated goal enteral rate well. With mental status improvement, he was advanced to a dysphagia diet.

On POD 39, the patient started a nocturnal enteral feeding regimen. GW was eating, but intake was inadequate to meet demands. Nocturnal enteral feeds met 100% of nutritional and fluid needs. The patient was discharged to a skilled nursing facility a few days later.

REFERENCES

1. Becher RD, Hoth JJ, Miller PR, Mowery NT, Chang MC, Meredith JW. A critical assessment of outcomes in emergency versus nonemergency general surgery using the American College of Surgeons National Surgical Quality Improvement Program database. *Am Surg*. 2011 July;77(7):951–959.
2. Becher RD, Hoth JJ, Miller PR, Meredith JW, Chang MC. Systemic inflammation worsens outcomes in emergency surgical patients. *J Trauma Acute Care Surg*. 2012 May;72(5):1140–1149.
3. Schiesser M, Müller S, Kirchhoff P, Breitenstein S, Schäfer M, Clavien P-A. Assessment of a novel screening score for nutritional risk in predicting complications in gastro-intestinal surgery. *Clin Nutr Edinb Scotl*. 2008 August;27(4):565–570.
4. Aoun JP, Baroudi J, Geahchan N. Prevalence of malnutrition in general surgical patients. *J Médical Liban Leban Med J*. 1993;41(2):57–61.
5. Howard L, Ashley C. Nutrition in the perioperative patient. *Annu Rev Nutr*. 2003;23(1):263–282.
6. Schwegler I, von Holzen A, Gutzwiller J-P, Schlumpf R, Mühlebach S, Stanga Z. Nutritional risk is a clinical predictor of postoperative mortality and morbidity in surgery for colorectal cancer. *Br J Surg*. 2009 December 10;97(1):92–97.
7. Andersen HK, Lewis SJ, Thomas S. Early enteral nutrition within 24h of colorectal surgery versus later commencement of feeding for postoperative complications. *Cochrane Database Syst Rev Online*. 2006;(4):CD004080.
8. Curtis CS, Kudsk KA. Enteral feedings in hospitalized patients: Early versus delayed enteral nutrition. *Pr Gastroenterol*. 2009 October;33:22–30.
9. Kudsk KA, Croce MA, Fabian TC, Minard G, Tolley EA, Poret HA et al. Enteral versus parenteral feeding. Effects on septic morbidity after blunt and penetrating abdominal trauma. *Ann Surg*. 1992 May;215(5):503–511; discussion 511–513.
10. Studley HO. Percentage of weight loss: A basic indicator of surgical risk in patients with chronic peptic ulcer. 1936. *Nutr Hosp Organo Of Soc Española Nutr Parenter Enter*. 2001 August;16(4):141–143; discussion 140–141.
11. Giger U, Büchler M, Farhadi J, Berger D, Hüsler J, Schneider H et al. Preoperative immunonutrition suppresses perioperative inflammatory response in patients with major abdominal surgery-a randomized controlled pilot study. *Ann Surg Oncol*. 2007 October;14(10):2798–2806.
12. Windsor JA. Underweight patients and the risks of major surgery. *World J Surg*. 1993 April;17(2):165–172.
13. White JV, Guenter P, Jensen G, Malone A, Schofield M, Academy Malnutrition Work Group et al. Consensus statement: Academy of Nutrition and Dietetics and American Society for Parenteral and Enteral Nutrition: Characteristics recommended for the identification and documentation of adult malnutrition (undernutrition). *J Parenter Enter Nutr*. 2012 April 24;36(3):275–283.
14. Perioperative total parenteral nutrition in surgical patients. The Veterans Affairs Total Parenteral Nutrition Cooperative Study Group. *N Engl J Med*. 1991 August 22;325(8):525–532.
15. Braga M, Gianotti L, Nespoli L, Radaelli G, Di Carlo V. Nutritional approach in malnourished surgical patients: A prospective randomized study. *Arch Surg Chic Ill 1960*. 2002 February;137(2):174–180.
16. Bozzetti F, Gianotti L, Braga M, Di Carlo V, Mariani L. Postoperative complications in gastrointestinal cancer patients: The joint role of the nutritional status and the nutritional support. *Clin Nutr*. 2007 December;26(6):698–709.
17. Klein S, Kinney J, Jeejeebhoy K, Alpers D, Hellerstein M, Murray M et al. Nutrition support in clinical practice: Review of published data and recommendations for future research directions. National Institutes of Health, American Society for Parenteral and Enteral Nutrition, and American Society for Clinical Nutrition. *JPEN J Parenter Enteral Nutr*. 1997 June;21(3):133–156.
18. Davis CJ, Sowa D, Keim KS, Kinnare K, Peterson S. The use of prealbumin and C-reactive protein for monitoring nutrition support in adult patients receiving enteral nutrition in an urban medical center. *J Parenter Enter Nutr*. 2012 March 1;36(2):197–204.

19. Jeejeebhoy KN, Detsky AS, Baker JP. Assessment of nutritional status. *JPEN J Parenter Enteral Nutr.* 1990 October;14(5 Suppl):193S–196S.
20. Kondrup J, Rasmussen HH, Hamberg O, Stanga Z. Nutritional risk screening (NRS 2002): A new method based on an analysis of controlled clinical trials. *Clin Nutr.* 2003 June;22(3):321–336.
21. McClave SA, Snider HL. Understanding the metabolic response to critical illness: Factors that cause patients to deviate from the expected pattern of hypermetabolism. *New Horizons Baltim Md.* 1994 May;2(2):139–146.
22. Hart DW, Wolf SE, Herndon DN, Chinkes DL, Lal SO, Obeng MK et al. Energy expenditure and caloric balance after burn. *Ann Surg.* 2002 January;235(1):152–161.
23. Villet S, Chiolero RL, Bollmann MD, Revelly J-P, Cayeux RNM-C, Delarue J et al. Negative impact of hypocaloric feeding and energy balance on clinical outcome in ICU patients. *Clin Nutr Edinb Scotl.* 2005 August;24(4):502–509.
24. Greenberg GR, Jeejeebhoy KN. Intravenous protein-sparing therapy in patients with gastrointestinal disease. *J Parenter Enter Nutr.* 1979 November 1;3(6):427–432.
25. Jeejeebhoy KN. Permissive underfeeding of the critically ill patient. *Nutr Clin Pr Off Publ Am Soc Parenter Enter Nutr.* 2004 October;19(5):477–480.
26. Powell NJ, Collier B. Nutrition and the open abdomen. *Nutr Clin Pract.* 2012 August 1;27(4):499–506.
27. López Hellín J, Baena-Fustegueras JA, Sabín-Urkía P, Schwartz-Riera S, García-Arumí E. Nutritional modulation of protein metabolism after gastrointestinal surgery. *Eur J Clin Nutr.* 2008 February;62(2):254–262.
28. Dickerson RN, Pitts SL, Maish GO, Schroeppel TJ, Magnotti LJ, Croce MA et al. A reappraisal of nitrogen requirements for patients with critical illness and trauma. *J Trauma Acute Care Surg.* 2012 September;73(3):549–557.
29. Singer P, Anbar R, Cohen J, Shapiro H, Shalita-Chesner M, Lev S et al. The tight calorie control study (TICACOS): A prospective, randomized, controlled pilot study of nutritional support in critically ill patients. *Intensive Care Med.* 2011 April;37(4):601–609.
30. Davis KA, Kinn T, Esposito TJ, Reed RL 2nd, Santaniello JM, Luchette FA. Nutritional gain versus financial gain: The role of metabolic carts in the surgical ICU. *J Trauma.* 2006 December; 61(6):1436–1440.
31. Frankenfield DC, Coleman A, Alam S, Cooney RN. Analysis of estimation methods for resting metabolic rate in critically ill adults. *JPEN J Parenter Enteral Nutr.* 2009 February;33(1):27–36.
32. Heyland DK, Dhaliwal R, Drover JW, Gramlich L, Dodek P. Canadian clinical practice guidelines for nutrition support in mechanically ventilated, critically ill adult patients. *JPEN J Parenter Enteral Nutr.* 2003 October;27(5):355–373.
33. De Jonghe B, Appere-De-Vechi C, Fournier M, Tran B, Merrer J, Melchior JC et al. A prospective survey of nutritional support practices in intensive care unit patients: What is prescribed? What is delivered? *Crit Care Med.* 2001 January;29(1):8–12.
34. Rice TW, Wheeler AP, Thompson BT, Steingrub J, Hite RD, Moss M et al. Initial trophic vs full enteral feeding in patients with acute lung injury: The EDEN randomized trial. *J Am Med Assoc.* 2012 February 22;307(8):795–803.
35. Casaer MP, Mesotten D, Hermans G, Wouters PJ, Schetz M, Meyfroidt G et al. Early versus late parenteral nutrition in critically ill adults. *N Engl J Med.* 2011 August 11;365(6):506–517.
36. McClave SA, Heyland DK, Martindale RG. Adding supplemental parenteral nutrition to hypocaloric enteral nutrition: Lessons learned from the Casaer Van den Berghe study. *JPEN J Parenter Enteral Nutr.* 2012 January;36(1):15–17.
37. Heidegger CP, Berger MM, Graf S, Zingg W, Darmon P, Costanza MC et al. Optimisation of energy provision with supplemental parenteral nutrition in critically ill patients: A randomised controlled clinical trial. *Lancet.* 2013 February 2;381(9864):385–393.
38. Alberda C, Gramlich L, Jones N, Jeejeebhoy K, Day AG, Dhaliwal R et al. The relationship between nutritional intake and clinical outcomes in critically ill patients: Results of an international multicenter observational study. *Intensive Care Med.* 2009 October;35(10):1728–1737.
39. Weijs PJM, Stapel SN, de Groot SDW, Driessen RH, de Jong E, Girbes ARJ et al. Optimal protein and energy nutrition decreases mortality in mechanically ventilated, critically ill patients: A prospective observational cohort study. *JPEN J Parenter Enteral Nutr.* 2012 January;36(1):60–68.
40. Jensen GL, Hsiao PY, Wheeler D. Nutrition screening and assessment. In *A.S.P.E.N. Nutrition Support Core Curriculum*, 2nd edn. Mueller, CM (ed.). American Society of Parenteral and Enteral Nutrition, Silver Spring, MD; 2012, pp. 155–170.

41. Cheatham ML, Safcsak K, Brzezinski SJ, Lube MW. Nitrogen balance, protein loss, and the open abdomen. *Crit Care Med.* 2007 January;35(1):127–131.
42. Wade C, Wolf SE, Salinas R, Jones JA, Rivera R, Hourigan L et al. Loss of protein, immunoglobulins, and electrolytes in exudates from negative pressure wound therapy. *Nutr Clin Pract.* 2010 October 20;25(5):510–516.
43. Wooley JA, Btaiche IF, Good KL. Metabolic and nutritional aspects of acute renal failure in critically ill patients requiring continuous renal replacement therapy. *Nutr Clin Pr Off Publ Am Soc Parenter Enter Nutr.* 2005 April;20(2):176–191.
44. Singer P. High-dose amino acid infusion preserves diuresis and improves nitrogen balance in non-oliguric acute renal failure. *Wien Klin Wochenschr.* 2007;119(7–8):218–222.
45. Krenitsky J, Rosner MH. Nutritional support for patients with acute kidney injury: How much protein is enough or too much? *Pr Gastroenterol.* 2011 June;35:28–42.
46. Wolfe RR, Allsop JR, Burke JF. Glucose metabolism in man: Responses to intravenous glucose infusion. *Metabolism.* 1979 March;28(3):210–220.
47. Van den Berghe G, Wouters P, Weekers F, Verwaest C, Bruyninckx F, Schetz M et al. Intensive insulin therapy in critically ill patients. *N Engl J Med.* 2001 November 8;345(19):1359–1367.
48. Finfer S, Chittock DR, Su SY-S, Blair D, Foster D, Dhingra V et al. Intensive versus conventional glucose control in critically ill patients. *N Engl J Med.* 2009 March 26;360(13):1283–1297.
49. Vanek VW, Seidner DL, Allen P, Bistrian B, Collier S, Gura K et al. A.S.P.E.N. Position paper clinical role for alternative intravenous fat emulsions. *Nutr Clin Pract.* 2012 April 1;27(2):150–192.
50. Reintam Blaser A, Malbrain MLNG, Starkopf J, Fruhwald S, Jakob SM, De Waele J et al. Gastrointestinal function in intensive care patients: Terminology, definitions and management. Recommendations of the ESICM Working Group on Abdominal Problems. *Intensive Care Med.* 2012 March;38(3):384–394.
51. Doig GS, Heighes PT, Simpson F, Sweetman EA, Davies AR. Early enteral nutrition, provided within 24 h of injury or intensive care unit admission, significantly reduces mortality in critically ill patients: A meta-analysis of randomised controlled trials. *Intensive Care Med.* 2009 December;35(12):2018–2027.
52. Willcutts K. Pre-op NPO and traditional post-op diet advancement: Time to move on. *Pr Gastroenterol.* 2010 December;34:16–27.
53. Lassen K, Soop M, Nygren J, Cox PBW, Hendry PO, Spies C et al. Consensus review of optimal perioperative care in colorectal surgery: Enhanced Recovery After Surgery (ERAS) Group recommendations. *Arch Surg Chic Ill 1960.* 2009 October;144(10):961–969.
54. Lassen K, Coolsen MME, Slim K, Carli F, de Aguilar-Nascimento JE, Schäfer M et al. Guidelines for perioperative care for pancreaticoduodenectomy: Enhanced Recovery After Surgery (ERAS(®)) Society recommendations. *World J Surg.* 2013 Feb;37(2):240–258, [cited September 11, 2012]; Available from: http://www.ncbi.nlm.nih.gov/pubmed/22956014.
55. Neumann DA, DeLegge MH. Gastric versus small-bowel tube feeding in the intensive care unit: A prospective comparison of efficacy. *Crit Care Med.* 2002 July;30(7):1436–1438.
56. White H, Sosnowski K, Tran K, Reeves A, Jones M. A randomised controlled comparison of early post-pyloric versus early gastric feeding to meet nutritional targets in ventilated intensive care patients. *Crit Care.* 2009;13(6):R187.
57. Davies AR, Morrison SS, Bailey MJ, Bellomo R, Cooper DJ, Doig GS et al. A multicenter, randomized controlled trial comparing early nasojejunal with nasogastric nutrition in critical illness. *Crit Care Med.* 2012 August;40(8):2342–2348.
58. Metheny NA, Stewart BJ, McClave SA. Relationship between feeding tube site and respiratory outcomes. *JPEN J Parenter Enteral Nutr.* 2011 May;35(3):346–355.
59. De Aguilar-Nascimento JE, Kudsk KA. Clinical costs of feeding tube placement. *JPEN J Parenter Enteral Nutr.* 2007 August;31(4):269–273.
60. Marderstein EL, Simmons RL, Ochoa JB. Patient safety: Effect of institutional protocols on adverse events related to feeding tube placement in the critically ill. *J Am Coll Surg.* 2004 July;199(1):39–47; discussion 47–50.
61. Koopmann MC, Kudsk KA, Szotkowski MJ, Rees SM. A team-based protocol and electromagnetic technology eliminate feeding tube placement complications. *Ann Surg.* 2011 February;253(2):287–302.
62. Holte K, Kehlet H. Postoperative ileus: A preventable event. *Br J Surg.* 2000;87(11):1480–1493.
63. Lassen K, Kjaeve J, Fetveit T, Tranø G, Sigurdsson HK, Horn A et al. Allowing normal food at will after major upper gastrointestinal surgery does not increase morbidity: A randomized multicenter trial. *Ann Surg.* 2008 May;247(5):721–729.
64. Warren J, Bhalla V, Cresci G. Postoperative diet advancement: Surgical dogma vs evidence-based medicine. *Nutr Clin Pract.* 2011 March 29;26(2):115–125.

65. Moore FA, Feliciano DV, Andrassy RJ, McArdle AH, Booth FV, Morgenstein-Wagner TB et al. Early enteral feeding, compared with parenteral, reduces postoperative septic complications. The results of a meta-analysis. *Ann Surg*. 1992 August;216(2):172–183.
66. Lewis SJ, Andersen HK, Thomas S. Early enteral nutrition within 24 h of intestinal surgery versus later commencement of feeding: A systematic review and meta-analysis. *J Gastrointest Surg Off J Soc Surg Aliment Tract*. 2009 March;13(3):569–575.
67. Weimann A, Braga M, Harsanyi L, Laviano A, Ljungqvist O, Soeters P et al. ESPEN guidelines on enteral nutrition: Surgery including organ transplantation. *Clin Nutr Edinb Scotl*. 2006 April;25(2):224–244.
68. McClave SA, Martindale RG, Vanek VW, McCarthy M, Roberts P, Taylor B et al. Guidelines for the provision and assessment of nutrition support therapy in the adult critically ill patient: Society of Critical Care Medicine (SCCM) and American Society for Parenteral and Enteral Nutrition (A.S.P.E.N.). *J Parenter Enter Nutr*. 2009 April 27;33(3):277–316.
69. Kleessen B, Hartmann L, Blaut M. Fructans in the diet cause alterations of intestinal mucosal architecture, released mucins and mucosa-associated bifidobacteria in gnotobiotic rats. *Br J Nutr*. 2003 May;89(5):597–606.
70. Spapen H, Diltoer M, Van Malderen C, Opdenacker G, Suys E, Huyghens L. Soluble fiber reduces the incidence of diarrhea in septic patients receiving total enteral nutrition: A prospective, double-blind, randomized, and controlled trial. *Clin Nutr Edinb Scotl*. 2001 August;20(4):301–305.
71. Barrett JS, Shepherd SJ, Gibson PR. Strategies to manage gastrointestinal symptoms complicating enteral feeding. *JPEN J Parenter Enteral Nutr*. 2009 February;33(1):21–26.
72. Halmos EP, Muir JG, Barrett JS, Deng M, Shepherd SJ, Gibson PR. Diarrhoea during enteral nutrition is predicted by the poorly absorbed short-chain carbohydrate (FODMAP) content of the formula. *Aliment Pharmacol Ther*. 2010 October;32(7):925–933.
73. Scaife CL, Saffle JR, Morris SE. Intestinal obstruction secondary to enteral feedings in burn trauma patients. *J Trauma*. 1999 November;47(5):859–863.
74. Moore EE, Jones TN. Benefits of immediate jejunostomy feeding after major abdominal trauma—A prospective, randomized study. *J Trauma*. 1986 October;26(10):874–881.
75. Klek S, Sierzega M, Szybinski P, Szczepanek K, Scislo L, Walewska E et al. The immunomodulating enteral nutrition in malnourished surgical patients—A prospective, randomized, double-blind clinical trial. *Clin Nutr Edinb Scotl*. 2011 June;30(3):282–288.
76. Di Carlo V, Gianotti L, Balzano G, Zerbi A, Braga M. Complications of pancreatic surgery and the role of perioperative nutrition. *Dig Surg*. 1999;16(4):320–326.
77. Marik PE, Zaloga GP. Immunonutrition in high-risk surgical patients: A systematic review and analysis of the literature. *JPEN J Parenter Enteral Nutr*. 2010 August;34(4):378–386.
78. Osland E, Hossain MB, Khan S, Memon MA. Effect of timing of pharmaconutrition (immunonutrition) administration on outcomes of elective surgery for gastrointestinal malignancies: A systematic review and meta-analysis. *JPEN*. 2014 January;38(1):53–69.
79. Dive A, Miesse C, Galanti L, Jamart J, Evrard P, Gonzalez M et al. Effect of erythromycin on gastric motility in mechanically ventilated critically ill patients: A double-blind, randomized, placebo-controlled study. *Crit Care Med*. 1995 August;23(8):1356–1362.
80. MacLaren R, Kuhl DA, Gervasio JM, Brown RO, Dickerson RN, Livingston TN et al. Sequential single doses of cisapride, erythromycin, and metoclopramide in critically ill patients intolerant to enteral nutrition: A randomized, placebo-controlled, crossover study. *Crit Care Med*. 2000 February;28(2):438–444.
81. Parrish C, McClave S. Checking gastric residual volumes: A practice in search of science? *Pr Gastroenterol*. 2008 October;32:33–47.
82. McClave SA, Snider HL. Clinical use of gastric residual volumes as a monitor for patients on enteral tube feeding. *JPEN J Parenter Enteral Nutr*. 2002 December;26(6 Suppl):S43–S48; discussion S49–S50.
83. Moore FA, Moore EE, Jones TN, McCroskey BL, Peterson VM. TEN versus TPN following major abdominal trauma—Reduced septic morbidity. *J Trauma*. 1989 July;29(7):916–922; discussion 922–923.
84. Kudsk KA, Minard G, Croce MA, Brown RO, Lowrey TS, Pritchard FE et al. A randomized trial of isonitrogenous enteral diets after severe trauma. An immune-enhancing diet reduces septic complications. *Ann Surg*. 1996 October;224(4):531–5540; discussion 540–543.
85. Berger MM, Pichard C. Best timing for energy provision during critical illness. *Crit Care*. 2012 March 20;16(2):215.

34 Nutritional Support during Systemic Inflammatory Response Syndrome and Sepsis

Mark H. Oltermann and Mary E. Leicht

CONTENTS

INTRODUCTION

The nutritional care of intensive care unit (ICU) patients that have systemic inflammatory response syndrome (SIRS) or are septic can be very challenging. Whether patients respond differently with nutritional manipulation depending on the disease state of sepsis versus SIRS is a matter of debate. For this chapter, the response of sepsis and SIRS will be considered similar, with differences noted where literature supports. Although some societies have given Grade A recommendations

TABLE 34.1
Grading of Recommendations Should be A Through E and not B Through F

Grading of recommendations

B. Supported by at least two level I studies
C. Supported by at least one level I study
D. Supported by level II investigations
E. Supported by level III investigations
F. Level IV or V evidence only

Grading of evidence

I. Large, prospective, randomized trials with little risk of false-positive or false-negative error
II. Small randomized trials with higher risks of false positives or false negatives
III. Nonrandomized trials with contemporaneous controls
IV. Nonrandomized trials with historical controls
V. Case series or expert opinion

for feeding ICU patients, not all societies agree on the subset of septic or SIRS patients. The more traditional grading system used by the Society of Critical Care Medicine (SCCM) and the American Society of Parenteral and Enteral Nutrition (ASPEN) (see Table 34.1, adapted from Ref. [1]) requires 2 level I studies for a Grade A recommendation. The Canadian Clinical Practice Guidelines (http://www.criticalcarenutrition.com/) use terms such as *strongly recommend, recommend, should be considered*, and *insufficient data* as opposed to letter grades based on the same definitions for level of evidence. Most recently, the Surviving Sepsis Campaign (SSC) Guidelines committee has come out with their 2012 international guidelines for the management of severe sepsis and septic shock [2]. The 2012 guidelines also have specific recommendations for nutritional manipulation in septic patients. These authors follow the principles of GRADE (Grading of Recommendations, Assessment, Development and Evaluation) system. These grades go from A to D (with no E) with similar definitions to the traditional method. The difference is also to offer a *strength of recommendation* as either strong (designated by the number 1) or weak (designated by number 2). A strong adjunct implies *we recommend* (the benefits of adherence will clearly outweigh the undesirable effects), and a weak adjunct implies *we suggest* (the benefits probably outweigh the risks).

There has been debate in the past whether ICU patients should be fed at all [3,4], but that is less emphasized today for ICU patients sick enough to still be there for more than 2–3 days. One of the reasons that there is still controversy is that nutrition studies (large enough to meet criteria for level 1) are difficult to produce and costly. Plus, enteral formulas are relatively inexpensive compared to pharmaceutical agents, so commercial companies are less likely to support large expensive trials because there is little profit to be made. Finally, many feel that to do a true placebo-controlled trial (bring a tray into the room to those randomized to placebo, regardless whether they can even attempt to eat) would be unethical.

But the stakes are high, especially for sepsis. There are three areas that make sepsis particularly important. First, it is estimated that there are more than 1,000,000 cases per year of sepsis in this decade, up from the much quoted number of 750,000 per year in 2001 [5]. The exact numbers are often debated because they usually come from retrospective chart codes, but most believe the numbers are increasing. However, projected sepsis numbers for the future may be woefully misjudged. The risk of sepsis increases with age and takes off exponentially after age 65 [6]. The *baby boomers* (born from 1946 to 1964) just started retiring in 2011. This means we may have a much higher rate of sepsis than we are prepared for. Second, mortality rates for sepsis remain high, often over 20%, although some facilities have had improved success following the SSC *bundles* [7]. Third, caring for septic patients is very costly due to extended ICU and hospital stays.

The purpose of this chapter will be to review the recommendations and the data for septic and SIRS patients, realizing that there is some overlap, and try to come to some conclusions on how to manage the nutrition support therapy in these complex patients.

DEFINITIONS

Nutritional manipulation will be defined as forced feeding of an enteral product via a feeding tube, parenteral nutrition, or a combination thereof. It will not include oral supplements or *special diets* that are expected to be taken spontaneously by mouth. However, it is of note that some of the cleanest data for the use of *immune modulating formulas* is in patients given preoperative supplementation for at least 7 days prior to major elective surgery-typically by mouth [8,9]. Nonetheless, the emphasis of this chapter will be on nutritional manipulation as defined earlier.

The SIRS is the host's nonspecific cascade of inflammatory events that occur in response to some type of insult (infection, trauma, burns, pancreatitis, and major surgery). For literature purposes, SIRS is defined by at least two of the following manifestations:

1. Temperature >38°C or <36°C
2. Heart rate >90 beats/min
3. Respiratory rate >20 breaths/min, or a $PaCO_2$ <32 mmHg
4. WBC count >12,000 cells/mm^3, <4000 cells/mm^3, or >10% immature forms

These criteria are very nonspecific. An athlete just finishing a race would meet SIRS criteria (heart rate and respiratory rate). To be more specific, the insult should be the initiator of the manifestations. It is important to note, however, that the manifestations themselves are felt to be caused by the host response to the insult via hormones, cytokines, and inflammatory cells. Sepsis is defined as SIRS that is due to infection (the invasion of normally sterile tissues by microorganisms and/or their products). Severe sepsis is defined as sepsis with at least one SIRS-induced organ dysfunction. Septic shock is severe sepsis that requires medical support of blood pressure in spite of the patient receiving *adequate* volume resuscitation (societies still debate how much fluid is adequate). If more than one organ is dysfunctional or failing, the terms multiple organ dysfunction syndrome (MODS) and multiple organ failure syndrome (MOFS) are used, respectively. MOFS is the leading cause of death in noncoronary ICUs today. The definition of dysfunctional organs has varied from author to author [10–12] in the past, but can generally be summarized as in Table 34.2, and these definitions are consistent with the 2012 SSC Guidelines.

TABLE 34.2
Organ Failure Definitions

1. Respiratory: acute lung injury (ALI) or adult respiratory distress syndrome (ARDS). ALI requires bilateral lung infiltrates, no evidence of heart failure, and PaO_2/FIO_2 ratio of less than 300 mmHg. ARDS is just more severe, with a PaO_2/FIO_2 ratio of less than 250 mmHg.
2. Renal: oliguria in spite of *adequate* volume replacement or an acute rise in serum creatinine.
3. Central nervous system: altered mental status or a Glasgow coma score of <15.
4. Hepatic: jaundice or an acute rise in liver enzymes.
5. Cardiovascular: hypotension in spite of *adequate* fluids or evidence of an acute dilated cardiomyopathy.
6. Gastrointestinal: stress ulcer bleeding.
7. Hematologic: low platelet count, or an increase in protime (PT), partial thromboplastin time (PTT), or an increase in D-dimer levels not explained by other diseases.
8. Systemic: lactic acid levels greater than two times normal.

The complexity of the sepsis patient is compounded by the fact that it not only is an aggressive inflammatory state but is an immunosuppressive one as well. Bone in 1996 [13] first described what he called the compensatory anti-inflammatory response syndrome (CARS), which today is used to describe dysfunctions in immunity characterized by macrophage paralysis, suppressed T-cell proliferation, and increased lymphocyte apoptosis, among others [14]. It was first believed that SIRS and CARS occurred sequentially, but it is now known that these two responses actually occur simultaneously for prolonged periods [15,16]. Despite improvements in the management of SIRS, which have decreased the incidences of late MOFS, we are now presented with what has recently been proposed by Gentile et al. [14] as the persistent inflammation–immunosuppression catabolism syndrome (PICS). PICS carries many nutritional implications characterized by continued protein catabolism resulting in loss of lean body mass, poor nutritional status, impaired wound healing, and recurrent infections that often lead to readmissions to the ICU. This presents the potential for nutrition to play a pivotal role in the recovery and management of these patients.

As noted earlier, sepsis is only one cause of SIRS (although usually the most common). It is the SIRS itself that appears to cause the organ dysfunction, not the infection per se. Matzinger in 2002 [17] described the occurrence of SIRS in the absence of microbial infection exaggerating the inflammatory response through the same mechanisms and produce similar SIRS–CARS response [18,19]. Hence, the question remains: Does the nutritional manipulation of the septic patient need to be different from the non-septic SIRS patient? Also, in the last few years, there have been much data specifically on the nutritional manipulation of the ARDS patient (sepsis generally being the most common cause of ARDS). Is the lung injury truly different than the other tissues, or does it just come to our attention much quicker? Patients may not seem too bad when not making urine for a day, but shortness of breath and hypoxemia almost always require more immediate action. Future studies should focus on sepsis regardless of which organ is failing.

NONNUTRITIONAL CARE OF THE SEPTIC AND/OR SIRS PATIENT

Before reviewing the nutritional literature, it is imperative to review the care of septic or SIRS patient in general. If there are multiple other *drivers* of mortality in ICU patients, then nonnutritional care must be standardized as much as possible while performing nutrition-focused studies in order to see the true treatment effect of nutrition. Optimal nutrition may not be able to overcome the deleterious effect of poor care in these other areas. Some of the older nutrition literature predates other ICU studies that have shown major effects on mortality with specific nonnutritional interventions. Yet these trials continue to be included in meta-analyses. And since nutrition studies are often smaller in patient numbers, there is not an opportunity for the variation in these other areas to equalize out over time in the *treatment* arm versus the *control* arm. This is in contradistinction to the cardiology literature that succeeds for two major reasons: one is that they often have large numbers enrolled (often over 10,000 patients), and second, they usually do a very good job of standardizing all the other evidenced-based care between the two groups being studied. Since nutritional studies tend to have small numbers and poor standardization, these studies' outcomes could easily be influenced by noncompliance in areas of care that have clearly been shown to independently improve survival. The following eight topics are important to optimize if nutrition is to have an opportunity in studies to show a change in outcomes.

RESUSCITATION

The first steps in the management of a septic/SIRS patient are the same as in all critically ill patients: airway, respiration, and organ perfusion. But the septic patient has been subjected to studies using a specific resuscitation strategy called early goal-directed therapy (EGDT) first put forth by Rivers et al. [20] in 2001. This original article randomized septic shock patients (defined as still hypotensive after fluid bolus or sepsis-induced lactate levels greater than 4 mmol/L) to *standard care* or EGDT for the first 6 h of emergency department (ED) care. This EGDT protocol not only included arterial lines and central lines for central venous pressure (CVP) monitoring (which was also part of the *standard* arm), but also added a specific central venous oxygen saturation ($ScvO_2$) goal of greater than 70% as a primary endpoint. To reach this primary endpoint, the EGDT arm patients ended up with more fluid, more inotropic support (dobutamine), and more red blood cell transfusions. The ICU physicians ultimately caring for the patient after leaving the ED were often unaware of the patient assignment, so in some ways, this trial was even *blinded.* Mortality was reduced with EGDT from 46.5% to 30.5% for controls. This 16% *absolute* reduction in mortality equates to a number needed to treat (NNT) of only seven (for every seven patients treated with this therapy, one additional life can be expected to be saved compared with the standard therapy). Subsequently, many institutions have adopted EGDT and have shown success compared to their previous mortality rates. This prompted the SSC to propose guidelines [21] and to sponsor a study educating hospitals and following the success of a *6 h bundle* (essentially the components of EGDT) and a *24 h bundle* on mortality rates [7]. This study documented an approximate 6% absolute reduction in mortality over 2 years when bundle compliance improved over the same time frame. The 2012 SSC Guidelines have dropped the *24 h bundle* and have added a *3 h bundle* for all sepsis patients. They have kept the *6 h bundle*, and the resuscitation endpoints are essentially the same as the EGDT of the Rivers trial.

Subsequent to the 2012 guidelines, an article was published that questions the value of EGDT for septic patients. The Protocolized Care for Early Septic Shock (ProCESS) trial published in 2014 [22] randomized *septic shock* patients (hypotensive after fluid- or sepsis-induced lactate levels >4) to one of three arms: classic EGDT typical of Rivers, a different resuscitation protocol that does not require a central line, or *physician discretion.* There was no statistically significant difference in mortality rates between the three groups (all around 20%). This has prompted a lot of discussion and may delay the SSC 2012 guidelines from becoming *mandates.* An important difference in these patients when reviewing the article is that to get into the trial, hypotensive patients had to *fail* only 1 L of fluid to be included. The standard today is failure of a 30 cc/kg crystalloid fluid bolus before declaring the patient an *EGDT candidate.* The implication is that the ProCESS patients may not be as critically ill as the original Rivers patients. Another notable finding in this article was that approximately 60% of the patients in the two arms that were not classic EGDT ultimately required central lines anyway. So it would seem that a *central line avoidance* strategy of resuscitation most of the time won't work anyway. And finally, the primary endpoint in the original Rivers EGDT trial was the $ScvO_2$. In their trial, there were significant numbers of patients in the *control* group that did not reach $ScvO_2$s of 70% (60.2% vs 94.9%). With today's more aggressive resuscitation strategies, regardless of whether EGDT is utilized, it is likely that the number of patients with $ScvO_2$s of less than 70% at the end of resuscitation is much smaller. The ProCESS trial did not comment on $ScvO_2$ levels in the approximate 60% of patients that ended up with central lines that were in the control group, so the true number is not yet known. But if in today's efforts of resuscitation, a goal of $ScvO_2$ of 70% can be reached >85% of time, even without a central line, it would take many more patients than 1341 patients enrolled in the ProCESS trial to prove a difference in mortality.

Source Control

Since SIRS is defined as the body's response to an insult, it makes sense that if anything can be done to reduce or remove the insult, it should have the potential to improve outcomes. Although patients have been known to have a chronic, smoldering abscess for weeks prior to getting attention, it has anecdotally been known for years that in patients *with severe sepsis* (at least one sepsis-induced organ dysfunction), delay in the removal of an easily reversible source of infection (collection of pus, obstructed urinary or biliary tracts, dead bowel, infected foreign body) leads to an increase in mortality [23]. Although not based on prospective randomized trials, for every hour that there is ongoing stimulation of the inflammatory cascade, the likelihood of the patient progressing to

MODS and MOFS increases. The SSC Guidelines recommend source control within the first 12 h if possible (1C). Zero hour is usually considered to be triage time in the ED.

Antimicrobials

The data to show increases in mortality with inadequate or delayed antibiotics for documented infection are not randomized, but nonetheless profound. Kollef et al. [24] showed a fourfold increase in mortality (12.2%–52.1%) for ICU patients receiving inadequate antibiotics. In ICU patients specifically noted to have bloodstream infection [25], Ibrahim documented that mortality increased from 28.4% to 61.9%. These two studies together equate to an approximate NNT of 3 and demonstrate the critical importance of proper antibiotic choices.

More recently, Kumar et al. [26] showed that for every hour in delay in starting antibiotics in patients that presented with hypotension due to infection, mortality increases by 8%. Similar to this, Gaieski et al. [27] demonstrated that in septic patients presenting to the ED meeting criteria for EGDT, mortality can be reduced by an absolute 14% if *appropriate* antibiotics can be infused within 1 h of presenting in shock. Sadly, 14.9% of patients in the Gaieski study got the wrong antibiotic initially. If this is truly the *standard of care* currently, and nutrition articles in septic patients don't standardize for which patients get appropriate or timely antibiotics, it is no wonder the nutrition literature in sepsis patients is so controversial. The SSC Guidelines recommend *effective* antimicrobials within 1 h of recognition of septic shock (1B).

Ventilator Management

Most septic/SIRS patients where nutritional manipulation is considered are on a ventilator. Ventilator management strategies can have an impact on mortality as demonstrated by the ARDS Network original prospective randomized trial [28] utilizing a low tidal volume (6 mL/kg of ideal body weight [IBW]) as compared to a *high* tidal volume of 12 mL. The *high* was not atypical of tidal volumes used in patients across the country at that time. Mortality was lowered from 39.8% to 31% (NNT = 11). Although many other ventilator modes have come and gone with varying success claimed, this is the only randomized prospective trial in print to date to show improved survivals. Yet rarely do nutrition trials standardize ventilator management in their studies. Smaller tidal volumes are one of the few areas that receive a Grade 1A recommendation by the SSC.

Manipulation of the Coagulation Cascade

In septic patients, there has been felt to be an overlap of the inflammatory and coagulation cascades. In February 2001, the results of a multicenter prospective trial [29] were published showing efficacy of activated protein C (drotrecogin alfa: Xigris®) for patients with severe sepsis. The FDA eventually approved the drug for a sicker subset of patients in the trial (those with an APACHE II score >25) where mortality in that subgroup was shown to be reduced from 43.7% to 30.9% (NNT = 8). Approximately one decade later, the drug has been voluntarily removed from the market based on a new prospective randomized controlled trial (PRCT), the PROWESS SHOCK trial, [30] which failed to show the benefit of activated protein C. The overall mortality was lower (approximately 25%) in this trial compared to the original in patients with similar severity of illness. This trial was noteworthy in that it demanded a more aggressive resuscitation strategy (although not exactly EGDT) in both arms of the study. It is possible that the more aggressive resuscitation strategy negated any benefits of the drug.

There may yet be data to support the manipulation of the coagulation cascade during sepsis. In the retrospective analysis [31] of two large sepsis trials (activated protein C and antithrombin III), it was noted that when looking just at the placebo arm patients, those who received deep venous thrombosis prophylaxis doses of subcutaneous heparinoid products (subcutaneous heparin or low-molecular-weight heparin) had a lowered mortality rate of 42% versus 32.8% (NNT = 11), compared to those who did not receive this type of prophylaxis. These results were unrelated to death from pulmonary embolism. Although this is a retrospective analysis of prospective data and not randomized, it remains very intriguing. Pharmacoprophylaxis against deep venous thrombosis is a Grade 1B recommendation by SSC Guidelines.

Corticosteroids

Early trials of high-dose steroids (pharmacologic, not physiologic) in sepsis patients have been negative. In 2002, Annane et al. [32] showed improved survival using physiologic doses of hydrocortisone in a subgroup (defined as *steroid responsive* based on a cosyntropin stimulation test) of severe sepsis patients. Mortality was reduced from 63% to 53% (NNT = 10). Subsequently, the CORTICUS trial [33] was unable to reproduce this. This trial had an overall lower mortality rate (around 32%) compared to the original Annane trial. Marik and Zaloga [34] suggest that a random cortisol level of <25 μg/dL in a septic shock patient be utilized as a threshold to treat. The optimum use of steroids in septic shock is still unsettled and controversial on whether there is actually improvement in survival. The SSC Guidelines suggest not doing a stimulation test (2B), and only using hydrocortisone when usual fluid and vasopressors are unable to restore hemodynamics (2C).

Aggressive Serum Glucose Control

Van den Berghe [35] randomized postoperative surgical patients to an aggressive serum glucose control protocol versus a more liberal protocol. Although not specifically a sepsis study, the greatest reduction in mortality involved deaths due to MOFS with a proven septic focus. In patients sick enough to remain in an ICU for >5 days, mortality was reduced from 20.2% to 10.6% (NNT = 10). Interestingly, aggressive glucose control also significantly reduced acute renal failure requiring dialysis, the number of red blood cell transfusions, and critical illness polyneuropathy. Thus, based on this one study in print by 2001, *tight glucose control* (80–110 mg/dL) became the standard, and even the SSC had glucose control as part of its 24 h bundle in 2004 [21]. Enthusiasm waned because these results could not be easily reproduced. The NICE-SUGAR trial [36] in 2009 randomized over 6000 medical and surgical patients and appeared to show worse outcomes with tight control (27.5% mortality vs 24.9%). This was possibly related to higher incidence of hypoglycemic episodes in the tight control group (6.8% vs 0.5%). The meta-analysis by Griesdale et al. [37] concluded no overall mortality benefit, increased risk of hypoglycemia, but possible benefit in the surgical subpopulation. The true benefit of glucose control is unclear. Most have *loosened* the goals in the 140–180 mg/dL level. Once continuous glucose monitoring becomes a standard so as to reduce the number of hypoglycemic events, these studies should be repeated. The range 80–110 mg/dL is considered *normal*. Is there really a survival benefit to being *abnormal*? Is there really a difference in medical and surgical patients, or is it the technology that is limiting us from realizing an absolute 10% improvement in survival? The SSC Guidelines recommend glucose levels <180 mg/dL as opposed to <110 mg/dL (Grade 1A).

Multidisciplinary, Intensivist-Led ICU Team

Without even discussing nutrition, areas have been addressed that significantly influence mortality of the septic/SIRS patient. Whether or not there is a formal nutrition support service/team, it is logical that full-time ICU physicians familiar with the critical care literature and leading a multidisciplinary team of nurses, therapists, dietitians, and pharmacists would improve outcomes. In a review article by Young and Birkmeyer [38], relative reductions in mortality rates for intensivist-model ICUs ranged from 15% to 60%. Conservative estimates were over 50,000 lives saved per year in the United States if intensivists were fully implemented. Although the studies were not prospectively randomized, there was enough evidence for the Leapfrog Group to make it a part of their hospital safety initiative [39]. A more recent study looking at unit dynamics [40] showed that improvements in survival were statistically related to two different areas: the first is whether the unit has a physician leader and a daily plan of care review. The second area was nurse staffing ratios.

GOALS OF NUTRITION

The ultimate goal of nutritional manipulation of the patient is to improve morbidity and mortality. Mortality is fairly objective, although the timing that correlates best with efficacy (ICU mortality, hospital mortality, 28 day mortality, or 6 month mortality) is still debated. Assuming that the intensivist-led team has fully addressed all of the previous issues in a timely fashion, does nutrition play a role? The absolute answer is unclear, but ranges from a possible worse survival [3,41] all the way to an absolute reduction in mortality of 19.4% [42]. This equates to an NNT of 5! Morbidity is harder to keep objective. ICU days, ventilator days, and hospital length of stay are influenced by many issues besides patient improvement. Early mortality influences numbers of patients that don't develop morbidity complications. Nosocomial infections, especially pneumonia, lack gold standard definitions. Other commonly cited intermediary goals of nutrition may not correlate well with improved morbidity and mortality. Weight gain may be limited to fat and water. Nitrogen balance studies are prone to error and primarily become positive when the patient is able to physically exercise more (restore skeletal muscle). Negative caloric balance over time tends to correlate with mortality. But is it really the calories that are important, or is it the protein that typically accompanies the calories? Most complications and mortality occur in patients that are in negative nitrogen balance [43]. Is this cause and effect, or are they in negative nitrogen balance *because* they are deteriorating? Although there are no specific inflammatory markers that identify patients at risk for malnutrition, it is increasingly recognized that malnutrition can, at least in part, be attributed to the inflammatory state due to the extreme metabolic stress on the human body [44]. Traditional nutrition screening/assessment tools do not fully recognize the impact of inflammation; thus, the Academy of Nutrition and Dietetics and ASPEN have proposed new etiologic-based definitions that consider the time and degree of inflammation [45].

NUTRITIONAL MANIPULATION VERSUS NOTHING BY MOUTH

Up until now, it has always been felt unethical to have a *true* placebo-controlled trial with nutrition in critically ill ICU patients. The *placebo* arm would involve bringing a tray to the patient's room and removing it after some arbitrary time. Even the ventilated, sedated patient would get only a *tray to the room* if randomized to the placebo arm. Newer data [46] might suggest that this type of trial may not be unreasonable, at least for limited time frames (less than 10 days), especially in previously well-nourished patients. Until then, we must extrapolate from data we do have.

The mortality rate of severe sepsis (with one organ dysfunction) is usually cited at 20%. If respiratory is the failing organ system, mortality increases to as high as 30% (ARDS Network data). The risk of nutritional manipulation (complications of tubes, lines, and metabolic derangements) is around 5%–10%. It would appear, then, that nutritional manipulation in these patients would have a favorable risk–benefit ratio. SIRS-induced respiratory failure patients are also likely to be NPO for >5 days and therefore at risk for starvation-related morbidity (nosocomial infections, delayed wound healing, pressure ulcers, and prolonged rehabilitation from massive lean body mass losses). It would seem that this subgroup of patients would benefit from nutrition. There are two studies worth mentioning, but neither is specifically in septic patients. The first, by Kudsk et al. [47], randomized severe trauma patients to receive a standard enteral formula ($n = 18$) or a study formula ($n = 17$). Patients who met the same entrance criteria but were not randomized because of lack of enteral access ($n = 19$) served as a *contemporaneous* control. Although not prospectively randomized to the control arm, they still provide insight to the natural progression of this illness with little nutritional manipulation (only 2 of 19 *control* patients received any nutrition prior to a complication). The control patients indeed had the worse outcomes, with higher septic complications, longer hospital stays, and higher costs. This is remarkable in light of the fact that one of the major reasons they didn't get enteral access was because they were thought to clinically *not be sick enough* to be entered into the trial.

The second article is based on subset analysis of Casaer et al. [46]. In this article, patients were randomized to early versus late parenteral supplementation of nutrition. Everyone was supposed to be on the same early enteral protocol that included a progression of rates. The *early* group got 20% dextrose on days 1 and 2 (caloric goals of 400 kcal on day 1 and 800 kcal on day 2); then, total parenteral nutrition (TPN) started on day 3 if enteral nutrition was not meeting 100% of the requirements. The *late* group got 5% dextrose at hydration doses only, and was not supplemented with TPN until day 7 if enteral nutrition was not meeting caloric goals.

There were 517 post hoc subgroup patients (about 11% of the total 4640 enrolled) felt to have surgical contraindications to enteral nutrition that were also enrolled in the trial. Essentially, this subset was 20% dextrose on days 1 and 2 then full TPN, versus 5% dextrose only until day 7 when TPN was started. The rate of infection was lower in the late group (29.9% vs 40.2%) and a 20% relative increase in the likelihood of being discharged alive. Based on these two imperfect studies, it would appear that in well-nourished patients, enteral nutrition is better than NPO, but NPO is better than TPN within the first 7 days, especially in hypermetabolic ICU patients. Most feel that malnourished patients may benefit from less time of NPO, but this has not been independently studied.

TIMING

It would seem that the timing of parenteral nutrition has been answered in the previous section: as long as the patient is well nourished at hospital admission, there is no rush in starting TPN and may possibly cause harm in starting too early. Reasons for this finding will be discussed in the next section. Whether malnourished patients benefit from earlier parenteral nutrition is still unclear.

For enteral nutrition, three separate areas of timing seem important. The first is initiating enteral nutrition in relation to admission. Most sepsis/SIRS ICU patients are hypermetabolic and will have exaggerated losses, so starting early could potentially minimize net losses. Also, the patients typically do not become anabolic for many weeks. So time lost by not providing nutrition cannot be made up until the patient is anabolic. Additionally, overfeeding cannot make up for lack of feeding, and there is concern that overfeeding hypermetabolic ICU patients may be harmful [48,49]. Bartlett et al. [50] demonstrated increased mortality once a total caloric deficit of 10,000 calories is reached. It may not just be caloric load as total calories may just be a *carrier* for protein balance noting that most complications occur in patients who are in negative nitrogen balance [43]. In critically ill patients, nitrogen balance responds more to protein loading than caloric loading [51].

Second, early enteral nutrition has the potential to modulate the inflammatory response itself if started within 24 h [52]. Cerra et al. [53] documented that *late* enteral nutrition (started at least 3 days after the start of hypermetabolism) compared to TPN did not influence the development of MOFS; therefore, it would appear that there is a finite time window for influencing the metabolic response. Since many patients come in at different time frames during their hypermetabolism, it would make sense to start as quickly as possible once the patient has been resuscitated appropriately.

Third, time to achievement of nutritional goals is an important consideration. If feeds are advanced too slowly, tolerance may be delayed, and this may exacerbate nutritional losses, and if advanced too quickly, feeding intolerance may be exacerbated resulting in potential complications. Ibrahim et al. [54] reported worse outcomes in mechanically ventilated patients fed early versus late (after 5 days). This study compared initiating feeds at goal rate with gastric feeds versus low-dose feeds for first 5 days then titrating to goal rate. The worse outcomes were primarily from ventilator-associated pneumonia (VAP). Rice et al. [55] randomized 200 patients on ventilators to either initial trophic feeds (averaging 15.8% of needs through day 6) to full-energy group (reach goal within 24 h).

There was no difference in the overall outcomes (mortality around 20%). This helped prompt the ARDS Network to do the EDEN trial [56], comparing initial trophic feeds (averaging 400 kcal/day) to full feedings with an advancement protocol similar to the Rice trial. Again, there was no difference in mortality (overall death rate of 22%). Based mostly on these three previous trials, the SSC Guidelines give a 2B recommendation to avoid an aggressive advancement rate in feeding during the first week. There seems to be an increase in gastrointestinal complication rate (if not VAP rate) and no improvement in survival. A compromise rate (that has not been independently studied compared to either trophic or *full*) would be to start early (within 24 h) and reach goal by day 3. In one study [57], this appeared to be a *therapeutic dose* that has the potential to improve outcomes.

ENTERAL VERSUS PARENTERAL

Chapter 11 provides greater detail of the benefits of enteral over parenteral. Essentially, every PRCT of enteral versus parenteral has always shown TPN to be worse in complication rates [58,59] but not necessarily mortality [60]. Yet many people with short bowel are alive today because of long-term TPN. Is it the TPN itself that is harmful, the patient, and/or timing (are ICU patients predisposed to harm during hypermetabolism), or a combination? The following are some of the issues that are likely to be important to the discussion:

1. It is much easier to overfeed utilizing TPN. Whatever is written gets given.
2. TPN does not have the opportunity to favorably influence the inflammatory cascade as enteral nutrition can.
3. TPN has been shown to worsen superior mesenteric artery (SMA) blood flow [61]. The first week of hypermetabolism may be a critical time when SMA flow is important.
4. Parenteral fat solutions utilized in the United States are typically high in ω-6 fatty acids, which may be proinflammatory [62].
5. Glucose control is typically worse with TPN.

GASTRIC VERSUS POST-PYLORIC

Gastric feedings are typically given through a large bore tube: nasal, oral, or percutaneous. Post-pyloric tubes are smaller and softer and reduce the incidence of regurgitation and microaspiration [63]. Gastric tubes allow quicker initiation of feeds, but post-pyloric tubes are more likely to reach goal rate in a timely fashion [64]. Since up to 75% of patients enrolled in enteral nutrition trials [57,65] do not get a *therapeutic dose* of enteral nutrition, more reliable and rapid post-pyloric access should be sought. If post-pyloric was just as quick and easy as gastric, this argument would be mute; most would agree that for ICU patients, post-pyloric would be preferred. However, the stomach is also a *safety valve* and is the first to stop working when the rest of the bowel is in jeopardy. To bypass the stomach puts the responsibility on the medical team to ensure that feeding the bowel is the appropriate therapy. Once the patient is resuscitated, low-dose small bowel feeds can be started even in patients on vasopressors [66–68]. Most nutrition studies today can make gastric feeds work by tolerating higher residuals and more rapid utilization of pro-kinetics [69]. The Ibrahim trial [54] mentioned earlier that documented worse outcomes of early versus late enteral feeding in ventilated patients was with the use of gastric access. There was a higher rate of VAP in gastric-fed patients.

TOTAL CALORIC REQUIREMENTS

The optimum total final caloric load for the severe sepsis/SIRS patient remains poorly studied. The usual equations don't work well in the ICU compared to indirect calorimetry (IC) [70]. But even with daily IC to guide caloric loads to match metabolism, outcomes have not been improved [71].

Much may depend on the *phase* of illness. Optimal daily calories may change from hypermetabolism during the first few days to stabilization and finally to anabolism. General recommendations typically range from 22 kcal/kg/day of IBW to as much as 35 or more kcal/kg/day of actual weight (some using a correction factor for obese patients). This produces wide variations and could be a doubling of caloric recommendations. There is growing evidence that overfeeding is harmful, leading to hyperglycemia and prolonged ventilator time. Some have even promoted *permissive underfeeding* [72] as a strategy to improve outcomes. As patients progress along the SIRS/MODS/MOFS pathway, their cells have impaired glucose uptake. Therefore, contrary to typical recommendations, as patients get sicker, they probably should be fed fewer total calories, not more. A goal of 25 total kcal/kg/day IBW may be a good place to start for most ICU patients. Higher loads should be reserved for patients not clinically responding to nutrition and objective evidence of higher metabolic needs (IC). *Not clinically responding* should have objective definitions such as patients remaining in negative nitrogen balance in spite of improvement in inflammatory markers, hand grip strength, wound healing, etc. IBW should be considered as it may be more representative of lean body mass.

MACRONUTRIENT MAKEUP

The optimal ratio of fat, carbohydrate, and protein in the septic/SIRS patient is also unknown from prospective randomized trials. Nitrogen balance in hypermetabolic patients is more likely to respond to protein loading than it is to caloric loading. Therefore, the first decision relates to protein needs. Most recommend 1.5 gm/kg/day. When dealing with IBW, this number comes closer to 2.0 gm/kg/day for most patients that are often overweight and maybe even higher in obese patients. Outcomes may be more related to protein deficit than total calorie deficit [71], so optimizing protein dose should be paramount. Abnormal protein losses should also be taken into account and added on the earlier value, 2.0 gm/kg/day. Some examples of abnormal losses would include large weeping wounds, continuous renal replacement therapies, protein-losing enteropathy, and nephrotic syndrome. Protein calories subtracted from total leaves nonprotein calories. Some institutions exclude protein calories from the formulas, but this potentially can lead to overfeeding.

The distribution of carbohydrate and lipid (nonprotein) calories warrants consideration. The typical recommendation of 15%–30% of total calories as fat (correlating to approximately 20%–40% of nonprotein calories) appears too wide. There is a trend toward high-fat diets in diabetics (to facilitate glucose control) and in patients on ventilators (to aid in weaning). These diets are not physiologic, and have not been vigorously studied to show improvements in meaningful outcomes. In fact, many believe that high-fat diets, especially those high in the ω-6 variety found in intralipid, may be harmful and stimulate proinflammatory cytokines [73]. Battistella et al. [74] showed that trauma patients given TPN that included IV fat (25% of total calories) had higher infection rates and longer lengths of stay than those given no lipids for the first 10 days. From the ventilator standpoint, there is no advantage to altering fat/carbohydrate ratios as long as the patient is not overfed [75]. In the Battistella article, the lipid patients actually had longer ventilator times. Therefore, for TPN patients, consider withholding IV fats completely for the first 10 days (in well-nourished patients) or giving low doses (5%–10% of nonprotein calories). Propofol has become a very common sedative in ICUs today. The carrier solution is 10% intralipid. At 20 mL/h, a relatively low dose when used alone as a sedative, propofol has as many fat calories per day as was utilized in the Battistella article. These calories need to be taken into account from the dietary standpoint. Propofol's prolonged use (>48 h) in high doses (>20 mL/h) should be discouraged in SIRS patients. The data for enteral products that may have a more favorable mixture of fat types (ω-6, ω-3, medium-chain triglycerides, fish oils, borage oils) are more complex as will be discussed in the next sections.

SPECIFIC ENTERAL FORMULAS

Still one of the greatest controversies today in critical care nutrition involves the area of specialty immune enteral formulas, particularly in the septic patient. Initially labeled *immune enhancing*, this was changed to *immune modulating* when it was theorized that the septic patient's immune system may already be overstimulated. Based on bench and animal research, many commercial companies have formulated products with a variety of additives purported to help the septic/SIRS/MODS/MOFS patient. Still many of the additives have not been studied individually in ICU patients; therefore, one criticism is that it is difficult to determine whether these are synergistic or antagonistic in the final formula. They usually contain one or more of the following: arginine, glutamine, nucleic acids, ω-3 fatty acids, or other specialty oils. Many articles show improvement in morbidity, but only in patient subsets. Few articles have shown improvement in survival [76] but have been criticized for *less rigorous* methodologies. Two of the larger older studies [57,65] have high *dropout* rates based on the inability to get an adequate dose of formula. It is unprecedented to have 75% of patients enrolled in a trial not receive therapeutic amounts of "drug." How reliable is an intent-to-treat analysis in this scenario? Does a meta-analysis make it more accurate? In more recent years, there has been a concentration on ARDS patients with formulas that alter inflammation based on the fat makeup of the product. The following reviews will be somewhat historical in nature and work through the articles up to current time. Be aware, however, that the SSC 2012 Guidelines gave a Grade 2C to using nutrition with NO specific immune-modulating supplements in patients with severe sepsis.

The starting point will be the Heyland meta-analysis [41] of 2001 reviewing the published and some unpublished data to that point. This was a strict intent-to-treat analysis and was one of the first to raise the question whether immunonutrition may actually be harmful in certain subsets of ICU patients. As this argument was debated after 2001, it seems to have capsulated to the septic patient who is at highest risk for harm, and the arginine content of the formula may be the culprit. Septic patients are often the most *inflamed*, and giving an immune stimulant could be harmful. It is possible that the SIRS of sepsis is different from non-sepsis SIRS (trauma, major surgery). The immune literature is much stronger in acute trauma and elective major surgery. This is an enticing theory, although it remains just that: theory.

The trend for the increase in mortality in the Heyland meta-analysis in critically ill patients (not just sepsis) is driven by three articles, and one was unpublished (Ross product). In the Ross study, presented at the SCCM Congress in 2003, there were significantly more deaths reported in the experimental formula (20/87, 23%) compared with the control formula (8/83, 9.6%, $p = 0.03$). The excess deaths were mostly found in septic patients (pneumonia at baseline). Ten of twenty-six pneumonia patients receiving the experimental formula died (38.5%), whereas no pneumonia patients died in the control group (0/9, 0%). This appears very dramatic, but hard to discuss without published data as to whether severity of illness was the same, and whether other *drivers* of mortality were equally applied. In addition, the arginine content of the Ross product (5 g/1000 kcal) is much lower than other immune formulas (about 12 g/1000 kcal).

In the trial by Bower et al. [65], there were more deaths in the experimental formula group (24/153, 15.7%) than in the control (12/143, 8.4%). This is nearly statistically significant with a p value of 0.055, which went unreported in the original study. The mortality was mostly seen in the septic subgroup. Of 44 septic patients receiving experimental formula, 11 died (25%), whereas only 4 of 45 (8.9%) control formula patients died. Again, this seems fairly dramatic. However, most of this difference is driven by the septic patients who were *unsuccessfully fed*. It is difficult to imagine how supplemental arginine is contributing to mortality, when the difference is primarily seen in those that didn't get much formula. In fact, all of the mortality difference in the Bower study is being driven by the *unsuccessfully fed* subgroup (see Table 34.3). Imagine for a moment that the Bower trial showed significant improvements in intent-to-treat survival rates, but

TABLE 34.3
Bower et al. Mortality Rates

Feeding Subgroup	Experimental Mortality	Control Mortality
79 unsuccessfully fed	13/47 (27.7%)	3/32 (9.4%)
200 successfully fed	10/100 (10%)	7/100 (7%)
20 unsuccessfully fed septic patients	5/15 (33%)	0/5 (0%)

the improvements were primarily driven by the subset of *unsuccessfully fed* patients. Surely, the article would have been heavily criticized for that reason.

In the Atkinson study [57], the third article to contribute significantly to the mortality data of the Heyland meta-analysis, there was a much higher overall mortality rate (46%) than was predicted based on APACHE II scores, and slightly higher in the experimental formula group (48% experimental, 44% control, not significant). Approximately 20% of the patients in the study were septic, but the study design did not allow endpoint separation based on sepsis or SIRS. The remarkable aspect of this study was that over 50% of the patients enrolled were either unstable transfers from the wards or emergency transfers from other hospitals. In light of the fact that timely resuscitation has one of the most profound influences on mortality, it is hard to determine whether nutrition is actually being studied as an independent variable in mortality determination.

So the theory at this point is that arginine is harmful in the septic patient. The SIRS from sepsis is different, and arginine gets converted to nitric oxide, which, as a vasodilator, makes the patient more hypotensive and detrimental on outcome. However, the Galban et al. paper, which was included in the Heyland meta-analysis, brought a different perspective [76]. Although included, it did not carry as much weight because it was not felt to be as *rigorous*. The trial looked only at ICU mortality and was not blinded. It also dropped some randomized patients and did not have a strict definition of sepsis. Nevertheless, the mortality rate was significantly lower ($p = 0.05$) in the experimental formula (17/89, 19.1%) compared to the control formula (28/87, 32.2%). And most pertinent to this discussion, it was a study specifically done in septic patients (pneumonia being the most common source) and utilized a formula high in arginine (12.5 g/1000 kcal free arginine). One other criticism of this article was that the improvement in survival was *only significant* [77] in the least sick patients (APACHE II scores of 10–15), and it is *not helpful* in more critically ill patients. This myth continues to be perpetuated. In reality, there was improved survival in those patients with APACHE II scores greater than 15, but as a subgroup, those numbers of patients were small and did not reach statistical significance by themselves. It is inappropriate to make conclusions on post hoc subgroup analysis.

One other paper that fueled this debate during this time was by Bertolini et al. [78] and randomized ICU patients to an immune enteral formula or TPN. Because of the concern in septic patients brought out by the Heyland meta-analysis, the septic subgroup was looked at separately associated with the planned interim analysis after a total of 237 patients were enrolled. They did indeed find a significant increase in mortality in the septic patients given the enteral formula versus TPN. However, there were only 39 septic patients of the total enrolled, and the experimental formula (different from Bower et al.) was actually low in added arginine (5 g/1000 kcal) and high in ω-6 fatty acids. In addition, similar to the Atkinson study [57], over 50% of the septic patients came to the ICU from a hospital ward, making the standardization of aggressive resuscitation unclear.

To summarize the arginine/sepsis controversy to this point, recommendations varied from a moratorium for septic patients because they shorten lengths of stay only by increasing mortality (Heyland meta-analysis), all the way to improving survival by an absolute amount of 13.1% (Galban).

This correlates to one life saved for every eight patients treated with an arginine enteral formula specifically in a septic cohort. Concerns with the arginine hypothesis are as follows:

1. The Heyland meta-analysis [41] admits that "we found a higher (trend in) mortality in patients receiving immunonutrition in the subgroup of studies using formulas *other than those of high arginine content*" (emphasis added).
2. There is some arginine present in all whole-protein formulas. Why is mortality higher in those patients only getting small doses of experimental formula, if it is truly due to high arginine content?
3. An article by Argaman et al. [79] in septic pediatric patients (6–16 years old) reports an increase in arginine oxidation to both nitric oxide and urea leading to negative arginine balance, suggesting that arginine is *conditionally essential* during sepsis.
4. Experimental data suggest that the production of nitric oxide during sepsis may limit inappropriate vasoconstriction, may inhibit leukocyte adhesion, and may inhibit activation of nuclear transcription factor kappa B (NF-κB), which increases proinflammatory cytokine production [80]. All of these would be favorable in severe sepsis.
5. The phase III placebo-controlled trial of a nitric oxide synthase inhibitor (to lower serum arginine levels) in septic patients was actually stopped early because of an increase in mortality in those patients receiving the experimental drug [81].
6. The 2008 article by Beale et al. [82] showed improved organ function scores specifically in septic patients utilizing an immune formula with added arginine (see more details later).

ARDS/SEPSIS FORMULAS

One of the early trials was by Gadek et al. [83] in 1999, and was not included in the Heyland meta-analysis. It specifically looked at ARDS patients, approximately half originated from sepsis. The experimental diet in this study is different from that utilized in the Bower, Atkinson, and Galban studies. It is a high-lipid formula (55.2% of total calories) but contains a wide variety of oils (not just the ω-6 variety) including ω-3 fatty acids. It also does not contain added arginine. Favorable outcomes that reached statistical significance included days of ventilatory support, ICU length of stay, and a decrease in the number of new organs failing. There was only a trend toward lower mortality. The only concern with this article is that the control formula also contains 55.2% of total calories as lipid, but essentially all of the ω-6 variety. Are the patients doing better only because of *worse* outcomes in the control formula?

Singer et al. [84] were similarly able to show improved ventilatory outcomes in ARDS patients utilizing the same formula. This article was pertinent in that the ventilator management was standardized (lung protective strategy) to limit ventilator-induced lung injury. But there was no breakdown on percent of patients that were specifically noted to be septic. The only breakdown was medical versus surgical.

Pontes-Arruda et al. [42] in 2006 looked specifically at septic patients requiring mechanical ventilation utilizing the high-fat ARDS product. One important point to make in this article was that the control formula, although the same commercial product (Pulmocare), had changed its makeup of fat. Although the same 55.2% of total calories come from fat, the Singer study's control had 96.8% corn oil, 3.2% soy lecithin as its source. This study's control fat was 55.8% canola oil, 14% corn oil, 20% medium-chain triglycerides, 7% high oleic safflower oil, and 3.2% lecithin, making a weaker argument that the *control* formula is harmful. This study also appeared to standardize resuscitation, ventilator management, and steroid use consistent with the SSC guidelines at that time [21], thereby truly trying to isolate nutrition as a single variable. Survival was dramatically improved in the *evaluable* population of patients (103 out of total of 165). The control group's mortality at 28 days was 52% compared with 33% in the experimental group. That is a 19.4% absolute reduction, correlating with an NNT of only 5. The intent-to-treat numbers were similar: 46% compared to 31% (NNT = 7).

The OMEGA trial came out in 2011 [85]. This was sponsored by the ARDS Network so all included patients were intubated patients with ALI/ARDS. Sepsis was felt to be the source of lung injury in about 75%, and overall mortality was 21.7% (lower than many of the other trials). Ventilator and fluid management were standardized based on previous ARDS Network trials. As opposed to previous nutrition trials, this was not one tube feeding product versus control product. The choice of tube feed was left to individual facilities as long as it was not an immune/fish oil product. Patients were randomized in a double-blind fashion to receive twice daily supplement of ω-3 fatty acid, γ-linolenic acid, and antioxidants compared to placebo. Plasma levels of ω-3 fatty acids were increased in the experimental group, although only measured in about 20% of all patients. The trial was stopped early by the independent review board for futility after the first 272 patients. There were more ventilator-free days and trend toward lower mortality in the placebo arm (26.6% mortality in supplemented group and 16.3% in the control). The placebo group had more protein in the supplement to make it isocaloric resulting in a net difference of about 16 g more protein per day in the placebo arm. Propofol infusion for sedation was allowed, and there was a trend toward higher propofol use in the experimental arm. By not standardizing the tube feeding component, it is unknown which patients may have received a formula with a less favorable fat mixture. Current formulas have a wide range of ω-6/ω-3 fat ratios. The real remarkable aspect of this study is the low mortality rate in this control group fed higher doses of protein (16.3%). The ARDSNet trials have never had a mortality rate that low before. These are all patients on ventilators with ALI/ARDS. Is protein the key to improved survival?

Finally, the INTERSEPT trial by Pontes-Arruda in 2011 [86] randomized early sepsis patients (non-intubated, non-ARDS) in a blinded fashion to the ARDS formula versus a standard formula lower in fat than previous studies (Ensure Plus-29% fat) to counter the argument of *control* causing more harm. There was no difference in 28-day mortality (overall 27%), but significant differences were found favoring the experimental formula in the areas of progression of sepsis to sepsis shock and new organ failures, specifically respiratory failure requiring ventilation and cardiovascular failure.

OTHER SEPSIS ARTICLES

In 2008, Beale et al. [82] randomized septic patients to receive an experimental enteral *supplement* (combined with an immune-modulated formula) versus control supplement (combined with standard formula). The experimental supplement had glutamine dipeptides, vitamins C and E, β-carotene, selenium, zinc, and butyrate. Both groups ended up with 30% total calories as fat, so this study did not use an ARDS-type formula in the experimental group. The experimental group's supplement was high in protein (72% of supplement calories from protein) of which 30 g was glutamine. The immune-modulated formula had added arginine (6.7 g/1000 kcal). The primary endpoint for this study was organ dysfunction assessed by daily total Sequential Organ Failure Assessment scores over the 10-day study period. Overall 6-month mortality was around 33% and not different between groups. The trial was designed to enroll 344 patients but was stopped early at the first interim analysis of only 50 patients because of benefit in the experimental arm. One of the major differences that must be taken into account is the protein content of the overall diets. The daily experimental *supplement* had 42.5 g of protein per day compared to 0 g in the control supplement. The immune formula that the experimental supplement was added to already had 22% total calories as protein, whereas the standard formula had only 15%. This leads to significantly different overall protein loads in the two different diets.

GLUTAMINE/ANTIOXIDANTS

Patients with sepsis experience a high level of oxidative stress. Antioxidant demand is increased coupled with a reduction in the body's antioxidant capacity. Studies demonstrate a reduction in antioxidant levels in sepsis, which correlates with increased mortality [87]. Selenium and glutamine play vital roles in many antioxidative pathways that occur during sepsis [88]. Thus, it would seem reasonable to conclude that supplementation of these nutrients may potentially improve clinical outcomes.

Glutamine is described as a conditionally essential amino acid during times of stress. Decreased plasma concentrations of glutamine have been associated with poor clinical outcomes [89]. Some studies report glutamine deficiencies in 25%–35% of critically ill patients [89,90]. Skeletal muscle exports significant quantities of glutamine for redistribution to other tissues, with an estimated turnover rate of up to 1 gram per kilogram per day [90], where it is utilized for a multitude of functions. Glutamine can act as a fuel source for enterocytes, as well as immune cells such as leukocytes and macrophages. It can also play a role in nucleic acid synthesis and facilitates acid–base balance in the kidneys. The majority of studies that have shown benefit with glutamine supplementation provide it in the parenteral form as part of a central parenteral nutrition prescription (as opposed to dosing separate from the nutrition plan). A small study by Griffith et al. [91] in 2002 showed an overall trend toward improved ICU survival with glutamine supplementation, 71% of which were septic. This trend became significant at 6 months. It was even more profound in the subgroup that was fed for at least 5 days. The enteral glutamine data are not as clear, but the Beale study mentioned earlier had glutamine supplementation as part of its cocktail. Enteral glutamine in appropriate dosing needs further study, but for parenteral, the NNT to save one life may be as low as 5 in the intent-to-treat analysis of 6-month mortality [81].

Selenium, a trace element, is a primary component of selenoproteins and glutathione peroxidase that has antioxidant and anti-inflammatory effects [92]. Patients with SIRS and severe sepsis have 40% lower selenium levels [93]. Again, it seems to be a prime area to study. Selenium has been studied alone and in combination with other antioxidants. Overall, studies have shown a reduction in mortality (up to 10% absolute) in critically ill patients including those with sepsis. Angstwurm et al. [94] showed that the sicker patients were ones most likely to benefit. A recent meta-analysis by Manzanares et al. [95] looking at antioxidants (with or without selenium) concluded that there are significant reductions in mortality in sicker ICU patients (mortality >10%) and that higher doses of selenium (>500 μg/day) were needed to maximize the benefit. In the SIGNET trial [96], Andrews et al. looked at glutamine- and selenium-supplemented TPN in ICU patients (around 55% sepsis). Although there was no difference in outcome in the intent-to-treat analysis, there was a significant reduction in infections in a predefined subgroup of patients that received TPN for ≥5 days.

However, a more recent paper reveals interesting results. The REDOXS trial [97] was a multicenter prospective randomized blinded trial employing a 2 × 2 factorial design looking at glutamine and antioxidants (selenium and vitamins). There were over 1200 patients enrolled, with approximately 300 in each of the four groups (placebo, glutamine only, antioxidants only, and both glutamine and antioxidants). This trial differed from others in that it supplemented glutamine both IV and enteral, and at doses much higher than other studies (30 g more per day than the maximum dose in previous studies). The selenium was also IV and enteral with total dose of 800 μg/day. Overall mortality was 29.8%, with a trend toward increased 28-day mortality in those who received glutamine. This trend became significant for in-hospital mortality and mortality at 6 months. And contrary to previous studies, antioxidants had no effect on study outcomes. The SSC 2012 Guidelines give a Grade 2C to NOT using supplemental selenium. There was no specific grade for glutamine alone in the guidelines.

The REDOXS trial has substantial differences compared to other glutamine trials besides the obvious high-dose of glutamine. The patients were sicker (as noted by the high overall mortality rate), and most were in shock at the start of the trial. They were all on ventilators, and two or more organ failure was part of entrance criteria. This means that many had renal and/or liver failure, patients often excluded from other nutrition trials that include major protein supplements. Supplements were given independent of the nutrition plan (other studies have glutamine as part of central parenteral nutrition). As noted by Bistrian [98], this could lead to amino acid profile imbalance. If a single amino acid is providing upward of 60% of the total dietary protein, the potential for toxicity is greater.

CONCLUSION

What recommendations can be made at this time for the nutritional manipulation of the SIRS patient, with sepsis as the most common cause of SIRS especially in the medical intensive care unit? Although nutrition has shown to be important, its effects can be overshadowed by poor compliance in other areas of sepsis care (resuscitation, early appropriate antibiotics, and ventilator management). As other therapies for sepsis have fallen through in the last few years (activated protein C, tight glucose control, steroid therapy), the nutrition literature for sepsis has become stronger (see Figure 34.1). The anti-arginine argument in sepsis is becoming weaker, although still needs a definitive trial. The literature favoring ARDS formulas for ALI and sepsis is strong with the one exception of the OMEGA trial by the ARDS Network. It is likely that twice daily supplements will not overcome the use of a standard formula already high in ω-6 fatty acids and the allowance of propofol as a sedative. Do fish oil capsules make a difference in people who continue to routinely eat fried food and red meat? Glutamine and antioxidant literature is favorable as individual supplements as well as just overall protein supplementation. The REDOXS trial looks unfavorably toward glutamine, but again, similar to the OMEGA trial, these are supplements given independent of the nutrition regimen, which is not necessarily physiologic. The following are suggestions for nutrition based on the current state of the literature for sepsis/SIRS.

Once the patient is well resuscitated and appropriate antibiotics have been given, focus should then be turned to enteral access, and preferably post-pyloric if the institution can gain that access quickly without significant delay in the initiation of feedings. Feedings should be started at moderate doses (20%–30% of needs), with protocols for automatic increases to reach goal by 72 h as long as this is tolerated. The formula should be an immune-modulating or an ARDS formula based on local protocols and local interpretation of the arginine argument. Protein supplement should be added at the start in hopes of at least reaching protein goals even if caloric goals are not achievable. Glutamine can be added enterally early in low doses. Avoid significant propofol use. Consider supplemental TPN use only after the first 7 days if the patient is well nourished. In malnourished patients, most feel that earlier parenteral supplementation improves outcome. If supplemental or full TPN is truly required, parenteral glutamine should be added as part of a TPN prescription if available, and not as a separate additive. High-dose lipids should be avoided. Concentrate on meeting protein needs. Separate antioxidants can be added if not already part of the formula. Local definitions and protocols should be defined for *success* or *failure* of nutrition in order to help decide when to increase protein and/or calorie dose. In other words, nutrition decisions should be *data driven*, no different than any other medical decision making in the ICU today. In fact, the data now suggest that nutrition may be as or more important for mortality outcomes as anything else we do for the septic patient.

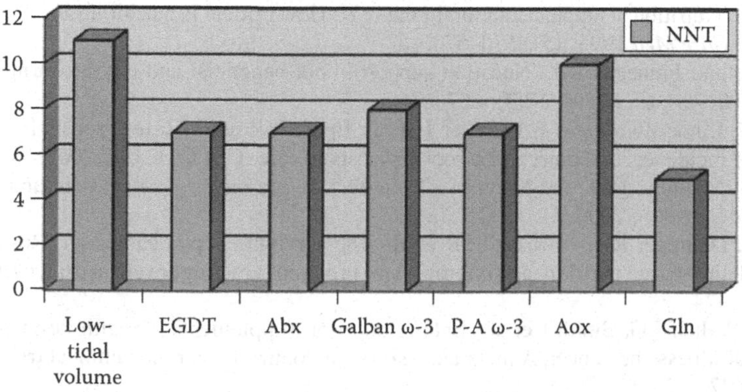

FIGURE 34.1 NNT, number needed to treat to save one life; EGDT, early goal-directed therapy; Abx, appropriate early antibiotics; Galban omega 3 supplemented (see Ref. [76]); P-A, Pontes-Arruda omega 3 supplemented (see Ref. [42]); Aox = antioxidant; Gln, parenteral glutamine.

CASE STUDY

RD was a 65-year-old male (5 foot 10 in., BMI of 28) admitted through the ED with presumed septic shock felt to be due to pneumonia. The patient remained hypotensive after his 30 cc/kg fluid bolus, so *code sepsis* was activated (code alert for an EGDT candidate). This prompted specific very broad-spectrum antibiotics that only *code sepsis* patients get as one-time doses in the ED. A central line was placed in ED, and all protocols for EGDT were followed, meeting CVP and $ScvO_2$ goals within 4 h of triage. The patient required intubation in the ED and was placed on low-tidal-volume ventilation. For persistent hypotension in spite of meeting CVP goals, vasopressors were started. CT scans were done during transportation from ED to the ICU, which showed moderate to large pleural effusion on the side of the pneumonia. Because of the concern for empyema (a potential reversible *source*), a chest tube was placed in the ICU at hour 8. After hemodynamic stabilization, a small bowel feeding tube was placed at bedside, and the patient was started on the ARDS/sepsis formula at 20 cc/h, in spite of still requiring vasopressors. Protein supplements were added, which included low-dose enteral glutamine. After taking a more thorough history from the family, it was felt that his illness was most consistent with community-acquired pneumonia, so his ICU antibiotics were tailored to that. The patient met goal nutrition (25 kcal/kg of IBW/day and 2 g/kg IBW of protein) by day 3. By day 6, patient remained on ventilator, but was off of vasopressors. C-reactive protein was decreasing, but prealbumin was not rising, so he underwent metabolic cart monitoring and empirically increased to 2.5 g/kg IBW of protein. Metabolic cart documented slight overfeeding, so total calories were decreased keeping the protein dose at the higher level. Over the next week, the patient gradually improved, and his prealbumin started to rise. He was extubated on day 10 of hospitalization, while tube feeds were continued since he had a small bowel tube. He underwent swallow evaluation the next day and was able to take thick liquids. He was transferred out of ICU on day 11. Tube feeds were reduced as he took in more calories by mouth. By day 14, he was meeting his nutrition goals orally, and tube feeds were discontinued. He was discharged doing well on day 16.

REFERENCES

1. Sackett DL.: Rules of evidence and clinical recommendations on the use of antithrombotic agents. *Chest* 1989; 95: 2S–4S.
2. Dellinger RP, Levy MM, Rhodes A et al.: Surviving sepsis campaign: International guidelines for management of severe sepsis and septic shock: 2012. *Crit Care Med* 2013; 41: 580–637.
3. Koretz RL.: Nutritional supplementation in the ICU. How critical is nutrition for the critically ill? *Am J Respir Crit Care Med* 1995; 151: 570–573.
4. Marino PL and Finnegan MJ.: Nutrition support is not beneficial and can be harmful in critically ill patients. *Crit Care Clin* 1996; 12(3): 667–676.
5. Angus DC, Linde-Zwirble WT, Lidicker J et al.: Epidemiology of severe sepsis in the United States: Analysis of incidence, outcome, and associated costs of care. *Crit Care Med* 2001; 29(7): 1303–1310.
6. Martin GS, Mannino DM, and Moss M.: The effect of age on the development and outcome of adult sepsis. *Crit Care Med* 2006; 34: 15–21.
7. Levy MM, Dellinger RH, Townsend SR et al.: The surviving sepsis campaign: Results of an international guideline-based performance improvement program targeting severe sepsis. *Crit Care Med* 2010; 38(2): 367–374.
8. Heys SD, Walker LG, Smith I et al.: Enteral nutrition supplementation with key nutrients in patients with critical illness and cancer: A meta-analysis of randomized controlled clinical trials. *Ann Surg* 1999; 229: 467–477.
9. Beale RJ, Bryg DJ, and Bihari DJ.: Immunonutrition in the critically ill: A systemic review of clinical outcome. *Crit Care Med* 1999; 27: 2799–2805.

10. Fry DE, Pearlstein L, Fulton RL et al.: Multiple system organ failure: The role of uncontrolled infection. *Arch Surg* 1980; 115: 136–140.
11. Marshall JC, Cook DJ, Christou NV et al.: Multiple organ dysfunction score: A reliable descriptor of a complex clinical outcome. *Crit Care Med* 1995; 23: 1638–1652.
12. Vincent JL, Moreno R, Takala J et al.: The sepsis-related organ failure assessment (SOFA) score to describe organ dysfunction/failure. *Int Care Med* 1996; 22: 707–710.
13. Bone RC.: Toward a theory regarding the pathogenesis of the systemic inflammatory response syndrome: What we do and do not know about cytokine regulation. *Crit Care Med* 1996; 24: 163–172.
14. Gentile LF, Cuenca AG, Efron PA et al.: Persistent inflammation and immunosuppression: A common syndrome and new horizon for surgical intensive care. *J Trauma Acute Care Surg* 2012; 72: 1491–1501.
15. Osuchowski MF, Welch K, Siddiqui J et al.: Circulating cytokine/inhibitor profiles reshape the understanding of the SIRS/CARS continuum in sepsis and predict mortality. *J Immunol* 2006; 177: 1967–1974.
16. Xiao W, Mindrinos MB, Seok J et al.: A genomic storm in critically injured humans. *J Esp Med* 2011; 208: 2581–2590.
17. Matzinger P.: The danger model: A renowned sense of self. *Science* 2002; 296: 301–305.
18. Zhang Q, Raoof M, Chen Y et al.: Circulating mitochondrial DAMPs cause inflammatory responses to injury. *Nature* 2010; 464: 104–107.
19. Pugin J.: Dear SIRS, the concept of "alarmins" makes a lot of sense. *Intensive Care Med* 2008; 34: 218–221.
20. Rivers E, Nguyen B, Havstad S et al.: Early goal-directed therapy in the treatment of severe sepsis and septic shock. *N Engl J Med* 2001; 345: 1368–1377.
21. Dellinger RP, Carlet JM, Mansur H et al.: Surviving sepsis campaign guidelines for management of severe sepsis and septic shock. *Crit Care Med* 2004; 345: 1368–1377.
22. A randomized trial of protocol-based care for early septic shock. The process investigators. *NEJM* 2014; 370: 1683–1693.
23. Jimenez Mf and Marshall JC.: Source control in the management of sepsis. *Int Care Med* 2001; 27: S49–S62.
24. Kollef MH, Sherman G, Ward S et al.: Inadequate antimicrobial treatment of infections. A risk factor for hospital mortality among critically ill patients. *Chest* 1999; 115(2): 462–474.
25. Ibrahim EH, Sherman G, Ward S et al.: The influence of inadequate antimicrobial treatment of bloodstream infections on patient outcomes in the ICU setting. *Chest* 2000; 118: 146–155.
26. Kumar A, Roberts D, Wood KE et al.: Duration of hypotension before initiation of effective antimicrobial therapy is the critical determinant of survival in human septic shock. *Crit Care Med* 2006; 34(6):1589–1596.
27. Gaieski DF, Mikkelsen ME, Band RA et al.: Impact of time to antibiotics on survival in patients with severe sepsis or septic shock in whom early goal-directed therapy was initiated in the emergency department. *Crit Care Med* 2010; 38(4): 1045–1053.
28. Ventilation with lower tidal volumes as compared with traditional tidal volumes for acute lung injury and the acute respiratory distress syndrome. The acute respiratory distress syndrome network. *N Engl J Med* 2000; 342: 1301–1308.
29. Bernard GR, Vincent JL, Laterre PF et al.: Efficacy and safety of recombinant human activated protein C for severe sepsis. *N Engl J Med* 2001; 344: 699–709.
30. Ranieri VM, Thompson BT, Barie PS et al.: Drotrecogin alfa (activated) in adults with septic shock. *NEJM* 2012; 366: 2055–2064.
31. Davidson BL, Geerts WH, and Lensing AWA.: Low-dose heparin for severe sepsis. (letter to editor). *N Engl J Med* 2002; 347 (13): 1036–1037.
32. Annane D, Sebille V, Charpentier C et al.: Effect of treatment with low doses of hydrocortisone and fludrocortisone on mortality in patients with septic shock. *JAMA* 2002; 288: 862–871.
33. Sprung CL, Annane D, Keh D et al.: Hydrocortisone therapy for patients with septic shock. *N Engl J Med* 2008; 358: 111–124.
34. Marik PE and Zaloga GP.: Adrenal insufficiency during septic shock. *Crit Care Med* 2003; 31: 141–145.
35. Van den Berghe G, Wouters P, Weekers F et al.: Intensive insulin therapy in the critically ill patient. *N Engl J Med* 2001; 345: 1359–1367.
36. The NICE-SUGAR study investigators: Intensive versus conventional glucose control in critically ill patients. *N Engl J Med* 2009; 360: 1283–1297.

37. Griesdale DE, de Souza RJ, van Dam RM et al.: Intensive insulin therapy and mortality among critically ill patients: A meta-analysis including NICE-SUGAR study data. *CMAJ* 2009; 180(8): 821–827.
38. Young MP and Birkmeyer JD.: Potential reduction in mortality rates using and intensivist model to manage intensive care units. *Effect Clin Pract* 2000; 3(6): 284–289.
39. Milstein A, Galvin RS, Delbanco SF et al.: Improving the safety of health care: The Leapfrog initiative. The Leapfrog group. *Effect Clin Pract* 2000; 5: 313–316.
40. Checkley W, Martin GS, Brown SM et al.: Structure, process, and annual ICU mortality across 69 centers: United States critical illness and injury trials group critical illness outcomes study. *Crit Care Med* 2014; 42: 344–356.
41. Heyland DK, Novak F, Drover JW et al.: Should immunonutrition become routine in critically ill patients? A systematic review of the evidence. *JAMA* 2001; 286(8): 944–953.
42. Pontes-Arruda A, Albuquerque AA, and Albuquerque JD.: Effects of enteral feeding with eicosapentaenoic acid, γ-linolenic acid, and antioxidants in mechanically ventilated patients with severe sepsis and septic shock. *Crit Care Med* 2006; 34(9): 2325–2333.
43. Church JM and Hill GL.: Assessing the efficacy of intravenous nutrition in general surgical patients: Dynamic nutritional assessment with plasma proteins. *JPEN* 1987; 11(2): 135–139.
44. Jensen GL.: Inflammation: An expanding universe. *Nutr Clin Pract* 2008; 23(1):1–2.
45. White JV, Guenter P, Jensen G et al.: Consensus statement: Academy of Nutrition and Dietetics and American Society for Parenteral and Enteral Nutrition: Characteristics recommended for the identification and documentation of adult malnutrition (undernutrition). *JPEN* 2012; 36: 275–283.
46. Casaer MP, Mesotten D, Hermans G et al.: Early versus late parenteral nutrition in critically ill adults. *N Engl J Med* 2011; 365: 506–517.
47. Kudsk KA, Minard G, Croce MA et al.: A randomized trial of isonitrogenous enteral diets after severe trauma: An immune-enhancing diet reduces septic complications. *Ann Surg* 1996; 224(4): 531–543.
48. Muller TF, Muller A, Bachem MG et al.: Immediate metabolic effects of different nutritional regimens in critically ill medical patients. *Intensive Care Med* 1995; 21: 561–566.
49. Patino JF, de Pimiento SE, Vergara A et al.: Hypocaloric support in the critically ill. *World J Surg* 1999; 23: 553–559.
50. Bartlett RH, Dechert RE, Mault JR et al.: Measurement of metabolism in multiple organ failure. *Surgery* 1982; 92: 771–779.
51. Coss-Bu JA, Klish WJ, Walding D et al.: Energy metabolism, nitrogen balance, and substrate utilization in critically ill children. *Am J Clin Nutr* 2001; 74: 664–669.
52. Lowry SF.: The route of feeding influences injury responses. *J Trauma* 1990; 30(12): S10–S15.
53. Cerra FB et al.: Enteral nutrition does not prevent multiple organ failure syndrome (MOFS) after sepsis. *Surgery* 1988; 104(4): 727–733.
54. Ibrahim EH, Mehringer L, Prentice D et al.: Early *versus* late enteral feeding of mechanically ventilated patients: Results of a clinical trial. *JPEN* 2002; 26(3): 174–181.
55. Rice TW, Morgan S, Hays MA et al.: Randomized trial of initial trophic versus full-energy enteral nutrition in mechanically ventilated patients with acute respiratory failure. *Crit Care Med* 2011; 39: 967–974.
56. Initial trophic vs full enteral feeding in patients with acute lung injury. The EDEN randomized trial. ARDS clinical trials network. *JAMA* 2012; 307: 795–803.
57. Atkinson S, Sieffert E, Bihari D et al.: A prospective, randomized, double-blind, controlled clinical trial of enteral immunonutrition in the critically ill. *Crit Care Med* 1998; 26(7): 1164–1172.
58. Moore FA, Moore EE, Jones TN et al.: TEN versus TPN following major abdominal trauma: Reduced septic morbidity. *J Trauma* 1989; 29(7): 916–923.
59. Perioperative total parenteral nutrition in surgical patients. The Veterans affairs total parenteral nutrition cooperative study group. *N Engl J Med* 1991; 325(8): 525–532.
60. Peter JV, Moran JL, and Phillips-Hughes J.: A meta-analysis of treatment options of early enteral versus early parenteral nutrition in hospitalized patients. *Crit Care Med* 2005; 33(1): 213–220.
61. Gatt M, MacFie J, Anderson A et al.: Changes in superior mesenteric artery blood flow after oral, enteral and parenteral feeding in humans. *Crit Care Med* 2009; 37(1): 171–176.
62. Umpierrez GE, Spiegelman R, Zhao V et al.: A double-blind, randomized clinical trial comparing soybean oil-based versus olive oil-based lipid emulsions in adult medical-surgical intensive care unit patients requiring parenteral nutrition. *Crit Care Med* 2012; 40: 1792–1798.
63. Heyland DK, Drover JW, MacDonald S et al.: Effects of postpyloric feeding on gastroesophageal regurgitation and pulmonary microaspiration: Results of a randomized controlled trial. *Crit Care Med* 2001; 29(8): 1495–1501.

64. Kearns PJ, Chin D, Meuller L et al.: The incidence of ventilator-associated pneumonia and success in nutrient delivery with gastric versus small intestinal feeding: A randomized clinical trial. *Crit Care Med* 2000; 28(6): 1742–1746.
65. Bower RH, Cerra FB, Bershadsky B et al.: Early enteral administration of a formula (Impact®) supplemented with arginine, nucleotides, and fish oil in intensive care unit patients: Results of a multicenter, prospective, randomized, clinical trial. *Crit Care Med* 1995; 23(3): 436–449.
66. Zaloga GP, Robert PR, and Marik P.: Feeding the hemodynamically unstable patient: A critical evaluation of the evidence. *Nutr Clin Pract* 2003; 18(4): 285–293.
67. Manci EE and Muzevich KM.: Tolerability and safety of enteral nutrition in critically ill patients receiving intravenous vasopressor therapy. *JPEN* 2013; 37: 641–651.
68. Yang S, Wu X, Yu W, and Li J.: Early enteral nutrition in critically ill patients with hemodynamic instability: An evidence-based review and practical advice. *Nutr Clin Pract* 2014; 29: 90–96.
69. Nguyen NQ, Chapman M, Fraser RJ et al.: Prokinetic therapy for feed intolerance in critical illness: One drug or two? *Crit Care Med* 2007; 35: 2561–2567.
70. Cooney RN and Frankenfield DC.: Determining energy needs in critically ill patients: Equations or indirect calorimeters. *Curr Opin Crit Care* 2012; 18(2): 174–177.
71. Weijs PJ, Stapel S, de Groot SD et al.: Optimal protein and energy nutrition decreases mortality in mechanically ventilated, critically ill patients: A prospective observational cohort study. *JPEN* 2012; 36: 60–68.
72. Zaloga GP and Roberts P.: Permissive underfeeding. *New Horizons* 1994; 2(2): 257–263.
73. Suchner U, Katz DP, Fürst P et al.: Effects of intravenous fat emulsions on lung function in patients with acute respiratory distress syndrome or sepsis. *Crit Care Med* 2001; 29(8): 1569–1574.
74. Battistella FD, Widergren JT, Anderson JT et al.: A prospective, randomized trial of intravenous fat emulsion administration in trauma victims requiring total parenteral nutrition. *J Trauma* 1997; 43(1): 52–60.
75. Talpers SS, Romberger DJ, Bunce SB et al.: Nutritionally associated increased carbon dioxide production: Excess total calories vs high proportion of carbohydrate calories. *Chest* 1992; 102(2): 551–555.
76. Galban C, Montejo JC, Mesejo A et al.: An immune-enhancing enteral diet reduces mortality rate and episodes of bacteremia in septic intensive care unit patients. *Crit Care Med* 2000; 28: 643–648.
77. Heyland DK.: Immunonutrition in the critically ill patient: Putting the cart before the horse? *Nutr Clin Pract* 2002; 17(5): 267–272.
78. Bertolini G, Iapichino G, Radrizzani D et al.: Early enteral immunonutrition in patients with severe sepsis: Results of an interim analysis of a randomized multicentre clinical trial. *Int Care Med* 2003; 29: 834–840.
79. Argaman Z, Young VR, Noviski N et al.: Arginine and nitric oxide metabolism in critically ill septic pediatric patients. *Crit Care Med* 2003; 31(2): 591–597.
80. Marik PE.: Cardiovascular dysfunction of sepsis: A nitric oxide and L-arginine-deficient state? *Crit Care Med* 2003; 31(2): 591–597.
81. López A, Lorente JA, Steingrub J et al.: Multiple-center, randomized, placebo-controlled, double-blind study of the nitric oxide synthase inhibitor 546C88: Effect on survival in patients with septic shock. *Crit Care Med* 2004; 32(1): 21–30.
82. Beale RJ, Sherry T, Lei K et al.: Early enteral supplementation with key pharmaconutrients improves sequential organ failure assessment scores in critically ill patients with sepsis: Outcome of a randomized, controlled, double-blind trial. *Crit Care Med* 2008; 36: 131–144.
83. Gadek JE, DeMichele SJ, Karlstad MD et al.: Effect of enteral feeding with eicosapentaenoic acid, γ-linolenic acid, and antioxidants in patients with acute respiratory distress syndrome. *Crit Care Med* 1999; 27(8): 1409–1420.
84. Singer P, Theilla M, Fisher H et al.: Benefit of an enteral diet enriched with eicosapentaenoic acid and gamma-linolenic acid in ventilated patients with acute lung injury. *Crit Care Med* 2006; 34: 1033–1038.
85. Rice TW, Wheeler AP, Thompson BT et al.: Enteral omega-3 fatty acid γ-linolenic acid, and antioxidant supplementation in acute lung injury. *JAMA* 2011; 306(14): 1574–1581.
86. Pontes-Arruda A, Martins LF, de Lima SM et al.: Enteral nutrition with eicosapentaenoic acid, γ-linolenic acid and antioxidants in the early treatment of sepsis: Results from a multicenter, prospective, randomized, double-blinded, controlled study: The INTERSEPT study. *Crit Care* 2011; 15: R144.
87. Heyland DK, Dhaliwal R, Suchner U et al.: Antioxidant nutrients: A systemic review of trace elements and vitamins in the critically ill patient. *Int Care Med* 2005; 31: 327–337.
88. Berger MM and Chiolero RL.: Antioxidant supplementation in sepsis and systemic inflammatory response syndrome. *Crit Care Med* 2007; 35[Suppl.]: S584–S590.

89. Oudemans-van Straaten HM, Bosman RJ, Treskes M et al.: Plasma glutamine depletion and patient outcome in acute ICU admissions. *Int Care Med* 2001; 27: 84–90.
90. Biolo G, Zorat F, Antonione R et al.: Muscle glutamine depletion in the intensive care unit. *Int J Biochem Cell Biol* 2005; 37: 2169–2179.
91. Griffiths RD, Allen KD, Andrews FJ et al.: Infection, multiple organ failure, and survival in the intensive care unit: Influence of glutamine-supplemented parenteral nutrition on acquired infection. *Nutrition* 2002; 18: 546–552.
92. Alhazzani W, Jacobi J, Sindi A et al.: The effect of selenium therapy on mortality in patients with sepsis syndrome: A systematic review and meta-analysis of randomized controlled trials. *Crit Care Med* 2013; 41: 1–10.
93. Forceville X, Laviolle B, Annane D et al.: Effects of high doses of selenium, as sodium selenite, in septic shock: A placebo-controlled, randomized, double-blind, phase II study. *Crit Care* 2007; 11: R73.
94. Angstwurm MW, Engelmann L, Zimmerman T et al.: Selenium in intensive care (SIC): Results of a prospective randomized, placebo-controlled, multi-center study in patients with severe systemic inflammatory response, sepsis and septic shock. *Crit Care Med* 2007; 35: 118–126.
95. Manzanares W, Dhaliwal R, Jiang X et al.: Antioxidant micronutrients in the critically ill: A systematic review and meta-analysis. *Crit Care* 2012; 16: R66.
96. Andrews PJ, Avenell A, Noble DW et al.: Randomized trial of glutamine, selenium, or both, to supplemental parenteral nutrition for critically ill patients. *BMJ* 2011; 342: D1542.
97. Heyland D, Muscedere J, Wischmeyer PE et al.: A randomized trial of glutamine and antioxidants in critically ill patients. *NEJM* 2013; 368: 1489–1497.
98. Bistrian BR.: Letter to the editor. *NEJM* 2013; 369: 482.

35 Nutrition Therapy in Patients with Cancer and Immunodeficiency

Vanessa Fuchs-Tarlovsky and Elizabeth Isenring

CONTENTS

NUTRITION AND CANCER

One of the most significant nutritional issues that can arise during cancer treatment is malnutrition. Malnutrition may result from the disease process, from the use of antineoplastic therapy, or both. Side effects related to common oncology therapies, including chemotherapy, radiation, immunotherapy, and surgery, are the key contributors in promoting deterioration in nutritional status. Additionally, deterioration in nutritional status has been found to predict outcome prior to the initiation of therapy [1]. Malnutrition reduces quality of life (QOL), decreases performance status, and increases morbidity and mortality. Malnutrition adversely affects tissue function and humoral and cellular immunity. It is not surprising that a significant proportion of patients with cancer end up being critically ill because of those factors [2]. Aggressive treatment and resulting complications such as infections can increase the degree of malnutrition increasing morbidity and mortality [3].

Patients with cancer tend to be immunosuppressed not only due to their illness but also due to the treatment needed for that purpose. The use of intensive nutritional therapy for some patients with cancer may promote weight gain and positive nitrogen balance, which increases the tolerance of cancer therapy and improves immune response. The benefits of nutrition therapy in patients with cancer may outweigh concerns of nutritional effects on tumor growth. The choice of nutritional therapy is dependent on the availability and access to a functional gastrointestinal tract, comfort and compliance for the patients, antineoplastic therapy toxicities, and site of radiation therapy [3].

Critical care of patients with cancer has progressed despite many challenges in recent decades. In the early 1980s, a cancer diagnosis was considered a contraindication for therapies, but improved supportive care and consumer demand initially validated benefits of critical care for these patients. A desire to peruse more aggressive therapies in search of enhanced patient outcomes also led to practice changes within the critical care environment in the 1990s [4].

The value of nutrition support in critically ill patients with cancer, HIV, and bone morrow transplantation is to provide exogenous substrates to meet protein and energy requirements, thereby protecting vital visceral organs and attenuating catabolic responses. Although improved clinical outcomes as a result of nutritional support have been studied inadequately, it seems logical that nutrition-related morbidity and mortality could be prevented or ameliorated by appropriate and timely interventions [2,5].

Metabolic Changes in Critically Ill Patients with Cancer

Nutritional problems associated with malignancy are important, ranging from localized effects induced by the tumor on the organ involved or adjacent structures, to systemic effects caused by metastasis or humoral factors produced by these tumor cells. Significant glucose intolerance, increased fat depletion, and protein turnover are common characteristics of a critically ill cancer patient. Additionally, the malnourished patient with cancer is also unable to conserve energy because of inefficient metabolism.

Several mediators are responsible for metabolic changes in patients with cancer, including hormones, cytokines, and growth factors. Table 35.1 lists cytokine effects on protein, carbohydrate, and lipid metabolism in cancer cachexia. Components associated with daily energy expenditure include basal metabolic rate, the thermogenic effect of exercise, and food intake. In critically ill patients, stress and illness are additional factors that increase energy expenditure [2]. There is usually a negative energy balance that results from a decreased energy intake due to anorexia and/or hypophagia and an energy expenditure that sometimes increases in absolute value and always fails to adapt to

TABLE 35.1
Cytokine Effects on Protein, Carbohydrate, and Lipid Metabolism in Cancer Cachexia

	Protein	Carbohydrate	Lipid
TNF-α	• Increased muscle proteolysis • Increased protein oxidation • Increased hepatic protein synthesis	• Increased glycogenolysis • Decreased glycogen synthesis • Increased glyconeogenesis • Increased glucose clearance • Increased lactate production	• Decreased lipogenesis • Decreased LPL in fat tissue
IL-1	• Increased hepatic protein synthesis	• Increased gluconeogenesis • Increased glucose clearance	• Increased lipolysis • Decreased LPL synthesis • Increased fatty acid synthesis
IL-6	• Increased hepatic protein synthesis		• Increased lipolysis • Increased fatty acid synthesis
IFN-γ			• Decreased lipogenesis • Increased lipolysis • Decreased LPL activity

Source: Findlay, M, Bauer, J, Brown, T, Head and Neck Guideline Steering Committee. Available from http://wiki.cancer.org.au/australia/COSA:Head_and_neck_cancer_nutrition_guidelines/Summary_of_recommendations. In: Head and Neck Guideline Steering Committee. Evidence-based practice guidelines for the nutritional management of adult patients with head and neck cancer. Sydney: Cancer Council Australia. Available from: http://wiki.cancer.org.au/australia/COSA:Head_and_neck_cancer_nutrition_guidelines.

TABLE 35.2
Metabolic Abnormalities in Cancer Patients

Carbohydrate
- Increased gluconeogenesis from amino acids, lactate, and glycerol
- Increased glucose disappearance and recycling
- Insulin resistance

Lipid
- Increased lipolysis
- Increased glycerol and fatty acid turnover
- Lipid oxidation noninhibited by glucose
- Decreased lipogenesis
- Decreased lipoprotein lipase activity
- Nonconstant increase in plasma levels of nonessential fatty acids (NEFA)
- Nonconstant increase in plasma levels of lipid

Protein
- Increased muscle protein catabolism
- Increased whole-body protein turnover
- Increased liver protein synthesis
- Decreased muscle protein synthesis

Source: Findlay, M, Bauer, J, Brown, T, Head and Neck Guideline Steering Committee. Available from http://wiki.cancer.org.au/australia/COSA:Head_and_neck_cancer_nutrition_guidelines/Summary_of_recommendations. In: Head and Neck Guideline Steering Committee. Evidence-based practice guidelines for the nutritional management of adult patients with head and neck cancer. Sydney: Cancer Council Australia. Available from: http://wiki.cancer.org.au/australia/COSA:Head_and_neck_cancer_nutrition_guidelines.

conditions of semi-starvation [6]. The rise in energy expenditure is usually slight (100–300 kcal/day), but, if not compensated by increased energy intake, can cause a loss of body fat (0.5–1 kg) or muscle mass (1–2.3 kg/month) (Table 35.2) [16].

Patients with solid tumors may require critical care when they present initially or if current bulky disease erodes vessels and tissues, or compresses body organs, causing hemorrhages and organ failure. These patients frequently undergo surgical resection, debulking, or reconstructive surgical procedures. Patients with solid tumors are also more likely to receive palliative surgical interventions such as stenting, embolization, catheter or shunt placement, and diverting procedures. The unique critical care needs of these patients vary based on location, initial size, stage of disease, and tumor growth rate, but principles of care are consistent. In all patients, possible and probable complications can be anticipated, and advance planning related to the extent of supportive interventions to be offered should be discussed with patients and their health-care decision-making teams [4].

Nutritional Screening and Assessment in Patients with Cancer

Due to the effects of the tumor and/or the anticancer treatment, patients with cancer are one of the diagnostic groups at greatest risk of developing malnutrition [6]. In the absence of nutrition risk screening, malnutrition may not be recognized or treated [7]. Nutrition risk screening is a quick and easy process to identify patients at malnutrition risk. Most of the tools consist of key items including unintentional weight loss and decreased dietary intake. Several valid and reliable nutrition screening tools for cancer patients exist, including the Malnutrition Universal Screening Tool (MUST), Malnutrition Screening Tool (MST), Nutrition Risk Screening 2002 (NRS-2002), and Mini Nutritional Assessment Short Form Revised (MNA-SFR) for older patients. In a recent review, NRS-2002 received a grade of I, and MST, MNA-SFR, and MUST received grade II evidence to support their use [8]. Clinicians are recommended to use a valid and reliable tool appropriate to their setting (e.g., person conducting the screening, resources available, and intervention protocols in place). Once a nutrition screening identifies an at-risk patient, a more thorough nutrition assessment can then contribute to a diagnosis of malnutrition. Nutrition assessment is more comprehensive than screening and includes a nutritional and medical history, review of dietary intake, nutrition impact symptoms, a physical examination, laboratory parameters, and anthropometric measures [8].

The scored Patient-Generated Subjective Global Assessment (PG-SGA) can be used as a nutrition screen, assessment, and/or outcome measure. However, because it needs to be conducted by a trained health professional, it is typically used as part of a comprehensive nutritional assessment [6]. PG-SGA is based on a combination of known prognostic indicators of weight loss and performance status as well as clinical aspects of dietary intake and its impediments (including nutrition impact symptoms), allowing the identification of malnutrition and assessment of nutritional status [6]. Other validated nutritional assessment tools include the Subjective Global Assessment (SGA) and MNA.

It is recommended that cancer patients be screened at planning or on commencement of anticancer therapy and rescreened regularly thereafter (weekly or every clinic visit) [9].

It is important to measure and record regular body weights as it is not always apparent when someone is losing weight as bulking effect and body changes related to the disease, for example, ascites, might mask lean body weight loss and composition changes. BMI has limitations as the sole measure of nutritional status as malnutrition can be overlooked in patients within *healthy* or *overweight* BMI ranges despite losing significant amounts of weight [6].

Indirect calorimetry (IC) is the standard to allow precise measurements of the daily caloric expenditure in the clinical setting. Ongoing monitoring of nutritional intake, biochemical parameters, body weight, and composition is important to evaluate patient outcomes. If IC is not available, PENN equation (2013) has been proved to reliably calculate energy requirements in critically ill patients. It is suggested to monitor biochemical parameters and body composition as well.

Nutritional Implications of Antineoplastic Therapy

Chemotherapy agents are classified based on their mechanism of action and are given either intravenously or orally. Certain chemotherapy agents have more toxic effects on kidney and liver due to their elimination or metabolism pathways. As these therapies are a systemic treatment, they affect the entire body. Due to potential damage to the epithelium and mucosa of the gastrointestinal tract, antineoplastic therapies may cause nausea, vomiting, diarrhea, altered gastric motility, and altered taste sensation. Continued nutritional intervention throughout cancer diagnosis and treatment can prevent or decrease complications and the severity of side effects [1].

Radiation therapy can affect healthy cells that are near the radiation field, leading to a number of side effects. Precisely which side effects arise will depend on the radiation dose, duration, and site. Additionally, nutrition-related impact symptoms may increase if radiation is given in conjunction with another oncologic therapy such as chemotherapy [1]. Immunotherapy may cause fever, nausea, vomiting, anorexia, and asthenia, which will also affect nutrition intake.

Depending on the site of surgery, nutritional status and function might also be affected. For instance, pharyngeal surgery may lead to chewing and swallowing difficulties. Gastrectomy can cause early satiety, malabsorption, vitamins D and B_{12} deficiencies, hypoglycemia, and dumping syndrome. Intestinal resections can lead to maldigestion and malabsorption of macro- and micronutrients as well as fluid and electrolytes.

Nutritional Management

Ideally, patients undergoing treatment for cancer will meet their nutritional needs to be managed orally. The oral route is physiologically superior and should be maintained as long as possible. Recommending modified textures, fortifying calories in liquids and soft solids, and spacing out eating times are important management tips to help the patient complete treatment with minimal nutrition compromise [10].

Attainable goals of nutrition support in the critically ill patient include the minimization of starvation effects with regard to energy and substrates, prevention of specific nutrient deficiencies, and the support of acute inflammatory response until the hypermetabolic response resolves and healing occurs. Calories sufficient to meet the energy needs of patients should be achieved.

Carbohydrates remain the primary source of energy in hypermetabolic patients and should comprise approximately 60% of nonprotein calories [11]. Exogenous insulin administration tends to be ineffective, increasing cellular uptake in septic patients because of inhibited glucose oxidation [12].

Protein demands are increased markedly in critically ill patients, as well as with oncology patients. The high catabolic rate is refractory to protein or glucose infusion, but protein synthesis is responsive to amino acid infusions making nitrogen balance possible. Protein requirements in septic or injured patients range from 1.2 to 2 g/kg/day [12]. The recommended nonprotein calorie–nitrogen ratio is usually 150:1, but highly stressed patients require a lower ratio of 80:1–100:1 [2]. Fluids and electrolytes should be supplied to maintain adequate urine output and normal serum electrolyte levels.

It is controversial to add antioxidants to medical nutrition therapy in cancer patients [13]. In a recent study, authors found that adding antioxidants in certain dosages during oncology treatment maintained hemoglobin levels [14] and improved QOL in a group of cervical cancer women in oncology therapy with cisplatinum and concomitant radiotherapy [15]. However, nutritional management guidelines for patients with head and neck cancer currently recommend that antioxidants should not be taken during chemotherapy or radiotherapy due to possible tumor protection and reduced survival. Therefore, further studies are required before standard recommendations regarding antioxidants can be made and professional judgment should be used [16].

Regular monitoring of laboratory profile including electrolytes, liver functions, and lipid panel can ensure adequate nutritional supplementation and prevent unwanted complications [2,3].

The timing of nutrition support is determined by the priorities in the care of the critically ill patient. Nutrition intervention is appropriate in the catabolic phase when hemodynamic stability has been attained. The transitions from one phase to another phase of convalescence require nutrition support especially in the phase soon after recovery from a state of hemodynamic instability [17].

Enteral versus Parenteral Nutrition

The general consideration is that "if the gut works, use it." The enteral route is preferred for the provision of nutritional support in the critically ill patient. The enteral route has several advantages over parenteral nutrition: easy administration, good tolerance, promotes mucosal growth and development, helps maintain the barrier function of GI tract, and is less costly. Limitations of enteral feeding are the risk for aspiration and its contraindication in patients with ileus or bowel obstruction. In an article published by Kirby et al., authors discuss the many advantages and changes that have occurred in the nutritional managements of critically ill patients, patients with gastrointestinal diseases, and patients with selected cancers. Mechanical obstruction is the only contraindication to enteral nutrition according to the authors [18].

NUTRITION FOR PATIENTS WITH HUMAN IMMUNODEFICIENCY VIRUS (HIV) AND ACQUIRED IMMUNODEFICIENCY SYNDROME (AIDS)

Nutritional problems have been a part of the clinical aspects of AIDS. The origin of nutritional abnormalities in AIDS patients is multifactorial. The complex mechanisms that cause malnutrition include disorders of metabolism, hypercatabolism, GI tract alterations, and drug–nutrient interactions. Additional factors are psychological, social, and economical issues [19]. Two main paradigms should be considered: cachexia and starvation [20]. The pathophysiologic hallmark of cachexia is a disproportionate loss of lean body mass (LBM), which comprises the body cell mass (CM) and connective tissues, over the losses of body fat mass, with relative preservation of the extracellular body water. These changes result from an increase in metabolic rates, with catabolism predominating over anabolism, and elevations in measured resting energy expenditure. This catabolic state is triggered by events that result in the production and release of cytokines, including interleukin-1 (IL-1), IL-6, tumor necrosis factor, and interferon alpha (IFN-α) [21].

In contrast, starvation results from voluntary or involuntary reduction in food intake or assimilation due to external factors, such as dieting, poverty, famine, or malabsorption.

Metabolic and Nutritional Consequences of HIV Infection

Since HIV infection was recognized, wasting (defined as >5% loss of body weight or BMI < 20.5 kg/m^2) has been a major clinical problem associated with both morbidity and mortality. The importance of wasting as a poor prognostic indicator has formally recognized adoption of unexpected weight loss as an AIDS-defining illness, *the AIDS-wasting syndrome*. Wasting arises from a variety of causes, including altered energy intake, and one of the most marked features of HIV is its ability to generate profound metabolic alterations even in the absence of clinically apparent disease [22].

- *Intestinal abnormalities*: Acute and chronic diarrhea and weight loss have become a part of the clinical diagnosis of AIDS in HIV-infected patients. A variety of causes have been defined; however, in many patients, the cause still remains uncertain. Mucosal changes not associated with documented infection have been called HIV enteropathy [23,24]. Malabsorption should be considered if intake meets the energy requirement, but not the desired effect (stabilization or recovery of weight).
- *Malnutrition*: Protein–energy malnutrition (PEM): given the prominent wasting in AIDS, it is natural that an analogy would be made to PEM as it exists in non-HIV patients. Evidence for PEM in AIDS includes the changes in LBM and decreases in circulating levels of export proteins like serum albumin, pre-albumin, and retinal binding protein in the presence of progressive weight loss [25].
- *Micronutrient deficiencies*: The acute phase response to infection, stress, and inflammation results in rapid shifts of micronutrients from plasma to tissues with intracellular sequestration, as occurs with iron, zinc, and vitamin A [26].

Vitamin levels have been measured in patients with various stages of HIV infections. A particularly compelling issue was the possibility that vitamin B_{12} or folate deficiencies might underlie some of the cognitive changes that occur in AIDS [27]. Vitamin B_6 (pyridoxine) deficiency is common in CDC stage III HIV patients.

Very high doses of vitamins and trace elements are used frequently by HIV-infected individuals, and most encouraging results have come from studies in rural Africa, where RDI has been brought up to 100% and not exceeded; therefore, administering very high doses of vitamins is not recommended [22,27].

The CDC defines the AIDS wasting syndrome as profound involuntary weight loss greater than 10% of baseline body weight plus either chronic diarrhea (at least two stools per day for more than 30 days) or chronic weakness and documented fever for greater than 30 days, intermittent or constant in the absence of concurrent illness, and documented fever for greater than 30 days, intermittent or constant in the absence of concurrent illness or conditions other than HIV infection that could explain findings like that in cancer, tuberculosis, cryptosporidiosis, or other specific enteritis [23,25].

Body weight, however, was demonstrated to be a poor indicator of malnutrition. Loss of fat-free mass is associated with poorer QOL and outcomes. In addition to AIDS, wasting is correlated with reduced survival in other diseases.

Nutritional Intervention

The major goal in HIV-infected patients is the maintenance of LBM. Nutrition support should be focused on optimal nutrition as well as QOL. Recommendations for nutrition interventions are

TABLE 35.3
Stepwise Approach to Optimal Nutrition Support for HIV Patients

Oral diet

- Oral nutrition ad lib without intervention if weight and condition remain stable. Goal is 30–35 kcal and 1.0–1.7 g protein/kg

Oral supplement

- Nutritional counseling by dietician with oral supplementation in case of malnutrition defined by weight loss of 10% in 6 months (this could increase energy intake in about 50% of malnourished HIV-infected patients)

Enteral nutrition

- Enteral nutrition with polymeric formula meeting the criteria of optimal nutrition in case the patient is unable to meet these criteria with oral supplements
- In case of diarrhea, oligomeric formula should be used to influence malabsorption
- The supplementation of sodium to the formula to an amount of 2400 mg/L could also influence the absorption of fluids
- Soluble fibers could be tested to influence diarrhea, but negative side effects should be considered

Parenteral nutrition

- TPN should be considered if enteral route is not available
- Most of AIDS patients using TPN suffer from severe gastrointestinal infections such as crypto- or microsporidiosis in which fecal fat and protein loss are over 20%
- In case of nontreatable infection, home TPN can be considered
- For persistent diarrhea, monitoring electrolytes and adjusting doses via IV are important

Source: McNally, K., *The AIDS Reader*, 8, 121, 1998.

TABLE 35.4
Efficacy and Risks of Drug Interventions on Fat Distribution Alterations in HIV Patients

	Effect over			
Intervention	**Lipoatrophy**	**Lipohypertrophy**	**Lipid Levels**	**Insulin Response**
Lifestyle (diet, exercise)	Unknown	Improve	Improve	Improve
Change ZDV or d4T for ABC or TDF	Improve	No changes	Improve	No changes
Pravastatin	Improve	No changes	↓ Cholesterol	No changes
Metformin	Negative effect	Improve	Improve	Improve
Glitazones	Improve	No changes	Negative effect	Improve
rGH	Negative effect	Improve	Negative effect	Negative effect
Uridine	Improve	Negative effect	↓Cholesterol HDL	No changes

Source: Kalinkovich, A. et al., *Clin. Exp. Immunol.*, 89, 351, 1992.
Abbreviations: ZDV, zidovudine; ABC, abstinence, be faithful, condomise; TDF, tenofovir disoproxil fumarate; HDL, high-density lipoprotein; rGH, growth hormone resurrects.

shown in Table 35.3 [28]. Effects of different drugs used for treating HIV patients and their effect on body composition and nutrition needs are shown in Table 35.4 [23].

An individual infected with HIV should be treated as a chronically infected patient. This means that optimum nutrition should be provided and given, ensuring also that malabsorption is not a problem. Optimum nutrition is described as 30–35 kcal/kg of actual body weight and 1.5–1.7 g of protein/kg actual body weight [22].

Micronutrient requirements should meet 100%–150% RDI, with special attention to antioxidants. If malabsorption is present, the micronutrient status should be evaluated and, if necessary, supplemented orally.

In overweight patients, the provision of protein should be based on current body weight, but energy intake should be adapted to the desired weight of the patient. Especially in patients with lypodystrophia, adequate protein intake should be ensured [22].

Because nutritional therapy has a beneficial effect on the clinical course of immunologic status of critically ill patients, one must not disregard the potential positive benefits of nutritional therapy in the treatment of malnourished HIV/AIDS patients. As a result of the escalating costs of treatment and the predicted AIDS endemic, HIV/AIDS nutritional therapy regimens must be simple to administer and cost-effective [28].

Prior to initiating therapy, some authors advice to interview each patient, perform a complete physical examination, conduct a nutritional assessment, evaluate gut function, and calculate daily caloric and protein requirements. The selection of oral, enteral, and parenteral therapies is crucial in the successful management of these patients [28].

Insufficient food supply, micronutrient deficits, dyslipidemia, insulin resistance, obesity, cardiovascular disease, and bone disorders complicate the treatment of HIV infection. Nutrition and exercise interventions can be effective in ameliorating symptoms associated with HIV and antiretroviral therapy (ART). Macronutrient supplementation can be useful in treating malnutrition and wasting. Multivitamin (vitamin B complex, vitamin C, and vitamin E) supplements and vitamin D may improve QOL and decrease morbidity and mortality [29].

Nutritional counseling and exercise interventions are effective for treating obesity, fat redistribution, and metabolic abnormalities. Physical activity interventions improve body composition, strength, and fitness in HIV-infected individuals. Taken collectively, the evidence suggests that a proactive approach to nutrition and physical activity guidance and interventions can improve outcomes and help abrogate the adverse metabolic, cardiovascular, and psychological consequences of HIV and its treatments [30].

Specific oral nutritional supplements have also been postulated to have beneficial effects on HIV and the wasting syndrome; individuals with higher levels of vitamins B1, B2, B6 and niacin have a survival advantage [31]. In a recent study with a goal to combine probiotics and micronutrients into an affordable and highly palatable nutritional supplement and assess outcomes in HIV-positive participants ($n = 21$) receiving highly active ART, authors found that all yogurt types caused an increase in the subject's energy level and ability to perform daily activity scores. According to the safety measures taken to assess the tolerance of the yogurt, there were no adverse events, and the yogurt was well tolerated. These preliminary findings suggest that micronutrient-supplemented probiotic yogurt may support immune function among people living with HIV [32].

ART and the introduction of the protease inhibitors pose nutritional challenges [33]. All of the protease inhibitors and a few of the nucleoside reverse transcriptase inhibitors have dietary requirements that facilitate absorption and subsequent pharmacologic action. Since most patients report many symptoms, including gastrointestinal disturbances, stomach pain, fatigue, and nausea (which are probably disease related but may be exacerbated by the drugs themselves), it is important to provide adequate dietary counseling to avoid frustration, depression, and poor adherence to the prescribe regimen [34].

Enteral feeding may be useful if the absorptive function of the GI tract remains intact. An elemental diet containing small peptides, branched-chain amino acids, or medium-chain triglycerides may be well tolerated if GI tract function is only partially intact. Low-residue, lactose-free preparations may limit the amount of diarrhea resulting from enteral feedings [35].

Enteral feeding by percutaneous endoscopic gastrostomy (PEG) tubes was studied prospectively [36]. Amino acids were supplied as small peptides, and 40% of the lipid was in the form of medium-chain triglycerides. Although weight gain did not reach statistical significance, there was a significant increase in body CM, fat content, and serum albumin concentrations. Recently, Nataraja et al. aimed to determine the complications of PEG placement in a pediatric HIV-positive population. They concluded that there is a low rate of serious complications with PEG insertion and that the rate was comparable to that seen in pediatric oncology patients. The minor complication rate is, however, higher than a nonimmune-compromised population, and careful patient follow-up is recommended so that the appropriate therapy can be promptly initiated [37].

Administration of total parenteral nutrition (TPN) has been studied in a few small-uncontrolled series of AIDS patients in attempts to facilitate weight gain and replete body CM. In a retrospective study of TPN in 22 patients with more than 10% loss of body weight, 15 patients gained weight and 9 returned to previous activity [36]. Kotler and colleagues [38] demonstrated weight gain in 12 patients with AIDS receiving intravenous TPN.

TPN has demonstrated a variable effect upon body composition, with repletion occurring in patients with eating disorders or malabsorption syndromes, and progressive depletion occurring in patients with serious systemic infections [13]. Enteral nutrition can also replete body mass in AIDS patients without severe malabsorption [35]. Crenn et al. [39] found that plasma citrulline is a reliable biomarker of enterocyte functional mass in HIV patients. Citrulline does not allow the etiologic diagnosis of enteropathy, but it can discriminate between protease inhibitor toxic diarrhea and infectious enteropathy and quantify the functional consequences, which makes it an objective tool for indicating the need for parenteral nutrition [39].

Some authors suggest considering combining both enteral and parenteral support with metabolic support in the acute phase of illness and between bouts of infections to facilitate patient care and to restore lean tissue [36].

Because all HIV/AIDS patients differ in the nutritional requirements, diet tolerance, and degree of intestinal dysfunction, there is no single nutritional therapy regimen that can be utilized in the treatment of all these patients. It is recommended to individualize oral diets combined with food supplements and enteral and parenteral nutrition in the treatment of HIV/AIDS patients [28].

Finally, a group of Spanish experts published recommendation guidelines on nutrition in the HIV patient, with an aim to provide recommendations on the approach to nutritional problems (malnutrition, cachexia, micronutrient deficiency, obesity, lipodystrophy) affecting HIV-infected patients. These recommendations have been agreed upon by a group of experts in the nutrition and care of HIV-infected patients, on behalf of the different groups involved. The latest advances in pathophysiology, epidemiology, and clinical care presented in studies published in medical journals or at scientific meetings were evaluated. The group found that there is no single method of evaluating nutrition status and body composition in these patients, so different techniques—computed tomography (CT scan), magnetic Resonance Imaging (MRI), and dual-energy x-ray absorptiometry (DXA)—must be combined. The energy requirements of symptomatic patients may increase by up to 20%–30%. There is no evidence to support the increase in protein or fat intake. Micronutrient supplementation is necessary only in special circumstances (vitamin A in children and pregnant woman). Aerobic and resistance exercise is beneficial both for cardiovascular health and for improving lean mass and muscular strength. It is important to follow the rules of food safety at every stage of disease. Therapeutic intervention in anorexia and cachexia must be tailored, by combining nutritional and pharmacological support (appetite stimulants, anabolic steroids, and, in some cases, testosterone). Artificial nutrition (oral supplementation, enteral or parenteral nutrition) is safe and efficacious, and improves nutritional status and response to therapy. In children, nutritional recommendations must be made early and are a necessary component of therapy [40].

NUTRITION IN BONE MARROW AND STEM CELL TRANSPLANTATION

The earliest report of therapeutic marrow infusion dates back to 1939, when a patient received intravenous marrow from his brother to treat aplastic anemia [41]. The diseases treated by bone marrow transplantation (BMT) include hematologic malignancies, solid tumors, and other pathologic conditions. These include acute myelogenous leukemia, chronic myelogenous leukemia, acute lymphocytic leukemia, myeloproliferative disorders, multiple myeloma, non-Hodgkins lymphoma, and Hodgkin disease. Solid tumors include breast cancer, testicular cancer, ovarian cancer, glioma, neuroblastoma, small-cell lung cancer, and non-small-cell lung cancer.

Patients with hematological malignancies present with different critical care issues from those with solid tumor malignancies. First, the nature of these malignancies is diffuse at diagnosis, producing general body responses to widespread malignancy such as capillary permeability syndrome, clotting, and catabolism that consequently triggers complications such as respiratory distress, hypotension, disseminated intravascular coagulation, renal insufficiency, and hepatic dysfunction [4,42].

Critical care admission may also be provided based on the use of specific therapies. For many years, the trajectory of hematopoietic stem cell transplantation required severely myelosuppressive, high-dose chemotherapy, or radiation followed by infusion of foreign antigenic material. Frequent admissions to the ICU for these patients occurred due to serious complication rates exceeding 20%–40%. Common reasons for ICU admission for patients with hematopoietic stem cell therapies include respiratory distress, severe bleeding, sepsis, rejection disorders including graft versus host disease (GvHD), and chemotherapy toxicities such as hepatic veno-occlusive disease (VOD) or renal failure [4].

At present, two types of BMT can be performed: allogeneic (allo-BMT) and autologous BMT (a-BMT). BMT involves the transfer of marrow from a donor to a recipient, and allo-BMT involves the use of the patient's own marrow.

High-dose conditioning (HDC) and adjunct peripheral blood stem cell transplantation (PBSCT) are globally accepted methods for the treatment of hematological malignancy (i.e., leukemia, lymphoma, and myeloma) [43]. The stem or progenitor cell transplant consists of antilogous or allogeneic infusion of hematopoietic cells collected from peripheral blood. The cells are collected after the administration of hematopoietic growth factors, with or without chemotherapy.

In BMT, stem cells are taken from the bone marrow, and in PBSCTs, stem cells are taken from the circulating blood. PBSCTs are performed more frequently than BMTs as the procedure is easier and the body can generate new stem cells faster.

Irrespective of the type of BMT, conditioning regimens have tremendous and deleterious consequences on the anatomical and functional integrity of the GI tract; the duration of profound neutropenia produces mucositis. Allo-BMT patients receive conditioning regimens combining high-dose chemotherapy with total-body irradiation to induce profound immunosuppression. Total-body irradiation is extremely toxic, inducing severe and prolonged mucositis.

Within 7–10 days after chemotherapy or chemoradiotherapy, patients almost invariably develop oroesophageal mucositis and GI toxicity. Both conditions may result in decreased oral intake, nausea, vomiting, diarrhea, decreased nutrient absorption, and loss of nutrients from the gut, especially amino acids, secondary to altered transmembrane transport of nutrients.

BMT has evolved as a treatment option for patients with end-stage disease and those at high risk for relapse. The consequences of BMT that affect patient's nutritional status include nutrition impact symptoms such as nausea, vomiting, mucositis, diarrhea, hepatic VOD, and GvHD [2].

Malnutrition is frequent in patients with solid tumors and impaired nutritional status before transplantation is a negative outcome prognostic factor after BMT [4]. Those assessed as malnourished prior to PBSCT have a longer hospital stay [44]. While many patients pre-PBSCT are well nourished, nutritional status often declines posttransplantation and can continue for some time. One prospective study suggested that up to 30% of the PBSCT survivors still experience eating difficulties at day +125 and up to 22% at 1-year post-PBSCT [45]. Weight gain is an unreliable indicator of nutritional status but is significant in considering hepatic VOD, especially in the presence of jaundice and an abnormal liver profile. Nutritional assessment tools such as the SGA or PG-SGA are valid measures of nutritional status in patients with cancer [9]. Metabolic abnormalities include increased protein catabolism, hyperglycemia, increased serum cholesterol and triglycerides, and vitamins (K, B_{12}, thiamine, E, b-carotene) and electrolyte (magnesium, zinc, selenium, copper) deficiencies. In recent years, indications for TPN have decreased in favor of enteral nutrition. However, TPN is still largely used in BMT/PBSCT, mainly because of GI sequelae associated with BMT (e.g., nausea, vomiting, and oroesophageal mucositis) making placement of nasogastric tubes poorly tolerated by BMT patients. Moreover, virtually all patients undergoing BMT/PBSCT have a dedicated central venous catheter in place through which TPN can be safely administered.

Although energy expenditure might differ between a-BMT and allo-BMT patients, consensus dictates that energy requirements in BMT recipients may reach 130%–150% of predicted basal energy expenditure [41]. Therefore, 30–35 kcal/kg body weight per day is usually recommended. Lipids may be safely given, providing 30%–40% of nonprotein energy. Protein needs are also increased and generally satisfied by provision of 1.4–1.5 g/kg body weight per day of a standard amino acid solution. TPN was not strictly *total* because patients may also tolerate oral food intake [46].

TPN is not routinely administered to a-BMT patients unless complications occur, such as prolonged mucositis [47]. Muscaritoli et al. report that TPN should be initiated on day 1 after allo-BMT and continue for 15–21 days according to the intensity and duration of mucositis; oral intake is not allowed during TPN period to minimize the risk of both gut contamination from food and diarrhea. TPN has rapidly moved from simple supportive care to adjunctive therapy because of the potential nutritional benefits of a specialized nutritional intervention, such as improvement of tolerance to chemo-radiotherapy, prevention or reduction of mucositis, reduction of septic complications, and maintenance of immunocompetence and modulation of biological responses.

The possibility that the administration of specific nutritional substrates, such as lipids and glutamine, during the delicate phase of aplasia and bone marrow reconstitution may influence outcome is an intriguing topic deserving further investigation in larger controlled clinical trials.

Glutamine

The rationale for administering glutamine-supplemented nutrition to BMT patients was initially based on the concept that glutamine is the primary fuel for rapidly dividing cells such as enterocytes and for gut-associated lymphoid tissue and that its administration enterally or parenterally could prevent or migrate treatment-induced gastrointestinal toxicity [48].

Glutamine administration after BMT has shown to exert positive effects on nitrogen balance, incidence of infectious complications, lymphocyte counts [49], survival duration of hospital stay, and need for TPN [50].

Nutritional support is considered an integral part of supportive care in BMT and PBSCT patients. TPN still represents the main tool for providing nutritional support to patients undergoing BMT/PBSCT, despite several attempts currently being made at different institutions to feed these patients enterally. The aim of TPN after BMT is to prevent secondary gastrointestinal toxicity and metabolic alterations induced by aggressive conditioning regimens. TPN easily allows for modulation of fluid, electrolyte, and micronutrient provision, which may be necessary considering the complexity and severity of the clinical conditions possible in the post-BMT period. The timing of nutritional support may also be critical in determining the short-term outcome of BMT patients, although controlled data are lacking [47]. HDC and adjunct PBSCT are associated with decreased nutritional status, QOL, and physical activity levels, with fat-free mass remaining below baseline levels at 100 days posttransplantation [50]. Further research is required to determine if a nutrition and exercise intervention program post hospital discharge may be beneficial for these patients.

CONCLUSION

In summary, patients with cancer undergoing BMT/PBSCT are at high nutritional risk and should be identified early through a validated nutrition-screening tool. Malnourished patients or those identified as at nutritional risk should receive appropriate nutrition intervention. This may include a modified texture or fortified diet to enable patients to receive adequate nutrition despite experiencing nutritional impact symptoms. High energy and protein supplements can also be used in addition to replacing an oral diet if not tolerated. If patients cannot meet their nutritional requirements orally and have a functional GI tract, then enteral tube feeding can be considered. Otherwise, TPN can be initiated if there are gastrointestinal problems. Regular rescreening and monitoring of nutritional status is required for best patient outcome. Early and appropriate nutrition intervention has been shown to demonstrate improved patient outcomes, and therefore it is important that the multidisciplinary team considers and manages the nutritional concerns of patients for best QOL and health outcomes.

CASE REPORT 1: Solid Tumor

The patient is a 43-year-old female with gastric cancer. Four months ago, she began experiencing nausea, vomiting, and early satiety. She was taken to the hospital where they ordered a CT scan in which a tumor was found. She was sent to the OR for a total gastrectomy with a gastrojejunoanastomosis and a palliative jejunostomy.

CLINICAL HISTORY

Mother deceased due to gastric cancer.

Father deceased with a history of hypertension.

Two weeks after surgery, she was transferred to a tertiary hospital due to a small bowel fistula, and vascular access for TPN was obtained. Two days later, she underwent fistula closure and was transferred to the ICU postoperatively. She continued with TPN (1500 Kcal), 1.6 g/kg/protein (75 g), which comprised 220 g carbohydrate, 45 g lipid, 75 g protein, plus vitamins and micronutrients.

Actual weight: 45 kg
Height: 155 cm
Glucose: 118 mg/dL (deciliter)
Urea: 56
Creatinine: 0.78
Total protein: 5.90
Albumin: 2.14
Globulin: 3.76
Total bilirubin: 0.78
Direct bilirubin: 0.34
Indirect bilirubin: 0.44

COMMENT

The incidence of gastrojejunal or duodenal stump fistulas following subtotal gastrectomy or total gastrectomy has been reported to be 1%–2% [29], with approximately 25% originating from the gastrojejunostomy. In this review, suture line failure accounted for 82% of all gastroduodenal fistulas. The causes of fistulas arising from the gastrojejunostomy may be related to the suture line containing tumor, ischemia of the gastric stump due to high ligation of the gastric artery and vasa previa, stomal obstruction, pancreatitis, or tension on the suture line.

In all clinical situations, if the gut is functional, then it should be used as the route for feeding. If a fistula develops distal to the site of enteral access, then TPN is indicated. Once the fistula develops, parenteral nutrition should be initiated as soon as possible, particularly in a high-risk malnourished patient. The route of parenteral nutrition should be formulated to meet the patient's calorie and protein goals. In all, nutritional support should be considered supplementation of macronutrients as well as micronutrients or trace elements. Gastrointestinal losses such as fistulas result in the deficiency of multiple trace elements, especially Zn and Se. Fistulas lead to loss of large volumes of protein-rich fluid each day and result in deficiencies of selenium and other trace elements.

CASE REPORT 2: Hematological Malignancy

Max is a male aged 51 years diagnosed with lymphoma.

Treatment: high-dose conditioning and autologous peripheral blood stem cell transplant.

Height: 176.5 cm

Length of hospital stay: 18 days. Following transplantation, Max experiences significant nutrition impact symptoms as shown in the following table. Due to a poor oral intake, Max is losing weight.

Nutritional Assessment Information

At 2 Weeks Pre-Hospital Admission	Discharge	100 Days Posttransplantation
Weight 79.1 kg	Weight 74.2 kg	Weight 78.4 kg
BMI 25.4 kg/m^2	BMI 23.6 kg/m^2	BMI 25.2 kg/m^2
PG-SGA global rating A (well nourished)	PG-SGA global rating B (moderately malnourished)	PG-SGA global rating A (well nourished)
PG-SGA score = 3	PG-SGA score = 18	PG-SGA score = 2
No nutrition impact symptoms. Energy level—*not the usual self*	Significant nutrition impact symptoms: No appetite Foods taste and smell funny Dry mouth, early satiety, fatigue, and lies in bed half of the day Decreased oral intake	No nutrition impact symptoms. Energy level—*not the usual self*
Energy intake 2100 kcal (~9000 kJ)	Energy intake 900 kcal (~3700 kJ)	Energy intake 2000 kcal (8400 kJ)
Protein 75 g	Protein 80 g	Protein 35 g

Nutrition Intervention

Session #1: Nutritional assessment 2 weeks prior to transplantation. Currently well nourished, no nutritional impact symptoms, and eating well.

Encouraged balanced diet and lifestyle in the lead up to the procedure.

Session #2: Days following transplantation

Nutritional diagnosis: Inadequate energy and protein intake as related to nutritional impact symptoms as evidenced by the presence of vomiting, diarrhea, mucositis, no appetite, and minimal oral intake

Goal

1. Minimize weight loss

Strategy

1. Initiate TPN

Session #3: 1 week posttransplant

Nutritional diagnosis: malnutrition as related to inadequate energy and protein intake secondary to nutritional impact symptoms as evidenced by diet history (providing <50% of requirements) and PG-SGA global rating of B

Goals

1. Maintain weight
2. Food safety

Strategies

1. Five to six meal/snacks per day, high energy, and protein options discussed
2. High energy and protein supplements twice daily
3. Safe food practice (education and materials provided)

Session #4: at discharge

Goal

1. Improving nutritional status

Strategies

1. Include protein source at each meal
2. Monitor oral intake and weight regularly
3. Education for healthy diet and lifestyle for home until review 100 days posttransplant

Session #5: 100 days posttransplantation

Goal

1. Maintain nutritional status

Strategies

1. Continue healthy eating and exercise strategies
2. Ongoing monitoring of weight

REFERENCES

1. Marian M, Roberts S. Introduction to the nutritional management of oncology patients. In: Marian M, Roberts S. (eds.), *Clinical Nutrition for Oncology Patients*. Jones & Bartlett Publishers, Boston, MA, 2010.
2. Wong P, Enriquez A, Barrera R. Nutrition support in critically ill patients with cancer. *Oncology and Critical Care*, 17(3):743–767, 2001.
3. Robuck JT, Fleetwood JB. Nutritional support of the patient with cancer. *Focus on Critical Care*, 19(2):129–130, 132–134, 136–138, 1992.
4. Shelton B. Admission criteria and prognostication in patients with cancer admitted to the intensive care unit. Intensive care of the cancer patient. *Critical Care Clinic*, 26(1):1–15, 2010.
5. Klein S, Kinney J, Jeejeeboy K et al. Nutritional support in clinical practice: Review of published data and recommendation for future research directions. *American Journal of Clinical Nutrition*, 66:683–706, 1997.
6. Isenring E, Cross G, Kellett E, Koczwara B, Daniels L. Nutritional status and information needs of medical oncology patients receiving treatment at an Australian public hospital. *Nutrition and Cancer: An International Journal*, 62(2):220–228, 2010.
7. Watterson C, Fraser A, Banks M, Isenring E, Miller M, Silvester C, Hoevnaars R, Bauer J, Vivanti A, Ferguson M. Evidence based practice guidelines for the nutritional management of malnutrition in adult patients across the continuum of care. *Nutrition and Dietetics*, 66(Suppl 3):S1–S34, 2009.
8. Skipper A, Ferguson M, Thompson K, Castellanos V, Porcari J. Nutrition screening tools: An analysis of the evidence. *JPEN*, 36(3):292–298, 2012.
9. Isenring E, Hill J, Davidson W et al. Evidence-based practice guidelines for the nutritional management of patients receiving radiation therapy. *Nutrition and Dietetics*, 65(Suppl. 1):S1–S18, 2008.
10. Whitman MM. The starving patient: Supportive care for people with cancer. *Clinical Journal of Oncology Nursing*, 4:121–125, 2000.
11. Singer P et al. ESPEN guidelines on parenteral nutrition: Intensive care. *Clinical Nutrition*, 28:387–400, 2009.
12. Cresci G. *Nutrition Support for the Critically Ill Patient A Guide to Practice*, CRC Press, Boca Raton, FL, 2005.
13. Fuchs-Tarlovsky V. Role of antioxidants in cancer therapy. *Nutrition*, 2013 Jan;29(1):15–21.
14. Fuchs-Tarlovsky V. Antioxidant supplementation has a positive effect on oxidative stress and hematological toxicity during oncology treatment in cervical cancer patients. *Support Care Cancer*. 2013 May;21(5):1359–1363.
15. Fuchs-Tarlovsky V, Bejarano M, Gutierrez SG, Casillas MA, López-Alvarenga JC, Ceballos G. Efecto de los suplementación con antioxidantes sobre el estrés oxidativo y la calidad de vida durante el tratamiento oncológico. *Nutrición Hospitalaria*, 26(4):819–826, 2011.
16. Cancer Council Australia: Cancer Guidelines Wiki http://wiki.cancer.org.au/australia/COSA (Accessed February 12, 2015.)
17. Bozzetti F. Nutritional support in cancer. In: Allison S, Fürst P et al. (eds.), *Basics in Clinical Nutrition*, 2nd edn., Galen, Prague, Czech Republic, 2000, pp. 239–242.
18. Kirby DF, Teran JC. Enteral feeding in gastrointestinal diseases and cancer. *Gastrointestinal Endoscopy Clinics of North America*, 8(3):623–643, 1998.
19. Fajardo A, Lara C. Intervención nutricional en VIH/SIDA, una guía práctica para su intervención y seguimiento. *Gac. Méd Mex*, 137(5):489–500, 2001.
20. Kotler DP. The wasting report 1996. In: *Eleventh International Conference on AIDS*, Vancouver, British Columbia.
21. Kalinkovich A et al. Elevated serum levels of TNF receptors (s TNF-R) in patients with HIV infection. *Clinical and Experimental Immunology*, 89:351–355, 1992.
22. Jonkers CF, Sauerwein HP. Nutrition support in AIDS. In: Allison S, Fürst P et al. (eds.), *Basics in Clinical Nutrition*, 2nd edn., Galen, Prague, Czech Republic, 2000, pp. 247–250.
23. Recomendaciones Sobre Alteraciones Metabólicas en Pacientes Con Infección Por el Vih (Marzo 2009). Grupo de expertos de GEAM, GESIDA y la Secretaría del Plan nacional sobre el sida. GEAM. Grupo de Estudio de Alteraciones Metabólicas en Sida GESIDA. Grupo de Estudio de Sida SPNS. Secretaría del Plan Nacional sobre el Sida.
24. Ramratnam B et al. A practical approach to managing diarrhea in the HIV-infected person. *The AIDS Reader*, 7(6):190–196, 1997.
25. Kotler DP et al. Wasting syndrome: Nutritional support in HIV infection. *AIDS Research and Human Retroviruses*, 10:931–934, 1994.

26. McNally K. Nutritional assessment and management for patients with HIV disease. *The AIDS Reader* 8(3):121–130, 1998.
27. Coodley GO et al. Micronutrient concentrations in the HIV wasting syndrome. *AIDS*, 7(12):1595–6000, 1993.
28. Hickey MS, Weaver KE. *Gastrointestinal Endoscopy Clinics of North America*, 17(3):545–561, 1988.
29. Acton QA. Issues in AIDS, HIV and STD research and treatment. *Schoraly Editions.* Altanta, GA. 2013. ISBN:978-1-490-10834-6: 77–139.
30. Botros D, Somarriba G, Neri D, Miller TL. Interventions to address chronic disease and HIV: Strategies to promote exercise and nutrition among HIV-infected individuals. *Curr HIV/AIDS Rep* 9:351–363, 2012.
31. Horn T et al. The wasting report: Current issues in research and treatment of HIV associated wasting and malnutrition. Treatment Action Group, 1996.
32. Hemsworth JC, Hekmat S, Reid G. Micronutrient supplemented probiotic yogurt for HIV-infected adults taking HAART in London, Canada. *Gut Microbes*, 3(5):414–419, 2012.
33. Achim S. HIV infection and malnutrition. *Current Opinion in Clinical and Metabolic Care*, 1:375–380, 1998.
34. Shevitz AH, Knox TA. Nutrition in the era of highly active antiretroviral therapy. *CID*, 32(15 June):1769–1775, 2001.
35. Kotler DP et al. Nutritional effects and support in the patients with AIDS. *Journal of Nutrition*, 122:723–727, 1992.
36. Singer P et al. Clinical and immunologic effects of lipid. Based parenteral nutrition in AIDS. *Journal of Parenteral and Enteral Nutrition*, 16:165–167, 1992.
37. Nataraja RM, Fishman JR, Nasser A et al. Percutaneous endoscopic gastrostomy placement in a human immunodeficiency virus-positive pediatric population leads to an increase in minor complications. *Journal of Laparoendoscopic & Advanced Surgical Techniques, Part A*, 21(2):171–175, 2011.
38. Kotler DP et al. Effect of home TPN on body composition in patients with AIDS. *Journal of Parenteral and Enteral Nutrition*, 14:454–458, 1990.
39. Crenn P, DeTruchis P, Neveux N. Plasma citrulline is a biomarker of enterocyte mass and an indicator of parenteral nutrition in HIV-infected patients. *American Journal of Clinical Nutrition*, 90(3):587–594, 2009.
40. Polo R, Gómez-Candela C, Miralles C et al. Recommendations from SPNS/GEAM/SENBA/SENPE/AEDN/SEDCA/GESIDA on nutrition in the HIV-infected patient. *Nutricion Hospitalaria*, 22(2):229–243, 2007.
41. Osgoog EE, Riddle MC, Matthews TJ. Aplastic anemia treated with daily transfusion and intravenous marrow. *Annals of Internal Medicine*, 13:357–367, 1939.
42. Bhatt V. Review: Drug-induced neutropenia pathophysiology, clinical features, and management. *Annals of Clinical & Laboratory Science* 34:131–137, 2004.
43. Gratwohl A et al. Hematopoietic stem cell transplantation a global perspective. *Journal of the American Medical Association*, 303(16):1617–1624, 2010.
44. Horsley P, Bauer J, Gallagher B. Poor nutritional status prior to peripheral blood stem cell transplantation is associated with increased length of hospital stay. *Bone Marrow Transplant*, 35(11):1113–1116, 2005; Ottery FD. The clinical guide to oncology nutrition. In McCallum P. Polisena C. (eds.), *Patient Generated Subjective Global Assessment*, American Dietetic Association, Chicago, IL, 2000, pp. 11–23.
45. Iestra, JA et al. Body weight recovery, eating difficulties and compliance with dietary advice in the first year after stem cell transplantation: A prospective study. *Bone Marrow Transplant*, 29(5):417–424, 2002.
46. Chamouard C, Chambrier VC, Michallet M et al. Energy expenditure during allogeneic and autologous bone marrow transplantation. *Clinical Nutrition*, 17:253–257, 1998.
47. Muscaritoli M, Grieco G, Capria S, Iori AP, Rossi Fanelli F. Nutritional and metabolic support in patients undergoing bone marrow transplantation. *American Journal of Clinical Nutrition*, 75:183–190, 2002.
48. Piccirillo N, De Matteis S et al. Glutamine-enriched parenteral nutrition after analogous peripheral blood stem cell transplantation: Effects on immune reconstitution and mucositis. *Haematologica*, 88(2):192–200, 2003.
49. Ziegler TR, Young LS, Benfell K et al. Clinical and metabolic efficacy of glutamine supplemented parenteral nutrition after bone marrow transplantation. A randomized double-blind, controlled study. *Annals of Internal Medicine*, 116:821–828, 1992.
50. Hung Y, Bauer J, Horsley P, Bashford J, Isenring E. Changes in nutritional status, body composition, quality of life, and physical activity level of cancer patients undergoing autologous peripheral blood stem cell transplantation. *Supportive Care in Cancer*, 21(6):1579–1586, 2013.

36 Nutrition Support in the Chronically Critically Ill Patient

Rifka C. Schulman and Jeffrey I. Mechanick

CONTENTS

INTRODUCTION

Chronic critical illness (CCI) defines an increasingly recognized unique subset of critically ill patients. While surviving the acute phase of severe illness, these patients are dependent on prolonged mechanical ventilation (PMV), artificial nutrition, and a host of multi-organ support for an extended period of time. The CCI syndrome (CCIS) describes a characteristic metabolic phenotype due to chronic inflammation, irrespective of the inciting acute illness (e.g., trauma, sepsis, or surgery). By consensus, CCI commences at the time of tracheotomy, typically performed after 10–14 days of mechanical ventilation, reflecting the view that the patient will neither die nor be weaned from the ventilator in the near future. While the ultimate goal is liberation from mechanical ventilation, attention to nutritional and metabolic parameters is now understood to play an integral role in the recovery process of CCI, as previously outlined by our group [1].

This growing patient population, fueled by technological advances in the intensive care unit (ICU), carries a tremendous burden of morbidity, mortality, and cost; fewer than 50% are liberated from the ventilator, and 1-year mortality rates are estimated at 48%–68% [2]. Interventions to ameliorate this burden are likely to have a significant impact. Early identification of those patients unlikely to recover and most fitting for a palliative care approach is important for patients and their families, in addition to minimizing excessive cost to hospitals.

METABOLIC MODEL OF CRITICAL ILLNESS

Critical illness can be understood as comprising distinct stages within the context of allostatic change. Why develop this model? It is hoped that identifying patient subsets based on a coherent physiological state can clarify clinical management strategies and interpretation of clinical research evidence.

While homeostasis is the capacity to maintain essential physiological parameters within a narrow range, allostasis refers to the adjustment of homeostatic set points in response to a stressor [3]. Allostasis is necessary for the survival of a threatened organism in the short term, but with recurrent stressors, allostatic load and ultimately overload occur consuming vital resources and organ reserve [4]. Four distinct metabolic phases of critical illness are constructed: acute critical illness (ACI), prolonged acute critical illness (PACI), CCI, and recovery from critical illness (RCI) [5].

ACI follows an inciting event triggering a programmed Darwinian adaptive *stress response*. This allostatic process is mediated by enhanced neuroendocrine activity, with a catecholamine and cytokine repertoire that confers a survival advantage [6]. The resulting hormonal milieu is associated with a state of insulin resistance and diverts substrate from anabolic to catabolic pathways. Certain cytokines (tumor necrosis factor-α, interleukin-1, and IL-6) shift reverse-phase reactants (e.g., albumin, transferrin, and cortisol-binding globulin) to acute-phase reactants (e.g., C-reactive protein and immunoglobulins) and stimulate skeletal muscle proteolysis [7]. Effects of acute illness on adipose tissue include enhanced lipolysis, recruitment of macrophages, reductions in anti-inflammatory adiponectin, and an increase in proinflammatory cytokines [8]. Increased gluconeogenesis and suppression of peripheral glucose uptake result in stress-induced hyperglycemia [9].

PACI, beginning at around day 3 of critical illness, constitutes a persistent state of heightened catabolism, inflammation, and insulin resistance. Immune–neuroendocrine (INA) output fails to downregulate in PACI, and as a result, tissue breakdown continues to provide needed substrates. This process of allostatic load accrual eventuates in a state of allostatic overload, which conceptually means that there exists a physiological debt that cannot be repaid. Life-preserving metabolic adaptations occurring early in ACI emerged through natural selection. These physiological networks are programmed, predictable, and constitute the lessons learned in formal medical education. However, once a patient depends on technology for life preservation, physiological networks have decayed into unpredictable and potentially detrimental processes that have had no evolutionary precedent.

CCI, beginning with tracheotomy at around day 10–14, represents a unique physiological state where independent of the inciting event, patients assume a common phenotype due to extensive allostatic loading: the CCIS. Classic features of the CCIS include (1) PMV requiring tracheostomy placement, (2) kwashiorkor-like malnutrition (3), stress hyperglycemia, (4) neuroendocrine dysfunction, (5) impaired wound healing, (6) compromised immune function, (7) metabolic bone disease, (8) critical illness myopathy and polyneuropathy, (9) neurocognitive dysfunction, and (10) excessive symptom burden [5,10]. Recently, we have subtyped CCI based on the inflammatory status of the patient. Type-1 CCI designates a fulminant, multisystem pathophysiology, propagated by allostatic overload or extensive allostatic loading. Type-2 CCI, or single-system CCI, describes patients with PMV unable to liberate from mechanical ventilation due to neuromuscular or anatomical reasons, but in whom allostatic unloading occurs with INA downregulation to near-normal levels [1].

RCI, if achieved, generally begins with successful liberation from mechanical ventilation and involves downregulation of inflammatory allostatic mechanisms and resumption of anabolic processes. Survivors of CCI frequently suffer from persistent organ dysfunction, disability, and impaired quality of life. This highlights a salient problem with this metabolic model: demarcations between sequential stages are blurred, necessitating more rigorous, evidence-based criteria.

Thus, two unanswered questions regarding the metabolic model are "how to validate this concept?" and "what are the best markers for each stage?" For now, validation is supported by the successful clinical application of these concepts in practice and research. Candidate markers are those reflecting INA activity, including humoral pulsatility and biorhythms.

MALNUTRITION OF CCI

One of the prototypical features of the CCIS is the presence of kwashiorkor-type malnutrition. A heightened state of inflammation, mediated via the action of cytokines, enhances proteolysis and inhibits hepatic synthesis of albumin, in the setting of increased cellular protein utilization [7]. Resultant hypoalbuminemia facilitates third-spacing and the development of anasarca, predisposing the CCI patient to pulmonary edema, skin breakdown, and malabsorption due to gut edema. Further loss of nitrogen commonly occurs through diarrhea, vomiting, wound drainage, ostomy output, and/or hemodialysis [11]. Muscle atrophy is exacerbated by immobilization, impaired neuroendocrine function (e.g., hypogonadotropic hypogonadism), and side effects of medications. Kwashiorkor-type malnutrition is differentiated from marasmic-type malnutrition, which follows simple starvation in the absence of heightened inflammation and hypoalbuminemia. Alternatively, newer terminology classifies malnutrition by etiology and increasing level of inflammation: starvation-related, chronic disease-related, or acute disease-related malnutrition [12].

Provision of timely nutrition support to the CCI population is essential to attenuate catabolism and loss of lean body mass, but has classically been associated with common pitfalls. Both over- and undernutrition have been frequently reported in the ICU, related to lack of knowledge or prioritization on the part of physicians, difficulties with the determination of energy and protein goals in the grossly edematous patient, impaired gastrointestinal (GI) function, and feeding interruptions for procedures or ventilator weaning trials. Underfeeding in the ICU, with a subsequent accumulation of an *energy debt*, has been associated with increased rates of nosocomial infection [13], prolonged dependence on mechanical ventilation [14], possibly related to atrophy of diaphragmatic muscles, and mortality [15]. Overfeeding is similarly harmful, also predisposing to infection and increased mortality via mechanisms of impaired glycemic control, liver dysfunction, hypertriglyceridemia, and azotemia [16].

The strategic goals for nutrition support in the CCI population include (1) decreasing the component of catabolism due to negative energy balance, while avoiding the detrimental effects of overfeeding; (2) suppression of cytokine-mediated inflammation; (3) optimization of nitrogen retention for preservation of lean body mass; (4) correction of any micronutrient deficiencies or functional insufficiencies; and (5) decreasing the amount of allostatic load so that allostatic overload dissipates (INA downregulates) with resultant improvement in organ function. This last point is somewhat nebulous at first impression, but we propose that allostatic load can, in fact, be reduced through meticulous attention to virtually every metabolic metric (clinical and biochemical) demonstrated. This is based on the premise that the CCI state is a complex network, where emergent clinical outcomes can be optimized by addressing every abnormal node (e.g., β-cell function, bone hyperresorption) or edge (e.g., insulin sensitivity, bisphosphonate sensitivity) [17]. This novel therapeutic paradigm undoubtedly requires validation as well.

NUTRITIONAL ASSESSMENT

Evaluation of the nutritional status of the CCI patient begins with a thorough history and physical examination. Assessment should identify preexisting malnutrition based on prehospital weight and body mass index (BMI), recent loss of weight or poor appetite, comorbidities, and status of the GI tract. If prehospital weight is unknown, admission weight is preferred to later weights, which typically follow large volume resuscitation and fluid shifts. Severity of disease and degree of inflammation are also important indicators of nutritional risk. Physical examination should take note of the presence or absence of sarcopenia, anasarca, signs of micronutrient deficiencies, nonhealing wounds, and other possible sources of nitrogen loss.

Review of biochemical parameters, including electrolytes, renal, and liver functions, is essential prior to the initiation of nutrition support, in order to design a safe and patient-specific formula. Hypoalbuminemia, an expected abnormality in the CCIS, is a reflection of the extent of inflammation, and not a direct indicator of nutritional status [18]. Interestingly, improvement in albumin levels has been shown to correlate with improved outcome in the CCI population [19]. Prealbumin, with a shorter half-life than albumin, may be a better indicator of short-term nutritional sufficiency, but has not been shown to correlate with outcome.

Use of various instruments for the determination of body composition, such as ultrasound, dual x-ray absorptiometry, magnetic resonance imaging, and bioelectrical impedance, has not been shown to be helpful in the CCI population. The cutaneous skin-fold assessment is considered inaccurate for these patients due to edema.

Various screening tools have been developed in order to objectively assess a patient's nutritional risk. The Nutritional Risk Screening (NRS 2002) is a widely used evidence-based tool, validated in the general population of hospitalized patients [20]. This semiquantitative tool utilizes a point system accounting for the degree of undernutrition (e.g., weight loss, BMI, and decreased oral intake) and severity of disease, with nutrition support recommended for patients with a combined score of ≥3 out of 7. This tool is problematic for discriminating severity of nutritional risk in a critically ill population, as nearly all ICU patients would qualify for ≥3 points. Recently, Heyland et al. [21] described the NUTRIC score, specifically validated in a population of medical-surgical ICU patients, remaining in the ICU for 3 days or longer (i.e., PACI + CCI + RCI). This scoring system incorporates markers of acute and chronic starvation, and acute and chronic inflammation, which were shown in this prospective observational study to correlate with worse outcome and most improvement with aggressive nutritional support. Because a risk assessment tool validated solely in the CCI population has not been designed, extrapolation from an ICU-specific tool, combined with clinical judgment, seems prudent to best evaluate the CCI patient for nutritional risk.

NUTRITION COMPONENTS

Accurate determination of energy goals in the CCI population is challenging. Indirect calorimetry, the *gold standard* for the calculation of energy requirements in the clinical setting, requires expertise and special equipment to operate, is expensive and unavailable at many institutions, and is associated with a number of potential confounding factors. Alternatively, numerous predictive equations have been designed to predict energy requirements, some adding a stress factor to reflect the hypermetabolism of critical illness. Despite multiple comparative studies, there is no consensus as to which equation is most accurate in the ICU population, and no formula validated solely in the CCI population. Furthermore, weight-based formulas are confounded by fluid status and body composition, with lean body mass being more metabolically active than fat mass. Therefore, adjustments should be made for the obese and the elderly, groups in which the ratio of lean to fat mass is typically decreased. One approach is to use the adjusted body weight (AjBW) in the obese population: AjBW = IBW + [(ABW − IBW) × correction factor], where ABW is the actual body weight, IBW is the ideal body weight, and the correction factor is between 0.25 and 0.50 [22].

The recent tight calorie control study (TICACOS) study, a prospective randomized trial of mechanically ventilated ICU patients, found a trend toward not only reduced hospital mortality but also an increase in the length of stay, duration of mechanical ventilation, and infection rate, in the subset of patients with nutrition requirements determined by frequent performance of indirect calorimetry, compared to those utilizing a predictive equation [23]. Determination of energy goals in the CCI patient is therefore controversial, and challenging, and benefits from clinical judgment in combination with the tool or formula used.

For convenience, a simple approach is to use 20–25 kcal/kg/day of dry, adjusted weight for the determination of energy requirements [24]. A minimum intake of about 100 g of dextrose per day and 1 g/kg/week of lipid is recommended to avoid starvation-related catabolism and essential fatty acid deficiency, respectively [25,26].

A paramount goal of nutrition support in the CCIS is to attenuate nitrogen loss and to maximally preserve lean body mass, which is catabolized through the natural course of critical illness. Therefore, the significance of providing adequate nitrogen, as the protein component of a nutrition support regimen, must be stressed in this patient population. Determination of nitrogen balance through urine collection studies is confounded by nitrogen loss via other routes (e.g., wounds, diarrhea, and hemodialysis) and is infrequently performed. Calculation of protein requirements is therefore reliant on predictive equations, generally accepted as 1.2–1.5 g/kg/day in the critically ill population [27], but must be tailored to the individual CCI patient based on clinical and biochemical factors. Consideration for providing up to 2.0 g/kg/day can be made on a case-by-case basis for patients identified with other routes of nitrogen loss, and especially following burns or trauma. A recent prospective observational study showed that attainment of target protein goals of at least 1.2 g/kg/day plus reaching target energy goals by indirect calorimetry in a cohort of critically ill patients was associated with a 50% reduction in 28-day mortality [28]. Patients achieving energy but not protein goals showed no association with mortality. Other research supports the notion of a positive correlation between energy intake and nitrogen balance, with adequate energy intake required to mitigate hypercatabolism [29].

MODE OF NUTRITION SUPPORT

The primary mode of nutrition in CCI, as in the general ICU population, is enteral nutrition (EN). Semi-elemental formulas, comprised of hydrolyzed protein, are preferred over whole-protein formulas, having been associated with improvements in diarrhea and visceral protein stores and a decreased length of stay in trauma and critically ill patients [30–32]. Clinical factors such as hyperglycemia, altered electrolytes, and fluid status should facilitate choice of an optimal patient-specific enteral formula. Standard use of high-fat, low-carbohydrate *pulmonary formulas* to decrease CO_2 generation from carbohydrate oxidation has not shown to be effective in ventilator management and may cause delayed gastric emptying due to high fat content [33].

Use of immune-enhancing EN, containing an increased ω-3:ω-6 fatty acid ratio and antioxidants, has been considered for potential benefit in the critically ill population. While conflicting data have previously been reported on this subject, the recent OMEGA study, a randomized placebo-controlled trial of patients with acute lung injury, showed no outcome benefit and possible harm (fewer ventilator-free days and more days with diarrhea) with immune-enhancing EN compared to control EN [34]. This form of nutrition has not been specifically studied in the CCI population and cannot be routinely recommended based on the available data.

All efforts to optimize the use of the enteral route are advocated, including the use of prokinetic agents, tolerance of higher volumes of gastric residuals up to 500 mL [35], and consideration for postpyloric feeding access. A prospective randomized study of *more severely ill* ICU patients (APACHE II score >20) showed an association with improved nutrition intake and nitrogen balance, and reduced EN-related complications and ICU length of stay, in patients utilizing nasojejunal versus nasogastric feeding routes [36]. No such association was seen in the *lesser severely ill* group, in whom nasogastric feeding is preferred. Recently, volume-based EN protocols, in which the total daily goal volume of nutrition guides the delivery rate, have been advocated to compensate for missed nutrition while feeds are held on standard protocols [37].

One question in the literature that has sparked much debate involves the indications for use of parenteral nutrition (PN) for the critically ill. CCI-specific data are not available in this area and must be extrapolated from the general ICU literature base. While use of EN as the primary mode of nutrition is widely accepted, many ICU patients cannot reach energy and protein targets due to impairment of the GI tract and holding of feeds prior to procedures and trials of ventilator weaning.

Supplemental parenteral nutrition (SPN), the addition of PN to maximally tolerated EN, is a potential mechanism to maximize the delivery of target nutrition. The appropriate timing of SPN differs across continents, with the American Society for Parenteral and EN recommending withholding of SPN for the first 7 days in the ICU in previously healthy patients [35] and the European Society for Clinical Nutrition and Metabolism endorsing the use of SPN in appropriate patients after day 2 in the ICU [25]. The disagreement emanates from methodological differences (prioritization of randomized controlled trials over prospective cohort studies) in prior studies of PN, documenting potential hazards such as increased rates of hyperglycemia and infection, and poorer outcomes. Importantly, these studies were performed in settings of overfeeding by the current standard, the absence of tight glycemic control, and before the institution of central line—associated bacteremia prevention protocols. Another potential mechanism of harm induced by PN involves an attenuation of autophagy, a protective pathway responsible for the removal of cellular debris, which is known to be impaired due to critical illness [38].

Recently, the multicenter randomized controlled EPaNIC trial [39] compared late versus early timing of the initiation of SPN, in the setting of tight glycemic control. Results found no mortality difference, but a decreased median ICU length of stay (3 vs 4 days) and reduced infectious rate in the late initiation group. However, a closer look reveals the relative health of the study population with a low ICU mortality of 6%, short ICU length of stay, and exclusion of severely malnourished patients from the study [40]. The NRS 2002 tool used in the trial to identify patients at nutritional risk, not validated in an ICU population, may have been suboptimal. One possible conclusion of these results is that early SPN is of no benefit and potentially harmful in lower nutritional risk patients, but for high-risk patients, potential benefit cannot be ruled out [41]. Other potential confounding factors in the EPaNIC trial include the use of standardized PN formulas, the large intravenous dextrose infusion used in the early SPN group over the first 48 h in the ICU, which may have been detrimental, and the absence of indirect calorimetry to substantiate nutritional targets. Of note, another recent randomized controlled trial from Geneva showed improved outcome with SPN, added after ICU day 3 in patients estimated to stay greater than 5 days in the ICU, and using indirect calorimetry for energy determination [42].

Based on the available ICU data, current understanding of the pathophysiology of the CCIS, and clinical experience caring for this burdened patient population, an approach should be taken to maximize delivery of nutrition, targeting energy (as dextrose and lipid), protein, and micronutrient goals. If nutrition goals cannot be met with EN, consideration for SPN should be made on a case-by-case basis. Of note, patients with CCI have by definition been in the ICU greater than 7 days and would qualify for use of SPN according to both American and European guidelines. The more important question lies in the initiation of nutrition support earlier in the ICU stay (during ACI or PACI) to attenuate catabolism and inflammation and *prevent* the transition to CCI.

MONITORING AND TROUBLESHOOTING

Once a nutrition support regimen is initiated, close monitoring of clinical and biochemical variables is imperative to ensure maximal benefit and to minimize harm to the CCI patient. Daily monitoring of electrolytes, glucose, renal, and liver function is recommended initially to assess tolerance and guide the adjustment of type and volume of enteral formula, or possibly of the components of PN. Monitoring of weights, *I's and O's*, sodium and BUN level, and the fluid status of the patient can guide the use of more or less concentrated formulas, and the provision of free water requirements. Albumin and prealbumin should be followed, but with an understanding that decreased levels are reflective of the degree of inflammation and may not directly reflect nutritional status.

Serum phosphorus levels should be monitored, with hypophosphatemia a common finding, and typically reflecting *refeeding hypophosphatemia*, a milder version of the well-described *refeeding syndrome*, or vitamin D deficiency, particularly common among CCI patients [43,44]. Phosphate supplementation is important to optimize diaphragmatic muscle strength needed for ventilator weaning. Refeeding syndrome may develop in chronically or severely malnourished patients in response to the reintroduction of carbohydrate to the starved metabolic state. In addition to hypophosphatemia, refeeding syndrome is characterized by hypokalemia, hypomagnesemia, fluid overload, and, in severe cases, multiorgan failure. If suspected, dextrose and fluid volume should be limited temporarily with close monitoring of electrolytes and fluid status.

Evidence of possible overfeeding (e.g., hyperglycemia, abnormal liver function, and azotemia) should prompt a temporary decrease in nutrition rate and further investigation for other etiologies. Furthermore, consideration of the total amount of calories received, including dextrose in intravenous fluids and lipid-based propofol infusions, should guide the nutrition support prescription.

Conversely, inability to attain target nutrition from the enteral route should encourage utilization of all possible strategies including SPN, if indicated. Consideration for intradialytic PN may be appropriate for supplementing nutrition in patients with end-stage renal disease [45].

Diarrhea frequently complicates the delivery of EN in the CCIS. In addition to simple intolerance of feeds, common etiologies include kwashiorkor-related gut edema, infection with *Clostridium difficile*, stool impaction, and sorbitol-containing medications. Possible consequences of untreated diarrhea include dehydration, electrolyte abnormalities, malabsorption, and skin irritation, predisposing to the development of decubiti ulcers. Once correctible etiologies, such as infection, have been excluded, potential therapies based on clinical experience, and not strong evidence, include the addition of bismuth/salicylate directly to EN (10–30 mL/500 cc bag) or 4 g of cholestyramine two to three times daily [5]. If tolerance to semi-elemental feeds cannot be accomplished, a diluted elemental formula can be trialed. The practice of adding prebiotics (inulin, oligofructosaccharides) or probiotics (*Bifidobacterium, Lactobacillus*) for CCI patients with recurrent *C. difficile* infection may be beneficial and is thought to confer minimal risk; the evidence on this practice remains inconclusive.

METABOLIC CONTROL

Metabolic control of glycemic status plays a significant role in the delivery of safe and effective nutrition support in the CCI population. As mentioned earlier, the inflammatory pathophysiology of the CCIS creates a metabolic milieu propagating insulin resistance and impaired glucose uptake mechanisms. Resultant *stress hyperglycemia* has been associated with a multitude of harmful effects, including oxidative tissue damage, proinflammatory effects, and endothelial dysfunction [9]. Sustained hyperglycemia has been linked to poor clinical outcomes, including increased rates of infection and impaired wound healing [46,47]. Furthermore, glycemic variability has been shown to be an independent predictor of mortality in the ICU [48,49].

The evidence base on tight glycemic control has put forth a pendulum of views in the ICU over the past decade. While traditional thinking considered stress hyperglycemia a benign response to critical illness, Van den Berghe et al. showed, in 2001, improved morbidity and mortality in the Leuven surgical ICU with tight glycemic control using intravenous insulin, targeting blood glucose 80–110 mg/dL, compared to the traditional approach (BG < 215 mg/dL) [50]. A subsequent similar study in the medical ICU by Van den Berghe showed improved morbidity but not mortality in the tight glycemic control group [51]. These proof-of-concept studies could not be replicated in subsequent years, culminating in 2009 with the Normoglycemia in Intensive Care Evaluation-Survival Using Glucose Algorithm Regulation (NICE-SUGAR) study, which showed an increased mortality and increased rate of severe hypoglycemia in the tight control group (80–108 mg/dL) compared to moderate control (140–180 mg/dL) [52]. A recent *post hoc* analysis of the NICE-SUGAR study database showed a strong association between moderate and severe hypoglycemia and the risk of death [53]. While a number of important differences in the Leuven and NICE-SUGAR study designs help with interpretation of the disparate results, of note is the delivery of nutrition to goal in the Van den Berghe studies (with the addition of SPN when needed), while patients in NICE-SUGAR were underfed: 19 versus 11 kcal/kg/day, respectively [54]. The ability to safely attain tight glycemic control without excessive risk of hypoglycemia appears to be linked to the delivery of adequate nutrition. Thus, the strong interplay between metabolic control and nutrition support is evident, with the two components both required for optimal outcome [55]. Another conclusion from the results of these studies is that the level of attainable safe glycemic control may vary by the capabilities and resources of the particular institution or hospital unit [56].

While application of the concepts of glycemic control for CCI have previously required extrapolation from the general ICU literature, recent work by our group at the Mount Sinai Hospital's respiratory care unit (RCU) has focused specifically on the CCI population. In our unit, point-of-care glucose testing every 6 h guides a subcutaneous insulin protocol of long and rapid-acting insulin, targeting 80–110 mg/dL. A retrospective review of blood glucose data on our unit (n = 58) demonstrated a

TABLE 36.1
RCU Insulin Dosing Protocol

Insulin Total Daily Dose	Standing Insulin	Correction Insulin
<20 units	Q24h basal peakless insulin (glargine, detemir)	Q6h rapid-acting insulin (lispro, aspart, glulisine)
20–40 units	Q12h basal peakless insulin (glargine, detemir)	Q6h rapid-acting insulin (lispro, aspart, glulisine)
41–80 units	Q6h intermediate acting insulin (NPH)	Q6h rapid-acting insulin (lispro, aspart, glulisine)
>80 units	Q6h intermediate acting insulin (NPH)	Q3h rapid-acting insulin (lispro, aspart, glulisine)

Source: Adapted from Hollander, J.M. and Mechanick, J.I., *Nutr. Clin. Pract.*, 21, 587, 2006.

Notes: After initial determination of a total daily dose of insulin (typically using a weight-based formula such as 0.3–0.6 units/kg), combinations of long/intermediate and rapid-acting insulin can be used in conjunction with enteral nutrition to optimize glycemic control in patients with CCI.

mean blood glucose of 128.4 mg/dL after the first 72 h in the RCU with concomitant low rates of hypoglycemia [57]. Table 36.1 outlines our approach to insulin dosing in CCI patients, based on the total daily dose of insulin, with every 6 h dosing of NPH insulin used for higher total daily doses. In the RCU, strategies employed to optimize tight but safe glycemic control include close monitoring of nutritional delivery, staff education of nurses and nurse practitioners regarding optimal glycemic management, and a bag of 10% dextrose at the bedside for use when tube feeds are interrupted to prevent hypoglycemia with insulin on board.

NUTRITION/ENDOCRINE PHARMACOLOGY

Aside from nutrition support and metabolic control, a variety of substances have been considered for adjunctive beneficial roles in the CCIS. Again, the majority of available evidence in this area is extrapolated from the general ICU population.

Glutamine, an amino acid that is frequently deficient in critical illness, has been posited to augment nitrogen retention and immune function. While smaller studies have shown improved outcome, including decreased length of stay and mortality [58,59], a recent randomized controlled trial administering short-term (up to 7 days) parenteral glutamine in the ICU found no effect on the incident rates of infection [60]. Potential benefits of longer-term supplementation or effects on other outcomes require further study. Possible adverse effects of glutamine supplementation, including azotemia and hyperammonemia, should be avoided with concomitant increases in the volume of free water flushes.

Non-healing decubiti ulcers are a significant problem in the CCI population. While delivery of sufficient nitrogen and prevention of hyperglycemia are essential factors in the optimization of skin health, other nutritional substances have been suggested to promote wound healing including zinc, vitamin C, multivitamins, vitamin A, and arginine. The available data on the use of these substances to promote wound healing remain inconclusive and have been reviewed in greater detail previously [1].

Supplementation to correct endocrine deficiencies in the CCIS has been suggested. Consideration for growth hormone replacement therapy to counteract the wasting and catabolic nature of CCI was shown detrimental in two large trials demonstrating increased morbidity and mortality [61]. Correction of hypogonadism in CCI patients with testosterone replacement, to preserve lean body mass and bone density, cannot be routinely recommended based on available data in the general ICU population [62].

Carnitine is a required factor for the transport of medium- and long-chain fatty acids into mitochondria for beta-oxidation [63]. Supplementation with carnitine for the correction of potential deficiency may be of benefit in patients with renal failure, especially on hemodialysis [64], unexplained hypoglycemia, impairment in gluconeogenesis, or using drugs that are known to deplete carnitine levels (e.g., valproate). It is our practice in the RCU to use 1 g twice daily via the enteral route or 1 g daily parenterally when supplementation is indicated.

CCI-related bone hyperresorption, an entity that has been identified as occurring frequently in this population, may predispose to osteoporosis, fractures, and a worsened quality of life in survivors of CCI [44]. A recent retrospective cohort study of ICU patients requiring ventilator support for 2 days or greater found an increased fracture risk in postmenopausal female study patients, compared to population-based controls [65]. Multiple contributing factors to bone hyperresorption in CCI include cytokine-mediated losses, vitamin D deficiency, immobilization, endocrine deficiencies, and medications. Supplementation with adequate calcium and vitamin D, combined with bisphosphonate therapy, has shown encouraging results in the CCI population to attenuate bone hyperresorption. The use of calcitriol in this patient population may be necessary to counteract impaired renal 1-α hydroxylase due to immobilization-related suppression of parathyroid hormone. A retrospective study of the use of calcitriol plus pamidronate (90 mg) versus calcitriol alone in CCI patients with hyperresorption found a significant decrease in urine N-telopeptide (NTx) [66]. A randomized, prospective controlled trial comparing ibandronate (3 mg) versus placebo in a cohort of CCI patients showed a 34% reduction in serum C-telopeptide (CTx) compared with a 13% increase for the control group on day 6 after therapy, and no increase in adverse events [67]. A retrospective study of potential effect on renal function following treatment with pamidronate did not find significant reductions in GFR or elevations in creatinine in CCI patients with or without CKD, compared to fluctuations in renal parameters in the general CCI population [68]. This stands in contrast to prevailing concerns about bisphosphonate therapy in patients with renal impairment.

It is our current practice in the RCU to routinely supplement CCI patients with calcium 1000–1500 mg elemental calcium, ergocalciferol 2000 international units daily, and calcitriol 0.25 μg daily, unless contraindicated. Urine NTx is routinely measured, and when elevated greater than 70 nmol BCE/mmol Cr, pamidronate 90 mg is administered intravenously, after at least 3 days of vitamin D supplementation to prevent subsequent development of hypocalcemia and hypophosphatemia.

CASE STUDY

A 64-year-old Caucasian female with a past medical history significant for hypertension, obesity, and osteoarthritis is being transferred from the medical ICU to the RCU. She was admitted to the hospital 12 days prior after she was noted to have fever, chills, and altered mental status. In the emergency department, she was hemodynamically unstable, requiring mechanical ventilation, pressor support, and transfer to the medical ICU. Intravenous fluids and antibiotics were given for presumed septic shock, later confirmed with gram-negative bacteremia and a urinary tract infection. Her hospital course was complicated by acute kidney injury, GI bleeding requiring blood transfusions, and inability to be liberated from the ventilator. EN with a standard whole-protein formula was started on ICU day 2, with variable tolerance and periods of NPO surrounding the GI bleeding episode. On ICU day 11, after discussion with her family, the ICU team opted for placement of a tracheostomy and gastrostomy tube, followed by transfer to the RCU for assistance in ventilator weaning.

Upon transfer to the RCU, the patient requires full ventilatory support via tracheostomy. Physical exam is significant for stable vital signs, a weight of 104 kg (prehospital weight 95 kg), height of 62 in., BMI 38.3 kg/m^2, delirium, generalized muscle weakness, anasarca, sarcopenia, and obesity. The whole-protein EN formula (1.2 kcal/cc) is running at 30 cc/h via the gastrostomy tube. The patient's nurse reports intermittent diarrhea and some early skin breakdown and erythema of the sacrum. Laboratory studies indicate normal serum electrolytes, glucose 245 mg/dL, creatinine 1.4 mg/dL, albumin 2.4 g/dL, prealbumin 14 mg/dL, normal liver function tests, phosphorus 1.8 mg/dL, 25-OH vitamin D 14 ng/mL, and 24 h urine NTx 94 nmol BCE/mmol Cr. Point-of-care glucose values over the past 24 h are 214, 266, 278, and 236 mg/dL. What nutrition-related interventions are needed to optimize this CCI patient for recovery and liberation from the ventilator?

1. *Nutrition support*
   a. *Nutrition assessment*: This patient is considered to be in CCI based on her requirement for PMV following critical illness and placement of a tracheostomy. She demonstrates the classic inflammatory phenotype of the CCIS, including anasarca, muscle wasting, weakness, skin breakdown, hypoalbuminemia, and hyperglycemia. She is at high nutritional risk given suboptimal nutrition intake over the past 12 days of hospitalization. Given the fulminant CCI picture, the patient can be subclassified as type-1 CCI.
   b. *Nutrition components*: Based on her prehospital weight of 95 kg and her ideal body weight of 50 kg, an AjBW can be determined as 68 kg for use in the calculation of energy and protein requirements: AjBW = IBW + [(ABW − IBW) × correction factor], using a correction factor of 0.4. If 25 kcal/kg/day is used (indirect calorimetry is unavailable), this patient's energy target is 1700 kcal/day. Her daily protein target is 102 g/day, using 1.5 g/kg/day. Her current EN regimen of 1.2 kcal/cc at 30 cc/h supplies 864 kcal/day, which is consistent with gross underfeeding at 12.7 kcal/kg/day.
   c. *Mode of nutrition support*: The patient was changed to a semi-elemental formula (1.2 kcal/cc), comprised of 35% carbohydrate (relatively low carbohydrate), with a goal rate of 60 cc/h, providing 1728 kcal/day and 109 g of protein daily. The patient did well on this formula, with resolution of her diarrhea, and reached the target nutrition rate within 1 day in the RCU.
   d. *Monitoring and troubleshooting*: Daily laboratory studies should be monitored on the first few days of her nutrition regimen. Since her serum phosphorus was low, this should be aggressively repleted with close monitoring of electrolytes and repletion with vitamin D to correct vitamin D deficiency. If refeeding syndrome is suspected, the rate of EN should be temporarily decreased with close monitoring.
2. *Metabolic control*: The patient's uncontrolled hyperglycemia must be addressed. Using a weight-based approach (0.5 units/kg) and her prehospital weight of 95 kg, she can be initiated on a total daily dose of 48 units of insulin. She should be started on NPH 12 units every 6 h, with a correction scale of rapid-acting insulin every 6 h as needed. Blood glucose should be followed closely with daily titration of the insulin regimen until blood glucose is stabilized. The precise target range of blood glucose should be dictated by the ability of the unit to safely achieve that target range while avoiding hypoglycemia (range: 80–110–140–180 mg/dL targets).
3. *Nutrition/endocrine pharmacology*: This patient was identified with CCI-related bone hyperresorption and vitamin D deficiency. She should be initiated on calcium and vitamin D supplementation, followed by treatment with pamidronate 90 mg intravenously over 4 h. Follow-up bone markers can be checked after 2 weeks to assess for improvement. Given the presence of an early-stage sacral decubitus ulcer, adjunctive supplementation with zinc, vitamin C, and a multivitamin may be considered.

CONCLUSIONS

CCI represents a unique subset of the general ICU population with a distinct phenotype regardless of the inciting acute illness and carrying a tremendous burden of morbidity, mortality, and impaired quality of life in survivors. The pathophysiology contributing to the CCIS, including a heightened and persistent inflammatory and catabolic metabolic milieu, is a manifestation of an allostatic overload state. This scientific understanding, combined with extrapolation from the large evidence base in the general ICU, the small but growing evidence base in the CCI population, and clinical experience with this patient group, is the foundation behind the principles outlined earlier. Intensive metabolic support refers to the therapeutic combination of nutrition support with metabolic control and nutritional pharmacology, as a three-component model, initiated early in the ICU stay to prevent and ameliorate the onset of CCI [69]. Figure 36.1 summarizes the key steps to optimizing nutrition support in the CCI patient, with the ultimate goals of liberation from mechanical ventilation, resolution of CCI, and improved quality of life in survivors.

Continuing to build on the evidence base focusing specifically on CCI will help foster an improved understanding of the optimal approach to nutrition support in this distinct population. An ongoing project of our group in the RCU involves the development of a predictive model for the prediction of likelihood to be liberated from mechanical ventilation based on clinical and biochemical variables to be identified. Once available, this model would help in focusing resources and guiding physicians, patients, and families, toward aggressive and costly medical therapy or toward a palliative care approach. It is our hope that a greater understanding and appreciation of this complex patient population fosters improved outcomes in the future.

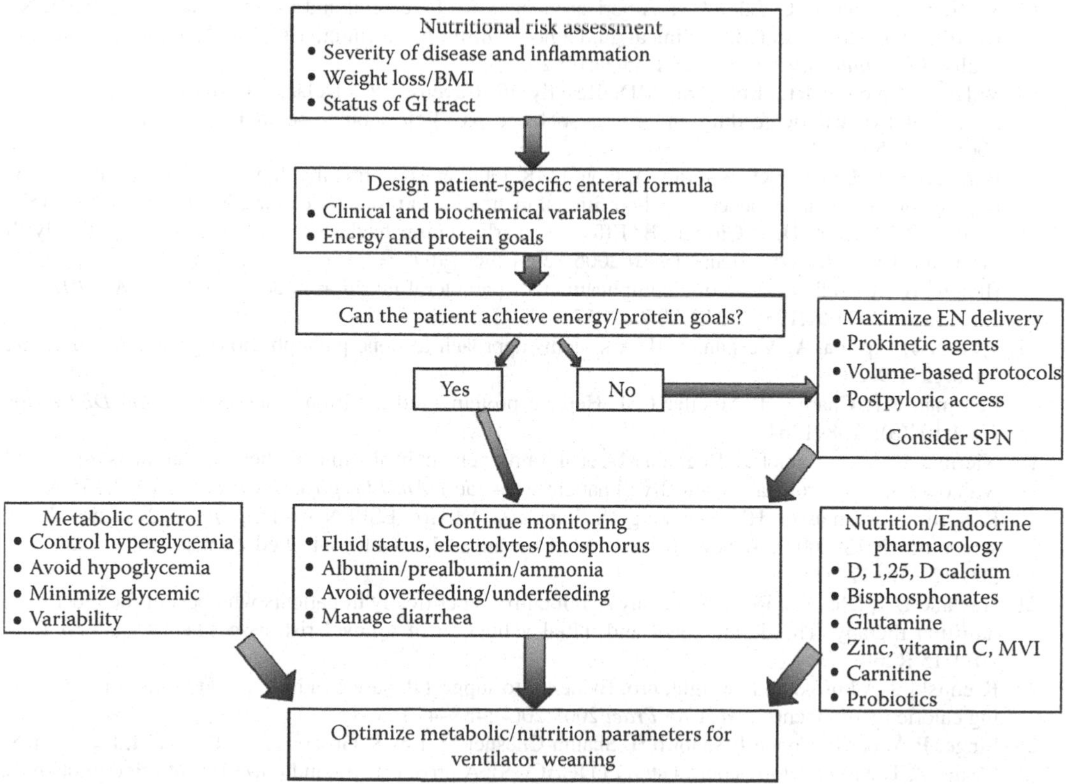

FIGURE 36.1 Flowchart demonstrating our approach to nutrition support in the chronic critical illness (CCI) patient. Following nutritional assessment, patients require optimization of energy and protein targets, followed by close monitoring and adjustments for common pitfalls (e.g., diarrhea). Concomitant with nutrition, attention to glycemic control and consideration for pharmacological supplementation is recommended to best ameliorate allostatic load and optimize patients for liberation from mechanical ventilation. BMI, body mass index; GI, gastrointestinal; EN, enteral nutrition; SPN, supplemental parenteral nutrition; D, vitamin D_2 or D_3 supplementation; 1,25-D, calcitriol supplementation; MVI, multivitamin.

REFERENCES

1. Schulman RC, Mechanick JI. Metabolic and nutrition support in the chronic critical illness syndrome. *Respir Care* 2012;57(6):958–977.
2. Nelson JE, Cox CE, Hope AA, Carson SS. Chronic critical illness. *Am J Respir Crit Care Med* 2010;182(4):446–454.
3. McEwen BS, Wingfield JC. The concept of allostasis in biology and biomedicine. *Horm Behav* 2003;43(1):2–15.
4. Brame AL, Singer M. Stressing the obvious? An allostatic look at critical illness. *Crit Care Med* 2010;38(10 Suppl.):600–607.
5. Hollander JM, Mechanick JI. Nutrition support and the chronic critical illness syndrome. *Nutr Clin Pract* 2006;21(6):587–604.
6. Singer M, De Santis V, Vitale D, Jeffcoate W. Multiorgan failure is an adaptive, endocrine-mediated, metabolic response to overwhelming systemic inflammation. *Lancet* 2004;364(9433):545–548.
7. Chang HR, Bistrian B. The role of cytokines in the catabolic consequences of infection and injury. *J Parenter Enteral Nutr* 1998;22(3):156–166.
8. Marques MB, Langouche L. Endocrine, metabolic, and morphologic alterations of adipose tissue during critical illness. *Crit Care Med* 2013;41(1):317–325.
9. Mechanick JI. Metabolic mechanisms of stress hyperglycemia. *J Parenter Enteral Nutr* 2006;30:157–163.
10. Nelson JE, Meier DE, Litke A, Natale DA, Siegel RE, Morrison RS. The symptom burden of chronic critical illness. *Crit Care Med* 2004;32(7):1527–1534.
11. Ziegler TR. Parenteral nutrition in the critically ill patient. *N Engl J Med* 2009;361(11):1088–1097.
12. Mueller C, Compher C, Ellen DM. American Society for Parenteral and Enteral Nutrition (A.S.P.E.N.) Board of Directors. A.S.P.E.N. clinical guidelines: Nutrition screening, assessment, and intervention in adults. *J Parenter Enteral Nutr* 2011;35(1):16–24.
13. Villet S, Chiolero RL, Bollmann MD, Revelly JP, Cayeux MC, Delarue J, Berger MM. Negative impact of hypocaloric feeding and energy balance on clinical outcome in ICU patients. *Clin Nutr* 2005;24(4):502–509.
14. Barr J, Hecht M, Flavin KE, Khorana A, Gould MK. Outcomes in critically ill patients before and after the implementation of an evidence-based nutritional management protocol. *Chest* 2004;125(4):1446–1457.
15. Artinian V, Krayem H, DiGiovine B. Effects of early enteral feeding on the outcome of critically ill mechanically ventilated patients. *Chest* 2006;129(4):960–967.
16. Btaiche IF, Khalidi N. Metabolic complications of parenteral nutrition in adults, Part1-2. *Am J Health Syst Pharm* 2004;61:1938–1949, 2050–2057.
17. Weiss AJ, Lipshtat A, Mechanick JI. A systems approach to bone pathophysiology. *Ann NY Acad Sci* 2010;1211:9–24.
18. Fuhrman MP, Charney P, Mueller CM. Hepatic proteins and nutrition assessment. *J Am Diet Assoc* 2004;104(8):1258–1264.
19. Nierman DM, Mechanick JI, Begonia MA et al. Improvement in albumin but not prealbumin is associated with outcome of chronically critically ill patients (abstract). *Am J Respir Crit Care Med* 1997;155:A774.
20. Kondrup J, Rasmussen HH, Hamberg O, Stanga Z. Ad Hoc ESPEN working group. Nutritional risk screening (NRS 2002): A new method based on an analysis of controlled clinical trials. *Clin Nutr* 2003;22(3):321–336.
21. Heyland DK, Dhaliwal R, Jiang X, Day AG. Identifying critically ill patients who benefit the most from nutrition therapy: The development and initial validation of a novel risk assessment tool. *Crit Care* 2011;15:R268.
22. Krenitsky J. Adjusted body weight, pro: Evidence to support the use of adjusted body weight in calculating calorie requirements. *Nutr Clin Pract* 2005;20(4):468–473.
23. Singer P, Anbar R, Cohen J, Shapiro H, Shalita-Chesner M, Lev S, Grozovski E, Theilla M, Frishman S, Madar Z. The tight calorie control study (TICACOS): A prospective, randomized, controlled pilot study of nutritional support in critically ill patients. *Int Care Med* 2011;37:601–609.
24. Kreymann KG, Berger MM, Deutz NE, Hiesmayr M, Jolliet P, Kazandjiev G, Nitenberg G et al. ESPEN Guidelines on enteral nutrition: Intensive care. *Clin Nutr* 2006;25(2):210–223.
25. Singer P, Berger MM, Van den Berghe G, Biolo G, Calder P, Forbes A, Griffiths R et al. ESPEN guidelines on parenteral nutrition: Intensive care. *Clin Nutr* 2009;28:387–400.
26. Mascioli EA, Lopes SM, Champagne C, Driscoll DF. Essential fatty acid deficiency and home total parenteral nutrition patients. *Nutrition* 1996;12:245–249.

27. Cerra FB, Benitez MR, Blackburn GL, Irwin RS, Jeejeebhoy K, Katz DP et al. Applied nutrition in ICU patients: A consensus statement of the American College of Chest Physicians. *Chest* 1997;111(3):769–778.
28. Weijs PJ, Stapel SN, de Groot SD, Driessen RH, de Jong E, Girbes AR, Strack van Schijndel RJ, Beishuizen A. Optimal protein and energy nutrition decreases mortality in mechanically ventilated, critically ill patients: A prospective observational cohort study. *J Parenter Enteral Nutr* 2012;36:60–68.
29. Japur CC, Monteiro JP, Marchini JS, Garcia RW, Basile-Filho A. Can an adequate energy intake be able to reverse the negative nitrogen balance in mechanically ventilated critically ill patients? *J Crit Care* 2010;25:445–450.
30. Brinson RR, Curtis WD, Singh M. Diarrhea in the intensive care unit: The role of hypoalbuminemia and he response to a chemically defined diet (case reports and review of the literature). *J Am Coll Nutr* 1987;6(6):517–523.
31. Brinson RR, Kolts BE. Diarrhea associated with severe hypoalbuminemia: A comparison of a peptide-based chemically defined diet and standard enteral alimentation. *Crit Care Med* 1988;16(2):130–136.
32. Meredith JW, Ditesheim JA, Zaloga GP. Visceral protein levels in trauma patients are greater with peptide diet than with intact protein diet. *J Trauma* 1990;30(7):825–829.
33. Doley J, Mallampalli A, Sandberg M. Nutrition management for the patient requiring prolonged mechanical ventilation. *Nutr Clin Pract* 2011;26(3):232–241.
34. Rice TW, Wheeler AP, Thompson BT, deBoisblanc BP, Steingrub J, Rock P. NHLBI ARDS clinical trials network. Enteral omega-3 fatty acid, gamma-linolenic acid, and antioxidant supplementation in acute lung injury. *JAMA* 2011;306(14):1574–1581.
35. Martindale RG, McClave SA, Vanek VW, McCarthy M, Roberts P, Taylor B, Ochoa JB, Napolitano L, Cresci G, American College of Critical Care Medicine, A.S.P.E.N. Board of Directors. Guidelines for the provision and assessment of nutrition support therapy in the adult critically ill patient: Society of Critical Care Medicine and American Society for Parenteral and Enteral Nutrition: Executive summary. *Crit Care Med* 2009;37:1757–1761.
36. Huang HH, Chang SJ, Hsu CW, Chang TM, Kang SP, Liu MY. Severity of illness influences the efficacy of enteral feeding route on clinical outcomes in patients with critical illness. *J Acad Nutr Diet* 2012;112(8):1138–1146.
37. Heyland DK, Cahill NE, Dhaliwal R, Wang M, Day AG, Alenzi A, Aris F, Muscedere J, Drover JW, McClave SA. Enhanced protein-energy provision via the enteral route in critically ill patients: A single center feasibility trial of the PEP uP protocol. *Crit Care* 2010;14:R78.
38. Vanhorebeek I, Gunst J, Derde S, Derese I, Boussemaere M, Guiza F, MartinetW, Timmermans JP, D'Hoore A, Wouters PJ, Van den Berghe G. Insufficient activation of autophagy allows cellular damage to accumulate in critically ill patients. *J Clin Endocrinol Metab* 2011;96:E633–E645.
39. Casaer MP, Mesotten D, Hermans G, Wouters PJ, Schetz M, Meyfroidt G, Van Cromphaut S et al. Early versus late parenteral nutrition in critically ill adults. *N Engl J Med* 2011;365:506–517.
40. McClave SA, Heyland DK, Martindale RG. Adding supplemental parenteral nutrition to hypocaloric enteral nutrition: Lessons learned from the Casaer Van den Berghe study. *J Parenter Enteral Nutr* 2012;36:15–17.
41. Schulman RC, Mechanick JI. Can nutrition support interfere with recovery from acute critical illness? *World Rev Nutr Diet* 2013;105:69–81. Doi: 10.1159/000341272.
42. Heidegger CP, Graf S, Thibault R, Darmon P, Berger M, Pichard C. Supplemental parenteral nutrition (SPN) in intensive care unit (ICU) patients for optimal energy coverage: Improved clinical outcome. *Clin Nutr Suppl* 2011;1:2–3.
43. Skipper A. Refeeding syndrome or refeeding hypophosphatemia: A systematic review of cases. *Nutr Clin Pract* 2012;27:34–40.
44. Nierman DM, Mechanick JI. Bone hyperresorption is prevalent in chronically critically ill patients. *Chest* 1998;114(4):1122–1128.
45. Scurlock C, Raikhelkar J, Mechanick JI. Impact of new technologies on metabolic care in the intensive care unit. *Curr Opin Clin Nutr Metab Care* 2009;12(2):196–200.
46. Fietsam R Jr, Bassett J, Glover JL. Complications of coronary artery surgery in diabetic patients. *Am Surg* 1991;57(9):551–557.
47. Furnary AP, Zerr KJ, Grunkemeier GL, Starr A. Continuous intravenous insulin infusion reduces the incidence of deep sternal wound infection in diabetic patients after cardiac surgical procedures. *Ann Thorac Surg* 1999;67(2):352–362.
48. Krinsley JS. Glycemic variability: A strong independent predictor of mortality in critically ill patients. *Crit Care Med* 2008;36(11):3008–3013.

49. Hermanides J, Vriesendorp TM, Bosman RJ, Zandstra DF, Hoek-Stra JB, DeVries JH. Glucose variability is associated with intensive care unit mortality. *Crit Care Med* 2010;38(3):838–842.
50. Van den Berghe G, Wouters P, Weekers F, Verwaest C, Bruyninckx F, Schetz M, Vlasselaers D, Ferdinande P, Lauwers P, Bouillon R. Intensive insulin therapy in the critically ill patients. *N Engl J Med* 2001;345:1359–1367.
51. Van den Berghe G, Wilmer A, Hermans G, Meersseman W, Wouters PJ, Milants I, Van Wijngaerden E, Bobbaers H, Bouillon R. Intensive insulin therapy in the medical ICU. *N Engl J Med* 2006;354:449–461.
52. NICE-SUGAR Study Investigators, Finfer S, Chittock DR, Su SY, Blair D, Foster D, Dhingra V et al. Intensive versus conventional glucose control in critically ill patients. *N Engl J Med* 2009;360:1283–1297.
53. NICE-SUGAR Study Investigators, Finfer S, Liu B, Chittock DR, Norton R, Myburgh JA, McArthur C et al. Hypoglycemia and risk of death in critically ill patients. *N Engl J Med* 2012;367(12):1108–1118.
54. Berger MM, Mechanick JI. Continuing controversy in the intensive care unit: Why tight glycemic control, nutrition support, and nutritional pharmacology are each necessary therapeutic considerations. *Curr Opin Clin Nutr Metab Care* 2010;13(2):167–169.
55. Scurlock CS, Raikhelkar J, Mechanick J. Parenteral nutrition in the critically ill patient (letter). *N Engl J Med* 2010;362(1):81; author reply 83–84.
56. Weiss AJ, Mechanick JM. Glycemic control: How tight in the intensive care unit? *Semin Thorac Cardiovasc Surg* 2011;23(1):1–4.
57. Schulman RC, Zhu C, Godbold J, Mechanick JI. Achieving tight glycemic control safely in patients with chronic critical illness (CCI) using a subcutaneous insulin protocol. *AACE 21st Annual Scientific and Clinical Congress*, Philadelphia, PA, May 2012, poster #221.
58. Griffiths RD, Jones C, Palmer TF. Six-month outcome of critically ill patients given glutamine-supplemented parenteral nutrition. *Nutrition* 1997;13(4):295–302.
59. Novak F, Heyland D, Avenell A, Drover JW, Su X. Glutamine supplementation in serious illness: A systematic review of the evidence. *Crit Care Med* 2002;30(9):2022–2029.
60. Andrews PJ, Avenell A, Noble DW, Campbell MK, Croal BL, Simpson WG et al. Randomised trial of glutamine, selenium, or both, to supplement parenteral nutrition for critically ill patients. *BMJ* 2011;342:d1542. Doi: 10.1136/bmj.d1542.
61. Takala J, Ruokonen E, Webster NR, Nielsen MS, Zandstra DF, Vundelinckx G, Hinds CJ. Increased mortality associated with growth hormone treatment in critically ill adults. *N Engl J Med* 1999;341(11):785–792.
62. Mechanick JI, Nierman DM. Gonadal steroids in critical illness. *Crit Care Clin* 2006;22(1):87–103.
63. Borum PR. Carnitine in parenteral nutrition. *Gastroenterology* 2009;137(Suppl. 5):S129–S134.
64. Emami Naini A, Moradi M, Mortazavi M, Amini Harandi A, Hadizadeh M, Shirani F, Basir Ghafoori H, Emami Naini P. Effects of oral L-carnitine supplementation on lipid profile, anemia, and quality of life in chronic renal disease patients under hemodialysis: A randomized, double-blinded, placebo-controlled trial. *J Nutr Metab* 2012;2012:510483.
65. Orford NR, Saunders K, Merriman E, Henry M, Pasco J, Stow P, Kotowicz M. Skeletal morbidity among survivors of critical illness. *Crit Care Med* 2011;39(6):1295–1300.
66. Nierman DM, Mechanick JI. Biochemical response to treatment of bone hyperresorption in chronically critically ill patients. *Chest* 2000;118(3):761–766.
67. Via MA, Potenza MV, Hollander J, Liu X, Peng Y, Li J et al. Intra-venous ibandronate acutely reduces bone hyperresorption in chronic critical illness. *J Int Care Med* 2012;27(5):312–318.
68. Schulman RC, Zhu C, Godbold J, Mechanick JI. Safety of intravenous pamidronate for bone hyperresorption in patients with chronic critical illness (CCI) and chronic kidney disease (CKD). *The Endocrine Society's 94th Annual Meeting and Expo*, Houton, TX, June 2012, poster #SAT-366.
69. Scurlock C, Raikhelkar J, Mechanick JI. Intensive metabolic support: Evolution and revolution. *Endocr Pract* 2008;14(8):1047–1054.

37 Nutrition Therapy for the Obese Critically Ill Patient

Britta Brown and Katherine Hall

CONTENTS

INTRODUCTION

The standard definition of obesity is based on the body mass index (BMI), which is a calculation of an individual's weight in kilograms divided by their height in meters squared. Currently, overweight is defined as a BMI of 25.0–29.9 and obesity is a BMI ≥30.0 [1]. In addition, obesity can be further classified as grade 1 (BMI 30 to <35), grade 2 (BMI 35 to <40), and grade 3 (BMI >40) [1]. The most recent National Health and Nutrition Examination Survey (NHANES) data from 2011 through 2012, cited the prevalence of obesity among adults more than 20 years old as 34.9% [2] with no significant change compared to data from 2003 through 2008 or 2009–2010 [2,3]. NHANES data from this same time period indicates the prevalence of grades 2 and 3 obesity was 14.5% and 6.4%, respectively [3]. Following this general trend, an estimated 25%–30% of ICU patients are obese [4]. Obese patients are predisposed to a variety of comorbid conditions that can be exacerbated during critical illness [5–9]. A well-established concept is that providing routine medical care can be more challenging for this patient population [9]. However, researchers have also coined the phrase *obesity ICU conundrum* to describe the surprising finding that critically ill obese patients often have equivalent or improved mortality rates compared with nonobese critically ill patients [9]. Obese ICU patients are often medically and metabolically complex. Critical care RDs must understand the medical complexities and metabolic issues affecting this patient population to implement nutrition support regimens that optimize clinical outcomes without exacerbating the harmful effects of over- or underfeeding.

COMORBID CONDITIONS ASSOCIATED WITH OBESITY AND CRITICAL ILLNESS

Obesity has been associated with a variety of chronic health issues that can become challenging for clinicians who care for this patient population (Tables 37.1 and 37.2).

MORBIDITY AND MORTALITY

Obesity has been linked to more than 60 comorbid medical conditions all of which can exacerbate critical illness and make caring for the critically ill obese patient a challenge [1]). Ventilation requirements are affected by excess adipose tissue. Increased intra-abdominal pressure has been shown to shift the diaphragm resulting in decreased lung volume, atelectasis, and reduced gas exchange [9,15,16]. The subsequent increased pressure requirements can reduce cardiac output and promote hypotension. Obese individuals requiring mechanical ventilation have been found to require longer duration and prolonged periods of weaning from mechanical ventilation compared to their non-obese counterparts [17]. Underlying obstructive sleep apnea (OSA) and providing excess energy (i.e., overfeeding), this patient population can result in hypercapnia, further prolonging respiratory compromise.

Altered skin integrity and pressure ulcers are also a concern among this patient population. A study conducted in 2008 found that patients with elevated BMI (35.8 ± 4.9 kg/m^2) and metabolic syndrome had decreased tissue perfusion and therefore may be more vulnerable to pressure ulcer development [18,19]. Frequent repositioning and use of off-loading devices is critical. However, as BMI increases, nursing staff find it increasingly more challenging to mobilize and regularly turn patients [9]. Lifting teams or specialized lifting equipment with higher weight limits may be

TABLE 37.1
Medical Conditions Associated with Obesity

Cardiovascular	*Pulmonary*	*Endocrine*
Hypertension	Obstructive sleep apnea	Diabetes
Coronary artery disease	Obesity hypoventilation syndrome	Infertility
Congestive heart failure	Restrictive lung disease	
Stroke		
Hyperlipidemia		
Skin and integument	*Gastrointestinal*	*Immune dysfunction*
Impaired wound healing	Gallstones	Nosocomial infections
Pressure ulcers	Gastroesophageal reflux (GERD)	
Cellulitis	Hepatic steatosis (NAFLD)	
Musculoskeletal	*Cancer*	*Psychosocial*
Osteoarthritis	Breast	Depression
Back pain/injuries	Endometrium	Social
Gout	Colon	Isolation/discrimination
	Prostate	Diminished quality of life
	Esophagus	
	Stomach	
	Liver	
	Kidney	

Sources: Hurt, R.T. and Frazier, T.H., Obesity, in: Mueller CM, Ed., *The A.S.P.E.N. Adult Nutrition Support Core Curriculum,* 2nd edn., American Society for Parenteral and Enteral Nutrition, Silver Spring, MD, 2012, pp. 603–619; Levi, D. et al., *Crit. Care Clin.*, 19, 11, 2003.

TABLE 37.2
Challenges Providing Care for Critically Ill Obese Patients

Respiratory	Mechanics of breathing
	CO_2 retention
	Obstructive sleep apnea (OSA)
	Increased risk of aspiration pneumonia
	Pulmonary embolism/deep vein thrombosis
	Safety of tracheostomy placement [10,11]
Cardiac	Increased blood volume, increased cardiac output, increased stroke volume
	Decreased left ventricular contraction, decreased ejection fraction
	Diastolic dysfunction related to ventricular hypertrophy
Pharmacological	Choosing a weight to use for medication dosing
	Lipophilicity of medication (i.e., sedatives)
	Decreased hepatic clearance of some medications
	Creatinine clearance for renal dosing
Vascular access	Difficulty placing and finding anatomical *landmarks*
Enteral access	Difficulty placing at bedside and confirming location
	Weight limits for fluoroscopy/endoscopy suites
	Safety of PEG placement [12,13]
Imaging	Weight limits for CT scans, MRI, fluoroscopy, interventional radiology
	Images obscured by adipose tissue
General patient care	Changing bed linens, bathing, repositioning
	Clean skin/wound care
	Fecal incontinence management
	Transporting patient out of the ICU (tests, procedures, surgery, etc.)
	Lack of equipment designed for bariatric ICU patients

Sources: Hurt, R.T. and Frazier, T.H., Obesity, in: Mueller CM, Ed., *The A.S.P.E.N. Adult Nutrition Support Core Curriculum,* 2nd edn., American Society for Parenteral and Enteral Nutrition, Silver Spring, MD, 2012, pp. 603–619; Levi, D. et al., *Crit. Care Clin.*, 19, 11, 2003; Shikora, S. and Naylor, M., Nutritional support for the obese patient, in: Shikora S, Martindale R, Schwaitzberg S, Eds., *Nutritional Considerations in the Intensive Care Unit: Science, Rationale, and Practice,* Kendall/Hunt Publishing Co., Dubuque, IA, 2002, pp. 209–217; Marik, P. and Varon, J. *Chest,* 113, 492, 1998; Kiraly, L. et al., *JPEN J. Parenter. Enteral Nutr.*, 35, 29S, 2011; El Solh, A.A. and Jaafar, W., *Crit. Care,* 11, R3, 2007; Aldawood, A.S. et al., *Anaesth. Intensive Care,* 36, 69, 2008; McGarr, S.E. and Kirby, D.F., *JPEN J. Parenter. Enteral Nutr.*, 31, 212, 2007; Wiggins, T.F. et al., *Nutr. Clin. Pract.*, 24, 723, 2009.

necessary even for frequent tasks such as bathing, toileting, and changing bed linens. Delay in any of these tasks will increase the risk of pressure ulcer development and skin tear infections.

Similar to nonobese patients, early initiation of nutrition support is recommended by clinical practice guidelines for the obese critically ill patient [20]. However, nutrition support may be delayed due to inability to gain feeding access. Imaging guidance for enteral access may not be accurate if a patient's weight exceeds 300 lb (136 kg), and subcutaneous adipose tissue can obstruct identification of central venous access sites for parenteral nutrition [4]. Obese patients may be at increased risk for developing complications after placement of long-term enteral access devices with increased risk of hernia, wound infection, and ileus [21,22]. However, two studies have indicated overall safety of percutaneous endoscopic gastrostomy placement for obese patients, particularly among clinicians who perform this procedure more frequently [12,13].

With the variety of comorbidities associated with obesity, one may assume that obesity would be an obvious risk factor for increased mortality in critical illness. However, multiple studies have been conducted to better understand the effects of obesity on mortality, and the results are quite mixed. Some studies have found an increased risk of death with obesity [17,23–28], while others have found improved outcomes among obese patients [29–37], and some have found no difference in mortality when comparing obese to nonobese critically ill patients [38–41]. These findings have led researchers to coin the phrase *ICU obesity conundrum* to describe the surprising finding that critically ill obese patients often have equivalent or improved mortality rates compared with nonobese critically ill patients [9].

There is more evidence of obesity adversely affecting outcomes among the critically ill obese trauma patients [25,28,42,43], but it is possible that factors other than obesity were associated with increased mortality rates. For example, a study of 1334 trauma patients initially found a 70% increase in mortality in the obese critically ill patients compared to the nonobese critically ill patients, but upon further review, it was noted that hyperglycemia (>150 mg/dL) on the day of admission, not obesity (BMI > 40), was actually the predictor of increased mortality [44]. It is also possible that adipose distribution on the body (i.e., abdomen versus lower extremities) determines one's risk of mortality. Paolini and colleagues examined 403 ICU patients and found that abdominal obesity, not BMI >30, increased mortality [45]. Due to the discrepancies in data, multiple investigators have conducted meta-analyses to better assess the data and hopefully come to a conclusion regarding the relationship between obesity and mortality in critically care. The authors of three recent meta-analyses that included trauma, medical, surgical, and mixed ICUs concluded that obese ICU patients have either equivalent or improved outcomes [46–48].

Researchers and clinicians have developed numerous hypotheses for the potential causative factors of the *ICU obesity conundrum* [9,47–49]. Some believe that the excess energy reserves are beneficial during the catabolic response of critical illness. Alternatively, the lower BMI group may have experienced weight loss or be underweight due to a chronic disease such as cancer or AIDS, and it may be their underlying chronic condition(s) at the time of admission that decreases survival in this group. Others have argued that some of the hormones secreted by the adipose tissue are actually protective. For example, obese patients have been found to have higher levels of leptin and interleukin-10 (IL-10). Elevated leptin levels have been associated with improved survival among septic patients [50]. IL-10 has anti-inflammatory properties and can prevent release of tumor necrosis factor and IL-6 [52]. It is also thought that critically ill obese patients receive a different standard of care by transferring to the ICU sooner or staying in the ICU longer due to more favorable nursing staffing ratios [9]. It may be more difficult to provide routine nursing care for an obese patient on a general medical or surgical ward, compared to that in an ICU setting.

The majority of studies do agree on one point; obesity does increase hospital length of stay and duration of mechanical ventilation [17,28,29,32,33,36,37,39,40,43]. Obesity has also been associated with greater utilization of resources and decreased functional status upon hospital discharge [37].

EFFECTS OF OBESITY ON IMMUNITY

In the past, adipose stores were believed to provide the body only with extra energy reserves. However, in 1999, investigators noted that C-reactive protein correlated independently with BMI, and some began to hypothesize that those excessive fat stores may produce a chronic inflammatory state [52–56]. The composition of fat stores changes dramatically with age. A newborn baby's fat stores are composed mainly of brown fat, which may be related to resting energy expenditure in adults, whereas adipose stores in adults are composed mainly of white adipose tissue [57–59]. The white adipose tissue is comprised of leukocytes, macrophages, pre-adipocytes, and adipocytes [60,61]. These macrophages and adipocytes secrete inflammatory mediators, such as angiotensinogen, tumor necrosis factor alpha (TNF-α), IL-6, and C-reactive protein, and create a chronic inflammatory state similar to that seen with trauma and sepsis [62,63]. The increase in angiotensinogen from fat cells appears to increase angiotensin and angiotensin II, which leads to volume expansion, sodium retention, and hypertension [62,64]. Elevated levels of TNF-α and IL-6 may result in dyslipidemia and insulin resistance and have prothrombotic effects, which increase an individual's risk of myocardial infarct and deep venous thrombosis [61,62,64]. These inflammatory markers appear to be most problematic when found in abdominal fat stores. The combination of excess visceral fat, dyslipidemia, elevated blood pressure, insulin resistance, proinflammatory state, and prothrombotic state has been used to diagnose the metabolic syndrome [65,66]. Interestingly, all of these inflammatory mediators have been shown to decrease with weight loss [52,62,66]. Some investigators also believe that the increased levels of leptin and IL-10 secreted from adipose tissue may actually decrease mortality and be one explanation for the *ICU conundrum*, as previously discussed [47].

METABOLIC ISSUES ASSOCIATED WITH OBESITY

Research by Jeevanandam and colleagues [67] suggests that this patient population is predisposed to metabolic alterations that can complicate the provision of nutrition support. A key finding from their study was that obese trauma patients experienced significantly higher net carbohydrate and protein oxidation rates and lower fat oxidation rates compared to nonobese patients. They concluded that obese patients could not take advantage of their abundant fat stores under stress conditions and had to depend on endogenous glucose synthesized from the breakdown of body protein. Once nutrition support is initiated, however, this no longer appears to be the case. Dickerson and associates found that if the patient's obligatory glucose needs and protein requirements are met via a hypocaloric, high-protein regimen, fat stores will be mobilized to provide additional energy requirements for nitrogen balance and adequate healing of wounds [68]. The exact amount of carbohydrate necessary to meet obligatory glucose needs varies in the literature. The Recommended Dietary Allowance for carbohydrate is 130 g/day for adults "based on the average minimum amount of glucose utilized by the brain" [69]. The components needed for wound healing such as granulation tissue, fibroblasts, and new epithelial cells also require additional glucose. The patients in Dickerson's study averaged 230 g of glucose daily (range of 100–350 g) with endogenous fat oxidation totaling approximately 68% of nonprotein energy expenditure [68]. All 13 of the patients studied had either an abscess with fistula or wound dehiscence on admission that required healing. The patients were able to demonstrate tissue healing on the hypocaloric high-protein TPN regimen they received.

Obese patients are also at increased risk for the deleterious effects of overfeeding, such as hyperglycemia, hypercapnia, and impaired weaning from mechanical ventilation [4–7]. Consequently, preexisting medical conditions combined with the stress response and metabolic changes associated with critical illness can create challenges for the RD in assessing nutritional status and developing appropriate plans of care for obese patients.

NUTRITION ASSESSMENT

To address the unique metabolic issues affecting critically ill obese patients, research has been published on predictive energy equations [70–88] and hypocaloric, high-protein feeding strategies for this unique patient population [89–99]. Table 37.3 summarizes current nutrition practice guidelines for critically ill obese patients published by the Society for Critical Care Medicine (SCCM) [20] and the American Society for Parenteral and Enteral Nutrition (ASPEN) [20,100], as well as the Academy of Nutrition and Dietetics [101].

ENERGY

Assessing the energy needs of critically ill obese patients has been a focus of debate for clinicians and researchers. Although it is recognized that indirect calorimetry is the *gold standard* for assessing energy needs, day-to-day variations in measured resting energy expenditure can occur. Furthermore, many facilities do not have access to indirect calorimetry, thus necessitating the use of predictive energy equations. The Academy of Nutrition and Dietetics systematic review of resting metabolic rate predictive equations for critically ill obese adults states "if indirect calorimetry is not available, the Registered Dietitian (RD) should use the Penn State University [PSU (2003b)] equation in critically ill mechanically

TABLE 37.3
Nutrition Practice Guidelines for Critically Ill Obese Patients

Society for Critical Care Medicine (SCCM) [20] and American Society for Parenteral and Enteral Nutrition (ASPEN) [20,100]	*Energy* Not to exceed 60%–70% *target energy requirements* OR 11–14 kcal/kg actual body weight per day OR 22–25 kcal/kg ideal body weight per day *Protein* ≥2.0 g/kg ideal body weight grade 1–2 obesity (BMI 30–40) ≥2.5 g/kg ideal body weight grade 3 obesity (BMI ≥ 40) *Overall grade: D* *Supported by at least two level III investigations* Level III evidence: nonrandomized, contemporaneous controls
Academy of Nutrition and Dietetics Evidence Analysis Library [101]	*Energy* Best method—nonobese and obese patients = indirect calorimetry (IC) If IC not available or not practical, what is the best way to estimate RMR? Penn State 2003—70% accuracy For patients ≥ 60 years old, modified Penn State 2010—74% accuracy *Protein* No specific recommendations
European Society for Parenteral and Enteral Nutrition (ESPEN) [103]	No specific recommendations for obese patients
Canadian Clinical Practice Guidelines	No specific recommendations

Note: Guideline of 20–25 kcal/kg actual body weight for patients receiving parenteral nutrition (PN).

ventilated adults with obesity who are less than 60 years of age. For obese patients 60 years or older, the PSU (2010) equation should be used" (fair, conditional recommendation) [102]. Recommended equations for predicting metabolic rate for obese critically ill adults are listed in Table 37.4.

The SCCM and ASPEN joint guidelines recommend a hypocaloric feeding strategy that "does not exceed 60%–70% of target energy requirements or 11–14 kcal/kg actual body weight per day (or 22–25 kcal/kg ideal body weight per day)" [20] (Table 37.3).

TABLE 37.4
Resting Metabolic Rate Predictive Equations for Obese Critically Ill Adults

Penn State equation (2003b) [80]

RMR (kcal per day) = Mifflin(0.96) + Ve(31) + Tmax(167) − 6212

Modified Penn State equation (2010) [83]

Critically ill obese (BMI ≥ 30) and ≥ 60 years old

RMR (kcal per day) = Mifflin(0.71) + Ve(64) + Tmax(85) − 3085

Notes

Mifflin St. Jeor equation

Men: RMR = (9.99 × weight) + (6.25 × height) − (4.92 × age) + 5

Women: RMR = (9.99 × weight) + (6.25 × height) − (4.92 × age) − 161

Weight = kg Height = cm Age = years

Tmax = max temp last 24 h, centigrade Ve = expired minute ventilation

Protein

Recent efforts have focused on better understanding the protein requirements for patients with obesity. Choban and Dickerson combined their data using hypocaloric, high-protein feeding studies and used regression analysis to determine that a minimum of approximately 1.9 g of protein per kilogram of ideal body weight (IBW) per day is needed to achieve nitrogen equilibrium in patients with grade 1 or 2 obesity who are receiving hypocaloric feedings, but a higher intake of approximately 2.5 g of protein per kilogram of IBW per day is likely needed for patients with grade 3 obesity [89]. These authors advocate weekly monitoring of nitrogen balance for patients receiving hypocaloric feedings and adjusting the protein intake as clinically indicated. They also advocate monitoring renal and hepatic tolerance to protein intake as well as indirect calorimetry for patients who are not achieving expected clinical outcomes. Choban and Dickerson concluded that more research is needed to define the optimal protein intakes of critically ill obese patients, especially those with grade 3 obesity. Nonetheless, their approach for assessing protein needs has been endorsed in the SCCM/ASPEN *Guidelines for the Provision and Assessment of Nutrition Therapy in the Adult Critically Ill Patient* guideline C5 [20] (Table 37.3).

Essential Fatty Acids

Investigators have found that additional lipid administration may not initially be necessary when patients are provided hypocaloric, high-protein, fat-free parenteral nutrition [68,103]. Dickerson and colleagues found that oxidation of fat stores was able to provide participants with approximately 68% of their nonprotein calorie expenditure [68]. In another study where lipids were withheld while obese patients received hypocaloric, high-protein, fat-free parenteral nutrition for a range of 14–58 days, no signs of essential fatty acid deficiency were found [103]. It is believed that human adipose contains approximately 10%–15% linoleic acid [104,105] thus supplying the body with daily requirements of linoleic acid as fat stores are mobilized. The extent of time that obese individuals can rely on their fat stores for essential fatty acid needs is unknown, and monitoring of the triene–tetraene ratio should be done regularly if lipids are withheld for an extended amount of time.

Vitamins and Minerals

The ideal vitamin and mineral intakes for this patient population remain unknown. It is generally accepted that clinicians should strive to provide 100% of the Dietary Recommended Intakes (DRI) of the major vitamins and minerals. Disease-specific consideration may be warranted for patients with acute kidney injury (AKI), chronic kidney disease, burns or altered skin integrity, altered GI function, or history of bariatric surgery. For example, obese patients who have had prior bariatric surgery may be deficient in iron, vitamin B_{12}, folate, thiamine, and vitamin D. Suggested nutrition monitoring guidelines have been published for this subgroup of patients [5,106].

Fluid

The fluid needs for critically ill obese patients can vary greatly based on their underlying medical conditions and the clinical course of their acute illness. It is not uncommon for these patients to experience volume overload due to diastolic dysfunction (ventricular hypertrophy) resulting from an increased preload needed to support the increased blood volume of their excess adipose tissue [9] (Table 37.2). Clinicians should monitor patients closely for clinical signs and symptoms of volume overload, and intake and output records should be followed closely. Critically ill obese patients may require a fluid-restricted enteral formula or a concentrated PN solution.

TABLE 37.5
ASPEN Obesity in Critical Care Summit Report

Summary of recommendations for monitoring nutrition therapy in the critically ill obese patient with obesity:

1. Frequent blood glucose monitoring
2. Check serum triglycerides before and during IV-lipid administration
3. Arterial blood gases (ABG) to check for nutrition-induced hypercapnia
4. Monitor for volume overload, intake, and output records[a]
5. Routine monitoring of electrolytes (especially K+, Mg, phosphorous, Ca++)
6. Serum urea nitrogen (especially if renal impairment)
7. Serial evaluation of AST, ALT, alk phos, and bilirubin during the recovery phase
8. Weekly prealbumin in the absence of new inflammation, stress, or infection may be useful
9. Nitrogen balance to evaluate adequacy of protein intake
10. Serial body weights are not useful in the acute phase due to fluid status, but may be useful long-term during recovery

Source: Dickerson, R.N. and Drover, J.W., *JEPN J. Parenter. Enteral Nutr.*, 35, 44S, 2011.

[a] To ensure that daily enteral intake is recorded and consistent with prescribed regimen.

NUTRITION MONITORING

Monitoring the efficacy and tolerance of nutrition support in this patient population has been challenging for clinicians. To date, the majority of research has focused on preventing the deleterious effects of overfeeding, including hyperglycemia, hypertriglyceridemia, hypercapnia/delayed weaning from mechanical ventilation, nonalcoholic fatty liver disease (NAFLD), and fluid overload [107]. However, Heyland and colleagues have suggested a possible association between not meeting caloric targets (despite acknowledging the lack of consensus in defining caloric targets) and increased mortality [108]. Therefore, diligent monitoring of actual nutrition intake is imperative to ensure patients receive their prescribed regimen. Traditional use of laboratory values (albumin, prealbumin, transferrin) and serial weights are not useful markers of nutritional efficacy [107]. The *ASPEN Obesity in Critical Care Summit Report* advocates focusing on clinical outcomes such as tissue granulation and wound healing, weaning from mechanical ventilation, recovery from or prevention of infectious complications, physical conditioning, recovery from critical illness, and discharge from the ICU [107], while recognizing that these outcomes can be difficult to quantify (Table 37.5).

CASE STUDY

The following case reviews the basic concepts of providing nutrition assessment, intervention, and monitoring for a critically ill obese patient. In this example, a 43-year-old female is admitted to the ICU with acute pancreatitis and AKI, necessitating continuous renal replacement therapy (CRRT). A jejunal feeding tube is placed at the bedside, and the medical team begins enteral nutrition support therapy. Tables 37.6 through 37.8 summarize this patient's case.

This case highlights the complexities and challenges of monitoring the tolerance and effectiveness of nutrition support therapy. Since this patient is experiencing AKI and is receiving CRRT, nitrogen balance studies are not feasible and body weights are highly variable. Routine laboratory monitoring of blood glucose, electrolytes, blood urea nitrogen, and liver enzymes is completed, in part, to monitor renal function, as well as tolerance to nutrition support therapy. Serial ABGs are completed to assist with ventilator monitoring and to assess for possible overfeeding. In this case, the most useful nutrition monitoring tools included serial completion of indirect calorimetry to assess energy needs, laboratory testing as previously mentioned, examination of intake and output records and clinical assessment for possible volume overload, diligent assessment for alterations in skin integrity, and overall signs of improvement in clinical status.

TABLE 37.6
Case Study: Anthropometric and Physical Assessment Data

Admission body weight	168 kg
Current body weight	177 kg
Usual body weight	165 kg (107% UBW)
Weight history	2005—136 kg 2009—148 kg 2010—155 kg
Ideal body weight	54.5 kg (±10%); (325% IBW)
Body mass index (BMI)	67.05 (Grade 3 obesity)
Height	5′4″ (162.6 cm)
Physical	Obese female, 2–3+ edema in bilateral lower extremities, stage 1 pressure ulcer—coccyx, yeast—abdominal pannus

TABLE 37.7
Case Study: Nutrition Assessment

Estimated energy needs	11–14 kcal/kg actual = 1947–2478 kcal 22–25 kcal/kg IBW = 1199–1362 kcal 60%–70% REE = 2292–2674 kcal Penn State 2003 = 3377 kcal
Measured energy needs	REE = 3820; RQ = 0.77
Estimated protein needs	≥2.5 g/kg IBW = 136 g
Estimated fluid needs	Providing ~2000 mL/day to match intake and output records while on CRRT
Vitamin and mineral needs	100% DRI (monitor renal function and duration of CRRT)
Nutritional risk factors and considerations	Altered skin integrity History of DM and risk for hyperglycemia CRRT—increased protein/vitamin needs, risk for electrolyte abnormalities Obesity Critical illness

TABLE 37.8
Case Study: Enteral Nutrition Plan

Initial goal: to provide 1200–1400 kcal/day, >135 g protein/day

Option #1	**Option #2**
Polymeric high-protein EN formula (1 kcal/mL; ~62 g protein/L)	"Bariatric" EN formula (1 kcal/mL; ~93 g protein/L)
Protein modular	Protein modular
Goal: EN at 40 mL/h + protein modular—2 packets TID.	*Goal*: EN at 50 mL/h + protein modular—1 packet BID
Provides: 1392 kcal, 150 g protein, ~800 mL free water	*Provides*: 1344 kcal, 141 g protein, ~1000 mL free water
EN volume does not meet DRI for vitamins and minerals	EN volume does not meet DRI for vitamins and minerals

CONCLUSION

As obesity rates continue to rise in the United States, clinicians will encounter obese patients more frequently in their practices. It is imperative that nutrition practitioners maintain their knowledge base regarding nutrition assessment, hypocaloric feeding strategies, medication issues, and general patient care issues associated with this population. Some practice guidelines currently address goals for feeding obese ICU patients, but many questions remain unanswered. Future research is needed to clarify current practice patterns and to evaluate clinical outcomes.

REFERENCES

1. Expert Panel in the Identification, Evaluation, and Treatment of Overweight in Adults. Clinical guideline on the identification, evaluation, and treatment of overweight and obesity in adults: Executive summary. *Am J Clin Nutr.,* 1998; 68:899–917.
2. Ogden CL, Carroll MD, Kit BK, Flegal KM. Prevalence of childhood and adult obesity in the United States, 2011–2012. *JAMA*. 2014; 311:806–814.
3. Flegal KM, Carroll MD, Ogden CL, Curtin LR. Prevalence and trend in obesity among US adults, 1999–2008. *JAMA,* 2010; 303:235–241.
4. Port AM, Apovian C. Metabolic support of the obese intensive care unit patient: A current perspective. *Curr Opin Clin Nutr Metab Care,* 2010; 13:184–191.
5. Hurt RT, Frazier TH. Obesity. In: Mueller CM, Ed. *The A.S.P.E.N. Adult Nutrition Support Core Curriculum,* 2nd edn. Silver Spring, MD: American Society for Parenteral and Enteral Nutrition; 2012: pp. 603–619.
6. Levi D, Goodman ER, Patel M, Savransky Y. Critical care of the obese and bariatric surgical patient. *Crit Care Clin.,* 2003; 19:11–32.
7. Shikora S, Naylor M. Nutritional support for the obese patient. In: Shikora S, Martindale R, Schwaitzberg S, Eds. *Nutritional Considerations in the Intensive Care Unit: Science, Rationale, and Practice*. Dubuque, IA: Kendall/Hunt Publishing Co.; 2002: pp. 209–217.
8. Marik P, Varon J. The obese patient in the ICU. *Chest,* 1998; 113:492–498.
9. Kiraly L, Hurt RT, Van Way CW. The outcomes of obese patients in critical care. *JPEN J Parenter Enteral Nutr.,* 2011; 35:29S–35S.
10. El Solh AA, Jaafar W. A comparative study of the complications of surgical tracheostomy in morbidly obese critically ill patients. *Crit Care,* 2007; 11:R3.
11. Aldawood AS, Arabi YM, Haddad S. Safety of percutaneous tracheostomy in obese critically ill patients: A prospective cohort study. *Anaesth Intensive Care,* 2008; 36:69–73.
12. McGarr SE, Kirby DF. Percutaneous endoscopic gastrostomy (PEG) placement in the overweight and obese patient. *JPEN J Parenter Enteral Nutr.,* 2007; 31:212–216.
13. Wiggins TF, Garrow DA, DeLegge MH. Evaluation of percutaneous endoscopic feeding tube placement in obese patients. *Nutr Clin Pract.,* 2009; 24:723–727.
14. Calle EE, Rodriquez C, Walker-Thurmond K, Thun MJ. Overweight, obesity and mortality from cancer in a prospectively studied cohort of U.S. adults. *N Engl J Med.,* 2003; 348(17):1625–1638.
15. Hess DR, Bigatello LM. The chest wall in acute lung injury/acute respiratory distress syndrome. *Curr Opin Crit Care,* 2008; 14(1):94–102.
16. Jubber AS. Respiratory complications of obesity. *Int J Clin Pract.,* 2004; 58:573–580.
17. El-Solh A, Sikka P, Bozkanat E, Jaafar W, Davies J. Morbid obesity in the medical ICU. *Chest,* 2001; 120(6):1989–1997.
18. Kraemer-Aguiar LG, Laflor CM, Bouskela E. Skin microcirculatory dysfunction is already present in normoglycemic subjects with metabolic syndrome. *Metabolism,* 2008; 57(12):1740–1746.
19. Redlin Lowe J. Skin integrity in critically ill obese patients. *Crit Care Nurs Clin N Am.,* 2009; 21:311–322.
20. American Society for Parenteral and Enteral Nutrition and Society of Critical Care Medicine. Guidelines for the provision and assessment of nutrition support therapy in the adult critically ill patient. *JPEN J Parenter Enteral Nutr.,* 2009; 33:277–316.
21. Alexander JW. Wound infections in the morbidly obese. *Obese Surg.,* 2005; 15(9):1276–1277.
22. Longcroft-Wheaton G, Marden P, Colleypriest B, Gavin D, Taylor G, Farrant M. Understanding why patients diet after gastrostomy tube insertion: A retrospective analysis of mortality. *JPEN,* 2009; 33:375–379.

23. Goulenok C, Monchi M, Chiche JD, Mira JP, Dhainaut JF, Cariou A. Influence of overweight on ICU mortality. *Chest,* 2004; 125(4):1441–1445.
24. Bercault N, Boulain T, Kuteifan K, Wolf M, Runge I, Fleury JC. Obesity related excess mortality rate in an adult intensive care unit: A risk-adjusted matched cohort study. *Crit Care Med.,* 2004; 32:998–1003.
25. Neville AL, Brown CR, Weng J, Demetriades D, Velmahos GC. Obesity is an independent risk factor of mortality in severely injured blunt trauma patients. *Arch Surg.,* 2004; 139:983–987.
26. Burnes MC, McDaniel MD, Moore MB, Helmer SD, Smith RS. The effect of obesity on outcomes amount injured patients. *J Trauma,* 2005; 58:232–237.
27. Nasraway SA Jr, Albert M, Donnelly AM, Ruthazer R, Shikora SA, Saltzman E. Morbid obesity is an independent determinant of death among surgical critically ill patients. *Crit Care Med.,* 2006; 34:964–971.
28. Bochicchio GV, Joshi M, Bochicchio K et al. Impact of obesity in the critically ill trauma patient: A prospective study. *J Am Coll Surg.,* 2006; 203:533–538.
29. Marik PE, Doyle H, Varon J. Is obesity protective during crucial illness? An analysis of a national ICU database. *Crit Care Shock,* 2003; 6:156–162.
30. Tremlay A, Bandi V. Impact of body mass index on outcomes following critical care. *Chest,* 2003 2003; 123:1202–1207.
31. Finkielman JD, Gajic O, Afessa B. Underweight is independently associated with mortality in post-operative and non-operative patients admitted to the intensive care unit: A retrospective study. *BMC Emerg Med.,* 2004; 4:3.
32. Garrouste-Orgeas M, Troche G, Azoulay E et al. Body mass index. An additional prognostic factor in ICU patients. *Intensive Care Med.,* 2004; 30:437–443.
33. Ray DE, Matchett SC, Baker K, Wasser T, Young MJ. The effect of body mass index on patient outcomes in a medical ICU. *Chest,* 2005; 127:2125–2131.
34. Ciesla DJ, Moore EE, Johnson JL et al. Obesity increases risk of organ failure after severe trauma. *J Am Coll Surg.,* 2006; 203:539–545.
35. Nasraway SA Jr, Albert M, Donnelly AM et al. Morbid obesity is an independent determinant of death among surgical crucially ill patients. *Crit Care Med.,* 2006; 34:964–970.
36. O'Brien JM Jr, Phillips GS, Ali NA et al. Body mass index is independently associated with hospital mortality in mechanically ventilated adults with acute lung injury. *Crit Care Med.,* 2006; 34:738–744.
37. Morris AE, Stapleton RD, Rubenfeld GD et al. The association between body mass index and clinical outcomes in acute lung injury. *Chest,* 2007; 131:342–348.
38. O'Brien JM JR, Welsch CH, Fish RHM, Ancukiewicz M, Kramer AM. Excess body weight is not independently associated with outcome in mechanically ventilated patients with acute lung injury. *Ann Intern Med.,* 2004; 140:338–345.
39. Peake SL, Moran JL, Ghelani DR, Lloyd AJ, Walker MJ. The effect of obesity on 12-month survival following admission to intensive care: A prospective study. *Crit Care Med.,* 2006; 34:2929–2939.
40. Alban RF, Lyass S, Marguiles DR, Shabot MM. Obesity does not affect mortality after trauma. *Am Surg.,* 2006; 72:966–969.
41. Newell MA, Bard MR, Goettler CE et al. Body mass index and outcomes in critically injured blunt trauma patients: Weighing the impact. *J Am Coll Surg.,* 2007; 204:1056–1061.
42. Choban PS, Weiretter LJ, Maynes C. Obesity and increased mortality in blunt trauma. *J Trauma,* 1991; 31(9):1253–1257.
43. Brown CV, Neville AL, Rhee P et al. The impact of obesity on the outcomes of 1,153 critically injured blunt trauma patients. *J Trauma,* 2005; 59:1048–1051.
44. Diaz JJ Jr, Norris PR, Collier BR et al. Morbid obesity is not a risk factor for mortality in crucially ill trauma patients. *J Trauma,* 2009; 66(1):226–231.
45. Paolini JM, Mancini J, Genestal M et al. Predictive value of abdominal obesity vs. body mass index for determining risk of intensive care unit mortality. *Crit Care Med.,* 2010; 38(5):1308–1314.
46. Hogue CW, Stearns JD, Colantuoni E. The impact of obesity on outcomes after critical illness: A meta-analysis. *Intensive Care Med.,* 2009; 35(7):1152–1170.
47. Akinnusi ME, Pineda LA, El Solh AA. Effect of obesity on intensive care morbidity and mortality: A meta-analysis. *Crit Care Med.,* 2008; 36(1):151–158.
48. Oliveros H, Villamor E. Obesity and mortality in critically ill adults: A systemic review and meta-analysis. *Obesity,* 2008; 16(3):515–521.
49. Hurt RT, Frazier TH, McClave SA, Kaplan LM. Summit report. Obesity epidemic: Overview, pathophysiology, and the intensive care unit conundrum. *JPEN,* 2011; 35(supplement 1):4S–13S.

50. Bornstein SR, Licinio J, Tauchnitz R, Engelmann L, Negrao AB, Gold P, Chrousos GP. Plasma leptin levels are increased in survivors of acute sepsis: Associated loss of diurnal rhythm in cortisol and leptin secretion. *J Clin Endrocrinol Metab.,* 1998; 83:280–283.
51. Fiorentiono DF, Zlotnik A, Mosmann TR, Howard M, O'Garra A. IL-10 inhibits cytokine production by activated macrophages. *J Immunol.,* 1991; 147:3815–3822.
52. Cottam DR, Schaefer PA, Shaftan GW, Velcu L, Angus G. Effect of surgically-induced weight loss on leukocyte indicators of chronic inflammation in morbid obesity. *Obesity Surg.,* 2002; 12:335–342.
53. Colwell GA. Inflammation and diabetic vascular complications. *Diabetes Care,* 1999; 22:1927–1928.
54. Visser M, Bouter LM, McQuillan GM, Wener MH, Harris TB. Elevated C-reactive protein levels in overweight and obese adults. *JAMA,* 1999; 282:2121–2135.
55. Yudkin JS, Stehouwer CD, Emeis JJ, Coppack SW. C-reactive protein in healthy subjects: Associations with obesity, insulin resistance, and endothelial dysfunction: A potential role for cytokines originating from adipose tissue? *Arterioscler Thromb Vasc Biol.,* 1999; 19:972–978.
56. Barinas-Mitchell E, Cushman M, Meilahn EN, Tracy RP, Kuller LH. Serum levels of C-reactive protein are associated with obesity, weight gain, and hormone replacement therapy in healthy postmenopausal women. *Am J Epidemiol.,* 2001; 153:1094–1101.
57. Lidell ME, Enerback S. Brown adipose tissue—A new role in humans? *Nat Rev Endocrinol.,* 2010; 6:319–325.
58. Van Marken Lichtenbelt WD, Vanhommerig JN, Smulders NM, Drossaerts JM et al. Cold-activated brown adipose tissue in healthy men. *N Engl J Med.,* 2009; 360:1509–1517.
59. Virtanen KA, Lidell ME, Orava J et al. Functional brown adipose tissue in healthy adults. *N Engl J Med.,* 2009; 360:1518–1525.
60. Marti A, Marcos A, Martinez A. Obesity and immune function relationships. *Obese Rev.,* 2001; 2:131.
61. Honiden S, McArdle JR. Obesity in the intensive care unit. *Clin Chest Med.,* 2009; 30:581–599.
62. Cottam DR, Mattar SG, Barinas-Mitchell E, Eid G, Kuller L, Kelley DE, Schauer PR. The chronic inflammatory hypothesis for the morbidity associated with morbid obesity: Implications and effects of weight loss. *Obesity Surg.,* 2004; 14:589–560.
63. Shipman AR, Millington GW. Obesity and the skin. *Br J Dermatol.,* 2011; 165:743–750.
64. Bray GA. Obesity is a chronic, relapsing neurochemical disease. *Int J Obesity,* 2004; 28:34–38.
65. Grundy SM, Brewer HB Jr, Cleeman JI, Smith SC Jr. Definition of metabolic syndrome: Report of the National Heart Lung and Blood Institute/American Heart Association Conference on scientific issues related to definition. *Circulation,* 2004; 109:433–438.
66. Doyle SL, Lysaght J, Reynolds JV. Obesity and post-operative complications in patients undergoing non-bariatric surgery. *Obesity Rev.,* 2009; 11:875–886.
67. Jeevanandam M, Young DH, Schiller WR. Obesity and the metabolic response to severe multiple trauma in man. *J Clin Invest.,* 1991; 87:262–269.
68. Dickerson RN, Rosato EF, Mullen JL. Net protein anabolism with hypocaloric parenteral nutrition in obese stressed patients. *Am J Clin Nutr.,* 1986; 44:747–755.
69. A Report of the Panel on Macronutrients, Subcommittees on Upper Reference Levels of Nutrients and Interpretation and Uses of Dietary Reference Intakes, Standing Committee on the Scientific Evaluation of Dietary Reference Intakes."6 Dietary Carbohydrates: Sugars and Starches." *Dietary Reference Intakes for Energy, Carbohydrate, Fiber, Fat, Fatty Acids, Cholesterol, Protein, and Amino Acids (Macronutrients).* Washington, DC: The National Academies Press; 2005.
70. Feurer ID, Crosby LO, Buzby GP, Rosato EF, Mullen JL. Resting energy expenditure in morbid obesity. *Ann Surg.,* 1983; 197:17–21.
71. Pavlou KN, Hoefer MA, Blackburn GL. Resting energy expenditure in moderate obesity: Predicting velocity of weight loss. *Ann Surg.,* 1986; 203:136–141.
72. Ireton-Jones CS, Turner WW, Liepa GU. Equations for the estimation of energy expenditures in patients with burns with special reference to respiratory status. *J Burn Care Rehab.,* 1992; 13:330–333.
73. Ireton-Jones C, Jones JD. Improved equations for predicting energy expenditure in patients: The Ireton-Jones equations. *Nutr Clin Pract.,* 2002; 17:29–31.
74. Liggett SB, St. John RE, Lefrak SS. Determination of resting energy expenditure utilizing the thermodilution pulmonary artery catheter. *Chest,* 1987; 91:562–566.
75. Amato P, Keating KP, Querica RA, Karbonic J. Formulaic methods of estimating calorie requirements in mechanically ventilated obese patients: A reappraisal. *Nutr Clin Pract.,* 1995; 10:229–232.
76. Cutts ME, Dowdy RP, Ellersieck MR, Edes TE. Predicting energy needs in ventilator-dependent critically ill patients: Effect of adjusting weight for edema or adiposity. *Am J Clin Nutr.,* 1997; 66:1250–1256.

77. Flancbaum L, Choban PS, Sambucco S, Verducci J, Burge JC. Comparison of indirect calorimetry, the Fick method, and prediction equations in estimating the energy requirements of critically ill patients. *Am J Clin Nutr.,* 1999; 69:461–466.
78. Glynn CC, Greene GW, Winkler MF, Albina JE. Predictive versus measured energy expenditure using limits-of-agreement analysis in hospitalized obese patients. *JPEN J Parenter Enteral Nutr.,* 1999; 23:147–154.
79. Barak Nir, Wall-Alonso E, Sitrin MD. Evaluation of stress factors and body weight adjustments currently used to estimate energy expenditure in hospitalized patients. *JPENJ Parenter Enteral Nutr.,* 2002; 26:231–238.
80. Frankenfield DC, Rowe WA, Smith JS, Cooney RN. Validation of several established equations for resting metabolic rate in obese and nonobese people. *J Am Diet Assoc.,* 2003; 103:1152–1159.
81. Frankenfield D, Smith JS, Cooney RN. Validation of 2 approaches to predicting resting metabolic rate in critically ill patients. *JPEN J Parenter Enteral Nutr.,* 2004; 28:259–264.
82. Frankenfield D, Hise M, Malone A, Russell M, Gradwell E, Compher C. Prediction of resting metabolic rate in critically ill adult patients: Results of a systematic review of the evidence. *J Am Diet Assoc.,* 2007; 107:1552–1561.
83. Frankenfield D, Coleman A, Alam S, Cooney RN. Analysis of estimation methods for resting metabolic rate in critically ill adults. *JPEN J Parenter Enteral Nutr.,* 2009; 33:27–36.
84. Frankenfield D. Validation of an equation for resting metabolic rate in older obese, critically ill patients. *JPEN J Parenter Enteral Nutr.,* 2011; 35:264–269.
85. Boullata J, Williams J, Cottrell F, Hudson L, Compher C. Accurate determination of energy needs in hospitalized patients. *J Am Diet Assoc.,* 2007; 107:393–401.
86. Weijs PJM. Validity of predictive equations for resting energy expenditure in US and Dutch overweight and obese class I and class II adults aged 18–65 y. *Am J Clin Nutr.,* 2008; 88:959–970.
87. Anderegg BA, Worrall C, Barbour E, Simpson KN, Delegge M. Comparison of resting energy expenditure prediction methods with measured resting energy expenditure in obese, hospitalized adults. *JPEN J Parenter Enteral Nutr.,* 2009; 33:168–175.
88. Frankenfield DC, Ashcraft CM, Galvan DA. Prediction of resting metabolic rate in critically ill patients at the extremes of body mass index. *JPEN J Parenter Enteral Nutr.,* 2013; 37:361–367.
89. Choban PS, Dickerson RN. Morbid obesity and nutrition support: Is bigger different? *Nutr Clin Pract.,* 2005; 20:480–487.
90. Choban PS, Flancbaum L. Nourishing the obese patient. *Clin Nutr.,* 2000; 19:305–311.
91. Dickerson RN. Specialized nutrition support in the hospitalized obese patient. *Nutr Clin Pract.,* 2004; 19:245–254.
92. Boitano M. Hypocaloric feeding of the critically ill. *Nutr Clin Pract.,* 2006; 21:617–622.
93. Burge JC, Goon A, Choban PS, Flancbaum. Efficacy of hypocaloric total parenteral nutrition in hospitalized obese patients: A prospective, double-blind randomized trial. *JPEN J Parenter Enteral Nutr.,* 1994; 18:203–207.
94. Choban PS, Burge JC, Scales D, Flancbaum L. Hypoenergetic nutrition support in hospitalized obese patients: A simplified method for clinical application. *Am J Clin Nutr.,* 1997; 66:546–550.
95. Dickerson RN, Boschert KJ, Kudsk KA, Brown RO. Hypocaloric enteral tube feeding in critically ill obese patients. *Nutrition,* 2002; 18:241–246.
96. Liu KJM, Cho MJ, Atten MJ, Panizales E, Walter R, Hawkins D, Donahue PA. Hypocaloric parenteral nutrition support in elderly obese patients. *Am Surg.,* 2002; 4:394–400.
97. McCowan KC, Friel C, Sternberg J, Chan S, Forse RA, Burke PA, Bistrian BR. Hypocaloric total parenteral nutrition: Effectiveness in prevention of hyperglycemia and infectious complications—A randomized clinical trial. *Crit Care Med.,* 2000; 28:3606–3611.
98. Choban P, Dickerson R, Malone A, Worthington P, Compher C; American Society for Parenteral and Enteral Nutrition. A.S.P.E.N. Clinical guidelines: nutrition support of hospitalized adult patients with obesity. *JPEN J Parenter Enteral Nutr.* 2013; Nov;37(6):714–744.
99. Dickerson RN, Medling TL, Smith AC et al. Hypocaloric, high-protein nutrition therapy in older vs younger critically ill patients with obesity. *JPEN J Parenter Enteral Nutr.,* 2013; 37:342–351.
100. American Society for Parenteral and Enteral Nutrition. Nutrition therapy of the severely obese, critically ill patient: Summation of conclusions and recommendations. *JPEN J Parenter Enteral Nutr.,* 2011; 35:88S–96S.
101. Kross EK, Sena M, Schmidt K, Stapleton RD. A comparison of predictive equations of energy expenditure and measured energy expenditure in critically ill patients. *J Crit Care.* 2012 Jun;27(3):321.e5–e12.

102. Guidelines and position papers from the European Society for Clinical Nutrition and Metabolism. ESPEN Website. http://www.espen.org/education/espen-guidelines (Accessed February 12, 2015.)
103. Parnes HL, Mascioli EA, LaCivita CL et al. Parenteral nutrition in overweight patients: Are intravenous lipids necessary to prevent essential fatty acid deficiency? *J Nutr Biochem.*, 1994; 5:243–247.
104. Phinney SD, Tang AB, Johnson SB, Holman RT. Reduced adipose 18:3 omega 3 with weight loss by very low calorie dieting. *Lipids*, 1990; 25:798–806.
105. Gelhorn A, Marks PA. The composition and biosynthesis of lipids in human adipose tissues. *J Clin Invest.*, 1961; 40:125–132.
106. Fujioka K, DiBaise JK, Martindale RG. Nutrition and metabolic complications after bariatric surgery and their treatment. *JEPN J Parenter Enteral Nutr.*, 2011; 35:52S–59S.
107. Dickerson RN, Drover JW. Monitoring nutrition therapy in the critically ill patient with obesity. *JEPN J Parenter Enteral Nutr.*, 2011; 35:44S–51S.
108. Heyland DK, Cahill N, Day AG. Optimal amount of calories for critically ill patients: Depends on how you slice the cake! *Crit Care Med.,* 2011; 39:2619–2626.

Section VIII

Professional Issues

38 Ethical Considerations in the Critically Ill Patient

Denise Baird Schwartz

CONTENTS

INTRODUCTION

Clinical ethics considerations in the critically ill will remain a case-by-case–based model, unless there is a change to a proactive, integrated, systematic process in health-care institutions and systems. An enlightened role of each individual's responsibility in advance care planning about end-of-life care is essential. This chapter provides a background of the problem and identifies solutions to develop a system that promotes preventive ethics and opens communication for patients and their family on this topic.

BACKGROUND

Health-care clinical ethics awareness has increased over the past four decades as evidenced by landmark adult ethics cases depicted in Table 38.1.[1,2] These cases have provided the opportunity to change how we approach end-of-life care and have been instrumental in giving other individuals the right to live and die with dignity. During this period, clinical ethics health care has evolved with interprofessional hospital bioethics committees, legislation aimed at promoting advance directives, palliative care team development, ethical guidelines, and ethics position and practice papers published by national health-care organizations.

Despite these advancements, there is a practice gap between clinical ethics and life-sustaining treatments, including nutrition therapy for the critically ill, compared to what is achievable on the basis of current knowledge. This is measurable based on the number of patients without advance directives in intensive care units (ICUs), designating the individual's wishes.[1] The lack

TABLE 38.1
Landmark Adult Ethics Cases and Court Outcome[1,2]

Individual	Court Case Outcomes
Karen Ann Quinlan 1954–1985 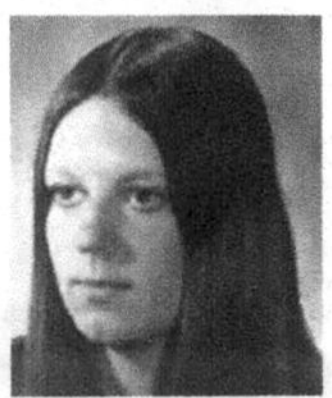 1975 21 years old at the time of brain injury Resulted in PVS 1976 Removed from ventilator Tube feeding continued	• New Jersey Supreme Court 1976 ruled ventilator, a life-sustaining measure, could be removed if prognosis existed of *no reasonable possibility of a patient returning to a cognitive, sapient state* and a hospital ethics committee could confirm such a conclusion • New Jersey Supreme Court: 1. Introduced *substitutional judgment* or *subjective test*, allowing a proxy to decide what the individual would have wanted 2. Provided for criminal and civil legal protection for all involved parties in decision-making process • Case helped establish hospital ethics committees and enactment of states' *living will* legislation
Nancy Beth Cruzan 1957–1990 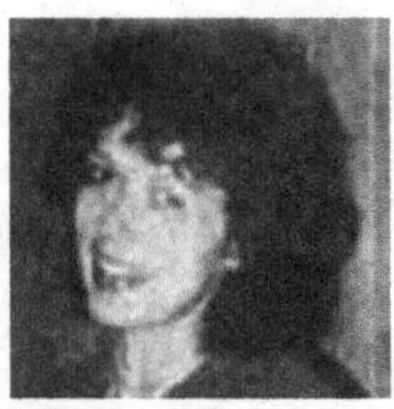 1983 25 years old at the time of car accident Resulted PVS 1990 Tube feeding discontinued	• Missouri Supreme Court 1990 determined feeding tube could lawfully be removed only if there was *clear and convincing evidence* that removal was in accordance with her wishes • US Supreme Court 1990: 1. Acknowledged constitutional right that grants a competent person a right to refuse lifesaving hydration and nutrition 2. Surrogate may act for patient in electing treatment withdrawal; evidence of incompetent person's wishes to withdraw treatment be proved by clear and convincing evidence to be an appropriate standard 3. Rejected co-guardians' contentions that the state must accept substituted judgment of close family members 4. Established ANH as life-sustaining, no different than ventilators and hemodialysis: they are medical treatments 5. Recommended use of DPAHC and living wills as valuable safeguards to patient's interest in directing medical care • Case stimulated increased use of health-care proxies or DPAHC and enactment of the Patient Self Determination Act of 1990
Theresa Marie (Terri) Schiavo 1963–2005 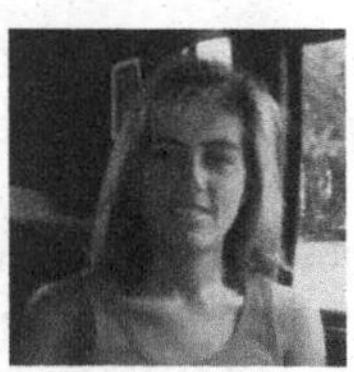 1990 26 years old at the time of cardiac arrest Resulted in PVS 2005 Tube feeding discontinued	• Florida 1998 spouse filed petition to have feeding tube removed on grounds that wife would not wish to be maintained in PVS. Her parents argued opposite position, resulting in a debate that spanned two feeding tube removals and reinsertions, four rejected appeals to the Supreme Court, intervention by Florida legislature and governor, Congress, and the president • 2005 federal district court refused to order reinsertion • Political reaction to the case resulted in refinement of living will legislation with regard to ANH in several states

Notes: PVS, persistent vegetative state; ANH, artificial nutrition and hydration; DPAHC, durable power of attorney for health care.

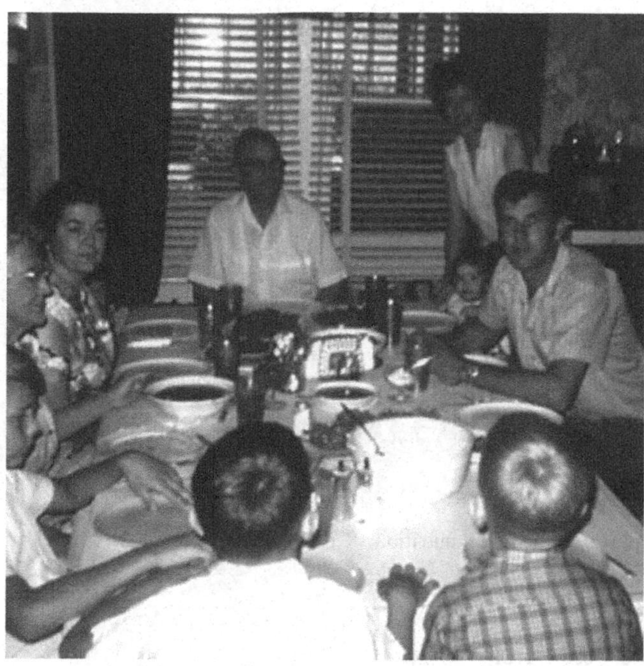

FIGURE 38.1 Patient/surrogate/family's concept of nutrition.

of communication between patients and their families concerning wishes for end-of-life care before the illness and health-care crisis is a challenging problem. The solution to this deficit will be multifactorial and will need a paradigm shift of all stakeholders. Critical care clinicians focus on nutrition support initiation and aspects of this therapy, such as route, timing, and substrates; yet, complexities of patient wishes are not always addressed. Nutrition support clinicians are in a prime position to promote culture change in clinical ethics to improve *whole* patient-centered care.

The importance of focusing on timely ethical decision-making is especially evident in practice settings where early nutrition intervention, especially critical care, is recommended to optimize health-care outcomes. Nutrition, whether administered orally or through tubes, can provide a sense of caring for individuals and their families and become more difficult to withdraw after being initiated, than to be withheld.[1] Patients/surrogate/family's concept of nutrition is different compared to the complexity of artificial nutrition, as exemplified in Figures 38.1 and 38.2.

Ethical dilemmas in the hospital entail nutrition therapy; often, this therapy is the first to start and the last to be stopped. The finality of the care goals is made apparent to both the family and the health-care professionals when nutrition is stopped.

INTEGRATING QUALITY OF LIFE GOAL SCREENING INTO CRITICAL CARE PRACTICE

Health-related quality of life (QOL) can be defined as the value assigned to the duration of life as modified by the impairments, functional states, perceptions, and social opportunities that are influenced by disease, injury, treatment, or policy. QOL is highly individual, and there are high levels of variability between individuals.[3] QOL goal screening needs to become an initial step for critical care professionals, before the nutrition care process (NCP) as indicated in Figure 38.3 and prior to starting nutrition support.[4]

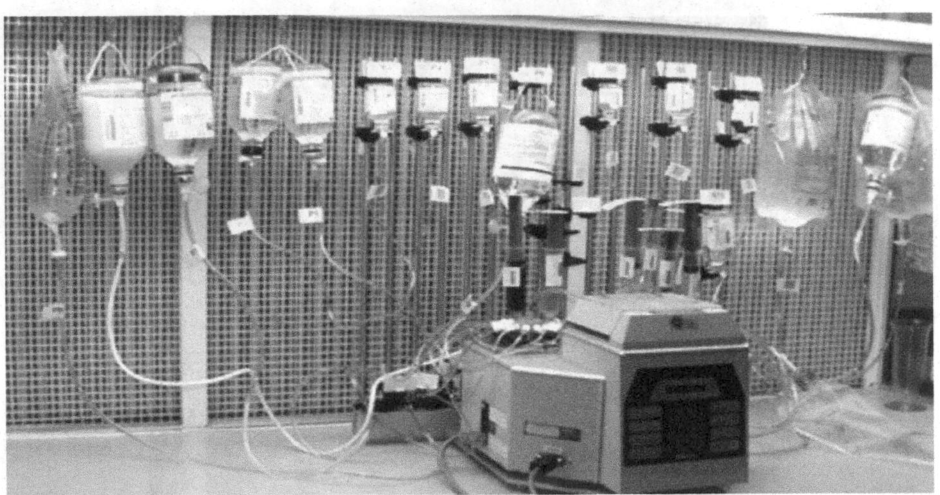

FIGURE 38.2 Complexity of artificial nutrition.

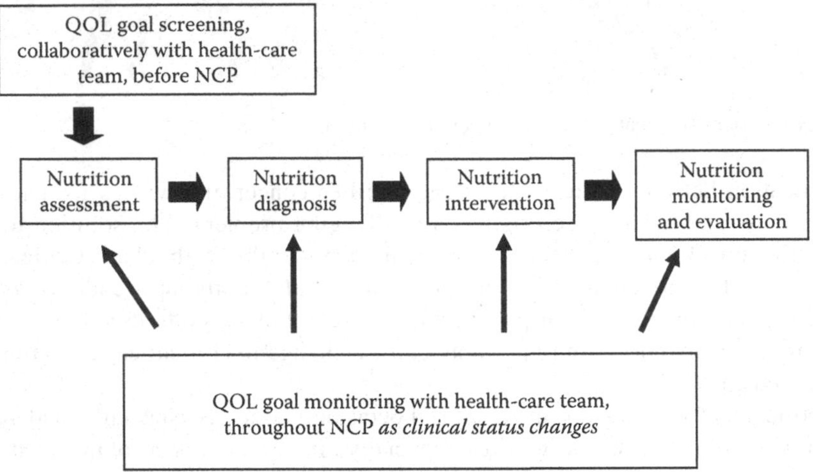

FIGURE 38.3 Screening and monitoring for quality of life (QOL) goals and nutrition care process (NCP).

NUTRITION CARE PROCESS

NCP is a systematic problem-solving method that registered dietitians (RDs) use to think critically and make decisions that address practice-related problems.[5] Just as nutrition screening is done before the NCP, QOL goal screening should be completed before NCP as it is essential to provide patient-centered care.

Assuring that this alternative health-care outcome is considered would facilitate changing the critical care clinician's focus to goal-oriented patient-centered care. The Institute of Medicine defines patient-centered care as "care that is respectful of and responsive to individual patient preferences, needs, and values" and that ensures "that patient values guide all clinical decisions."[6] This definition emphasizes the importance of clinicians and individuals working together to produce the best outcomes possible, rather than a disease-outcome-based paradigm.[7]

Various sources can be used by the critical care clinician to screen for the individual's QOL goals to facilitate patient-centered decision-making for initiation and continued use of artificial nutrition. Table 38.2 provides sources in the individual's chart, communication with the individual and their

TABLE 38.2
Sources for Screening and Monitoring for Quality of Life Goals for Artificial Nutrition Decision-Making

1. Advance directive (indicating surrogate decision-maker and health-care treatment preferences)
2. Durable power of attorney for health care (DPAHC)
3. Physician orders for life-sustaining treatment (POLST)
4. Medical orders for life-sustaining treatment (MOLST)
5. Interprofessional unit rounds
6. Discussion with health-care professionals, including physician, dietitian, nurse, social worker, chaplain, case manager, and palliative care team members
7. Comments from individuals and their family members when assessing nutrition status and during nutrition support education
8. Futility of treatment based on individual's overall clinical status as assessed by physician

family/surrogate/decision-maker, and discussion with other health-care professionals that could add to the screening process for QOL goals.

UNDERSTANDING CULTURAL VALUES AND RELIGIOUS DIVERSITY

Critical care clinician's understanding of cultural and religious diversity is necessary to best meet the needs of a heterogeneous patient population. This diversity awareness provides the clinician the ability to tailor information for patients, families, and significant others that promote understanding of decision-making dealing with the use of aggressive life-sustaining treatments, including artificial nutrition. Table 38.3 provides a sample of religious and cultural perspective diversity for end-of-life care decisions.

These perspectives are not meant to be inclusive for everyone in that religious or cultural group, but are presented to facilitate a better understanding of the individualized perspective diversity in clinical ethics.[4]

IMPROVING HEALTH LITERACY AND TEACH-BACK METHOD

Nutrition, even delivered by a feeding tube, represents the bridge between a therapy that gives a sense of normalcy for patients and families and the technology-driven health-care system. Initiation of artificial nutrition may result in patients and families/significant others accepting therapies, such as mechanical ventilation, cardiopulmonary resuscitation, and other advanced treatments that may not be in congruency with the patient's wishes.[1] Use of evidence-based practice guidelines such as from the Academy of Nutrition and Dietetics is beneficial in providing appropriate information.[17] Medical treatment decisions require a critical appraisal of the potential benefit and harm of the options, within the context of the patient's characteristics, conditions, and preferences.[18] Nutrition support clinicians should be a part of the interprofessional collaborative collegial process that can facilitate improved health literacy in clinical ethics.

Health literacy is defined as the degree to which individuals obtain, process, and understand basic health information and services to make appropriate health decisions. Health literacy involves a range of social, cultural, and individual factors. Poor health literacy affects all levels of health care, from individuals, to providers, to health-care environments.[19]

The teach-back technique is an effective method to ensure that individuals understand what they have been told. It involves asking the individual to explain or demonstrate what they were taught. If the individual does not explain correctly, the assumption is that the information was not presented in an understandable way. The information then would be retaught using an alternative approach.[19]

TABLE 38.3
Religious and Cultural Perspectives on End-of-Life Decisions

African-American, Black	Prefer more life-sustaining treatment compared to white patients Feel that patient should be primary decision-maker in end-of-life care May view overly individualistic focus as disrespectful to family heritage Perceive suffering as spiritually meaningful, and life as always having some value Ceasing aggressive therapies may be equated with giving up Perspective that end of life is in God's hands[8–11]
Asian (specific ethnic group not designated)	Value physician's obligation to promote patient welfare by encouraging patient hope, even in terminal illness Special status of elderly should not be burdened with bad news Illness is considered a family event rather than individual occurrence Family members and physicians share decisional duties[12]
Bosnian	Prefer physician, due to expert knowledge, make independent decisions to reduce burden on individuals and families Expect physician to maintain individual's optimism by not revealing terminal diagnosis[12]
Buddhism	Not mandatory or moral obligation to preserve life at all costs No specific teachings on individuals in persistent vegetative state; nutrition support keeps person alive artificially, which is not mandatory Terminal care should be available, and hospice movement is supported[13]
Catholicism	Person has a moral obligation to use ordinary or proportionate means of preserving his or her life Person may forgo extraordinary or disproportionate means of life Medically assisted nutrition and hydration become morally optional when they cannot reasonably be expected to prolong life or when they would be excessively burdensome for individual or would cause significant physical discomfort, for example, resulting from complications in the use of means employed Free and informed judgment made by a competent adult individual concerning the use or withdrawal of life-sustaining procedures should always be respected and normally complied with, unless it is contrary to Catholic moral teaching[14]
Caucasian, White (non-Hispanic)	Prefer less life-sustaining treatment than black patients Feel that patient should be primary decision-maker for end-of-life care Concerned about dying individuals undergoing needless suffering[8,9,11]
Chinese	Hope is considered very important in care of dying, as hope prevents suffering by avoiding despair; prefer family-centered decision-making Food represents more than source of energy; it embodies family, love, and caring Much distress in terminal persons can be attributed to or related to anorexia and cachexia Medical decision is usually based on best interests of person; treatment utility is often open to interpretation Family members protect terminally ill individuals from knowledge of condition Individuals and families do not discuss possible death due to belief that direct acknowledgement of morality may be self-fulfilling[12,13]
Confucian	Death is good if one has fulfilled one's moral duties in life, and resistance to accepting terminal illness or insisting on futile treatment may reflect individual's perception of unfinished business[13]
Eastern European	Tradition of physician-centered, paternalistic decision-making Physician rather than person or family often determines a person's level of life support[12]
Filipino	May not want to discuss end-of-life care because these exchanges demonstrate lack of respect for belief that individual fate is determined by God[13]

(Continued)

TABLE 38.3 (*Continued*)
Religious and Cultural Perspectives on End-of-Life Decisions

Greek Orthodox	Withholding or withdrawing of artificial nutrition is not allowable even if there is no prospect of recovery[13]
Hinduism and Sikh	Duty-based rather than rights-based and believe in karma, a casual law where all acts and human thoughts have consequences
	Death is viewed as a passage to a new life; the way you die is important
	A do-not-attempt-resuscitation order is usually accepted or desired because death should be peaceful[13]
Hispanic	Prefer less aggressive, comfort-focused end-of-life care
	Favor family-centered decision-making and limited patient autonomy
	Family members actively protect terminally ill person from the knowledge of condition
	Consider family members, rather than individual alone, as holding decision-making power regarding life support
	May be reluctant to formally appoint a specific family member to be in charge because of concerns about isolating these persons or offending other relatives
	Consensually oriented decision-making approach appears to be more acceptable[12,15]
Islamic	Premature death should be prevented, but treatments can be withheld or withdrawn in terminally ill individuals when physicians are certain about inevitability of death and that treatment in no way will improve condition or quality of life
	The intention must never be to hasten death, only to abstain from overzealous treatment[13]
Judaism	Withdrawal of continuous life-sustaining therapy is not allowed, but withholding further treatment is allowed as part of dying process, if it is an intermittent life-sustaining treatment and if it was a clear wish of the patient
	Food and fluid are regarded as basic needs and not treatment
	It is permissible to withhold food and fluid if this is the individual's expressed wishes, when individual approaches final days of life, when food and even fluids may cause suffering and complications[13]
Korean	Consider family members, rather than individual alone, as holding the decision-making power regarding life support[12]
Lebanese	With every interaction at end of life, importance given to the role of family
	Loyalty to family is first in importance, even before religion, nationality, or ethnicity
	Important to acknowledge family-oriented outlook and make family one of the central elements in communication protocol[16]
Native American	Words should be chosen carefully because once spoken, they may become a reality
	Negative words and thoughts about health can become self-fulfilling
	Prominent value on thinking and speaking in a positive way[12]
North American	Emphasis placed on autonomy and openly discuss treatment decisions; norm is for individual medical care decision-making[12,13]
Pakistani	Family members protect terminally ill individuals from the knowledge of condition
	Physicians may be adopted into family unit and addressed as parent, aunt, uncle, or sibling; this family status provides physician with role sanctioning involvement in intimate discussions[12]
Protestantism	Most will, if there is little hope of recovery, accept and understand the withholding or withdrawal of therapy[13]
Taoism	Philosophical Taoism acceptance is only an appropriate response when facing death and artificial measures contradicts natural events
	Religious Taoism death may lead to an afterlife torture in endless hell, where a Taoist might cling to any means of extending life to postpone that possibility[13]

In addition to verbal communication, readability is a significant factor affecting the potential impact of the message. A fifth-grade reading level or less is recommended for information material and has been identified as criterion for low literacy.[20]

PREVENTIVE ETHICS CONCEPTS

Preventive ethics proposes that ethical conflict is largely predictable and can be avoided with proactive interventions aimed at the organization, unit, and individual levels.[21] The goals of preventive ethics are to use a proactive approach to identify common triggers of ethical conflict and to address these triggers before they contribute to conflict. Preventive ethics represents a dramatic shift from the traditional ethics approach, which uses a case-by-case approach, reacting to ethically challenging patient situations as they arise in the clinical setting or when a consultation is requested. Common triggers for possible ethical conflict are presented in Table 38.4.

Once common triggers are identified, specific interventions can be planned to prevent the ethical conflict from occurring, which are identified in Table 38.5.

PARADIGM SHIFT

To achieve optimum preventive clinical ethics for critically ill patients, a paradigm shift is required by the individual/patient, family, surrogate decision-maker, health-care professional, and health-care facilities. These paradigm shifts are presented in Table 38.6.

The paradigm shift process would be greatly enhanced if conversations about end-of-life care preferences occurred between the individual and their family members before the illness and hospitalization. Organizations are involved in trying to facilitate this paradigm shift by health-care professionals with guidelines, position, and practice papers, non-health-care individuals have the opportunity and responsibility to be informed and act.

RECOMMENDATIONS FOR DEVELOPING POLICIES AND PROCEDURES

Development and implementation of a policy and procedure for artificial nutrition ethical decision-making at health-care facilities requires consideration of the patient population, cultural diversity, and religious affiliation, where applicable. The published recommendations and guidelines from national organizations should be included as a foundation in the policy and procedure. Implementation of the policy and procedure requires education of all individuals involved in the process. Format for a sample acute care policy and procedure is shown in Table 38.7.

TABLE 38.4
Common Triggers for Possible Ethical Decision-Making Conflict

Patient/Surrogate/Family Triggers	Patient Unit and System Triggers
Vulnerability—elderly, very young, non-English speaking, incapacitated	Lack of health-care team consensus or conflict
Lack of social support	Inconsistent health-care providers
End-of-life situation	Strong hierarchical/power structures
Disagreement with health-care providers	Ineffective shift report or handoff procedures of health-care team members
Unrealistic treatment expectations by patient/surrogate/family	Late or absent family health-care meetings
	False hope or difficult discussion avoidance

Source: Epstein, E.G., *Am. Assoc. Crit. Care Nurs.*, 23, 217, 2012.

TABLE 38.5
Interventions to Prevent Ethical Decision-Making Conflict

Patient/Surrogate/Family Triggers	Intervention Options
Unrealistic expectations	Discuss with patient/family reasons for expectations
	Frequent, consistent discussion with patient/family
Religious beliefs conflicting with reality	Discuss/document important aspects of beliefs
	Ask to meet with patient/family religious leader to better understand foundations of beliefs
	Hospital chaplain visits
	Consistent care by health-care team members with similar beliefs
Infrequent visits by family	Determine reason
	Alleviate fear of hospital setting
	Assist with transportation, if possible, such as taxi vouchers
Lack of social support	Identify a small cohort of nurses for consistent care
	Institute a point-contact system: particular family member or a specific provider serves as a contact who can more easily identify providers who can answer family's questions
Cultural beliefs that are unfamiliar to providers	Research culture and beliefs
	Ask patient/family to describe culture: what should team know about the culture; what would help family members
Patient Unit and System Triggers	
Family meetings initiated late	Identify patients in intensive care unit who remain critically ill 48 h after admission to unit
	Develop a procedure for initiating an early health-care team meeting to discuss current plan and initial and regularly scheduled follow-up family meetings
Lack of consensus	Construct a process for scheduling health-care team meetings to discuss different perspective about care of patients with complex problems

Source: Epstein, E.G., *Am. Assoc. Crit. Care Nurs.*, 23, 217, 2012.

Critical care clinicians could use this sample format to expand the important considerations section with recommendations and guidelines from the organizations listed and other organizations pertinent to the patient population in which the policy and procedure would be used.[1] Also, modification of the procedure section should be done collaboratively in each institution. Concepts in Table 38.8 dealing with important ethical considerations developed by the American Society for Parenteral and Enteral Nutrition could be used to enhance the sample policy and procedure for artificial nutrition decision-making.

DESIGNING AND IMPLEMENTING QUALITY IMPROVEMENT PROJECTS AND BENCHMARKING DATA

A quality improvement project in clinical ethics and artificial nutrition identifying if there is adequate documentation to determine that individuals and their family have been involved in the decision-making process dealing with artificial nutrition for patients in the ICU would be valuable. The number of patients on artificial nutrition, with and without an advance directive (designating surrogate decision-maker and treatment preferences) on the chart should be measured. Information gathered could include the individual's age, gender, religion, culture,

TABLE 38.6
Stakeholders and Paradigm Shifts

Stakeholders	Paradigm Shift
Individual/patient	To recognize the need to address health-care wishes prior to an illness or hospitalization with a person who will be able to follow through with hard decisions, rather than ignore inevitability of this period in one's life
	To provide detailed aspects of health-care wishes to assist surrogate/family decision-maker and health-care providers, rather than vague concepts and generalities about end-of-life care
Family members	To be active member in this paradigm shift by starting conversation with family members about wishes for end-of-life care, rather than never discussing the topic
	Completing documents that provide specific information about end-of-life care, selecting a person as decision-maker, rather than not taking the time to plan and formalize these decisions
Surrogate decision-maker	To recognize they represent the patient, not themselves in the decision-making process
	To have a conversation between the individual and the surrogate decision-maker and detailed written documentation about end-of-life care is required, not just be listed as a durable power attorney for health care without discussion
Health-care professional	To be part of an interprofessional health-care team approach to clinical ethics, rather than the responsibility of only one or two professions, with a sense of territory limitations
	To become knowledgeable in health-care decision-making concepts and issues, rather than it is other health-care professional's role
Health-care facilities	To develop systems that focus on *whole* patient-centered care based on patient's wishes for end of life, rather than facility mortality rate and impact on reimbursement
	To implement a preventative ethics model with the goal to have a proactive, integrated, systematic process that prevents ethical problems, rather than deals with the ethics problem on a case-by-case basis, after it has occurred
	To increase use of palliative care consults, for quality of life goal assistance for patients and their families and not only consider it for end of life on the last day or hours of an individual's life
	To increase use of hospice consults for appropriate individuals rather that omit this service that can assist patients and their families
	To develop in the facility an atmosphere of collegial, interprofessional health-care team approach to clinical ethics, rather than the responsibility of only one or two professions, with a sense of territory limitations

language preference, and presence of family/decision-maker. Additional useful information might incorporate the number of family care conferences, palliative care, and bioethics consults during the hospitalization.

Critical care nutrition support clinicians could design and lead this project in collaboration with other health-care team members, including physicians, nurses, social workers, chaplains, and palliative care team members. This information could serve as a baseline before implementing any processes, such as development and implementation of a policy and procedure to improve and standardize the procedures of communication between the patient, family, and health-care providers on artificial nutrition. Analyzing the problems and determining the root causes of these issues would help define the improvement goals.

After implementing the improvement plan, remeasuring a sample size would facilitate determining if measurable goals were achieved and if the process change is sustainable. Incorporating a standardized process in clinical ethics and artificial nutrition could then be shared between health-care facilities to benchmark best practice and translate ethical decision-making for artificial nutrition into clinical practice. A sample quality improvement project is depicted in Table 38.9.

TABLE 38.7
Sample ICU Artificial Nutrition Health-Care Choices Communication Policy and Procedure

Policy

The policy is to provide ethically and medically appropriate artificial nutrition, based on published evidence-based guidelines and recommendations of recognized authorities and translate these guidelines and recommendations into patient-centered care.

Purpose

The purpose is to promote health literacy and written documentation in the medical record concerning health-care decisions for artificial nutrition. The intent is to provide early communication between health-care providers, patients, and families/surrogate and designation of a decision-maker, with attention to spiritual/faith and cultural diversity.

Important considerations

Include components from the following organizations and other organizations as appropriate for the individual population, culture, and religious affiliation

a. Academy Nutrition and Dietetics (AND) Position Paper and Practice Paper on Ethical and Legal Issues in Feeding and Hydration
b. American Academy of Pediatrics Clinical Report
c. American College of Physicians Ethics Manual
d. American Medical Association Policy on Provision of Life-Sustaining Medical Treatment dealing with nutrition
c. American Society for Parenteral and Enteral Nutrition Ethics Position Paper

Procedure

1. One member of the health-care team, with approval of patient's physician, discusses with patient/family about health-care choices, which include artificial nutrition, based on patient's wishes/quality of life goals during the first 2–3 days of admission to ICU.
2. A letter of introduction to ICU and health-care choices would be given to the patient/family/decision-maker during the earlier-mentioned discussion, as a tool for health literacy in this discussion. Cultural diversity component would be achieved by having the letter in appropriate language on the back side of the letter in English, as needed. Translation phone service would be used as appropriate.
3. Health-care clinicians would be involved in training sessions dealing with communication, spiritual and cultural diversity, difficult subjects and role-playing, and teach-back method.
4. A designated group of medical, spiritual, and cultural diversity advisors would be identified to review the process and content of the information.
5. An evaluation tool would be used by the health-care team member prior to visiting the patient/family, and the assessment tool would be completed after the discussion. This tool would incorporate both the health-care professional evaluation and patient/family evaluation. The results would be evaluated for revisions and reevaluated periodically for changes needed.
6. Communication process through medical record; written and verbal would be done with the information obtained about the patient's health-care choices concerning artificial nutrition.
7. Patients in ICU ≥3 days should be screened for supportive care needs by palliative care team members based on a system of defined screening criteria, as developed by the palliative care team. Patients would be identified during ICU rounds at high risk for palliative care team involvement to help with health-care choices for patient quality of life goals, including the use of artificial nutrition.
8. Family care conferences recommended for patients in ICU 5–7 days or less, incorporating a discussion on artificial nutrition. Document in progress notes family care conference outcome/recommended plan.

ADVANCE CARE PLANNING INITIATIVES

Numerous initiatives have been developed and promote concepts that help individuals and their family better understand advance care planning. Table 38.10 provides resources for health-care providers and the public to increase their knowledge in this important aspect of health care that would be useful when determining the appropriate use of artificial nutrition.

TABLE 38.8
Important Considerations in American Society for Parenteral and Enteral Nutrition (ASPEN) Ethics Position Paper

1. To extent possible, decisions regarding artificial nutrition and hydration (ANH) should be based on evidenced-based medicine (EBM), best practices, and clinical experience and judgment in discussion with the patient, family, or significant others.
2. From a scientific, ethical, and legal perspective, there should be no differentiation between withholding and withdrawing of ANH; the term *forgoing* is used for both, recognizing that withdrawing is more emotionally laden than withholding, especially within specific cultures.
3. Decisions regarding forgoing ANH should incorporate a benefit–risk–burden analysis based on EBM and best practices in discussion with the patient, family, or significant others.
4. Limited time trials are an acceptable alternative when the benefits of ANH are questionable, and trial nature of ANH is communicated and consented to by patients and family prior to its initiation.
5. Scientific evidence on physiology of patients with brain death, in a coma, or in a persistent vegetative state (PVS), indicates these patients do not experience thirst or hunger and therefore are not likely to suffer.
6. ANH may not provide benefit and may have associated risks in patients with severe dementia or in a PVS.
7. Artificial hydration of terminally ill patients can lead to discomfort due to fluid overload, pulmonary and generalized edema, shortness of breath, etc., and may be discontinued on clinical and ethical grounds provided such discontinuation is not in conflict with existing laws, institutional policies, and consent/consensus of decision-makers.
8. Forgoing ANH in infants and children at end of life may be ethically acceptable when competent parents and medical team concur that intervention no longer confers a benefit to the child or creates a burden that cannot be justified.
9. Religious, cultural, and ethnic background of patients and families need to be respected to the extent it is consistent with other ethical principles and duties.
10. Consent, respect, and preservation of dignity should be paramount during ethical and legal deliberations regarding ANH.
11. Many states in the United States require *clear and convincing evidence* to forgo ANH in decisionally incapacitated patients without documented ANH preferences.
12. Patients with decision-making capacity and authority should be appropriate moral agents to make choices regarding ANH based on evidence-based information qualified practitioners present to them.
13. For patients lacking decision-making capacity, health-care professional has an ethical legal obligation to reference an advance directive or discussion with authorized surrogate decision-maker, whether appointed through mechanisms of a durable power of attorney for health-care directive, court, or statutory processes.
14. Surrogate decision-makers (including but not limited to family members and/or significant others) should be given same considerations as individual patients with decision-making capacity.
15. Health-care professionals should not be ethically obligated to offer ANH if in their clinical judgment there is not adequate evidence for therapy or burden or risk of intervention far outweighs its benefit.
16. Establishment of interdisciplinary teams and conference with patient and family is highly encouraged; interdisciplinary ethics committees or panels should be consulted when involved parties cannot resolve the ethical dilemma.
17. Care should continue until conflict regarding ANH is resolved; if unable to resolve conflicts, even with the ethics consultation, orderly transfer of care assuring continuity of care is recommended to an equally and willing practitioner and or institution; at no time should patients or families feel abandoned.

Source: Barrocas, A. et al., *Nutr. Clin. Pract.*, 25, 672, 2010.

CASE STUDY

An 84-year-old male was admitted with altered mental status. At the assisted living facility, prior to admission, the individual's food intake had decreased over the past 3 months, which resulted in a 10% unintentional weight loss. Declining mental status during the past several months was reported by his daughter. The patient's wife had passed away several years earlier.

After diagnostic procedures showed a bleeding cerebral aneurysm and after discussion with the physician as to the diagnosis and risk/benefits to a procedure, the daughter agreed to an

TABLE 38.9
Sample Quality Improvement Project

Gather members of health-care team dealing with nutrition support of critically ill patients
Determine number and percent of patients on nutrition support that have an advance directive on chart in intensive care unit
Collect patient data of all individuals receiving nutrition support and analyze with interprofessional health-care team
Develop and implement policy and procedure for ethical decision-making for artificial nutrition, collaboratively with health-care team
Remeasure population to determine change and sustainability
Share best practice between health-care institutions and organizations of clinical ethics and nutrition support

TABLE 38.10
Resources for Advance Care Planning Decision-Making

Advance Care Planning Information Sources	Focus of Initiative, Campaign, and Programs
Consider the Conversation, http://www.considertheconversation.org/	Using film to inspire person-centered care Goal: to inspire culture change that results in end-of-life care that is more person-centered and less system-centered
The Conversation Project, http://www.theconversationproject.org	Developed in collaboration with Institute for Healthcare Improvement Goal: to have every person's end-of-life preferences expressed and respected Provides Starter Kit to help gather thoughts on the process and then have conversations with a loved one on wishes for end-of-life care
Five Wishes—Aging with Dignity, http://www.agingwithdignity.org/five-wishes.php	Written in everyday language Helps start and structure important conversations about care in times of serious illness Useful guide and documentation tool of individual's wishes
National Healthcare Decisions Day, http://www.nhdd.org	Goal: to inspire, educate, and empower the public and providers about the importance of advance care planning Collaborative effort of national, state, and community organizations in the United States Provides specific resources for activities to promote National Healthcare Decisions Day Resources are provided as templates and can be adapted to include local contact and other information as needed Held annually on April 16
Physician Orders for Life-Sustaining Treatment (POLST), http://www.polst.org	Paradigm program Designed to improve the quality of care people receive at the end of life Based on effective communication of patient wishes, documentation of medical orders on a brightly colored form, and a promise by health-care professionals to honor these wishes
Speak Up campaign, http://www.advancecareplanning.ca	Campaign to promote advance care planning in Canada Developed to raise awareness of importance of advance care planning, as well as issues related to an aging population, a strained health-care system, and end-of-life care Speak Up campaign kit contains material to promote advance care planning

Source: Schwartz, D.B., *Clin. Nutr. Insight,* 2012; 38:4–5.

interventional neurosurgery. The daughter appeared to be the appropriate surrogate decision-maker; no other family was present at the hospital. Although the patient had another daughter, she was not involved in her father's health care. There was no durable power of attorney for health care (DPAHC), physician orders for life-sustaining treatment (POLST), or other documents indicating the patient's wishes or authorized decision-maker, in the chart initially.

The patient's registered nurse (RN) presented the case during the ICU walking daily interprofessional rounds on the first day post admission. After rounds, the RD received a physician consult order for the initiation of enteral tube feeding. Post extubation, the patient exhibited dysphagia, which was confirmed by the speech-language pathologists. The RD discussed the planned initiation of the enteral tube feeding with the daughter, including reason for this therapy, monitoring aspects, and goals for the nutrition intervention. The patient's daughter was receptive to the information and expressed appreciation for the thorough explanation of the intervention, and the RD provided written material and contact information if the daughter had any further questions.

The following day, the RD saw the daughter in the ICU and asked how she was doing with her father's illness and if there were any more questions that could be addressed concerning her father's nutrition care. The patient's daughter indicated that she did not know if she was making the right decisions on behalf of her father for all of his medical treatments. The RD encouraged the daughter to express her concern with her father's physician and nurse. Additionally, the RD indicated that the focus of all health-care clinicians in the hospital was to provide patient-centered care based on the patient's wishes.

Due to the timeliness and sensitivity of the discussion, the RD indicated that a licensed clinical social worker (LCSW) might be of benefit to provide further information on how to proceed with the daughter's concerns and discuss decision-making. Although the patient's daughter indicated she did not want to bother anyone, the RD indicated she could call the LCSW and determine her availability to speak with her. The patient's daughter requested that the discussion with the LCSW not occur in her father's hospital room, even though he did not appear to be alert.

The LCSW came immediately to meet with the patient's daughter and took her to a small meeting room in the ICU to have the discussion and talk through her own feelings about her father's future care. By incorporating health literacy components, rather than using medical language (such as advance directive, DPAHC, POLST, living will), the LCSW asked if there was any written document that her father had that indicated what he wanted if he came to the hospital. At that point, the daughter shared a detailed advance directive (designating a decision-maker and specific health-care wishes) that she had in her purse; this document indicated his QOL goals and that there were to be no heroics if specific minimum standards were not met.

Following this discussion, the LCSW contacted the patient's physician, RN, and RD and advised them of the patient's wishes. The advance directive was placed in the chart and a family conference was scheduled for the next day. That same afternoon, the neurosurgeon examined the patient, after which he met with the daughter to discuss that there had been a stroke and that her father would not be likely to ever eat or engage in meaningful interaction. A neurology consult confirmed this diagnosis, the same day. After discussion with the patient's daughter, the primary care physician ordered, "'Do not attempt resuscitation,' palliative care, and hospice consults." The patient's daughter requested the physician to initiate comfort care immediately for her father. The enteral tube feeding was discontinued due to the burdens exhibited with fluids and increased secretions. Chaplain visits were provided for emotional support for the daughter. The palliative care team met with the daughter to provide support and bereavement information to her, following her request.

Throughout this process, health-care team members verbally communicated and documented electronically in the medical record. The patient expired the next day with his daughter at the bedside. The palliative care team followed up with the daughter over the next few days to assist with the coping process and to provide support as needed.

This case study exemplifies an effective health-care team communication process in the ICU, by working collaboratively to provide *whole* patient-centered care, based on the patient's wishes. It demonstrated how the process started with a *conversation* about artificial nutrition, between the RD and the daughter/surrogate decision-maker, and resulted in critical information dissemination to appropriate health-care providers to assist in the decision-making process. The patient's nurse was kept informed of the process, and the physician provided up-to-date information on the patient's clinical status for informed health-care decision-making by the patient's daughter. Early communication, during the hospitalization, concerning the patient's expressed QOL goals between the health-care team members and the patient/surrogate/family decision-makers, is essential to develop a relationship that facilitates whole patient-centered care, rather than dealing with often segmented disease-focused care and therapies in a crisis mode.

An important concept, in this case study, is that any health-care team member during interaction with the patient/surrogate/family decision-maker may be provided with the opportunity to receive information on the topic of patient-centered care/patient wishes. This information should then be communicated to appropriate health-care team members (physician, nurse, clinical social worker) that can move the information along in an effective manner. Both verbal and written documentation in the medical record resulted in a timely and uniform process to keep all health-care team members informed to prevent providing mixed messages to the patient/surrogate/family decision-makers about goals of care.

Another aspect of this case involves the role of health literacy. The patient's daughter did not recognize medical jargon, such as advance directive, living will, DPAHC, and POLST, but understood a simple question, "Had your father written any information or instructions before he came to the hospital?" It was not until that simple question to help start the conversation did the patient's daughter share a document that was very detailed in her father's QOL goals and was able to assist with *in-the-moment* decisions. Often, without that detailed input from the individual, the surrogate/family member decision-maker may say, "I hope I did the right thing," either way, whether treatments were provided for comfort care or aggressive medical interventions that prolonged the dying process.

FACILITATING CHANGE IN THE CLINICAL ETHICS HEALTH-CARE MODEL

Change is required to improve the current clinical ethics health-care model. Figure 38.4 lists components of the current model and includes aspects of the future model that would result in improvement.

To achieve these changes, the integration of an altered model has three different levels: individual and clinical, professional organizations, and society and global. These three levels are shown in Figure 38.5.

A rapid change in improving the current system would be achieved by targeting these three areas with knowledge and action steps to achieve change and facilitate sustainability of this improvement in the clinical ethics health-care model.

This chapter is aimed at changing the clinicians' practice to improve the clinical ethics health-care model. Yet, part of the problem remains with the individual, the non-health-care professional. The importance of starting the conversation by individuals and family to prevent the clinical ethics health-care dilemmas cannot be overstated. Resources are available to help individuals begin dialogue with family members about end-of-life health-care decisions, as indicated in Table 38.10. An additional resource is *Breathe* by Anne Bland, written for both the non-health-care professional and the health-care clinician, to serve as an example of how intertwining intimate stories dealing with family relationships, faith, and values can be a tool to start this sensitive conversation.[24]

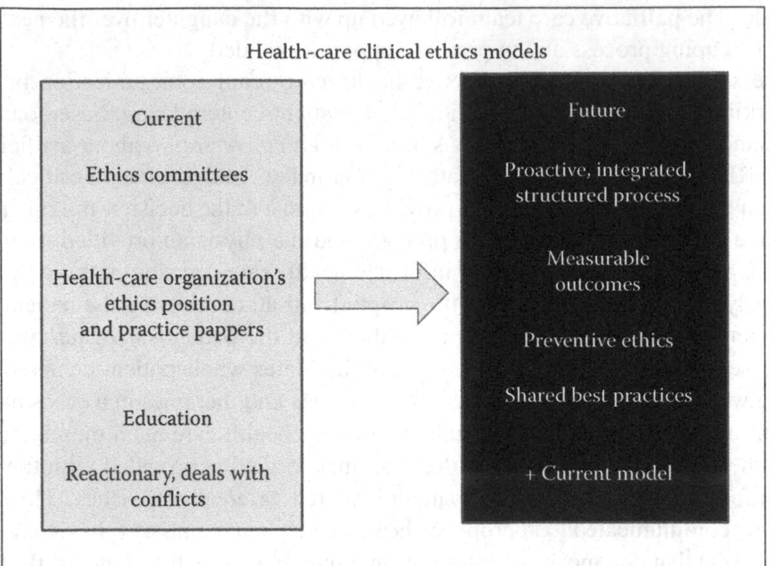

FIGURE 38.4 Changing the clinical ethics health-care model.

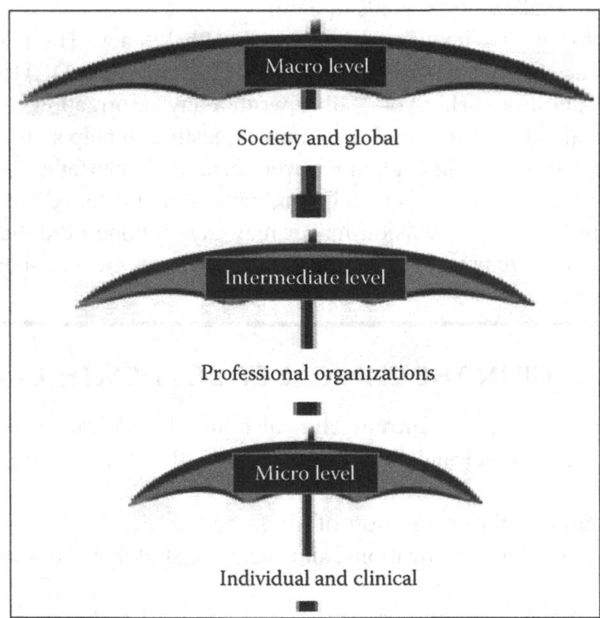

FIGURE 38.5 Levels for integrating change with clinical ethics health care.

SUMMARY

Critical care clinicians should work collaboratively to achieve a clinical ethics health-care model that promotes a proactive, integrated, structured process, with measurable outcomes, and encourages shared best practices throughout health-care systems. The goals of this chapter are presented in Table 38.11 to promote change in critical care nutrition support practice by incorporating preventive clinical ethics. Engaging and empowering patients and their family in the decision-making process involving artificial nutrition is essential in ethical considerations in the critical care setting.

TABLE 38.11
Ethical Considerations in the Critically Ill Patient Chapter Goals

Inspire and Empower Nutrition Support Critical Care Clinicians to
Screen for quality of life goals before feeding tubes
Understand cultural and religious diversity in clinical ethics
Improve health literacy and use teach-back method with clinical ethics patient education for artificial nutrition
Develop hospital policies and procedures collaboratively to incorporate preventive ethics in critical care nutrition support practice
Design quality improvement projects in artificial nutrition and clinical ethics, benchmark data
Share best practice with other facilities and clinicians
Bring awareness of advance care planning initiatives, that is, National Healthcare Decisions Day, Physicians Order for Life-Sustaining Therapy, Speak Up campaign, the Conversation Project

REFERENCES

1. Geppert CMA, Barrocas A, Schwartz DB. Ethics and law. In: Mueller C, Kovacevich D, McClave S, Miller S, Schwartz DB, eds. *The A.S.P.E.N. Adult Nutrition Support Core Curriculum,* 2nd edn. Springfield, MD: American Society for Parenteral and Enteral Nutrition, 2012, pp. 656–676.
2. Mittleman LR. The legal implications of withholding and withdrawing nutrition support. *Support Line,* 1992; 14:1–5.
3. Netuveli G, Blane D. Quality of life in older ages. *Br Med Bull.,* 2008; 85:113–126.
4. Schwartz DB, Posthauer ME, O'Sullivan Maillet J. Practice paper of academy and dietetics: Ethical and legal issues of feeding and hydration. *J Acad Nutr Diet.* June 2013. http://www.eatright.org/positions (accessed February 12, 2015.)
5. Writing Group of the Nutrition Care Process/Standardized Language Committee. The nutrition care process and model part 1. The 2008 update. *J Am Diet Assoc.,* 2008; 108:1113–1117.
6. Barry MJ, Edgman-Levitan S. Shared decision making—The pinnacle of patient-centered care. *N Engl J Med.,* 2012; 366:780–781.
7. Reuben DB, Tinetti ME. Goal-oriented patient care—An alternative health outcomes paradigm. *N Engl J Med.,* 2012; 366:777–779.
8. Bayer W, Mallinger JB, Krishman A, Shields CG. Attitudes toward life-sustaining interventions among ambulatory black and white patients. *Ethn Dis.,* 2006; 16:914–919.
9. Phipps E, True G, Harris D, Chong U, Tester W, Chavin SI, Braitman LE. Approaching the end of life: Attitudes, preferences, and behaviors of African-American and white patients and their family caregivers. *J Clin Oncol.,* 2003; 21:549–554.
10. Torke AM, Garas NS, Sexson W, Branch WT. Medical care at the end of life: Views of African American patients in an urban hospital. *J Palliat Med.,* 2005; 8:593–602.
11. Volandes AE, Paasche-Orlow M, Gillick MR, Cook EF, Shaykevich S, Abbo ED, Lehmann L. Health literacy not race predicts end-of-life care preferences. *J Palliat Med.,* 2008; 11:754–762.
12. Searight HR, Gafford J. Cultural diversity at the end of life: Issues and guidelines for family physicians. *Am Fam Physician,* 2005; 71:515–522.
13. Preedy VR, ed. *Diet and Nutrition in Palliative Care.* Boca Raton, FL: CRC Press, 2011.
14. *Ethical and Religious Directives Issued by the United States Conference of Catholic Bishops,* 5th edn. November 17, 2009.
15. Kelley AS, Wenger NS, Sarkisian CA. Opiniones: End-of-life care preferences and planning. *J Am Geratr Soc.,* 2010; 58:1109–1116.
16. Gebara J, Tashjian H. End-of-life practices at a Lebanese hospital: Courage or knowledge? *J Transcult Nurs,.* 2006; 17:381–388.
17. Gallagher-Allred CR. Communication and education for families dealing with end-of-life decisions. *J Acad Nutr Diet.,* 2012; 112:309–310.
18. Gabriel SE, Normand ST. Getting the methods right—The foundation of patient-centered outcomes research. *New Eng J Med.,* 2012; 367:787–790.
19. Carbone ET, Zoellner JM. Nutrition and health literacy: A systematic review to inform nutrition research and practice. *J Acad Nutr Diet.,* 2012; 112:254–265.

20. Weiss BD. *Health Literacy and Patient Safety: Help Patients Understand Manual for Clinicians,* 2nd edn. American Medical Association Foundation, 2007. http://www.ama-assn.org/ama1/pub/upload/mm/367/healthlitclinicians.pdf (accessed February 12, 2015.)
21. Epstein EG. Preventive ethics in the intensive care unit. *Am Assoc Crit Care Nurs.,* 2012; 23:217–224.
22. Barrocas A, Geppert G, Durfee SM, O'Sullivan Maillet J, Monturo C, Mueller C, Stratton K, Valentine C, A.S.P.E.N. Board of Directors. *Nutr Clin Pract.,* 2010; 25:672–679.
23. Schwartz DB. Three steps for improving end-of-life nutrition care. *Clin Nutr Insight,* 2012; 38:4–5.
24. Bland A. *Breathe—A True Story of Letting Go of My Parents Gracefully, For I Will See Them Again.* Bloomington, IN: Xlibris, 2009. http://breathe-annebland.com/ (accessed February 12, 2015.)

39 Instituting Professional Nutrition Practice Guidelines and Protocols

In the Intensive Care Unit

Malissa Warren, Robert Martindale, and Mary S. McCarthy

CONTENTS

INTRODUCTION

Critical care providers may be overcome with an abundance of information on a daily basis. In a 1998 editorial titled "Bringing Evidence to the Clinic," the authors point out that physicians must read 19 articles a day, 365 days per year to remain current in their clinical practice (Davidoff et al. 1995). A broad search for critical care nutrition results in nearly 4000 records. Roughly 250 clinical trials related to early enteral nutrition (EN) and parenteral nutrition (PN) in critically ill patients combined have been published over the past year. Remaining current with the proliferation of clinical literature can create a daunting task for health-care providers. Decision support tools such as guidelines and protocols in most cases are developed by expert review of systematic research and can provide guidance to the clinician to translate evidence at the bedside. The Canadian Clinical Practice Guidelines (Heyland et al. 2003), the Guidelines for the Provision and Assessment of Nutrition Support Therapy in the Adult Critically Ill Patient (Martindale et al. 2009), and the European Society for Parenteral and Enteral Nutrition Guidelines (Kreymann et al. 2006, Bozetti and Forbes 2009) offer comprehensive recommendations for optimal nutrition therapy in the intensive care unit (ICU). The guidelines are disseminated and revised periodically, serving as an excellent foundation upon which to build evidence-based practice. Numerous nutrition therapy protocols have been established to improve the nutritional adequacy of critically ill patients; yet, observational studies comparing guideline implementation to bedside practice indicate a significant gap in translating knowledge into performance. The practice guidelines may act to filter the plethora of information for critical care providers and teams; however, the heterogeneity and complexity of critical illness and the rapid evolution of nutrition therapy over the past few decades are significant factors impacting nutrition therapy.

Feeding the critically ill patient has progressed from supportive measures traditionally regarded as a means to prevent protein energy malnutrition and preserve lean body mass to time-sensitive therapy intended to attenuate the detrimental metabolic influences of severe stress. Critically ill patients are in a dynamic state of inflammation and immune suppression taking weeks to months for complete resolution. Upon admission to the ICU, multiple factors including timing of insult, prestress comorbidities, and nutritional status will influence the duration and degree of the hyper-dynamic inflammatory response. The prevalence of malnutrition in the hospitalized patient is well documented, identifying one-third of patients as malnourished upon admission and another two-thirds of patients with additional deterioration of their nutritional status during the hospital course (Tappenden et al. 2013). Patients in the ICU are at significant risk for iatrogenic malnutrition due to the obligatory catabolic effects of severe illness, cumulative energy and protein deficits, and patient immobility and lack of muscle function that characterize the ICU setting (Gruther et al. 2008). For these reasons, poorly nourished critically ill patients are at significantly increased risk for more infections, poor wound healing, prolonged mechanical ventilation, longer hospital stays, decreased quality of life, and higher mortality rates than their better nourished counterparts (Braunschweig et al. 2000, Doig et al. 2008, Faisy et al. 2009, 2011). The necessity to address malnutrition in hospitalized patients has also been highlighted recently by the 2012 Academy of Nutrition and Dietetics and the American Society for Parenteral and Enteral Nutrition Consensus Statement: Characteristics Recommended for the Identification and Documentation of Adult Malnutrition (Undernutrition) (White et al. 2012).

Nutrition therapy when given appropriately can mitigate the metabolic response to stress and to a degree prevent devastating energy and protein deficits that can result in hospital-associated malnutrition. Obtaining maximal benefit from nutrition therapy requires prompt and in some cases specialized nutrient delivery. The optimal nutrition regimen for hospitalized patients is best administered utilizing feeding protocols. Critical care nutrition protocols have evolved over time with the shifting of evidence in critical care nutrition practice giving way to changes in recommendations such as route of delivery, source of nutrition, patient selection, and dose and timing of nutrition. Four decades ago, PN was established as a viable source of nutrition for hospitalized patients to ameliorate the devastating effects of malnutrition often associated with chronic disease and critical illness. By the 1990s, the dogma of nutrition support was changing when results of the Veterans Affairs Total Parenteral Nutrition Cooperative Study revealed PN to be beneficial for the most severely malnourished patient but detrimental for the mild-to-moderately malnourished patient contributing to increased risk of complications and potentially greater mortality (The Veterans Affairs Cooperative Study Group 1991). Additional studies to date have confirmed the importance of stratifying the use of PN to malnourished patients who are unable to tolerate an enteral source of nutrition and/or will undergo major surgery (Bozetti et al. 2001, Braunschweig et al. 2001, Gramlich et al. 2004, Marik and Zaloga 2004, Sena et al. 2008, Martindale et al. 2009, Casaer et al. 2011, Doig et al. 2013). In addition, the consequences of hypercaloric feeding and poor glycemic control were also exposed. Feeding standards continued to evolve, reducing doses of PN to 30 kcal/kg versus 60 kcal/kg and improving blood glucose control to normoglycemia with the use of continuous insulin drip protocols (McCowen et al. 2000, van den Berghe et al. 2001). Thereafter, prospective randomized controlled trials provided promising outcomes supporting mortality benefits for early and adequate enteral feeding (Taylor et al. 1999, Heyland et al. 2003, Barr et al. 2004, Martin et al. 2004, Doig et al. 2008). The evidence for early EN to attenuate the metabolic response in ICU patients continues to grow making early enteral feeding a primary foundation of critical care and postoperative nutrition protocols in ICUs today (Lewis et al. 2001, Marik and Zaloga 2004, Heyland et al. 2003, Doig et al. 2009, Lewis et al. 2009, Barlow et al. 2011, Doig et al. 2011, Osland et al. 2011, Marimuthu et al. 2012). Thus, the primary goals of feeding protocols are to synthesize evidence-based guidelines for optimal nutrition practice and improve the provision of early enteral feeding in the ICU, reduce morbidity and mortality, and decrease malnutrition-associated hospital costs.

REVIEW OF THE EVIDENCE FOR ENTERAL AND PARENTERAL FEEDING PROTOCOLS

Evidence clearly suggests that feeding protocols improve the delivery of nutrition to critically ill patients by promoting early initiation and enhanced adequacy of EN (Martindale et al. 2009). Since the early 2000s, major nutrition societies have published critical care nutrition guidelines providing consensus for best practices in critical care nutrition. Yet, despite concurrence among various critical care nutrition guidelines and evidence for the benefits of nutrition therapy, this agreement has not translated into adequate nutrition delivery in the critically ill patients with most major studies reporting only 30%–60% of goal calories being delivered (Alberda et al. 2009, Heyland et al. 2010b, Cahill et al. 2011). Villet and colleagues observed caloric deficits greater than 12,000 calories during the first week of ICU care, which correlated with increased infectious complications (Villet et al. 2005). Unfortunately, attempt to compensate later for deficits occurring in the first week was not associated with reduced complications likely indicating the importance of early adequate nutrition. In 2009, Faisy et al. conducted an observational study of ICU patients requiring prolonged mechanical ventilation and revealed that a negative energy balance in the first 14 days in the ICU was an independent factor of mortality (Faisy et al. 2009). In another large multicenter multinational observational study, Alberda and colleagues detected a reduction in mortality and ventilator-free days for every 1000 cal increase in energy provision and additional 30 g in protein provision, particularly for patients at the extremes of body mass index (Alberda et al. 2009). In a recent international prospective observational cohort study, the effect of enteral feeding protocols was evaluated in nearly 6000 patients. Hospitals utilizing evidence-based feeding protocols used more EN, started EN approximately 16 h earlier, and used more prokinetic agents in cases of elevated gastric residual volumes (GRVs) compared with sites that did not use a feeding protocol (Heyland et al. 2010b). Overall nutritional adequacy and intake from EN were higher at protocol sites versus nonprotocol sites.

Taylor and colleagues performed a prospective, randomized, controlled trial in mechanically ventilated patients following head injury to determine the effect of early enhanced EN on clinical outcome (Taylor et al. 1999). EN was initiated at goal rate in the intervention group versus titrating from 15 mL/h over time in the control group. By starting EN at goal infusion rate, the intervention group received almost twice the percentage of goal calories compared to the control group and had significantly lower incidence of infectious complications, 61% versus 85% in controls. Patients in the intervention group also demonstrated a trend toward enhanced neurological recovery at 3 months. A prospective study by Woien & Bjork evaluated the impact of a nurse-led nutrition support algorithm on the delivery of EN and PN in a convenience sample of ICU patients. When compared to controls (n = 21), patients in the intervention group (n = 21) were prescribed and received a significantly greater amount of nutrients, with a larger proportion delivered by EN. The algorithm also led to greater consistency in bedside nursing practices including monitoring GRV and incremental increases in the rate of enteral feeding (Woien and Bjork 2006).

In a prospective study of patients with major trauma, Kozar et al. established the success of a standardized enteral protocol focusing on the management of intolerance to EN. The protocol provided specific guidance in the event of vomiting, abdominal distention, diarrhea, high nasogastric output, and medication contraindications with feeding such as inotropic agents and paralytics. The majority of patients managed by the standardized protocol exhibited tolerance as defined by EN advancement per protocol with few patients requiring reduction in EN infusion rate or holding of EN feeding (Kozar et al. 2002).

In a large Australian study, Doig et al. evaluated whether nutritional guidelines can improve ICU feeding practices and reduce mortality in ICU patients. In this cluster randomized controlled trial, ICUs following guidelines fed patients earlier and achieved caloric goals more often. However, hospital mortality, the primary outcome of the study, was not different between the guideline and control ICUs. Control ICUs were initiating EN in 1.37 days versus 0.75 days at study sites.

Clearly, both sites were meeting guideline recommendations for early feeding practices, but the effect was not large enough to influence clinical outcome (Doig et al. 2008). Many before-and-after studies have evaluated the impact of feeding protocols on nutrition practice in the ICU and consistently demonstrate that these protocols are associated with increased use and/or infusion of EN. Evaluating the impact of nutrition protocols on increasing nutrient delivery, Spain and colleagues reported improved EN delivery with implementation of a nutrition protocol. EN was titrated to goal faster, and patients received 82% of goal volume when providers used the study infusion protocol versus only 66% of goal volume in the control group (Spain et al. 1999).

Mackenzie and colleagues also showed that implementation of an evidence-based feeding protocol improved EN delivery from 20% before implementing the feeding protocol to 80% post-protocol implementation. In addition, PN use was reduced in the post-implementation group (Mackenzie et al. 2005). In a similar prospective before and after protocol implementation study, Barr et al. demonstrated that a feeding protocol initiating feeding within 48 h of admission was associated with more patients receiving EN. Clinical outcomes of this study included shortened duration of mechanical ventilation and a reduction in mortality associated with EN protocol utilization in the study patients (Barr et al. 2004). In a recent retrospective study, Kiss et al. investigated the impact of implementing a nutrition support algorithm based on Society of Critical Care Medicine/American Society of Parenteral and Enteral Nutrition Guidelines and the European Society of Parenteral and Enteral Nutrition Guidelines. The study included pre- and post-implementation phases in a medical–surgical ICU in Switzerland without a dietitian or nutrition support team. The use of EN and the provision of nutrition increased post-implementation of the nutrition support algorithm (Kiss et al. 2012).

The successful application of feeding protocols extends beyond the critical care environment. A recent single-center retrospective chart review highlighted the benefits of protocol-driven nutrition therapy in patients over 65 years of age with percutaneous endoscopic gastrostomy (PEG) tubes (n = 109) (Ichimaru et al. 2013). Overall, the application of a feeding protocol after PEG placement in older adults was associated with shorter length of stay, greater energy and protein intake, and a lower incidence of oxygen desaturation events for patients receiving supplemental oxygen therapy when compared to nonprotocol patients.

ELEMENTS OF FEEDING PROTOCOLS

To encourage optimal utilization and timely initiation, feeding protocols should be incorporated into the ICU admission orders. Feeding protocols enable the bedside nurse along with the entire critical care team to initiate and improve the delivery of EN in a timely manner, minimizing delays that commonly occur in the ICU setting. Protocols may be préprinted order sets, algorithms, or computerized templates that facilitate protocol implementation. The elements of feeding protocols typically include guidance for the timing of feeding, route of feeding (EN versus PN), selection of

TABLE 39.1
Common Elements of Nutrition Protocols

Route of feeding—enteral versus parenteral
Location of enteral feeding—gastric versus small bowel
Timing of feeding
Enteral formula selection and adjuvant modulars
Laboratory monitoring
Blood glucose monitoring
Gastric residuals and prokinetic agents
Strategies to minimize holding of enteral nutrition for tests and procedures

feeding formula (immune enhancing versus standard EN formula), titration schedules, strategies for optimizing administration such as modifications in therapy for elevated GRVs, or minimizing time patients spend nil per os (NPO). In addition, protocols describe strategies to reduce risks of feeding such as aspiration, over- or underfeeding, and poor glycemic control. Table 39.1 provides some common elements of feeding protocols as well as specific examples from written feeding protocols.

BARRIERS TO ADEQUATE ENTERAL NUTRITION AND PROTOCOL COMPLIANCE

Provider and System-Related Barriers

Franklin and colleagues articulately point out the lack of scientific evidence to support the traditional practice of placing patients NPO throughout their hospital stay, particularly upon admission, when diagnostic tests are ordered, or in the early postoperative period (Franklin et al. 2011). This is problematic for critically ill patients for whom a narrow window of opportunity for the initiation of enteral feeding can lead to improved outcomes. The possibility of gut dysmotility, infectious complications, or other comorbid conditions during critical illness presents challenges to successful nutrition therapy if not implemented within 36–48 h (Fruhwald et al. 2007). The prospective observational cohort study by Franklin et al. involved documentation of reasons by the multidisciplinary nutrition team why patients remained NPO for 3 days or longer. Inappropriate NPO orders were those where insufficient evidence existed for ileus, waiting 24 h after percutaneous gastrostomy placement before feeding, severe pancreatitis, routine bedside procedures, and spinal precautions with prone positioning. The most common reason for NPO status documented in the medical record was concern for ileus (29.7%); however, medical staff continued to await the *return of bowel function* in the absence of objective findings. Other reasons for keeping patients NPO stated or written by physicians included patient instability, need for mechanical ventilation and related to this was the possibility of early weaning, and nausea with and without vomiting. Overall, one-fifth of the study patients ($n = 262$) were NPO for a mean of 5.2 ± 3.7 days. Even when the MNT entered specific nutrition recommendations in the patient's medical record, compliance with the notes, written every 3 days, never exceeded 59.5% (Franklin et al. 2011). After analyzing reasons why enteral feedings were withheld in mechanically ventilated patients, Rice et al. (2005) found that giving patients *nothing by mouth for procedures* accounted for 41% of the interruptions, although no justification could be found in 21% of the cases. Gastrointestinal intolerance and anticipated extubation were appropriate cessations. The best solution to the problem of unnecessary NPO status is an enteral feeding protocol that will identify patients who should be fasting but provide guidance for the progression of nutrition therapy as soon as practical. Kim et al. (2012) point out the lack of such protocols that specifically address the barriers to adequate enteral intake and provide strategies to overcome the barriers and mitigate the negative consequences of sustained undernutrition (Kim et al. 2012). Table 39.2 provides examples of common barriers to achieving adequate

TABLE 39.2
Potential Barriers to Adequate Nutrition Therapy

Lack of feeding access
Lack of bowel sounds or other signs of gastrointestinal function
Delay in initiation of nutrition orders
Feeding at *trickle or trophic* rates (10–20 mL/h)
Frequent holding of enteral nutrition for routine bedside care, tests, and procedures
Ill-defined gastric residual volume thresholds
Lack of knowledge regarding practice guidelines for nutrition therapy
Lack of dedicated registered dietitian in the ICU

nutrition in the ICU. In addition to unnecessary NPO diet orders, underprescribing of EN by critical care providers, slow titration, and frequent interruptions of administration for a variety of reasons including radiologic and operative procedures as well as routine nursing care are all common reasons for stopping or holding tube feeding (McClave et al. 1999, Adam and Batson 1997). Many of the obstacles may stem from a lack of ICU team education regarding the importance and safety of nutrition therapy in the ICU setting. Several recent surveys of ICU physicians indicate a significant lack of knowledge regarding evidence-based nutrition guidelines. Moreover, ICU physicians and nurses are focusing on multiple evidence-based protocols or tasks that they may view as a higher priority than nutrition care in the ICU (Heyland et al. 2010b, Marshall et al. 2012, Cahill et al. 2012). These obstacles commonly lead to a lack of compliance with feeding protocols by critical care clinicians, limiting protocol effectiveness. Spain et al. (1999) measured a 42% protocol noncompliance rate by critical care providers in the study described previously. Barr and colleagues illustrated similar problems with protocol adherence (Barr et al. 2004).

Adherence to feeding protocols is subject to the same factors affecting adherence to any protocol: staff motivation, education, engagement, and resources. In a study performed by Dobson and Scott, a nurse-led ICU enteral feeding algorithm was evaluated for its safety and efficacy, and for adherence to the detailed algorithm. This unique algorithm developed with multidisciplinary input enabled nurses to set safe and nutritionally adequate feeding goals based on patient weight. In addition, patients identified as being at nutritional risk were referred to a dietitian for further assessment. A 3-month prospective audit examined formula selection, infusion rate, volume received, frequency of GRV monitoring, and use of prokinetic medication. Audit results revealed that while dietitian referrals were appropriate 90% of the time, only 60% of patients were receiving the correct feeding regimen. Appropriate energy prescription based on accurate documented body weight occurred in only 2% of the sample. Efforts to improve adherence to protocols must include education outreach to all clinicians, active involvement in protocol development and revisions, and engagement in the recurring auditing process (Dobson and Scott 2007).

Monitoring Gastric Residual Volumes

Checking GRVs to determine tolerance of enteral feeding has been a routine nursing practice for many years. High GRV is one of the most frequent reasons cited for holding or reducing the rate of EN administered to critically ill patients (Hurt and McClave 2010). Although little evidence to date validates GRV as a measure of gastric emptying, gastric intolerance, risk of emesis, aspiration, or other adverse outcomes, the practice of monitoring GRVs continues to be a significant barrier to adequate EN. Pinilla et al. compared gastrointestinal tolerance using two enteral feeding protocols with differing GRV thresholds and the use of prokinetics. In this prospective randomized controlled trial, enteral feeding intolerance was reduced by an increased GRV threshold of 250 mL compared to 150 mL with the addition of prokinetics (Pinilla et al. 2001). In the study by Taylor and colleagues, patients randomized to the protocol with a higher cutoff value for GRV received nearly twice the volume of EN than control subjects (59% versus 36% goal volume). The study results revealed a significant reduction in the incidence of infection (85% versus 61%, respectively; $P < 0.05$) and a nonsignificant reduction in the incidence of pneumonia (63% versus 44%, respectively) compared with controls (Taylor et al. 1999). More recently, studies have examined the feasibility of forgoing GRV checks altogether. In a prospective before-and-after study, Poulard et al. compared the impact of no routine monitoring of gastric residuals with standard gastric residual checks in critically ill patients. After elimination of GRV checks, the study patients had a lower incidence of infection, higher infusion of EN, and no difference in vomiting and ventilator-associated pneumonia (VAP) compared to the patients who had routine GRV checks (Poulard et al. 2010). Most recently, Reignier and colleagues randomized nearly 450 patients to a protocol that directed adjustments to the rate of feeding if GRVs exceeded 250 mL or to an intervention protocol without GRV checks and rate of feeding adjustment only in the event of vomiting. Though the intervention group had a significantly higher incidence of vomiting, they did not have a higher rate of VAP (Reignier et al. 2013). These results should encourage the critical care provider to scrutinize the use of GRVs in protocols, applying current best evidence to select GRV thresholds and determine appropriate conditions and patient populations. Figure 39.1 provides an example of a sample protocol that incorporates guidelines for timing, route, and gastric residual monitoring.

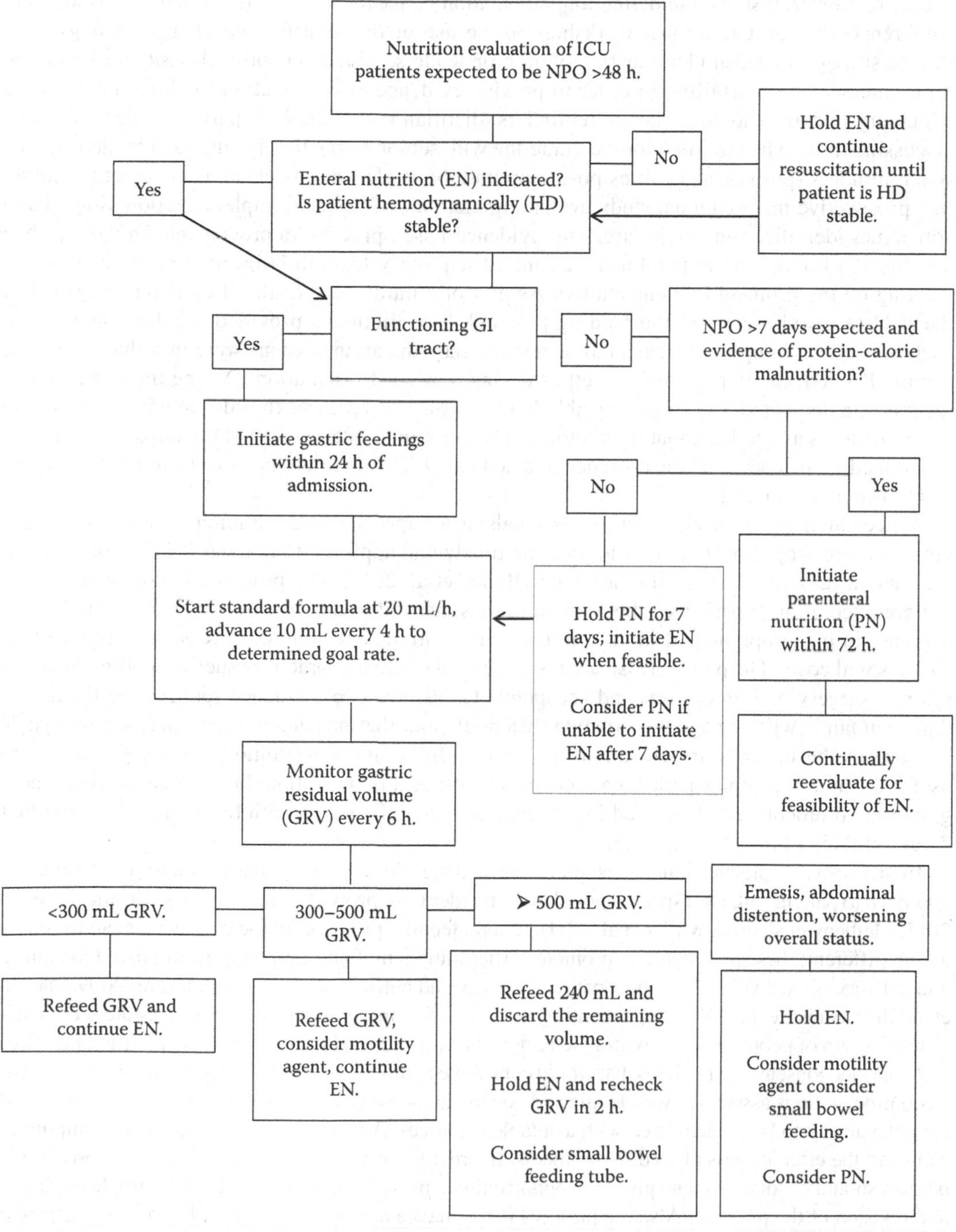

FIGURE 39.1 Sample critical care nutrition feeding protocol.

Achieving Protocol Compliance

Studies on protocol compliance conclude that in order to maintain success of protocols at the bedside, critical care teams must have ongoing involvement in protocol modifications and improvement. In addition, protocol compliance and performance should be routinely assessed and measured with timely feedback directly to the clinicians utilizing the protocols. Doig et al. achieved significant practice change with an extensive guideline implementation strategy in their cluster randomized study. Guideline implementation consisted of a 2-day guideline development conference with an educational workshop on the use of the multifaceted change strategy. The change strategy included identification of opinion leaders, education outreach visits for guideline initiation, academic detailing in order to provide evidence or information to clinicians who are reluctant to adopt guidelines, active reminders (dietitian reviewing ICU patients twice daily and discussing those who qualified for the guideline with senior staff), timely audit and feedback, passive reminders (posters, algorithms posted around the ICU), and in-servicing (Doig et al. 2008). In a prospective interventional study evaluating methods of protocol implementation, Soguel and colleagues identified nine major areas for evidence-based practice improvement. The group then developed a bottom-up protocol using an interdisciplinary team to build reference materials for training on the protocol implementation. As part of a multiphase trial, all clinicians working in the ICU received a copy of the feeding protocol. Two dietitians provided regular education to each ICU clinician upon implementation, and regular education sessions were introduced into the routine ICU education program as well as during new staff orientation. During the last phase of the study, a dedicated and knowledgeable ICU dietitian was present in order to advise other ICU team members as needed about the protocol. The combined intervention of the ongoing evidence-based feeding protocol and the presence of a dedicated ICU dietitian improved caloric delivery by 31.6% (Soguel et al. 2012).

A dedicated group of nutrition professionals at a large Northwest trauma center developed a nutrition support protocol in order to promote timely and appropriate EN and PN therapies first in the trauma ICU and then in all other ICUs (Bailey et al. 2012). The protocol, in conjunction with the presence of an experienced dietitian on rounds, has led to an increase in the use of EN and a decrease in inappropriate and short-term use of PN with a concomitant decrease in complications and hospital costs. The protocol also addresses several confusing practices such as holding feedings prior to surgery and procedures and acceptable GRVs. Protocol guidance reduces the likelihood that each nurse will manage the situation differently and that patients will not meet feeding goals because of the unnecessary cessation of feedings. In addition, institution-specific protocols are useful for highly complex patient care environments; at this institution, both an antioxidant and a glutamine protocol were developed for trauma patients and patients with burn injuries for the first 7 days of their admission to the ICU.

Evidence-based practice guidelines, protocols, and algorithms have all been used to standardize the approach to patient care for a specific population in order to improve patient outcomes (Gustafsson et al. 2012, Metheny et al. 2010, Miller et al. 2011). Enteral feeding protocols in the critical care environment are no different; these protocols can promote earlier initiation of nutrition therapy, improved tolerance, and delivery of goal volumes to meet patients' energy and nutrient needs (Pousman et al. 2009, Sheean et al. 2012, Singer et al. 2011). Implementing successful feeding protocols requires an astute multidisciplinary group of people who are willing to review the weaknesses in current bedside nutrition practices and consider consensus guidelines that would contribute to improved nutritional outcomes in their ICUs. Recommendations associated with feeding protocols should be easily interpreted and cost effective and have the ability to be implemented with available resources. As noted earlier, protocol noncompliance can limit the effectiveness of feeding protocols. In order to overcome resistance to protocol use, stakeholders should be identified and given the opportunity to provide input and feedback for implementation and revision of the protocol. Also the protocol performance and adherence must be routinely assessed with direct feedback to the clinicians implementing the protocols. As previously mentioned, feedback through audits and benchmarking reports on performance of key elements in critical care nutrition guidelines may significantly improve the use and adequacy of EN and PN when appropriate. Annual international quality improvement studies including the International Nutrition Survey by the Clinical Evaluation Research Unit in Canada and Nutrition Day Worldwide developed in Austria provide great opportunities for audit and feedback regarding the use of critical care nutrition protocols.

CONCLUSION

The supportive data are overwhelming for the development of evidence-based guidelines to standardize feeding practices of critically ill patients and improve patient outcomes. However, the current decade has seen advances in our understanding of the science of nutrition therapy and has brought much debate surrounding current nutrition practices in critically ill patients. A recent randomized controlled trial has raised controversy regarding the appropriate dose for nutrition therapy. In contrast to previous studies showing the consequences of caloric deficit, Rice and colleagues observed initial trophic feeding to be no different in terms of patient outcomes than providing goal caloric feeding in the first week of ICU stay (Rice et al. 2011). A closer look at the patient population indicates that many of the very ill patients and those with organ failure were excluded from the study group. It is important to understand that the remaining patients in the study were previously well nourished with ALI/ARDS, and therefore the results of this study, though an excellent, well-designed ICU study, cannot be extrapolated to all ICU patients. Two additional trials were published in the past 2 years revealing different outcomes regarding the use of supplemental PN to minimize caloric deficits in critically ill patients (Caesar et al. 2011, Heidegger et al. 2013). In a large, multicenter, randomized, controlled trial, Caesar and colleagues evaluated the use of early PN (starting on day 2 according to ESPEN recommendations) compared to late initiation of PN (on day 8 according to ASPEN/SCCM guidelines) in the Early Parenteral Nutrition Completing Enteral Nutrition in Adult Critically Ill Patients (EPaNIC) study. Patients who received PN late had fewer complications and shorter ICU stays than patients who received PN on day 2 (Caesar et al. 2011). In contrast, the Swiss trial conducted by Heidegger and colleagues demonstrated that patients who received supplemental PN to match caloric needs as determined by indirect calorimetry had fewer infections and fewer ventilator days than patients who did not receive supplemental PN (Heidegger et al. 2013). However, it is important to note that malnourished patients were excluded from the EPaNIC trial, and most of the included patients were elective surgical admissions not typically indicated for PN feeding. Though published guidelines and consensus statements over the past 15 years have allowed us to evaluate and benchmark our progress in critical care nutrition, discrepancy in practice still exists in nutrition therapy around the world. Clearly, hospitals with feeding protocols tended to perform significantly better in quality improvement studies, feeding patients earlier and more adequately than hospitals without feeding protocols. However, current controversies in critical care nutrition that highlight discrepancies in the literature have experts and researchers asking for studies based on *high-risk patients* and *a broader range of outcomes* to determine which patients will benefit most from nutrition therapy protocols (Heyland 2013). The critical care setting is heterogeneous and complex; therefore, it is not surprising that discrepancy in research results exists. Understandably, critical care providers who are attempting to apply evidence-based medicine in their ICU nutrition practice may experience confusion and skepticism regarding the plethora of literature and diverging results. Protocols have become a foundational tool for hospitals to translate evidence-based guidelines into bedside application and can guide complex decision making in order to close gaps between knowledge and practice. Nevertheless, to be effective, nutrition therapy protocols must target the right patients to successfully optimize the quality of patient care, improve patient outcomes, and decrease hospital costs. Last, protocols and guidelines do not take into consideration all circumstances in an intensive care setting; a provider's clinical judgment remains an essential component to patient care.

CASE PRESENTATION AND DISCUSSION

A 56-year-old male with recently diagnosed non-small-cell lung cancer was admitted to the surgical ICU following a right pulmonary lobectomy. History includes smoking, COPD, chronic pain, constipation, and a recent 7-day admission to the hospital for post obstructive pneumonia. He has lost 10 pounds (lbs) unintentionally in the past month. He is 5 ft 10 in. tall and now weighs 145 lbs. His BMI was 20.8 on admission. The ICU early feeding protocol was used as it promotes enteral feeding within 24–48 h for patients that are expected to remain ventilated for more than 24 h. The surgical team determined that the patient was not ready for extubation on postoperative day (POD) 1 and ordered EN according to the protocol via an orogastric tube. A standard enteral formula containing 1.2 cal/mL was started at 20 mL/h, and a nutrition consult was ordered. The nurse raised concerns about advancing tube feeding in the absence of bowel sounds and his history of dependence upon narcotics for chronic pain. The team decided to order an abdomen/chest/pelvic x-ray. The x-ray findings were not consistent with obstruction; however, there was some concern for pneumonia. The patient was treated for his pneumonia. On POD 5, the team decided that they will attempt extubation the following morning. The patient was successfully extubated on POD 6. The patient was seen by speech pathology following extubation and was cleared for a mechanical soft diet.

Question: In addition to type of formula and nutrition consult for recommended interventions by the unit dietitian, what other protocol elements may be important to promote early and adequate feeding for this patient?

Comments: Abdominal distention and elevated gastric residuals are common reasons for the interruption of EN. The feeding protocol should include specifics regarding monitoring EN tolerance and rationale for holding EN. The patient is at increased risk for delayed gastric emptying due to recent anesthesia and surgery, ongoing stress of postop recovery, and history of bowel dysmotility (constipation) related to narcotic dependence for chronic pain. An interdisciplinary discussion regarding feeding strategies to address any apprehension for protocol compliance early in this patient's ICU course will be beneficial. Observational data undoubtedly indicate that ongoing involvement of the ICU team members in protocol feedback and improvement is imperative to promote protocol compliance and improve nutrition-related outcomes. Committed stakeholders will promote the goals of EN. First, early initiation of EN may help mitigate postoperative ileus. Second, If GRVs are consistently under 500 mL in the absence of abdominal distention or signs of obstruction, the feeding protocol may direct the provider to continue feeding the patient and order pro-motility agents. If residuals remain elevated despite pro-motility agents, placing a feeding tube distal to the stomach with simultaneous gastric decompression may be necessary. Newer data would support not routinely measuring GRVs in select patients (Reignier et al. 2013). Titration schedule promoting goal feeding within 24 h, water flushes, and a bowel regimen are additional protocol elements that when initiated early can promote adequate GI function, maintain feeding tube patency, and minimize holding of EN. The protocol should give a specific titration schedule achieving goal feeding within 24–48 h. Another common interruption to enteral feeding is procedures both at the bedside and in the operating room. In this patient's case, it is possible that the team may request tube feeding to be held at midnight the evening prior to extubation. It is likely the tube feeding will be held for at least 8 h. Instead, stopping tube feeding and removing gastric residuals prior to extubation minimize time that feedings are held. Feeding protocols should address interruptions of feeding for procedures, minimizing the holding of feeds to no more than 2 h for procedures that require NPO status. If the patient is expected to go to surgery requiring anesthesia, the time frame for holding feeds may be extended to 2–4 h. Again, it will be important for stakeholders to support the protocol and promote compliance among providers involved in all steps of the patient's care for continued success of the protocol.

REFERENCES

Adam S and Batson S. 1997. A study of problems associated with delivery of enteral feed in critically ill patients in five ICUs in the UK. *Intensive Care Medicine*, 23, 262–266.

Alberda C, Gramlich L, Jones N et al. 2009. The relationship between nutritional intake and clinical outcomes in critically ill patients: Results of an international multicenter observational study. *Intensive Care Medicine*, 35, 1728–1737.

Bailey N, Clark M, Nordlund M, Shelton M, Farver K. 2012. New paradigm in nutrition support. Using evidence to drive practice. *Critical Care Nursing Quarterly*, 35(3), 255–267.

Barlow R, Price P, Reid TD et al. 2011. Prospective multicentre randomised controlled trial of early enteral nutrition for patients undergoing major upper gastrointestinal surgical resection. *Clinical Nutrition*, 30(5), 560–566.

Barr J, Hecht M, Flavin KE, Khorana A, Gould MK. 2004. Outcomes in critically ill patients before and after the implementation of an evidence based nutritional management protocol. *Chest*, 125, 1446–1457.

Bozetti F, Braga M, Gianotti L, Gavazzi C, Mariani L et al. 2001. Postoperative enteral versus parenteral nutrition in malnourished patients with gastrointestinal cancer: Randomised multicentre trial. *Lancet*, 358, 1487–1492.

Bozetti F and Forbes A. 2009. The ESPEN clinical practice guidelines on PN: Present status and perspectives for future research. *Clinical Nutrition*, 28(4), 359–364.

Braunschweig C, Gomez S, Sheean P. 2000. Impact of declines in nutritional status on outcomes in adult patients hospitalized for more than 7 days. *Journal of American Dietetic Association*, 100(11), 1316–1322.

Braunschweig C, Levy P, Sheean PM, Wang X. 2001. Enteral compared to parenteral nutrition: A meta-analysis. *American Journal of Clinical Nutrition*, 74(4), 534–542.

Cahill NE, Murch L, Cook D, Heyland DK. 2012. Barriers to feeding critically ill patients: A multicenter survey of critical care nurses. *Journal of Critical Care*, 6, 727–734.

Cahill NE, Murch L, Jeejeebhoy K et al. 2011. When early enteral feeding is not possible in critically ill patients results of a multicenter observational study. *Journal of Parenteral and Enteral Nutrition*, 35(2), 160–168.

Casaer MP, Mesotten D, Hermans G et al. 2011. Early versus late parenteral nutrition in critically ill adults. *New England Journal of Medicine*, 365, 506–517.

Davidoff F, Haynes B, Sackett D, Smith R. 1995. Evidence based medicine: A new journal to help doctors identify the information they need. *British Medical Journal*, 310, 1085–1086.

Dobson K and Scott A. 2007. Review of ICU nutrition support practices: Implementing the nurse-led enteral feeding algorithm. *Nursing Critical Care*, 12(3), 114–123.

Doig GS, Simpson F, Finfer S et al. 2008. Effect of evidence-based feeding guidelines on mortality of critically ill adults: A cluster randomized controlled trial. *Journal of the American Medical Association*, 300(23), 2731–2741.

Doig GS, Heighes PT, Simpson F, Sweetman EA, Davies AR. 2009. Early enteral nutrition provided within 24 h of injury or intensive care unit admission, significantly reduces mortality in critically ill patients: A meta-analysis of randomised controlled trials. *Intensive Care Medicine*, 35(12), 2018–2027.

Doig GS, Heighes PT, Simpson F, Sweetman EA. 2011. Early enteral nutrition reduces mortality in trauma patients requiring intensive care: A meta-analysis of randomised control trials. *Injury*, 42(1), 50–56.

Doig GS, Simpson F, Sweetman EA et al. 2013. Early parenteral nutrition in critically ill patients with short term relative contraindications to early enteral nutrition: Randomized controlled trial. *Journal of American Medical Association*, 309(20), 2130–2138.

Faisy C, Candela Llerena M, Savalle M, Mainardi JL, Fagon JY. 2011. Early ICU energy deficit is a risk factor for staphylococcus aureus ventilator associated pneumonia. *Chest*, 140(5), 1254–1260.

Faisy C, Lerolle N, Dachraoui F et al. 2009. Impact of energy deficit calculated by a predictive method on outcome in medical patients requiring prolonged acute mechanical ventilation. *British Journal of Nutrition*, 101, 1079–1087.

Franklin GA, McClave SA, Hurt RT et al. 2011. Physician-delivered malnutrition: Why do patients receive nothing by mouth or a clear liquid diet in a university hospital setting. *Journal of Enteral and Parenteral Nutrition*, 35(3), 337–342.

Fruhwald S, Holzer P, Metzler H. 2007. Intestinal motility disturbances in intensive care patients pathogenesis and clinical impact. *Intensive Care Medicine*, 33, 36–44.

Gramlich L, Kichian K, Pinilla J, Rodych NJ, Dhaliwal R, Heyland DK. 2004. Does enteral nutrition compared to parenteral result in better outcomes in critically ill adult ICU patients: A systematic review of the literature. *Nutrition*, 20, 843–848.

Gruther W, Benesch T, Zorn C et al. 2008. Muscle wasting in intensive care unit patients: Ultrasound observation of M. quadriceps femoris muscle layer. *Journal of Rehabilitation Medicine*, 40(3), 185–189.

Gustafsson UO, Scott MJ, Schwenk W et al. 2012. Guidelines for perioperative care in elective colonic surgery: Enhanced recovery after surgery ERAS society recommendations. *Clinical Nutrition*, 31, 783–800.

Heidegger CP, Berger M, Graf S et al. 2013. Optimisation of energy provision with supplemental parenteral nutrition in critically ill patients. *Lancet*, 381, 385–393.

Heyland DK, Cahill NE, Dhaliwal R, Sun X, Day AG, McClave SA. 2010b. Impact of enteral feeding protocols on enteral nutrition delivery: Results of a multicenter observational study. *Journal of Parenteral and Enteral Nutrition*, 34(6), 675–684.

Heyland DK, Dhaliwal R, Drover JW, Gramlich L, Dodek P. 2003. Canadian clinical practice guidelines for nutrition support in mechanically ventilated critically ill adult patients. *Journal of Parenteral and Enteral Nutrition*, 27(5), 355–373.

Heyland DK. 2013. Critical care nutrition support research: Lessons learned from recent trials. *Current Opinion in Clinical Nutrition and Metabolic Care*, 16, 176–181.

Hurt RT and McClave SA. 2010. Gastric residual volumes in critical illness: What do they really mean? *Critical Care Clinics*, 3, 481–490.

Ichimaru S, Amagai T, Shiro Y. 2013. The application of a feeding protocol in older patients fed through percutaneous endoscopic gastrostomy tubes by the intermittent or bolus methods: A single center, retrospective chart review. *Asia Pacific Journal of Clinical Nutrition*, 22(2), 229–234.

Kim H, Stotts NA, Froelicheer ES, Engler MM, Porter C. 2012. Why patients in critical care do not receive adequate enteral nutrition: A review of the literature. *Journal of Critical Care*, 27, 702–714.

Kiss CM, Byham-Gray L, Denmark R, Loetscher R, Brody RA. 2012. The impact of implementation of a nutrition support algorithm on nutrition care outcomes in an intensive care unit. *Nutrition in Clinical Practice*, 6, 793–801.

Kozar RA, McQuiggan MM, Moore EE, Kudsk KA, Jurkovich GJ, Moore FA. 2002. Postinjury enteral tolerance is reliably achieved by a standardized protocol. *Journal of Surgical Research*, 104, 70–75.

Kreymann KG, Berger MM, Deutz NE et al. 2006. ESPEN guidelines on enteral nutrition: Intensive care. *Clinical Nutrition*, 25(2), 210–223.

Lewis SJ, Andersen HK, Thomas S. 2009. Early enteral nutrition within 24 hours of intestinal surgery versus later commencement of feeding: A systematic review and meta-analysis. *Journal of Gastrointestinal Surgery*, 3, 569–575.

Lewis SJ, Egger M, Sylvester PA, Thomas S. 2001. Early enteral feeding versus "nil by mouth" after gastrointestinal surgery: A systematic review and meta analysis of controlled trials. *British Journal of Medicine*, 323(7316), 773–776.

Mackenzie SL, Zygun DA, Whitmore BL, Doig CJ, Hameed SM. 2005. Implementation of a nutrition support protocol increases the proportion of mechanically ventilated patients reaching enteral nutrition targets in the adult intensive care unit. *Journal of Parenteral and Enteral Nutrition*, 29(2), 74–80.

Marik P and Zaloga G. 2004. Meta-analysis of parenteral and enteral nutrition in patients with acute pancreatitis. *British Medical Journal*, 328, 1407–1410.

Marimuthu K, Varadhan KK, Ljungqvist O, Lobo DN. 2012. A meta-analysis of the effect of combinations of immune modulating nutrients on outcome in patients undergoing major open gastrointestinal surgery. *Annals of Surgery*, 255(6), 1060–1068.

Marshall A, Cahill N, Gramlich L et al. 2012. Optimizing nutrition in intensive care units: Empowering critical care nurses to be effective agents of change. *American Journal of Critical Care*, 21(3), 186–194.

Martin CM, Doig GS, Heyland DK et al. 2004. Multicentre, cluster-randomized clinical trial of algorithms for critical care enteral and parenteral therapy (ACCEPT). *Canadian Medical Association Journal*, 170(2), 197–204.

Martindale RG, MCClave SA, Vanek VW et al. 2009. Guidelines for the provision and assessment of nutrition support therapy in the adult critically ill patient: Society of critical care medicine (SCCM) and American society for parenteral and enteral nutrition (A.S.P.E.N.). *Journal of Parenteral and Enteral Nutrition*, 33(3), 277–316.

McClave SA, Sexton LK, Spain DA et al. 1999. Enteral tube feeding in the intensive care unit: Factors impeding adequate delivery. *Critical Care Medicine*, 27(7), 1252–1256.

McCowen KC, Friel C, Sternberg J, Chan S et al. 2000. Hypocaloric total parenteral nutrition: Effectiveness in prevention of hyperglycemia and infectious complications a randomized controlled trial. *Critical Care Medicine*, 11, 3606–3611.

Metheny NA, Davis-Jackson J, Stewart BJ. 2010. Effectiveness of an aspiration risk-reduction protocol. *Nursing Research*, 59(1), 18–25.

Miller KR, Kiraly L, Lowen CC, Martindle RG, McClave SA. 2011. "CAN WE FEED" A mnemonic to merge nutrition and intensive care assessment of the critically ill patient. *Journal of Parenteral and Enteral Nutrition*, 35(5), 643–659.

Osland E, Yunus RM, Khan S, Memon MA. 2011. Early versus traditional postoperative feeding in patients undergoing resectional gastrointestinal surgery: A meta-analysis. *Journal of Parenteral and Enteral Nutrition*, 35(4), 473–487.

Pinilla JC, Samphire J, Arnold C, Liu L, Thiessen B. 2001. Comparison of gastrointestinal tolerance to two enteral feeding protocols in critically ill patients: A prospective randomized controlled trial. *Journal of Parenteral and Enteral Nutrition*, 25, 81–86.

Poulard F, Dimet J, Martin-Lefevre L, Bontemps F et al. 2010. Impact of not measuring residual gastric volume in mechanically ventilated patients receiving early enteral feeding: A prospective before-after study. *Journal of Parenteral and Enteral Nutrition*, 34(2), 125–130.

Pousman RM, Pepper C, Pandharipande P et al. 2009. Feasibility of implementing a reduced fasting protocol for critically ill trauma patients undergoing operative and nonoperative procedures. *Journal of Parenteral and Enteral Nutrition*, 33(2), 176–180.

Reignier J, Mercier E, Le Gouge A et al. 2013. Effect of not monitoring residual gastric volume on risk of ventilator associated pneumonia in adults receiving mechanical ventilation and early enteral feeding. *Journal of American Medical Association*, 309(3), 249–255.

Rice T, Swope T, Bozeman S et al. 2005. Variation in enteral nutrition delivery in mechanically ventilated patients. *Nutrition*, 21, 786–792.

Rice TW, Mogan S, Hays MA, Bernard GR, Jensen GL, Wheeler AP. 2011. Randomized trial of initial trophic versus full-energy enteral nutrition in mechanically ventilated patients with acute respiratory failure. *Critical Care Medicine*, 39(5), 967–974.

Sena MJ, Utter GH, Cuschieri J et al. 2008. Early supplemental parenteral nutrition is associated with increased infectious complications in critically ill trauma patients. *Journal of the American College of Surgeons*, 207, 459–467.

Sheean PM, Peterson SJ, Zhao W, Gurka DP, Braunschweig CA. 2012. Intensive medical nutrition therapy: Methods to improve nutrition provision in the critical care setting. *Journal of the Academy of Nutrition and Dietetics*, 112, 1073–1079.

Singer P, Anbar R, Cohen J et al. 2011. The tight calorie control study (TICACOS): A prospective, randomized, controlled pilot study of nutritional support in critically ill patients. *Intensive Care Medicine*, 37, 601–609.

Soguel L, Revelly JP, Schaller MD, Longchamp C, Berger MM. 2012. Energy deficit and length of hospital stay can be reduced by a two-step quality improvement of nutrition therapy: The intensive care unit dietitian can make the difference. *Critical Care Medicine*, 40(2), 412–419.

Spain DA, McClave SA, Sexton LK et al. 1999. Infusion protocol improves delivery of enteral tube feeding in the critical care unit. *Journal of Parenteral and Enteral Nutrition*, 23(5), 288–292.

Tappenden KA, Quatrara B, Parkhurst ML, Malone AM, Fanjiang G, Ziegler TR. 2013. Critical role of nutrition in improving quality of care: An interdisciplinary call to action to address adult hospital malnutrition. *Journal of Parenteral and Enteral Nutrition*, 37(4), 482–497.

Taylor S, Fettes SB, Jewkes C, Nelson RJ. 1999. Prospective, randomized, controlled trial to determine the effect of early enhanced enteral nutrition on clinical outcome in mechanically ventilated patients suffering head injury. *Critical Care Medicine*, 27(11), 2525–2531.

The Veterans Affairs Cooperative Study Group. 1991. Perioperative total parenteral nutrition support in surgical patients. *New England Journal of Medicine*, 325, 525–532.

van den Berghe G, Wouters P, Weekers F et al. 2001. Intensive insulin therapy in critically ill patients. *New England Journal of Medicine*, 345(19), 1359–1367.

Villet S, Chiolero RL, Bollmann MD et al. 2005. Negative impact of hypocaloric feeding and energy balance on clinical outcome in ICU patients. *Clinical Nutrition*, 24(4), 502–509.

White JV, Guenter P, Jensen G et al. 2012. Consensus statement: Academy of Nutrition and Dietetics and American Society for Parenteral and Enteral Nutrition: Characteristics recommended for the identification and documentation of adult malnutrition (Undernutrition). *Journal of Parenteral and Enteral Nutrition*, 36(3), 275–283.

Woien H and Bjork I. 2006. Nutrition of the critically ill patient and effects of implementing a nutritional support algorithm in ICU. *Journal of Clinical Nursing*, 15(2), 168–177.

40 Quality and Performance Improvement in the Intensive Care Unit

Mary Krystofiak Russell

CONTENTS

In the early 1990s, Graham described health-care quality as "the optimal achievable result for each patient, the avoidance of iatrogenic complications, and the attention to patient and family needs in a manner that is cost-effective and reasonably documented" [1]. The Institute of Medicine (IOM) defines quality in health care as "the degree to which health services for individuals and populations increase the likelihood of achieving desirable outcomes and the degree to which they are consistent with current professional knowledge" [2]. The IOM further states that health care should be safe, patient-centered, timely, efficient, and equitable. Quality care should be a given for all health-care customers; to assure that it is, regulatory oversight is required.

In the United States, several accrediting organizations have been granted *deeming authority* by the Centers for Medicare and Medicaid Services (CMS) to survey all hospitals for compliance with the Medicare Conditions of Participation and Coverage. These organizations include The Joint Commission (TJC), the Healthcare Facilities Accreditation Program (HFAP), and Det Norske Veritas (DNV). The organizations are described briefly later in text. Detailed information about standards for each organization is available only to subscriber facilities. Each organization places a high value on quality and performance improvement in various aspects of health-care practice.

The TJC is an *independent, not-for-profit organization* that "accredits and certifies more than 20,000 health care organizations and programs in the United States. Joint Commission accreditation and certification is recognized nationwide as a symbol of quality that reflects an organization's commitment tomeeting certain performance standards" [3].

The HFAP is authorized by the CMS to survey all hospitals for compliance with the Medicare Conditions of Participation and Coverage. Created in 1945 to conduct an objective review of services provided by osteopathic hospitals, the HFAP has maintained deeming authority since the inception of the CMS in 1965 and provides accreditation to hospitals, ambulatory care/surgical facilities, mental health facilities, physical rehabilitation facilities, clinical laboratories and critical access hospitals, and primary stroke centers [5].

The HFAP strives to assist facilities in achieving and maintaining high-quality, safe patient care. This is done in part by extracting the hospital's core measure data from the Hospital-Compare website. The data are aggregated and used during the survey process to allow hospitals to see how they measure compared to their previous reporting period as well as to other HFAP-accredited hospitals nationwide [6].

The DNV Accreditation Standards US (NIAHO) [7] were created in 2008 for hospitals in the United States and integrate the ISO 9001:2008 quality management approach [8]. The ISO 9001:2008 standard is based on quality management principles including a strong customer focus, motivation and involvement of top management, and continual improvement. DNV offers disease-specific certifications such as primary stroke center and cancer center certifications, adapting high-level quality and certification processes to different types of health-care organizations [7].

This chapter will provide an overview of the nutrition quality improvement (QI) literature, emphasize projects that improve the work of nutrition support practitioners in intensive care units (ICUs), describe the importance to quality care of implementation of a structured operational excellence program such as LEAN, and highlight the value to quality practice of clinical guidelines and standards. Although intensive care hospital settings are used as examples, many of the tools and techniques can be applied to any health-care setting.

QUALITY IMPROVEMENT

QI must be an integral part of the management and direction of a health-care organization. QI supports the mission, vision, values, and strategic plan and must be collaborative across disciplines. Deeming organizations charge the leadership of the organization with setting QI priorities and identifying how the priorities are adjusted in response to urgent or unusual events, providing sufficient staff and resources, and tracking effectiveness of QI through measurement, assessment, monitoring, and analysis to identify opportunities for improvement. QI standards focus on collection of data, aggregation, and analysis (including internal and external comparisons and identification of undesirable patterns and trends), identifying and managing events, use of analysis to drive change, and maintenance of an ongoing, proactive QI program to develop and implement appropriate corrections. QI has grown out of the relatively recent observation of the major, and unfortunately persistent, gaps between evidence-based and actual practice [9]. In the United States, the resources devoted to quality (the application of research) are far fewer than the resources devoted to the primary research projects themselves. The Agency for Healthcare Research and Quality (AHRQ) receives only about 1% of the financial and other resources provided to the National Institutes of Health [9].

Health-care spending in the United States, in 2010, was $8233 per capita, which far exceeds the world's per capita average [10]. To help manage this issue, the Patient Protection and Affordable Care Act of 2010 [11] was created; one of its tenets was to allow for financial incentives for well-defined, coordinated, high-quality care, rather than the traditional *fee for service* care of the past [12]. Three strategies created by the CMS as on outgrowth of this program reward health-care organizations that promote value. These strategies include accountable care organizations (ACOs), value-based purchasing (VBP), and penalties levied on practices that lead to poor outcomes such as hospital-acquired conditions and readmission of patients within 30 days of discharge [12].

ACOs, at the present time, have only a small presence in the U.S. hospitals [13] and are therefore not a major consideration in QI, particularly in nutrition care. VBP is a financial plan that links payments to providers for improved performance by that provider. At this time, four patient conditions are considered in the VBP arena: heart failure, pneumonia, postsurgical recovery, and acute myocardial infarction [12]. Nutrition is not specifically mentioned or involved in these measures; however, more measures will be added in the future. The CMS intends for the VBP programs to improve care as they contain costs; it is likely that nutrition measures may be added as a result of clearly defined QI initiatives, such as early nutrition intervention and support across the continuum of care for patients at risk for pneumonia.

Hospital readmission reduction programs aim to lower the excessive cost of readmission events [12]. Although ICU nutrition QI programs have yet to focus on the nutrition plan as part of the continuum of care, it is feasible that in the future, early ICU nutrition intervention programs, followed by aggressive nutrition intervention programs on the intermediate care units and in the skilled nursing/home care environments, could have a markedly positive effect on the readmission statistics and hence reimbursement profiles of forward-thinking hospitals. The nutrition support/care teams in these organizations are poised to have a far more *front and center* position than they have had in the past, with careful consideration and initiation of appropriate nutrition care QI programs.

Malnutrition and its effect on chronic disease complications and health-care costs have achieved high visibility thanks to the publication of several high-profile articles and creation of an interdisciplinary alliance program (Alliance to Advance Patient Nutrition) aimed at addressing hospital malnutrition and assuring that nutrition therapy is *a critical component of patient care* [14–16]. ICU implementation of the various components of the Alliance to Advance Patient Nutrition care model and toolkit [16] is highly feasible and would be an appropriate starting place for a robust QI, and performance measurement, initiative.

Principles to transform the ICU and broad hospital environment include creating an institutional culture where nutrition is viewed as a priority for improving quality care and cost, empowering all clinicians to address barriers and collaborate on nutritional decisions, and leveraging the electronic health record to standardize nutrition documentation [16]. Principles to guide clinician action include screening, assessment, and diagnosis of all patients at risk for malnutrition, establishment, and enforcement of a policy to provide nutrition intervention within 24 h of an *at-risk* screening and incorporation of nutrition counseling into the discharge plan [16]. The latter component would not be an immediate part of an ICU QI program but could easily be incorporated into an *all-hospital* program to position nutrition therapy as a crucial part of the *plan the stay, plan the day* approach to highly effective hospital care.

The U.S. Department of Health and Human Services Health Information Technology and Quality Improvement website offers and references a wealth of information and tools that may be effective in assisting ICU nutrition QI teams with project planning [17]. These tools include the FADE process (discussed later), PDSA (described in the section "Operational Excellence"), Six Sigma (using the DMAIC principles [define, measure, analyze, improve, control]), Continuous Quality Improvement, and Total Quality Management.

FADE provides the structure for problem-solving and PI. This process, developed by Organizational Dynamics Incorporated, consists of four steps:

1. *Focus* includes development of a problem statement, including the impact and desired outcome of the project.
2. *Analyze* involves collection of baseline data to determine how bad (or good) things actually are.
3. *Develop* includes asking what steps are needed to correct the problem.
4. *Execute* involves implementing the plan, monitoring results, and returning to *Analyze* if the results are not as hoped for.

See [18] for the detailed graphic describing all of the components of the process.

The Pathway model [19] describes two different *agendas* that use measurement to set the stage for QI. Both techniques require the use of clear purpose, focused goals, and valid, reliable performance metrics. Beyond that, they differ significantly.

Pathway I, or the *Selection* model [19], uses the act of selection itself to improve quality. In this nutrition-focused example, a patient who is anticipating an ICU stay following a major surgical procedure may do research and choose a surgeon and a care team who are dedicated to providing preoperative nutrition assessment (and support, if appropriate) and early, aggressive postoperative nutrition care including enteral (and if appropriate parenteral) nutrition with composition and at goal rates consistent with national evidence-based guidelines. Thus, the patient is thought to "improve(s) the outcomes of care by shifting business to the caregivers with better outcomes" [19]. This pathway contains inherent barriers, including the absence of the information the patient needs to make the best choice, the desire to *stick with* a certain physician and care team because of previous good experiences, the cost of care in various settings and the limitations set by the insurance plan (if applicable), and the inability or lack of desire of the patient to apply medical outcome measures to their own experience [19]. According to Berwick and colleagues, "selection itself involves skills not yet well developed in health care." Yet this tool, which relies almost completely on the people and organizations that do not directly provide care, may be very helpful for achieving the best outcomes from currently available performance.

Pathway II, the *Change* model, may actually move the distribution of performance. This pathway directly involves the providers of care (in this discussion, those who direct, provide, manage, and evaluate nutrition support of ICU patients). Berwick and colleagues note that the core of this pathway is the fact that "every system is perfectly designed to achieve the results it gets" [20]. It also involves measurement for improvement and then branches into analyzing the process and results of care (rather than the performance of the care itself). In the ICU nutrition example, the organization would use the electronic health record (HER) to collect information about the preoperative care, surgical procedures, and postoperative ICU nutrition care of all patient undergoing a certain procedure (process data) and the outcomes of the procedures including specific measures of nutritional status and nutrition quality of life. The results of these analyses would be transmitted to departmental and organizational leaders and then to the care delivery terms and practitioners.

An example from the published literature of this type of approach was published by Peterson and colleagues [21]. The team conducted a retrospective cohort study of patients at a tertiary care medical center who received parenteral nutrition (PN) before and after the initiation of PN order-writing privileges for registered dietitians (RDs). They used an existing QI database of PN information, including patient demographics, diagnoses, past medical history, and anthropometric measurements. A second database included information about PN prescriptions, patient medications, and vital signs. During a 4-year period, 1080 patients were started on PN before the RDs received order-writing privileges, and 885 were started after privileges were granted. The investigators found that patients prescribed PN after the RDs gained order-writing privileges were significantly more likely (27% vs. 45% previously) to receive PN appropriately (based on American Society for Parenteral and Enteral Nutrition [ASPEN] guidelines). In addition, the cost of RD-ordered PN was 20% less than that of the PN ordered before the change in privileges, resulting in a $300,000 cost reduction to the organization [21].

A different but similarly focused process, Goldratt's Theory of Constraints [22], was applied to the analysis of barriers to optimum nutrition care by Klein, Stanek, Wiles, and other interdisciplinary team members in a trauma center in Baltimore [23]. The goal of the process was to improve care systems and thus outcomes for trauma patients by providing them with nutrition support appropriate to their risk levels and clinical conditions. The objective was to identify the problem in the care process that, if corrected, would yield the greatest positive chance in outcomes, and to create and implement a realistic solution to the problem. Four steps defined this process:

1. Identify symptoms of the problem
2. Identify what to change
3. Identify what to change to
4. Define how to cause the change

At the end of a year-long process, monitoring and reassessment of nutritional status were identified as the *weakest links* in the nutrition care process, and a nutrition support care map was constructed [23]. Following implementation, the care map was expected to improve compliance with TJC (then JCAHO) standards and reduce adverse outcomes related to nutrition care.

James [24] presciently noted in 2002 that frontline data collections systems should "collect data once, as close to the point of generation as possible" and "use patient registries for chronic disease" to establish denominators for key criteria. A "standardized outcomes tracking system that spans the nation," as recommended by McGlynn, remains to be achieved and will be of incredible value for understanding the effectiveness of, and modifying the approach to, clinical interventions of all kinds [25], including ICU nutrition care. Without consistently collected and assiduously monitored data that measure appropriate biological parameters and preferably clinical outcomes, these goals will remain elusive.

To illustrate the difficulty of tracking appropriate nutrition outcomes for critically ill patients using frequently available laboratory tests, consider the recent systematic review of randomized controlled trials designed "to assess whether commonly used anthropometric, biochemical, and clinical nutrition indicators are predictive of patient outcomes in the critically ill" [26]. Ferrie and Allman-Farinelli extracted from the literature randomized clinical trials of nutrition interventions in critically ill patients that reported any nutrition indicator (e.g., serum albumin, prealbumin, transferrin) after baseline and meaningful clinical outcome variables (e.g., ICU length of stay, ventilator days, infectious complications). Of 223 studies identified, two independent reviewers determined that 51 studies met eligibility criteria. After analysis, the authors concluded that 30 studies reported no difference in clinical outcomes. The number of studies that reported a statistical relationship between specific nutrition indicator(s) and outcome was equal to those that reported no such relationship. The authors concluded that "no commonly used anthropometric or biological indicator consistently predicts outcomes in ICU patients, and advocated for priority development of indicators of nutritional efficacy that "are more closely linked to the patient's clinical progress" such as wound healing and physical function [25]. Current work on the relationship of protein intake to lean body mass, and its effect on ICU outcomes, may help develop such an indicator.

OPERATIONAL EXCELLENCE

High-performing organizations typically have three key characteristics: a distinct process for improvement, a clear understanding of customer expectations, and a high level of employee engagement. The lean QI philosophy and set of principles for cultural transformation and operational excellence were created at the Toyota Motor Company [27]. It is designed to develop organizations that excel in all of the characteristics named earlier. Relevant to quality and performance improvement, lean techniques strive to develop workflows that promote efficiency, quality, and safety and evolve an organizational culture that strives for continuous learning and improvement. Lean is [27]

- An attitude of continuous improvement
- Value-creating
- Unity of purpose
- Respect for the people who do the work
- Visual
- Flexible regimentation

All of these principles may be applied to ICU nutrition quality and QI; one of the most relevant is the last. Flexible regimentation includes the concept of *standard work*: developing a common process for performing a specific service based on the best available evidence and continually working to improve the standard process. A nutrition support team may develop a standard workflow for receiving a consult for PN, assessing the patient, and, if PN is indicated, writing and transmitting the order. The team may also work in an interdisciplinary fashion with the pharmacy and the nursing staff to develop and implement processes for order receipt and delivery/administration of the PN solution. Data collection at every stage of this process is important to its continuous improvement. The backbone of the process is the *standard work*, which allows for regular data collection and monitoring in order to identify process concerns, process outliers, and outcomes. The monitoring process uses the classic QI circular process PDSA: Plan, Do, Study, Act [28, 29].

PDSA involves several steps:

- Setting aims
- Establishing measures
- Selecting changes
- Testing changes
- Implementing changes
- Spreading changes

In an example cited in the second edition of the ASPEN Adult Nutrition Support Core Curriculum, Cahill [8] describes how the PDSA cycle could improve timeliness of enteral nutrition (EN) initiation in the ICU. The PLAN phase includes a team brainstorming meeting organized by the unit dietitian (RD), which results in several suggestions for improving the timeliness of EN initiation. The DO phase involves adding a *nutrition category* to the daily rounding checklist and assuring that the RD is present on rounds as many days per week as feasible. The STUDY phase is the data collection and review, after which it's determined that the checklist was completed only 60% of the time and the RD could attend rounds only twice weekly. The ACT phase involves the entire team agreeing to continue and work harder on the changes, increasing staff education, and working toward the goal of adding EN orders to the ICU admission order set [8]. A second PDSA cycle begins to evaluate this change with audit results suggesting reduction in time for the initiation of EN and increase in the number of patients receiving EN within 24–48 h of admission.

An exploratory study of the oral intake of critically ill patients following extubation did not specifically call out a QI methodology, yet review suggests that the PDSA methodology may have been at work. Peterson and colleagues conducted a prospective observational study of 50 adult medical or surgical ICU patients who received mechanical ventilation for at least 24 h, never received PN or EN, and were advanced to an oral diet post-extubation [30]. Prior to conducting the study, the team had internally validated the nutritional status evaluation tool, Subjective Global Assessment (Detsky et al.), for ICU patients. Adequacy of oral intake was assessed using a modified multiple-pass 24 h recall. The investigators found inadequate intake in all patients, regardless of age, severity of illness, nutritional status, location in the hospital, ICU and hospital length of stay, and days on mechanical ventilation. They assumed that weakness, therapeutic diet prescription, underappreciation of the importance of nutrition, and barriers to intake were key contributors to their findings. They challenged their own colleagues and others to implement protocols involving nutritional supplementation and intense mealtime monitoring and to verify the effect of oral intake post-extubation on clinical outcomes [30].

CLINICAL PRACTICE GUIDELINES AND PRACTICE STANDARDS

Worldwide, clinical practice guidelines exist for a variety of health-care procedures and team members. TJC and other deeming organizations encourage hospitals to use guidelines (such as those from the AHRQ, the National Guideline Clearinghouse, and professional organizations) when designing or improving processes. Guidelines must be appropriate to the organization, with criteria consistent with its mission, vision, and values, and must be reviewed, revised, adapted, and approved by leadership before implementation. To fully benefit from guideline use, organizations must evaluate the outcomes of patients treated and refine the guidelines as necessary.

In 1996, Schwartz published the results of a performance improvement process applied to enteral and parenteral practice and outcomes that were enhanced using standards and guidelines available at that time. The article includes a nutrition support decision tree and patient outcome statements [31], citing some of the guidelines and standards created by ASPEN. Since publication of the article, ASPEN has created or revised guidelines for the use of nutrition support in critically ill adult [32] and pediatric [33] patients, standards for nutrition support of hospitalized adult [34] and pediatric [35] patients, standards of practice and professional performance for dietitians in nutrition support [36], and standards for nutrition support nurses, pharmacists, and physicians [37–39]. Clinician leaders and organizational administrators must incorporate these standards into clinical competency checklists for practitioners to help to assure that clinicians are providing the best and safest care to patients, demonstrate staffing effectiveness, and continuously reset the bar for quality health-care outcomes.

CONCLUSION

The consumers of the twenty-first century demand cost-effective and efficacious health. Regulatory agencies require collection and analysis of data for performance improvement, documentation of the competence of health-care providers, and use of appropriate standards and protocols to assure patient safety and clinical quality. Consumers access data from these agencies and others when making decisions about where to seek health care. Nutrition support professionals in ICUs, and indeed all practice settings, must continuously evaluate and improve their practice, to provide optimal nutrition care and assure the best possible outcome for patients.

REFERENCES

1. Graham NO. *Quality Assurance in Hospitals*. Aspen Publishers, Rockville, MD, 1990, pp. 3–13.
2. Kohn LT, Corrigan JM, Donaldson MS. Committee on quality of healthcare in America, Institute of Medicine. *To Err Is Human-Building a Safer Health System.* National Academy Press, Washington, DC, 2000 and http://www.iom.edu/Global/News%20Announcements/Crossing-the-Quality-Chasm-The-IOM-Health-Care-Quality-Initiative.aspx, accessed October 30, 2013.
3. The Joint Commission. http://www.jointcommission.org/about_us/about_the_joint_commission_main.aspx, accessed June 30, 2013.
4. The Joint Commission Organization. http://www.jcrinc.com/The-Joint-Commission-Organization/, and http://store.jcrinc.com/2014-hospital-accreditation-standards/, accessed November 30, 2013.
5. Healthcare Facilities Accreditation Program. Overview. http://www.hfap.org/about/overview.aspx, accessed June 30, 2013.
6. Heathcare Facilities Accreditation Program. Resources. Quality. http://www.hfap.org/resources/quality.aspx, accessed June 30, 2013.
7. DNV GL. http://www.dnvusa.com/industry/healthcare/, accessed November 30, 2013.
8. International Organization for Standardization. http://www.iso.org/iso/iso_9000, accessed November 30, 2013.
9. Cahill N. Quality improvement. In *The A.S.P.E.N. Adult Nutrition Support Core Curriculum*, 2nd edn. Mueller C, Kovacevich D, McClave S, Miller S, Schwartz D, Eds., American Society for Parenteral and Enteral Nutrition, Silver Spring, MD, 2012, pp. 677–692.
10. KaiserEDU.org. US healthcare costs. 2012. http://www.kaiseredu.org/Issue-Modules/US-Health-Care-Costs/Background-Brief.aspx, accessed May 15, 2013.
11. Office of the Legislative Counsel. Compilation of patient protection and affordable care act. 2012. http://legcounsel.house.gov/
12. Rosen BS, Maddox PJ, Ray N. A position paper on how cost and quality reforms are changing healthcare in America: Focus on nutrition. *J Parenter Enteral Nutr.* Published online 13 June 2013; 37(6):796–801. http://pen.sagepub.com/content/early/2013/06/11/0148607113492337.
13. Audet AM, Kenward K, Patel S, Joshi MS. Hospitals on the path to accountable care: Highlights from a 2011 national survey of hospital readiness to participate in an accountable care organization. *Issue Brief (Commonw Fund).* 2012; 22:1–12.
14. White JV, Gunter P, Jensen G, Malone A, Schofield M. Consensus statement: Academy of Nutrition and Dietetics and American Society for Parenteral and Enteral Nutrition: Characteristics recommend for identification and documentation of adult malnutrition (undernutrition). *J Parenter Enteral Nutr.* 2012; 36:275–283.
15. Jensen GL, Mirtallo J, Compher C et al. Adult starvation and disease-related malnutrition: A proposal for etiology-based diagnosis in the clinical practice setting from the International Consensus Guideline Committee. *J Parenter Enteral Nutr.* 2012; 34:156–159.

16. Alliance to Advance Patient Nutrition. http://malnutrition.com/alliance, accessed June 30, 2013.
17. US Department of Health and Human Resources: Health Resources and Services Administration. http://www.hrsa.gov/healthit/toolbox/HealthITAdoptiontoolbox/QualityImprovement/whatisqi.html, accessed November 30, 2013.
18. Patient Safety Quality Improvement. The FADE wheel. http://patientsafetyed.duhs.duke.edu/module_a/methods/fade.html (accessed January 11, 2015.)
19. Berwick DM, James B, Cove MJ. Connections between quality management and improvement. *Med Care.* 2003; 41(Suppl):I-30–I-38.
20. Juran JM (ed.). *Juran's Quality Control Handbook*, 4th edn. McGraw Hill, New York, 1988.
21. Peterson S, Chen Y, Sullivan S et al. Assessing the influence of registered dietitian order-writing privileges on parenteral nutrition use. *J Am Diet Assoc.* 2010; 110:1703–1711.
22. Dettmer HW. *Goldratt's Theory of Constraints: A Systems Approach to Continuous Improvement.* ASQC Quality Press, Milwaukee, WI, 1997.
23. Klein CJ, Stanek GS, Wiles CE. Nutrition support care map targets monitoring and reassessment to improve outcomes in trauma patients. *Nutr Clin Pract.* 2001; 16:85–97.
24. James B. Information systems concepts for quality measurement. *Med Care.* 2002; 41(Suppl):I-71–I-79.
25. McGlynn EA. An evidence-based quality measurement and reporting system. *Med Care.* 2002; 41(Suppl):I-8–I-15.
26. Ferrie S, Allman-Farinelli M. Commonly used "nutrition" indicators do not predict outcome in the critically ill: A systematic review. Nutr Clin Prac. Published online 3 June 2013; 28(4):463–484. DOI: 10.1177/0884533613486297.
27. Toussaint JS, Berry LL. The promise of lean in health care. *Mayo Clinic Proc* 2013; 88:74–82.
28. Langley GJ, Moen RM, Nolan KM, Nolan TW, Norman CL, Provost LP. *The Improvement Guide: A Practical Approach to Enhancing Organizational Performance*, 2nd edn. Jossey-Bass, San Francisco, CA, 2009.
29. Institute for Healthcare Improvement. How to Improve. http://www.ihi.org/knowledge/Pages/HowtoImprove/default.aspx (accessed January 11, 2015.)
30. Peterson S, Tsai A, Scala C et al. Adequacy of oral intake in critically ill patients 1 week after extubation. *J Am Diet Assoc.* 2010; 110:427–433.
31. Schwartz DB. Enhanced enteral and parenteral nutrition practice and outcomes in an intensive care unit with a hospital-wide performance improvement process. *J Am Diet Assoc.* 1996; 96:484–489.
32. McClave SA, Martindale RG, Vanek VW et al. Guidelines for the provision and assessment of nutrition support therapy in the adult critically ill patient: Society of critical care medicine (SCCM) and American society for parenteral and enteral nutrition (A.S.P.E.N.). *J Parenter Enteral Nutr.* 2009; 33:277–316.
33. Mehta N, Compher C, and the A.S.P.E.N. Board of Directors. A.S.P.E.N. Clinical Guidelines: Nutrition support of the critically ill child. *J Parenter Enteral Nutr.* 2009; 33:260–276.
34. Ukleja A, Freeman K, Gilbert K, Kochevar M, Kraft M, Russell M, Shuster M. Task Force on Standards for Nutrition Support: Adult Hospitalized Patients, and the American Society for Parenteral and Enteral Nutrition Board of Directors. Standards for nutrition support: Adult hospitalized patients. *Nutr Clin Pract.* 2010; 25:404–414.
35. Corkins M, Griggs C, Groh-Wargo S, Han-Markey T, Helms R, Muir M, Szeszycki E. Task Force on Standards for Nutrition Support: Pediatric Hospitalized Patients, and the A.S.P.E.N. Board of Directors. Standards for nutrition support: Pediatric hospitalized patients. *Nutr Clin Pract.* 2013; 28:263–276.
36. Joint Standards Task Force of A.S.P.E.N. and the American Dietetic Association Dietitians in Nutrition Support Dietetic Practice Group; Russell M, Stieber M, Brantley S et al. American Society for Parenteral and Enteral Nutrition (A.S.P.E.N.) and American Dietetic Association (ADA): Standards of practice and standards of professional performance for registered dietitians (generalist, specialty, and advanced) in nutrition support. *Nutr Clin Pract.* 2007; 22:558–586.
37. American Society for Parenteral and Enteral Nutrition (A.S.P.E.N.) Board of Directors and Nurses Standards Revision Task Force, DiMaria-Ghalili R, Bankhead R, Fisher A, Kovacevich D, Resler R, Guenter P. Standards of practice for nutrition support nurses. *Nutr Clin Pract.* 2007; 22:458–465.
38. American Society for Parenteral and Enteral Nutrition (A.S.P.E.N.) Task Force for Revision of Nutrition Support Pharmacist Standards, Rollins C, MS, Durfee S, Holcombe B, Kochevar M, Nyffeler M, Mirtallo J. *Nutr Clin Pract.* 2008; 23:189–194.
39. Mascarenhas M, August D, DeLegge M, Gramlich L, Iyer K, Patel V, Schattner M. Task Force on Standards for Nutrition Support Physicians, American Society for Parenteral and Enteral Nutrition Board of Directors. 2012 standards of practice for nutrition support physicians. *Nutr Clin Pract.* 2012; 27:295–299.

Index

F

G

H

N

Q

R

S

T

U

V

W

Printed in the United States
by Baker & Taylor Publisher Services